Cardiological Society of India

CARDIOLOGY

UPDATE 2024

Cardiological Society of India

CARDIOLOGY

UPDATE 2024

Volume 1

Editor-in-Chief

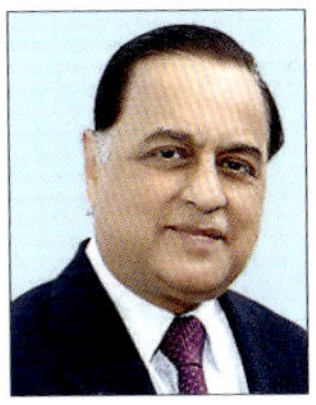

Sanjay Tyagi

MD(Medicine) DM(Cardiology) FAMS FICP FCSI FICA FRCP(Edinburgh) FSCAI FESC FACC(USA)

Dr BC Roy National Awardee

Senior Consultant, Academic Advisor (HOD) and Clinical Director Cardiology

Apollo Hospitals, Northern Region, New Delhi, India

President-Elect, Cardiological Society of India

Secretary General (India), International College of Cardiology (USA)

National Coordinator, Cardiology and Interventional Cardiology, National Board of Examination

Formerly

Director General Health Services, Govt of India

Dean, Maulana Azad Medical College, New Delhi

Director, Professor and HOD Cardiology

GB Pant Institute of Postgraduate Medical Education and Research

Co-Editors

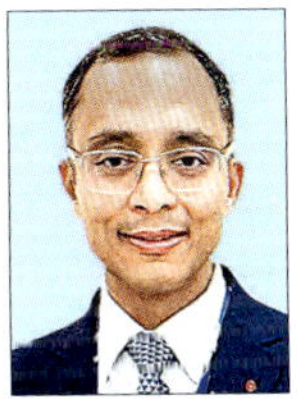

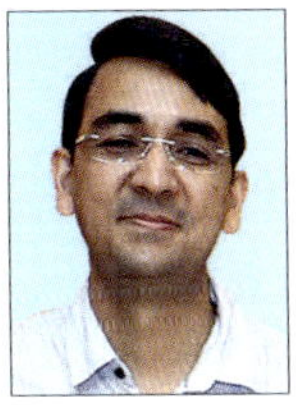

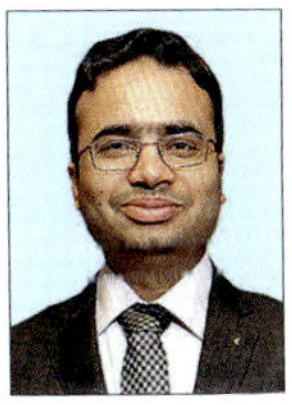

Mohit D Gupta MD DM FAMS FACC(USA)

Director–Professor, Department of Cardiology

GB Pant Institute of Postgraduate Medical Education and Research

New Delhi, India

Saurabh Kumar Gupta MD DM

Professor, Department of Cardiology

All India Institute of Medical Sciences

New Delhi, India

Ankit Bansal MD DM(Cardiology)

Professor, Department of Cardiology

GB Pant Institute of Postgraduate Medical Education and Research

New Delhi, India

Foreword

M Khalilullah

JAYPEE

JAYPEE BROTHERS MEDICAL PUBLISHERS

The Health Sciences Publisher

New Delhi | London

Jaypee Brothers Medical Publishers (P) Ltd

Headquarters
EMCA House
23/23-B, Ansari Road, Daryaganj
New Delhi 110 002, India
Landline: +91-11-23272143, +91-11-23272703
+91-11-23282021, +91-11-23245672
E-mail: jaypee@jaypeebrothers.com

Corporate Office
Jaypee Brothers Medical Publishers (P) Ltd.
4838/24, Ansari Road, Daryaganj
New Delhi 110 002, India
Phone: +91-11-43574357
Fax: +91-11-43574314
E-mail: jaypee@jaypeebrothers.com

Overseas Office
JP Medical Ltd.
83, Victoria Street, London
SW1H 0HW (UK)
Phone: +44-20 3170 8910
Fax: +44(0)20 3008 6180
E-mail: info@jpmedpub.com

Website: www.jaypeebrothers.com
Website: www.jaypeedigital.com

Inquiries for bulk sales may be solicited at: jaypee@jaypeebrothers.com

CSI Cardiology Update 2024 (Volume 1) / Sanjay Tyagi

First Edition: **2025**

ISBN: 978-93-6616-795-4

Printed at: Samrat Offset Pvt. Ltd.

DEDICATION

We dedicate this book to our parents and teachers for their inspiration, unwavering support, guidance and making us believe that we can overcome any challenges.

We are indebted to wives and children for their encouragement and most importantly sparing us the invaluable time required for this arduous task.

We owe our deepest gratitude to our patients for their trust and being part of our journey.

Contributors

Editor-in-Chief

Sanjay Tyagi MD(Medicine) DM(Cardiology) FAMS FICP FCSI FICA FRCP(Edinburgh) FSCAI FESC FACC(USA)
Dr BC Roy National Awardee
Senior Consultant, Academic Advisor (HOD) and Clinical Director Cardiology
Apollo Hospitals, Northern Region, New Delhi, India
President-Elect, Cardiological Society of India
Secretary General (India), International College of Cardiology (USA)
National Coordinator, Cardiology and Interventional Cardiology, National Board of Examination

Formerly
Director General Health Services, Govt of India
Dean, Maulana Azad Medical College, New Delhi
Director, Professor and HOD Cardiology
GB Pant Institute of Postgraduate Medical Education and Research

Co-Editors

Mohit D Gupta MD DM FAMS FACC(USA)
Director–Professor
Department of Cardiology
GB Pant Institute of Postgraduate
Medical Education and Research
New Delhi, India

Saurabh Kumar Gupta MD DM
Professor
Department of Cardiology
All India Institute of Medical Sciences
New Delhi, India

Ankit Bansal MD DM(Cardiology)
Professor
Department of Cardiology
GB Pant Institute of Postgraduate
Medical Education and Research
New Delhi, India

Contributing Authors

Aarya A Naik MBBS
PGY1 MD (Medicine)
University of Tennessee Medical
Center
Memphis, Tennessee, USA

Abhilasha MD
Senior Resident
SRM Medical College
SRM Institute of Science and
Technology
Chennai, Tamil Nadu, India

Abhinav Aggarwal MD(Medicine)
DNB(Medicine)
Senior Resident
Department of Cardiology
VMMC and Safdarjung Hospital
New Delhi, India

Abhinay Tibdewal MD DNB DM FSCAI
Consultant Interventional Cardiologist
Medica Superspeciality Hospital
Kolkata, West Bengal, India

Abhishek Chaturvedi MD
Interventional Cardiology Fellow
Georgetown University MedStar
Washington Hospital Center
Washington DC, USA
International Fellow
Center for Chronic Disease Control
(CCDC)
New Delhi, India

Lt Col (Dr) Abhishek Mallick MD(Pediatrics) DNB(Pediatrics) DM(Pediatric Cardiology)
Senior Resident
Department of Cardiology
Advanced Cardiac Center
Postgraduate Institute for Medical Education and Research
Chandigarh, India

Abhishek Garg MD DM
Resident, Department of Cardiology
Dayanand Medical College and Hospital
Unit-Hero DMC Heart Institute
Ludhiana, Punjab, India

Abhishek Goyal MD DM
Professor
Department of Cardiology
Dayanand Medical College and Hospital
Unit-Hero DMC Heart Institute
Ludhiana, Punjab, India

Abhishek Kumawat MD
3rd Year (DM)
ABVIMS and DR RML Hospital
New Delhi, India

Abraham Oomman MD DM(Cardiology)
Senior Consultant Interventional Cardiologist
Apollo Main Hospital
Chennai, Tamil Nadu, India

Abraham Paul MD DM(Cardiology)
Consultant, Aster Medcity
Kochi, Kerala, India

Achukatla Kumar Pharm D
Senior Research Consultant
Apollo Hospitals
Indore, Madhya Pradesh, India

AD Arun Mohan MD DrNB(Cardiology)
Resident, Meenakshi Hospital
Thanjavur, Tamil Nadu, India

Aditi A Naik MBBS
3rd Year
NHL Medical College and VS Hospital
Ahmedabad, Gujarat, India

Aditya Kapoor MD DM
Professor and Head
Department of Cardiology
Sanjay Gandhi Postgraduate Institute of Medical Sciences
Lucknow, Uttar Pradesh, India

Advait Akash MD DM(Cardiology)
Cardiologist
Heart Hospital
Patna, Bihar, India

Aftab Khan MD(Medicine) DM(Cardiology) DNB(Cardiology)
Consultant Interventional Cardiologist
Department of Cardiology
Director, Electrophysiology Services
Apollo Multispeciality Hospitals
Kolkata, West Bengal, India

Aishwarya Gaur DNB(General Medicine)
Resident
Department of Medicine
ESIC Model Hospital
Jaipur, Rajasthan, India

Aishwarya Vyas MD DM
Resident
Department of Cardiology
SMS Medical College
Jaipur, Rajasthan, India

Ajay Bahl FRCP DM
Professor
Postgraduate Institute of Medical Education and Research
Chandigarh, India

Ajay Kumar Sinha MD PhD FRCP(Edinburgh) FACC FESC FCSI FICC FAPSCC
Director
Department of Clinical Cardiology and Research
Jai Prabha Medanta Superspecialty Hospital
Patna, Bihar, India

Ajay M Naik MD DM DNB FACC FHRS
Cardiac Electrophysiologist
Marengo CIMS Hospital
Ahmedabad, Gujarat, India

Ajay S Chaurasia MD DM(Cardiology)
Professor and Head
Department of Cardiology
Topiwala National Medical College and BYL
Nair Charitable Hospital
Mumbai, Maharashtra, India

Ajit Desai MD DM(Cardiology) DNB(Cardiology) FACC
Additional Director
Department of Cardiology
Jaslok Hospital
Mumbai, Maharashtra, India

Ajit D Pai BA MPH
Data Scientist
Cardiovascular Specialists of Redlands and Inland Empire
Redlands, CA, USA

Ajit Kumar Valaparambil MD DM
Senior Consultant
Kerala Institute of Medical Science
Former Dean and Head
Department of Cardiology
Sree Chitra Tirunal Institute
Thiruvananthapuram, Kerala, India

Ajit S Mullasari MD DM
Chairman and Head
Department of Cardiology
Institute of Cardio Vascular Diseases
The Madras Medical Mission Hospital
Professor of Practice
Indian Institute of Technology – Madras
Chennai, Tamil Nadu, India

A Kader Sahib MD DrNB MRCP(London)
Consultant Cardiologist
Apollo Hospitals
Trichy, Tamil Nadu, India

Akash Gopi MD DNB(Cardiology)
Cardiologist
Fortis Hospitals
Bengaluru, Karnataka, India

Akash Shah MD(Medicine)
3rd Year DM Cardiology Resident
Bombay Hospital
Mumbai, Maharashtra, India

Akhilesh Kumar MD(Medicine) DrNB(Cardiology)
Senior Resident
Fortis Escort Heart Institute
New Delhi, India

AK Pancholia MD FACC FESC FCSI FISH FIMSA MAMS
Head
Department of Medicine, Clinical and Preventive Cardiology
Arihant Hospital
Indore, Madhya Pradesh, India
BC Roy and Charak Awardee of MPIMA

Amal Khan MD MNAMS DM
Former Professor
Department of Cardiology
WBMES
Visiting Consultant
Manipal Hospital, Salt Lake
Kolkata, West Bengal, India

Amartya Khan MD(Anesthesiology) DrNB
Critical Care Medicine Trainee
RN Tagore International Institute of Cardiac Sciences
Kolkata, West Bengal, India

Amitabha Chattopadhyay DCH DNB
Fellowship in Pediatric Cardiology (Australia)
Chief Pediatric Cardiologist and Clinical Lead Eastern India
Department of Pediatric Cardiology
Narayana Superspeciality Hospital
Howrah, West Bengal, India

Amit Aggarwal DNB MNAMS FIACM FICP
Senior Specialist
Department of Medicine
ABVIMS and Dr RML Hospital
New Delhi, India

Amit Garg MD(Radiodiagnosis)
Senior Consultant
Department of Imaging
Fortis Escort Heart Institute
New Delhi, India

Amit Malviya MD DM
Additional Professor
Department of Cardiology
NEIGRIHMS
Shillong, Meghalaya, India

Amit Mittal MD DM(Cardiology)
Senior Consultant
Department of Cardiology
Indraprastha Apollo Hospital
New Delhi, India

A Muruganathan MD
Chairman
Shristi AG Hospital
Tirupur, Tamilnadu, India
Director Elect – API Physicians Research Foundation

(Col) Anil Dhall Sena Medal MD(Medicine) DM(Cardiology) FACC FESC FAHA FRCP(Edinburgh) FSCAI FHRS FCSI
Professor and Head
Department of Cardiology
Janakpuri Super Speciality Hospital
New Delhi, India

Anil Sharma MD DM(Cardiology) FAPSC FSCAI FACC
Professor and Head
Department of Cardiology
Bombay Hospital
Mumbai, Maharashtra, India

Anil Sivadasan Radha MD DNB(Pediatrics) DNB(Cardiology) EPGB
Senior Consultant Interventional Pediatric Cardiologist
Lisie Hospital
Kochi, Kerala, India

Animesh Mishra MD DM
Senior Professor and Head
Department of Cardiology
NEIGRIHMS
Shillong, Meghalaya, India

Anindya Mukherjee MD DM
Senior Clinical Fellow
Adult Congenital Heart Disease
Bristol Heart Institute
United Kingdom

Anirban Das MD DM
Senior Resident
Burdwan Medical College
Burdwan, West Bengal, India

Anish Bhargav MD DM
Senior Resident and EP Fellow
JIPMER
Puducherry, India

Anish Keepanasseril MD(Obstetrics and Gynecology) DNB(Obstetrics and Gynecology) MNAMS MRCPI(Obgyn) MSc Epidemiology(LSHTM, UK)
Professor, Department of Obstetrics and Gynecology, JIPMER
Puducherry, India

Anish Kumar Khan DM(Cardiology) MD(Pulmonary Medicine) FCCP(USA) DAA(CMC Vellore) EDARM(HERMES)
Consultant Interventional Cardiologist and Pulmonologist
Visiting Consultant
Manipal Hospital, Salt Lake
Kolkata, West Bengal, India

Anita Saxena MD DM FACC
Vice Chancellor
Pt BD Sharma University of Health Sciences
Rohtak, Haryana, India

Ankit Bansal DM(Cardiology)
Professor
Department of Cardiology
GB Pant Institute of Postgraduate Medical Education and Research
New Delhi, India

Ankit Garg MS FNB
Assistant Professor
Department of Pediatric Cardiology
Pediatric Super-Specialty Wing
Amrita Institute of Medical Sciences
Faridabad, Haryana, India

Ankit Kumar Sahu MD DM
Associate Professor
Department of Cardiology
Sanjay Gandhi Postgraduate Institute of Medical Sciences
Lucknow, Uttar Pradesh, India

Ankur Handa MD DM
Senior Resident
Department of Cardiology
Cardiothoracic Sciences Centre
All India Institute of Medical Sciences
New Delhi, India

Anne Princy Steaphen MD DM
Assistant Professor
Department of Cardiology
Tamil Nadu Government Multi Super Speciality Hospital
Chennai, Tamil Nadu, India

AN Patnaik MD DM DNB FACC
Senior Consultant Cardiologist
Star Hospitals
Hyderabad, Telangana, India

Anuja Gadre MD DM(Cardiology)
Senior Resident
Department of Cardiology
Postgraduate Institute of Medical Education and Research
Chandigarh, India

Anuj Gupta MBBS
Student, All India Institute of Medical Sciences, Bhopal
Bhopal, Madhya Pradesh, India

Anupam Srivastava MD(Medicine)
Senior Resident
Department of Cardiology
Assam Medical College and Hospital
Dibrugarh, Assam, India

Anushree Kumbhalkar MD DM(Cardiology)
Senior Resident
Department of Cardiology
All India Institute of Medical Sciences, Nagpur
Nagpur, Maharashtra, India

Archit Dahiya MD(Medicine) DM(Cardiology)
Senior Interventional Cardiologist
Holy Heart Hospital
Rohtak, Haryana, India

Arif Mustaqueem MD(Medicine) DNB(Cardiology)
Associate Director
Department of Cardiology
Max Super Specialty Hospital
Saket, New Delhi, India

Arijit Ghosh MD DM
In-charge Cath Lab
Manipal Hospital
Kolkata, West Bengal, India

Arijit Kumar Ghosh MD DM FACC FESC FSCAI FAPSIC FAPVS FICC FCSI
Professor and Head
Department of Cardiology
All India Institute of Medical Sciences, Nagpur
Nagpur, Maharashtra, India

Arjun Mali MD DM(Cardiology)
Assistant Professor
Department of Cardiology
Topiwala National Medical College and BYL
Nair Charitable Hospital
Mumbai, Maharashtra, India

Arpita Katheria MD
Assistant Professor
Department of Cardiology
Sanjay Gandhi Postgraduate Institute of Medical Sciences
Lucknow, Uttar Pradesh, India

Arun Arul David MD
DrNB Cardiology Registrar
Department of Cardiology
Apollo Speciality Hospital, Vanagaram
Chennai, Tamil Nadu, India

Arun Mohanty MD DM FESC FACC
Professor
Sir Ganga Ram Hospital
New Delhi, India

Arup Dasbiswas MD DM(Cardiology) FCSI FICC FIAE FIAMS FICP FSCAI(USA) FACC(USA) FESC(Europe) FAPVS(Asia)
Emeritus Professor (Cardiology)
PKG Medical College and Hospital
Ex-Director, ICVS, IPGMER
Ex-Professor and Head
Department of Cardiology
IPGMER and SSKM Hospital
Kolkata, West Bengal, India

Arvind Kumar Jaiswal MD DM
Consultant Cardiologist
Shekhar Hospital
Lucknow, Uttar Pradesh, India

Arvind Kumar MD DM(Cardiology) FESC FICC FACC
Senior Consultant Cardiologist
Jeevak Heart Hospital
Patna, Bihar, India

Arya Subhadra DNB DM DrNB
Consultant Cardiology
St Gregorios Medical Mission Hospital
Parumala, Kerala, India

Aseem Basha MD
Assistant Professor
Department of Cardiology
All India Institute of Medical Sciences
New Delhi, India

Asha Moorthy MD DM FCCP FIACM FICP FIMSA FICC
Professor and Head
Department of Cardiology
Saveetha Medical College
Chennai, Tamil Nadu, India

Asharam Panda MD DM
Assistant Professor
Department of Cardiology
Dreams University and Health Sciences and Padmini Care Hospital
Cuttack, Odisha, India

Ashish Deshpande MD DM(Cardiology) FACC
Consultant Interventional Cardiologist
Department of Cardiology
Oriion Citicare Superspeciality Hospital
Ex-Professor and Head, MGM Medical College and Hospital
Aurangabad, Maharashtra, India

Ashish Jai Kishan MD(Medicine) DNB(Cardiology)
Senior Consultant
Fortis Escort Heart Institute
New Delhi, India

Ashish Kumar Jain MD DNB(Cardiology)
Associate Consultant Cardiologist
Sir Ganga Ram Hospital
New Delhi, India

Ashish Kumar Jha MD DM(Cardiology) FACC FSCAI
Cardiologist, Heart Hospital
Patna, Bihar, India

Ashish Kumar MD DM
Associate Consultant
Division of Interventional Cardiology
Medanta Heart Institute
Medanta – The Medicity
Gurugram, Haryana, India

Ashmit Bhardwaj MBBS
Medical Student
University of Leeds
Leeds, United Kingdom

Ashok Seth FRCP FACC MSCAI FAPSIC DSc
Chairman
Fortis Escorts Heart Institute
New Delhi, India

Ashwani Mehta DM(Cardiology)
Senior Consultant Cardiologist
Sir Ganga Ram Hospital
New Delhi, India

Ashwin Mahesh MD
Cardiovascular Disease Fellow
University of Pittsburgh Medical Center (UPMC)
Harrisburg, PA, USA

A Sreenivas Kumar MD DM FACC
Senior Consultant Cardiologist and Director
Department of Cardiology and Clinical Research
Apollo Hospital, Jubilee Hills
Hyderabad, Telangana, India

Atul Mathur MD(Medicine) DM(Cardiology)
Chairman and Head
Department of Cardiology
Fortis Escort Heart Institute
New Delhi, India

Avani Jain MD
Medical Officer
DNS Hospital
Indore, Madhya Pradesh, India

Avinash Mani MD DM(Cardiology)
Consultant
Department of Cardiology
Fortis Escorts Heart Institute
New Delhi, India

Avishkar Agrawal MD
Senior Resident
Department of Cardiology
All India Institute of Medical Sciences
New Delhi, India

Awadesh Kumar Sharma MD DM
Associate Professor
LPS Institute of Cardiology
Kanpur, Uttar Pradesh, India

Ayush Malhotra MD(Medicine) DrNB(Cardiology)
Specialist Grade
Department of Cardiology
Janakpuri Super Speciality Hospital
New Delhi, India

Ayush Shukla MD DM FAPSIC FSCAI
Assistant Professor
Department of Cardiology
King George's Medical University
Lucknow, Uttar Pradesh, India

Babu Reddy MD DM
Associate Professor
Department of Cardiology
Sri Jayadeva Institute of Cardiovascular Sciences and Research
Bengaluru, Karnataka, India

Balachander Jayaraman MD DM
Professor (Retired)
JIPMER
Puducherry, India

Balbir Singh MD DM
Chairman Cardiac Sciences
Max Hospital
Saket, New Delhi, India

Barun Kumar DM(Cardiology)
Additional Professor
Department of Cardiology
All India Institute of Medical Sciences, Rishikesh
Rishikesh, Uttarakhand, India

BC Srinivas MD DM(Cardiology)
Former Professor and Head
Department of Cardiology
Sri Jayadeva Institute of Cardiovascular Sciences and Research
Bengaluru, Karnataka, India

BG Vinodkumar MD
Junior Registrar
Billroth Hospital
Chennai, Tamil Nadu, India

Bhanu Duggal DM(Cardiology)
Professor and Head
Department of Cardiology
All India Institute of Medical Sciences, Rishikesh
Rishikesh, Uttarakhand, India

Bharat Dalvi MD DM
Consultant Cardiologist
Sir HN Reliance Hospital and Glenmark Cardiac Centre
Mumbai, Maharsahtra, India

Bhavuk Jaiswal MD(Medicine) DNB(Medicine) DM(Cardiology)
Associate Consultant
Fortis Escort Heart Institute
New Delhi, India

Bhushan Shah MD DNB(Cardiology)
Assistant Professor
Department of Cardiology
All India Institute of Medical Sciences, Bhopal
Bhopal, Madhya Pradesh, India

Bhushan Tile DM(Cardiology)
Senior Resident
ABVIMS and Dr RML Hospital
New Delhi, India

B Hygriv Rao MD DM FACC FESC
Director
Division of Pacing and Electrophysiology
KIMS Group of Hospitals
Hyderabad, Telangana, India

Bidyut Roy MD(Medicine) DM(Cariology)
Senior Resident
Department of Cardiology
IPGMER
Kolkata, West Bengal, India

Biraja Prasad Beura MD
Senior Resident Cardiology
MKCG Medical College
Berhampur, Odisha, India

Biswajit Majumder MD DM FACC FESC FSCAI FCSI FICP FAPSIC
Professor and Head
Department of Cardiology
RG Kar Medical College and Hospital
Kolkata, West Bengal, India

Biyanka Jaltotage MBBS(Hons) MSc
Cardiologist, Fiona Stanley Hospital
Perth, Western Australia, Australia

Blessvin Jino MD DM FNB
Consultant Interventional Cardiologist
Meditrina Hospital
Kollam, Kerala, India

BR Mishra MD DM FCSI FIAE FICC
Senior Consultant Cardiologist
Max Diagnostic
Cuttack, Odisha, India

B Shukti MBBS Dip GO MSc Medicine(Cardiology)(UK) FHEA(UK)
Senior Lecturer University/FE College
Senior Trust Doctor
United Kingdom

BS Yadav MD DM(Cardiology) FCSI FACC FSCAI
Professor and Head
Department of Cardiology
LN Medical College
Former Professor and Head
Department of Cardiology
Gandhi Medical College
Bhopal, Madhya Pradesh, India

Chandan Kumar Das MD(Medicine) DNB(Cardiology)
Super Specialist (Cardiology)
JLN Hospital and Research Center
Bhilai, Chhatisgarh, India

Chandra Bhan Meena MD DM FACC FSCAI FESC MHRS MAPHRS
Senior Professor
Department of Cardiology
SMS Medical College
Jaipur, Rajasthan, India

Chhabi Satpathy MD DM FACC FSCAI FESC FCSI FICC FIAE
Professor and Head
Division of Cardiology
MKCG Medical College
Berhampur, Odisha, India

CM Nagesh MD DM
Professor
Department of Cardiology
Sri Jayadeva Institute of Cardiovascular Sciences and Research
Bengaluru, Karnataka, India

C Rohit Swaminathan MD DM
DM Resident
Department of Cardiology
Amrita Institute of Medical Sciences
Kochi, Kerala, India

C Venkata S Ram MD MACP FACC FASH
Director
Apollo Institute for Blood Pressure Management
Apollo Group of Hospitals
Hyderabad, Telangana, India
Professor of Internal Medicine
University of Texas Southwestern Medical Center
Dallas, TX, USA

D Anuradha MD DNB
Junior Consultant Cardiologist
Apollo Hospitals Health City
Visakhapatnam, Andhra Pradesh, India

Dayasagar Rao V DM(Cardiology) FRCP(Canada) FRCP(Edinburgh)
Consultant Cardiologist
KIMS Hospital
Secunderabad, Telangana, India

Debabrata Biswas DNB(Medicine)
Postdoctoral Trainee
Department of Cardiology
NH-RTIICS
Kolkata, West Bengal, India

Debabrata Roy MD DM(Cardiology) FACC FESC FSCAI FAHA
Senior Consultant Interventional Cardiologist and Academic Co-ordinator
NH-RTIICS
Kolkata, West Bengal, India

Debasish Mohapatra MD(General Medicine) DM
Interventional Cardiologist
BM Birla Heart Hospital
Kolkata, West Bengal, India

Debayan Sarkar MBBS
Junior Specialist Doctor
University Hospitals
Biringham, United Kingdom

Debdatta Bhattacharyya MD MRCP CCST(Cardiology, UK)
Senior Consultant and Chief of Cath-lab
NH-RTIICS
Kolkata, West Bengal, India

Deepanjan Bhattacharya MD DM
Assistant Professor
Department of Cardiology
All India Institute of Medical Sciences, Kalyani
Kalyani, West Bengal, India

Deepa S Kumar MD DM(Cardiology) PDF(Pediatric Cardiology)
Additional Professor
Department of Cardiology
Sree Chitra Tirunal Institute for Medical Sciences and Technology
Thiruvananthapuram, Kerala, India

Deepthi Kodati MD DM FESC
Consultant Cardiologist
Trust Health Care
Durgabai Deshmukh Hospital
Hyderabad, Telangana, India

Deepti Chopra DTCD MD MAMS ACME FAIMER(2nd year)
Professor and Head
Department of Pharmacology
All India Institute of Medical Sciences, Bilaspur
Bilaspur, Himachal Pradesh, India

Devanu Ghosh Roy MD DM
Senior Consultant
Department of Cardiology
Peerless Hospital and BK Roy Research Centre
Kolkata, West Bengal, India

Dev B Pahlajani DNB(Medicine) DNB(Cardiology) FSCAI
Head
Department of Cardiology
Breach Candy Hospital
Mumbai, Maharashtra, India

Devesh Kumar DM(Cardiology)
Assistant Professor
Department of Cardiology
VMMC and Safdarjung Hospital
New Delhi, India

Dhananjay Kumar MD
Additional Director
Fortis Escorts Heart Institute
New Delhi, India

Dharmendra Jain DM
Professor
Department of Cardiology
Institute of Medical Sciences
Banaras Hindu University
Varanasi, Uttar Pradesh, India

Dhiman Kahali MD Dip(Cardiology) DM(Cardiology)
Senior Consultant and Director
BM Birla Heart Research Centre
Kolkata, West Bengal, India

Dibya Kumar Baruah MD DM FACC FSCAI FAPSC FCSI
Senior Consultant and Director
Catheterization Laboratory
Apollo Hospital, Health City
Visakhapatnam, Andhra Pradesh, India

Dilip Kumar MD DM FACC FRCP(Glasgow) FSCAI FESC FICC FHRS FHFA Certified Cardiac Device Specialist(CCDS, HRS, USA)
Director – Cardiac Cath Lab Services
Senior Consultant Interventional Cardiologist and Electrophysiologist
Chief Academic Co-ordinator
Medica Institute of Cardiac Science
Kolkata, West Bengal, India

Dipankar Das MD DM FAPSIC
Head
Department of Cardiology
Hayat Super Speciality Hospital
Guwahati, Assam, India

Dipankar Ghosh Dastidar DCH MD(Medicine) DM(Cardiology) FACC FESC FCSI FICP FSCAI
Associate Professor and Head
Department of Cardiology
Burdwan Medical College
Burdwan, West Bengal, India

Disha Shetty MD DM
Assistant Professor
Department of Cardiology
Sri Jayadeva Institute of Cardiovascular Sciences and Research
Bengaluru, Karnataka, India

Dixit Goyal MD DM(Cardiology)
Assistant Professor
GB Pant Institute of Postgraduate Medical Education and Research
New Delhi, India

Dorairaj Prabhakaran MD DM(Cardiology) MSc FRCP FNASc FNA DSc(Honoris Causa)
Executive Director
Centre for Chronic Disease Control (CCDC)
Distinguished Professor – Public Health Foundation of India (PHFI)
New Delhi, India

DP Sinha MD DM FSCAI FJCS
Head
Department of Cardiology
ILS Hospital
Dum Dum, West Bengal, India

Ferooz Ahmad Banday MD(Medicine) DM(Cardiology)
Resident
Department of Cardiology
IPGMER
Kolkata, West Bengal, India

Ganesan Karthikeyan MD DM
Professor
Department of Cardiology
All India Institute of Medical Sciences
New Delhi, India

Gaurav Singhal DM(Cardiology)
Head
Department of Cardiology
ESIC Model Hospital
Jaipur, Rajasthan, India

Gaurav Tripathi MD DM FSCAI
Consultant and Head
Department of Cardiology
Suyash Hospital
Raipur, Chattisgarh, India

Gautam Sharma MD DM
Professor
Department of Cardiology
Professor-In-Charge
Centre for Integrative Medicine and Research
All India Institute of Medical Sciences
New Delhi, India

Gautam Singal MD DNB
Associate Professor
Department of Cardiology
Dayanand Medical College and Hospital
Unit-Hero DMC Heart Institute
Ludhiana, Punjab, India

Ghanshyam Sharma MD(Medicine)
Associate Professor
Department of Medicine
RD Gardi Medical College
Ujjain, Madhya Pradesh, India

Girish Dwivedi MD DM MRCP(UK) PhD(UK) FRACP FASE FESC FCSANZ FSCCT
Professor and Senior Cardiologist
Department of Cardiology
Fiona Stanley Hospital
Harry Perkins Institute of Medical Research
School of Medicine
The University of Western Australia
Perth, Western Australia, Australia

Girish MP MD DM
Professor
Department of Cardiology
GB Pant Hospital
New Delhi, India

Gopalakrishnan A DM
Additional Professor
Sree Chitra Tirunal Institute
Thiruvananthapuram, Kerala, India

Gopal Chandra Ghosh DM(Cardiology) FACC FESC
Consultant Cardiologist
GitaRam Hospital and RN Thakur Hospital
Berhampore, West Bengal, India

Gourav Bhattacharya MD DM(Cardiology)
Senior Resident
Department of Cardiology
Burdwan Medical College and Hospital
Burdwan, West Bengal, India

Goutam Datta MD DNB DM MRCP(UK) FESC FSCAI
Professor
IPGMER
Kolkata, West Bengal, India

G Ravi Kiran MD MRCP DM
Assistant Professor
Department of Cardiology
Nizamabad Medical College
Interventional Cardiologist
Medicover Hospital
Nizamabad, Telangana, India

Gurpreet S Wander MD DM FACC FAMS
Principal and Professor
Department of Cardiology
Dayanand Medical College and Hospital
Unit-Hero DMC Heart Institute
Ludhiana, Punjab, India

G Venkateshwara Reddy MD DM
Head
Department of Cardiology
Star Pinnacle Heart Centre
Visakhapatnam, Andhra Pradesh, India

Haresh Mehta MD(Medicine) DNB(Cardiology) FACC FESC FSCAI
Director – Interventional and Structural Cardiology,
SL Raheja – Fortis Hospital
Mumbai, Maharashtra, India

Harikrishnan S DM FACC FRCP FAMS
Professor and Head
Department of Cardiology
Sree Chitra Tirunal Institute for Medical Sciences and Technology
Thiruvananthapuram, Kerala, India

Harinder K Bali MD DM
Chairman Cardiac Sciences
Livasa Hospital
Mohali, Punjab, India

Harshit Khare MD DM(Cardiology)
Assistant Professor
Department of Cardiology
Sanjay Gandhi Postgraduate Institute of Medical Sciences
Lucknow, Uttar Pradesh, India

Harsh Wardhan MD(Medicine) DM(Cardiology)
Principal–Director, Cardiac Sciences
Supreme Hospital
Faridabad, Haryana, India

Hemant Kumar Satpathy MD
Maternal-Fetal- Medicine (MFN) Specialist
Methodist Women's Hospital
Omaha, NE, USA

Hem Chandra Kalita MD(Medicine) DM(Cardiology)
Professor
Department of Cardiology
Assam Medical College and Hospital
Dibrugarh, Assam, India

Hetan C Shah MD DNB(Cardiology) FACC FESC FSCAI
Professor
Department of Cardiology
Seth GS Medical College and KEM Hospital
Mumbai, Maharashtra, India

Himanshu Dabral MD DM
Director
Division of Interventional Cardiology
Medanta Heart Institute
Medanta – The Medicity
Gurugram, Haryana, India

Himanshu Jindal MD(General Medicine) DNB(Cardiology)
Resident
Max Super Speciality Hospital
Patparganj, New Delhi, India

HK Chopra MD DM FRCP FACC FISC FISCU FASE FCSI FIAE FIMSA
Senior Consultant Cardiologist
Medanta Moolchand Heart Institute
Chairman
CME Moolchand Medcity
New Delhi, India
Past President – National CSI

Ilayaraja U MD DM
Cardiologist
Billroth Hospital
Chennai, Tamil Nadu, India

I Sathyamurthy MD DM FACC FRCP DSc(Honoris Causa)
Senior Interventional Cardiologist
Department of Cardiology
Apollo Main Hospitals
Chennai, Tamil Nadu, India

Jacob Jose MD DM(Cardiology) FACC FASE FCCP MS
Consultant Cardiologist
Naruvi Hospitals
Vellore, Tamil Nadu, India

Jagdish Chander Mohan MD DM
Interventional Cardiologist
Department of Cardiology
Institute of Heart and Vascular Diseases
Jaipur Golden Hospital
Rohini, Delhi, India

Jaideep C Menon DM(Cardiology) MPH
Professor
Adult Cardiology and Public Health
Amrita Institute of Medical Sciences and Research Center
Amrita Vishwa Vidyapeetham
Kochi, Kerala, India

Jaideep Dey MD(General Medicine) DNB(Cardiology)
Associate Director
Department of Cardiology
BLK-Max Super Specialty Hospital
New Delhi, India

Jaishankar Krishnamoorthy MD DM FIAMS
Director and Clinical Lead of Cardiology and Electrophysiology
Director – Cath Lab Services
Medway Heart Institute
Chennai, Tamil Nadu, India

Jamal Yusuf MD DM(Cardiology) FSCAI FESC FNAMS
Director–Professor
GB Pant Institute of Postgraduate Medical Education and Research
New Delhi, India

Jayagopal PB MD DM DNB FACC FICC FCSI FESC FSCAI FRCP(E)
Director, Head and Senior Interventional Cardiologist
Lakshmi Hospital
Palakkad, Kerala, India

Jayranganath M MD DM(Cardiology)
Professor and Head
Sri Jay Deva Institute of Cardiovascular Science and Research
Bengaluru, Karnataka, India

Jenu Rose Jose E MD DNB DM(Cardiology) PDF(Pediatric Cardiology)
Consultant Pediatric Cardiologist
Lisie Hospital
Kochi, Kerala, India

Jesu Krupa MD DM(Cardiology)
Faculty
Department of Cardiology
Christian Medical College
Vellore, Tamil Nadu, India

John Jose E MD DM Fellowship in Interventional Cardiology
Professor and Head
Department of Cardiology Unit-2
Cardiac Valve and Structural Heart Disease
Christian Medical College Hospital
Vellore, Tamil Nadu, India

Joyal J Kandathil MD DM
Consultant Cardiology
St Gregorios Medical Mission Hospital
Parumala, Kerala, India

Joy M Thomas MD DM
Senior Consultant
Interventional Cardiology and Cardiac Electrophysiology
Department of Cardiology
Apollo Speciality Hospital, Vanagaram
Chennai, Tamil Nadu, India

JPS Sawhney DM FESC FACC FRCP
Chairperson
Department of Cardiology
Dharma Vira Heart Center
Sir Ganga Ram Hospital
New Delhi, India

JS Thomas Xavier Paulsingh DM FNB(Interventional Cardiology)
Associate Consultant and Interventional Cardiologist
Meenakshi Mission Hospital and Research Centre
Madurai, Tamil Nadu, India

Juan Lu BSc MPE PhD
AI Scientist
Harry Perkins Institute of Medical Research
School of Medicine
The University of Western Australia
Perth, Western Australia, Australia

Juhi Singh MD DNB(Medicine)
Senior Resident
Department of Cardiology
Sir Ganga Ram Hospital
New Delhi, India

Justin Paul Gnanaraj MD DNB(Medicine) DM DNB(Cardiology) FACC FESC FSCAI
Professor
Institute of Cardiology
Madras Medical College
Chennai, Tamil Nadu, India

Kabir Sethi MD DM
Department of Structural Heart Interventions
University Hospital of Mainz
Germany

Kajal Ganguly MD DM FACC
Consultant Interventional Cardiologist
Manipal Hospital
Kolkata, West Bengal, India

Kamal K Sethi MD DM FACC FHRS FCSI FISE
Director
Department of Cardiology
Chairman and Managing Director
Delhi Heart and Lung Institute
New Delhi, India

Kanika Kukreja MD(Medicine)
Senior Resident (Academic)
Department of Cardiology
All India Institute of Medical Sciences, Rishikesh
Rishikesh, Uttarakhand, India

Karthikeyan R MD
Senior Resident
ABVIMS and Dr RML Hospital
New Delhi, India

Kartik Pandurang Jadhav MD DM
Interventional Cardiologist
Department of Cardiology
Apollo Hospital
Hyderabad, Telangana, India

K Arun Kumar MD DM
Research Scholar
Department of Cardiology
Institute of Medical Sciences
Banaras Hindu University
Varanasi, Uttar Pradesh, India

Kaushik Manna MD(General Medicine) DM(Cardiology)
Consultant Interventional Cardiologist
NH-RTIICS
Kolkata, West Bengal, India

Kavita Tyagi MS DNB(Anatomy) DNB(Medicine) DNB(Cardiology) FNB(Interventional Cardiology)
Consultant Cardiologist
Sir Ganga Ram Hospital
New Delhi, India

Kayan Siodia MD FACC FSCAI
Interventional Cardiologist
Breach Candy Hospital
Mumbai, Maharashtra, India

Kiran Gaur MSc PhD
Associate Professor and Head
Department of Statistics, Mathematics and Computer Science
Government SKN Agriculture University
Jaipur, Rajasthan, India

KK Talwar MD DM FAMS FNA FACC DSc(Honoris Causa)
Chairman – Heart Institute
PSRI Hospital
New Delhi, India

KN Srinivasan MD DNB(Cardiology) FCSI FESC FSCAI
Senior Interventional Cardiologist
Department of Cardiology
Apollo Main Hospitals
Chennai, Tamil Nadu, India

Kranthi Kumar Gedala MD(General Medicine)
Senior Resident in Adult Cardiology
Amrita Institute of Medical Sciences and Research Center
Amrita Vishwa Vidyapeetham
Kochi, Kerala, India

Krishnamoorthy KM DM DNB
Professor
Sree Chitra Tirunal Institute
Thiruvananthapuram, Kerala, India

K Sivaprasad MD DM DNB FESC FSCAI
Professor and Head
Department of Cardiology
Government Medical College
Thiruvananthapuram, Kerala, India

Kumar Himanshu MD DM
Assistant Professor
LPS Institute of Cardiology
Kanpur, Uttar Pradesh, India

Lakshmi Durga Kumaraguruparan MD(Pediatrics) DNB(Pediatrics) DM
Resident
Department of Cardiology
Sri Ramachandra Institute of Higher Education and Research
Chennai, Tamil Nadu, India

Lekha Adik Pathak MD(Medicine) DM(Cardiology) FRCP(Edinburgh)
Director and Head
Department of Cardiology
Nanavati Max Super Speciality Hospital
Mumbai, Maharashtra, India

Louie Fischer MD DM MRCP(UK) FRCP(Edinburgh) FACC FSCAI FESC
Professor and Chief Interventional Cardiologist
MOSC Medical College Hospital
Kochi, Kerala, India

Maddury Jyotsna MD DM FACC FESC FICC
Professor and Head (Retired)
Department of Cardiology
Nizam's Institute of Medical Sciences
Hyderabad, Telangana, India

Madhu Shukla MBBS PhD
Head of Noninvasive Cardiology
Department of Cardiology
Institute of Heart and Vascular Diseases, Jaipur Golden Hospital
Rohini, New Delhi, India

Madhu Sreedharan MD DM MRCP(UK) FRCP FACC
Director
NIMS Heart Foundation
Thiruvananthapuram, Kerala, India

Madhuvanthi Rajendran DCH DNB
Registrar in Cardiology
Kovai Medical Centre Hospital
Coimbatore, Tamil Nadu, India

Mahendra Chouhan DNB(Medicine) DrNB
Senior Resident
Department of Cardiology
Janakpuri Super Speciality Hospital
New Delhi, India

Mahesh Nalin Kumar MD DrNB FACC FESC
Head and Senior Consultant Cardiology
St Gregorios Medical Mission Hospital
Parumala, Kerala, India

Mainak Mandal MBBS
Postgraduate Trainee
Department of General Medicine
KPC Medical College
Kolkata, West Bengal, India

Mainak Mukhopadhyay MD MRCP DM FESC CCDS
Consultant Interventional Cardiologist
Manipal Hospital
Kolkata, West Bengal, India

Manish Bansal MD DNB(Cardiology)
Senior Director Clinical and Preventive Cardiology
Medanta – The Medicity
Gurugram, Haryana, India

Manish Narang PhD MPharm
Director Medical Affairs
Asia Pacific and Japan
Abott Vascular
New Delhi, India

Manjira Sinha PhD
Senior Scientist
TCS Research
Kolkata, West Bengal, India

Manju Bhargav BR MD
Senior Resident
Department of Cardiology
Government Medical College
Thiruvananthapuram, Kerala, India

Manoj Kumar Agarwala MD(PGI) DM(PGI) FACC
Consultant Cardiologist
Department of Cardiology
Apollo Hospital, Jubilee Hills
Hyderabad, Telangana, India

Manojkumar Rohit MD DM(Cardiology) MNAMS
Professor
Department of Cardiology
Postgraduate Institute of Medical Education and Research
Chandigarh, India

Manoranjan Mandal MD Dip Card DM
Professor and Head
Department of Cardiology
NRS Medical College
Kolkata, West Bengal, India

Manu Gupta MBBS
Resident
Department of Medicine
PCMS and RC
Bhopal, Madhya Pradesh, India

Manu R MD DM
Senior Interventional Cardiologist
Meditrina Hospital
Kollam, Kerala, India

Mayank Shami MD
Senior Resident
Department of Cardiology
MAMC and GIPMER
New Delhi, India

Meenakshi Kadiyala MD(General Medicine) DM(Cardiology)
Professor and Head
Department of Cardiology
Saveetha Medical College
Chennai, Tamil Nadu, India

Meenu Nair MD DM
Resident
Department of Cardiology
Amrita Institute of Medical Sciences
Kochi, Kerala, India

Milind Kharche MD DM(Cardiology) FACC FESC FSCAI
Chief Interventional Cardiologist
Care CIIGMA Hospital
Aurangabad, Maharashtra, India

Milind Phadke MD DM
Additional Professor
Lokmanya Tilak Municipal Medical College and General Hospital
Mumbai, Maharashtra, India

Mohit D Gupta MD DM FAMS FACC(USA)
Director–Professor
Department of Cardiology
GB Pant Institute of Postgraduate Medical Education and Research
New Delhi, India

Mohit M Bhagwati DNB(Cardiology) FSCAI MNAMS
Incharge
Acute Cardiac Care and Heart Failure Clinic
Consultant
Department of Cardiology
Holy Family Hospital
New Delhi, India

Mohsin Raj Mantoo MD DM
Post-DM Senior Resident
Department of Cardiology
All India Institute of Medical Sciences
New Delhi, India

Mona Bhatia MD FRCR(UK) FSCMR(USA) FSCCT(USA)
Principal–Director and Head
Department of Imaging
Fortis Escort Heart Institute
New Delhi, India

Monika Bhandari MD DM FACC FESC FSCAI APSIC
Additional Professor
Department of Cardiology
King George's Medical University
Lucknow, Uttar Pradesh, India

Monika Jain MD
Final Year Resident Doctor
Department of Medicine
RD Gardi Medical College
Ujjain, Madhya Pradesh, India

Monika P Jawanjal MD DM
Assistant Professor
Department of Cardiology
Kasturba Medical College, Manipal
Manipal, Karnataka, India

MPS Chawla MD FACP FRCP FICP FIACM FISC FIMSA
Senior Professor and Former Head
Department of Medicine
ABVIMS and Dr RML Hospital
New Delhi, India

Mrinal Kanti Das MD DM FICP FICC FCSI FACC FESC
Consultant Cardiologist
CK Birla Hospitals (BMB/CMRI)
Kolkata, West Bengal, India

M Shanmathi MBBS
Duty Medical Officer
Meenakshi Hospital
Thanjavur, Tamil Nadu, India

MS Prashant MD
Resident
Department of Cardiology
Apollo Hospital
Hyderabad, Telangana, India

MS Ravi MD DM(Cardiology)
Former Director
Department of Cardiology
Madras Medical College and Rajiv Ghandhi Government General Hospital
Chennai, Tamil Nadu, India

Mukesh Goel MS MCh(CTVS)
Senior Consultant
Indraprastha Apollo Hospital
New Delhi, India

Mukund Prabhu MD DM PDF(Electrophysiology)
Associate Professor, Department of Cardiology (EP Division)
Kasturba Medical College, Manipal
Manipal, Karnataka, India

Muralidharan TR MD DM
Professor and Director
Institute of Cardiac Sciences
SRM GLOBAL Hospitals
SRM Institute of Science and Technology
Chennai, Tamil Nadu, India

Nadeem Akhtar MD
Senior Resident
Department of Cardiology
SP Medical College and HRMC Centre
Bikaner, Rajasthan, India

Nagaraj Desai MD DM(Cardiology) FACC
Director
Namana Medical Centre
Bengaluru, Karnataka, India

Nagendra Boopathy Senguttuvan MD DM FACC FSCAI Fellowship in Interventional Cardiology and Structural heart disease Interventions(USA)
Professor
Clinical Lead – Structural Heart Diseases Interventions
Department of Cardiology
Sri Ramachandra Institute of Higher Education and Research
Chennai, Tamil Nadu, India

Nakul Sinha MD DM
Chairman – Cardiology
Max Hospital
Former Professor and Head
Department of Cardiology
Sanjay Gandhi Postgraduate Institute of Medical Sciences
Lucknow, Uttar Pradesh, India

Nandhakumar Vasu MD DNB(Cardiology) FNB(Interventional Cardiology)
Senior Consultant
Department of Cardiology
Institute of Cardio Vascular Diseases
The Madras Medical Mission Hospital
Chennai, Tamil Nadu, India

Narra Lavanya MD(General Medicine) DrNB(Cardiology)
Consultant Interventional Cardiologist
KIMS Hospitals
Hyderabad, Telangana, India

Navanil Biswas MD(General Medicine) DrNB(Cardiology)
Consultant Interventional Cardiologist
Apollo Multispeciality Hospital
Kolkata, West Bengal, India

Navdeep Singh Sidhu MD DM FAPSIC FACC
Assistant Professor
Department of Cardiology
All India Institute of Medical Sciences, Bilaspur
Bilaspur, Himachal Pradesh, India

Naved Aslam MD DM
Professor
Department of Cardiology
Dayanand Medical College and Hospital
Unit-Hero DMC Heart Institute
Ludhiana, Punjab, India

Navjyot Kaur MD DNB MRCP DM
Assistant Professor
Department of Cardiology
Command Hospital (Air Force)
Bengaluru, Karnataka, India

Neeraj Awasthy MD FNB(Pediatric Cardiology)
Director
Department of Pediatric and Congenital Heart Disease
Fortis Escorts Heart Institute
New Delhi, India

Nikhil Borikar MD DM(Cardiology)
Associate Professor
Department of Cardiology
Topiwala National Medical College and BYL
Nair Charitable Hospital
Mumbai, Maharashtra, India

Nilesh Giri MD(Medicine) DM(Cardiology)
Resident
Department of Cardiology
IPGMER
Kolkata, West Bengal, India

Nirat Beohar MD FACC FSCAI
Professor of Medicine
Columbia University Medical Center
Director, Cardiac Catheterization Laboratory, Structural Heart Disease and Interventional Cardiology Fellowship
Columbia University Division of Cardiology
Mount Sinai Medical Center
Miami Beach, FL, USA

Nirmal Ghati MD DM
Assistant Professor
Department of Cardiology
Cardiothoracic Sciences Centre
All India Institute of Medical Sciences
New Delhi, India

Nishad Chitnis MD MRCP DNB
Consultant Cardiologist
Heart Care Clinic
Karveer Cardiac Centre
Kolhapur, Maharashtra, India

Nitin K Kabra MD DM FACC
Professor and Head
Department of Cardiology
Gandhi Medical College Hospital
Secunderabad, Telangana, India

Nitish Prasad MD DrNB
Consultant Cardiologist
Apollo Hospitals
Bhubaneswar, Odisha, India

NK Mohanty MD DM
Professor
Department of Cardiology
SCB Medical College
Cuttack, Odisha, India

NN Khanna MD DM FRCP(London Glasgow, Edinburgh) FACC FSCAI FESC FAPSIC FCCP FEISI FICC FCSI
Senior Consultant Cardiologist
Indraprastha Apollo Hospital
New Delhi, India
Advisor – Apollo Group of Hospitals in India

OP Yadava MS DNB
CEO and Chief Cardiac Surgeon
National Heart Institute
New Delhi, India

Oruganti Sai Satish MD DM(Fellowship in EP and Pacing)
Senior Professor and Head Unit 1
Department of Cardiology
Nizams Institute of Medical Sciences
Hyderabad, Telangana, India

Padma Madhab Bisoi MD(General Medicine)
Postdoctoral Trainee
BM Birla Heart Hospital
Kolkata, West Bengal, India

Panchanan Sahoo MD(Medicine) DM(Cardiology) FACC FESC FICC FISE
Professor, Senior Consultant and Electrophysiologist
Department of Cardiology
Kalinga Institute of Medical Sciences
Bhubaneswar, Odisha, India

Pankaj Harkut MD DM(Cardiology) FACC FESC
Consultant Interventional Cardiologist
Swasthyam Superspeciality Hospital
Nagpur, Maharashtra, India

Pankaj Kashyap MD DM(Cardiology)
Assistant Professor
Department of Cardiology
Topiwala National Medical College and BYL Nair Charitable Hospital
Mumbai, Maharashtra, India

Pankaj Manoria MD DM FACC FESC
Director
Manoria Heart and Critical Care Hospital
Bhopal, Madhya Pradesh, India

Parag Barwad MD DM FESC FSCAI CEPS-AC
Additional Professor
Department of Cardiology
Postgraduate Institute of Medical Education and Research
Chandigarh, India

Parayaru Kottayil Asokan MD DM FRCP FCSI FACC FESC FSCAI FICC
Chief Consultant Interventional Cardiologist
Department of Cardiology
Fathima Hospital
Kozhikode, Kerala, India

Paul V George MD DM
Senior Professor
Department of Cardiology Unit-2
Christian Medical College Hospital
Vellore, Tamil Nadu, India

Pawan Sharma MD(General Medicine) DM(Cardiology)
Senior Interventional Cardiologist
Associate Director and Unit-Head Cardiology
Max Superspeciality Hospital
Patparganj, New Delhi, India

P Chakradhar MD DM
Consultant Cardiologist
Apollo Hospitals Health City
Visakhapatnam, Andhra Pradesh, India

P Chandrasekhar MD DM FACC
Head and Professor
Department of Cardiology
Kurnool Medical College
Kurnool, Andhra Pradesh, India

PC Manoria MD DM FACC FESC FCAPSC
Director, Manoria Heart and Critical Care Hospital
Bhopal, Madhya Pradesh, India

PC Rath MD DM FICC FESC FACC FRCP(London) FRCP(Edinburgh)
Senior Consultant Cardiologist and Head
Department of Cardiology
Apollo Hospital, Jubilee Hills
Hyderabad, Telangana
Apollo Hospital
Bhubaneshwar, Odisha, India

Pintu Nahata MD DM(Cardiology) FACC FSCAI FESC FCI
Senior Professor and Head
Department of Cardiology
SP Medical College and HRMC Centre
Bikaner, Rajasthan, India

Pooja Sharma Gupta MBBS
Resident
Department of Dermatology
PCMS and RC
Bhopal, Madhya Pradesh, India

Prabahakar Koregol MD DM(Cardiology) FSCAI
Senior Consultant Cardiologist
Department of Cardiology
Fortis Hospitals and Namana Medical Centre
Bengaluru, Karnataka, India

Pradeep Kumar Mustepally MD DNB
Consultant Cardiologist
Apollo Hospital, Jubilee Hills
Hyderabad, Telangana, India

Pradyumna Kumar Singh MD
Senior Resident
Department of Cardiology
ABVIMS and Dr RML Hospital
New Delhi, India

Prakas Chandra Mondal MD MRCP(UK, Ireland) MRRCPS(Glasgow) DM(Cardilogy) DNB(Cardiology) FACC(USA)
Consultant Interventional Cardiologist and Head
Department of Cardiology
Apolo Multispeciality Hospital
Kolkata, West Bengal, India

Prasant Kr Sahoo MD DM FRCP FACC FSCAI FESC FAPSIC FCSI FICC
Director Interventional Cardiology
Apollo Hospitals
Bhubaneswar, Odisha, India
Chairman CSI NIC 2021-25

Prashant Bobhate MD(Pediatrics) FNB(Pediatrics Cardiology) FPVRi Fellowship in Pulmonary Hypertension(Canada)
Consultant Pediatric Cardiologist
Childrens Heart Center
Kokilaben Dhirubai Ambani Hospital
Mumbai, Maharashtra, India

Prashant Moorthy MD(FRCR)
Assistant Professor
Saveetha Medical College
Chennai, Tamil Nadu, India

Prashant Panda MD DM
Associate Professor
Department of Cardiology
Postgraduate Institute of Medical Education and Research
Chandigarh, India

Prasit Maity DNB
Consultant
Department of Imaging
Fortis Escort Heart Institute
New Delhi, India

Prathap Kumar N MD DM FIC
Chief Interventional Cardiologist
Meditrina Hospital
Kollam, Kerala, India

Pratishtha Mehra PhD
Senior Research Associate
Department of Cardiology
GB Pant Institute of Postgraduate Medical Education and Research
New Delhi, India

Praveen Arumugam MD
Senior Resident
Department of Cardiology
Cardiothoracic Sciences Centre
All India Institute of Medical Sciences
New Delhi, India

Pravin K Goel MD DM FACC FSCAI
Director – Interventional Cardiology
Medanta Heart Institute
Lucknow, Uttar Pradesh, India

Preetam Krishnamurthy MD DM PDF CCDS
Assistant Professor and Consultant Electrophysiologist
Sri Ramachandra Institute for Higher Education and Research
Chennai, Tamil Nadu, India

Preethi Caleb Harris MD DCH
Senior Resident
Department of Cardiology
NEIGRIHMS
Shillong, Meghalaya, India

Preeti Gupta MD(Internal Medicine) DrNB(Cardiology) FACC FESC FSCAI FICC FCSI
Professor
Department of Cardiology
VMMC and Safdarjung Hospital
New Delhi, India

Preetish Rath PhD
Candidate (Computer Science)
Tufts University, Medford
Massachusetts, USA

Priya Jagia MD DNB
Professor and Head
Department of Cardiovascular Imaging and Endovascular Interventions
Cardiothoracic Sciences Centre
All India Institute of Medical Sciences
New Delhi, India

PS Banerjee MD DM(Cardiology) FACC
Chief Interventional Cardiologist
Manipal Hospital
Former Head
Department of Cardiology
Medical College
Kolkata, West Bengal, India
Past President – Cardiological Society of India

Puneet Rastogii MD DM
Professor and Head
Department of Cardiology
GR Medical College
Gwalior, Madhya Pradesh, India

Punitha Lakxmi Ramesh MD
Senior Resident
Department of Cardiology
Sree Chitra Tirunal Institute for Medical Sciences and Technology
Thiruvananthapuram, Kerala, India

Purneshwar Pandey MD DM(Interventional Cardiology)
Consultant
Department of Cardiology
Fortis Hospital
Vasant Kunj, New Delhi, India

Purushotham Reddy Ramireddy Gari MD
Resident in Cardiology
Nizams Institute of Medical Sciences
Hyderabad, Telangana, India

Raghav R Nagpal MD
Consultant – Interventional and Structural Cardiology
SL Raheja – Fortis Hospital
Mumbai, Maharashtra, India

Rahul Nijhawan DM(Cardiology) PDF(Electrophysiology)
Assistant Professor
Department of Cardiology
GB Pant Institute of Postgraduate Medical Education and Research
New Delhi, India

Raja J Selvaraj MD DNB PDF EP
Professor
JIPMER
Puducherry, India

Rajeev Agarwal MD DM
Consultant Cardiologist
Jaswant Rai Speciality Hospital
Meerut, Uttar Pradesh, India

Rajeev Garg MD(Medicine) Dip Card(NIMS) DNB(Cardiology) MNAMS FSCAI FESC FACC Diplomate National Board
Senior Consultant Interventional Cardiologist
Aware Gleneagles Global Hospital
Hyderabad, Telangana, India

Rajeev Gupta MD PhD
Chair Preventive Cardiology and Medicine
Eternal Heart Care Centre and Research Institute
Jaipur, Rajasthan, India

Rajeev Gupta MD DM(Cardiology)
Professor and Head
Department of Cardiology
Gandhi Medical College
Bhopal, Madhya Pradesh, India

Rajendra Kumar Jain MD DM FACC DIU(Paris)
Founder and Director
KIMS Group of Hospitals
Hyderabad, Telangana, India

Rajesh Sharma MD DM
Associate Professor
Department of Cardiology
Indira Gandhi Medical College and Hospital
Shimla, Himachal Pradesh, India

Rajesh Thachathodiyil MD DM FACC
Head
Department of Cardiology
Amrita Institute of Medical Sciences
Kochi, Kerala, India

Rajesh Vijayvergiya MD DM FSCAI FACC FESC FISES
Professor
Department of Cardiology
Advanced Cardiac Centre
Postgraduate Institute of Medical Education and Research
Chandigarh, India

Rajiv C MD DM(Cardiology)
Senior Consultant
Aster Medcity
Kochi, Kerala, India

Rajiv Passey DNB(Medicine) DM(Cardiology) MNAMS FICP FESC
Senior Consultant Interventional Cardiologist
Co-Director Cath Lab and In-charge CCU
Dharma Vira Heart Centre
Sir Ganga Ram Hospital
New Delhi, India

Rajneesh Jain MD DM
Senior Consultant
Director – Cathlab and Vice Chairperson
Sir Ganga Ram Hospital
New Delhi, India

Rajneesh Kapoor MD DNB FACC
Chairman
Division of Interventional Cardiology
Medanta Heart Institute
Medanta – The Medicity
Gurugram, Haryana, India

Rajpal Prajapati DM
Associate Professor
Department of Cardiology
Institute of Medical Sciences
Banaras Hindu University
Varanasi, Uttar Pradesh, India

Rakesh Maurya MD DM
Consultant Cradiologist
Jaswant Rai Speciality Hospital
Meerut, Uttar Pradesh, India

Rakesh Yadav MD DM
Professor
Department of Cardiology
All India Institute of Medical Sciences
New Delhi, India

Ramakrishna J MD DM
Consultant Cardiologist
Apollo Hospital, Jubilee Hills
Hyderabad, Telangana, India

Ramdas G Pai MD FACC FRCP(Edinburgh)
Professor
California University of Science and Medicine
Colton, CA, USA

Ranjit K Nath MD DM FACC FSCAI FESC FCSI
Director–Professor and Head
Department of Cardiology
ABVIMS and Dr RML Hospital
New Delhi, India

Rathindra Nath Karmakar MD DM
Consultant
Department of Cardiology
Narayana Multispeciality Hospital
Kolkata, West Bengal, India

Ratul Ghosh MD
Resident
Department of Cardiology
RG Kar Medical College and Hospital
Kolkata, West Bengal, India

Ravikishore Amancharla MD DM FACC
Head and Senior Consultant
Cardiologist and Electrophysiologist
Health City
Cayman Islands

Ravikumar Rathnagiri MD DM FESC
Senior Consultant and Clinical Lead
Institute of Heart and Lung Transplant
MGM Healthcare
Chennai, Tamil Nadu, India

Ravi R Kasliwal MD DM(Cardiology)
Chairman Clinical and Preventive Cardiology
Medanta – The Medicity
Gurugram, Haryana, India

Ravi Vishnu Prasad MD(Medicine) DM(Cardiology)
Professor and Head
Department of Cardiology
Indira Gandhi Institute of Medical Sciences (IGIMS)
Patna, Bihar, India

Rishika Mehta MD(Pediatrics) DrNB(Pediatric Cardiology)
Pediatric Cardiologist
Department of Pediatric Cardiology
Narayana Superspeciality Hospital
Howrah, West Bengal, India

Rishi Sethi MD DM FACC FESC FRCP(Edinburgh, London) FSCAI FAPSIC FAMS FCSI FISC
Professor, Department of Cardiology
King George's Medical University
Lucknow, Uttar Pradesh, India

Rohan Naik MD
Assistant Professor
Department of Medicine
West Virginia University Heart and Vascular Institute
Morgantown, West Virginia, USA

Ronak Sheth MD FNB(Pediatric Cardiology)
Consultant Pediatric Cardiologist
Fortis Hospital
Mumbai, Maharashtra, India

Ronak V Ruparelia DNB(Medicine) DNB(Cardiology)
Interventional Cardiologist
Bankers Super Speciality Hospital
Vadodara, Gujarat, India

Roopa Salwan MD DM
Senior Director
Myocardial Infarction Program
Senior Consultant
Cardiology and Interventional Cardiology
Max Super Speciality Hospital
Saket, New Delhi, India

Roshan Rao MD DM FACC FESC FSCAI
Senior Interventional Cardiologist and Head
Department of Cardiology
Apollo Hospitals
Indore, Madhya Pradesh, India

R Rameshwar MD(General Medicine)
PG in DM(Cardiology)
Saveetha Medical College
Chennai, Tamil Nadu, India

Ruchi Sharma MD MD
Resident
ESIC Hospital
Faridabad, Haryana, India

Rufus Demel X MD DNB(Cardiology) FNB(Interventional Cardiology)
Chief Consultant Cardiologist
Devaki Heart Center
Madurai, Tamil Nadu, India

Rupendra Nath Saha MD
Senior Resident (Academic)
Department of Cardiology
All India Institute of Medical Sciences, Rishikesh
Rishikesh, Uttarakhand, India

Sabyasachi Pandey MD(Pediatrics) DM(Pediatric Cardiology)
Resident
Sri Jay Deva Institute of Cardiovascular Science and Research
Bengaluru, Karnataka, India

Sachin Maggo MD
Senior Resident
Department of Cardiology
Indira Gandhi Medical College and Hospital
Shimla, Himachal Pradesh, India

Sachin Ralya MD(Radiodiagnosis)
Department of Imaging
Fortis Escort Heart Institute
New Delhi, India

Safal MD DM
Professor
Department of Cardiology
MAMC and GIPMER
New Delhi, India

Sajan Narayanan MD(Internal Medicine) DM(Cardiology) FESC
Senior Consultant and Interventional Cardiologist
Little Flower Hospital and Research Institute
Kochi, Kerala, India

Sakshi Sachdeva MD DM
Assistant Professor – Pediatric Cardiology
ABVIMS and Dr RML Hospital
New Delhi, India

Sameer Shrivastava MD(General Medicine) DM(Cardiology)
Principal–Director and Chief of Noninvasive Cardiology
Max Super Specialty Hospital
Saket, New Delhi, India

Samshad Alam MD(Medicine) DM(Cardiology)
Associate Direrctor
Jai Prabha Medanta Superspecialty Hospital
Patna, Bihar, India

Samuel Jebavaram MD DNB
Senior Registrar, Billroth Hospital
Chennai, Tamil Nadu, India

Sandeep Kamat MD DM(Cardiology)
Assistant Professor
Department of Cardiology
Topiwala National Medical College and BYL
Nair Charitable Hospital
Mumbai, Maharashtra, India

Sandeep Seth DM(Cardiology)
Professor
Department of Cardiology
All India Institute of Medical Sciences
New Delhi, India

Sandeep Singh MD DM
Professor
Department of Cardiology
All India Institute of Medical Sciences
New Delhi, India

Sandipta Ray MD DM
Consultant Interventional Cardiologist
Manipal Hospital
Kolkata, West Bengal, India

Sangeeta Dhir MDS(Periodontology) Fellow(Implantology)
Consultant Dentistry and Clinical Research
Max Hospital
Saket, New Delhi, India

Sanjay Mehrotra MD DM
Consultant and Interventional Cardiologist
NH Institute of Cardiac Sciences
Bengaluru, Karnataka, India

Sanjay Tyagi MD(Medicine) DM(Cardiology) FAMS FICP FCSI FICA FRCP(Edinburgh) FSCAI FESC FACC(USA)
Dr BC Roy National Awardee
Senior Consultant, Academic Advisor (HOD) and Clinical Director Cardiology
Apollo Hospitals, Northern Region, New Delhi, India
President-Elect, Cardiological Society of India
Secretary General (India), International College of Cardiology (USA)
National Coordinator, Cardiology and Interventional Cardiology, National Board of Examination
Formerly
Director General Health Services, Govt of India
Dean, Maulana Azad Medical College, New Delhi
Director, Professor and HOD Cardiology
GB Pant Institute of Postgraduate Medical Education and Research

Sanjeev Asotra MD DM
Professor
Department of Cardiology
Indira Gandhi Medical College and Hospital
Shimla, Himachal Pradesh, India

Sanjeev Hanumantacharya Naganur MD(Pediatrics) DM(Cardiology) FICC FSCAI FPICS
Associate Professor
Department of Cardiology
Advanced Cardiac Center
Postgraduate Institute for Medical Education and Research
Chandigarh, India

Sanjeev Kathuria DM(Cardiology)
Professor
Department of Cardiology
GB Pant Institute of Postgraduate Medical Education and Research
New Delhi, India

Sanjeev Kumar MS MCh(Cardiothoracic and Vascular Surgery)
Professor and Head
Department of Cardiothoracic and Vascular Surgery (CTVS)
All India Institute of Medical Sciences, Patna
Patna, Bihar, India

Sankar Chandra Mandal MD(Medicine) DM(Cardiology) FACC(USA) FSCI FESC
Professor
Department of Cardiology
IPGMER
Kolkata, West Bengal, India

Sarita Rao MD DM FACC FSCAI
Senior Interventional Cardiologist and Director, Cath Lab
Apollo Hospitals
Indore, Madhya Pradesh, India

Saroj Mandal MD(Medicine) DM(Cardiology) FRCP(Edinburgh) FRCP(Glasgow) FACC(USA) FSCAI(USA) FESC(EURO)
Professor
Department of Cardiology
Institute of Cardiovascular Sciences
IPGMER
Kolkata, West Bengal, India

Sarumathi Thangavel MD FACC
Consultant Cardiologist
Lakshmi Hospital
Chennai, Tamil Nadu, India

Sateesh Reddy DNB(General Medicine) DM(Cardiology)
Senior Resident
Kalinga Institute of Medical Sciences
Bhubaneswar, Odisha, India

Satish K Parashar MD FACC
Senior Consultant Cardiologist and Director
Non-Invasive Cardiac Laboratory
Heart Centre
New Delhi, India

Satish Kumar MD(Pediatrics)
Senior Resident
Childrens Heart Center
Kokilaben Dhirubai Ambani Hospital
Mumbai, Maharashtra, India

Satya Sahitya Mandava MD DM
Senior Resident
Postgraduate Institute of Medical Education and Research
Chandigarh, India

Satya S Mandava MD DM
Fellow, Department of Cardiology
Advanced Cardiac Centre
Postgraduate Institute of Medical Education and Research
Chandigarh, India

Satyavan Sharma MD DM(Cardiology) MNAMS(Cardiology)
Honorary Consultant Cardiologist
Department of Cardiology
Bombay Hospital
Mumbai, Maharashtra, India

Satyavir Yadav MD DM
Associate Professor
Department of Cardiology
All India Institute of Medical Sciences
New Delhi, India

Satyendra Tewari MD DM(Cardiology) FACC FSCAI FCAPSC FESC FCSI FICC
Professor
Department of Cardiology
Sanjay Gandhi Postgraduate Institute of Medical Sciences
Lucknow, Uttar Pradesh, India

Saumitra Ray MD FRCP FESC FACC FSCAI FCSI FICP
Consultant
Woodlands Hospital
Kolkata, West Bengal, India

Saurabh Bhardwaj MD DrNB(Cardiology)
Junior Consultant Cardiologist
Indraprastha Apollo Hospitals
Sarita Vihar, New Delhi

Saurabh Dhumale MD DrNB(Cardiology)
Consultant Interventional Cardiologist
NH-RTIICS
Kolkata, West Bengal, India

Saurabh Kumar Gupta MD DM
Professor
Department of Cardiology
All India Institute of Medical Sciences
New Delhi, India

Saurav Mishra MD DM
Consultant – Interventional Cardiology
Medanta Heart Institute
Lucknow, Uttar Pradesh, India

Seenu Prasanth A MD(General Medicine) DM(Cardiology)
Senior Resident
Department of Cardiology
All India Institute of Medical Sciences, Nagpur
Nagpur, Maharashtra, India

Shabbir Ali Shaik MD DM FNB
Fellow Interventional Cardiologist
Department of Cardiology
Apollo Hospital, Jubilee Hills
Hyderabad, Telangana, India

Sharad Chandra DM FACC FESC FSCAI FAPSIC FCSI
Professor
Department of Cardiology
King George's Medical University
Lucknow, Uttar Pradesh, India

Shibba Takkar Chhabra MD DM
Professor
Department of Cardiology
Hero DMC Heart Institute
Dayanand Medical College and Hospital
Ludhiana, Punjab, India

Shinjan Patra MD(Internal Medicine) DM(Endocrinology)
Assistant Professor and Consultant Endocrinologist
Department of Endocrinology and Metabolism
All India Institute of Medical Sciences, Nagpur
Nagpur, Maharashtra, India

Shirisha Reddy Kommareddy MD DM
Consultant Cardiologist
KIMS Hospital
Hyderabad, Telangana, India

Shitij Chaudhary MD
Senior Resident
Department of Cardiology
All India Institute of Medical Sciences
New Delhi, India

Shivangi Tiwari MD
Final Year Resident Doctor
Department of Medicine
RD Gardi Medical College
Ujjain, Madhya Pradesh, India

Shivani Rao MD DM
Associate Professor
Department of Cardiology
ABVIMS and Dr RML Hospital
New Delhi, India

Shreyak P Kadu MD DM(Cardiology)
Assistant Professor
Department of Cardiology
Topiwala National Medical College and BYL
Nair Charitable Hospital
Mumbai, Maharashtra, India

Shreya Rani MBBS
Medical Officer
Jai Prabha Medanta Superspecialty Hospital
Patna, Bihar, India

Shridhar Dwivedi MD PhD FAMS FRCP(UK) FIACS(Canada)
Senior Consultant Cardiologist and Head, Academics
National Heart Institute
New Delhi, India

Shubhanshu Pal MD(Medicine)
Postdoctoral Trainee (3rd year)
Institute of Cardiovascular Sciences
IPGMER
Kolkata, West Bengal, India

Shyam Prasad Sahoo MBBS
Student
SRM Medical College
Chennai, Tamil Nadu, India

Siddhartha Pandey MD DM
Senior Resident
Department of Cardiology
SCB Medical College
Cuttack, Odisha, India

Sidhartha Chattopadhyay MRCP(1&2, UK)
Registrar
Department of Cardiology
Ruby General Hospital Limited
Kolkata, West Bengal, India

Sivashanmuganathan Velu MD DM
Consultant Cardiologist
Medway Heart Institute
Chennai, Tamil Nadu, India

Sivasubramanian Ramakrishnan MD DM
Professor
Department of Cardiology
All India Institute of Medical Sciences
New Delhi, India

SK Dwivedi MD DM FACC FESC FSCAI
Professor and Head
Department of Cardiology
King George's Medical University
Lucknow, Uttar Pradesh, India

Smit Shrivastava MD PGDHHM DM(Cardiology) FACC FSCAI FESC FICP FIMSA FICN FISE
Professor and Head
Advance Cardiac Institute
Pt JNM Medical College and Dr BRAM Hospital
Raipur, Chhattisgarh, India

S Murugarajan MD DM
Senior Assistant Professor
Department of Cardiology
National Centre of Ageing
Madras Medical College
Chennai, Tamil Nadu, India

Sneha Garg MD DM
Associate Consultant
Department of Cardiology
Max Hospital
Saket, New Delhi, India

Snehal Kulkarni MD DrNB FACC
Director – Pediatric Cardiac Sciences
Fortis Healthcare
Mumbai, Maharashtra, India

SN Routray MD DM FACC FESC FSCAI
Professor
Department of Cardiology
SCB Medical College
Cuttack, Odisha, India

Somnath Maji MD
Resident
Department of Cardiology
RG Kar Medical College and Hospital
Kolkata, West Bengal, India

Somnath Mukhopadhay MD DM(Cardiology) FESC
Consultant
Nightingale Hospital
Kolkata, West Bengal, India

Sonal Jain MD DrNB(Cardiology)
Resident
Sir Ganga Ram Hospital
New Delhi, India

Soormpally Vijay MD DM
Fellow in Electrophysiology
Department of Cardiac Electrophysiology, AIG Hospital
Hyderabad, Telangana, India

Soumik Ghosh DM
Associate Professor
Department of Cardiology
Institute of Medical Sciences
Banaras Hindu University
Varanasi, Uttar Pradesh, India

Soumya Patnaik MD
Assistant Professor
Department of Cardiology
University of Texas
Houston, Texas, USA

S Radhakrishnan MD DM
Professor and Head
Department of Pediatric Cardiology
Pediatric Super-Specialty Wing
Amrita Institute of Medical Sciences
Faridabad, Haryana, India

S Ramesh MD DM FACC FSCAI FESC
Professor and Senior Consultant
Sri Ramachandra Insitute of Higher Education and Research
Chennai, Tamil Nadu, India

SR Sharath Shanmugam MD(General Medicine)
PG in DM(Cardiology)
Sri Ramachandra Medical College
Chennai, Tamil Nadu, India

Sreelal Thazhathu Veettil MD DM
Resident, Department of Cardiovascular Imaging and Endovascular Interventions
Cardiothoracic Sciences Centre
All India Institute of Medical Sciences
New Delhi, India

Sridhar Kasturi MD DM FACC FESC FSCAI FICC
Head
Department of Cardiology and Cardiothoracic Surgery
KIMS – Sunshine Hospitals, Begumpet
Secunderabad, Telangana, India

Srina Ray MBBS
Senior House Officer
Scunthorpe General Hospital
United Kingdom

Srinivas Rao Maddury MD DM
Senior Interventional Cardiologist and Head
Department of Cardiology
Apollo Hospital
Hyderabad, Telangana, India

Sriram Easwaran MD DM
Assistant Professor
Lokmanya Tilak Municipal Medical College and General Hospital
Mumbai, Maharashtra, India

S Selvamani DNB(Cardiology)
Senior Consultant and Interventional Cardiologist
Meenakshi Mission Hospital and Research Centre
Madurai, Tamil Nadu, India

S Shanmugasundaram MD DM
Cardiologist
Department of Cardiology
Billroth Hospital
Chennai, Tamil Nadu, India

SS Iyengar DM(Cardiology) FRCP(Edinburg)
Consultant Cardiologist
Manipal Hospital
Bengaluru, Karnataka, India

SS Mishra MD FAIMS MCAM DoCM FCCP FIAE FICC FCSI
Professor and Director
SOA University, Bhubaneswar
Professor and Director
Dreams Health Sciences and Padmini Care Hospital
Director, Med 'n' Heart Clinic
Cuttack, Odisha, India

Subhasis Roy Chowdhury MD DM FSCAI
In-charge Cath Lab
Manipal Hospital
Kolkata, West Bengal, India

Subrahmanya Murti V MD DM
Senior Specialist Cardiology
Aster CMI Hospital
Bengaluru, Karnataka, India

Subrat Kumar Muduli DM(Cardiology)
Associate Professor
Department of Cardiology
GB Pant Institute of Postgraduate Medical Education and Research
New Delhi, India

Subroto Mandal MD DM DC FACC FICC FCPCI FSCAI
Professor and Head
Department of Cardiology
Director, Cath Lab
Ubuntu Heart and Super Specialty Hospital
Bhopal, Madhya Pradesh, India

Sudeep Verma MD FNB(Pediatric Cardiology)
Consultant
Department of Pediatric Cardiology
Krishna Institute of Medical Sciences (KIMS)
Secunderabad, Telangana, India

Sudeshna Jana MTech
Researcher
TCS Research
Kolkata, West Bengal, India

Sudhir Chandra Sinha MD DM FACC
Senior Consultant Cardiologist
Star Pinnacle Heart Centre
Visakhapatnam, Andhra Pradesh, India

Sudipta Mondal MD DM
Postdoctoral Fellow in Electrophysiology
Sree Chitra Tirunal Institute (SCTIMST)
Thiruvananthapuram, Kerala, India

Sujatha Vipperla MD DM FIC FSCAI
Consultant Cardiologist
Indus Hospitals
Visakhapatnam, Andhra Pradesh, India

Sulabh Chandrakar MD DM FSCAI
Director and Consultant Cardiologist
Prathmesh Hospital
Raipur, Chattisgarh, India

Suman Bhandari MD DM FACC FESC FSCAI FIMSA
Director
Department of Cardiology
Fortis Escorts Heart Institute
New Delhi, India

Sunandan Sikdar MD DM FACC
Consultant
Department of Cardiology
Narayana Multispeciality Hospital
Kolkata, West Bengal, India

Sundaram Chandrashekhar MD DM
Assistant Professor
Department of Cardiology
Trichy SRM College
Tiruchirappalli, Tamil Nadu, India

Sunil Kumar S MD DM(Cardiology) FESC FSCAI
Professor and Head
Department of Cardiology
JSS Medical College and Hospital
Mysuru, Karnataka, India

Sunita Kumbhalkar MD(Medicine) DNB(Cardiology)
Professor and Head
Department of General Medicine
All India Institute of Medical Sciences, Nagpur
Nagpur, Maharashtra, India

Supraja Moorthy MD DNB(FRCR)
Assistant Professor
Saveetha Medical College
Puducherry, India

Sura Kishore Mishra MD DM(Cardiology)
Professor and Head
Department of Cardiology
SCB Medical College
Cuttack, Odisha, India

Suvro Banerjee MD FRCP(London) FRCP(Edinburgh) FICC FCSI FSCAI FACC FESC
Senior Consultant
Department of Cardiology
Apollo Multispeciality Hospital
Kolkata, West Bengal, India

Suyash Tripathi DM
Associate Professor
Department of Cardiology
Institute of Medical Sciences
Banaras Hindu University
Varanasi, Uttar Pradesh, India

Tamagna Ghosh MD DM(Cardiology)
Assistant Professor
Department of Cardiology
Seth GS Medical College
KEM Hospital
Mumbai, Maharashtra, India

Tanmay Mukhopadhyay MD DM(Cardiology) FESC FSCAI
Associate Professor
Department of Cardiology
Burdwan Medical College and Hospital
Burdwan, West Bengal, India

Tanmoy Majee MD DM(Cardiology)
Consultant
Department of Cardiology
Ruby General Hospital Limited
Kolkata, West Bengal, India

Tanuja Makhani MD
Senior Resident
Department of Cardiology
Postgraduate Institute of Medical Education and Research
Chandigarh, India

Tarun Kumar MD DM FSCAI FACC
Professor
Department of Cardiology
ABVIMS and DR RML Hospital
New Delhi, India

T Govindan Unni MD DM(Cardiology)
Professor and Head
Department of Cardiology
Jubilee Mission Medical College and Research Institute
Thrissur, Kerala, India

Tharun David Varghese M MD DM
Consultant Interventional Cardiologist
MOSC Medical College Hospital
Kochi, Kerala, India

Thomas Alexander MD DM
Head, Department of Cardiology
Kovai Medical Centre Hospital
Coimbatore, Tamil Nadu, India

Tiny Nair MD DM FACC FRCP
Head, Department of Cardiology
PRS Hospital
Thiruvananthapuram, Kerala, India

Tirthankar Dasgupta PhD
Senior Scientist
TCS Research
Kolkata, West Bengal, India

Tom Devasia MD DM FACC FSCAI FESC PGDD MBA
Professor and Unit-Head
Department of Cardiology
Kasturba Medical College, Manipal
Manipal, Karnataka, India

Trinath Kumar Mishra MD DM FCSI FACC
Professor
Department of Cardiology
MKCG Medical College
Berhampur, Odisha, India

Umesh K Pandey DM
Associate Professor
Department of Cardiology
Institute of Medical Sciences
Banaras Hindu University
Varanasi, Uttar Pradesh, India

Umesh Tripathi MD DM
Assistant Professor
Department of Cardiology
King George's Medical University
Lucknow, Uttar Pradesh, India

Umeshwar Pandey MD DM
Professor and Head
LPS Institute of Cardiology
Kanpur, Uttar Pradesh, India

Upendra Kaul MD DM FCSI FSCAI FAPSIC FACC FAMS
Awarded Padmashiri and
Dr BC Roy Award
Chairman – Cardiology and
Dean- Academics and Research
Batra Hospital and Medical Research Center
New Delhi, India

Vaibhav Shukla MD DM
Senior Interventional Cardiologist
Apollo Hospitals
Indore, Madhya Pradesh, India

Valakkada J DM
Associate Professor
Sree Chitra Tirunal Institute
Thiruvananthapuram, Kerala, India

Vardhini Vijaykumar BDS MDS
Medical Advisor
Hyderabad, Telangana, India

Vibhav Sharma MD DM
Assistant Professor
Department of Cardiology
Amrita Institute of Medical Sciences
Faridabad, Haryana, India

Vidyut Jain MD FRCP(UK) FSCAI FESC FACC
Consultant Cardiologist
Choithram Hospital and Research Center
Indore, Madhya Pradesh, India

Vijaya Kumar Varada MD DM(Cardiology)
Post DM Senior Resident
Department of Cardiology
All India Institute of Medical Sciences, Rishikesh
Rishikesh, Uttarakhand, India

Vijay Bang MD DM FCSI FESC FSCAI FACC
Senior Interventional Cardiologist
Lilavati Hospital and Research Center
Honorable Professor and Head
Grant Medical College and
Sir JJ Group of Hospitals (Former)
Mumbai, Maharashtra, India

Vijay Garg MD FIAE FICP FCSI FICA(USA) FISE FACC(USA) FACP(USA) FIMSA FISC FESC(Europe)
Professor, Department of Medicine
RD Gardi Medical College
Ujjain, Madhya Pradesh, India

Vijay Kumar Chopra MD DM FESC FHFA FCSI
Senior Cardiologist
Max Super Speciality Hospital
Saket, New Delhi, India

Vijay Kumar MD DM
Associate Professor
Department of Cardiology
Sri Jayadeva Institute of
Cardiovascular Sciences and Research
Bengaluru, Karnataka, India

Vijay Kumar MD DNB(Cardiology)
Director
Department of Cardiology
Fortis Escorts Heart Institute
New Delhi, India

Vimal Mehta MD DNB(Medicine) DM(Cardiology) FESC FACC
Director–Professor
Department of Cardiology
Head of Unit-III
GB Pant Institute of Postgraduate Medical Education and Research
New Delhi, India

Vinayaga Pandian DNB DrNB FSCAI
Consultant Cardiologist
Health City
Cayman Islands

Vinayak Agrawal MD DM
Senior Director and Head
Clinical Cardiology and Cardiac Imaging
Fortis Memorial Research Institute (FMRI)
Gurugram, Haryana, India

Vinit Kumar MD DM(Cardiology) FESC FSCAI FAPSIC
Cardiologist
Department of Cardiology
Heart Hospital
Patna, Bihar, India

Vinod Sharma MD DM(Cardiology) FRCP(London) FACC MBA(Healthcare Administration)
Vice-CEO and Head
Department of Cardiology Services
National Heart Institute
East of Kailash, New Delhi, India

Vinutha Rajesh MD FACC
Assistant Professor
Loma Linda University School of Medicine
Loma Linda, CA, USA

Vipin Kumar MD DM(Cardiology) FACC FSCAI
Senior Consultant Cardiologist
Ruban Memorial Hospital
Patna, Bihar, India

Vishal Batra MD DM
Professor
Department of Cardiology
GB Pant Institute of Postgraduate Medical Education and Research
New Delhi, India

Vishal Gavali MD(General Medicine)
Senior Registrar
Department of Cardiology
Jaslok Hospital
Mumbai, Maharashtra, India

Vishal Rastogi MD DM(Cardiology)
Director
Department of Cardiology
Fortis Escorts Heart Institute
New Delhi, India

Viveka Kumar MD DM FACC FSCAI FCSI
Director
Department of Cardiology
Max Hospital
Saket, New Delhi, India

Vivekanand S Gajapati MD DM
Consultant Cardiologist
SDM Narayana Heart Centre
Dharwad, Karnataka, India

Vivek BS MD DM
Senior Consultant
Director – Clinical Cardiology and Non-Invasive Imaging
Sir Ganga Ram Hospital
New Delhi, India

Vivek Chaturvedi MD DM FACC
Senior Consultant Cardiologist and Head
Department of Cardiology
Amrita Insitute for Medical Sciences and Research
Faridabad, Haryana, India

Vivek Kumar MD DM(Cardiology)
Senior Consultant
Department of Cardiology
Indraprastha Apollo Hospital
New Delhi, India

Vivek Narasimha V DNB(General Medicine) DrNB(Cardiology)
Fellow in Cardiology
KIMS Hospital
Secunderabad, Telangana, India

Vivudh Pratap Singh MD DM(Cardiology)
Senior Consultant – Interventional Cardiology
Fortis Escorts Heart Institute
New Delhi, India

Vinay Kumar Bahl MD DM(Cardiology)
Director – Cardiac Sciences
MS Ramaiah Medical College
Bengaluru, Karnataka, India

Yash Lokhandwala MD DM
Visiting Faculty
LTMG Hospital
Mumbai, Maharashtra, India

Yash Paul Sharma MD DM
Professor and Head
Department of Cardiology
Postgraduate Institute of Medical Education and Research
Chandigarh, India

Foreword

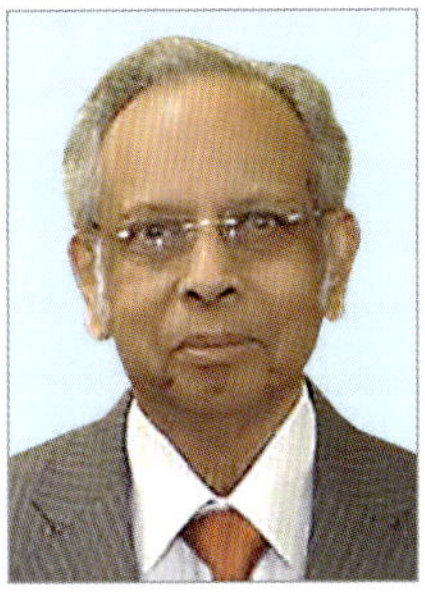

M Khalilullah
Padam Shree, Padam Bhushan, Dr BC Roy Awardee
Director and Senior Consultant Cardiologist
The Heart Centre, New Delhi, India
Former President, Cardiological Society of India
Director, GB Pant Institute of Postgraduate Medical Education and Research
New Delhi, India

It is with immense pride and respect for our profession that I introduce the *"CSI Cardiology Update 2024"*, an authoritative guide to the latest advancements and research in cardiovascular medicine, presented by the Cardiological Society of India. This annual volume, unveiled at the National Conference, reflects our continued commitment to elevating cardiology practice and enriching the knowledge of clinicians who dedicate themselves to the care of heart patients around the world.

The chapters in this edition are authored by some of the finest minds in cardiovascular medicine and interventional cardiology, each bringing a wealth of experience and insight into critical areas of our field. Their collective contributions span a remarkable range of topics, addressing everything from preventive strategies, advanced diagnostic approaches, medical management to innovative interventions. Together, they provide an invaluable resource for specialists, physicians, and fellows at all levels, seeking to keep pace with the rapid developments in cardiology and refine their approach to patient care.

As we stand at the forefront of cardiovascular healthcare, facing both the promise of new technologies and the persistent challenge of widespread cardiovascular disease, this book serves as a reminder of our shared mission: To improve the health and lives of those we serve. The knowledge contained in these pages is a testament to the dedication, expertise, and collaborative spirit that define our fraternity of cardiologists.

I extend my deepest gratitude to each contributor and to the editorial team for their hard work in bringing this volume to fruition. It is my hope that this update will not only inform but also inspire our readers to continue striving for excellence in their practice. May the insights found here empower you to make a meaningful difference in the lives of your patients and in the broader landscape of cardiovascular care.

Preface

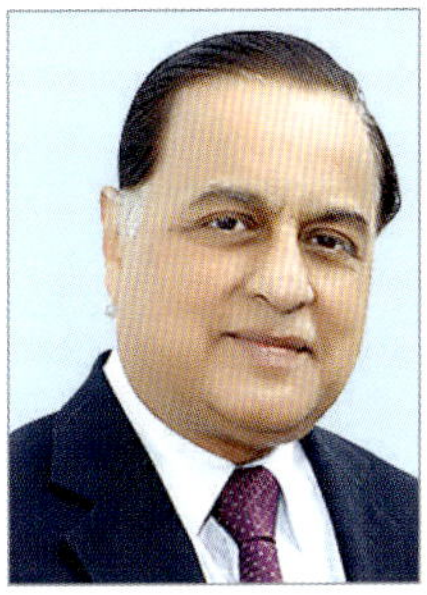

Sanjay Tyagi MD(Medicine) DM(Cardiology) FAMS FICP FCSI FICA FRCP(Edinburgh) FSCAI FESC FACC(USA)
Dr BC Roy National Awardee
Senior Consultant, Academic Advisor (HOD) and Clinical Director Cardiology
Apollo Hospitals, Northern Region, New Delhi, India
President-Elect, Cardiological Society of India
Secretary General (India), International College of Cardiology (USA)
National Coordinator, Cardiology and Interventional Cardiology, National Board of Examination
Formerly
Director General Health Services, Govt of India
Dean, Maulana Azad Medical College, New Delhi
Director, Professor and HOD Cardiology
GB Pant Institute of Postgraduate Medical Education and Research

A very warm greetings from the Cardiological Society of India (CSI).

It is an honor and a privilege to present the "*Cardiology Update 2024*" on behalf of CSI. It is a thoughtfully curated collection of the latest advances, research insights, and clinical practices in cardiovascular medicine. This edition, launched in conjunction with the Annual National Conference of the CSI, serves as a testament to the remarkable progress in our field and the relentless pursuit of excellence by cardiologists worldwide.

The updated book, largest till date, is divided into two volumes. It has been edited into 21 sections and 226 chapters written by eminent national and international authors. The chapters in this volume represent the contributions of distinguished experts, each a leader in their respective domain of cardiovascular care and research. This book addresses a wide spectrum of topics, from state-of-the-art interventional procedures and diagnostic innovations to the evolving paradigms in preventive cardiology, artificial intelligence, and complex disease management. Every chapter is crafted to ensure relevance and applicability to practicing cardiologists, merging latest in evidence-based research with real-world clinical insight.

Our aim is to provide cardiologists with a comprehensive, latest resource that enhances their clinical practice and supports them in delivering optimal care. With cardiovascular diseases remaining a leading cause of morbidity and mortality globally, the need for shared knowledge and refined clinical approaches is more critical than ever. It is our hope that this book will become an essential reference for clinicians, researchers, and healthcare providers dedicated to advancing cardiovascular science and patient outcomes.

I am deeply grateful to the galaxy of reputed national and international faculty for their expertise, commitment, and dedication to this project. Their work is the cornerstone of this book, reflecting the highest standards in cardiovascular medicine. I would also like to extend my appreciation to the CSI Scientific Committee and Executive Committee, especially Dr PC Rath, Dr Debabrata Roy, and Dr DP Sinha, whose support and organization were invaluable in bringing this publication to fruition. I would like to express my gratitude to my colleagues, Professor Jamal Yusuf, Professor Girish MP, Professor Vishal Batra, and Dr Subrat Kumar Muduli for their support. I would also like to place on record my sincere gratitude for Jaypee Brothers Medical Publishers, specially Ms Nedup for working tirelessly with the authors and compiling this book.

I dedicate this Update to my teachers, parents, patients, students, and family—wife Dr Mamta, son Dr Dhruv, and daughter Dr Swati—for being eternally supportive and encouraging throughout my journey.

May "*CSI Cardiology Update 2024*" inspire you, deepen your knowledge, and empower your practice as we all work toward a future of healthier hearts and lives.

Contents

VOLUME 1

SECTION 1: GENERAL CARDIOLOGY

SECTION 2: ECHOCARDIOGRAPHY/IMAGING

SECTION 3: ARTIFICIAL INTELLIGENCE IN CARDIOLOGY

SECTION 5: HYPERTENSION

SECTION 6: HEART FAILURE

SECTION 8: CARDIO-OBSTETRICS

SECTION 9: CONGENITAL HEART DISEASE

SECTION 10: VALVULAR HEART DISEASE/MISCELLANEOUS

SECTION 11: PULMONARY VASCULAR DISEASE

VOLUME 2

SECTION 12: CHRONIC CORONARY SYNDROMES

SECTION 13: ACUTE CORONARY SYNDROME

SECTION 15: STRUCTURAL INTERVENTION

Scan the QR code to access references of all the chapters.

SECTION 1

General Cardiology

Section Outline

CHAPTER

1

Cardiovascular Disease Epidemic in India

Debabrata Biswas, Debabrata Roy

ABSTRACT

India is currently in early stage of cardiovascular disease epidemic transition characterized by lower cardiovascular death as compared to communicable, maternal, neonatal, and nutritional deaths taken together. Recent trends have demonstrated an epidemic reversal in prevalence of cardiovascular disease and its risk factors with highest prevalence shifting from the uppermost to the lowest socioeconomic strata. Cardiovascular disease prevention in India is affected by various issues such as poor awareness and control, variation in risk factors and accessibility, and affordability of and skill gap in healthcare service.

Keywords: Cardiovascular disease, communicable, maternal, neonatal, deaths

INTRODUCTON

India is experiencing a shift from a pandemic to an epidemic of cardiovascular disease, yet its mortality rates are lower than those of infectious, maternal, newborn, and nutritional diseases. Lack of information, risk factors, accessibility, pricing, and skill shortages in healthcare, all make prevention difficult.

PROBLEM STATEMENT OF CARDIOVASCULAR DISEASES EPIDEMIC: GLOBAL AND ASIAN

Cardiovascular diseases (CVD) are the leading cause of death globally.[1] According to the "Global Burden of Disease Study" nearly 18.6 million CVD deaths occurred worldwide in 2019, among which 58% occurred in Asia. Nearly 39% of these CVD deaths were premature, i.e., age <70 years.[2] There has been a rapid rise in CV deaths in Asia over the past 30 years, from 23% in 1990 to 35% in 2019. The proportion of premature CV deaths was around 39% in Asia in 2019, compared to 23% in the U.S. and 22% in Europe.[3] The CV epidemic in Asia exhibits gross geographic heterogeneity with different transition stages in different countries:[4]

- *Early stage:* In lower-middle income countries such as India, Nepal, and Pakistan. The mortality pattern is characterized by lower CV death rate but a higher proportion of premature CV deaths and deaths due to communicable, maternal, neonatal, and nutritional diseases.
- *Stage of rapid increase:* In China and most Asian countries. It is characterized by high CV death rate that exceeds the cancer-related death rate.
- *Stage of degenerative disease:* In Japan and South Korea characterized by lower CV death rate and premature deaths but a higher rate of cancer- and dementia-related deaths.

INDIA AS A SUBSET OF SOUTH ASIA

South Asians constitute around 25% of the world's population but contribute to >50% of global CVD deaths. Among Asians living in the US, the highest age-standardized mortality rates from ischemic heart disease was found in Asian Indians (men and women). Since 2011, Asian-Indian is the only race/ethnicity for which that rate is increasing.[4]

South Asian population has many unique characteristics that highlight the need for unique CV risk assessment and reduction strategies as recognized in the MASALA (Mediators of Atherosclerosis in South Asians Living in America) study initiated in 2010.[5] Some key insights are:

- Younger age at onset of type 2 diabetes and at a lower body mass index (BMI) which predisposes to premature

ASCVD. UK Biobank prospective cohort study has reported that type 2 diabetes might explain 22% of the risk of future ASCVD events in South Asians versus 7% in Europeans.[6]

- Greater proportion of hypertensives in the population as evidenced by >40% prevalence of hypertension among adults in India and Nepal and greater CV event rates with each level of systolic blood pressure.
- Elevated risk of ischemic heart disease in South Asians even at a much lower LDL-C level compared with other ethnic groups, attributable to a higher LDL-C particle burden at a given LDL-C level and a complex metabolic milieu of elevated triglyceride and dysfunctional high-density-lipoprotein cholesterol.
- South Asians have the highest concentration of Lp(a) which magnifies CAD risk 16 times in diabetics and by 25 times in those with raised TC:HDL ratio.
- Central adiposity; higher waist-hip ratio at similar BMI as Europeans and a typical "high level body fat-normal BMI-low muscle mass" phenotype.
- Highest age-standardized rates of death and disability attributable to ambient particulate air pollution.

In recognition of the above facts current US clinical practice guideline for cholesterol management has considered South Asian ancestry to be a "risk enhancing" clinical factor in those with borderline (5.0 to <7.5%) and intermediate (7.5 to <20.0%) 10-year ASCVD risk.[7]

NATIONAL TRENDS IN CARDIOVASCULAR DISEASES EPIDEMIC IN INDIA

Total death in India attributable to CVD has risen from 15.2% in 1990 to 28.1% in 2016 and disability adjusted life years (DALY) has also increased from 6.9 to 14.1%.[9] More than half of the total CVD deaths in India in 2016 were in people younger than 70 years.[8]

The number of cases of ischemic heart disease increased from 10.2 million in 1990 to 23.8 million in 2016, and cases of stroke from 2.8 million in 1990 to 6.5 million in 2016. The age-standardized prevalence of rheumatic heart disease decreased in India by 10.8% from 1990 to 2016.

The age-standardized DALY rate due to CVD in India was 1.3 times the global average in 2016, that of ischemic heart disease was 1.6 times the global average, rheumatic heart disease was 2.4 times the global average, and the age-standardized DALY rate due to stroke were comparable to the global average.[9]

When the risk factors were analyzed contributing to DALYs due to CVD in India in 2016, dietary risks, high systolic blood pressure, air pollution, high total cholesterol, tobacco use, high fasting plasma glucose, and high BMI stand out to be the most important ones.

Behavioral Risk Factors

The leading behavioral risk factors that contributed to the CVD DALYs in 2016 were dietary risks (low consumption of fruits, vegetables, grains, and nuts, and high consumption of sodium, trans fat, and red meat), followed by tobacco use and low physical activity.[10]

Metabolic Risk Factors

Among metabolic risk factors, high blood pressure and high total cholesterol, followed by high fasting blood glucose level and high BMI, were the major contributors to the CVD DALYs in India.

Analysis based on two consecutive nationally representative cross-sectional household surveys from India, the NFHS-4 (from 2015 to 2016) and the NFHS-5 (2019 to 2021), revealed interesting national trends and transition in socioeconomic gradients of various risk factors.[11]

- *Diabetes*: Changing trend of diabetes across different socioeconomic strata showed a substantial flattening in the wealth gradients and a reversal in education gradients between 2015–2016 and 2019–2021. By 2019–2021 the prevalence of diabetes increased by 0.3 percentage points (relative increase of 24.2%) for those in the bottom wealth quintile compared to a 0.3 percentage points decrease (relative decrease of 7.8%) for those in the top wealth quintile. Regarding education versus diabetes trend, 0.5 percentage points increase (relative increase of 21.2%) in diabetes among the uneducated group has been observed, whereas prevalence among people with more than secondary education remained virtually unchanged.[12]
- *Unhealthy weight*: Over the period of 6 years (from 2015 to 2021) unhealthy weight, which includes overweight, obesity and morbid obesity, showed the largest absolute increase in prevalence. Overweight increased by 17% from a baseline prevalence of 20%, and obesity by 28.4% from a baseline prevalence of 4.1%. The magnitude of the change in overweight was substantially higher among people with low socioeconomic status compared to people with high socioeconomic status. Rising trend of overweight was also seen in those without education compared to the educated population.
- *Hypertension*: Between NFHS-4 and 5, hypertension slightly decreased by 1.1 percentage points nationally. Hypertension increased by 1.4 percentage points for those without education but decreased by 3.3 percentage points for those with the highest level of education. Prevalence of hypertension is now higher among those in the poorest wealth quintile compared to those in the top wealth quintile.

These socioeconomic trends substantiate the "reversal hypothesis" which states that as countries develop, CVD risk shifts from being disproportionately high among the rich to disproportionately high among the poor. India is currently evolving through this epidemic reversal phase. The magnitude of these epidemiologic shifts tends to be higher among women.

POPULATION LEVEL CHANGES IN INDIA INFLUENCING CARDIOVASCULAR DISEASES EPIDEMIC

Higher cardiovascular disease burden in India can be partly explained by six population level changes:[13]

1. *Epidemiological transition from communicable to noncommunicable diseases*: As of 2016, all states in India have an epidemiological transition ratio (ratio of communicable to noncommunicable disease) of <0.75 favoring noncommunicable diseases largely CVD.
2. *Demographic shift*: Life expectancy of the Indian population has increased from 49.7 years (50.5 years for males and 49 years for females) in 1973 to 67.9 years (66.4 years for males and 69.6 years for females) in 2012. The rapidly aging population adds to the high propensity of CVD.
3. *Nutritional transition*: This is characterized by a decrease in intake of healthy foods such as coarse cereals, pulses, fruits and vegetables, and increase in intake of animal products, processed and ready-to-eat fast foods that are energy dense and having high salt content.

4 and 5:

Sociocultural and economic transitions: Industrialization and urbanization have led to decline in physical activity and increase in sedentary lifestyle, stress, substance abuse, and novel risk factors like air pollution.

6. *Environmental transition*: Recently, persistent exposure to household air pollutants have been implicated for the rising prevalence of disease burden in India.

ISSUES IN PREVENTION

Awareness and Control

Awareness generation on health hazards of important risk factors such as growing fast food intake, physical inactivity, tobacco use, and indoor air pollution is of utmost importance.

- *Fast food intake*: Health hazards of fast foods need to be taught at schools in order to minimize its consumption. Parents can play a great role in setting an example by not eating fast foods themselves and encouraging home foods.[13]
- *Physical inactivity and unhealthy diet*: Poddar V et al.[14] investigated the patterns of physical activity in India, stratified by zones, BMI, urban-rural areas, and gender, and found that 57% of the population did not meet physical activity regimen of WHO. Physical inactivity is more common among females and urban population. More than 90% did no recreational physical activity.
- *Tobacco and alcohol use*: The Global Adult Tobacco Survey (GATS) 2, a nationally representative survey for systematically monitoring adult tobacco use has found that in India, prevalence of tobacco use has decreased from 34.6% in GATS 1 (2009–2010) to 28.6% in GATS 2 (2016–2017).[10]

Though there is a relative decrease in smoking there has been a steady increase in drinking among young which when superimposed on adverse factors operating since childhood causes CVD. Adolescent health education, particularly targeting tobacco and alcohol, should be incorporated in school education program. Study on the impact of anti-tobacco awareness programs has shown significantly higher mean knowledge scores of study subjects after conducting awareness programme.[15] Fast food and tobacco companies pay crores in "surrogate advertisement" to promote unhealthy habits by integrating them with healthy activities and sports, which create an impediment to such awareness programs.

VARIABILITY OF RISK FACTORS

State Wise Variability

In a country of 1.3 billion people with cultural and lifestyle diversities, CVD epidemic pattern differs from state to state. *India State-level Disease Burden Initiative CVD Collaborators* group has placed states into four groups based on *epidemiological transition level (ETL),* defined by the ratio of DALYs from communicable diseases to those from noncommunicable diseases and injuries combined, with a low ratio denoting high ETL and vice versa **(Table 1)**.[8] ETL is a marker of socioeconomic status.

The prevalence of CVD in 2016 was highest in Kerala, Punjab, and Tamil Nadu (high ETL state group), followed by Andhra Pradesh, Himachal Pradesh, Maharashtra, Goa, and West Bengal (high and higher-middle ETL state groups).[8]

There was an increasing gradient of prevalence of ischemic heart disease from the low to the high ETL state groups, with the highest prevalence in Kerala, Punjab, Tamil Nadu (high ETL state group).[8]

Punjab and Tamil Nadu (high ETL state) showed the highest DALY rate of ischemic heart disease followed by Haryana, Andhra Pradesh, Karnataka (higher-middle ETL). The DALY rate of stroke varied 6.2 times between the states in 2016 highest being in West Bengal and Odisha in the east, Tripura and Assam in the northeast, and Chhattisgarh in central India.[8]

Although the prevalence of ischemic heart disease and stroke in 2016 was highest in the high ETL state groups, the increase in the age-standardized prevalence of ischemic heart disease since 1990 was higher in the low and lower-middle ETL state groups, that are home to 55% of India's population.[8]

TABLE 1: Grouping of the states of India as per Epidemiological Transition Level (ETL).

Low ETL	Lower-middle ETL	Higher-middle ETL	High ETL
• Bihar	• Arunachal Pradesh	• Haryana	• Himachal Pradesh
• Jharkhand	• Mizoram	• Delhi	• Punjab
• Uttar Pradesh	• Nagaland	• Telangana	• Tamil Nadu
• Rajasthan	• Uttarakhand	• Andhra Pradesh	• Goa
• Meghalaya	• Gujarat	• Jammu and Kashmir	• Kerala
• Assam	• Tripura	• Karnataka	
• Chhattisgarh	• Sikkim	• West Bengal	
• Madhya Pradesh	• Manipur	• Maharashtra	
• Odisha		• Union territories other than Delhi	

The age-standardized prevalence of stroke increased in all ETL state groups from 1990 to 2016 duration but age-standardized DALY rate declined in all ETL state groups, the smallest decrease being in the low ETL state group. This decreasing trend of age-standardized DALY rate may indicate improving healthcare in general but the increase in the DALY rate of ischemic heart disease and the relatively lower improvements in rates of DALYs due to stroke in resource-poor low ETL states indicate the lack of appropriate preventive and therapeutic healthcare facilities for CVD in these states.[12]

Both the age-standardized prevalence of rheumatic heart disease as well as DALY rate due to rheumatic heart disease has decreased from 1990 to 2016 in all ETL state groups, indicating improvement in public health in general but the very fact that the DALY rate of rheumatic heart disease in 2016 was highest in the relatively less developed low ETL state group demands greater focus on healthcare resource allocation in these states.

Urban–Rural Gradients

Rural areas experienced a faster increase in the prevalence of CVD risk factors between 2015–2016 and 2019–2021. Overweight increased by 29.6% in rural compared to 8.6% in urban areas; diabetes increased by 14.4% in rural compared to 2.6% in urban areas; hypertension decreased by 2.2% in rural compared to 12.1% decrease in urban areas.[12]

A pooled analysis of three nation-wide cross-sectional surveys examined the variation in seven cardiovascular health (CVH) markers, including smoking, diet, physical activity, BMI, blood pressure, fasting glucose, and total cholesterol, in metropolitan and small cities and rural parts of India and stratified the participants with ≥6, 4–5, and ≤3 ideal CVH metrics as having good, moderate, and poor CVH, respectively.[16]

The distribution of good, moderate, and poor CVH stratified by residence were 3.9%, 41.0%, and 55.1% for metropolitan cities; 7.8%, 49.2% (95% CI 47.8%, 50.7%), and 43.0% for smaller cities; and 10.4%, 60.9%, and 28.7% in rural villages, respectively, after adjusting for age, sex, education, and asset tertiles.[16] This clearly demonstrates the inverse relationships between urbanization and CVH.

Large numbers in the population are moving from rural areas to cities and towns due to economic transition exposing them to various ill-effects of urban living such as ease of access to energy-dense fast foods, unhealthy foods, higher use of motorized transports, mechanization of manual work, mental stress, difficult access to leisure-time physical activity, and environmental risks like air pollution. Therefore, urban population especially the urban poor, are more predisposed to CVD.

Regional Trends of Cardiovascular Disease Risk Factors

Unhealthy weight, diabetes, and hypertension were highest in prevalence in South India in both 2015–2016 and 2019–2021. Overweight burden was disproportionately high in the South compared to the other regions which has become even more pronounced over the years. Smoking remains highest in the Northeastern region though all regions experienced decreasing smoking trend.[11] Empowered action group (EAG) of states was constituted by the Government of India in 2001, with the aim of fostering development in India's less developed states. EAG states include Bihar, Chhattisgarh, Jharkhand, Madhya Pradesh, Orissa, Rajasthan, Uttarakhand, and Uttar Pradesh.[17] Study has shown rising trend of hypertension and overweight in EAG member states.

Household Clustering

Apart from macro-disparity, understanding the clustering of CVD risk factors at small socio-geographic levels (household, community, district, and state) is crucial for targeting appropriate intervention and policy making. Studies have found that for most of the CVD risk factors except smoking, the level of clustering was highest for households, followed by communities, districts, and then states.[18] Therefore, health promotion interventions aimed at reducing CV risk might be especially effective when targeted at household level instead of targeting higher levels or the general population.

Small Area Variability

A study on small area variability in CVD risk factors (hypertension, diabetes, and obesity) in India showed that small areas contributed the most to geographic variability. Hence, small areas should be taken into consideration when designing preventive strategies and policies to prevent and manage CVD risk factors in India.[19]

Dietary Diversity

A balanced diet that includes an essential quantity of calories, protein, fat, micronutrients, and dietary fibers is more likely to reduce the risk of CVD. Dietary diversity at the regional level in India is determined by several factors, such as geographical availability of foods, accessibility to markets, purchasing capacity, level of education, individual tests, and preferences, etc., and this diversity influences occurrence of CVD.

A study by Dolui et al.[20] on dietary diversity from NFHS-4 data calculated Dietary Diversity Scores (DDS) based on a 24-hour recall period by summing the number of food groups consumed on the last day. Nine food groups were included: (1) Milk or curd, (2) Pulses or beans, (3) Dark green leafy vegetables, (4) Fruits, (5) Eggs, (6) Fish, (7) Chicken or meat, (8) Fried foods, and (9) Aerated drinks. The food groups were weighted by level of consumption frequencies: Never-0; Occasional-1; Weekly-2; and Daily-4; The DDS was classified as low ≤12; moderate 13–25; and high ≥26 for further analysis. A moderate dietary diversity score significantly decreases the likelihood of heart disease (OR 0.88 with $p < 0.10$) for adult men compared to a lower score of dietary diversity. Also, the participants in the highest quartile of dietary diversity score were less likely to have diabetes and hypertension compared to those at the lowest quartile. Daily consumption of fish, eggs, and chicken has been positively correlated with diabetes, heart disease, and cancer.[20]

In the CARRS study, following three dietary patterns were noted:[21]

1. *Prudent*: Fruits, green leafy vegetables and raw vegetables, nuts
2. *Indian*: Refined grains, cooked vegetables, fish, coffee
3. *Nonvegetarian*: Meat, poultry, egg, fish

The CARRS study has showed that adults without CVD are more likely to follow relatively unhealthy Indian and nonvegetarian diet pattern. Misra et al.[22] showed that improper dietary behavior also penetrated rural areas.

ACCESSIBILITY, AFFORDABILITY, AND SKILL GAP

Healthcare system in India faces major challenges of quality, accessibility, and affordability for a large section of the population, especially rural population. There is a shortage of qualified doctors, nurses, technicians, and infrastructure. India is currently having 0.76 doctors and 2.09 nurses per 1,000 population which is far from WHO recommendations of 1 doctor and 2.5 nurses per 1,000 population, respectively. Glaring disparity in healthcare accessibility between rural and urban India is evidenced by availability of only 33% doctors to serve the rural population which constitute 66% of the total Indian population.[23]

Affordability remains a major problem with around 70% of total healthcare expenses being borne by private expenditure, of which about 62% is out-of-pocket expenditure.[24]

To address the skill-gap training of informal healthcare providers has been studied in a randomized controlled trial. Training increased correct case management by 7.9 percentage points (14.2%) without affecting the use of unnecessary medicines and antibiotics.[25]

INHERENT BIOLOGICAL RISK AMONG INDIANS: THE LIFE COURSE APPROACH

High ecological differences between South Asian and European countries in terms of CVD risk have been attributable to Barker's hypothesis of "fetal origins of adult disease" or "thrifty phenotype" hypothesis which emphasizes the effects of physical and social exposures at various stages of life, from gestation to adult life, on chronic disease risk.[13]

Complex interplay of prenatal (maternal and paternal) as well as postnatal factors, ranging from birth to childhood, adolescence, and young adulthood, compounded by the population level transitions culminate into the high prevalence of CVD in India **(Fig. 1)**.[13]

CONCLUSION

The CVD in South Asia can no longer be considered a problem of the affluent part of society. The CVD prevention efforts should target lower socioeconomic group which form the majority of India's massive population yet have much higher difficulty in accessing care and treatment. Small geographic areas and household clustering needs attention during formulation of CVD prevention policies. AI can play an important role in addressing skill gap in an affordable manner.

Burgeoning CVD epidemic in South Aasia: Life course approach

- **Maternal nutrition:**
  ↑ Fat intake at 18 weeks
  ↑ Plasma glucose at 28 weeks
  ↑ Folate and ↓ Vitamin B12 level
- **Fetal and neonatal: (Genetically predetermined)**

Glucose metabolism:
↑ Hepatic glucose output and localized hepatic IR
↑ Insulin and plasma leptin; ↓ IGFBP-1
↑ Glucocorticoid action

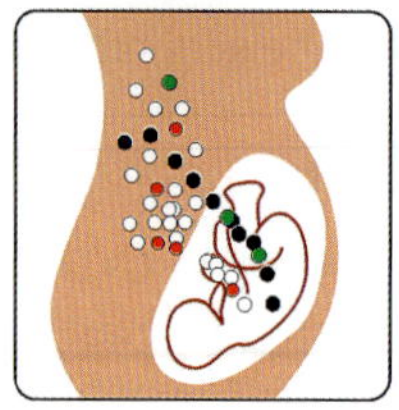

Early life- ↓threshold for RF to produce CVD

Body composition and body fat:
↓ Subcutaneous adipose tissue storage → fat stored in visceral adipose tissue
↑ Atherogenic dyslipidemia (↑transmembrane FFA flux in visceral adipocytes)
↓ Adiponectin, ↑ proinflammatory cytokine release

Inflammtory state:
↑CRP, homocysteine, leptin, IL-6, TNF-α

Lipid metabolism:
↓HDL2b in >90%; small dense LDL; Lp(a)-magnifies CAD risk 16× in DM, 25× in ↑TC:HDL

↓

Transitions: Increase propensity to develop cardiac risk factors

Epidemiological
CD to NCD

Nutritional
- ↓ Coarse cereals, pulses, vegetables
- ↑ Meat, processed food, energy dense high salt food

Socio-cultural and economic
- Agrarian → Industrialized
- Manual → Mechanized (HTN, DM, dyslipidemia, physical inactivity, stress, substance abuse, air pollution)

Environmental
Air pollution, noise pollution, plastics, organic pollution

FIG. 1: Life course approach.
Source: Adapted from Kalra A, et al. (2023).[13]

ONLINE REFERENCES

Please scan the QR code provided at the end of the table of contents for References of this chapter.

CHAPTER

2

Epidemiology of Coronary Heart Disease in India and Important Risk Factors: Recent Evidence

Rajeev Gupta, Kiran Gaur

ABSTRACT

Coronary heart disease (CHD) is an epidemic in India and has emerged as one of the more important causes of death and disability. The Global Burden of Disease (GBD) study and India State-Level Disease Burden Initiative have systematically collated data from diverse data-sources from India and have calculated the number of individuals dying from CHD, estimated burden of CHD using disability-adjusted life years (DALYs) lost, and prevalence of the disease using meta-regression techniques. In the most recent iteration of the GBD study (2024), national data on these three metrics are available and show increasing trends in the absolute number of women and men dying of CHD as well as increasing burden of the disease estimated using DALYs and prevalence rates from the years 2000 to 2021. An important finding is a high burden of premature CHD (age 15–49 years) and a rapidly increasing burden among the middle-aged (age 50–69 years) women and men. Risk factors for CHD in India have been studied in two large international studies, case–control INTERHEART study and population-based prospective Prospective Urban Rural Epidemiology (PURE) study. Both the studies show that standard lifestyle risk factors (viz., smoking/tobacco, unhealthy diet, sedentary habits, psychosocial stress, depression, indoor air pollution, and low educational status) and biological risk factors (viz., hypertension, dyslipidemias, diabetes, abdominal obesity, and frailty) are important. Strategies for CHD prevention should commence in adolescents and young individuals to prevent the epidemic of premature and middle-aged CHD in India.

Keywords: India, risk factors, premature CHD, GBD, epidemic

INTRODUCTION

Coronary heart disease (CHD) has emerged as the most important cause of death and disability in India, measured as either disability-adjusted life years (DALYs) lost or years of life lost (YLLs) in recent decades.[1] The India State-Level Disease Burden Initiative, a joint venture of the Indian Council of Medical Research (ICMR) and the United States-based Institute for Health Metrics and Evaluation (IHME), analyzed data on noncommunicable diseases and communicable diseases using locally and globally available resources from the years 1990 to 2015.[2] It was reported that in the 1990s, the most important causes of death across the country were communicable and maternal and child health conditions; this changed in the 2010s and presently the most important causes of deaths and DALYs are noncommunicable diseases across the country.[2] According to the recent Global Burden of Disease (GBD) study, deaths from CHD in India increased by 20.5% from 2011 to 2021 along with an increase in many other noncommunicable diseases; on the other hand, deaths from communicable diseases (barring COVID-19) declined, e.g., diarrheal deaths decreased by 25.0% in the same period.[3] Studies have reported that this change is associated with demographic and epidemiological transition and increased aging and standard CHD risk factors in the country.[4-11] Some of these risk factors are summarized in **Box 1**.

Data from nationally available risk factor evaluation studies in India have shown that almost all the classical CHD risk factors are increasing in India.[6,7] Serial National Family Health Surveys (NFHS) have reported an increase in obesity, hypertension, diabetes, and other nonlaboratory markers.[11] The causes-of-causes, the social determinants, are also increasing.[10,12,13] In this chapter, we focus on changing trends in CHD mortality in India using data from the GBD study published in 2024.[14-16] The study has compiled data

BOX 1 Important CHD risk factors in India.

Macrolevel determinants	Microlevel risk factors
• Urban and rural infrastructure • Social organization, stress • Illiteracy • Work environment, unemployment, job stress • Transportation • Social support, cohesion • Food, agriculture • Unhealthy food promotion • Poverty, social exclusion, minorities • Social patterning • Sanitation • Healthcare financing • Universal health care • Healthcare infrastructure • Facilities for physical activity, beneficial health behaviors	• Age • Family history • Smoking • Physical inactivity • Dietary factors (trans fats, saturated fats, refined carbohydrates) • Excessive salt intake • Low fruit and vegetable intake • Ambient (outdoor, indoor) air pollution • Raised BP and hypertension • Raised LDL cholesterol • Low HDL cholesterol • Raised triglycerides • Diabetes • Insulin resistance, metabolic syndrome • *Inflammatory markers*: Infections, C-reactive protein, interleukins • Early life events, maternal and child health • Genetic factors

up to the year 2021. We also focus on age-related differences in absolute numbers, mortality rates, and DALYs. State-level data are not yet available in the latest iteration of GBD study and are not reported. We also discuss the important CHD risk factors in India identified using the case-control INTERHEART study[17,18] and the prospective Prospective Urban Rural Epidemiology (PURE) study,[19,20] and the contribution of these risk factors to CHD events and deaths.

GLOBAL BURDEN OF DISEASE STUDY

Harmonization of mortality data across the globe according to causes of death is important, and for decades, reliable data on cause-specific numbers of deaths have been missing. The World Health Organization initiated this process following the publication of the *World Health Report* (1993). This led to the publication of the first GBD report in 1997.[21] Unsurprisingly, cardiovascular diseases (CVDs—CHD and strokes) emerged as the most important cause of death globally. However, what was surprising was that CVDs were also the principal cause of deaths in lower-income countries including India. Subsequent GBD studies have continued to report cause-specific deaths across the globe and currently, data from 204 countries are available.[22] Detailed methods for calculation of deaths, DALYs, and prevalence rates are available at the GBD website.[22] In this chapter, we have analyzed trends in CHD deaths and disability in India. Data for different states in the country are not yet available and are not reported.

Subsequent cycles of GBD have also focused on risk factors and their association with causes of death. From the initial focus on a limited number of risk factors, principally behavioral and metabolic, the more recent iterations have analyzed global data according to 87 risk factors.[16] The risk factors have been classified according to hierarchy from level 1 to level 4. Level 1 risks are an aggregate of environmental and occupational risks, behavioral risks, and metabolic risks. At level 2, there are 20 risk categories such as air pollution, child and maternal malnutrition, and high body mass index. Level 3 risks include more specific factors such as particulate matter pollution and dietary factors, while level 4 risks include household air pollution from solid fuels and child stunting. The metabolic risk aggregate is not inclusive of level 3 or 4 risks. We have not focused on GBD risk factors for the present study and provide only a general commentary on important risk factors in India with a particular focus on India-specific studies such as the INTERHEART and PURE for CHD risk factor associations.[17-20]

CORONARY HEART DISEASE MORTALITY TRENDS

Sparse data on national mortality trends have been available in India before the publication of GBD studies.[23] Older data from the Registrar General of India clubbed all CHD deaths with diseases of the circulatory system and were based on data from rural regions and selected urban regions of the country.[6] CHD deaths were not well reported.[6] There were other limitations of the Indian data as reported earlier by our group and others.[6,7,23] In the GBD study, annual trends in deaths from CHD are available from 1990, but for this chapter, we have included data from the year 2000 to the most recent **(Table 1)**.[22] The absolute number of deaths has increased from 0.75–0.85 million in the early years of the present century (2000–2004) to >1.6 million in more recent years (2018–2021). The absolute number of individuals dying of CHD in India currently is the highest in the world, more than any other large country including China, the United States, and Brazil.[1] Moreover, while the absolute number of individuals as well as rates of men and women dying from CHD is declining in most parts of the developed world, it is increasing in India.[1] *India is truly the coronary capital of the world.*

The absolute number of men and women dying from CHD is given in **Table 1**. In the year 2021, CHD led to 1.63 million deaths (men 1.01 million and women 0.62 million). **Figure 1** shows the trends in absolute number of men and women dying of CHD from the years 2000 to 2021. There is a significant increase, and this is observed among both men and women. There are significantly more deaths due to CHD in men as compared to women, and comparative

TABLE 1: Annual trends in CHD mortality from the year 2000 to 2021 in terms of absolute numbers and rate/100,000 population among men and women in India in Global Burden of Disease Study.

	Death, absolute number			Rate (deaths/100,000)		
Year	**Men**	**Women**	**Both**	**Men**	**Women**	**Both**
2000	477,121	279,089	756,210	89.0	56.2	73.2
2001	497,621	288,176	785,797	91.2	56.9	74.7
2002	510,587	301,537	812,124	91.9	58.4	75.7
2003	533,038	309,522	842,560	94.2	58.8	77.1
2004	546,712	308,191	854,902	95.0	57.4	76.8
2005	558,663	320,162	878,826	95.4	58.5	77.6
2006	584,333	345,365	929,698	98.1	61.9	80.6
2007	625,770	368,088	993,858	103.3	64.8	84.7
2008	657,435	383,740	1,041,175	106.8	66.4	87.2
2009	674,520	390,598	1,065,118	107.8	66.4	87.8
2010	712,388	404,723	1,117,111	112.2	67.6	90.6
2011	755,381	433,795	1,189,176	117.2	71.3	94.9
2012	784,798	477,579	1,262,377	120.0	77.3	99.3
2013	822,380	506,016	1,328,396	124.1	80.7	103.0
2014	864,889	534,605	1,399,493	128.8	84.0	107.0
2015	855,051	537,281	1,392,332	125.7	83.3	105.1
2016	872,823	566,503	1,439,326	126.8	86.7	107.3
2017	887,319	570,473	1,457,792	127.4	86.2	107.3
2018	932,430	595,587	1,528,018	132.4	89.0	111.2
2019	968,674	611,084	1,579,758	136.1	90.3	113.8
2020	993,277	615,489	1,608,766	138.3	90.0	114.7
2021	1,012,118	620,764	1,632,882	139.7	89.9	115.4

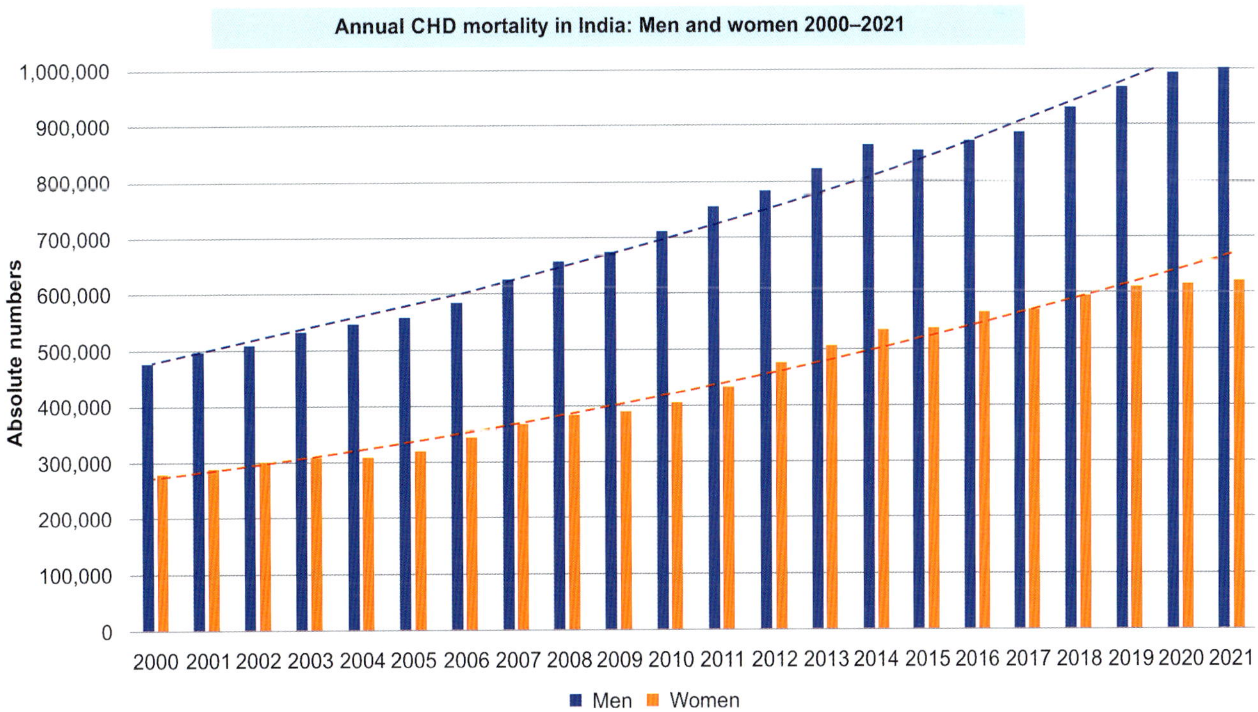

FIG. 1: Trends in absolute number of CHD deaths in men and women from 2000 to 2021 (GBD study).

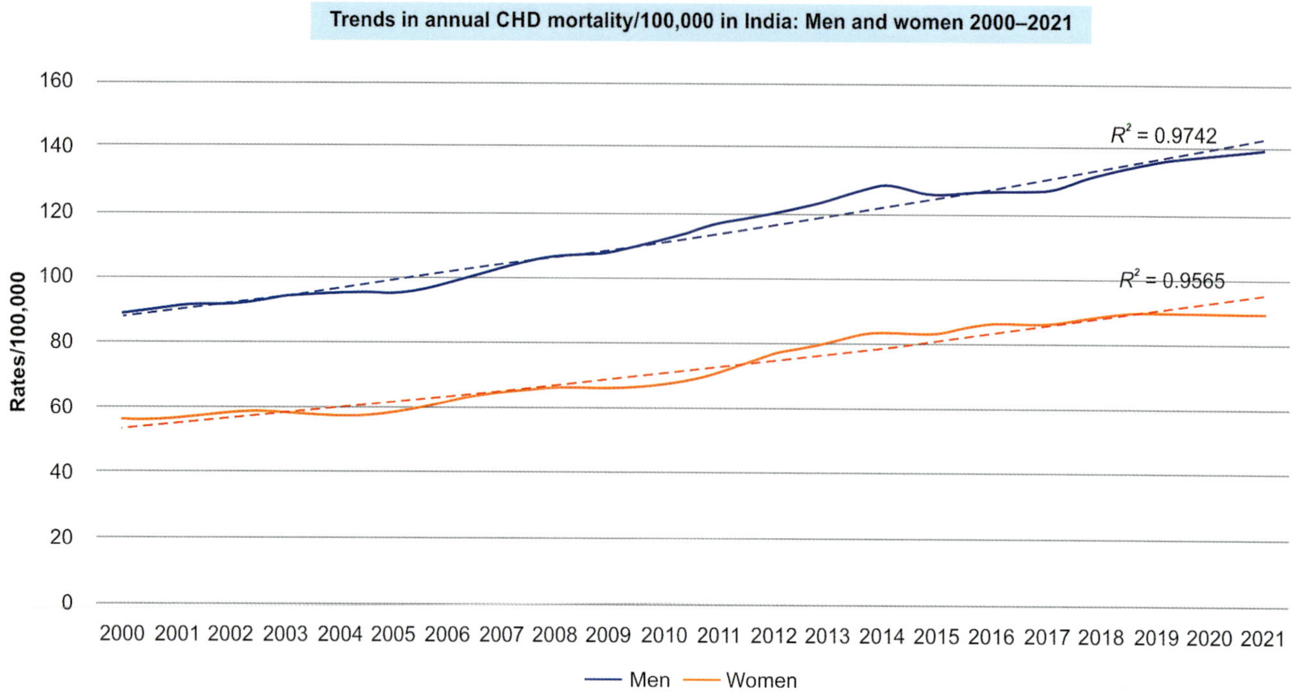

FIG. 2: Trends in CHD death rates/1,000 in men and women from 2000 to 2021 (GBD study).

trends show that the rate of increase is slightly more rapid in men (R^2 = 0.984) as compared to women (R^2 = 0.974). The rates of deaths from CHD in India (total 115.4/100,000, men 139.7/100,000, women 89.9/100,000) **(Table 1)** are lower than many countries in Central Asia, East and Central Europe, and South Asia.[1] However, these are substantially more than the developed countries of the Global North.[1,22] A comparative graph of trends in CHD deaths among men and women in numbers/1,000 is shown in **Figure 2**. This shows an increase in mortality rates from CHD. This is different from most high- and middle-income countries where these rates have substantially declined in the past 20 years.

Age-related Trends

We also obtained data for age-group-specific CHD deaths in India from the GBD database.[22] The age groups were classified as (1) premature CHD deaths (15–49 years), (2) middle-aged CHD deaths (50–69 years), and (3) older CHD deaths (≥70 years) for both men and women. Trends in absolute numbers of CHD deaths in various age categories are shown in **Figure 3**. Most of the CHD deaths in India occur in the middle-aged groups (50–69 years) for both men and women. There is a steeper increase in absolute CHD deaths in the older age group for both men and women, while the trends are the slowest for premature CHD deaths in the age group 15–49 years **(Fig. 3)**.

These trends show that while the number of premature deaths has remained almost flat over the past 20 years, the number of middle-aged and older people dying from CHD has increased substantially. Population-level policy changes that have resulted in a decline in smoking rates and tobacco consumption, and transfat intake along with better clinical control of important cardiovascular risk factors, i.e., hypertension, dyslipidemias, and diabetes, could be responsible for these trends.[7,23]

Rapidly increasing trends in CHD death rates for older individuals (70+ years) as compared to those for middle-aged and young men and women are shown in **Figures 4A and B**. This is important and shows that while the CHD death rates have remained flat for premature CHD deaths for both men and women (R^2 men 0.015, women 0.070), the increase is much more rapid in the middle-aged men than in women (R^2 men 0.448, women 0.187). In the older age group, the increase is more in women (0.077) than in men (0.075). Age-associated differential rates of increasing deaths from CHD are important for a prevention perspective. While the prevention efforts should continue to be focused on the younger and middle-aged, they need to be escalated for the older women and men.

DISEASE BURDEN DATA (DALYS)

Disability-adjusted life years lost is an important metric for the calculation of the burden of disease in a given population. It is a mathematical summation of YLLs due to premature mortality from a given cause in a person (ideal age is in countries with the longest life expectancy, e.g., Japan, Spain) and the years of healthy life lost due to disability (YLDs) and was developed in the WHO *World Health Report* (1993).

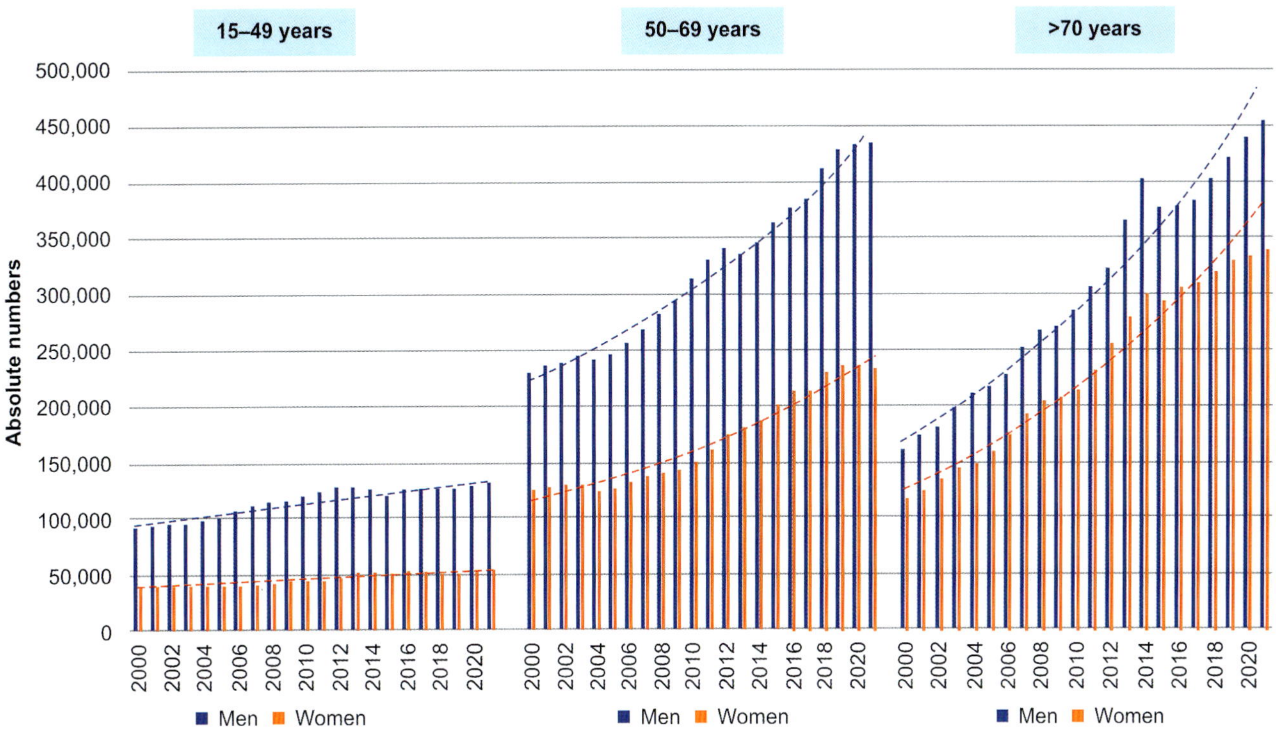

FIG. 3: Trends in CHD deaths in different age categories among men and women in India.

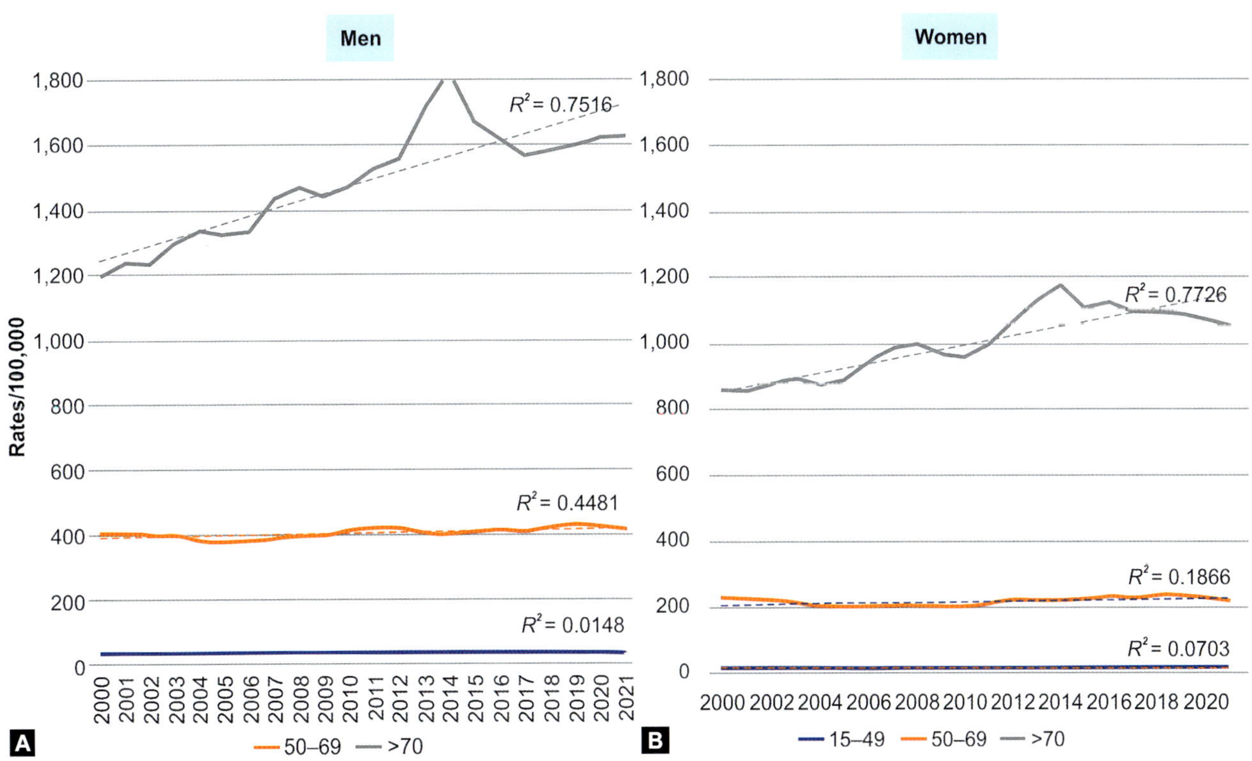

FIGS. 4A AND B: Annual trends in CHD deaths in (A) men and (B) women in different age groups.

TABLE 2: Annual trends in DALYs due to CHD in India from the year 2000 to 2021 in terms of numbers and rates/100,000 in men and women in India in Global Burden of Disease study.

	Absolute numbers			Rate per 100,000		
Year	**Men**	**Women**	**Both**	**Men**	**Women**	**Both**
2000	14,133,727	7,651,533	21,785,260	2,637.6	1,540.5	2,109.9
2001	14,573,398	7,802,264	22,375,662	2,670.6	1,540.2	2,126.4
2002	14,904,488	8,046,432	22,950,920	2,682.4	1,557.6	2,140.5
2003	15,335,056	8,127,557	23,462,613	2,711.0	1,543.0	2,147.8
2004	15,616,242	8,011,289	23,627,530	2,712.5	1,491.8	2,123.4
2005	15,931,702	8,207,673	24,139,375	2,719.6	1,499.6	2,130.3
2006	16,621,995	8,699,722	25,321,717	2,789.4	1,560.1	2,195.1
2007	17,640,236	9,151,243	26,791,479	2,911.5	1,611.4	2,282.5
2008	18,454,403	9,486,511	27,940,913	2,997.1	1,641.0	2,340.4
2009	18,948,528	9,671,164	28,619,692	3,029.3	1,644.0	2,357.9
2010	19,884,357	10,026,830	29,911,187	3,130.4	1,675.7	2,424.8
2011	20,962,086	10,637,745	31,599,830	3,251.7	1,748.9	2,522.1
2012	21,702,006	11,604,420	33,306,427	3,319.0	1,878.1	2,619.0
2013	22,098,213	12,091,283	34,189,496	3,333.8	1,928.0	2,650.3
2014	22,619,035	12,636,610	35,255,645	3,368.1	1,986.4	2,695.9
2015	22,655,934	12,845,535	35,501,469	3,331.3	1,991.8	2,679.4
2016	23,357,532	13,577,512	36,935,043	3,392.8	2,078.0	2,752.6
2017	23,796,999	13,618,593	37,415,592	3,416.4	2,058.6	2,755.0
2018	24,854,784	14,175,337	39,030,121	3,528.9	2,117.7	2,841.3
2019	25,634,248	14,443,587	40,077,835	3,601.7	2,133.8	2,886.2
2020	26,175,467	14,547,318	40,722,785	3,643.3	2,127.1	2,903.9
2021	26,637,413	14,679,265	41,316,678	3,678.0	2,126.6	2,920.9

It is useful for policymakers and health bureaucrats to calculate the burden and develop policies to reduce it. For example, in the last two decades, DALYs from infectious and maternal conditions have declined with a dramatic increase in burden from noncommunicable diseases including CVD and CHD.[2,4] The GBD study has provided recent data on DALYs in India **(Table 2)** and shows increasing DALYs in India, in both absolute numbers and rate or DALYs/100,000.[22] A doubling of absolute numbers from the years 2000 to 2021 (21.8 to 41.3 million) is observed in both men (14.1 to 26.6 million) and women (7.6–14.7 million). The corresponding rates for DALYs/100,000 have also increased exponentially.

Data on trends in DALYs in men and women in different age groups are shown in **Figure 5**. There are increasing secular trends in DALYs across all age groups. The trends are steeper in the middle-aged CHD (50–69 years) as compared to the younger and older age groups. Unsurprisingly, the disease burden calculated as DALYs is significantly more among younger and middle-aged men and women (<70 years) as compared to among those in the 70+ year age group **(Fig. 5)**. This is because YLLs and YLDs are significantly more in the younger individuals. A younger person loses more years of life (YLL) than an older individual; for example, a young man dying from CHD at 40 years has YLLs of 45 years (85 – 40 = 45) as compared to 10 years if CHD death occurs at 75 years (85 – 75 = 10). This finding should shift the prevention focus to younger age groups. If CHD prevention is focused on premature and middle-age deaths, the efforts should start two to three decades earlier, i.e., in adolescence and young adulthood.

The secular trends for DALY/100,000 in men and women are shown in **Figures 6A and B**. In terms of rates of DALYs lost, the burden is significantly higher in the older individuals compared to other age groups. The decline is more apparent among women aged 15–49 years (R^2 = 0.338) than men aged 15–49 years (R^2 = 0.086). An interesting observation is a decline in DALYs due to CHD among women in recent years. This finding needs more exploration as this is different from the previous GBD data.[1]

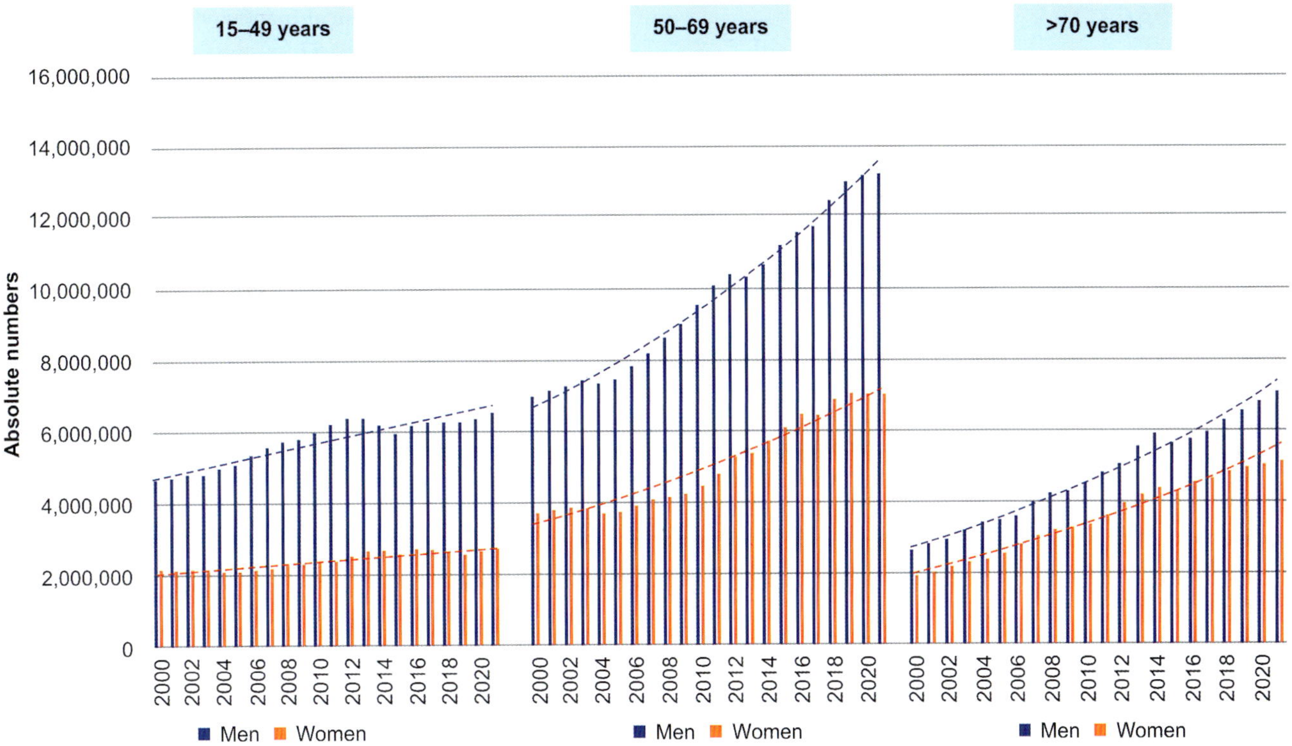

FIG. 5: Trends in CHD DALYs in different age categories among men and women.

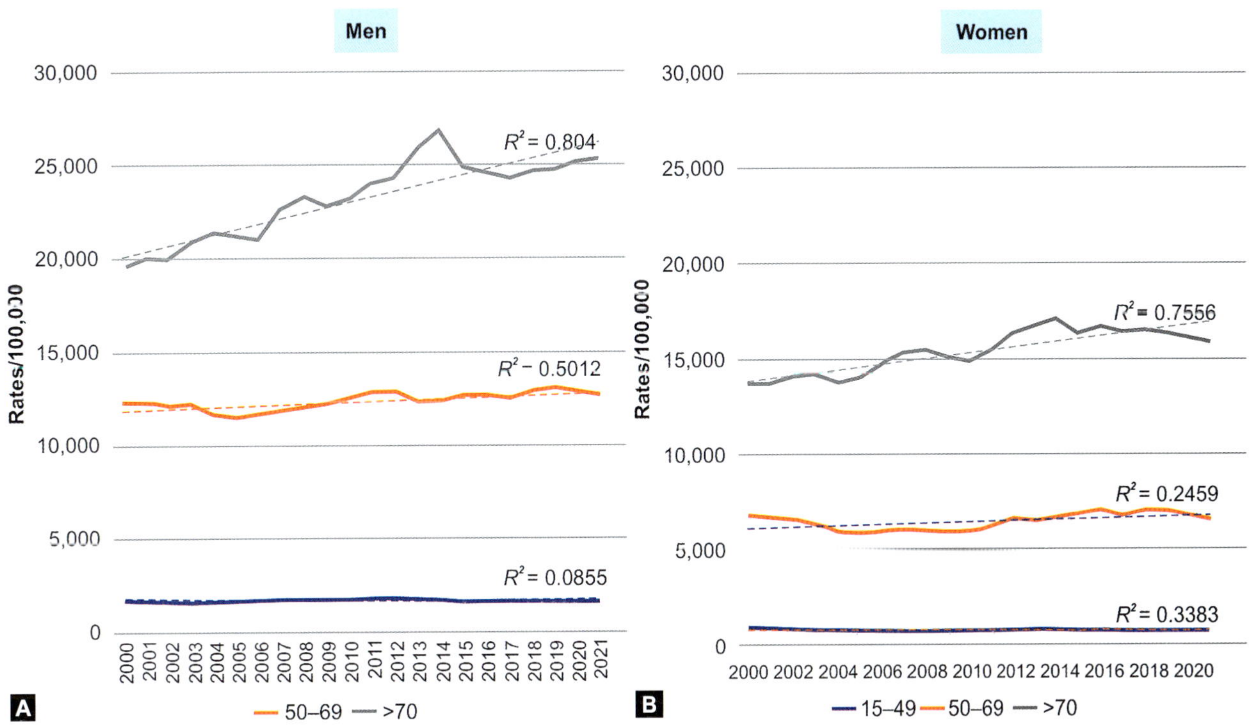

FIGS. 6A AND B: Annual trends in CHD DALYs/100,000 in men and women in different age groups.

RISK FACTORS

The study of causal risk factors for CHD in India has had a circuitous path.[24] In the early and mid-twentieth century, there were multiple theories and hypotheses to explain premature occurrence of CHD in Indians. The risk factors proposed were genetics, obesity, stress, and other social factors.[4,5] Early case-control studies in India reported unhealthy lifestyles (smoking, poor diet, stress, smokeless tobacco, etc.) and obesity-related factors (hypertension, diabetes, insulin resistance, and dyslipidemias) as important.[7,23] Studies that evaluated urban-rural differences in CHD risk factors reported the importance of standard modifiable risk factors (smoking, hypertension, diabetes, and dyslipidemias).[25] However, more recent studies have re-turned attention to genetic factors and dyslipidemias—specifically apolipoprotein B and lipoprotein(a)—as important.[24] Two large studies—the case-control INTERHEART study and the prospective PURE study—provide critical insights.[15-18]

INTERHEART Study

This large international case-control study was conducted in 52 countries in all the continents and was developed and initiated in India.[26] More than 15,000 men and women (n = 15,152) hospitalized with first myocardial infarction and matching controls (n = 14,820) were recruited in the international study. Case-control comparison showed that nine common modifiable risk factors were responsible for >90% of acute myocardial infarctions.[17] Five South Asian countries (India, Pakistan, Bangladesh, Nepal, and Sri Lanka) participated in the study with 1,732 cases and 2,204 controls.[18] Risk factors important in South Asian patients were dyslipidemias (increased apolipoprotein B/A_1 ratio), smoking, hypertension, diabetes, abdominal adiposity, psychosocial factors, physical inactivity, and low fruit and vegetable consumption **(Fig. 7)**.

An important finding in the INTERHEART study was a 10-year gap in the age of first myocardial infarction in South Asians compared to other countries; the mean age of presentation among participants in South Asian countries was 51 years compared to 61 years in the more developed countries. This study also reported that the CHD risk factors occurred earlier in South Asian participants as compared to developed countries, commensurate with earlier onset of acute coronary events. Thus, this study confirmed the importance of all the classical CHD risk factors for occurrence of an acute coronary event in India with the main difference being earlier (premature) occurrence of risk factors. This finding of premature occurrence of CHD risk factors has been confirmed in more recent national studies on hypertension and other risk factors.[7,11,27,28]

PURE Study

The PURE study is the first large-scale population-based prospective study to identify cardiovascular risk factors in lower-income countries, including India.[29] The study began in urban and rural locations in Bengaluru with about 30,000 participants and is presently being conducted in 26 countries across the globe with more than 200,000 participants. The PURE study has identified that 12 common risk factors are responsible for 65–70% of incident CVD and CAD events in the South Asian cohort **(Figs. 8A and B)**.[19,20] The 10 important risk factors identified in the PURE study for CVD were hypertension, non-HDL cholesterol, diabetes, low educational status, abdominal obesity, indoor air pollution, smoking/tobacco use, sedentary lifestyle, frailty, and depression. For the incident acute coronary event, raised non-HDL cholesterol (>120 mg/dL) was the most important risk factor followed by indoor air

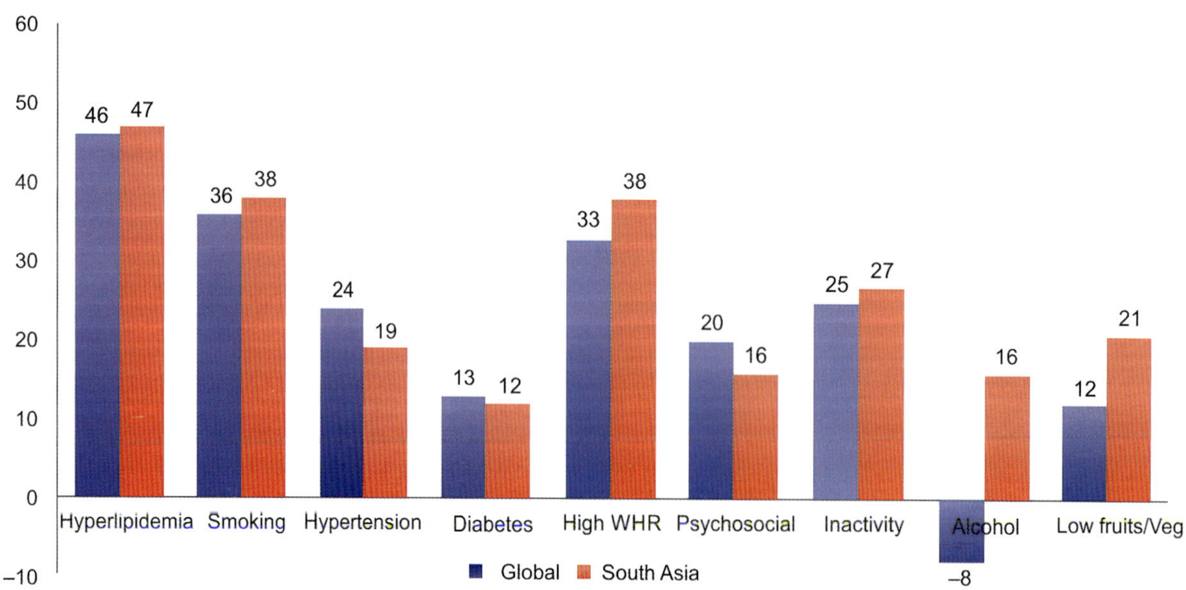

FIG. 7: Coronary risk factors in INTERHEART study: population attributable factors (%) and comparison of South Asians and global data.

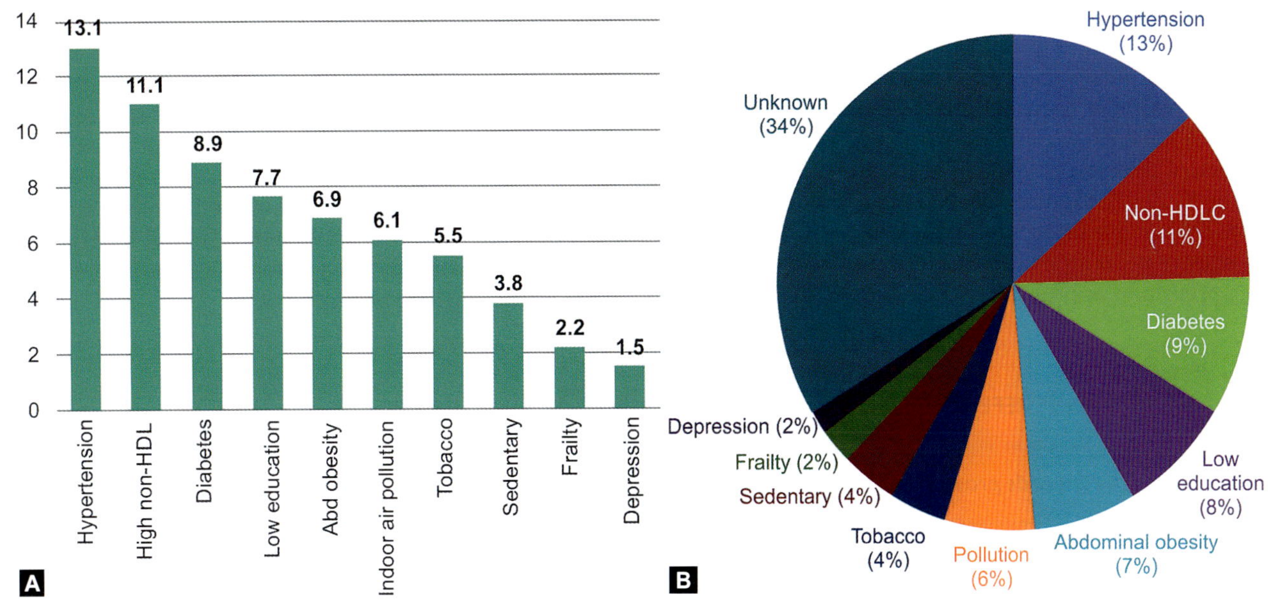

FIGS. 8A AND B: Proportionate attributable fractions (%) for various cardiovascular risk factors and incidence of cardiovascular diseases in the PURE South Asian cohort (*n* = 33,583; median follow-up 11.5 years).

BOX 2 **Risk factors identified as important in the PURE study. Cardiovascular diseases include CAD, stroke, and peripheral arterial disease. Numbers in parentheses are population attributable fractions.**

Cardiovascular diseases (CVD)	Coronary artery disease (CAD)
Hypertension (22%)	High non-HDL cholesterol (17%)
High non-HDL cholesterol (8%)	Hypertension (13%)
Household air pollution (7%)	Tobacco use (12%)
Tobacco use (6%)	Abdominal obesity (11%)
Poor diet (6%)	Diabetes (8%)
Low education (6%)	Low education (7%)
Abdominal obesity (6%)	Low grip strength (7%)
Diabetes (5%)	Household pollution (5%)
Low grip strength (3%)	Poor diet (4%)
Low physical activity (2%)	Low physical activity (<1%)
Depression (<1.0%)	Depression (<1%)
Excessive alcohol (<1.0%)	Excessive alcohol (<1%)

pollution, hypertension, and diabetes **(Box 2)**.[18] All these risk factors are similar to those in the INTERHEART study. An important difference was that while the INTERHEART study attributed 90% of the population-attributable risk to nine common risk factors, in the PURE study, only two thirds of population-attributable fraction was attributable to them. This difference is due to variation in statistical methods used in the two studies.

Risk Factor Trends

There are no nationwide studies that have evaluated trends in all coronary risk factors in India. The United Kingdom-based NCD-RISC collaboration has reported trends in four major risk factors—obesity (body mass index), hypertension, diabetes, and hypercholesterolemia (total, non-HDL, and LDL-cholesterol and triglycerides)—in all global regions.[30] This study has utilized data from disparate sources in the country including national, regional, and local studies and performed a meta-regression. Data are available only for many large countries including India. Trends show that while body mass index, obesity, hypertension, and diabetes are increasing rapidly, levels of various cholesterol subfractions and triglycerides have increased slowly.[30] The NCD-RISC reports that the global epicenters of hypertension, diabetes, and dyslipidemia have shifted to South Asia, especially India.[31-34] Increasing trends in various risk factors have also been reported in Jaipur Heart Watch studies. Over a 25-year period (1991–2016), using a time-interrupted study design with multiple cross-sectional studies, we reported a significant increase in obesity, hypertension, diabetes, and dyslipidemias in the Jaipur urban population.[35,36] All these findings have important implications for preventive cardiology in India. Control of these risk factors shall involve tackling socioeconomic, commercial, political, and health-system determinants of health with major changes in policy using a health-in-all-policy approach, better health, and medical education among all subsets of medical professionals and improving health literacy.[12,37]

CONCLUSION

This chapter shows that CHD has emerged as the most important cause of death and disability in India. Premature CHD is a concern and is associated with a high absolute number of deaths **(Fig. 3)**. Western European countries and the United States that suffered from premature CHD in the mid-twentieth century have been successful in delaying the onset of heart attacks from the early 40s to the late 70s using preventive approaches with the promotion of healthy environment with ambient and indoor pollution control, urban planning, etc., better general and health literacy, healthy lifestyles (pollutant-free healthy diet; promotion of physical activity—walking and cycling; and strict control of tobacco, smoking, and alcohol) and control of important risk factors including raised blood pressure, cholesterol, and diabetes.[12,38] We need to translate lessons learnt from scientific studies conducted in India and other parts of the globe, develop our own policies, and strictly implement them in the public and healthcare domains.

ONLINE REFERENCES

Please scan the QR code provided at the end of the table of contents for References of this chapter.

CHAPTER

3

Recent Trials in Cardiology

Subrahmanya Murti V, Vinay Kumar Bahl

ABSTRACT

This chapter reviews several cardiology trials that have significantly impacted patient management, highlighting the impact of these trials on patient care.

Keywords: Trials, patients, management

INTRODUCTION

Recently many cardiology trials have been published which have made an impact on management of patients. Few of these trials have been reviewed in this chapter.

ORBITA-2: A PLACEBO-CONTROLLED TRIAL OF PERCUTANEOUS CORONARY INTERVENTION FOR STABLE ANGINA[1]

Background

In patients with chronic coronary disease (CCD), the current guidelines recommend percutaneous coronary intervention (PCI) for those having lifestyle limiting angina despite maximal guideline directed medical therapy (GDMT) (Class 1 recommendation).[2] However, what is not known is whether PCI in itself can cause angina relief in CCD patients on no antianginal therapy. This study was done to evaluate whether PCI reduces angina symptoms as compared to a sham procedure in patients of CCD on minimal or no antianginal therapy.

Methods

Sham controlled double blinded randomized controlled trial. All selected patients first had a 2-week symptom assessment phase after antianginal drugs were stopped. A total of 301 patients underwent randomization into PCI and sham groups after 2 weeks.

Inclusion criteria were suitability for PCI as determined by the heart team, presence of angina or equivalent, anatomic evidence of severe coronary stenosis as determined by invasive or computed tomography (CT) coronary angiography and evidence of ischemia based on noninvasive testing or invasive physiology.

Exclusion criteria were acute coronary syndromes (ACSs) in the last 6 months, previous coronary bypass graft surgery, severe left ventricular systolic dysfunction (EF <35%), severe valvular disease, left main disease, and chronic total occlusions (CTOs).

Follow-up period was 12 weeks. The primary endpoint was angina symptom score calculated on the basis of angina episodes and use of antianginal medicines reported via a smartphone app. Secondary endpoints were frequency of angina, treadmill exercise time, stress echo score, and quality of life (QoL) scores.

Results

Mean age of the study population was 64 years. 150 patients were assigned to the sham group and 151 to the PCI group. A majority of the patients were in Canadian cardiovascular society (CCS) class II or III. 80% patients had single territory ischemia. At 12-week follow-up, the mean angina symptom score was 2.9 in the PCI group and 5.9 in the sham group (OR 2.21; $p < 0.001$). Among the secondary endpoints, there was a nonsignificant increase in exercise treadmill time. The mean exercise treadmill time was 700.9 seconds in the PCI arm versus 641.4 seconds in the placebo arm (OR 3.76).

There was also a nonsignificant increase in QoL score [indexed as per the Kansas City cardiomyopathy questionnaire (KCCQ)]. Six patients in the sham group had spontaneous (type 1) myocardial infarction (MI). Two patients had stroke in the PCI group as opposed to none in the sham group. Only 1 patient in the placebo group required unblinding due to unacceptable angina.

Interpretation and Limitations

The PCI as a monotherapy in patients of CCD resulted in a lower angina score as compared to a sham procedure. The duration of follow-up was small—12 weeks. However, the effect of PCI was sustained. The trial required cessation of antianginal medications which is contrary to guidelines. 80% of patients had single vessel territory ischemia. An interesting point to note—the effect of PCI on treadmill exercise time in ORBITA-2 was still 37 seconds less than the exercise treadmill time achieved by balloon angioplasty in the ACME trial[3] done in 1992—in an era without stents. Further, as compared to placebo, PCI had a 59.5 second increase in treadmill exercise time, which is almost similar to the roughly 55 seconds improvement noted by maximal dose of a single antianginal.

EMPACT-MI: EMPAGLIFLOZIN AFTER ACUTE MYOCARDIAL INFARCTION[4]

Background

Empagliflozin has already been evaluated in heart failure (HF)—both preserved and reduced ejection fraction irrespective of the presence of diabetes mellitus (DM) (EMPEROR-Preserved[5] and EMPEROR-Reduced[6]). Among the patients with diabetes, it was one of the first drugs to show efficacy in reducing cardiovascular events (EMPA-REG[7]). The EMPACT-MI trial was done to determine the effect of addition of sodium-glucose cotransporter-2 inhibitor (SGLT-2i) empagliflozin to the treatment of acute MI as regards to future mortality and HF in patients at high risk of the same.

Methods

Randomized double blinded trial. Patients with acute MI and at high risk of HF were randomized to either 10 mg empagliflozin or placebo within 14 days of hospital admission (about 3,260 patients in each arm). Patients aged 18 or more with ST elevation or non-ST elevation MI ACSs were included. High risk for HF was defined as—signs and symptoms of congestion requiring medical treatment with a newly depressed ejection fraction <45%. Additionally, the patient required to have more than one of the following high-risk features—age >65 years, new LVEF <35%, prior MI, estimated glomerular filtration rate (eGFR) <60 mL/min/1.73 m^2, atrial fibrillation, type 2 DM, elevated B-type natriuretic peptide (BNP) or NT-proBNP, uric acid >7.5 mg/dL, pulmonary artery systolic pressure >40 mm Hg, no revascularization, three-vessel coronary artery disease (CAD), and peripheral artery disease. Patients with severe valvular disease, planned coronary artery bypass surgery, systolic blood pressure <90 mm Hg, prior history of chronic HF and cardiogenic shock (CS) in the 24 hours preceding randomization were excluded.

Results

The difference in primary outcome (composite of HF hospitalization or all cause death) for empagliflozin compared to placebo was statistically insignificant [5.9 vs. 6.6 events per 100 patient years. Hazard ratio (HR) 0.90; $p = 0.21$]. The difference in secondary outcomes between the two groups was also statistically insignificant. These included (for empagliflozin compared to placebo)—all cause mortality (5.2% vs. 5.5%; HR 0.96), first HF hospitalization (2.6 vs. 3.4 events per 100 patient-years; HR 0.77; $p = 0.031$) and total HF hospitalization (2.4 vs. 3.6 adjusted events per 100 patient-years; incident rate ratio 0.67; $p = 0.006$). Safety outcomes for empagliflozin to placebo (in events per 100 patient-years) were as follows—adverse event causing drug cessation (2.0 vs. 3.0), hypotension (0.8 vs. 0.9), and acute kidney injury (0.7 vs. 1.1).

Interpretation and Limitations

In EMPACT-MI, early addition of empagliflozin after acute MI did not show any impact on all cause death or HF hospitalization. Similarly, the DAPA-MI[8] trial to evaluate dapagliflozin in a similar subset did not show any improvement in cardiovascular mortality. However, there was a positive impact on cardiometabolic outcomes.

ULTIMATE-DAPT: TICAGRELOR ALONE VERSUS TICAGRELOR PLUS ASPIRIN FROM MONTH 1 TO MONTH 12 AFTER PERCUTANEOUS CORONARY INTERVENTION IN PATIENTS WITH ACUTE CORONARY SYNDROMES: A RANDOMIZED, PLACEBO-CONTROLLED, DOUBLE-BLIND CLINICAL TRIAL[9]

Background

In patients with ACSs who have undergone PCI, present guidelines recommend 12 months of dual antiplatelet therapy (DAPT).[10] In this background, several trials have investigated a shortened DAPT (3-month DAPT in TICO[11] and TWILIGHT[12]). The ULTIMATE-DAPT trial aims to evaluate a 1-month DAPT duration followed by a comparison of ticagrelor monotherapy versus DAPT.

Methods

Randomized, double-blinded, placebo-controlled trial. All patients were started on 100 mg acetyl salicylic acid (ASA) and 90 mg per oral (PO) twice daily (BID) dose of ticagrelor before PCI. 1 month after PCI, patients were randomly assigned 1:1 to continue ASA + ticagrelor for an additional 11 months or to ticagrelor monotherapy with placebo for 12 months. Patients who had major bleeding events [Bleeding Academic Research Consortium (BARC) types 3 or 5], or adverse ischemic events were excluded. The primary endpoints were—superiority endpoint of occurrence of clinically relevant bleeding (BARC 2, 3, or 5) and noninferiority endpoint of 4-point major adverse cardiovascular and cerebrovascular events (MACCE).

Results

There were 1,700 patients in each arm. The primary superiority endpoint of clinically significant bleeding was seen in 2.1% treated with ticagrelor monotherapy versus 4.6% treated with ticagrelor plus ASA (HR 0.45; $p < 0.0001$). Numbers needed-to-treat (NNT) were 48 to prevent one clinically significant bleeding event and 100 to prevent one BARC type 3 or 5 bleeding event. Patients treated with ticagrelor monotherapy had similar rates of adverse ischemic events as compared to those on DAPT. The primary noninferiority endpoint of MACCE occurred in 3.6% treated with ticagrelor monotherapy and 3.7% treated with ticagrelor plus ASA (HR 0.98; p noninferiority <0.0001; p superiority = 0.89).

Interpretation and Limitations

In patients with an ACS treated with PCI followed by 1 month of ASA with ticagrelor, follow-up treatment with ticagrelor monotherapy for an additional 11 months reduced clinically relevant bleeding without an accompanying increase in MACCE, compared with follow-up treatment with ticagrelor and ASA (DAPT) for an additional 11 months.

TRANSCATHETER AORTIC VALVE IMPLANTATION IN LOW-RISK TRICUSPID OR BICUSPID AORTIC STENOSIS: THE NOTION-2 TRIAL[13]

Background

Transcatheter aortic valve implantation (TAVI) is now considered the first choice in treating older patients with symptomatic severe aortic stenosis (AS) across the spectrum of surgical risk. The Nordic Aortic Valve Intervention (NOTION)-2 trial aimed to compare TAVI with SAVR in low-risk patients ≤75 years of age with severe symptomatic AS, including both tricuspid and bicuspid AS.

Methods

Prospective, multicenter, randomized controlled trial comparing TAVI with SAVR in low surgical risk (STS score <4%) patients aged ≤75 years with severe symptomatic AS (aortic valve area <1.0 cm^2 or <0.6 cm^2/m^2 and mean transvalvular gradient >40 mm Hg or peak jet velocity >4.0 m/s). Patients with an ascending aorta ≥45 mm or CAD not suitable for both PCI and coronary artery bypass graft (CABG) surgery were excluded. In case of need for coronary artery revascularization in the TAVI arm, PCI was performed prior to or concomitant with TAVI. The primary endpoint was a composite risk of death of any cause, stroke, or rehospitalization (related to the procedure, valve, or HF) at 1 year after the procedure. Secondary endpoints included death of any cause, stroke, major or life-threatening bleeding, new-onset atrial fibrillation, need for permanent pacemaker implantation, valve endocarditis, valve thrombosis, need for valve reintervention, and valve performance as assessed by transthoracic echocardiography at 1 month and 1 year after the procedure.

Results

A total of 370 patients were included, 187 patients in the TAVI arm and 183 patients in the SAVR arm. The mean age of the patients was 71.1 years and the median STS score was 1.1%. 27% patients had a native bicuspid aortic valve confirmed by cardiac computed tomography. In the TAVI group, 72.7% patients were implanted with a self-expanding valve, the rest balloon expandable. 5.9% of patients in the TAVI arm also underwent PCI. In the surgery arm, 9.8% also underwent concomitant CABG. At 1 year, the primary endpoint was 10.2% in the TAVI group and 7.1% in the SAVR group, with an absolute risk difference between the two arms of 3.1% ($p = 0.3$) which was statistically nonsignificant. At 1 year, the cumulative incidence rates in the TAVI group compared with the SAVR group were lower for major or life-threatening bleeding (4.8% vs. 17.5%; HR 0.3) and new-onset atrial fibrillation (3.2% vs. 41.7%; HR 0.06) and higher for nondisabling stroke (3.7% vs. 0.5%; HR 7.0) and permanent pacemaker implantation (15.1% vs. 8.0%; HR 2.0). The risk of major vascular complications and MI were similar between the two groups. In the overall study population, 270 patients had a tricuspid AS and 100 patients a bicuspid AS. In the tricuspid cohort, the risk of the primary endpoint was 8.7% in the TAVI and 8.3% in the SAVR group, resulting in an absolute risk difference of 0.4% ($p = 0.9$). In the bicuspid cohort, the risk of the primary endpoint was 14.3% in the TAVI and 3.9% in the surgery group, resulting in an absolute risk difference of 10.4% ($p = 0.07$). The risk of death or disabling stroke at 1 year was 6.1% in the TAVI and 2.0% in the surgery group, resulting in an absolute risk difference of 4.1% ($p = 0.3$). Regarding valve performance, there was a markedly higher rate of moderate or greater paravalvular regurgitation (PVR) in the bicuspid TAVI cohort as compared to the bicuspid surgery cohort, resulting in an absolute risk difference of 9.1% (95% CI 0.6–17.6%), which is thrice the same difference in the tricuspid group.

Interpretation and Limitations

The study shows that in younger patients with severe symptomatic AS, TAVI and SAVR are comparable. However, overall primary outcome event rate is lesser in the SAVR group. Stroke and pacemaker implantation rates were higher in the TAVI arm. Bicuspid valve outcomes for TAVI were worse compared to SAVR underscoring two important points—first, SAVR still remains the better option and second, need for more trials in the bicuspid subset.

REDUCE-AMI: β-BLOCKERS AFTER MYOCARDIAL INFARCTION AND PRESERVED EJECTION FRACTION[14]

Background

In patients with acute myocardial infarction (AMI), particularly those with preserved ejection fraction, the role of long-term β-blockers has not been tested in large scale trials. Most of the trials for β-blockers are in the context of HF whether preserved or reduced. In the AMI setting, only one large trial has been done—the METOCARD-CNIC,[15] which also focused on intravenous β-blocker in an AMI setting and not on long-term maintenance. The REDUCE-AMI trial aimed to evaluate the benefit of β-blockade following AMI in patients with preserved left ventricular ejection fraction (LVEF).

Methods

Registry based, randomized, open-label, international multicentric trial. Patients with AMI with preserved LVEF (≥50%) were 1:1 randomized to receive oral β-blocker (n = 2,508) with oral metoprolol succinate or bisoprolol tartrate titrated to a target dose ≥100 mg daily or ≥5 mg daily, respectively, or to usual care (n = 2,512).

Results

The mean age of the study population was 63 years. Median follow-up was 3.5 years. 35% of the patients had ST-elevation MI and 96% underwent PCI. The primary outcome, composite of all-cause death or nonfatal AMI, for the β-blocker arm compared to usual care was: 7.9% versus 8.3%, HR 0.96; p = 0.64. Secondary outcomes for β-blocker arm compared to usual care were: (1) *All-cause death:* 3.9% versus 4.1%, HR 0.94; p = 0.66, (2) *AMI:* 4.5% versus 4.7%, HR 0.96; p = 0.74, and (3) *HF hospitalization:* 0.8% versus 0.9%, HR 0.91; p = 0.76. Safety outcomes for β-blocker arm compared to usual care were: (1) *Hospitalization for bradyarrhythmia, hypotension, or syncope:* 3.4% versus 3.2%; HR 1.08; p = 0.64, (2) *Asthma/COPD hospitalization:* 0.6% versus 0.6%, HR 0.94 (95% CI 0.46–1.89); p = 0.86, and (3) *Stroke hospitalization*: 1.4% versus 1.8%; HR 0.78 (95% CI 0.51–1.21); p = 0.35. As regards to β-blocker adherence, in the β-blocker arm it was 90.6% at 6–10 weeks and 81.9% at 11–13 months; and 11.3% at 6–10 weeks and 14.3% at 11–13 months in the usual care arm.

Interpretation and Limitations

The clinical benefit of β-blockers post AMI, particularly with preserve LVEF is unclear in the contemporary era of early revascularization. REDUCE-AMI showed that β-blocker therapy in the post-MI population with preserved LVEF did not show any reduction in all-cause mortality or recurrent AMI. One of the important drawbacks of the trial was that there was significant crossover between groups at 1 year which may have influenced the overall result. The increased β-blocker use in the usual care arm over time may indicate the treatment of common problems after AMI, including stable angina, atrial fibrillation, hypertension, or subsequent onset of reduced LVEF. Further, the design was open-label and endpoint data was collected from registry data.

PREVENTIVE PERCUTANEOUS CORONARY INTERVENTION VERSUS OPTIMAL MEDICAL THERAPY ALONE FOR THE TREATMENT OF VULNERABLE ATHEROSCLEROTIC CORONARY PLAQUES (PREVENT): A MULTICENTER, OPEN-LABEL, RANDOMIZED CONTROLLED TRIAL[16]

Background

The primary cause of ACS is now understood to be the rupture of a "vulnerable plaque"[17]—either a lipid rich plaque, a thin cap fibroatheroma[18] [thin-cap fibroatheroma (TCFA)—cap thickness <65 μm over a lipid rich plaque] and even sometimes a calcific plaque. These have now been associated with a trend toward higher major adverse cardiovascular events (MACE) events. However, the effect of presence of these vulnerable plaques in nonflow limiting and nonischemic lesions (by angiography, intravascular imaging, and coronary physiology) on MACE events is unclear. The PREVENT trial sought to assess the impact of preventive PCI on MACE among patients presenting with high-risk, nonflow-limiting vulnerable plaques identified through intracoronary imaging.

Methods

Following PCI of the culprit lesions in patients with ACS and chronic coronary syndrome (CCS), any untreated nonculprit lesions showing an angiographic diameter stenosis of 50% or more, were first assessed for physiology using fractional flow reserve (FFR). Intermediate lesions with an FFR >0.80 were further analyzed using intracoronary imaging techniques such as gray-scale intravascular ultrasonography (IVUS), radiofrequency IVUS, a combination of gray-scale IVUS and near-infrared spectroscopy (NIRS), or optical coherence tomography (OCT), based on the discretion of experienced operators. Vulnerable plaques were identified as lesions meeting at least two of the following criteria: (1) Minimal lumen area (MLA) of <4.0 mm^2 by IVUS or OCT; (2) Plaque burden exceeding 70% by IVUS; (3) Presence of a lipid-rich plaque by NIRS [(maxLCBI4mm) >315]; and (4) TCFA detected by RF-IVUS or OCT.

Eligible patients with one or two nonflow-limiting vulnerable plaques were randomly assigned 1:1 to either undergo PCI along with optimal medical therapy (OMT) or receive OMT alone. PCI of vulnerable plaques was performed with bioresorbable vascular scaffolds and everolimus eluting stents. The primary outcome was a composite of death from cardiac causes, target-vessel MI, ischemia-driven target-vessel revascularization, or hospitalization for unstable or progressive angina, all at 2 years after randomization. Secondary outcomes were the individual components of the primary composite outcome.

Results

The study enrolled 1,606 randomly assigned patients with a total of 1,672 qualifying lesions. Among them, 803 patients (with 831 lesions) were allocated to the preventive PCI plus OMT group, while 803 patients (with 841 lesions) were designated to receive OMT alone. The median FFR value of the 1,672 target lesions was 0.86, with a mean diameter stenosis of 54.5%. At 2 years, the primary outcome occurred in 0.4% patients in the preventive PCI group and in 3.4% patients in the OMT group (HR 0.11; $p = 0.0003$). Further, rates for each component of the composite primary endpoint were also lower in the PCI group, as were the composite rate of death from any cause or target-vessel MI or any revascularization. At 2 years, four patients (0.5%) in the PCI group had died compared to 10 (1.3%) in the OMT group. Nine (1.1%) patients had an MI in the PCI group versus 13 (1.7%) patients in the OMT group. Serious clinical or adverse effects did not differ between the two groups. During a median follow-up of 4.3 years (maximum up to 7.9 years), patients who underwent PCI had a consistent reduction in cumulative primary endpoint. Preventive PCI also reduced the composite patient-oriented risk of all-cause death, all MIs, or any repeat revascularization. Posthoc as-treated analysis showed that drug eluting stents may be better as compared to bioresorbable scaffolds as regards outcomes.

Interpretation and Limitations

Preventive PCI to treat vulnerable plaques resulted in a decrease in the composite primary endpoint at the 2-year mark as also across the full 7-year follow-up period. A major limitation is that the majority of patients had CCSs. The vulnerable plaques can be more dynamic in patients with ACS.

A DOUBLE-BLIND, RANDOMIZED, PLACEBO-PROCEDURE-CONTROLLED TRIAL OF AN INTERATRIAL SHUNT IN PATIENTS WITH HFREF AND HFPEF: PRINCIPAL RESULTS FROM THE RELIEVE-HF TRIAL[19]

Background

In patients with symptomatic HF (both preserved LVEF–heart failure with preserved ejection fraction (HFpEF) and reduced LVEF–HFrEF despite GDMT and recurrent hospitalization (one or more) for HF, interatrial shunt devices have been examined to provide some symptomatic benefit by unloading the preload of the left ventricle (LV). In this background, the RELIEVE-HF examined the benefit of the Ventura device as regards HF outcomes and LV parameters.

Methods

A placebo-procedure controlled trial of interatrial shunting (with the Ventura shunt) in patients with HFrEF and HFpEF randomized 508 patients to a shunt ($n = 250$) or placebo procedure ($n = 258$). All participants had symptomatic HF despite taking medications at maximally tolerated doses and one or more hospitalizations for HF. About 40% of participants had HFrEF and 60% had HFpEF.

Results

There was no significant difference between groups for the primary endpoint—a composite of all-cause death, need for heart transplant or left ventricular assist device, recurrent HF hospitalizations and change in QoL (using the KCCQ). There was also no difference between the groups as regards risk of annual cardiovascular events (55.7/year vs. 56.0/year; $p = 096$). There was an increase in QoL across both the groups, suggesting a placebo effect. An analysis comparing outcomes by baseline LVEF suggested that the shunt may be beneficial in patients with HFrEF, who had improvements in all parameters (though not statistically significant), and worsen outcomes in patients with HFpEF, who experienced increased rates of death and HF hospitalizations. In addition, for the primary safety outcome, no device-related or procedure-related major adverse cardiovascular or neurologic events were observed in either group.

Interpretation and Limitations

An interatrial shunt can unload up to 1 L/min from left to right. This likely leads to an improvement in patients with HFrEF. However, there was no benefit in patients with HFpEF likely due to a stiffer noncompliant both ventricles. This trial has not shown any difference in hard endpoints, but paves the way for future trials particularly among the HFrEF subset.

DANGER SHOCK TRIAL: MICROAXIAL FLOW PUMP OR STANDARD CARE IN INFARCT-RELATED CARDIOGENIC SHOCK[20]

Background

The Impella system is a centrifugal pump meant to unload the heart in CS or in the setting of protected PCI. In the setting of CS, this system now carries a class IIa recommendation[21] in the 2021 European Society of Cardiology guidelines. Previous trial results have only been equivocal at best as shown in the ISAR-SHOCK series of trials. The DanGer shock trial aimed to assess the effect of use of Impella CP on mortality among patients with ST-segment elevation myocardial infarction (STEMI) complicated by CS.

Methods

The trial aimed to compare the safety and efficacy of Impella CP on top of standard care with standard care alone among patients with STEMI and CS. Patients were randomized in a 1:1 manner to either Impella CP with standard care (n = 179) or standard care alone (n = 176). In the patients assigned to receive the Impella CP, the device was to be placed immediately after randomization and run at the highest possible performance level for at least 48 hours unless complications occurred. In the event of further hemodynamic compromise, treatment could be escalated to additional mechanical circulatory support after randomization in either trial group. In the Impella CP group, treatment could be escalated to the placement of an Impella 5.0, Impella RP device, or extracorporeal life support (ECMO). In the standard care group, ECMO was recommended, although placement of an Impella 5.0 device was allowed. The inclusion criteria were age ≥18 years having STEMI with CS. The exclusion criteria included: shock duration >24 hours; other causes of shock; shock due to mechanical complication to MI; severe aortic valve regurgitation/stenosis; severe peripheral arterial obstructive disease that would preclude Impella device placement; mechanical aortic valve prosthesis; left ventricular thrombus; shock due to right ventricular failure; out-of-hospital cardiac arrest with persistent Glasgow coma scale <8 after return of spontaneous circulation; and a life expectancy of <1 year due to comorbidities.

Results

Median age of the study population was 68 years with 79% males. The median LVEF was 25%, 20% required resuscitation before randomization, 72% patients had anterior wall MI, 96% had immediate PCI, and 44% also underwent nonculprit vessel PCI. Median duration of Impella CP support was 60 hours. The primary endpoint of all-cause mortality at 6 months for Impella CP + standard care versus standard care alone was: 45.8% versus 58.5% (HR 0.74; $p = 0.04$). Key secondary outcomes for Impella CP + standard care versus standard care alone were: (1) Composite at 6 months [escalation of treatment to additional mechanical circulatory support (short- or long-term), heart transplantation, or death of any cause]: 52.5% versus 63.6% (HR 0.72); (2) Composite safety endpoint (occurrence of severe bleeding, limb ischemia, hemolysis, device failure, or worsening aortic regurgitation): 24.0% versus 6.2% (HR 4.74); (3) Moderate or severe bleeding: 21.8% versus 11.9% ($p < 0.05$); (4) Limb ischemia: 5.6% versus 1.1% ($p < 0.05$); and (5) Need for renal replacement therapy (RRT) 41.9% versus 26.7% ($p < 0.05$).

Interpretation and Limitations

The trial shows that implantation of Impella CP with standard care is better than standard care alone in reducing 6-month mortality among patients of STEMI with CS. Risk of complications including bleeding, limb ischemia, need for RRT, and sepsis were all higher with Impella CP. Other mechanical circulatory support devices such as IABP and VA-ECMO have failed to show a benefit with routine use in STEMI with CS. One important point is that it took 10 years to enroll 355 patients across three countries. This trial supports the use of Impella CP among selected patients presenting with STEMI and CS.

STEP-HFPEF: SEMAGLUTIDE IN PATIENTS WITH HEART FAILURE WITH PRESERVED EJECTION FRACTION AND OBESITY[22]

Background

The burden of HFpEF is steadily increasing and many have an obese phenotype, which is also a part of scoring systems for HFpEF diagnosis. HFpEF with obesity phenotype is characterized by greater symptom severity, worse functional capacity, and a higher risk for HF hospitalization.[23] This study aimed to study the efficacy of treatment with semaglutide (a GLP-1 receptor agonist) on symptoms, physical limitation, exercise function, and weight loss in patients with HFpEF, and obese phenotype.

Methods

A total of 529 patients were randomized to subcutaneous semaglutide 2.4 mg once-weekly for 52 weeks or placebo. Semaglutide treatment was started at a dose of 0.25 mg once-weekly for the first 4 weeks. The dose was then escalated every 4 weeks to reach the maintenance dose (2.4 mg) by week 16. Randomization was stratified according to baseline body mass index (BMI) <35 kg/m^2 versus ≥35 kg/m^2. Inclusion criteria were: Age ≥18 years, LVEF of ≥45%, BMI of ≥30 kg/m^2, New York Heart Association (NYHA) functional class II, III, or IV symptoms, QoL measure—KCCQ-Clinical Summary Score (KCCQ-CSS) <90 points, and a 6-minute walk distance (6MWD) of ≥100 m. Further, at least one of the following findings were required: Elevated LV filling pressures, elevated natriuretic peptide levels plus echocardiographic abnormalities, or hospitalization for HF in the 12 months before screening plus ongoing treatment with diuretics or echocardiographic abnormalities. Exclusion criteria were mainly patient-reported change in body weight of >5 kg within 90 days before screening and a history of diabetes.

Results

Median age was 69 years. The median body weight was 105.1 kg and the median BMI was 37 kg/m^2. As regards to baseline medications 80.7% were on diuretics, 34.8% were on mineralocorticoid receptor antagonists, and 3.6% were on SGLT-2i. The coprimary endpoints for semaglutide versus placebo from baseline to week 52: (1) *Change in KCCQ-CSS:* 16.6 versus 8.7 ($p < 0.001$) and (2) *Percentage change in body weight:* –13.3 versus –2.6 ($p < 0.001$). The key secondary outcomes for semaglutide versus placebo: (1) *Change in 6MWD from baseline to week 52:* 21.5 versus 1.2 m ($p < 0.001$) and (2) *Percentage reduction from baseline to week 52 in NT-proBNP:* –20.9 versus –5.3 ($p < 0.05$); *hospitalization or urgent visit for HF:* 1 versus 12 events ($p < 0.05$). The median KCCQ-CSS was 59 points. Treatment with semaglutide (vs. placebo) improved all three KCCQ summary domains. Of patients treated with semaglutide, 37.9% experienced an increase in KCCQ-CSS of ≥20 points, compared with 26.6% treated with placebo. Conversely, 4.9% of patients treated with semaglutide experienced a decrease in KCCQ-CSS of ≥10 points, compared with 11% in the placebo group.

Interpretation and Limitations

Among obese patients with HFpEF, once weekly subcutaneous semaglutide was better than placebo in improving body weight, QoL outcomes including KCCQ-CSS and 6MWD at 52 weeks. There were improvements in HF-related symptoms, physical limitations, and exercise function, regardless of baseline health status or sex. One important limitation of this trial is that very few patients were on SGLT-2i at baseline. It is also unclear if the improvements in HF-related QoL measures were driven by weight loss (suggesting that other weight loss measures could be considered and potentially beneficial) or independent of this. The number of nonwhite participants was low, which may limit the generalizability of results. Further, the trial was overall underpowered.

ILUMIEN IV: OPTIMAL PERCUTANEOUS CORONARY INTERVENTION—OPTICAL COHERENCE TOMOGRAPHY GUIDED CORONARY STENT IMPLANTATION COMPARED WITH ANGIOGRAPHY: A MULTICENTER RANDOMIZED TRIAL IN PERCUTANEOUS CORONARY INTERVENTION[24]

Background

Intravascular imaging is now commonly utilized to guide PCI. OCT has a superior resolution but poor depth of penetration. Apart from identifying plaque morphology, it now commonly used to optimize the result of PCI in terms of stent sizing, expansion, apposition, and geographical miss/coverage. In this background, the ILUMIEN IV trial attempted to compare OCT-guided and angiographically-guided PCI in terms of short- and long-term outcomes.

Methods

This was a prospective, single-blind, randomized trial conducted at 80 sites in 18 countries in which patients with evidence of myocardial ischemia considered to be at high-risk or had high-risk coronary-artery lesions were randomized to undergo OCT- or angiography-guided PCI. A high-risk patient was defined as a patient with DM who was treated with medication, whereas a high-risk coronary-artery lesion was defined as that which was considered responsible for a recent MI, long or multiple lesions requiring stents longer than 28 mm, a dedicated two stent bifurcation lesion, lesion with heavy calcification, CTO, and complex in-stent restenosis. The main exclusion criteria included an ST-segment elevation MI ≤24 hours, creatinine clearance ≤30 mL/min/1.73 m^2, hemodynamic instability or CS, HF (Killip class ≥2 or NYHA class ≥3), LVEF ≤30%, and ventricular arrhythmias. The primary imaging endpoint was the final minimum stent area after PCI as assessed with OCT, while the primary clinical endpoint was target-vessel failure at 2 years, defined as a composite of death from cardiac causes, target-vessel MI, or ischemia-driven target-vessel revascularization. The major secondary endpoint was target-vessel failure, excluding periprocedural MI.

Results

A total of 2,487 patients were randomized to undergo OCT-guided PCI (1,233 patients, 1,353 lesions) or angiography-guided PCI (1,254 patients, 1,409 lesions). The mean age was 65.6 years. 42% of patients had DM, 17.9% had a creatinine clearance <60 mL/min, and mean LVEF was 55.2%. 42.5% of patients underwent PCI for silent ischemia or stable angina and 51.8% for unstable angina or non-ST-segment elevation MI. Only a minority (5.7%) had an ST-segment elevation MI. Maximum stent diameter per lesion, total stent length per patient, lesion postdilation, maximum inflation pressure per lesion, duration of fluoroscopy per patient, radiation dose per patient, and contrast media volume per patient were higher in the OCT-guided PCI group compared with the angiography-guided PCI. The primary imaging endpoint of mean minimum stent area after PCI was higher in the OCT-guided PCI group compared with the angiography-guided group (5.72 ± 2.04 mm^2 vs. 5.36 ± 1.87 mm^2; $p < 0.001$). OCT-guided PCI compared to angiography-guided PCI also had better stent expansion, and a significant reduction in major dissection, major malapposition, and major tissue protrusion. At a median follow-up of 729 days, the primary clinical endpoint of target-vessel failure was not significantly different between OCT- and angiography-guided PCI (7.4% vs. 8.2%; HR 0.90; $p = 0.45$). Consistently, the composite endpoint of target lesion failure was not significantly different between OCT- and angiography-guided PCI (6.4% vs. 7.1%; HR 0.89). As regards to the individual components of the primary clinical endpoint between OCT- and angiography-guided PCI, cardiac death (0.8% vs. 1.3%; HR 0.57), target-vessel MI (2.5% vs. 3.3%; HR 0.77); and ischemia-driven target-vessel revascularization (5.6% vs. 5.6%; HR 0.99) were not significantly different between the two groups. Definite or probable stent thrombosis occurred in 0.5% of patients assigned to OCT-guided PCI and 1.4% of patients assigned to angiography-guided PCI (HR 1.05; $p = 0.02$).

Interpretation and Limitations

The main conclusion from the ILUMIEN IV trial is that while OCT-guided PCI is associated with better angiographic, imaging, and procedural outcomes when compared to angiography-guided PCI, these results do not have a significant impact on long-term clinical outcomes or end-points except for stent thrombosis rates.

CONCLUSION

Clinical trials are the backbone of evidence-based medicine. Cardiology of all the sciences is highly evidence driven with new data coming at a rapid pace. The trials summarized herein are the most pivotal ones to come out recently, with the potential to change clinical practice guidelines. The good physician/interventionist is the one who knows what not to do, and knowledge of the same come from hard clinical evidence in the form of trials.

ONLINE REFERENCES

Please scan the QR code provided at the end of the table of contents for References of this chapter.

CHAPTER

4

Genetic Testing in Cardiovascular Disorders

Ajay Bahl

ABSTRACT

Genotyping plays an important role in the evaluation of inherited cardiac single-gene disorders. The most common disorders are cardiomyopathies, inherited channelopathies, and aortopathies involving the thoracic aorta. Genotyping is carried out using next-generation sequencing platforms, either disease-specific panels or whole exome sequencing. This is followed by cascade screening of family members using Sanger sequencing. Genotyping is also useful in young individuals who are victims of unexplained sudden death and for prenatal diagnosis.

Keywords: Genotyping, cardiomyopathy, inherited arrhythmic disorders, aortopathy

INTRODUCTION

Genotyping is now widely available and plays an important role in the evaluation of various inherited cardiac disorders caused by mutations in a single gene. These include cardiomyopathies, inherited arrhythmic disorders, and connective tissue disorders like Marfan's syndrome. In addition, genetic testing has a limited role in patients with congenital heart disease and dyslipidemias.

Genotyping is useful for single Mendelian gene disorders. Autosomal dominant pattern is the most common. X-linked, autosomal recessive, and mitochondrial inheritance is present in a small number. Most arrhythmic disorders and cardiomyopathies are a result of a single mutation. However, a small number may be due to two or more mutations. Individuals carrying more than one mutation often have early onset disease and more severe disease.

APPROACH TO GENOTYPING

Inherited cardiovascular disorders are caused by mutations spread across several genes. Next-generation sequencing (NGS) has permitted simultaneous screening of a large number of genes. NGS includes specific gene-oriented panels, whole exome sequencing, and whole genome sequencing **(Flowchart 1)**. Comprehensive gene-specific panels screen the genes known to be associated with the disease phenotype. Being focused, they give good coverage and are thus preferred. Whole exome sequencing covers a much larger proportion of the genome and is an alternative. Whole genome sequencing generates a huge amount of data and is mainly used for research purposes. Whole genome sequencing has a very limited role in a clinical setting.[1]

Variants detected on sequencing may be classified as pathogenic, likely pathogenic, variants of uncertain significance, likely benign, and benign.[2] As a result of advances in sequencing technologies, identification of sequence variations has become easy. However, due to the paucity of clinical data, the significance of a large number of variants is not clear. These are classified as variants

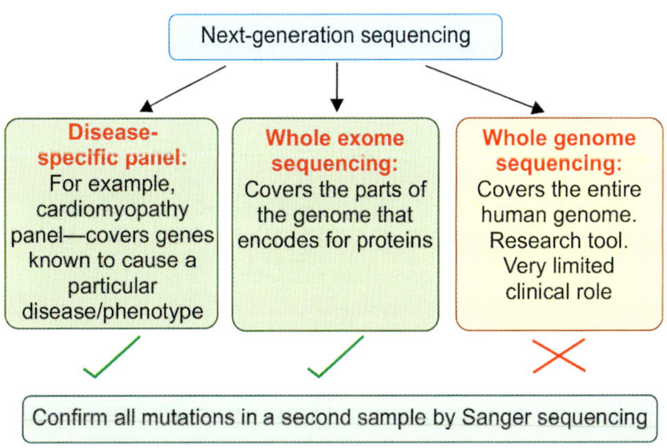

FLOWCHART 1: Next-generation sequencing.

of uncertain significance. Interpretation of many of the variants remains a big challenge. Only pathogenic and likely pathogenic variants are considered to be of significance and are actionable. Mutations have implications not only for the individual but also for the entire family and future generations. Thus, all mutations should be confirmed in a second sample by Sanger sequencing.

Once a mutation is confirmed in the proband, family members may be offered genetic screening **(Flowchart 2)**. Family members only need to be screened for the particular mutation(s) identified within the family. This is carried out using Sanger sequencing. If the family member does not carry the mutation, he/she is not at risk of developing disease in the future. Genetic screening of phenotypically normal family members is only possible if a mutation has been identified in the proband/family. Only clinical screening can be offered in case a disease-causing mutation has not been identified in the family. Many of these disorders have incomplete age-related penetrance. A normal clinical evaluation only indicates the absence of disease at the time of screening. Future development of disease and transmission to future generations is possible in phenotypically normal mutation carriers. Genotyping thus is advantageous. A family member who does not carry the mutation is not at risk of disease in the future and his/her children are also not at risk. However, mutation carriers remain at risk of disease and need regular follow-up to allow for early detection and management.

Once a mutation is identified in a family member, the screening is extended to his/her first-degree relatives, thus extending the screening to the entire family. This is called cascade screening.

The data on many sequence variations in disease-causing genes is sparse. As clinical data accumulates, the classification of these variants may change. As an example, a variant of uncertain significance may get reclassified as a benign or pathogenic variant or vice versa. Thus, the significance of identified variants should be periodically reassessed.

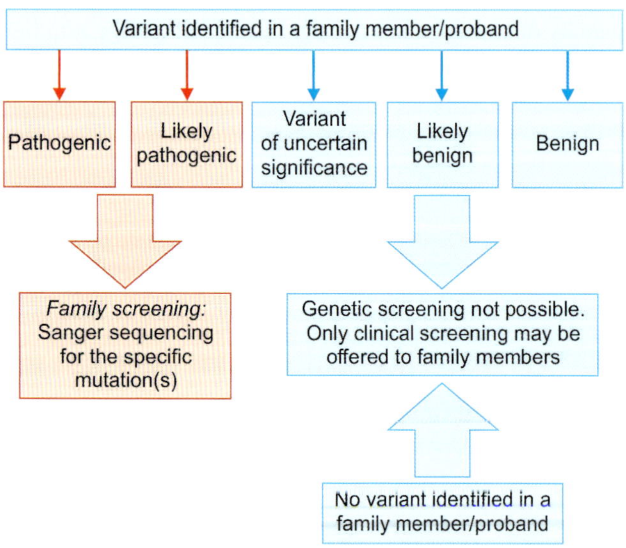

FLOWCHART 2: Screening of family members.

Genetic counseling is essential while planning genetic screening. It includes pre-test counseling, reaching a decision and consent, explanation of test result, and post-test counseling.

INDIAN DATA

All inherited disorders start with a de novo mutation in an individual called the founder. This person can then transmit the mutation to his/her descendants. Since individual founders are unique to each population, the spread of mutations is likely to differ across populations. Even though individual mutations differ, the disease-causing genes remain the same. Over a third of all sequence variations in Indians are reported to be novel.[3] The most common variant associated with cardiomyopathies in Indians is a 25 bp intronic deletion in *MyBPC3* which is seen in over 4% of all Indians. This variant is estimated to have developed in a founder 33,000–23,000 years ago. Over thousands of years, this variant spread in this individual's descendants and now involves millions of individuals.[4] Developing Indian and regional databases within the country is thus important.[5]

CARDIOMYOPATHIES

Genotyping plays an important role in the evaluation of patients with cardiomyopathies. These are caused by mutations spread across a large number of genes. Hypertrophic cardiomyopathy (HCM) is largely due to mutations in sarcomeric genes. The spectrum of mutations in dilated cardiomyopathy (DCM) is wider involving a larger number of genes including those encoding for sarcomeric and cytoskeletal proteins. Titin (*TTN*) truncating mutations are the most common cause of DCM.[6]

Cardiomyopathies have variable and age-related penetrance. The age of the first manifestation varies from the fetal stage (rare) to old age. Because thousands of mutations cause cardiomyopathies, it is not possible to accurately predict penetrance in an individual case. However, some data is available that can guide patient counseling. Patients carrying the HCM mutation have almost complete penetrance by 60 years of age.[7] Individuals carrying *TTN* truncating mutations that result in DCM have >95% penetrance by 40 years of age. Mutations causing arrhythmogenic right ventricular cardiomyopathy (ARVC) manifest disease phenotype in 60% of individuals by 70 years. There is variable expressivity. There is heterogeneity in disease manifestations and severity in individuals carrying the same mutation.

Genotyping plays an important role in family screening and counseling and may help in establishing the diagnosis in case of an uncertain phenotype. Genotyping has only a limited role in patient management.

Genotyping provides greater certainty as compared to clinical screening. If a relative does not carry the mutation, he/she is not at risk of disease in the future. Clinical screening does not provide this certainty. If a family member is phenotypically normal, it only indicates that the person does not have disease at that time. This does not predict the future development of the disease. Long-term and possibly lifelong clinical screening is hence required.

HYPERTROPHIC CARDIOMYOPATHY

Hypertrophic cardiomyopathy is caused by mutations in several sarcomeric genes. The most common genes involved are β-myosin heavy chain (*MYH7*) and the myosin binding protein C (*MYBPC3*). On comprehensive screening, 40–50% of individuals with HCM will be found to carry a mutation.

Hypertrophic cardiomyopathy is a heterogeneous disease often without a good genotype–phenotype correlation. Genotyping thus cannot be used to predict the phenotype or the risk of sudden death.[8,9] Genotyping may help in clarifying an uncertain diagnosis and identifying phenocopies like Fabry disease, Noonan syndrome, and glycogen storage disorders.

DILATED CARDIOMYOPATHY

Mutations are identified in 15–25% of DCM patients.[2] *TTN* is the most commonly affected gene.[6] The genotype usually does not predict the disease severity and cannot be used to guide therapy. The exceptions are some mutations in lamin A/C (*LMNA*), sodium channel protein type 5 subunit alpha (*SCN5A*), desmin (*DES*), filamin C (*FLNC*), RNA-binding protein 20 (*RBM20*), and tafazzin (*TAZ*) that are associated with a higher risk of sudden death.

RESTRICTIVE CARDIOMYOPATHY

Idiopathic restrictive cardiomyopathy is a common cause of restrictive cardiomyopathy (RCM) and overlaps with the HCM spectrum. Mutations, most commonly in sarcomeric genes, have been reported in 33–66% of idiopathic RCM patients. Mutations in the troponin I (*TNNI3*) gene are over-represented in idiopathic RCM.[10,11] *DES* mutations cause RCM along with conduction system disease. Transthyretin (*TTR*) and hemochromatosis (*HFE*) mutations may also cause RCM.

ARRHYTHMOGENIC RIGHT VENTRICULAR CARDIOMYOPATHY

Mutations are detected in 50–60% of ARVC patients. ARVC is caused by mutations in genes encoding desmosomal proteins of which plakophilin-2 (*PKP2*) is the most common. ARVC is an autosomal dominant disorder. The exceptions are ARVC associated with skin manifestations—Naxos disease and Carvajal syndrome that have an autosomal recessive transmission.

INHERITED ARRHYTHMIC DISORDERS

These include long QT syndrome (LQTS), Brugada syndrome, catecholaminergic polymorphic ventricular tachycardia (CPVT), and short QT syndrome. In addition, pre-excitation, conduction system blocks, bizarre QRS complexes, and atrial fibrillation may be seen with mutations in *SCN5A, LMNA, GLA, PRKAG2*, and *LAMP2*.

Genotyping plays an important role in the management of LQTS. This is because the precipitating factors and response to drug therapy differ in various forms of LQTS. LQTS1 usually has an excellent response to beta-blockers, while mexiletine has a role in the management of LQT3. Mutations are detected in around 75% of LQTS patients. The three most common forms LQT1, LQT2, and LQT3 are caused by mutations in *KCNQ1, KCNH2*, and *SCN5A*, respectively.

Brugada syndrome is clinically heterogeneous with marked male preponderance. Mutations are detected in only 20% of cases in *SCN5A*. Several other genes have been implicated; however, their role has not been definitely proven. CPVTs are associated with exercise or emotion-induced ventricular tachyarrhythmias. Mutations are detected in around 75% of patients in the cardiac ryanodine receptor (*RYR2*) or the cardiac calsequestrin-2 gene (*CASQ2*) genes.

AORTOPATHIES

Aneurysms and dissections can occur in both thoracic and abdominal aorta. Thoracic aortic aneurysms may have a genetic component whereas abdominal aortic aneurysms are more related to traditional risk factors and are not caused by specific mutations. Thoracic aortic aneurysms may occur as isolated disorders or may form part of a syndrome like Marfan syndrome, Ehlers–Danlos syndrome, or Loeys–Dietz syndrome. Even isolated thoracic aortic aneurysms that are familial may be a monogenic disorder. 20–30% of thoracic aortic aneurysms have a known genetic cause. Mutations in a large number of genes have been implicated in thoracic aortic aneurysms.

PRENATAL DIAGNOSIS

Prenatal diagnosis is important in families with severe disease manifestations where the parents want to prevent disease transmission to future generations. The role in families with milder phenotypes is unclear.[12] Prenatal screening is possible only if the disease-causing mutation in the family is known. Prenatal diagnosis can be achieved through two possible approaches. One is in vitro fertilization with preimplantation genetic screening. The second is prenatal genetic screening using chorionic villous biopsy or amniocentesis followed by possible medical termination of pregnancy in case the fetus carries the mutation, if the patient demands so.

VICTIMS OF SUDDEN DEATH

Sudden death in a young individual is a tragic event. Many sudden deaths in young persons are due to inherited disorders, most commonly cardiomyopathies and inherited arrhythmic disorders. Genotyping using an NGS platform should be carried out in all young sudden death victims who have an inherited disorder, unexplained cause of death, or a normal autopsy. Disease-causing mutations are identified in over a fourth of young sudden-death victims.[13] In such cases, family members who inherit the mutation are also at risk. Sudden death may be the first manifestation of these disorders. Genotyping allows family screening and early diagnosis, management, and prevention of sudden death in family members.

CONCLUSION

Genotyping plays an important role in the evaluation of inherited cardiac disorders caused by mutations in a single gene. The most common disorders are cardiomyopathies, inherited channelopathies, and aortopathies involving the thoracic aorta. Genotyping is carried out using NGS platforms, either disease-specific panels or whole exome sequencing.

ONLINE REFERENCES

Please scan the QR code provided at the end of the table of contents for References of this chapter.

CHAPTER

5

Cardiovascular Symptoms: Assessment and Interpretation

Vivek Narasimha V, Dayasagar Rao V

ABSTRACT

Evaluation of major symptoms perceived by patient as cardiac is the first step in suspecting the presence of cardiovascular disease. Chest discomfort is the cardinal symptom of CAD and appropriate evaluation of its type, severity, and frequency will help in assessing the pretest probability of obstructive coronary artery disease. Diseases other than CAD, such as dissecting aneurysm and pericarditis, should be considered when other appropriate investigations are negative for CAD. Structural heart disease can also lead to dyspnea, syncope, and palpitation, and appropriate evaluation is key to differentiate cardiac disease from other noncardiac problems.

Keywords: Chest pain, dyspnea, edema, palpitation, syncope, claudication

INTRODUCTION

Cardiovascular disease can be present without symptoms and be discovered as an incidental abnormality while being evaluated for other medical problems, such as heart disease during pregnancy. Most of the time, cardiac disease is suspected and evaluated following symptoms perceived by the patient as related to heart disease. Many symptoms are related to cardiovascular disease but major ones (but not limited to) include the following:

- Chest pain
- Dyspnea
- Edema
- Palpitation
- Syncope
- Fatigue
- Claudication

CHEST PAIN

Chest pain (discomfort) is considered synonymous with cardiac disease, with ominous prognosis and often rush to the emergency room of hospitals. It is regarded as a cardinal symptom of coronary artery disease but more popular; often, it is due to noncardiac diseases. The classic description of angina—chest pain due to obstructive coronary artery disease—was first made by William Heberden, the famous English physician of 18th centuries.

William Heberden published his first article on angina in 1772 and his description of symptom has stood test of time. The typical description of angina is retrosternal chest pressure or squeezing, burning, or heaviness with frequent radiation to neck, jaw, left arm, interscapular, epigastrium, and shoulders. It is often precipitated by factors like physical activity, eating, emotional stimulation, and cold environment and is generally relieved by rest or sublingual short-acting nitrates.

Atypical descriptions of chest pain that reduce the likelihood of myocardial ischemia include "sharp pain with respiratory variation, pain localized with a fingertip, pain lasting for hours or more or lasting for few seconds, and pain radiating to lower extremities."

Duration of pain is important in evaluation of chest pain. Angina generally lasts for <5 minutes and is relieved by rest or NTG—response to NTG is not a reliable marker of angina as it also occurs in noncardiac states like esophageal spasm. Not infrequently, a patient instead of describing chest discomfort in words, expresses symptoms by gestures such as clenched first over the sternum, indicating site and type of chest discomfort. This has been highlighted by Samuel A. Levine (Levine sign), an influential American cardiologist (1891–1966). Very infrequently, physical examination during an episode of chest discomfort may reveal areas of abnormal precordial cardiac pulsation (due to dyskinetic LV wall motion) or presence of apical systolic murmur (papillary muscle dysfunction), which disappear after relief of angina.

The precipitating factors—physical exercise, emotional stress, etc.—often result in increase of heart rate, blood pressure, and contractility that increases the myocardial oxygen demand, which is not met by increased coronary blood flow due to obstructive coronary artery disease. Combining history of angina with conventional risk factors for CAD helps in assessing pretest probability of CAD, as is presence of occlusive vascular disease in other areas, such as PAD and CVA.

Variations of Angina

Warm-up angina: A patient develops angina during initiation of walk and with continued walk angina disappears. It is postulated that a patient had coronary spasm initially that got relieved spontaneously with relief of angina. An alternative explanation is that coronary collaterals, which were dormant, opened up in response to exercise that relieved angina.

Second-wind angina is a term used to describe patients who after a period of rest, to relieve first angina, can walk a much longer distance or walk subsequently without any angina. This is attributed to the phenomenon of ischemic preconditioning, which makes the myocardium more resistant to ischemia after a brief period of ischemia.

Nocturnal angina: It occurs during sleep and has been observed in patients with syphilitic aortitis but is also observed in patients with severe aortic regurgitation. During sleep, the bradycardia that occurs results in worsening of aortic regurgitation leading to increase in LV EDV and thus precipitates angina. It is worth remembering that nocturnal angina is manifestation of incipient LVF, and a mild dose of diuretic in evening hours will relieve nocturnal angina.

Anginal Equivalents

Anginal equivalents are symptoms of myocardial ischemia other than classical chest discomfort. These include dyspnea (including flash pulmonary edema), dizziness, syncope, and extreme fatigue which are due to dysfunctional but viable myocardium consequent to myocardial ischemia.

Silent Ischemia

Silent ischemia is presence of objective evidence of myocardial ischemia in absence of angina or its equivalent. These include dynamic ECG changes, RWMA, and perfusion defects (on MPI).

Variable Threshold

An essential feature of variable threshold angina is variation in the degree of physical activity that induces angina; this is attributed to superadded coronary spasm on top of fixed obstruction and demands pharmacotherapy to counteract vasospasm.

Prinzmetal Angina

Also known as "vasospastic angina/angina inversa", prinzmetal angina always occurs at rest, usually between midnight and early morning. It is usually severe but can be relieved by taking sublingual nitrates. The most characteristic feature is ST elevation on ECG during episodes of angina indicating transmural ischemia.

Postprandial angina[1] is precipitation of angina following a large meal, which starts 20–30 minutes after meal and is relieved by nitrates.

During an episode of postprandial angina, there is an increase in the heart rate but no significant increase in blood pressure. The rate pressure product (RPP)–an indirect index of myocardial oxygen consumption—was not significantly different compared to control state. Postprandial angina develops characteristic symptoms within 20–30 minutes of meal and in some it may be associated with ECG changes during episodes of angina. Postprandial angina occurs in nearly 10% patients with chronic CAD and is often associated with severe degree of coronary artery disease, LMCA, and TVD.[2] Direct noninvasive measurements of blood flow indicate that whole heart blood flow increases to the same extent in postprandial angina as in control subjects. The myocardial ischemia results from redistribution of blood flow from stenotic arteries to nonstenotic coronary arteries, secondary to sympathetic system activation due to meal. This sympathetic nerve activation results in coronary vasodilation of normal coronary vessels but not in coronary vessels with >80% diameter stenosis as their coronary vasodilator reserve is exhausted. This results in "steal" of blood from ischemic territories to the nonobstructed coronary territory, with precipitation of angina.

Postprandial angina should not be confused with abdominal angina, which is ischemia of abdominal viscera that occurs after a meal and lasts for hours. It is due to ostial disease of mesenteric vessels. A CT angiogram of abdominal visceral vessels is gold standard for the diagnosis of abdominal angina.

Functional Assessment of Angina

Various classifications for functional assessment of angina were proposed, of which the Canadian Cardiovascular Society Classification (CCSC), Seattle Angina questionnaire (SAQ), and Braunwald classification of unstable angina are commonly used.

Thus, the symptom of chest discomfort must be evaluated appropriately to suspect the presence and severity of occlusive CAD.

Other Important Causes of Chest Pain

- Pericarditis
- Dissecting aneurysm of aorta

Aortic Dissection

Chest pain from aortic dissection is very sudden, severe, and maximal at onset in more than 90% of patients unlike cardiac ischemic discomfort which gradually builds up over a period of minutes. Chest pain is more common in type A dissection compared to type B (85% vs. 67%), whereas back pain is less frequent (43% vs. 70%). In rare cases, it may be classical ischemic chest pain when dissection involves the coronary artery, most commonly the right coronary artery.

Dissection of aorta should be considered in the presence of severe, uncontrolled hypertension or in the presence of conditions that predispose to dissection, including connective tissue disorders (Marfan syndrome, etc.), family history of aortic disease, known aortic valve disease, known thoracic aortic aneurysm, and previous aortic manipulation (including cardiac surgery).

Assessment of three clinical variables—sudden severe chest pain, mediastinal/aortic widening on chest X-ray, and pulse/BP differential (SBP > 20 mm Hg)—has identified them as independent predictors and can be used as an aid in improving patient care in aortic dissection. D-dimer value[3] of <500 ng/mL is a negative predictor of dissecting aneurysm within the first 24 hours after symptom onset.

Pericarditis

Pain of pericarditis usually has a gradual onset, is precordial in location, is worsened by breathing and coughing, and relieved by sitting and leaning forward. Rarely, discomfort spreads to the trapezial area of chest and shoulders, which may lead to musculoskeletal cause of pain. Most of the time, it is associated with audible pericardial rub, which is classically triphasic and often accentuated during inspiration. Finally, many patients with pericarditis shall have classical ECG changes (ST elevation in most of leads) of acute pericarditis, with regression of ECG over a period of weeks.

DYSPNEA

Dyspnea refers to a subjective experience of breathing discomfort that consists of quantitatively distinct sensations that vary in intensity. Various attempts were made to standardize symptoms, which includes NYHA, Borg visual analog scale, Goldman's specific activity scale, CCSC, WHO classification-modified from NYHA for PAH, and Perloffs' functional classification for dyspnea in congenital heart disease. Dyspnea on exertion in cardiac disease is mostly a symptom of left heart dysfunction, although patients with right heart conditions, such as primary PAH, can also have dyspnea as a presenting symptom. Positional changes are important to document, such as orthopnea, paroxysmal nocturnal dyspnea (PND), trepopnea platypnea, and bendopnea. Orthopnea is worsening of dyspnea on lying flat (consequence of worsening of filling pressures, secondary to shift of volume of blood from dependent position to central area). In cases of PND, there is a time lag of few hours between sleep and onset of breathlessness, secondary to shift of fluid from interstitial space to intravascular space, which increases in filling pressures. This volume shift results in dyspnea, secondary to movement of fluid into interstitial space of lung, due to increase in hydrostatic pressure, thus making it more rigid with more respiratory efforts needed to expand lung, manifesting as dyspnea.

The mechanism of dyspnea in pure right heart disease is more complex like in PAH. Limited contractile reserve of RV during exercise leads to impaired filling of left ventricle, leading to suboptimal systemic flow and pressure. This results in early anaerobic metabolism, increased CO_2 production, and hyperventilation, which are perceived as dyspnea. Skeletal muscle dysfunction and chronic deconditioning may also contribute to dyspnea of right heart disease.

Bendopnea, defined by Thibodeau et al. in 2014, refers to shortness of breath within 30 seconds of bending forward while sitting and is mediated by increased filling pressure during bending, which exacerbate already high filling pressure. This is purely subjective and not uncommon in individuals who are obese and elderly. The prevalence of bendopnea in the heart failure population is 21% and indicates hemodynamic congestion which precedes clinical congestion by weeks. Thibodean demonstrated that subjects with bendopnea had higher median capillary wedge pressure when sitting (19–30 mm Hg) compared to those without (8–22 mm Hg). The bending maneuver induced a substantial increase in PCWP in both groups. A more objective way of quantification of hemodynamics[4] during bending is a change in O_2 saturation during bending [falls by 3% bending oxygen saturation index (BOSI)]. This index, BOSI 3%, has predictive power of identifying recurrent worsening of heart failure (WHF). This simple clinical tool should be included in home monitoring of heart failure patients, along with periodic measurements of weight, to predict future congestive events and adjust pharmacotherapy accordingly.

PALPITATIONS

Palpitation is the subjective awareness of heart beat and occurs in two types of cardiac patients: (1) With cardiomegaly due to volume unloaded ventricles, where it is constant throughout day, and (2) patients with new onset of rapid heart action, which in younger age is likely to have paroxysmal SVT in younger individuals. In elderly, palpitations are a result of AF with fast ventricle rate and ventricular tachycardia, which are more often associated with structural heart disease. The onset, offset, duration, and associated symptoms, such as chest discomfort, syncope, or near syncope, as well as potential triggers are important for diagnosis and management. It is helpful to ask a patient to reproduce the cadence of their heart by tapping their fingers on a table-fast and irregular beating indicates AF. Sometimes, patients say that during palpitation, there is concomitant neck pulsation, which frequently occurs in AV re-entrant tachycardia, as in the occurrence of diuresis associated with termination of tachyarrhythmia, such as PSVT.

A thorough history is helpful in diagnosing the cause of palpitation and is important in triaging which patients need further evaluation. A 2-week continuous event monitor has the highest diagnostic yield to cost ratio and is considered the test of choice. For evaluation of paroxysmal tachycardia when using ambulatory ECG[5] monitoring, Holter monitoring for 24 hours has a limited role in evaluating palpitation and should be used when symptoms reliably occur at least once every 24 hours. Consumer-grade wearable devices, such as smart watches, have potential for medical use but current data shows variable accuracy and a high likelihood of detecting clinically irrelevant abnormalities.

CLAUDICATION

Claudication is characterized by fatigue, discomfort, cramping, or pain of muscles of extremities that is consistently induced by exercise and relieved by rest (usually within 10 minutes).

Arterial, venous, and neurogenic claudication are three distinct entities with clinical overlap of symptoms and subtle differences; however, differentiation is important as therapeutic options are totally different.

Arterial Claudication

In most patients with claudication, the blood flow at rest is normal but becomes insufficient during exercise, presenting clinically as cramping of muscles and relieved by rest. Usually, there is objective evidence of obstructive arterial disease like ankle brachial index (ABI) which if <0.9 has a sensitivity of >95% and specificity approaching 100% compared to angiography. In patients where values are borderline, measurement of ABI during or immediately after exercise (with affected limb) results in worsening of ABI values (0.9–0.7) as arterial blood flow cannot match the fall in vascular resistance due to obstructive arterial disease. Furthermore, ABI is a good predictor of disease progression—patients with ABI < 0.5 have a two-fold risk of requiring revascularization or major amputation as compared to patients with ABI > 0.5. The muscle group affected during exercise or walking is useful in determining the site of occlusion-claudication in buttocks or thighs indicates iliac vessel obstruction while femoropopliteal disease typically affects the calf muscles Infrapopliteal occlusion manifests as claudication in sole of foot.

Lumbar Canal Stenosis

A key feature of neurogenic claudication is its relationship to a patient's posture where lumber extension increases pain and lumber flexion decreases pain. This is responsible for better tolerance to climbing uphill compared to downhill walking. Pain relief occurs with sitting or forward flexion at waist, such as squatting or leaning forward. In most cases, symptoms occur in both legs and involve the entire leg. Occasionally, radicular pain due to nerve compression from lateral recess compression is a dominant symptom. Five repetitions of sit-to-stand test (5R-STS) in 10 seconds practically rules out spinal canal stenosis. Pathophysiology includes vascular (venous) obstruction and mechanical compression.

Venous Claudication

Venous claudication is an important symptom of venous outflow obstruction, generally a residual of old venous thrombosis. Under normal circumstances, during exercise, increased arterial inflow to legs is matched by an increased outflow via the venous system. In patients with venous claudication, balance between inflow and outflow is disrupted due to venous obstruction, resulting in swelling of leg and pain, consequent to a rise in venous pressure. The time to return to pre-exercise level is prolonged compared to normal (39.1 + 14.4 seconds vs. 1.1 + 1.1 seconds). The discomfort in leg is due to venous congestion, which is relived faster by lifting the leg to a higher level and takes a long time for the symptoms to fully resolve-more than 10 minutes.

SYNCOPE

Syncope is defined as transient loss of consciousness due to cerebral hypoperfusion, leading to inability to maintain postural tone. It is abrupt and brief, with no residual sequel or symptoms. It is often preceded by prodromal symptoms such as nausea, diaphoresis, epigastric distress, unsteadiness (light headiness), and blurring of vision. Presyncope is a term used to describe the occurrence of prodromal symptoms without loss of consciousness. Syncope should be distinguished from other causes of transient loss of consciousness like seizure disorder, hypoglycemia, falls, or functional episodes (pseudosyncope).

The most frequent cause of syncope is reflex syncope (58%) followed by cardiac cause (23%) and unexplained cause (19%). Reflex syncope (neurogenic syncope) is the most frequent entity and occurs in young and the clinical picture can be dominated by bradycardia (cardioinhibitory), hypotension due to vasodilation (vasodepressor), or combination of these symptoms. These are reproducible by the head-up tilting test in majority of patients. This vasovagal syncope has a benign course, though body injures due to syncope are not uncommon. Cardiac syncope is associated with increased mortality and should be suspected and evaluated appropriately in older patients with history of cardiac disease who experience episodes without any warning signs. Cardiac arrhythmias are the most common cause of cardiac syncope. Exertional syncope is classically seen in LVOT obstruction and less frequently in RVOT obstruction. The cause of syncope in these is related to a combination of a suboptimal increase in cardiac output and inappropriate vasodilatation, secondary to stimulation of mechanoreceptors in endocardium. Orthostatic hypotension is a common cause of syncope in elderly and occurs in nearly 20% of patients over the age of 75 years. Thus, measurement of postural changes in blood pressure is very important in initial evaluation of these patients.

EDEMA

Edema of lower limbs is a common symptom of cardiac patients, especially with right heart failure. Edema–increase in interstitial fluid in the cardiac patients–is due to rise in central venous pressure (hydrostatic pressure) over and above oncotic pressure, which drives fluid into interstitial space. Infrequently, a decrease in oncotic pressure (decrease in plasma protein) can worsen the edema. Cardiac edema is bilateral, pitting, and nontender that occurs in a dependent area with no significant diurnal variation unlike the edema of venous insufficiency, which occurs at the end of day. It is worth remembering that some of cardiac (calcium channel blockers and vasodilators) and noncardiac drugs (NSAIDs) cause retention of water resulting in edema. Sometimes, fluid retention is manifested by ascites and pleural effusion, especially in patients with severe right heart failure. Rarely, ascites may precede onset of leg edema (ascites precox), particularly in patients with constrictive pericarditis that should be distinguished from primary liver disorder by markedly elevated CVP in primary cardiac diseases.

CONCLUSION

Evaluating symptoms related to cardiovascular disease–chest pain, dyspnea edema, and palpitation–will identify the presence, type, and severity of cardiac disease, which will direct to appropriate investigation, for final cardiovascular diagnosis.

ONLINE REFERENCES

Please scan the QR code provided at the end of the table of contents for References of this chapter.

CHAPTER

6

Dynamic Auscultation

Mohit D Gupta, Dixit Goyal, Girish MP

ABSTRACT

Murmurs are crucial physical examination findings in patients, and cardiac auscultation is a vital tool for diagnosing them. With sensitivity and specificity reaching 70% and 98% in trained individuals, physicians can create a concise list of differential diagnoses. Dynamic auscultation, which alters circulatory dynamics, aids in better detection and differentiation of confusing murmurs, helping in better diagnosis and reducing morbidity and mortality. Healthcare providers should master these techniques.

Keywords: Murmurs, dynamic auscultation, maneuvers

INTRODUCTION

Murmurs are pivotal findings in clinical examination that can point toward likelihood of a diagnosis. Cardiac auscultation is a lost art nowadays. The knowledge of basic sciences such as anatomy, physiology, and underlying physics, with comprehensive and sincere clinical examination, can detect many pathologies and guide further management. The art of thorough clinical assessment is an important tool in cardiology and directs all further diagnostic tests and treatment. To note, the sensitivity and specificity for murmurs can reach up to 70% and 98%, respectively among trained cardiologists.[1] The murmurs usually have enough distinguishing qualities which along with patient's history frames differential diagnosis.[2] The dynamic variation in quality of murmurs is a useful phenomenon that aids in identifying a specific condition. The timely detection of cardiac murmurs can reduce the morbidity and mortality, and hence mastering these murmurs and their common etiologies, becomes essential. The method of changing circulatory dynamics by pharmacological and physiological interventions and monitoring how these changes affect heart sounds and murmurs is known as dynamic auscultation. This chapter offers a description of evaluation of dynamic auscultation.

BUT WHEN TO PERFORM THESE MANEUVERS?

Dynamic auscultation should only be performed during confusion among the heart sounds or when murmur is not heard properly, and we want to differentiate between two murmurs. Although it is an essential tool, it should not be viewed as the exclusive gold standard but rather as a component of the overall clinical picture.

DYNAMIC AUSCULTATION: METHODS

The three categories of dynamic auscultation include postural, pharmacological, and physiological techniques **(Table 1)**.

PHYSIOLOGICAL MANEUVERS

Valsalva Maneuver

The Valsalva maneuver consists of two phases: a straining period followed by a relaxation period.[3] The maneuver involves a deep breath followed by exhaling against tubing connected to a manometer, to maintain an intraoral pressure of 40 mm Hg during 20s of strain.[4] In practice, this can be

TABLE 1: Methods of dynamic auscultation.

Physiological maneuvers	Pharmacological		Postural changes
Valsalva	Vasodilator	Vasoconstrictor	Left lateral (MS)
Muller	Amyl nitrite	Phenylephrine	Sitting up and leaning forward (AR)
Isometric exercise			Sudden standing
Transient arterial occlusion	Others		Passive leg elevation
	Propranolol		Sudden squatting
	Isoprenaline		

TABLE 2: Stages of Valsalva maneuver.

Phases	Description	BP	HR
I: Onset of straining (1st 10 seconds)	Pulmonary vasculature empties into the left atrium and ventricle, causing a small rise in arterial pressure	↑	↓
II: Continued expiration (10–20 seconds)	Higher intrathoracic pressure inhibits venous return, decreasing cardiac output, and systemic blood pressure	↓	↑
III: End of expiration	Release of straining normalizes intrathoracic pressure, rapidly increasing ventricular filling and output	↓	↑↑
IV: Recovery 5–10 seconds after stopping expiration	Reflex vasoconstriction and tachycardia cause a further rise in blood pressure, leading to reflex bradycardia	↑	↓

achieved by instructing the patient to take a deep breath and then exhale forcefully for 20 seconds while keeping the glottis closed. The examiner may place the flat of their hand on the patient's abdomen to provide resistance for the patient to strain against. There are four stages of Valsalva maneuver **(Table 2 and Fig. 1)**.

The normal blood pressure response **(Fig. 2)** to the Valsalva maneuver consists of reductions in systolic and diastolic blood pressure during straining followed by a hypertensive overshoot after the release of the strain (type A response). In subjects with moderate heart failure the blood pressure response is characterized by an absent post-training hypertensive overshoot (type B response)[5,6] or by a maintenance of an elevated blood pressure during straining in subjects with more severe heart failure (type C response).[6]

HOW DOES VALSALVA DIFFERENTIATE MURMURS? (FIG. 3)

Most cardiac murmurs become less intense during the Valsalva maneuver as ventricular filling and cardiac output decrease. The intensity of murmurs associated with mitral regurgitation and aortic stenosis decreases, while those related to hypertrophic subaortic stenosis and mitral valve prolapse become louder. When the Valsalva maneuver is released, there is a quick increase in right and then left ventricular filling and output. The temporal difference in the filling of the right and left sides of the heart can be used to determine whether heart murmurs and noises originate on the right or left side. Murmurs originating on the right side of the heart, such as tricuspid stenosis or regurgitation or pulmonary stenosis or regurgitation, normally recover to baseline severity soon after straining is released within 1-4 cardiac cycles. On the other hand, left-sided murmurs typically take 5-10 beats to return to baseline intensity.[8]

SPECIFIC CONDITION AND VALSALVA MANEUVER

Hypertrophic obstructive cardiomyopathy (HOCM) has dynamic left ventricular outflow tract (LVOT) obstruction and gradient during systole as a result of interventricular septal hypertrophy and systolic anterior leaflet motion of the mitral valve. On performing Valsalva maneuver, during systole the left ventricular volume is reduced (Valsalva maneuver), the septum and mitral valve move closer to each other, resulting in increased gradient and a high intensity murmur. The diagnostic value of Valsalva Maneuver for HOCM: Sensitivity—65%, specificity 96%, positive predictive value—81%, and negative predictive value—92%.[10]

The murmur of *mitral valve prolapse* is limited to late systole and may intensify and lengthen during the Valsalva maneuver. The critical volume at which prolapse begins is when the contracting ventricle reaches 75 mL.[11] Then, this systolic murmur normally lengthens and frequently intensifies due to the earlier prolapse of the leaflet(s) during systole made possible by the reduction in left ventricular volume brought on Valsalva.

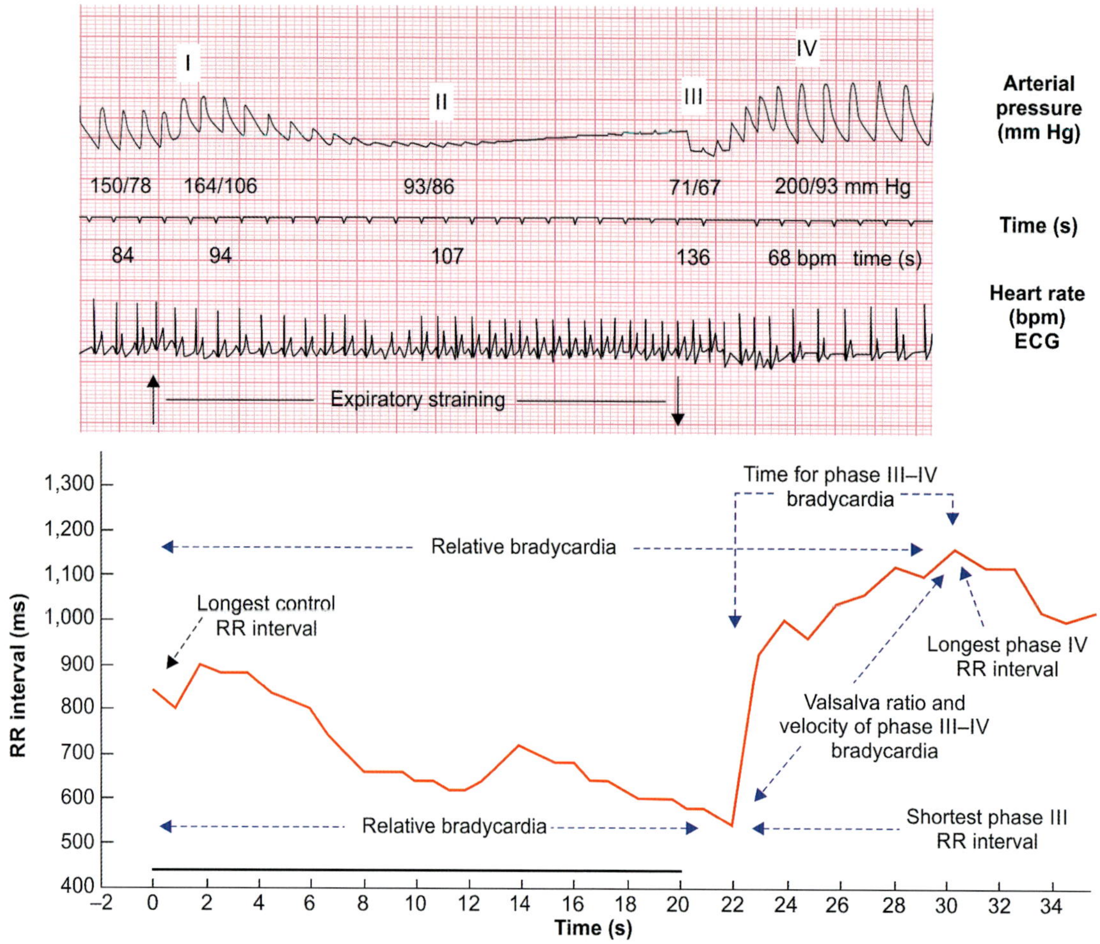

FIG. 1: Recordings of a typical normal pattern of heart rate or heart interval baroreflex responses to arterial pressure changes associated with phases I–IV of Valsalva maneuver performed during 20s of expiratory strain.[4]

When performing the Valsalva maneuver, the diastolic murmur of *mitral stenosis* (MS) frequently does not soften. The tachycardia that occurs during straining, causes delay in left atrial (LA) emptying and preserves the pressure gradient between the left atrium and ventricle. As a result, MS can have variable response to the Valsalva maneuver.[3]

Where to Avoid Valsalva Maneuver?

Since there is a rise in intraocular and intra-abdominal pressure, therefore the test must be avoided in patients with retinopathy and intraocular lens implantation.[12]

MULLER MANEUVER

It is opposite to Valsalva maneuver.

Methods to Elicit

Close nose with finger in mouth → suck the finger with closed glottis.

Another method is to generate 40–50 mm Hg of negative pressure by sucking on a mouthpiece connected to a manometer.

Increases right heart flow for longer periods compared to respiration.

Clinical implication: All right-sided murmurs increase except pulmonary ejection click.

POSTURAL CHANGE

Squatting (Fig. 4)

Method

From a standing position, have patient squat down bringing knees to the axilla region. Auscultate as the patient remains squatting for approximately 30 seconds. This is most easily done while the physician sits beside the patient, so as to reduce movement and allow for better concentration. These maneuvers are best used to distinguish HOCM and mitral valve prolapse.

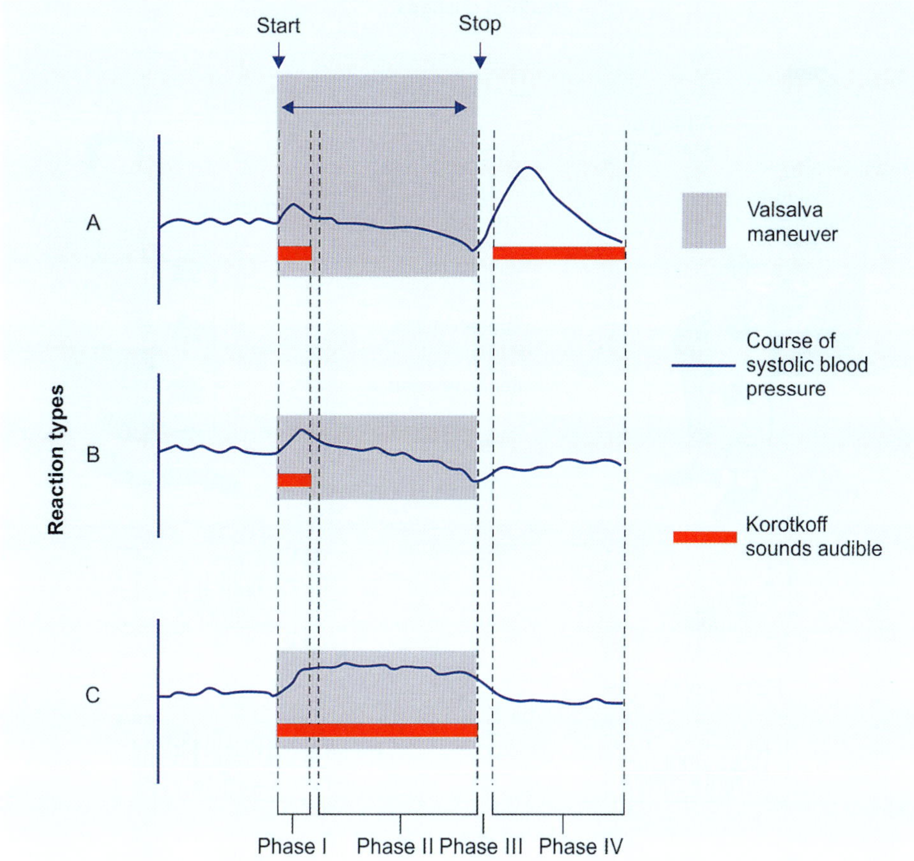

FIG. 2: Types of response patterns of the systolic blood pressure during execution of a Valsalva maneuver.[7]

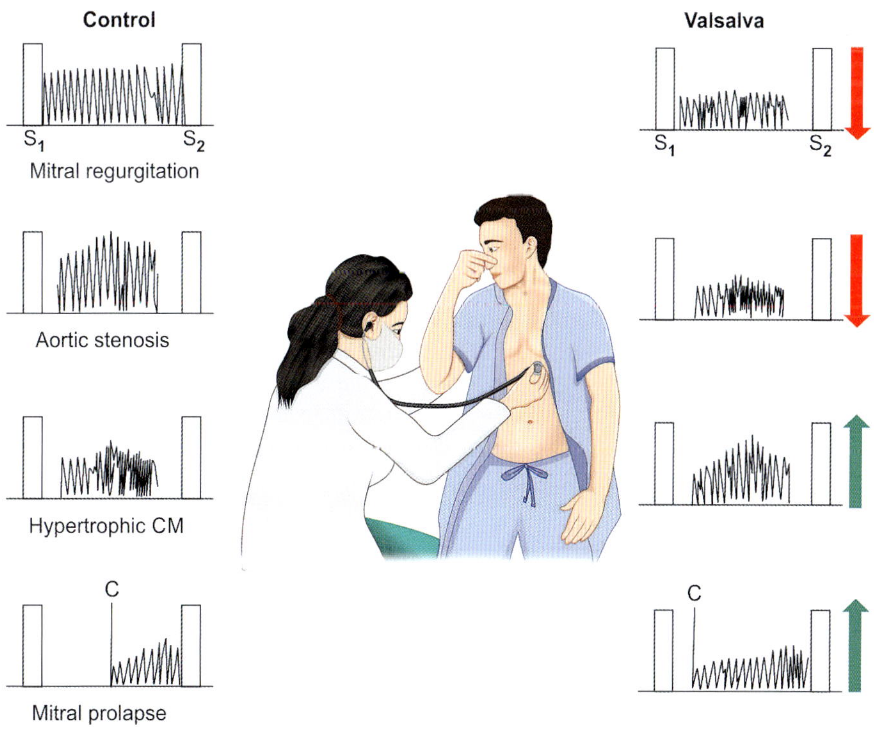

FIG. 3: Phase 1 of the Valsalva maneuver showing dynamic changes in left-sided murmurs.[9]

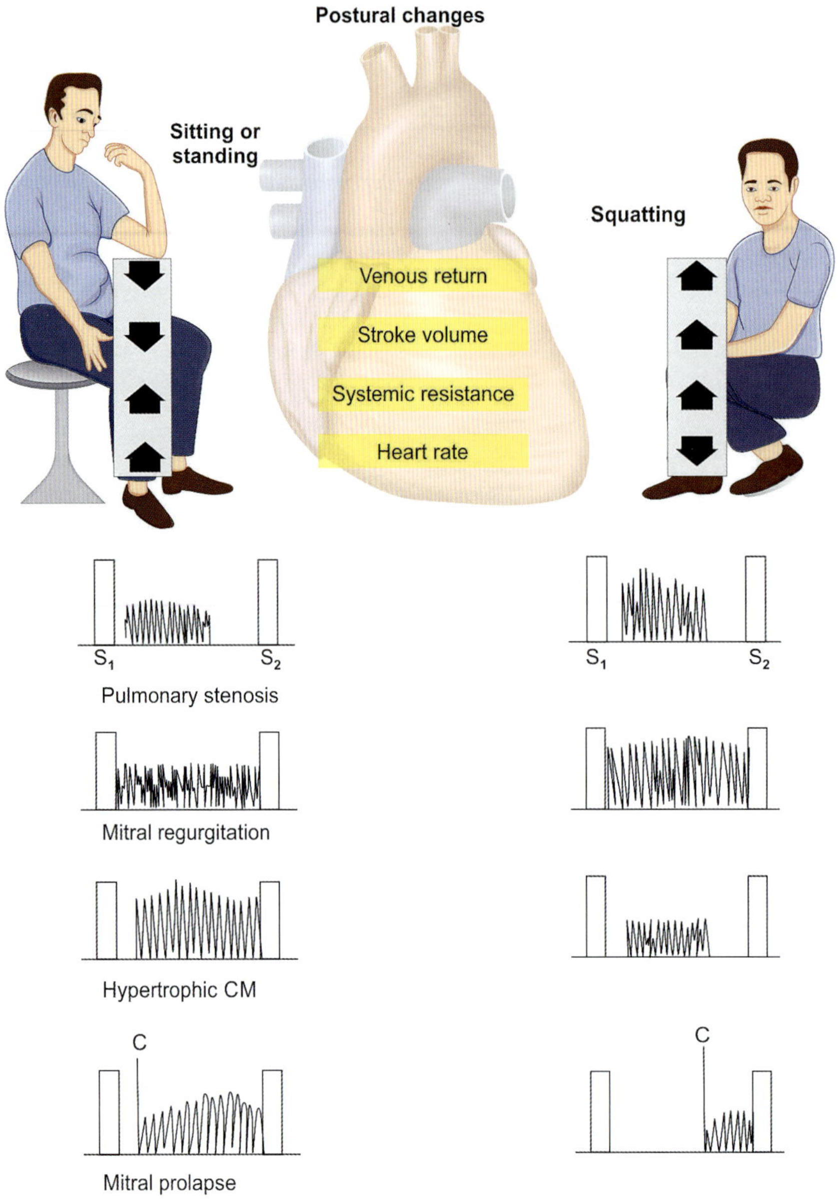

FIG. 4: Effect of squatting on murmurs.[3]

Physiological Response

Most systolic murmurs become more intense when one squats because it raises total peripheral resistance and the venous return to the heart, with reduction in heart rate allowing left ventricle filling. More intense S3, S4, and louder murmurs of PS, AS, TS, and MS are caused by the higher stroke volume due to the enhanced venous return. The increase in the murmurs of tetralogy of Fallot (TOF), patent ductus arteriosus (PDA), AR, MR, and VSD is attributed to the increased peripheral resistance. Increased preload and afterload together cause the HOCM murmur intensity to rise, the MVP click to be delayed, and the MVP murmur to shorten.[9]

Standing from squatting will have opposite effect causing reduced venous return and peripheral resistance and increased heart rate. This leads to attenuation of systolic murmurs and augmentation of murmur of HOCM and MVP.

PASSIVE LEG RAISE

Method

Make patient sit at 45° head up semirecumbent position then lower patient's upper body to horizontal and passively raise legs at 45° up maximal effect occurs at 30–90 seconds.

Physiological Response

It increases the venous return to the heart intensifying all the murmurs except HOCM and MVP.

ISOMETRIC EXERCISE

Many forms of dynamic maneuvers involving straining, might not be possible among deconditioned or unwilling hospitalized patients. Therefore, one of the easiest ways to support a physical examination at the bedside is to perform an isometric exercise, like a continuous handgrip.

Handgrip

The examiner's finger or a rolled towel, can be squeezed as tightly as possible by the patient with one or both hands. It is important to make sure the patient does not strain during hand grip since the Valsalva maneuver will obscure the findings. The force imparted by the handgrip can be measured in more formal research by using a calibrated dynamometer.

Usually, no discernible change in blood pressure or heart rate occurs for at least 60–90 seconds.

Clinical Implications

The heart rate, cardiac output, and both the systolic and diastolic blood pressure rise quickly when using a handgrip.[13] The increase in BP is more and that of HR and CO is less as compared to dynamic exercise.[14] The left ventricle's pressure gradient with the lower pressure chambers during systole is emphasized by the rise in systemic arterial pressure, which exacerbates the MR and VSD murmurs **(Fig. 5)**. The late systolic murmur of MVP is enhanced by a handgrip and functions similarly to mitral regurgitation.[13] The murmur of aortic regurgitation will get louder during a handgrip due to the increased diastolic blood pressure in the aorta.[8] In MS the LA pressure rises, the diastolic filling time of the left ventricle is shortened, and the opening snap (OS) moves closer to the A2 as a result of the elevated heart rate.[3] Murmurs of aortic stenosis and hypertrophic cardiomyopathy will decrease or show no change because the higher aortic pressure decreases the aortic valve gradient along with the opposing effect of increased heart rate.[3] Pregnant patients with suspected cardiac disease has amplification of left-sided regurgitant murmurs with isometric exercise. Left-sided regurgitant murmurs typically softens or disappear during pregnancy due to the reduction in systemic vascular resistance.[15]

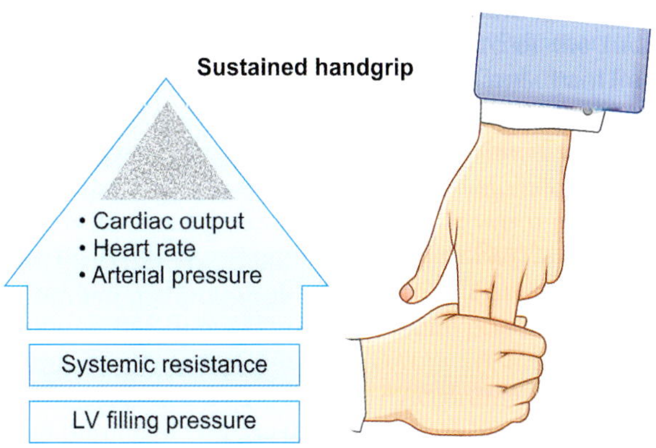

FIG. 5: Hemodynamic effects of isometric handgrip exercise.[9]

PHARMACOLOGICAL MANEUVERS

Amyl Nitrite

Procedure

In supine position, patient is made to inhale vapors of amyl nitrite which is broken over a piece of gauze. The patient is instructed to inhale deeply for three cycles. Its onset of action is within 10–30 seconds after inhalation.[16] Amyl nitrite causes vasodilation, an immediate drop in the systemic arterial pressure within 15 seconds but lasts only 30 seconds.[17] This is followed by a reflex tachycardia within 30–60 seconds after inhalation, enhancing the cardiac output in the second stage **(Fig. 6)**. It takes 1–2 minutes for mean arterial pressure (MAP) to return back to normal.[18]

Clinical Implication

Amyl nitrite increases the murmurs of AS and HOCM by increasing the gradient across aortic and decreasing the afterload, and accentuates MS and TS, due to reflex tachycardia. On the contrary, it decreases the murmurs of AR, MR, VSD, PDA, and TOF as a result of decreased aortic pressure. Amyl nitrite increases blood flow to the right heart and intensifies right-sided murmurs like that of tricuspid regurgitation. There is also an increase in the "innocent"

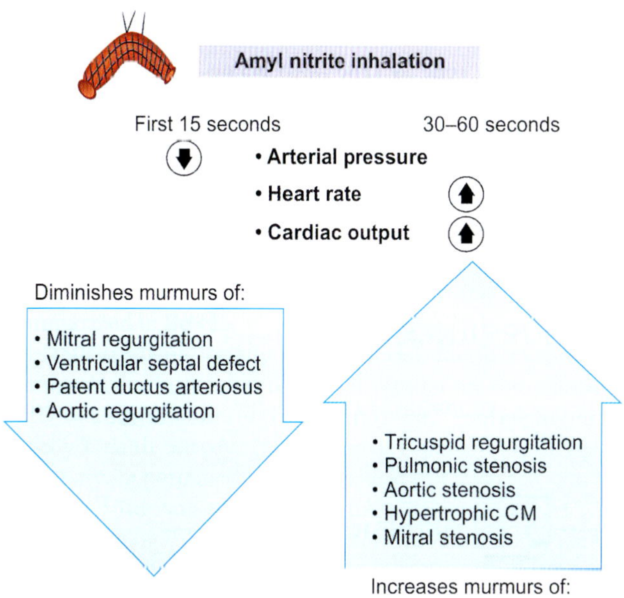

FIG. 6: Early and late hemodynamic and auscultatory changes in various murmurs during inhalation of amyl nitrite.

pulmonary flow murmur and the murmur of pulmonic stenosis. Notably, amyl nitrite has far less of an impact and offers minimal assistance in diagnosis in patients with congestive heart failure.[18]

Amyl nitrite is particularly helpful in distinguishing between the following:

- Austin flint murmur of AR versus mid-diastolic murmur (MDM) of MS (AR is decreased and MS is exaggerated due to tachycardia).
- TOF versus isolated PS (there is decreased murmur of TOF and enhanced murmur of PS).
- MR versus TR (MR softens and TR murmur intensifies).
- AR versus PR (PR murmur remains unchanged while AR murmur decreases).

Amyl nitrite also helps in differentiating congenital heart disease. Because of the reduced shunting over the septum or via the ductus caused by an increased systemic flow, the pansystolic murmur of a ventricular septal defect and the continuous murmur of a PDA will diminish. It causes a right-to-left shunting from the right ventricle to the aorta in the TOF, which lowers right ventricular forward flow and softens the murmur. Increased venous return, as previously noted, heightens the murmur of solitary pulmonic stenosis.[16]

PHENYLEPHRINE

Phenylephrine hydrochloride is an adrenergic agonist. The standard intravenous dose is 0.3–0.5 mg, which is formulated by mixing 10 mg of phenylephrine hydrochloride in 250 cc of normal saline.[8,16] It takes around 3 minutes to reach a systolic blood pressure elevation of 20–30 mm Hg.[8] The hemodynamic response includes an increase in MAP due to increased afterload with a reflex bradycardia and a variable decrease in cardiac output and stroke volume.

Clinical Implications

Phenylephrine acts in opposite manner to that of amyl nitrite. The intensity of murmurs of MR, AR, small VSDs, and PDA increase in intensity. In HOCM, due to a decrease in the dynamic outflow gradient and an increase in left ventricular volume, the murmur softens. These dynamic responses are often best evaluated in the cardiac catheterization or echocardiography laboratory with the objective gradients measurements.

PROPRANOLOL

Intravenous β-blocker has the opposite effect to that of phenylephrine. The outflow pressure gradient will be diminished by slowing the heart rate and decreasing left ventricular contractility.

Isoprenaline

Isoproterenol will increase the contractile force, heart rate, and consequently the outflow tract pressure gradient while accentuating the systolic murmur.

TRANSIENT ARTERIAL OCCLUSION

It might occasionally be challenging to get the patient to actively participate in procedures because of musculoskeletal disorders or altered mental states. Unwillingly, some patients may simultaneously execute two procedures with diametrically opposed hemodynamic outcomes. Patients often do the Valsalva technique, for instance, when squatting or doing an isometric handgrip exercise as highlighted previously in discussion of handgrip. Therefore, a technique that does not involve the patient's active interference has been developed.

The BP cuff is wrapped around the upper limbs of both arms during transient arterial occlusion (TAO), and the cuffs are concurrently inflated to 20–40 mm Hg above the patient's systolic blood pressure for 20 seconds. This procedure increases aortic impedance but does not raise aortic pressure.[19] This accentuates the murmurs on the left side such as AR, MR, and ventricular septal defects.

Diagnostic Value

Lembo et al.[20] demonstrated that TAO was superior to squatting in terms of intensifying left-sided regurgitant lesions and produced fewer false-positive diagnoses. Additionally, the sensitivity of this new maneuver for the identification of left-sided regurgitant murmurs was comparable to that of amyl nitrite inhalation or isometric handgrip exercise.

CONCLUSION

Dynamic auscultation is a critical component of cardiovascular examination, offering valuable insights into the functional status of the heart and great vessels. By altering physiological states through maneuvers such as inspiration, expiration, Valsalva maneuver, squatting, or standing, clinicians can uncover changes in heart sounds and murmurs that may otherwise go unnoticed in a static examination. These maneuvers help differentiate between various cardiac conditions.

ONLINE REFERENCES

Please scan the QR code provided at the end of the table of contents for References of this chapter.

CHAPTER

7

Biomarkers in Cardiovascular Medicine: Toward Precision Medicine

Ashish Kumar Jha, Advait Akash, Vinit Kumar

ABSTRACT

Biomarkers are transforming cardiovascular medicine by enabling more precise diagnosis, risk assessment, and treatment. This review explores the role of biomarkers in advancing cardiovascular precision medicine, emphasizing their applications in risk stratification, disease management, and pharmacogenomics. Diagnostic biomarkers, such as cardiac troponins and B-type natriuretic peptide (BNP), are crucial for early detection and accurate diagnosis of cardiovascular diseases (CVDs), including myocardial infarction and heart failure. Prognostic biomarkers, like high-sensitivity C-reactive protein (hs-CRP) and NT-proBNP, provide insights into disease progression and patient outcomes, guiding clinical decision-making and intervention strategies. Therapeutic biomarkers assist in personalizing treatment by monitoring therapeutic responses and predicting drug efficacy, as seen with LDL-C levels and genetic variants influencing clopidogrel metabolism. Technological advancements in genomics, proteomics, metabolomics, and imaging have significantly enhanced biomarker discovery and application. Genomics and proteomics enable the identification of novel biomarkers associated with CVD, while metabolomics provide a snapshot of metabolic changes related to disease states. Imaging techniques, such as MRI and PET, offer valuable insights into biomarker localization and function. Bioinformatics and computational biology further integrate and analyze complex data, supporting the identification and validation of biomarkers. Despite these advances, several challenges persist, including technical variability, reproducibility issues, and high costs of biomarker testing. Accessibility remains a barrier, particularly in resource-limited settings. Ethical and regulatory considerations also impact the development and application of biomarkers, necessitating robust frameworks for data protection and informed consent. Biomarkers hold great promise for enhancing cardiovascular care through personalized medicine. Continued research, technological innovation, and collaborative efforts are essential to overcome current challenges and maximize the potential of biomarkers in improving patient outcomes and advancing the field of cardiovascular medicine.

Keywords: Cardiovascular biomarkers, precision medicine, risk stratification, disease management, pharmacogenomics

INTRODUCTION

Biomarkers are measurable indicators of biological states or conditions, such as molecules, genes, or characteristics. In cardiovascular medicine, biomarkers are essential for diagnosing, prognosing, and monitoring cardiovascular diseases (CVD), allowing for timely diagnoses, better patient outcomes, and targeted therapies.

Cardiovascular diseases, including coronary artery disease, heart failure, stroke, and hypertension, are major causes of morbidity and mortality globally. CVD accounts for approximately 17.9 million deaths annually, making it a significant public health concern.[1] Effective prevention, early detection, and management strategies are crucial to addressing this burden.

Precision medicine tailors medical treatment to individual characteristics, considering genetic, environmental, and lifestyle factors. In cardiovascular health, precision medicine leverages biomarkers to provide personalized care, leading to more accurate diagnoses, risk assessments, and therapeutic strategies, thus improving patient outcomes and reducing healthcare costs.

The use of biomarkers in cardiovascular medicine has evolved from early indicators like cholesterol levels to more specific markers like troponins, which revolutionized the diagnosis of acute myocardial infarction in the 1990s.[2] This evolution reflects the increasing complexity and utility of biomarkers in cardiovascular care.

Technological advancements in genomics, proteomics, metabolomics, and imaging have significantly enhanced biomarker discovery. High-throughput screening, bioinformatics, and machine learning have accelerated the identification of novel biomarkers, improving the understanding and management of cardiovascular diseases.

Common biomarkers in cardiovascular medicine include troponins for diagnosing acute myocardial infarction, B-type natriuretic peptide (BNP) for assessing heart failure, and C-reactive protein (CRP) for indicating inflammation and cardiovascular risk. These biomarkers are integral to clinical decision-making in managing cardiovascular conditions **(Fig. 1)**.

TYPES OF BIOMARKERS IN CARDIOVASCULAR MEDICINE

Diagnostic Biomarkers

Diagnostic biomarkers are crucial tools in the early detection and accurate diagnosis of cardiovascular diseases (CVDs). These biomarkers are biological indicators that signal the presence of a disease or condition. For example, troponins, specifically cardiac troponin I (cTnI) and troponin T (cTnT), are proteins that become elevated in the blood following myocardial infarction (heart attack), providing a highly specific marker for this acute condition.

Another example is B-type natriuretic peptide (BNP) and its precursor, NT-proBNP, which are released in response to ventricular stretching and pressure overload, making them valuable for diagnosing heart failure. C-reactive protein (CRP) is another diagnostic biomarker; its elevated levels indicate inflammation and are associated with an increased risk of cardiovascular events, such as myocardial infarction and stroke.

The use of these biomarkers allows for timely identification of acute conditions, differentiation between various types of heart diseases, and insights into the underlying pathophysiology, guiding clinicians in selecting appropriate diagnostic tests and treatments.

Prognostic Biomarkers

Prognostic biomarkers provide vital information about the likely course or outcome of a disease, helping to predict disease progression and patient prognosis. For instance, N-terminal proB-type natriuretic peptide (NT-proBNP) not only aids in diagnosing heart failure but also predicts outcomes such as mortality and hospitalization rates in affected patients. Similarly, high-sensitivity C-reactive protein (hs-CRP) levels correlate with a higher risk of recurrent cardiovascular events, including heart attacks and strokes.

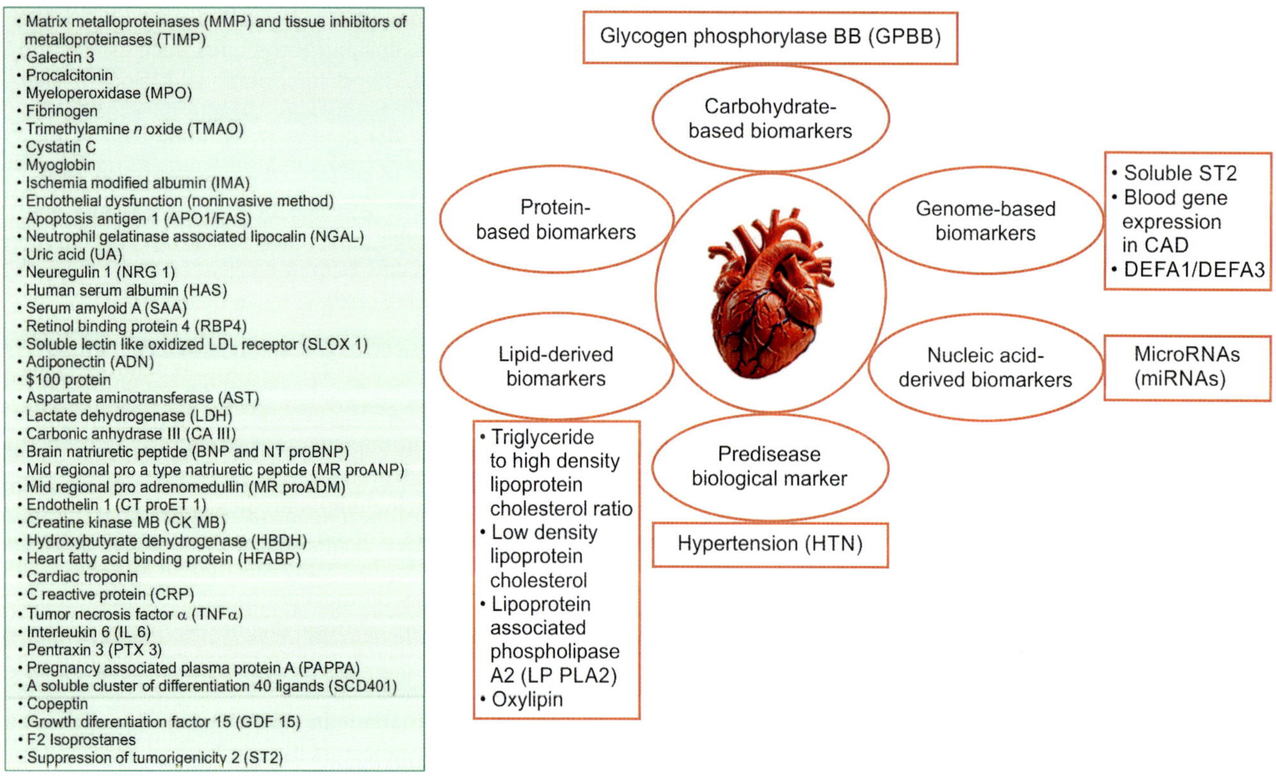

FIG. 1: Various biomarkers for cardiovascular disease.

Source: Thupakula S, Nimmala SSR, Ravula H, et al. Emerging biomarkers for the detection of cardiovascular diseases. Egypt Heart J. 2022;74;77.

Another important prognostic biomarker is galectin-3, which is associated with cardiac fibrosis and remodeling, and its elevated levels predict worse outcomes in heart failure patients.[3] These biomarkers enable healthcare providers to stratify patients based on their risk of adverse outcomes, allowing for more personalized and proactive management strategies. By monitoring disease progression, prognostic biomarkers also help identify patients who may benefit from more aggressive or targeted therapeutic interventions, informing clinical decision-making and guiding appropriate follow-up care.

Therapeutic Biomarkers

Therapeutic biomarkers, also known as predictive biomarkers, play a significant role in guiding treatment decisions and monitoring therapy responses. These biomarkers help tailor treatment plans to individual patients' needs, ensuring the most effective therapies with minimal side effects. For example, low-density lipoprotein cholesterol (LDL-C) levels guide the use of lipid-lowering therapies, such as statins, to reduce cardiovascular risk. Measurement of PCSK9 protein levels can help identify patients who might benefit from PCSK9 inhibitors, a class of drugs that lower LDL-C.

Additionally, genetic testing for *CYP2C19* variants can predict the response to clopidogrel, an antiplatelet medication, helping to optimize antithrombotic therapy. By personalizing treatment plans based on individual biomarker profiles, therapeutic biomarkers ensure that patients receive the most appropriate and effective treatments. They also enable monitoring of treatment efficacy, allowing for timely adjustments in therapy to achieve optimal outcomes, and identify patients who may not respond adequately to standard treatments, facilitating the exploration of alternative or adjunctive therapies.

TECHNOLOGIES AND METHODS FOR BIOMARKER DISCOVERY

Genomics, Proteomics, Metabolomics

Advances in genomics, proteomics, and metabolomics have significantly enhanced the discovery and understanding of biomarkers in cardiovascular medicine. *Genomics* involves the study of the complete set of genes or genetic material within an organism. By analyzing genetic variations, researchers can identify genetic predispositions to cardiovascular diseases and discover novel biomarkers associated with disease susceptibility and progression. Techniques such as genome-wide association studies (GWAS) and next-generation sequencing (NGS) have been pivotal in uncovering genetic variants linked to cardiovascular conditions.

Proteomics focuses on the large-scale study of proteins, including their functions, structures, and interactions.[3] By examining the proteome—the complete set of proteins expressed in a cell or tissue—researchers can identify protein biomarkers that are indicative of cardiovascular disease states. Mass spectrometry and protein microarrays are commonly used in proteomic studies to profile proteins and their post-translational modifications, revealing potential biomarkers for diagnosis and therapeutic targets.

Metabolomics involves the comprehensive analysis of metabolites, the small molecules produced during metabolic processes. This approach provides a snapshot of the metabolic state of an organism and can identify biomarkers associated with cardiovascular diseases. Techniques such as nuclear magnetic resonance (NMR) spectroscopy and mass spectrometry are used to analyze metabolic profiles, helping to understand disease mechanisms and discover new biomarkers for early detection and monitoring.

Imaging Techniques

Imaging techniques are essential for visualizing and quantifying biomarkers within the body, offering insights into disease processes and treatment effects. Advances in imaging technologies, such as magnetic resonance imaging (MRI), computed tomography (CT), and positron emission tomography (PET), have improved the ability to detect and monitor biomarkers related to cardiovascular health. For instance, cardiac MRI can assess myocardial tissue characteristics, while PET imaging can evaluate metabolic activity and receptor binding. These imaging modalities provide valuable information on the anatomical and functional changes associated with cardiovascular diseases, aiding in the discovery and validation of biomarkers.

Bioinformatics and Computational Biology

Bioinformatics and *computational biology* play a crucial role in the analysis and interpretation of complex biological data generated from genomics, proteomics, and metabolomics studies. Bioinformatics involves the use of software and algorithms to manage, analyze, and interpret large datasets. Computational biology applies mathematical models and simulations to understand biological systems and processes. Together, these fields facilitate the identification of potential biomarkers by integrating and analyzing data from various sources, such as genetic sequences, protein expressions, and metabolic profiles. Advanced data analytics, machine learning, and artificial intelligence are increasingly used to uncover patterns and correlations, leading to the discovery of novel biomarkers and the development of predictive models.

Multiomics Approaches

Multiomics approaches integrate data from genomics, proteomics, metabolomics, and other omics disciplines to provide a comprehensive understanding of biological systems. By combining information from multiple layers of biological data, researchers can gain a more holistic view of disease mechanisms and identify biomarkers that may not be apparent from a single omics perspective. This integrative approach enhances the ability to discover and validate biomarkers with greater accuracy and relevance. Multiomics studies often involve sophisticated analytical tools and data integration techniques to correlate findings across different omics layers, leading to the identification of biomarkers with improved specificity and sensitivity for cardiovascular diseases.

CLINICAL APPLICATIONS OF CARDIOVASCULAR BIOMARKERS

Risk Stratification

Risk stratification involves assessing an individual's likelihood of developing cardiovascular diseases (CVD) or experiencing adverse events. Cardiovascular biomarkers are instrumental in identifying high-risk individuals and refining risk assessment models. For instance, biomarkers such as high-sensitivity C-reactive protein (hs-CRP) and B-type natriuretic peptide (BNP) help identify patients at an elevated risk for cardiovascular events, even before clinical symptoms manifest.

These biomarkers can indicate underlying inflammation or cardiac stress that may predispose individuals to future cardiovascular issues. By integrating biomarker data with traditional risk factors (e.g. age, cholesterol levels, blood pressure), healthcare providers can develop personalized risk assessment models that offer a more nuanced evaluation of an individual's cardiovascular risk. This tailored approach enhances the ability to predict and prevent adverse cardiovascular events, allowing for more targeted and proactive interventions.

Disease Management

Disease management involves the continuous monitoring and treatment of patients with cardiovascular conditions. Biomarkers play a crucial role in tailoring treatment plans based on individual biomarker profiles. For example, patients with heart failure may have their treatment adjusted based on levels of B-type natriuretic peptide (BNP), with higher levels indicating worsening disease and necessitating changes in therapy.[4] Additionally, biomarkers such as cardiac troponins are used to monitor the effectiveness of interventions in acute coronary syndrome. By providing real-time insights into a patient's condition, biomarkers enable healthcare providers to make informed decisions about adjusting treatments, optimizing therapeutic regimens, and avoiding potential complications.

Monitoring disease progression and therapeutic efficacy is another critical application of biomarkers in disease management. Regular measurement of biomarkers can help track how well a patient's condition is responding to treatment and whether there is any progression of the disease. For example, changes in levels of biomarkers like NT-proBNP can signal improvements or deteriorations in heart failure, guiding treatment adjustments. This ongoing monitoring allows for a dynamic and responsive approach to managing cardiovascular diseases, ensuring that patients receive the most appropriate care based on their evolving health status.

Pharmacogenomics

Pharmacogenomics, the study of how genes affect an individual's response to drugs, is an emerging field that utilizes biomarkers to personalize pharmacotherapy for cardiovascular conditions. By identifying genetic variations that influence drug metabolism and efficacy, pharmacogenomics helps tailor medications to the individual patient's genetic profile. For instance, genetic testing for variants in the *CYP2C19* gene can predict a patient's response to clopidogrel, an antiplatelet medication used to prevent cardiovascular events.[5] Patients with certain genetic variants may not metabolize clopidogrel effectively, requiring alternative therapies or dosage adjustments to achieve optimal therapeutic outcomes.

Biomarkers in drug response prediction enhance the precision of pharmacotherapy by identifying patients who are likely to benefit from or experience adverse effects from specific medications. This personalized approach minimizes trial-and-error prescribing, reduces the risk of adverse drug reactions, and improves overall treatment efficacy. For example, biomarkers related to drug metabolism, such as those affecting statin therapy for cholesterol management, can guide the choice and dosage of lipid-lowering agents, ensuring that patients receive the most effective treatment with the least risk of side effects.

CHALLENGES AND LIMITATIONS

Technical and Methodological Challenges

The discovery and application of cardiovascular biomarkers face several technical and methodological challenges. One significant challenge is the complexity of biomarker measurement and validation. Biomarkers can be influenced by a variety of factors, including biological variability, sample handling, and assay performance.[5] Developing assays that are both sensitive and specific enough to reliably detect biomarkers at clinically relevant levels is often difficult. Additionally, the integration of different types of omics data (genomics, proteomics, metabolomics) into cohesive and interpretable results requires sophisticated analytical methods and high-quality data. Ensuring that these technologies are applied consistently across different laboratories and studies is crucial for achieving reliable and reproducible results.

Variability and Reproducibility Issues

Variability and reproducibility issues are major concerns in biomarker research and clinical application. Biological variability can lead to differences in biomarker levels among individuals, complicating the interpretation of results and potentially affecting diagnostic accuracy. Moreover, technical variability in laboratory procedures, such as differences in assay methods or equipment calibration, can lead to inconsistent results. Reproducibility of biomarker findings across different populations and settings is essential for validating their clinical utility. Addressing these issues requires rigorous standardization of biomarker assays, careful study design, and validation in diverse cohorts to ensure that biomarkers are both reliable and generalizable.

Cost-effectiveness and Accessibility

The cost-effectiveness and accessibility of biomarkers pose significant challenges, particularly in resource-limited settings. Advanced technologies used in biomarker discovery and measurement, such as high-throughput sequencing and mass spectrometry, can be expensive to implement and maintain. This can limit the availability of biomarker testing, especially in low- and middle-income countries where healthcare resources may be constrained. Additionally, the cost of developing and validating new biomarkers can be high, impacting their integration into routine clinical practice. To address these issues, there is a need for cost-effective biomarker assays and strategies that make biomarker testing more accessible to a broader population. Efforts to streamline and reduce the costs associated with biomarker discovery and testing are crucial for improving healthcare outcomes and equity.

Ethical and Regulatory Considerations

Ethical and regulatory considerations are important aspects of biomarker research and application. The use of biomarkers involves the collection and analysis of biological samples, which raises concerns about privacy and consent. Ensuring that patients provide informed consent and that their data are handled securely is essential for maintaining ethical standards. Additionally, the regulatory landscape for biomarker testing varies across countries, with differing requirements for the approval and use of diagnostic and prognostic tests. Navigating these regulatory requirements and ensuring compliance with standards for clinical validation, data protection, and ethical practices is crucial for the responsible development and application of biomarkers. Addressing these considerations helps build trust in biomarker-based technologies and ensures that they are used ethically and effectively in clinical settings.

CONCLUSION

Biomarkers have emerged as pivotal tools in cardiovascular medicine, offering significant advances in risk stratification, disease management, and pharmacogenomics. The integration of biomarkers into clinical practice has the potential to transform cardiovascular care by enabling personalized approaches to diagnosis, treatment, and monitoring. Through advancements in genomics, proteomics, metabolomics, and imaging technologies, as well as the application of bioinformatics and multiomics approaches, the field has made remarkable strides in understanding and utilizing biomarkers for cardiovascular health.

ONLINE REFERENCES

Please scan the QR code provided at the end of the table of contents for References of this chapter.

CHAPTER

8

Role of Pollution in Cardiovascular Diseases

Abhishek Chaturvedi, Dorairaj Prabhakaran

ABSTRACT

Cardiovascular diseases (CVDs) are the leading cause of morbidity and mortality globally, disproportionately affecting low- and middle-income countries (LMICs) such as India. Despite advances in awareness and treatment, progress in reducing CVD mortality has been uneven. Environmental pollutants such as air pollution, traffic noise, and contamination of water, soil, and food with metals and chemicals can partly explain this slower progress in LMICs. Of all the air pollutants described, particulate matter (PM)2.5 is the most important CVD risk factor linked to significant premature mortality. Traffic noise and metal/chemical pollution have also been implicated in the development of CVDs. The proposed mechanisms by which most of these pollutants increase the risk of CVDs include oxidative stress, systemic inflammation, endothelial dysfunction, autonomic dysfunction, vasoconstriction, platelet activation, and hypercoagulability. The complex interplay of these environmental factors with CVD underscores the need for comprehensive strategies to mitigate pollution and its impact on cardiovascular health, especially in resource-limited settings.

Keywords: Air pollution, cardiovascular diseases, metal pollution, PM2.5, traffic noise

INTRODUCTION

Cardiovascular diseases (CVDs) remain the leading cause of morbidity and mortality, affecting 621 million people worldwide and causing approximately 20.5 million deaths annually, 80% of which occur in low- and middle-income countries (LMICs).[1] In India, the age-standardized CVD-related death rates and disability-adjusted life years (DALYs) are 1.2 and 1.3 times higher than the global averages, with about 62% of these deaths being premature.[2,3] In 2017, CVD accounted for 26.6% of total deaths and 13.6% of total DALYs in India, up from 15.2% and 6.9% in 1990. With better awareness, prevention, and treatment of traditional CVD risk factors, global age-adjusted CVD mortality has improved over the past three decades. However, the progress has been uneven, with faster improvements in high-income countries compared to LMICs.[1] Environmental pollution related to air, noise, and metals has emerged as an important CVD risk factor that disproportionately impacts LMICs and could partly explain this suboptimal improvement in CVD mortality in LMICs. Although often overlooked, it is estimated that of the 9 million global deaths that were directly attributable to environmental pollution in the year 2019, 61.9% of these were due to CVD.[4] This chapter presents a comprehensive review of the evidence linking environmental pollution to CVDs, underlying mechanisms, prevention strategies, and way forward.

AIR POLLUTION

Air pollution is one of the most studied and discussed environmental CVD risk factors globally. It is now ranked fourth among the risk factors for mortality, with more attributable deaths than fasting glucose, low-density lipoprotein cholesterol, body mass index, kidney dysfunction, or alcohol use.[5] In 2019, around 12% of global deaths were attributed to air pollution, including 4.2 million from outdoor and 2.9 million from household sources.[4] Studies suggest that ambient particulate matter (PM)-related CVD deaths have been steadily increasing since 1990.[6] South and East Asia regions account for 59% of total ambient PM pollution-related deaths, and together with sub-Saharan Africa, they bear the burden of 8–15% of global air pollution-related DALYs. On the other hand, the United States, Canada, and Australia each share <2% burden of air pollution-related

DALYs.[4] In 2017, a study suggested that air pollution was responsible for 1.24 million deaths (12.5% of the total deaths) in India, with ambient air pollution contributing to 0.67 million and indoor air pollution to 0.48 million deaths.[7] This state-level disease burden study estimated that air pollution reduced average life expectancy in India by 1.7 years.[7] In 2019, 17.8% of deaths in India were attributed to air pollution, resulting in an economic loss of $36.8 billion.[8] This economic loss amounts to 1.4% of India's gross domestic product, in comparison to its total health expenditure of 3.8%, highlighting the negative impact of air pollution on India's health, economy, and growth. A recent analysis of 3.6 million deaths in India showed that a 10-point increase in PM2.5 was associated with a 1.4% increase in daily mortality even at concentrations well below the current Indian PM2.5 standards (<60 μg/m³ daily).[9]

Markers of Air Pollution

Ambient air pollution is a complex mixture of chemicals in gaseous and particulate forms and some gaseous copollutants that can occur in a particulate phase.[10,11] The most common gaseous pollutants include ozone, nitrogen oxides, carbon monoxide, sulfur dioxide, and benzene. The PM comprises elemental and organic carbon particles, transition metals, hydrocarbons, sulfates, nitrates, alkenes, alkanes, dioxins, furans, microbes, and lipopolysaccharides.[12,13] PM fractions of air pollution are broadly categorized by aerodynamic diameter: <10 μm [thoracic particles (PM10)], 2.5–10 μm [coarse particles (PM2.5–10)], <2.5 μm [fine particles (PM2.5)], and <0.1 μm (ultrafine particles). The reason for measuring PM based on size is primarily related to the ease of quantitative assessment of each fraction. Ultrafine particles are generally short-lived species and stay airborne for a few hours. Coarse and thoracic PM tend to settle in the upper and larger airways, primarily from processes such as mechanical grinding, agriculture, landfills, and wind-blown dust from roads, mines, biomass/coal burning in households, and construction sites.[14] Even though recent studies support the adverse health effects of ozone, ultrafine, and coarse/thoracic PM, there is overwhelming evidence to suggest that PM2.5 is the principal air pollutant posing the greatest threat to cardiovascular health globally.[12,15]

PM2.5 is an amalgam of primary (elemental carbon) and secondary (aerosols, sulfates, nitrates, transition metals, organic compounds, microbes, lipopolysaccharides) pollutants released from domestic fuel combustion, industrial activities, power generation, and road transport.[16,17] These particles are large but still smaller than the diameter of a human hair, stay airborne for a few days, and can be transported hundreds of miles depending upon the weather conditions.[18,19] The overall risk varies depending on the individuals affected as well as sources, composition, and temporal and spatial characteristics of PM2.5.[17] For example, road traffic-related air pollution peaks during rush hours and varies in composition within short distances; meteorological conditions can alter the propagation of particles and subsequent exposure; and significant differences exist in rural and urban concentrations of pollutants originating from fuel combustion. Additionally, climate change events such as wildfires, volcanic eruptions, dust storms, floods, and drought are associated with increased pollutant exposure and worse social conditions, thereby accelerating the impact of air pollution on cardiovascular health.[20,21]

Global Air Quality Trends and How India Measures Up

The World Health Organization (WHO)'s recommended limit of PM2.5 <10 μg/m³ annually and <25 μg/m³ daily was lowered to <5 μg/m³ annually and <15 μg/m³ daily in 2021.[22] In 2019, 99% of the global population was exposed to PM2.5 levels exceeding 2021 WHO recommendations. LMICs experience high household air pollution levels from open fires and inefficient stoves using kerosene, biomass, and coal, with indoor PM10 levels ranging from 200 to 2,000 μg/m³, sometimes exceeding 30,000 μg/m³ during cooking.[23,24] Compared to Western countries such as the United States and Canada, where PM2.5 levels routinely average <12 μg/m³, mean exposure to ambient PM2.5 in India is about 90 μg/m³, with peak daily levels sometimes exceeding 250 μg/m³.[18,19,25] In fact, these levels are well above the Indian National Air Quality Standards recommended limit of PM2.5 <40 μg/m³ annually and <60 μg/m³ daily.[9] Higher PM2.5 concentration in a closed environment has been reported to be 10 times more harmful than a similar outdoor concentration.[26] This is concerning because studies suggest that Indians spend 80% of their time indoors, and PM2.5 levels in most households range from 86 to 882 μg/m³.[27,28] Recent data suggest that there has been a 64% drop in household air pollution-related deaths in India from 1990 to 2019, however the 115% and 139% increase in ambient PM- and ozone pollution-related deaths remain a matter of concern.[8]

Association of Particulate Matter2.5 with Cardiovascular Risk Factors and Diseases

Air pollution has been linked to biomarkers and precursors of atherosclerosis, including carotid intima-media thickness, carotid plaques, coronary artery calcium, cardiac afterload, left ventricular hypertrophy, diastolic dysfunction, alteration in coronary flow reserve, and myocardial fibrosis.[29-32] Globally, air pollution contributes to an average loss of life expectancy of 20 months, which is as high as that for tobacco use (22 months).[5] The rise in ambient PM2.5 concentrations had been linked to an elevation in blood pressure (BP) by 1–3 mm Hg over the ensuing few days.[19] Studies have shown an 11% increased risk of hypertension and a 39% increased risk of type 2 diabetes per 10-point increase in PM2.5.[33-35] In the context of the Indian population, our group has demonstrated a temporal association between high ambient

PM2.5 levels, higher systolic BP, and incident hypertension.[36] In another analysis of >10,000 participants from India, we showed that ambient PM2.5 levels were associated with increased low-density lipoprotein cholesterol and total cholesterol and decreased high-density lipoprotein cholesterol.[37]

Short- and long-term PM2.5 exposures above recommended levels have been implicated in many CVDs.[12,13,17,38,39] The strongest epidemiological evidence exists with regard to ischemic heart disease (IHD). A German study reported a 2.9 times increased risk of myocardial infarction (MI) with traffic exposure within the past hour.[40] A meta-analysis involving 100,166 individuals showed that for every 5-point increase in PM2.5, there was a 13% increase in MI risk even at exposure levels below the annual European PM2.5 limit (25 µg/m^3).[41] For patients who have already suffered MI, higher PM2.5 exposure leads to poorer quality of life and a 20% increased risk of non-accidental mortality.[42,43] In stable coronary artery disease patients undergoing elective percutaneous coronary intervention, higher PM2.5 exposure increases the risk for future cardiac events and shortens life span by 1–2 years.[44]

Similar findings extend to other cardiac conditions such as heart failure (HF) and arrhythmias.[45-47] Studies show that with every 10-point increase in PM2.5 levels, there is an increase in HF hospitalization (plus associated mortality) risk by 2.1% (the strongest association being on the day of exposure), atrial fibrillation risk by 0.9%, out-of-hospital cardiac arrest risk by 2.2% (over the next 2 days), and stroke risk (plus associated mortality) by 1.1% for short-term exposure.[46-49] In another study, a long-term increase in PM2.5 concentration by 10 points increased stroke risk by 35% and stroke mortality by 83%.[50] While most studies are from high-income countries, similar trends are seen in LMICs, where a 10-point increase in PM2.5 increases the risk of stroke by 12–13% and MI by 11%, even after accounting for individual, household, and geographical covariates.[51,52]

Association of Particulate Matter2.5 with Cardiovascular Mortality

The components of PM2.5, including sulfates, nitrates, and organic and elemental carbon have been consistently linked with all-cause and CVD mortality.[53-55] Interestingly, ozone at higher concentrations (>23–25 parts per billion) may strengthen the association between PM2.5 and CVD mortality.[56] Short-term rise in PM2.5 by 10 points translates to a 0.3% and 0.63% excess risk of CVD mortality in regions with lower (<35 µg/m^3) and higher levels of daily PM2.5 exposure, respectively.[17,57] A 10-point rise in PM levels is linked to a 1.8% increase in short-term CVD mortality and a 9–12% increase in long-term CVD mortality, with women experiencing a 76% greater long-term risk.[12,50,52,58] In patients with concomitant cancer (especially socially vulnerable and minority populations), long-term exposure to high PM2.5 levels increased CVD mortality by 10.5%.[59]

In India, 49.2% of deaths from air pollution are due to CVD and diabetes, and a study from New Delhi showed that a 25-point increase in PM2.5 raises daily non-accidental mortality by 0.8%, and by 1.5% for those over 60 years of age.[8,60] Models indicate that improved air quality could potentially prevent 24% of IHD deaths and 18.5% of stroke deaths in India.[61] The recently published 10-city study in India estimates that even in cities with lower levels of air pollution, there was a 7.2% excess mortality attributable to air pollution.[9]

Dose–Response Relationship and the Time Frame of Exposure

The relationship between PM2.5 from various sources and CVD mortality is best described by a nonlinear exposure–response curve with steep increases at low exposure levels and some flattening at higher levels.[18,62] The WHO states that exceeding a PM2.5 concentration of 35 µg/m^3 increases mortality by 15%, while reducing levels to 25 µg/m^3 and 15 µg/m^3 decreases mortality by 6% each, but there is no safe lower limit.[18,19] Some studies have reported mortality risk at PM2.5 levels as low as 2 µg/m^3.[19,63-65]

Apart from the impact of actual PM2.5 levels, the time frames of exposure required to mediate acute CVD events are represented by exposure–response curves that demonstrate increased mortality risk even with short-term exposure to PM2.5 and ozone.[19,65] A recent study reported that air pollution could trigger MI within 1 hour of exposure.[66] This points to the concept of "vulnerability," in which a series of events spatially clustered around a time frame combine to precipitate an acute event. A 10-point daily increase in PM2.5 exposure raises hospitalizations for stroke by 0.8%, IHD by 0.4%, arrhythmias by 0.6%, and HF by 1.3%, with same-day effects seen for stroke, arrhythmia, and HF, but a 2-day delay for IHD.[67] Chronic PM2.5 exposure leads to changes in plaque burden, its vulnerability, posing greater CVD risks.[12,19,68] Additionally, air pollution-related deaths might occur in individuals whose health is already compromised, a concept known as the "harvesting effect" or "mortality displacement."[69]

Pathophysiology of Particulate Matter2.5-induced Cardiovascular Diseases

When inhaled, PM2.5 penetrates the lower respiratory tract, deposits deep within alveoli, interacts with and activates local cells (e.g., macrophages, dendritic cells, alveolar endothelial cells), and modifies endogenous structures (e.g., cell membranes, surfactant lipids, antioxidants). In addition, mediators of oxidative stress directly generated by particulate compounds or those produced in response to biological intermediates (e.g., modified phospholipids) can instigate a local inflammatory response.[19]

These initial events then mediate cardiovascular injury via six potential mechanisms **(Fig. 1)**: (1) endothelial

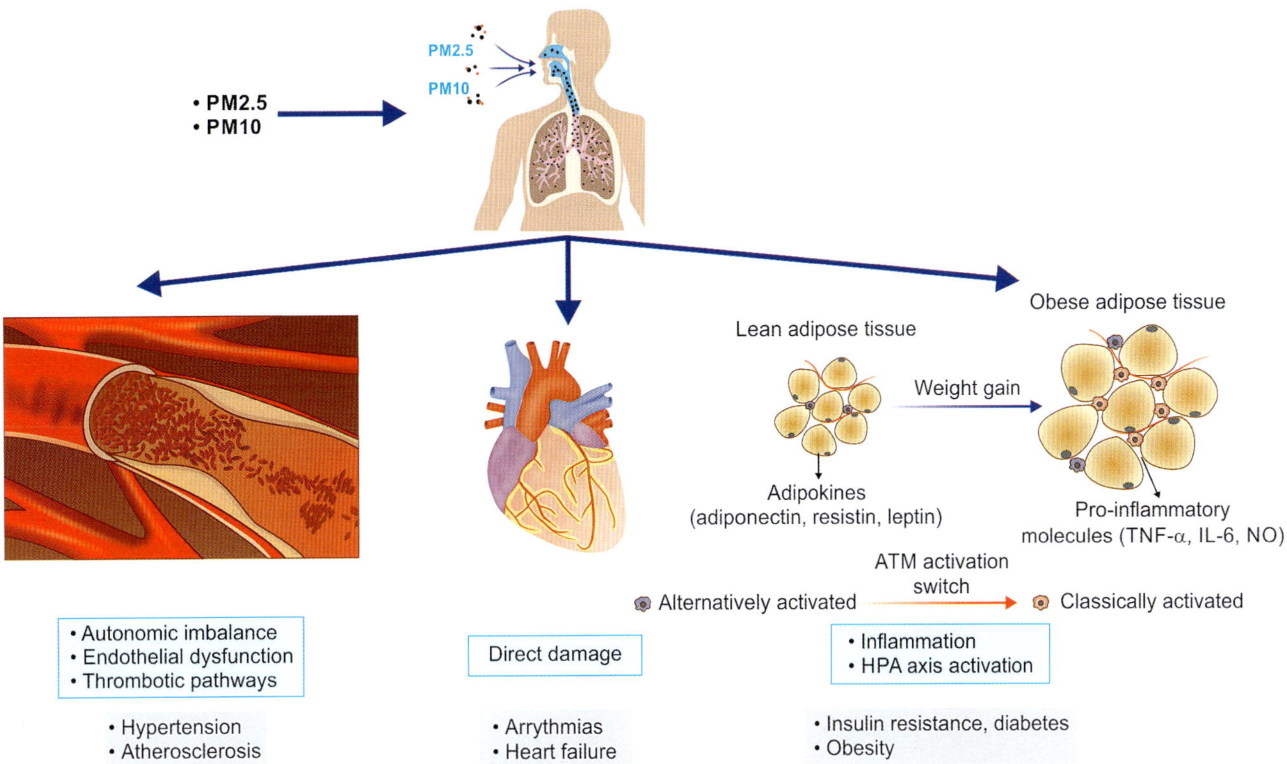

FIG. 1: Biological mechanisms linking PM2.5 and cardiovascular diseases.
(HPA: hypothalamic–pituitary–adrenal; PM: particulate matter; TNF: tumor necrosis factor; IL: interleukin; NO: nitric oxide)

dysfunction, (2) systemic inflammation, (3) prothrombotic milieu, (4) autonomic imbalance with increased sympathetic tone, (5) central nervous system effects on the metabolism and hypothalamic-pituitary-adrenal axis activation, and (6) epigenomic changes. These mechanisms eventually lead to increased reactive oxygen species, reactive nitrogen species, smooth muscle proliferation, adhesion molecule expression on endothelial cells, vasoconstriction, rhythm disturbances, monocyte infiltration, macrophage activation, rise in inflammatory cytokines, and stress hormones. Some pathways have more relevance to short-term exposures and are likely to factor mostly in a triggering role (e.g., autonomic imbalance evidenced by changes in BP and heart rate variability in response to PM exposures). Others likely play a more long-term role (e.g., hypothalamic-pituitary-adrenal axis activation leading to brown adipose dysfunction, white adipose inflammation, and insulin resistance). Although systemic inflammation and vasoconstriction have the strongest epidemiological evidence supporting their role in instigating and triggering CVD events, these pathways can still have considerable overlap depending upon underlying susceptibility due to biological risk factors (advanced age, prior CVD, traditional CVD risk factors, pulmonary disease, cancer, and/or immunosuppression) and social determinants of health (income inequality, poor housing, reduced tree cover, structural racism, and food deserts can increase a person's susceptibility to PM2.5).[12,19]

TRAFFIC NOISE

The evidence linking noise pollution with CVD is growing. The WHO reported that yearly, over 1.6 million healthy life-years are lost from transportation-related noise in Western Europe and that at least 20% of the population in Europe lives in areas where traffic noise is harmful.[70] Although transportation noise has been directly attributed to 48,000 new cases of IHD and 12,000 premature deaths, it is unfortunately not addressed in international guidelines for CVD prevention.[70-72]

Studies suggest a link between traffic noise and unhealthy behaviors such as reduced physical activity, alcohol use, and smoking.[70] Long-term exposure to noise increases the risk of hypertension, diabetes, and obesity.[73-76] Diabetes risk increases by 6% per 5 dB(A) rise in all-traffic noise, by 20% per 10 dB(A) increase in aircraft noise, and by 11% per 10 dB(A) rise in road noise.[70,77] The strongest link between noise exposure and CVD is with IHD, and a 10 dB(A) increase in road traffic noise raises incident IHD by 8%, and HF by approximately 12%.[74,78] Aircraft noise levels > 50 dB(A) increase CVD mortality from IHD, HF, and arrhythmia.[79]

Similarly, studies have shown a link between traffic noise and the risk of atrial fibrillation and ischemic stroke, though findings on stroke are mixed.[70,80-82]

The mechanisms by which noise exposure leads to CVD can be understood by the "noise-reaction" model. The elevated noise levels [>50 dB(A)] can disrupt routine activities and sleep, leading to emotional stress responses such as annoyance or anger and causes neurohormonal activation via the hypothalamic-pituitary-adrenal axis, sympathetic nervous system, and renin-angiotensin-aldosterone system.[83,84] This results in increased oxidative stress, circulating stress hormones, and chronic inflammation, which promote endothelial dysfunction, hypertension, insulin resistance, dyslipidemia, and activation of the coagulation system, eventually leading to IHD, stroke, HF, and arrhythmia.[83,85,86] Additionally, disrupted circadian rhythm and sleep disturbance (as a result of nighttime noise) itself is associated with obesity, hypertension, diabetes, and acute CVD events.[87] While the CVD effects of traffic noise and air pollution often overlap, an epigenome-wide association study found that traffic noise and air pollution independently affect DNA methylation, with distinct and shared enrichments for pathways related to inflammation, cellular development, and immune responses.[88]

METAL POLLUTION

Chronic exposure to low levels of nonessential metals found in daily life, such as lead, cadmium, arsenic, and mercury, have been previously linked to cancer, neurobehavioral disorders, and gastrointestinal and kidney diseases, but a growing body of evidence suggests that these metals increase the risk of CVD as well, with IHD being the principal one.[89,90] Lead (pathological range—plasma: >10 µg/dL, urine: >30 µg/g creatinine) is found in old paint, water pipes, contaminated food, and some kitchenware.[91] Cadmium (pathological range—plasma: >5 µg/L, urine: >5 µg/g creatinine) is found in batteries, pigments, plastics, ceramics, fertilizers, and burning fossil fuels.[91] Cigarettes contain both lead and cadmium. Arsenic (pathological range—plasma: >50 µg/L, urine: >150 µg/g creatinine) exposure mainly comes from contaminated groundwater.[91] Mercury (pathological range—plasma: >20 µg/L, urine: >10 µg/g creatinine) exposure occurs via fossil and biomass combustion, artisanal gold mining, deforestation, pesticides, and dental amalgams.[91] Lower-income communities, as well as those living near industrial sources, major roads, or in older homes with poor environmental regulation, are at disproportionately higher risk for metal-induced CVD.

Lead, cadmium, and arsenic are linked to subclinical atherosclerosis and various CVDs. Lead is a known risk factor for hypertension and has been associated with all-cause and CVD mortality even when blood lead levels are <3 µg/dL.[92-94] Cadmium exposure is associated with hypertension, carotid plaque vulnerability, stroke, and dilated cardiomyopathy, even at exposures as low as <0.5 µg/g creatinine.[95-98] Arsenic exposure shows dose-dependent associations with atherosclerosis, hypertension, diabetes, coronary artery disease, peripheral artery disease (e.g., black foot disease in Taiwan), stroke, and arrhythmias.[92,99-102] Mercury has also been associated with atherosclerosis, hypertension, IHD, arrhythmias, carotid disease, and CVD-related mortality.[102,103]

Although the mechanisms by which heavy metals cause toxic effects on cardiovascular health are not fully understood, it is proposed that contaminant metals disrupt antioxidant pathways, resulting in oxidative stress and chronic inflammation, which in turn leads to endothelial dysfunction, disturbances in lipid metabolism and ion homeostasis, and epigenetic dysregulation.[89,102] The application of chelation or antioxidants can potentially prevent and treat metal-induced CVD. A study in post-MI patients receiving ethylenediaminetetraacetic acid (EDTA) showed an 18% reduction in composite endpoint (death, MI, stroke, coronary revascularization, or hospitalization for angina) over 5 years.[104] The benefit of EDTA was even greater (41% risk reduction) for MI patients with diabetes.[105] Similar benefits of EDTA chelation therapy have been suggested in patients with peripheral artery disease and diabetes.[106]

CHEMICAL POLLUTION

Over the past few decades, the production of chemicals such as halogenated hydrocarbons, perfluoroalkyl substances, and plastic-associated chemicals has surged, leading to widespread environmental contamination and human exposure.[91] These substances, often persistent and bio-accumulative, have been linked to increased risks of CVD. Halogenated hydrocarbons, found in contaminated meat and fish, can cause insulin resistance, dyslipidemia, and obesity.[107] Perfluoroalkyl substances, used in water repellants and fire-fighting foams, are associated with obesity and diabetes.[107] Plastic-associated chemicals such as bisphenol A and phthalates, found in personal care products, pharmaceuticals, and food preservatives, disturb endocrine pathways and have been linked to diabetes and obesity.[108]

MITIGATION STRATEGIES

Pollution disproportionately impacts cardiovascular health in LMICs that have an enormous share of vulnerable populations and often lack the resources to address these issues. There is ample evidence to suggest that controlling various forms of pollution can not only dramatically reduce the morbidity and mortality associated with CVDs, but also ease the economic burden associated with it.[36,43,47,48,61,89,109,110] The first step toward prevention is recognizing pollution as a major, preventable risk factor in medical practice, public health strategies, and international societal guidelines. Additionally, comprehensive and coordinated actions across various sectors are required for the greatest impact.

Patient-level Strategies

Physicians should assess a patient's exposure to ambient air pollution, traffic noise, and metal/chemical contamination based on the residence and household sources (e.g., solid fuel combustion, poor ventilation, nearby highways/railways/airports), risk stratify based on pre-existing CVDs and comorbid conditions, and then advise on avoidance measures, such as minimizing outdoor activities on high pollution days, mask use, using portable air filters, avoiding known sources of air, noise, metal/chemical pollution, personal sound protection devices, soundproofing windows, regular exercise, and plant-based (antioxidant rich) diet, and chelation therapy if applicable.[89,91,111,112]

Policy-level Strategies

For air pollution, public health policies should focus on transitioning to renewable energy via educational campaigns, reducing energy consumption by energy-intensive industries, regulating industrial emissions, developing low-cost monitoring systems, facilitating management of agricultural residues, upgrading vehicles to more fuel-efficient standards, enhancing the availability of public transport, and incorporating green spaces and walkable trails into urban infrastructure. Governments, especially in LMICs, should promote innovative and scalable strategies to mitigate the negative impact of air pollution on cardiovascular health. For example, the PURI-HF (Air Purifiers on Heart Failure) trial aims to test the feasibility and effectiveness of portable air filters in improving indoor PM2.5 levels and functional capacity of HF with reduced ejection fraction patients in India.[113]

For noise pollution, governments should adopt urban redesign to reduce noise, enforce noise regulations for vehicles, implement soundproofing measures in residential and workspaces, adjust flight and railway paths, relocate road traffic, and promote innovations to build cost-effective solutions such as quiet road surfaces and low-noise tires. For metal and chemical pollution, stricter regulations on harmful chemicals, public health efforts to reduce water, food, and air contamination, and research to devise novel chelation therapies are crucial for lowering associated CVD risks.

WAY FORWARD

Although the evidence linking various forms of pollution and CVDs is growing, the results of observational studies lack uniformity and generalizability. For example, ambient air pollution exposure assessment in India has relied on source distribution, emission inventories, satellite remote sensing, and land-use regression techniques; however, large parts of rural India do not have air pollution monitors, challenging our reliance on monitoring networks for capturing country-wide patterns.[114,115] A potential solution is to deploy low-cost stationary and portable sensor systems in areas without monitoring, which would also help extend existing networks' spatial and temporal resolution.[116] Another strategy is to develop robust models of air pollution assessments and their impact on cardiovascular health longitudinally. The project "GEOHealth (Global Environmental and Occupational Health) India Hub" leverages publicly available information on air quality, meteorological variables, satellite data, land use, and emission inventories to build an exposure assessment model linking air pollution to health outcomes in existing, longitudinal study cohorts.[114,117-119] The evaluating effects of air pollution across the lifespan, particularly among sensitive groups and vulnerable populations through a modified life-course approach (across pregnancy, infancy, childhood, adolescence, adulthood, and old age), as outlined by GEOHealth-HEALS (GEOHealth Health Effects of Selected Environmental Exposomes Across the Life CourSe) study could help better understand the link between air pollution, socioeconomic status, lifestyle, and health outcomes and inform policy interventions.[120] Such models can serve as a comprehensive resource for future studies on exposure and health effects and generate new actionable evidence needed for policy reforms in India and similar regions around the world such as Asia and Africa.

CONCLUSION

Recognizing environmental pollution as a modifiable CVD risk factor presents opportunities for effective prevention and control. This awareness alone can guide patients, clinicians, and health authorities in developing strategies that integrate pollution prevention into the management of CVDs. Addressing environmental pollution through targeted interventions, such as a shift toward renewable energy, stricter emission regulations, improved urban planning, noise mitigation strategies, and enhanced monitoring of metal and chemical exposures, would not only promote overall cardiovascular health but also prevent health and economic losses attributable to pollution-related CVDs. Future research should focus on refining exposure metrics and understanding the impact of various co-pollutants and confounders, which can help devise comprehensive prevention strategies.

ONLINE REFERENCES

Please scan the QR code provided at the end of the table of contents for References of this chapter.

CHAPTER

9

Frailty in Cardiac Intensive Care Units: Assessment and Impact on Management

Ajay Kumar Sinha, Sanjeev Kumar, Samshad Alam, Shreya Rani

ABSTRACT

Frailty is a clinical syndrome characterized by reduced cognitive, physical, and physiological reserves, resulting in increased vulnerability to adverse health outcomes. This condition is becoming a significant concern in the cardiac intensive care unit (CICU). Frailty not only contributes to higher morbidity and mortality rates but also exacerbates complications associated with cardiovascular diseases. Notably, there is a bidirectional relationship between frailty and cardiovascular conditions, making it a critical area of focus in the CICU.

Prevalence and demographics: Frailty is particularly prevalent among older adults admitted to the CICU, with estimates suggesting that up to 63% of these patients exhibit signs of frailty. While frailty predominantly affects the elderly, it is also observed in younger patients under 65 years of age, with approximately 30% of this demographic admitted to the CICU being frail. This indicates that frailty is not solely an age-related issue but can also impact younger individuals, especially those with acute cardiovascular illnesses.

Frail patients in the CICU tend to have a greater burden of comorbidities and are often less likely to receive optimal treatment for their acute cardiovascular conditions. Recognizing the importance of this geriatric syndrome, this review will concentrate on the assessment, clinical outcomes, and interventions, aiming to determine appropriate strategies for evaluating, managing, and allocating resources for frail patients during and following their CICU stay.

Keywords: Aging, frailty, older adults, cardiovascular disease, cardiac critical illness

INTRODUCTION

Frailty is prevalent among older adults and patients admitted with acute cardiovascular illness. Defined as a clinical syndrome of increased vulnerability, frailty manifests as diminished cognitive, physical, and physiological reserves. It increases morbidity, mortality, and complications, and often has a bidirectional relationship with cardiovascular disease (CVD).[1] Frailty is common among older adults admitted to the CICU, with an estimate as high as 63% Although traditionally associated with older adults, frailty has been observed in up to 30% of younger patients admitted to the cardiac intensive care unit (CICU).[2]

Frail patients are more likely to be admitted due to acute medical illnesses following elective surgery and are more frequently transferred to medical or surgical ICUs postelective general surgery. Additionally, frail patients tend to have "do not resuscitate" (DNR) and "do not intubate (DNI)" orders and higher scores on illness severity scoring systems such as the Acute Physiology and Chronic Health Evaluation (APACHE) and the Sequential Organ Failure Assessment (SOFA).[3] Given the increased vulnerability of frail patients in the CICU, it is crucial to examine this geriatric syndrome in the context of cardiac critical illness. This review focuses on assessment, clinical outcomes, and interventions, aiming to establish appropriate strategies for assessment, management, and resource utilization in frail patients following CICU admission **(Figs. 1 and 2)**.

ASSESSMENT OF FRAILTY

Several tools have been developed to assess frailty in clinical settings. These tools vary in complexity, from simple physical performance tests to comprehensive evaluations incorporating multiple domains of health which include:

- *Fried frailty phenotype*: This tool assesses frailty based on five criteria—(1) unintentional weight loss, (2) exhaustion, (3) weakness (grip strength), (4) slow walking speed, and (5) low physical activity. Patients meeting three or more criteria are classified as frail.

- *Rockwood frailty index*: This index considers a broad range of health deficits, including diseases, disabilities, and laboratory abnormalities. It provides a continuous frailty score based on the proportion of deficits present.
- *Braden skin score*: Originally developed to predict pressure ulcer risk, this score has been adapted to assess frailty by evaluating mobility, activity, and sensory perception.
- *Clinical frailty scale (CFS)*: The CFS is a simple, easy-to-use tool that categorizes patients into nine levels of frailty based on their physical fitness and dependence on others.
- *Other tools*: Additional tools such as the Edmonton Frail Scale and the Groningen Frailty Indicator include cognitive and social dimensions to provide a comprehensive assessment of frailty. Automated machine-learning tools represent the likely future of frailty measurement and should be automated and incorporated into the patient's EMR, just as body mass index is.

The most commonly used is the clinical frailty score developed by the Canadian Study on Health and Ageing (CSHA) (**Table 1**).[4]

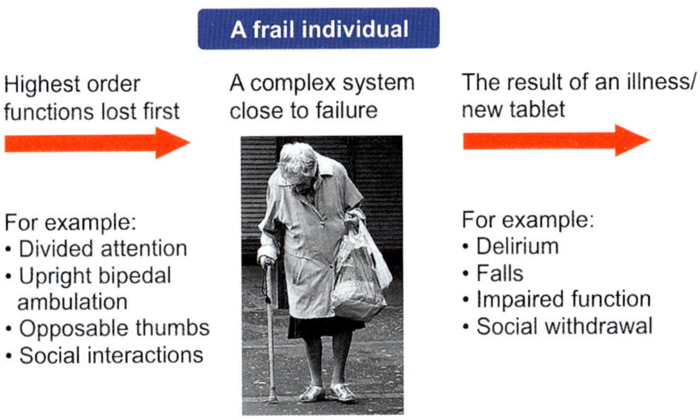

FIG. 1: Impacting quality of life.

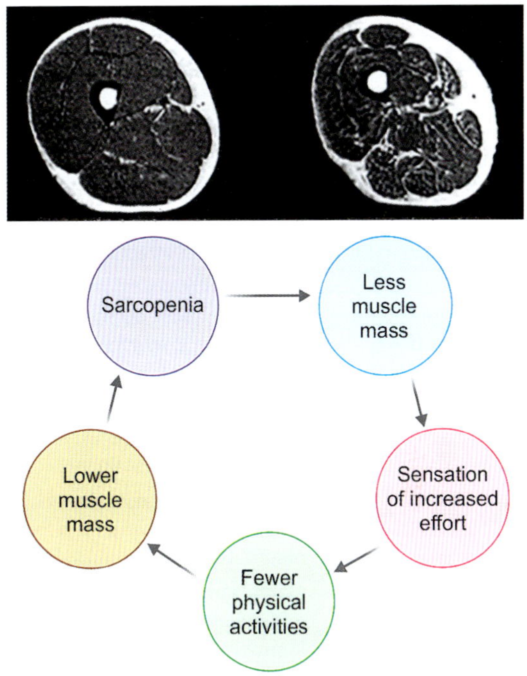

FIG. 2: Cycle of functional decline.

TABLE 1: Clinical frailty score developed by the Canadian study.

Score	Condition	Description
1	Very fit	People who are robust, active, energetic, and motivated. These people commonly exercise regularly. They are among the fittest for their age
2	Well	People who have no active disease symptoms but are less fit than category 1. Often, they exercise or are very active occasionally, e.g., seasonally
3	Managing well	People whose medical problems are well controlled, but are not regularly active beyond routine walking
4	Vulnerable	While not dependent on others for daily help, often symptoms limit activities. A common complaint is being "slowed up", and/or being tired during the day
5	Mildly frail	These people often have more evident slowing, and need help in high order IADLs (finances, transportation, heavy housework, and medications). Typically, mild frailty progressively impairs shopping and walking outside alone, meal preparation, and housework
6	Moderately frail	People need help with all outside activities and with keeping house. Inside, they often have problems with stairs and need help with bathing and might need minimal assistance (cuing and standby) with dressing
7	Severely frail	Completely dependent for personal care, from whatever cause (physical or cognitive). Even so, they seem stable and not at high risk of dying (within ~6 months)
8	Very severely frail	Completely dependent, approaching the end of life. Typically, they could not recover even from a minor illness
9	Terminally ill	Approaching the end of life. This category applies to people with a life expectancy <6 months, who are not otherwise evidently frail

CHALLENGES IN FRAILTY ASSESSMENT IN THE CARDIAC INTENSIVE CARE UNIT (TABLE 2)

Frail patients account for one-third of critical care admissions and face a significantly higher risk of developing new CVDs.

TABLE 2: Gaps in knowledge and future directions for management of frailty in the CICU.

Gaps in knowledge	Future directions
Lack of a gold-standard measurement tool for frailty in the CICU	A standardized frailty instrument is needed to establish the diagnosis and help manage frailty during acute cardiovascular disease
Frailty's interaction with prognostic factors in CICU is unclear	Study how illness severity and comorbidities affect frailty to tailor interventions
Limited outcome's data on older frail patients during acute CV illness	Research patient outcomes during and post-CICU to inform targeted treatments
The interaction of frailty and delirium among older patients in CICU is unclear	Investigate CICU's role in delirium and frailty to develop focused prevention and treatment plans
Unknown medication tolerance in frail CICU patients	Research pharmacological management optimization for frail older CICU patients
Impact of early mobilization on frailty in CICU is promising	Clarify early mobilization and rehabilitation programs in improving frailty during acute cardiovascular illness in CICU
Social support's impact on long-term outcomes of frailty is underexplored	Examine social support in long-term outcomes of frail older patients alongside biomedical therapies

Although multiple effective tools are used to assess frailty, a universally accepted gold-standard measure is still absent.

IMPACT ON MANAGEMENT (FLOWCHART 1)

Knowledge of a patient's frailty status can potentially improve clinical decision-making regarding procedural interventions and guide conversations about goals of care.

Understanding and identifying frailty in CICU patients is crucial for tailoring management strategies to improve outcomes. The presence of frailty necessitates a more individualized approach to care.

CLINICAL OUTCOMES IN THE CARDIAC INTENSIVE CARE UNIT

Duration of Stay

In the CICU, only two studies have examined the relationship between frailty and length of stay (LOS).[5] Goldfarb et al. evaluated the impact of early mobility in frail versus nonfrail patients admitted with acute cardiovascular conditions, revealing that frail patients had a longer median hospital LOS. Additionally, a German multicenter study linked frailty to an extended LOS among ICU patients aged 80 years or older.[6]

Resource Use

Preliminary studies indicate that frail patients tend to need prolonged mechanical ventilation and have a reduced likelihood of successful extubation. The organizational characteristics in critical care study, which analyzed one of the largest datasets of critically ill patients (over 100,000),

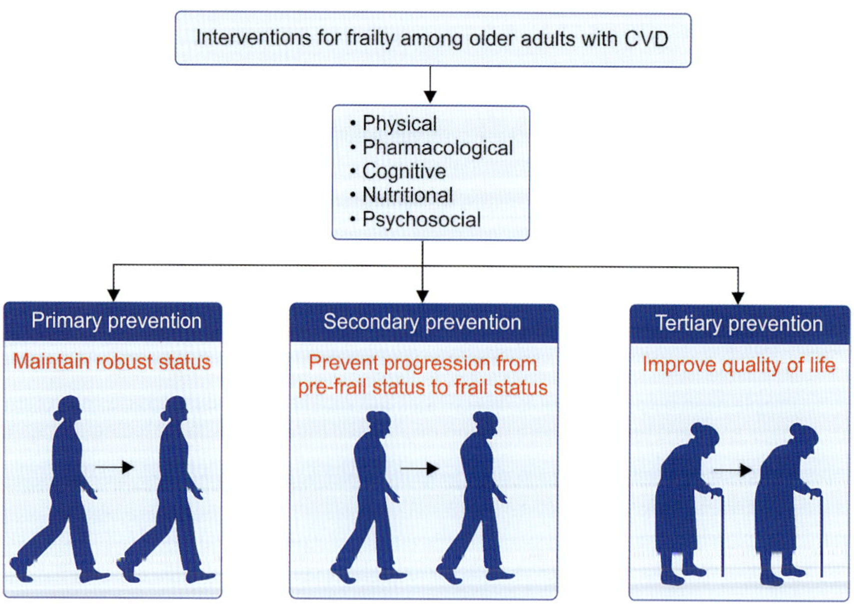

FLOWCHART 1: Interventions aimed to prevent or reverse frailty.

revealed that frail individuals consistently required greater levels of organ support.[7]

Mortality Rates in the Cardiac Intensive Care Unit and Hospital

Goldfarb et al.[5] reported that frail patients admitted to the CICU had more than double the mortality rate compared to nonfrail patients (6.7% vs. 2.9%). In general ICUs, frail patients exhibited an ICU mortality rate approaching 60%. Similarly, a retrospective analysis by Fernando et al.[8] of over 8,000 patients aged 18 and older found that frail patients had significantly higher odds of ICU mortality (OR 1.24, 95% CI 1.10–1.40). The FRAIL-FIT study further confirmed that frail individuals were less likely to survive in the ICU.[9] This trend is particularly evident in older adults, where frailty is associated with significantly higher mortality rates.[10]

COMPLICATIONS

In critical care, the link between frailty and a higher risk of major adverse events, such as bleeding, is well documented. The severity of bleeding tends to increase with the degree of frailty. Multiple studies have confirmed this, with one reporting that frail patients had 1.5 times higher odds of experiencing major adverse cardiovascular events (MACE) during their hospital stay compared to nonfrail patients.[11]

HOW DOES FRAILTY INFLUENCE THE MANAGEMENT?

Several studies have investigated sedative use in critically ill patients, highlighting its comparative effectiveness and potential consequences. However, there is limited data on optimal sedation practices specifically for frail patients in the CICU. International evidence-based guidelines universally recommend a protocol-driven, multidisciplinary approach that minimizes sedation while ensuring effective management of ventilatory desynchrony, anxiety, and pain.

This approach is facilitated by tools and strategies such as the Richmond Agitation-Sedation Scale (RASS), the Critical-care Pain Observation Tool (CPOT), spontaneous breathing trials, sedation vacations, delirium screening, and care bundles like the ABCDEF bundle.

For prevention and treatment, nonpharmacological interventions have proven effective, including cognitive and emotional stimulation, prevention of sensory impairments through hearing aids, vision optimization with glasses, reorientation and reassurance protocols, noise reduction, sleep optimization, early mobilization (EM), and the involvement of family, caregivers, or friends. Shortening the duration of critical care and ventilation is also essential for these patients.

Early Mobilization

Frail patients benefit significantly from EM programs that aim to preserve muscle mass and function, reducing the risk of functional decline.

Myopathy and neuropathy are other major complications that can arise during critical illness. They are linked to higher mortality rates, longer ventilation periods, extended hospital stays, decreased functional capacity and independence, and diminished quality of life (QoL). These complications, in turn, can lead to the onset or worsening of frailty.[12,13] EM, which may range from passive range of motion exercises to walking at least 50 feet, is crucial in the care of critically ill adults.

How Important is Rehabilitation?

After being admitted to critical care, many patients experience postintensive care syndrome (PICS), characterized by fatigue, neuropathy, muscle atrophy, malnutrition, cognitive impairments, and psychological issues. PICS affects about 64% of patients at 3 months and 56% at 12 months.[14] Postillness rehabilitation is essential for these patients, as it helps restore optimal function, preserves independence, and prevents the onset or worsening of frailty.

Nutritional Optimization

Malnutrition is common among frail patients. Implementing nutritional support plans, including protein supplementation and dietary modifications, can enhance recovery.

Some frail patients may experience reduced appetite, increased catabolism, and muscle or tissue wasting, highlighting the need for adequate nutrition to prevent malnutrition and further deterioration of frailty. Key strategies include minimizing feeding interruptions, frequently reassessing nutritional status, and initiating enteral nutrition within 48 hours of CICU admission. The European Society for Clinical Nutrition and Metabolism recommends appropriate macronutrient intake to reduce the incidence of frailty in critically ill older adults. A recent registry based randomized trial involving 1,329 critically ill patients with frailty found that higher protein intake (≥2.2 g/kg/day) was associated with a lower rate of discharge survival (46.1% vs. 50.2%, 95% CI 0.77–1.07, $p = 0.27$) and higher 60-day mortality (34.6% vs. 32.1%, 95% CI 0.92–1.26) compared to the standard protein dose (≤1.2 g/kg/day).

Do's and Dont's in Medication Management

Polypharmacy and inappropriate medication use can exacerbate frailty. Regular medication reviews and adjustments are essential to avoid adverse drug reactions and interactions. Polypharmacy and improper medication use can worsen frailty. To prevent adverse drug reactions and interactions, regular medication reviews and adjustments are crucial. Patients in the CICU often receive several new medications simultaneously, particularly frail older individuals with multiple comorbidities. These older, frail patients in the CICU are also at a higher risk of receiving inappropriate treatments.

FUTURE CRITICAL CARE PROTOCOLS

- There is no documented pharmacological intervention for treating or reversing frailty. Although some medications, such as alfacalcidol, teriparatide, piroxicam, testosterone, metformin, recombinant human chorionic gonadotropin, and capromorelin, show potential benefits, their impact on frailty is not yet clearly established. The use of delirium and sedation scales can improve care quality and outcomes for frail patients in critical care settings.
- Digital health technologies can aid in assessing and detecting frailty and can provide reminders for healthcare workers to implement early interventions.
- Including frailty assessments in critical care randomized controlled trials (RCTs) fosters the development of innovative interventions and improves the accuracy and efficiency of frailty detection.
- Electronic health records can be enhanced by establishing and promoting clear guidelines for multidisciplinary team consultations and by measuring frailty using hospital frailty risk scores.
- It is crucial to improve training and education to better identify frailty and postcritical care syndromes in the CICU.
- Involving palliative care for frail patients in critical care settings can support patient-centered decision-making, prevent unnecessary and futile interventions, and facilitate discussions about care goals.

Palliative Care

For severely frail patients with limited life expectancy, integrating palliative care principles can improve the QoL by focusing on symptom management and psychosocial support.

CONCLUSION

Frailty is a critical factor affecting outcomes in CICU patients. Effective assessment and management of frailty can lead to improved patient outcomes, including reduced mortality, shorter hospital stays, and decreased readmission rates. While multiple frailty assessment tools are available, selecting the most appropriate one for the clinical setting is essential. Comprehensive management strategies that address the unique needs of frail patients can enhance recovery and overall quality of care in CICUs. As the population ages, the focus on frailty in cardiac care will continue to grow, highlighting the need for ongoing research and development of best practices in this area. Focus on machine learning may help in future.

Frailty is prevalent among older patients admitted to the CICU and is linked to increased risks of both short- and long-term adverse outcomes. This often necessitates adjustments to standard CICU management practices. With the growing number of older patients being admitted to the CICU, a multimodal approach is essential for screening, diagnosing, and implementing evidence-based comprehensive treatment plans **(Figs. 3 and 4)**.

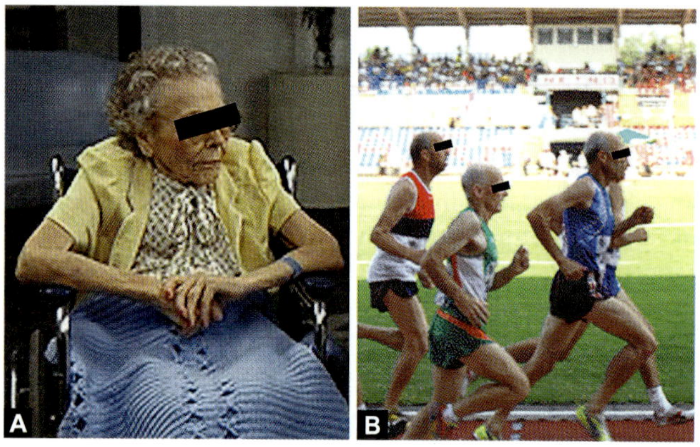

FIGS. 3A AND B: Frailty lies outside the comfort zone of guideline-based medicine.

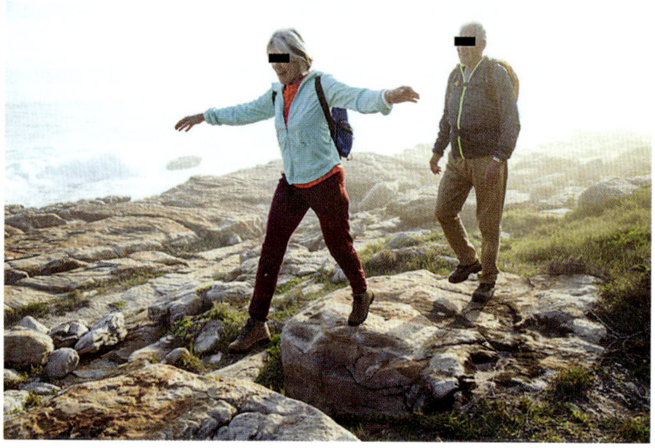

FIG. 4: Better balance prevents falls, builds confidence, and fosters independence.

ONLINE REFERENCES

Please scan the QR code provided at the end of the table of contents for References of this chapter.

SECTION

2

Echocardiography/Imaging

Section Outline

CHAPTER

10

Speckle-derived Strain: Technique, Applications, and Pitfalls

Manish Bansal, Ravi R Kasliwal

ABSTRACT

Speckle-tracking echocardiography (STE) is a grayscale-based technique used for quantifying myocardial deformation. Originally developed for left ventricular (LV) strain measurement, the technique has been expanded to other cardiac chambers also, especially the right ventricle and the left atrium. For each cardiac chamber, the STE-derived strain measurements have been shown to be more sensitive than the conventional echocardiographic parameters for detecting early cardiac dysfunction. These strain measurements have stronger prognostic value also. For these reasons, STE-based strain imaging is becoming an increasingly popular diagnostic modality. However, the lack of outcome studies showing the benefit of strain-guided management is currently the most important limitation of this technique.

Keywords: Global longitudinal strain, right ventricular strain, left atrial strain, reservoir strain

INTRODUCTION

Left ventricular (LV) systolic function is one of the most important prognostic factors in almost all forms of cardiac disorders. Hence, assessment of LV systolic function is an important goal of every echocardiographic examination performed, regardless of the indication. Ejection fraction (EF) is currently the most used parameter of LV systolic function in clinical practice. There are robust data to support its utility as a parameter with immense diagnostic, therapeutic, and prognostic implications. Despite this well-established utility, LVEF has several limitations.[1] Most important, it is not a true measure of myocardial contractile function. Instead, it just represents the proportion of the blood ejected from the left ventricle during each systole.

The search for a parameter that could allow direct assessment of the myocardial contractile function led to the advent of strain imaging. Although strain too is load dependent, it has distinct advantages over LVEF. Most important, it allows recognition of subclinical LV systolic dysfunction, which has considerable prognostic significance. For this reason, LV strain imaging has become an increasingly popular modality, finding its utility in several cardiac conditions. Although developed initially for the assessment of LV systolic function, strain imaging has now been extended to the other cardiac chambers also, especially the right ventricle and the left atrium. This chapter describes the basic technique of myocardial strain imaging, its applications, and the pitfalls.

WHAT IS MYOCARDIAL STRAIN?

In simple terms, myocardial strain refers to the percentage change in the length of a myocardial segment during any given phase of the cardiac cycle. Thus, if a 15-mm-long segment contracts and shortens to 10 mm, then the strain would be –33% (minus sign because of the reduction in the length). Conversely, if the same segment undergoes stretch and becomes 18 mm in length, then the strain would be +20%. The rate at which this shortening or lengthening occurs is known as the strain rate. In clinical practice, strain rate is not much used because of its poor signal-to-noise ratio.

HOW IS MYOCARDIAL STRAIN MEASURED?

Broadly, there are two main techniques of strain imaging—Doppler-based strain imaging and grayscale-based strain imaging or speckle-tracking echocardiography (STE). The Doppler-based strain has many limitations such as dependency on the angle of insonation, cumbersome measurement process, and poorer signal-to-noise ratio and is, therefore, not used.

Speckle-tracking echocardiography is currently the main echocardiographic modality used for strain imaging. It is a grayscale-based technique, which identifies the acoustic speckles present within an ultrasound image and tracks their motion over time. These acoustic speckles form because of the interaction of the ultrasound beam with the tissue as it traverses through the myocardium. By tracking the motion of these speckles during the cardiac cycle, the speckle-tracking software is able to analyze the pattern and the extent of the myocardial deformation. From these data, a comprehensive assessment of myocardial strain can be performed.

LEFT VENTRICULAR STRAIN IMAGING

The LV myocardium has a multilayered architecture with the myofibers arranged in different directions in the different layers. This arrangement of the myofibers allows the left ventricle to undergo a complex, multidimension deformation that is essential to its normal systolic and diastolic function. During systole, the left ventricle undergoes shortening in longitudinal and circumferential directions and thickens in the radial direction. In addition, it also undergoes rotation and twist. Each of these components can be quantified using STE.

Measurement of the Left Ventricular Strain

For measurement of the LV longitudinal strain, three apical views—namely apical four chamber, two chamber, and three chamber—are required.[2] Once good-quality images have been acquired, they are analyzed in the software available either on the echocardiography machine or on a stand-alone workstation. Once the image is opened in the software, the software typically displays the end-systolic frame with yo-yoing by a few frames before and after it. The first step now is to mark the LV endocardial border. The current generation systems can do this automatically, but if not available, then the border can be traced manually also. The border is traced from the basal segment of the LV myocardial wall near the mitral annulus to the other end of the mitral annulus near the base. The software then generates a region-of-interest (ROI), which is a few millimeters thick. The thickness of the ROI should be adjusted to include the full thickness of the myocardium, without extending into the pericardium. Once this adjustment is done, the software analyzes myocardial deformation and displays a cine loop showing the myocardial tracking. If the ROI appears to be tracking the myocardium properly, the tracking is accepted, and the software generates strain curves. Each LV view is divided into six segments and therefore six strain curves corresponding to each myocardial segment are displayed **(Fig. 1)**. Once this process is repeated with all the three apical views, the software generates a bull's-eye plot depicting the peak strain of each LV myocardial segment in a color-coded manner and provides the average of all the segmental strain values **(Fig. 2)**. This average is known as global longitudinal strain (GLS), which is clinically the most useful LV strain parameter.

In a similar manner, LV circumferential strain, radial strain, rotation, and twist can also be calculated **(Fig. 3)**.[2] For this, three short-axis views acquired at the LV base and mid and apical levels are required. The subsequent steps involved in the image analysis are same as for the longitudinal strain. Since the LV shortens in circumferential direction and thickens in the radial direction, circumferential strain has a negative value, and the radial strain has a positive value. In addition, the left ventricle undergoes rotation also, around its long axis, during each cardiac cycle. When viewed from the apical side, the LV apex rotates in an anticlockwise direction and the base rotates in the clockwise direction. By convention, the anticlockwise rotation is assigned a positive value and the clockwise rotation a negative value. Subtracting basal rotation from the apical rotation (which effectively means adding the two because of the opposite signs) yields the LV twist. Unlike strain, rotation and torsion are measured in degrees.

Avoiding Pitfalls

For accurate measurement of LV strain, careful attention to certain technical details is required:

- Good-quality grayscale images are essential for accurate strain analysis. All efforts must be made to optimize the images before acquiring them. Foreshortening of the images should be avoided.
- ECG gating is a must. A minimum of three cardiac cycles for each view should be acquired so that at least one untruncated cardiac cycle (the middle one) is always available for analysis.
- At normal heart rates, optimum frame rate for STE is in the range of 50–80 frames/s. Faster heart rates would need higher frame rates.
- While analyzing the images, the ROI width should be sufficient to cover the entire wall thickness but not too thick to extend beyond the myocardium.
- The ROI should follow the contour of the LV wall. It should not extend into the left atrium or the aortic root.
- Tracking should be proper and should follow the myocardial motion.

Clinical Applications of Left Ventricular Strain

As mentioned previously, the LV myocardium has a multilayered architecture. The longitudinal shortening is governed predominantly by the subendocardial fibers, whereas the mid-myocardial and subendocardial fibers

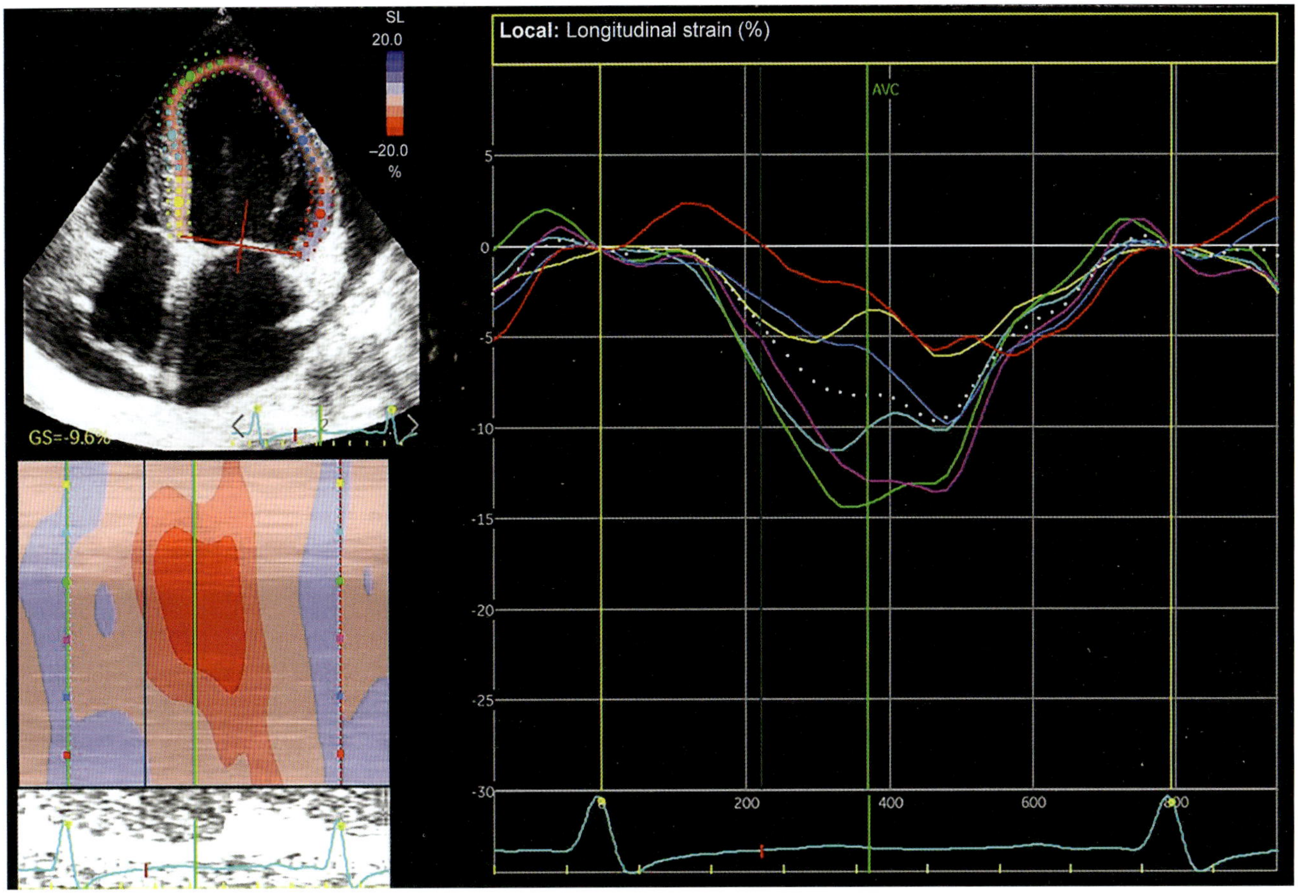

FIG. 1: Measurement of left ventricular longitudinal strain in an apical four-chamber view. The segmental strain curves are depicted.

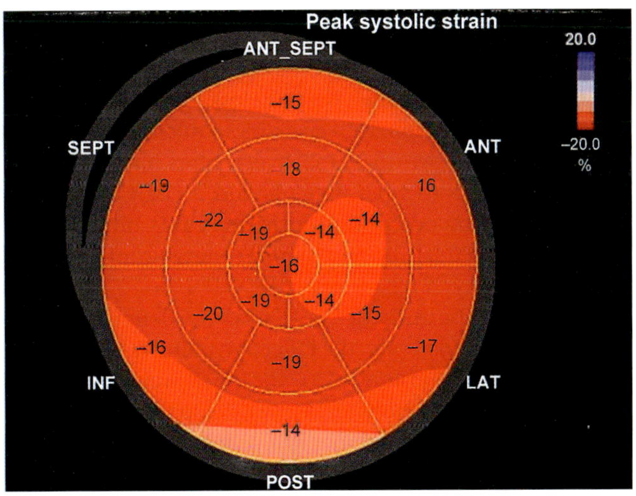

FIG. 2: The left ventricular longitudinal strain bull's-eye plot.

control the radial thickening, circumferential shortening, rotation, and twist.[2,3]

Since the subendocardial layer is the most susceptible to injury, longitudinal strain is generally the earliest to get impaired. For this reason, GLS has emerged as a reliable tool for detection of subclinical LV systolic dysfunction. Importantly, such subclinical LV systolic dysfunction manifesting as reduced GLS despite preserved LVEF has been shown to have significant negative prognostic value in a wide range of cardiac disorders. Hence, detection of subclinical LV systolic dysfunction has emerged as the most important application of LV strain imaging. The prognostic value of left ventricular global longitudinal strain (LVGLS) is supported by the observations that it correlates well with the extent of LV myocardial fibrosis as assessed using cardiac magnetic resonance (CMR) imaging or histopathology.[4,5]

An added advantage of LVGLS is that it is highly reproducible. The reproducibility of GLS is much superior to that of LVEF.[6] Unfortunately, the reproducibility of segmental longitudinal strain and the short-axis deformation parameters (i.e., radial and circumferential strain, rotation, and twist) is quite suboptimal rendering them unsuitable for routine clinical application.

Thus, LVGLS is the main LV strain parameter used for clinical purposes. Any cardiac condition in which detection of subclinical LV systolic dysfunction could be of relevance is a potential application for LV strain imaging. The most common uses of LV strain imaging are described below.

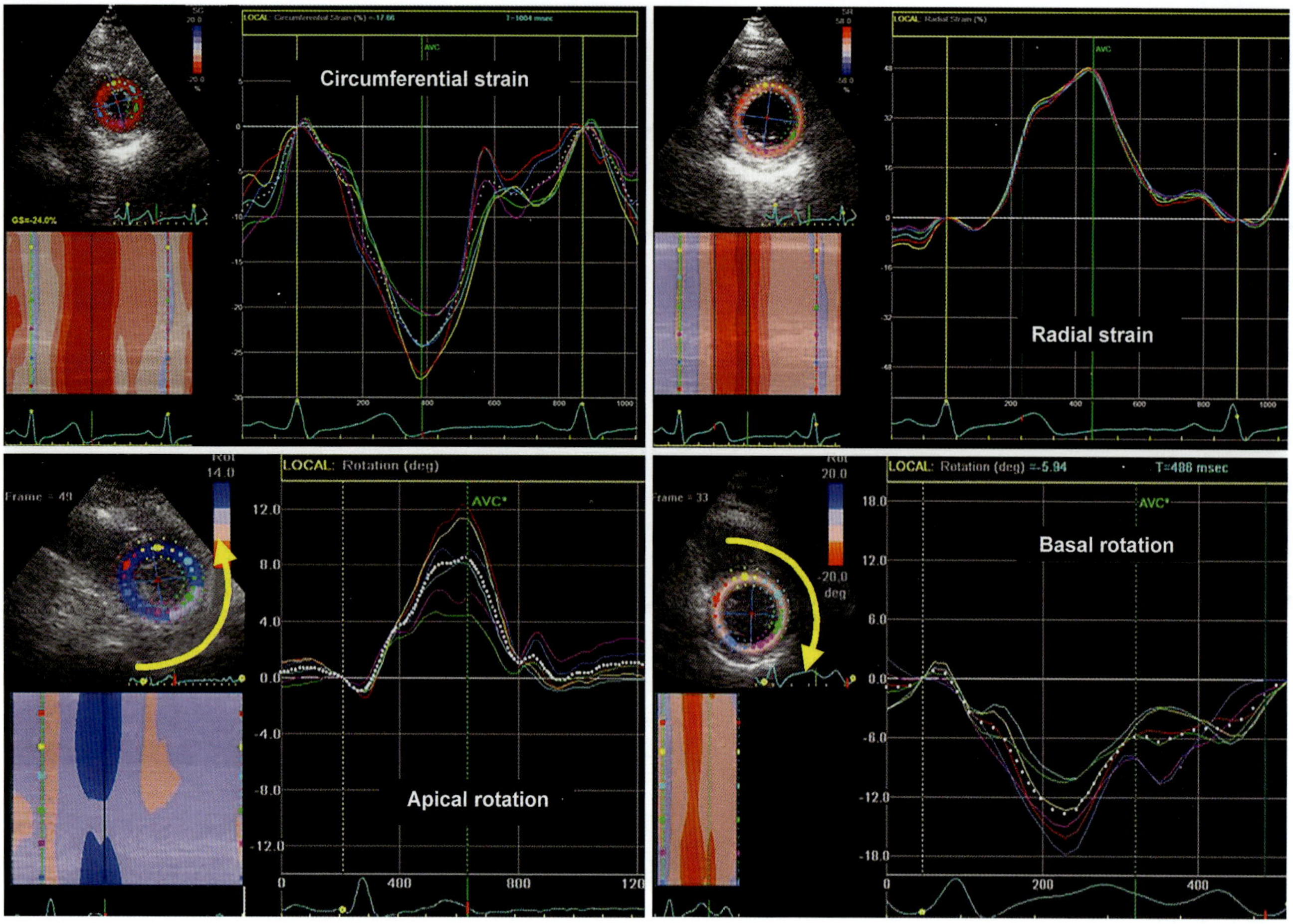

FIG. 3 Measurement of the short-axis deformation of the left ventricle using speckle-tracking echocardiography. Strain values are measured in percentages and rotation in degrees. Basal rotation is clockwise (when viewed from the left ventricular apex) and is assigned a negative value, whereas the apical rotation is counterclockwise and is assigned a positive value.

Valvular Heart Diseases

In patients with severe aortic stenosis (AS), aortic regurgitation (AR), and mitral regurgitation (MR), the two main class I indications for surgical intervention are symptoms and LV systolic dysfunction (LVEF < 60% for MR and <50% for AS and AR). It is now well recognized that both these events occur late in the course of the disease and do not represent the ideal threshold for intervention.[7]

Many recent studies have shown that LVGLS can detect ongoing myocardial damage in these valve lesions and identify the patients at increased risk for adverse events.[4,8-12] The use of LVGLS may therefore improve patient selection for intervention. A meta-analysis of 10 studies which included 1,067 patients with asymptomatic severe AS with preserved LVEF (LVEF >50%) showed that LVGLS was strongly associated with the adverse events. The all-cause mortality rose sharply as the LVGLS decreased below –14.7%.[9] This indicates that LVGLS below –14.7% may be used for referring patients for aortic valve intervention. Unfortunately, no randomized study is currently available to support this approach and hence, translating this into clinical practice has remained a challenge. Nonetheless, reduced LVGLS in patients with asymptomatic severe AS should at least prompt a more careful follow-up. Some investigators have suggested performing CMR in such patients and if CMR also shows significant LV myocardial fibrosis, then this may provide a stronger justification for offering intervention to these patients.[13]

The prognostic utility of LVGLS has been demonstrated in AR and MR also. However, the inflection point in AR has been demonstrated to be around –19% and in MR around –21%.[11,12] The patients having worse GLS than these thresholds have worse outcomes if treated medically. In contrast, in patients with better GLS, the outcomes are same regardless of whether they are treated medically or are subjected to surgery.

Cardio-oncology

Certain cancer therapeutic agents such as anthracyclines, trastuzumab, and alkylating agents have the potential to cause LV myocardial dysfunction. Early detection of such myocardial dysfunction is important to allow timely intervention. Addition of cardioprotective agents and modifying the chemotherapy regimen (minimizing the dose, using alternative agents) are the potential options.[14]

Left ventricular global longitudinal strain has been shown to be useful for early detection of cancer therapy-related cardiac dysfunction.[15] A 15% relative reduction in GLS from the baseline is considered significant.[14] Many observational studies have shown that in patients with cancer therapy-induced subclinical LV systolic dysfunction, treatment with cardioprotective agents such as beta-blockers may prevent further myocardial damage and the development of frank cardiac dysfunction and heart failure.[16] Unfortunately, a recent randomized study [Strain Surveillance of Chemotherapy for Improving Cardiovascular Outcomes (SUCCOUR)] of 331 patients at risk for cardiotoxicity failed to show the benefit of strain-based approach in preventing overt cardiac dysfunction.[17] However, in this study, the overall incidence of cardiotoxicity was low and this may have been the reason why strain imaging did not prove to be helpful.

Heart Failure

Heart failure with preserved EF (HFpEF) is becoming an increasingly common form of heart failure. Although LV diastolic dysfunction is the dominant cardiac abnormality in these patients, studies using strain imaging have shown that nearly half of all patients with HFpEF have evidence of subclinical LV systolic dysfunction.[18] Furthermore, LVGLS has been shown to be associated with the risk of heart failure hospitalization and cardiovascular death in this setting.[18,19] Based on these observations, reduced LVGLS is included as one of the echocardiographic criteria for diagnosing HFpEF.[20]

Even in patients with heart failure with reduced EF (HFrEF), LVGLS has prognostic value which is incremental to LVEF.[21,22] In a study of >4,500 patients hospitalized with acute heart failure, LVGLS was a stronger predictor of 5-year all-cause mortality than LVEF. It could predict all-cause mortality regardless of whether the LVEF was <40%, ≥40% to <50%, or ≥50%.[22]

Lastly, LVGLS is also helpful in detecting stage B heart failure which refers to a condition in which LV myocardial diseases is present, but clinical heart failure has not occurred. LVGLS can predict adverse events in these patients and may help guide the management.[23-25]

Cardiomyopathies

Cardiomyopathies, by definition, are primary diseases of the myocardium. Hence, some degree of myocardial dysfunction is ubiquitous in cardiomyopathies. Absolutely normal LVGLS argues against the diagnosis of LV cardiomyopathy, regardless of whether it is dilated cardiomyopathy, hypertrophic cardiomyopathy (HCM), restrictive cardiomyopathy (RCM), or arrhythmogenic cardiomyopathy. For this reason, LVGLS can be used for differentiating various cardiomyopathies from other conditions that may phenotypically mimic them (e.g., hypertensive heart disease and athlete's heart mimicking HCM and constrictive pericarditis mimicking RCM) **(Fig. 4)**.[1,26] In addition, in some cases, the pattern of myocardial dysfunction may also help in identifying the underlying etiology. Cardiac amyloidosis is a classic example in which relative LV apical sparing or the so-called "cherry-on-top" appearance of the LVGLS bull's-eye plot is a characteristic finding (albeit not very specific) **(Fig. 5)**.[27]

Apart from the diagnostic role as described above, LVGLS is also a strong predictor of clinical outcomes in all forms of cardiomyopathies.[1,26]

Other Disorders

Left ventricular global longitudinal strain can be used for detecting subclinical LV systolic dysfunction in a wide variety of noncardiac conditions.[28] These include systemic

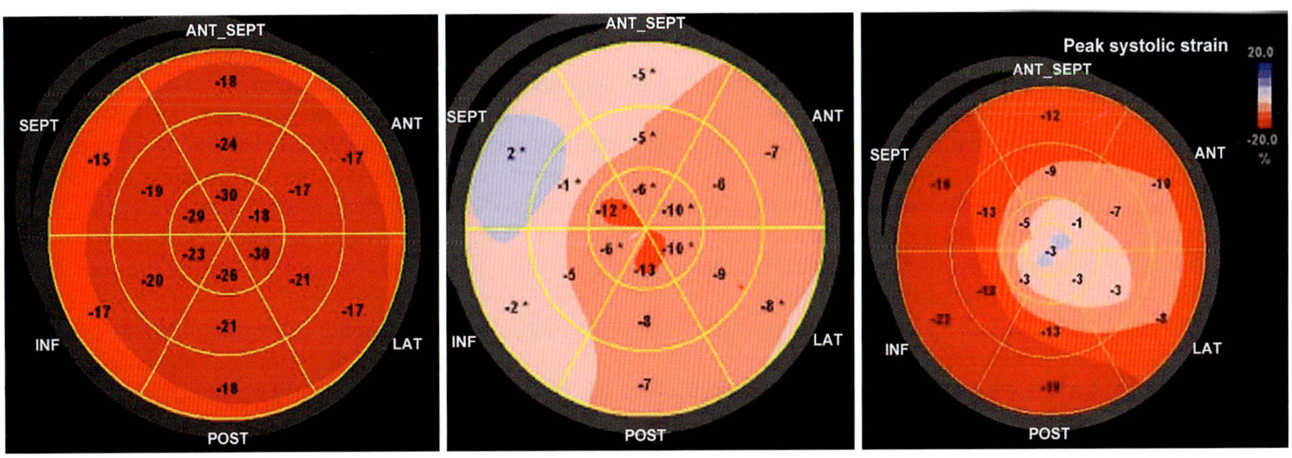

FIG. 4: The left ventricular longitudinal strain bull's-eye plots in athlete's heart (left image), a patient with hypertrophic cardiomyopathy with asymmetrical septal hypertrophy (center image), and a patient with apical hypertrophic cardiomyopathy (right image). Note how the strain values are reduced in the abnormal myocardium in hypertrophic cardiomyopathy but are normal in the athlete's heart.

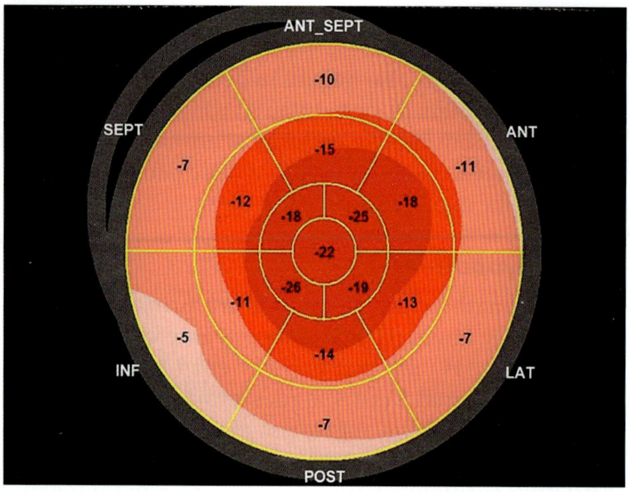

FIG. 5: Relative apical sparing of the left ventricular longitudinal strain giving rise to the "cherry-on-top" appearance in the bull's-eye plot in a patient with cardiac amyloidosis.

diseases such as obesity, hypertension, diabetes, obstructive sleep apnea, chronic liver disease, chronic kidney disease, viral infections such as dengue fever and coronavirus disease 2019, connective tissue diseases such as systemic lupus erythematosus, and hematological diseases such as thalassemia and sickle cell anemia.

Limitations of Left Ventricular Global Longitudinal Strain

Although LVGLS had emerged as a useful measure of LV myocardial function with significant diagnostic, prognostic, and therapeutic implications, it has some limitations that need to be borne in mind:

- The most important limitation of LVGLS is that at present, there are no outcome data available to show that strain-guided management truly improves clinical outcomes as compared to the conventional approach. This type of validation is essential for strain imaging to become widely adopted in clinical practice. As mentioned above, SUCCOUR is the only randomized study that has compared LVGLS-based management with LVEF-based management. This trial, unfortunately, did not show benefit with strain imaging, though the low event rates in this study likely compromised the power of the study.[17]
- STE is heavily dependent on image quality and therefore, careful attention to technical details is necessary, as described above.
- Just like any other imaging modality, STE also requires sufficient technical expertise for accurate results. Although the learning curve with STE is relatively short, the importance of requisite training and experience should not be overlooked.[29]
- One of the major limitations of LVEF is that it is influenced by the loading conditions. Unfortunately, LVGLS tool is load dependent. Strain rate is relatively load independent. Myocardial work, which is derived using STE-based longitudinal strain, is currently the closest echocardiographic measure of myocardial contractile function.[30]
- Strain imaging has generally been software dependent with different STE software and even the different versions of the same software providing different results. However, this vendor and software dependency has now considerably reduced due to collective efforts of the leading echocardiography societies and the various industry partners.[31] Nevertheless, it is still desirable to use the same software and version for serially following up the patients.

RIGHT VENTRICULAR STRAIN

The assessment of RV systolic function is even more challenging than that for the left ventricle. The right ventricle has a teapot-like shape because of which it is impossible to image it in any single echocardiographic projection. As a result, RV volumes and EF cannot be measured with two-dimensional echocardiography. Three-dimensional echocardiography overcomes this challenge but requires very good-quality images and is not easily available. Hence, the assessment of RV systolic function at present is limited to parameters such as tricuspid annular plane systolic excursion (TAPSE), tricuspid annular systolic velocity (TASV), and fractional area change (FAC), all of which have their own limitations. RV longitudinal strain offers an excellent solution to this problem because of its ease of measurement and the ability to quantify myocardial contraction without getting affected by the tethering or translational effects.

Measurement of Right Ventricular Strain

Unlike the left ventricle, the right ventricle contracts mainly in the longitudinal direction and hence, only longitudinal strain is measured for the right ventricle.

For RV strain measurement, an RV-focused apical four-chamber view should be acquired.[32,33] The conventional apical four-chamber view provides lower values of RV strain.[34] ECG gating, good image quality, and avoiding artifacts are all very important, as outlined for the left ventricle. The image is then analyzed using the dedicated RV strain tool available on the system. An ROI is created which extends from the base of the RV free wall near the lateral tricuspid annulus to the base of the interventricular septum. The ROI width should be optimum to cover the full thickness of the RV free wall (~5 mm). A too thick ROI underestimates RV strain, whereas a too thin ROI overestimates it. The software then analyzes the RV deformation and displays a cine loop showing the tracking. Once satisfactory tracking is confirmed, segmental RV strain curves are generated. The software also provides the average of the peak systolic strain of the three segments of the RV free wall [RV free wall longitudinal strain (RVFWLS)] as well as an average of all the six segments [RV four-chamber longitudinal strain (RV4CLS)] **(Fig. 6)**. The RVFWLS has a higher value than RV4CLS and is the recommended measurement for clinical use.[35]

The RVFWLS values vary according to the age, gender, software/vendor, echocardiographic view (RV focused or conventional), and analysis technique (dedicated software, free wall vs. four-chamber strain). A meta-analysis of studies involving 1,143 subjects and using EchoPAC software (developed by the General Electric) reported mean RVFWLS as 28.5 ± 4.8% with lower limit of normal being 20.2%.[32]

Clinical Applications

Right ventricular strain has been shown to be a sensitive marker of RV systolic dysfunction and often provides incremental information above the conventional measures of RV systolic function. Any cardiac or noncardiac condition that can lead to RV systolic dysfunction has a use for RV strain.

Pulmonary Hypertension

In patients with pulmonary hypertension (PH), RVFWLS can detect RV systolic dysfunction earlier than other parameters such as TAPSE and is an independent predictor of adverse outcomes **(Figs. 7A to D)**. In a study of 57 patients with PH and RV dysfunction but with normal TAPSE, RVFWLS ≥–20% (i.e., less negative than 20%) was a significant predictor of all-cause mortality (hazard ratio 3.76, 95% confidence interval 1.02–13.92) at approximately 28-month follow-up.[36] There are several other studies that have shown that RVFWLS predicts all-cause mortality and other adverse cardiovascular events in patients with PH and is superior to TAPSE, TASV, and RV FAC for this purpose.[37-40] A meta-analysis of 11 studies with 1,169 patients with PH confirmed that a relative reduction of RVFWLS of 19% was a predictor of the composite end point of all-cause mortality and PH-related events, whereas a relative reduction of 22% predicted all-cause mortality.[41]

Right ventricular free wall longitudinal strain can also be used for monitoring disease progression and treatment response in PH. In a study of 50 patients receiving treatment for PH, it was found that the persistence of or progression to a severe reduction in RVFWLS (<–12.5%) at 6 months was associated with greater disease severity and worse survival. Conversely, a 5% or more improvement in RVFWLS was associated with more than sevenfold lower mortality risk at 4 years.[42]

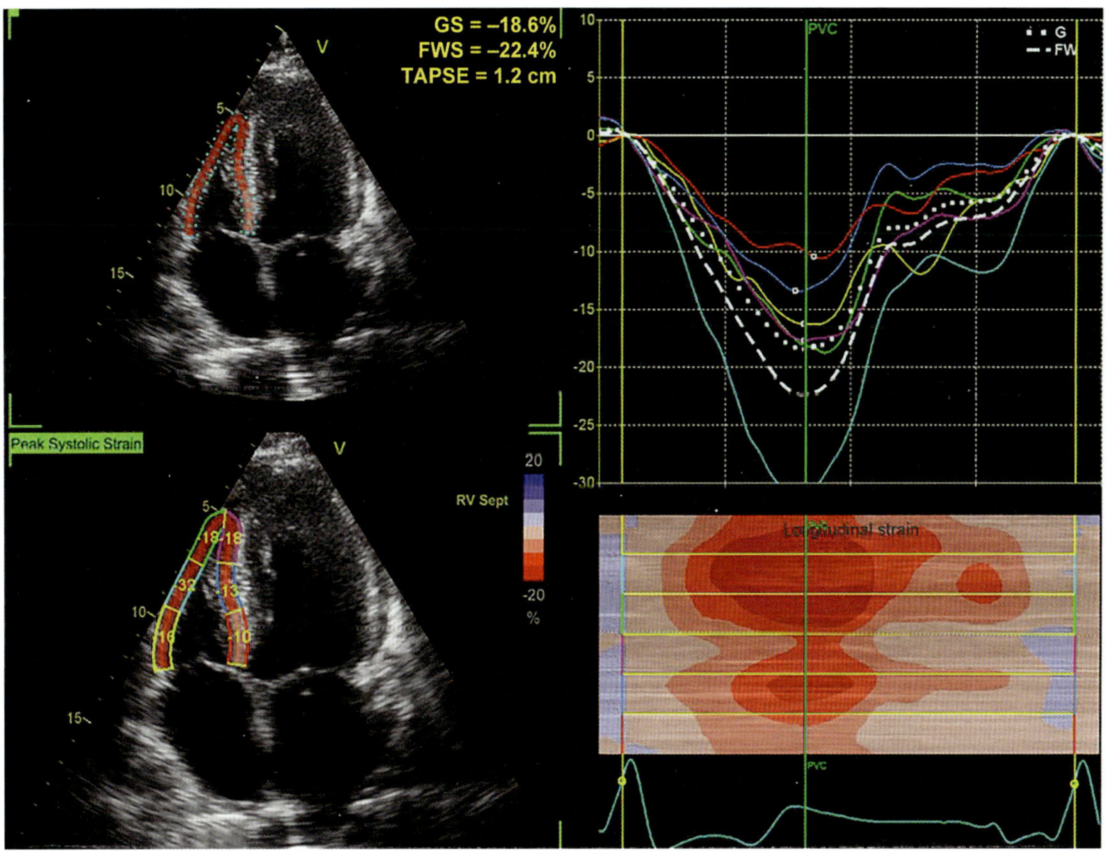

FIG. 6: Measurement of right ventricular (RV) longitudinal strain.

(FWS: RV free wall strain; GS: global longitudinal strain referring to the RV four-chamber strain; TAPSE: tricuspid annular plane systolic excursion)

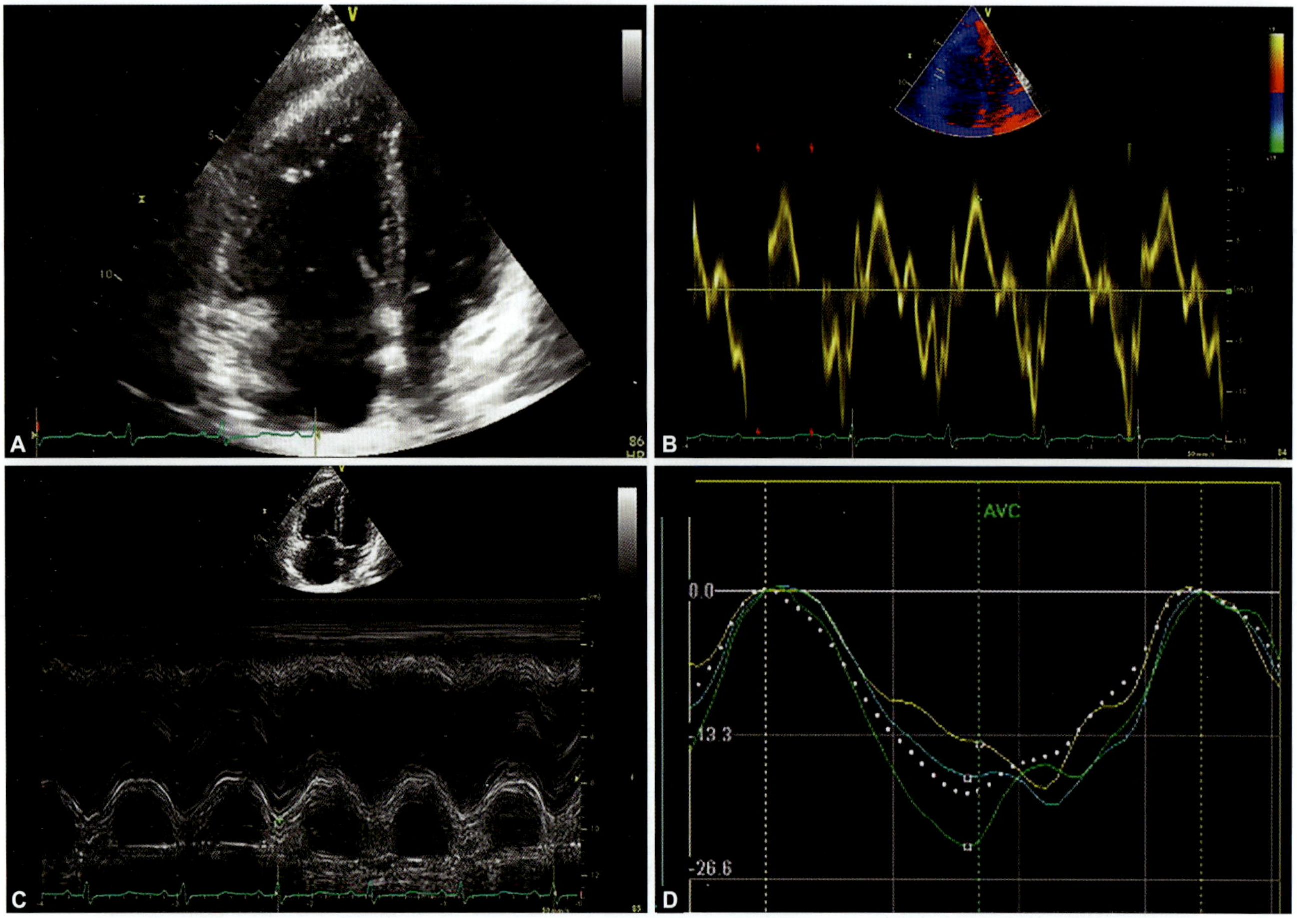

FIGS. 7A TO D: Fallacy of the conventional measures of the right ventricular systolic function. (A) Dilated right ventricle; (B) Near-normal tricuspid annular systolic velocity; (C) Near-normal tricuspid annular plane systolic excursion; (D) Significantly reduced (16–17%) right ventricular free wall strain.

Heart Failure

Both RVFWLS and RV4CLS are commonly reduced in patients with HFrEF and HFpEF.[43] RV strain can detect subclinical RV systolic dysfunction in these patients and is associated with symptomatic status and functional class.[43,44] It is also a predictor of heart failure hospitalization, all-cause mortality, and other adverse outcomes.[45-47] RV strain is also helpful in predicting adverse outcomes in heart transplant recipients.[48]

Tricuspid Regurgitation

Right ventricular free wall longitudinal strain is a strong predictor of all-cause mortality in patients with tricuspid regurgitation. Its predictive accuracy is superior to that of RV FAC and TASV and independent of the comorbidities and the functional status.[49,50]

Congenital Heart Diseases

There has been an increasing interest in using RV strain for assessing RV function in patients with congenital heart diseases associated with RV overload. A few studies have used RVFWLS to diagnose RV systolic dysfunction and to predict outcomes in patients with repaired tetralogy of Fallot.[51-54]

Limitations

All the limitations of STE apply to RV strain measurement also. In fact, RV strain measurement is more challenging than LV strain measurement, because of the thinner RV wall, poor endocardial delineation, and presence of multiple trabeculae. The use of the conventional apical four-chamber view instead of the RV-focused four-chamber view also adds to the measurement error.

LEFT ATRIAL STRAIN

The left atrium is in direct continuity with the LV cavity during the diastole. Hence, any abnormality of LV diastolic function adversely affects the left atrium, leading to left atrial (LA) remodeling. The degree of such LA remodeling serves as a surrogate measure of the LV diastolic dysfunction. LA remodeling also occurs in atrial fibrillation (AF), rheumatic heart disease, and atrial cardiomyopathy, which directly affect the LA structure and function, without the involvement of the left ventricle. Traditionally, the LA size (previously LA diameter, and more recently, LA volume) has been used for this purpose, but it has many limitations. LA strain imaging has emerged as a useful alternative with many advantages.

Measurement and Interpretation of Left Atrial Strain

The overall principles of the LA strain imaging are same as those for LV and RV strain imaging. Like the right ventricle, only longitudinal strain is measured for the left atrium also.

For LA strain imaging, the LA-focused apical four- or two-chamber view is required. A good-quality image with ECG gating is necessary. The image is then analyzed using the STE software. The LA endocardial border is traced from one end of the mitral annulus to the other without entering the pulmonary veins and the LA appendage. The ROI for LA strain is thinner (usually 3 mm) than the one used for LV strain analysis.[33,55]

Figure 8 shows a typical LA strain curve with QRS as the reference point. The left atrium undergoes stretching during the ventricular systole resulting in a positive wave. This is followed by a reduction in LA strain once the mitral valve opens and the left atrium ejects blood into the left ventricle. The peak LA strain which coincides with the T wave on the ECG represents the reservoir strain and is known as LA reservoir strain (LARS) or the peak atrial longitudinal strain (PALS). Clinically, this is the most important LA strain parameter.

The normal value of LARS has been shown to be around 39% (95% confidence interval 38–41%)[56] with 22–23% being considered the lower limit of the normal.[57]

Clinical Applications

Left atrial volume index (LAVI) is the currently recommended echocardiographic parameter for assessing LV diastolic function and LV filling pressure (LVFP). However, the increase in LA size occurs only with a sustained elevation in LVFP. In contrast, LA strain is a more sensitive measure of raised LVFP.[58] Hemodynamic and CMR studies have shown good correlation between LARS and invasively measured LVFP and LA myocardial fibrosis, respectively.[59,60] LARS also correlates with the postexercise LVFP.[61]

Many studies have shown that LARS is impaired in patients with LV diastolic dysfunction who have normal LAVI.[62-64] It is also able to more accurately distinguish between the different grades of LV diastolic dysfunction.[63] For these reasons, the incorporation of LARS either in addition to or in place of LAVI, in the algorithm proposed by the American Society of Echocardiography for diagnosing LV diastolic dysfunction, significantly improved the diagnostic accuracy of the algorithm.[62]

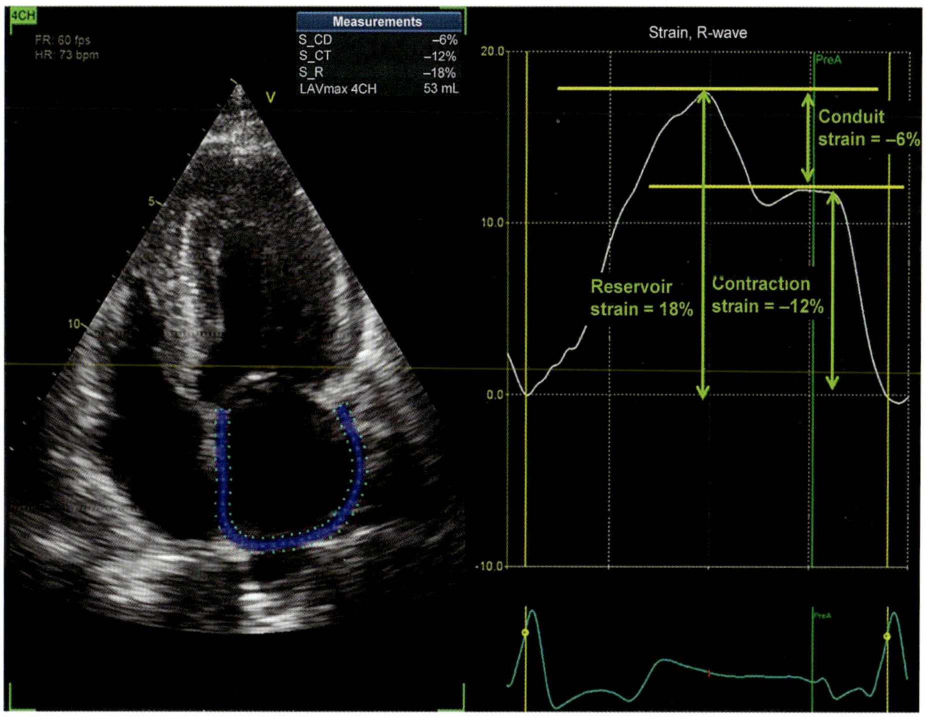

FIG. 8: Left atrial strain measurement using QRS as the reference point. There is an initial positive wave during ventricular systole which is followed by reduction in strain during early rapid filling phase and subsequently during active atrial contraction. The reservoir strain was calculated as 18%, conduit strain as 12–18 = –6%, and contraction strain as 0–12% = –12%.

(LAVmax 4CH: left atrial volume in the four-chamber view; S_CD: conduit strain; S_CT: contraction strain; S_R: reservoir strain)

Left atrial reservoir strain also correlates well with the symptoms and the overall functional status of the patients with LV diastolic dysfunction and HFpEF,[65-68] and can distinguish between noncardiac and cardiac causes of dyspnea. It shows good agreement with or even superior accuracy than the currently recommended algorithms for diagnosing HFpEF.[61,64,69-72]

It is also of interest that impaired LARS does not merely have diagnostic value but is also a marker of increased risk of adverse cardiac events. It is associated with the risk of AF, stroke, myocardial infarctions, heart failure hospitalization, and cardiovascular as well as all-cause mortality.[62,73-78]

The role of LARS in predicting AF and stroke is especially important. LARS predicts AF in many clinical settings, including after cardioversion or catheter ablation.[73-75,79-88] For prediction of stroke risk in AF, LARS has incremental value over CHA_2DS_2-VASc score.[76,77]

Limitations

There are several technical challenges in accurate LA strain measurement. The presence of the left atrium in the far field of the image sector, thin LA wall, mobility of the interatrial septum, and echocardiographic dropouts due to fossa ovalis, pulmonary veins, and LA appendage all tend to compromise the accuracy of LA strain measurement. In addition, more data are needed to establish the utility of LA strain for routine clinical adoption.

CONCLUSION

Speckle-tracking echocardiography is a useful modality for assessing myocardial deformation. The STE-derived LVGLS, RVFWLS, and LARS have been shown to be more sensitive for detecting respective cardiac chamber dysfunction than the conventional echocardiographic parameters. These strain measurements also have stronger prognostic value. However, the lack of outcome data showing the superiority of strain-guided management is currently the main reason limiting their wider use. In addition, it is also important to pay careful attention to the technical details and training requirements for accurate strain measurement.

ONLINE REFERENCES

Please scan the QR code provided at the end of the table of contents for References of this chapter.

CHAPTER

11

Impact of Bedside Echocardiography in Clinical Cardiology

Vibhav Sharma, Satyavir Yadav

ABSTRACT

A bedside screening echocardiographic examination is an indispensable adjunct to managing patients in critical care units, more so in cardiac ICUs. It is a rapid and widely available investigation, which not only provides a quick overview of cardiac function but also helps diagnose a variety of life-threatening conditions like acute coronary syndromes, cardiac tamponade, acute pulmonary embolism, aortic dissection, etc. A thorough hemodynamic assessment, aptly known as "echodynamics" that has shown fair positive correlation with invasive hemodynamic assessment can also be performed.

Keywords: Myocardial infarction, cardiac tamponade, pulmonary embolism, hemodynamics, aortic dissection

INTRODUCTION

A bedside echocardiogram that is synonymous with POCUS (point-of-care ultrasound) is a valuable tool that is easily and freely accessible in cardiac ICUs and provides rapid diagnostic and prognostic information in critically ill cardiac patients. A cardiac POCUS is performed by a broad range of practitioners, not just cardiologists, and is a promising tool for diagnosing several cardiac conditions in emergency as well as ICU settings. Traditionally, impetus has been on focused assessment of the parameter in question rather than a detailed two-dimensional echocardiography. Predominantly, the focus has been on identification of "vital" findings like ventricular function, regional wall motion abnormalities, tamponade physiology, and pulmonary embolism. This chapter aims to summarize current evidence regarding its use in contemporary critical care cardiology. Since this chapter is aimed at discussing the updates, we will limit our discussion to recent evidence supporting the use of bedside cardiac echocardiography in cardiac emergencies like myocardial infarction (MI), cardiogenic shock and heart failure, cardiac tamponade, pulmonary embolism, and aortic dissection without going into the details of performing a cardiac ultrasound.

MYOCARDIAL INFARCTION

A bedside echocardiogram is not a mandatory requirement before proceeding to emergent reperfusion therapy to avoid unnecessary delay in institution of such therapies; however, it is helpful in patients presenting with acute chest pain where an ECG and troponin are negative and presence of wall motion abnormalities weigh in favor of coronary artery disease. Similarly, assessment of cardiac function may be done in acute coronary syndrome (ACS) setting to guide further management.

With the widespread adoption of prompt reperfusion therapy, the incidence of mechanical complications of MI has come down significantly. Bedside echocardiography will continue to remain an essential diagnostic tool for prompt diagnosis of such complications, namely, acute mitral regurgitation (MR) secondary to papillary muscle rupture, LV free wall rupture and pseudoaneurysms, and rupture of the interventricular septum.

Acute Mitral Regurgitation Secondary to Papillary Muscle Rupture

Acute mitral regurgitation with severity varying between mild to severe is common after acute MI. Underlying mechanisms include basal inferior wall hypokinesia or akinesia and posterior mitral leaflet tethering secondary to LV dilation. But papillary muscle rupture causing acute severe MR leads to sudden worsening of hemodynamics and has, in general, a poor prognosis. Bedside echocardiography helps in identifying the various mechanisms of MR and papillary muscle rupture. If not identified on transthoracic echocardiography, a transesophageal echocardiography examination may be warranted. Partial- or complete-thickness tear of the papillary muscles may be identified leading to flail leaflets with attached chordae moving to and fro with each heartbeat. In the absence of preexisting heart disease, left chamber dimensions will typically be normal despite presence of hemodynamically severe regurgitation. Eccentric jets on color Doppler are frequently underestimated and quantitative measures of regurgitation like regurgitant volume, vena contracta, etc., are not reliable in presence of clinical instability. Pulmonary vein systolic flow reversal denotes severe MR and continuous wave Doppler profile usually has a velocity <5 cm/s owing to sudden rise in left atrial pressure, is triangular in shape, and shows an early peaking.

Ventricular Septal Rupture

Septal ruptures following an anterior wall MI tend to be apical and simple, whereas those following an inferior infarct are usually basally located and lead to tunneled defects, occasionally giving the appearance of ventricular septal dissections. Color Doppler examination allows identification of turbulent jets traveling from LV to RV. LV-to-RV gradient can be calculated by the help of continuous wave Doppler and pulmonary artery (PA) pressures can be estimated, giving indirect evidence of the volume of shunting.

Free Wall Rupture

Free wall rupture is detected by accumulation of echogenic fluid within the pericardial cavity. This may or may not be associated with features of cardiac tamponade. Color Doppler helps in identifying free flow of blood into the pericardial space and helps localize the site of rupture. In cases of RV free wall rupture, agitated saline helps confirm the diagnosis.

LV Pseudoaneurysm and Aneurysm

It is important to differentiate pseudoaneurysms from true aneurysms. Pseudoaneurysms usually have a narrow neck, which is less than half the maximum diameter of the aneurysm whereas true aneurysms usually are broad-based. Pseudoaneurysms are usually associated with an obvious defect on echocardiography overlying which a layered clot or echogenic pericardial fluid may be appreciated.

LV Clot

After an acute MI, LV clots are usually seen at LV apex following a large anterior infarct and in posterobasal areas following an inferior infarct. Early detection is important to institute prompt anticoagulation to prevent systemic embolism.

OPTIMIZING MANAGEMENT OF CARDIOGENIC SHOCK

A knowledge of invasive hemodynamics helps in phenotyping patients with acute decompensated heart failure (ADHF) with cardiogenic shock and guide patient management. However, invasive assessment is rarely feasible in these critically ill patients. Following are some bedside echocardiographic parameters that have been recently shown to correlate fairly with invasively measured parameters of diagnostic and prognostic significance.

- *RV contraction pressure index (RVCPI)*: It is an echo-Doppler-derived measurement of RV function, which was shown to have a sensitivity and specificity of 92% and 85%, respectively to identify reduced invasively derived RV stroke work index (RVSWI) with a cutoff <400 mm·mm Hg. It correlated well with reduced RVSWI in a prospective study of 94 patients with severe left ventricular (LV) dysfunction and NYHA IV heart failure.[1] Simplified RVCPI is calculated as TAPSE × (RV – RA pressure gradient), and RVSWI is calculated as stroke volume index × (mPAP – mRAP).
- *RV to PA coupling*: A low TAPSE/PASP ratio (<0.38 mm/mm Hg) strongly predicts maladaptive left and right ventricular (RV) remodeling and a poor prognosis. This cutoff was derived in a validation cohort of 111 patients with ischemic and nonischemic cardiomyopathy.[2]
- *PA pulsatility index*: It is the ratio of the PA pulse pressure to right atrial pressure. A heterogeneous subset of 8,285 consecutive patients undergoing right heart catheterization was prospectively followed up for 6.7 ± 3.3 years and stratified into quartiles with median values of 1.7, 2.8, 4.2, and 8.7, respectively. Those in the lowest quartile had highest risk of MACE and heart failure hospitalizations.[3]
- *Cardiac output (CO) assessment on echocardiography*: Thermodilution remains the gold standard for measurement of CO. Echocardiographically, CO can be assessed by: (a) CO = left ventricular outflow tract (LVOT) cross-sectional area × LVOT VTI × HR and (b) CO = (End-diastolic volume – end-systolic volume measured by Simpson's method) × HR. Previous studies had contradictory results with some showing echocardiographic CO to be a rapid and accurate measure whereas others showing a poor correlation with invasively measured CO. However, in a 2019 meta-analysis of 41 studies comprising 1,522 subjects, there was no significant difference in CO measured by echocardiography versus thermodilution. On subgroup analysis, no significant difference was found between transthoracic and transesophageal echocardiography. However, the reliability goes down in presence of a high CO states, sedation, and presence of structural heart disease.[4]

In a prospective observational study from Italy,[5] 101 consecutive heart failure patients with cardiogenic shock patients underwent echocardiographic hemodynamic assessment 30 minutes prior to cardiac catheterization. Following echocardiographic parameters were measured (prefix *e* denotes echocardiographic):

- *Mean estimated RA pressure (eRAP)*: Average of eRAP derived from three parameters: (1) IVC diameter and collapse, (2) hepatic venous flow pattern, and (3) Tricuspid E/e' ratio
- *Systolic PA pressure (eSPAP)*: Peak tricuspid regurgitation (TR) pressure gradient plus eRAP
- *Diastolic PA pressure (eDPAP)*: 4 × squared end-diastolic PR velocity + eRAP
- *Pulmonary vascular resistance (ePVR)*: Peak TR velocity/ RVOT VTI
- *PA pulsatility index (ePAPi)*: (sPAP - dPAP)/eRAP
- *Simplified ePAPi*: Peak TR pressure gradient/eRAP
- *RVCPI*: TAPSE/TR pressure gradient
- *Echocardiographic wedge pressure (eWP)*: TR peak gradient/2 (in patients without known pulmonary arterial hypertension).
- *Echocardiographic cardiac output (eCO)*: LVOT VTI × LVOT area × heart rate

These echocardiography-derived parameters showed a good correlation with invasively-measured parameters **(Table 1)**.

This study also showed good correlation between echocardiography and invasive hemodynamics in classifying shock phenotypes into LV predominant, RV predominant, or biventricular types (71% of the patients were correctly identified), whereas 60% of patients were correctly classified into clinical phenotypes based on the Diamond-Forrester classification. An overestimation of wedge pressure by echocardiography was mostly responsible for misclassifying dry patients into a wet phenotype. Reduced ePAPi was significantly associated with increased 60-day mortality. There was a good correlation between ePAPi and iPAPi at lower values of ePAPi, in which range it was useful to discriminate LV predominant heart failure from biventricular failure, but this correlation became weaker at higher values. This study is the first prospective study to validate the prognostic significance of echodynamic parameters against the invasive hemodynamic gold standard in the setting of acute cardiogenic shock complicating ADHF. Previously, studies conducted in ADHF patients have demonstrated reliability of these parameters.

TABLE 1: Correlation between echocardiographically-derived and invasively-measured hemodynamic parameters in 101 patients with ADHF–cardiogenic shock.[5]

Parameter	Correlation coefficient (r)	Sensitivity	Specificity
Cardiac index	0.88 ($p < 0.001$)	97%	73%
Systolic PA pressure	0.91 ($p < 0.001$)	87%	63%
Right atrial pressure	0.86 ($p < 0.001$)	90%	83%
Cardiac power output	0.82 ($p < 0.001$)	76%	85%
Pulmonary artery pulsatility index	0.67 ($p < 0.001$)	89%	92%
Wedge pressure	0.34 ($p = 0.01$)	84%	55%

ECHOCARDIOGRAPHY IN ACUTE PULMONARY EMBOLISM

Echocardiography has a prognostic and diagnostic role in pulmonary embolism. Its main role is in risk stratification, with a rather limited role in diagnosis when pretest probability of PTE is high and CT is not immediately feasible. With both, a sensitivity of ~50% and a NPV of ~50%, it has a limited role as a screening tool.[6] Its role in risk stratification of confirmed PTE is well established—a hemodynamically stable patient with elevated troponin is classified into sub-massive high or sub-massive low-risk categories based on the presence or absence of RV dysfunction, respectively.

- *RV dilation and dysfunction:* The prevalence of RV dysfunction in normotensive patients with acute PTE is 31%.[7] Normal RV measures <two-thirds the LV in apical four-chamber view. Dimensions greater than 41 and 35 mm, respectively at basal and mid RV as well as the cardiac apex formed by RV in the same view suggest RV dilation. TAPSE <17 mm correlates well with RV dysfunction in acute PTE. RV Tei index >0.43, RV fractional area change <35%, RVS' <10 cm/s, and RV global strain <–20% are all suggestive of RV dysfunction. An important point to remember is that measures of longitudinal RV function such as TAPSE and RVS' may be falsely normal due to regional RV dysfunction in acute PTE and measures of global RV function such as Tei index and fractional area change are hence more reliable. RV free wall strain, Tei index, and RV global and longitudinal strains more reliably predict a poor prognosis.[8,9]
- *Measures of stroke volume:* A LVOT VTI <15 cm/s was shown to be associated with 6 times greater likelihood of death and 23 times greater likelihood of shock and need for reperfusion in a retrospective study.[10] RVOT VTI <9.5 cm/s predicts low-indexed CO and increased risk of mortality.[11] There should be no outflow tract obstruction and pulsed-wave Doppler should be well aligned with the direction of flow with an angle no greater than 20°to avoid measuring falsely low VTI.
- *RA–PA coupling:* Whenever RV afterload increases, contractility increases appropriately till a certain point where RV failure occurs. TAPSE/PASP ratio measures this phenomenon and a value <0.4 denotes high risk of hemodynamic collapse in acute PTE.[12] This ratio tends to be even lower in cases of CTEPH, as the afterload builds

up slowly and RV has been able to adapt to generate greater PASP.

- *PASP/LV stroke volume ratio:* In a prospective observational study of 215 patients, a PASP/LV stroke volume ratio >1 reliably predicted the primary outcome of inhospital mortality, cardiac arrest, and need for advanced therapies.[13]
- *Thrombus in transit:* In a minority of patients, a thrombus in transit can be documented in its course from IVC to RA and RV and has a diagnostic and prognostic significance.
- *McConnell's sign*: It indicates RV mid free wall akinesia with preserved RV apical function. Initial descriptions of this sign have shown it to be highly specific for acute PTE but later studies show a sensitivity between 70–77% and a specificity between 57–71%[14,15] and similar findings can also be observed in acute coronary syndromes, especially RVMI and ARDS.
- *60/60 sign:* It is a combination of TR gradient <60 mm Hg and PA acceleration time <60 ms. When combined with McConnell's sign, it has a 94% specificity in diagnosing pulmonary embolism.[16]
- *Early systolic notching* in pulsed wave Doppler of RVOT is suggestive of raised PVR.

ECHOCARDIOGRAPHY IN CARDIAC TAMPONADE

Cardiac tamponade is an acute emergency, which can lead to rapid hemodynamic worsening and cardiovascular collapse if not tackled immediately. A bedside echocardiogram is a handy tool for a swift diagnosis and management **(Table 2)**. Although a cardiac tamponade can be diagnosed clinically with reasonable accuracy based on presence or absence of a "palpable" pulsus paradoxus and examination findings popularly known as the Beck's triad, an echocardiogram is essential to quantify the amount of pericardial fluid and study its hemodynamic effects on the heart. Echocardiographic features in cardiac tamponade are as follows:

- *Chamber collapse:* Diastolic collapse of the right-sided chambers is commonly seen. RA end-diastolic collapse occurs when the pericardial pressure rises above RA pressure, which is minimum at end diastole when the atria are relaxing. Brief diastolic collapse may be normally seen, but a duration of collapse greater than one-third of the cardiac cycle has a greater sensitivity and specificity for cardiac tamponade (sensitivity 94%, specificity 100%, and PPV 100%).[17] RV collapse occurs in early diastole and is less sensitive but highly specific for tamponade except in cases of elevated RV diastolic pressure due to various reasons. LA collapse that is seen in a quarter of hemodynamically unstable patients is a highly specific finding.[18]
- *Respiratory flow variation:* More than 25% variation across the mitral valve and greater than 40% variation across the tricuspid valve are suggestive of tamponade but are also seen in constrictive pericarditis and should not be taken as suggestive of tamponade in isolation, in the absence of chamber collapse and abnormal flow in the hepatic veins.
- *IVC diameter:* An IVC diameter greater than 2 cm with <50% respiratory flow variation reflects the increased central venous pressure but is not specific for tamponade.
- *Hepatic venous doppler:* Systolic flow predominance is seen.[19]

TABLE 2: Sensitivity and specificity of various echocardiographic findings in cardiac tamponade.

Parameter	Sensitivity	Specificity
Any chamber collapse	90%	65%
Abnormal hepatic venous flow	75%	91%
RA and RV collapse	–	98%

ECHOCARDIOGRAPHY IN AORTIC DISSECTION

Acute aortic dissections are uncommon but life-threatening conditions requiring emergent evaluation and management. In critically ill patients when immediate CT angiography, which is the reference standard, is not feasible, bedside echocardiography has an important role for diagnosing proximal dissections. Untreated ascending aortic dissections have a mortality rate ranging from 36–72% and a surgical mortality rate of 4.4% in the first 48 hours. A 2023 meta-analysis[20] assessing the diagnostic accuracy of a bedside transthoracic echocardiography found an overall sensitivity and specificity of 62.4% and 87.5%, respectively. Identification of an intimal flap or tear and an intramural hematoma significantly increases the accuracy increasing the specificity to 96.6% and a high positive likelihood ratio of 20.04%. Besides identifying the dissection, a swiftly done echocardiogram can also identify serious complications of dissection such as acute aortic regurgitation and cardiac tamponade **(Table 3)**.

However, transthoracic echocardiography remains inferior to transesophageal echocardiography for diagnosis of aortic dissection.[21] Transthoracic echocardiography had higher false negative and positive rates as compared to transesophageal echocardiography (28.6% and 18.6% vs. 4.3% and 2.4%, respectively) **(Table 4)**.

ASSESSING FLUID RESPONSIVENESS: IVC ASSESSMENT

Assessment of fluid responsiveness is important in patients with hypotension as timely correction of fluid status increases stroke volume and improves blood pressure. There are several noninvasive measures of fluid responsiveness used by critical care physicians to assess the hydration status of ICU patients. IVC diameter and its variation with

TABLE 3: Pooled diagnostic odds ratio, positive, and negative likelihood ratios of echocardiographic findings in aortic dissection.[20]

	Pooled diagnostic odd's ratio	Positive likelihood ratio	Negative likelihood ratio
Any echocardiographic feature	25.2	3.28	0.30
Intimal tear, flap, or intramural hematoma (IMH)	61.9	20.04	0.05
Dilation of aorta	5.7	3.03	0.33
Pericardial effusion	15.3	9.0	0.11
Aortic regurgitation	12.0	5.7	0.18

TABLE 4: Diagnostic performance of transthoracic echocardiography (TTE) as compared to transesophageal echocardiography (TEE) for aortic dissection.[21]

	Stanford A		Stanford B	
	Sensitivity	Specificity	Sensitivity	Specificity
TTE	85.35%	84.51%	45.89%	87.05%
Contrast TTE	93.30%	97.60%	83.60%	94.50%
TEE	93.64%	95.50%	99.80%	99.87%

inspiration is a handy tool for the bedside assessment of hydration status. Several small studies and meta-analyses have critically reviewed the reliability of this parameter.

Potential confounders in measuring IVC diameter are given as follows:

- The exact point along the course of the vessel where its diameter should be measured is not exactly defined.
- Measurements should be taken perpendicular to the course of the vessel.
- Respiratory variation exactly does not happen in the sagittal plane.
- Significant interobserver variability
- Not reflective of fluid responsiveness in cases of intra-abdominal pathology leading to raised intra-abdominal pressure
- Unreliable in presence of right heart failure, chronic constrictive pericarditis, severe TR, restrictive cardiomyopathy, etc.
- Varies with intrathoracic pressure changes, variability is exaggerated in patients taking deep breaths and underestimated with rapid shallow breathing. In mechanically ventilated patients, it is dependent on applied PEEP and set tidal volume.
- IVC may be chronically dilated in elite athletes and sometimes in presence of prominent Eustachian valves.

The available evidence on the matter is heterogeneous comprising of poorly conducted small studies with methodological limitations. In a large study of 540 mechanically ventilated patients with a set tidal volume, IVC diameter had the worst diagnostic performance when compared to SVC diameter, pulse pressure variation, and maximum velocity on pulse-wave Doppler of the LVOT.[22] A meta-analysis of 20 studies also pointed toward the nonreliability of IVC diameter as a measure of fluid responsiveness.[23] If we look at individual studies, there are as many studies with a negative result as there are positive studies on the topic, in both spontaneously breathing as well as mechanically ventilated patients. To conclude, at present, the reliability of IVC assessment as a predictor of fluid responsiveness remains controversial and further research is needed.

CONCLUSION

A bedside echocardiographic examination remains a rapid, handy, and reliable diagnostic modality in cardiac ICUs to diagnose a variety of conditions and their complications. Echodynamics helps in identifying overall hemodynamics of the patient and has been shown to have a fair correlation with invasive hemodynamics. A bedside echocardiography is very useful in situations in which there is a high clinical suspicion of a pulmonary thromboembolism, but a CT is not feasible due to unstable hemodynamics; in fact, it is the only circumstance where an echocardiography assumes a guideline-directed diagnostic role as opposed to its predominant role as risk stratifying tool in pulmonary thromboembolism. Its role in diagnosis as well as immediate management of cardiac tamponade cannot be overemphasized. It also has a role in assessing hydration status of a patient, diagnosing emergencies like aortic dissection, and mechanical complications of MI.

ONLINE REFERENCES

Please scan the QR code provided at the end of the table of contents for References of this chapter.

CHAPTER

12

Echocardiographic Guidance in Percutaneous Approaches to Primary and Secondary Mitral Regurgitation

Sameer Shrivastava, Arif Mustaqueem, Jaideep Dey

ABSTRACT

Mitral regurgitation is a major valvular heart disease seen frequently among cardiac patients. Due to advances in transcatheter interventional therapy, many such patients with comorbidities are eligible for nonsurgical mitral valve treatment. Echocardiography forms the imaging backbone in such situations. Transesophageal echocardiography with three-dimensional imaging is critical for procedural success and avoidance of complications. In this chapter, we discuss the stepwise echocardiographic approach and the necessary views required for transcatheter mitral repair/replacement.

Keywords: Primary mitral regurgitation, secondary mitral regurgitation, septal puncture, transesophageal echocardiography, 3D imaging

INTRODUCTION

Isolated mitral regurgitation (MR) is the third most common form of valvular heart disease (VHD) after rheumatic heart disease (RHD) and aortic stenosis, with an estimated worldwide prevalence of 24.2 million people as of 2022.[1] In India, despite RHD being by far the most prevalent form of VHD, a substantial number of patients with degenerative and secondary MR are encountered in clinical practice. Due to the long asymptomatic phase in the course of the natural history of MR, patients often present late with marked diminution of cardiac function and associated comorbidities. Transcatheter mitral valve interventions (TMVI) offer a viable and safer option for such high-risk patients.[2] Echocardiographic imaging support is critical during TMVI as the native mitral valve (MV) apparatus is not visualized on fluoroscopy alone. Being a venous access procedure, it is of paramount importance to achieve an ideal interatrial transseptal puncture site so that the device and hardware can be advanced across and implanted appropriately. Procedural success and possible complications can also be diagnosed early using a combination of both 2D and 3D imaging. In this chapter, we will briefly discuss the applied anatomy of MV with respect to TMVI and echocardiographic criteria for severity of MR and suitability for transcatheter intervention. Finally, we provide an approach to sequentially image the relevant structures echocardiographically during TMVI.

DISCUSSION

Anatomy of Mitral Valve Apparatus

The MV apparatus **(Fig. 1)** consists of mitral leaflets (anterior and posterior), mitral annulus, chordae tendinae, papillary muscles, and associated left atrial (LA) and left ventricular (LV) walls.[3] Abnormalities in any one or more of these components may lead to MR.

Mitral leaflets **(Fig. 2)** are asymmetrical in size, with the anterior mitral leaflet (AML) larger in surface area compared to the posterior mitral leaflet (PML). However, the PML has a larger attachment to the annulus (covering two-thirds of the MV annulus) compared to the AML. Normally, the mitral leaflets coapt at a depth of 5–7 mm from the mitral annular plane with a leaflet overlap (coaptation length) of at least 5 mm.[4] The junction point of the two leaflets is known as commissures (anterolateral and posteromedial). The PML is divided into three scallops (P1, P2, and P3 lateral to medial) due to two indentations. The corresponding abutting segments of AML are labeled as A1, A2, and A3 with A1 scallop in proximity to the left atrial appendage and A3 scallop near the interatrial septum (IAS).

The fibrous annulus is saddle-shaped and contributes to valvular competence due to contraction during ventricular systole. The annular size may reduce by up to 25% during ventricular systole, which explains the susceptibility to

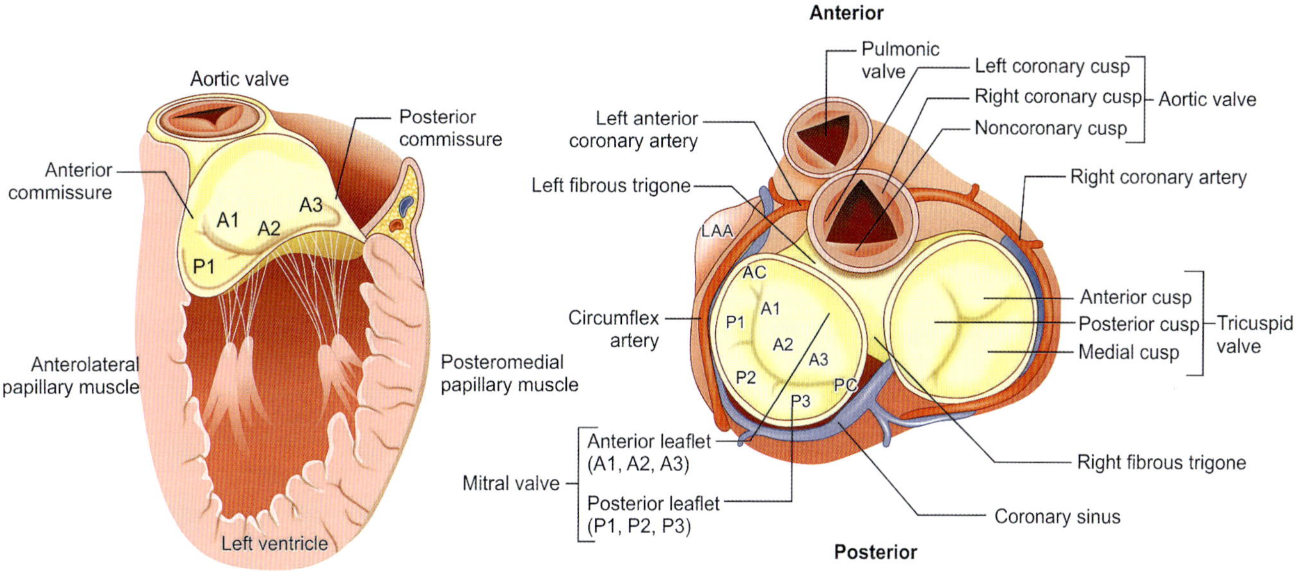

FIG. 1: Mitral valve anatomy: Showing components of mitral valve apparatus and its relationship to surrounding structures.

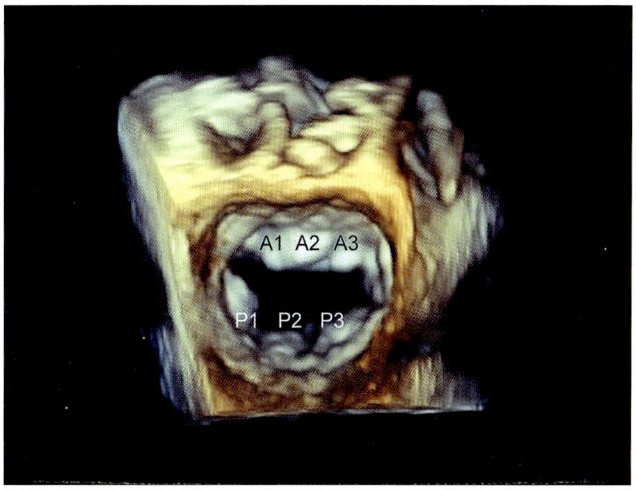

FIG. 2: Mitral leaflets consisting of anterior and posterior mitral leaflets that are divided into three parts named 1–3 from lateral to medial.

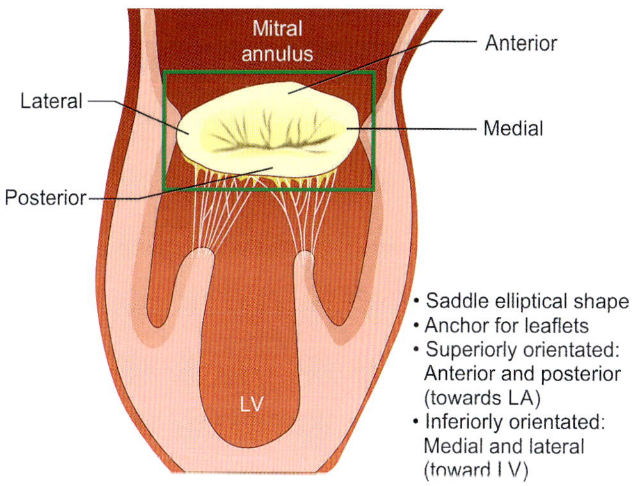

FIG. 3: Mitral annulus showing its various components.

valvular incompetence during contractile dysfunction states.[4] The anterior annulus is much more compact and in continuity with the aortic annulus. The posterior annulus is composed of comparatively loose connective tissue and is in continuation with the LA endocardium. This makes the posterior annulus more susceptible to dilatation and calcification in pathologic states. With progressive LV dilatation, the annulus assumes a more spherical shape **(Fig. 3)**.

The chordae tendinae are fibrous cords that connect the mitral leaflets to the underlying papillary muscles. The primary chordae are attached to the free edges of leaflets while the secondary chordae attach to the ventricular aspect of the mitral leaflets. Disruption of chords leads to leaflet prolapse or getting flail with resultant acute MR **(Figs. 4A and B)**.

The two papillary muscles, anterolateral and posteromedial, arise from the distal thirds of the ventricular myocardium. The former has a dual blood supply from the left anterior descending (LAD) and left circumflex (LCx) coronary arteries while the latter has a single blood supply from either right coronary (RCA) or LCx artery. This makes the posteromedial papillary muscle more prone to ischemic

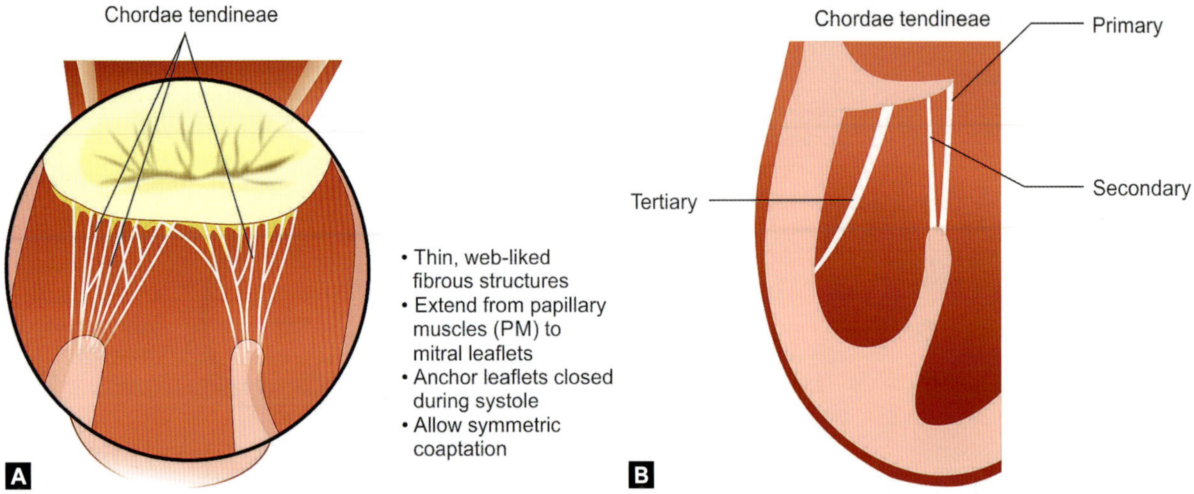

FIGS. 4A AND B: (A) Chordae tendinae, its fine structure, and (B) Distribution into primary, secondary and tertiary chordae.

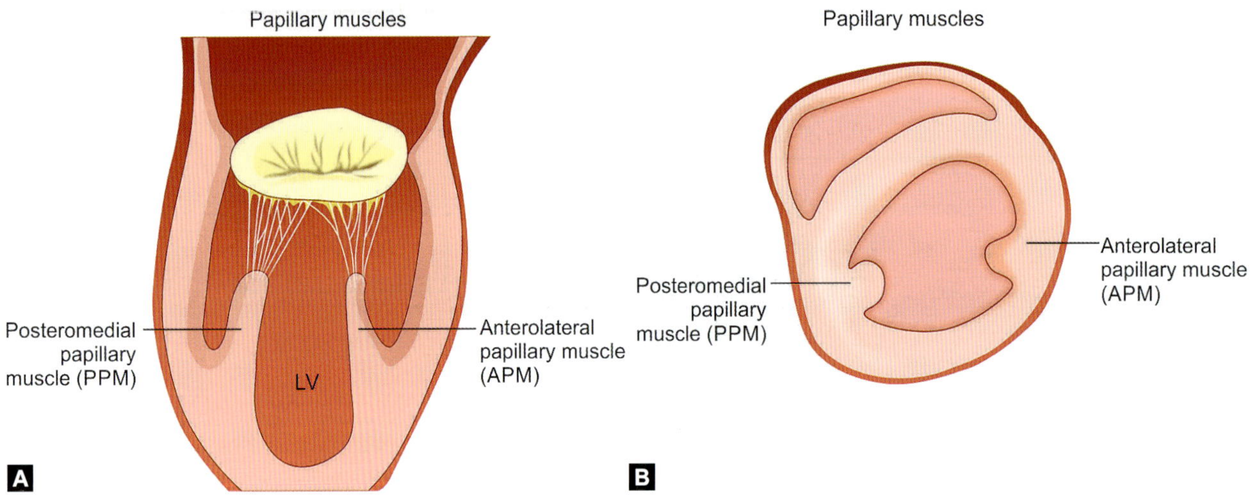

FIGS. 5A AND B: Papillary muscles and their components.

injury as compared to anterolateral papillary muscle. LV dilatation due to any cause leads to apical displacement of the papillary muscles with stretching of chordae. The resulting tethering of mitral leaflets and apical displacement of the zone of coaptation leads to MR **(Figs. 5A and B)**.

Assessment of Mechanism and Etiology of Mitral Regurgitation

The Carpentier classification, first proposed in 1983, is the most commonly applied classification system for MR, due to corroboration of mechanism with etiology. More recently, a modification of the previous classification **(Table 1)** has been proposed, considering advances in MV repair techniques and utilization of 3D echocardiography **(Fig. 6)**.[5]

Echocardiography is the initial investigation of choice in the assessment of MR severity, mechanism, and suitability for TMVI. Transthoracic echocardiography (TTE), transesophageal echocardiography (TEE) supplemented with 3-dimensional imaging (3D), and exercise stress echocardiography provide a comprehensive means for MR assessment. Exercise echocardiography is useful in the evaluation of patients with discordance in symptoms and resting MR (latent MR) and assessment of stress induced LV function and pulmonary artery systolic pressures (PASP).[6] The indications for valvular intervention in severe MR are outlined in various consensus guidelines published in recent years.[6,7]

The echocardiographic criteria for MR severity assessment are summarized in **Table 2** and **Figures 7A and B**.

TABLE 1: Modified Carpentier classification of mitral regurgitation.[5]

MR type		Mechanism	Etiology
I		Normal leaflet motion	• Annular dilatation • Infective endocarditis • Leaflet perforation
II		Increased leaflet motion	• Flail leaflet • Prolapsed leaflet
III		Restricted leaflet motion	
	IIIa	Restricted leaflet opening and closure	• Rheumatic heart disease • Inflammatory valvulopathies
	IIIb	Restricted leaflet closure (systolic restriction with symmetric tethering)	• Dilated cardiomyopathy • Chronic global ischemic cardiomyopathy
	IIIc	Restricted leaflet closure (systolic restriction with asymmetric tethering)	Posterior LV wall motion abnormality (isolated PML tethering)
IV		Systolic anterior motion of leaflet(s)	
	IVa	Hypertrophic cardiomyopathy	
	IVb	Post MV repair	
	IVc	Hypovolemic state and hyperdynamic LV	
V		Hybrid mechanism	Any combination of abovementioned categories

Note: Some of the patients with mitral regurgitation types I, II, IIIb, and IIIc are candidates suitable for transcatheter mitral valve interventions.

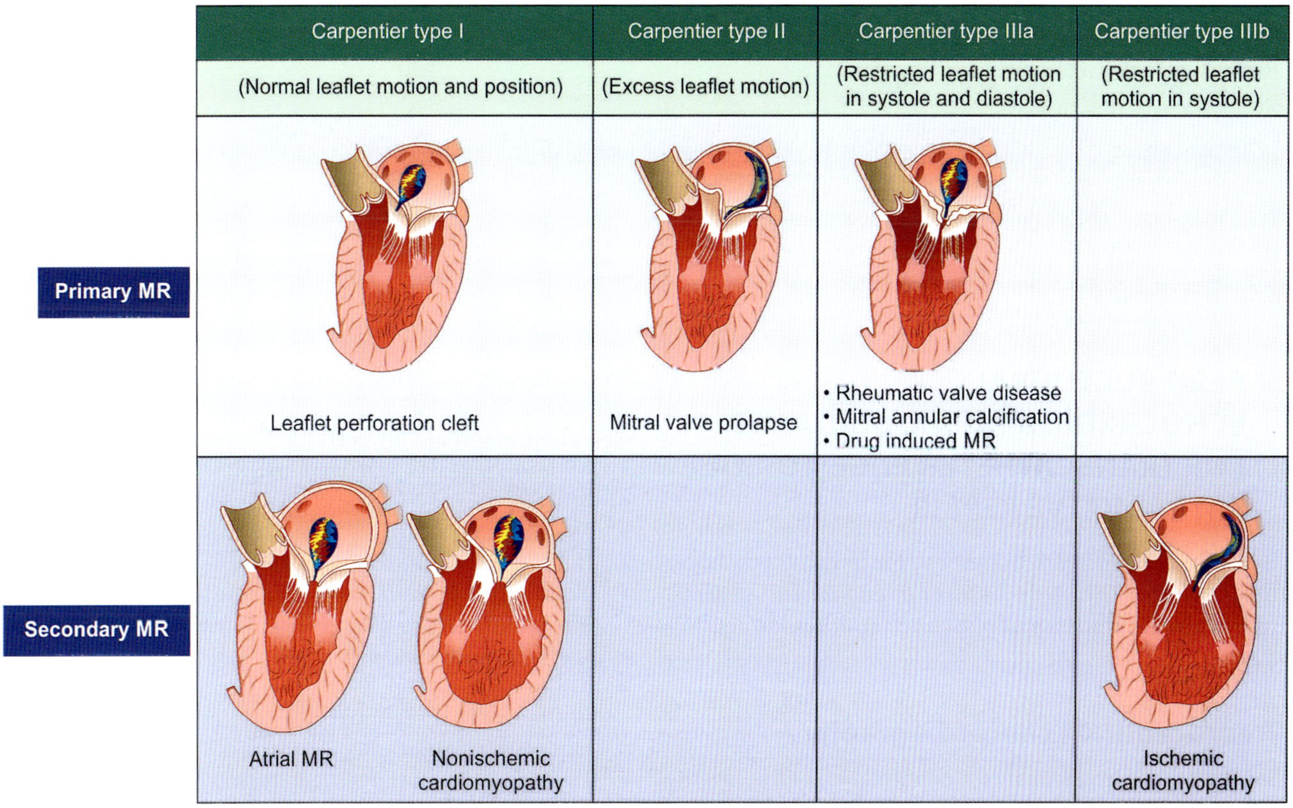

FIG. 6: Classification of MR into primary and secondary and further subdivisions.

Source: El Sabbagh A, Reddy YNV, Nishimura RA. Mitral valve regurgitation in the contemporary era: Insights into diagnosis, management, and future directions. JACC Cardiovasc Imaging. 2018;11(4):628-43.

TABLE 2: Echocardiographic parameters for assessment of severity of mitral regurgitation.[6,8,9]

Parameter	Primary severe MR	Secondary severe MR
Qualitative		
Valve morphology	• Flail leaflet • Ruptured papillary muscle • Large perforation • Retracted leaflets	Leaflets morphologically normal with tethering and loss of coaptation
Color flow jet area	Large central jet occupying >50% of LA area or eccentric wall impinging jet of variable size (Coandă effect)	Large central jet occupying >50% of LA area or eccentric wall impinging jet of variable size (Coandă effect)
Flow convergence zone	Large throughout systole	Large throughout systole
Continuous wave Doppler signal	Dense/holosystolic/triangular	Dense/holosystolic/triangular
Semiquantitative		
Vena contracta width (mm)	≥7, ≥8 (biplane)	≥7, ≥8 (biplane)
Pulmonary vein flow	Systolic flow reversal	Systolic flow reversal
Mitral inflow	E dominant (>1.2 m/s)	E dominant (>1.2 m/s)
Mitral TVI/aortic TVI	>1.4	>1.4
3D vena contracta area (VCA, mm^2)*	>41	>43
Quantitative		
Effective regurgitant orifice area (EROA) (mm^2)	≥40	≥40 (≥30 if elliptical orifice)
Regurgitant volume (mL)	≥60	≥60 (≥45 in low flow conditions)
Regurgitant fraction (%)	≥50	≥50
Associated supportive findings		
LV/LA dimensions	Dilated (LVESD ≥40 mm, LA maximum diameter ≥55 mm/LA volume ≥60 mL/m^2)	Dilated
Pulmonary artery systolic pressure (PASP)	Usually elevated	Usually elevated

*Investigational, not currently endorsed in recent guidelines.

PERIPROCEDURAL ECHOCARDIOGRAPHIC GUIDANCE FOR TRANSCATHETER EDGE-TO-EDGE MITRAL VALVE REPAIR

Currently, two devices are approved for transcatheter edge-to-edge repair (TEER); the *MitraClip*® and *Pascal*® systems. Both require a transseptal puncture for access to the MV apparatus.

Preprocedural Echocardiography

The TTE is usually adequate for confirmation of the severity and mechanism of MR. However, TEE views are required to evaluate the MV in patients with limited acoustic window and suitability for TEER. Stringent inclusion and exclusion criteria need to be fulfilled prior to the procedure.[8,10] The TEE views required **(Figs. 8A to D)** are:

- Midesophageal 0° four-chamber view
- Midesophageal 40–60° short-axis view
- Midesophageal 90–110° long-axis view
- Midesophageal 120° long-axis view
- Transgastric 0° short-axis view at the level of MV

The parameters to be assessed for a successful TEER are as follows (primary/secondary MR):

- MR originates **(Figs. 9A and B)** from the central portion of the valve. If secondary jets are noted, they must be clinically insignificant.
- Flail gap <10 mm (largest gap between leaflets measured in two views; ME 0° four-chamber view and ME 120° long-axis view on TEE)

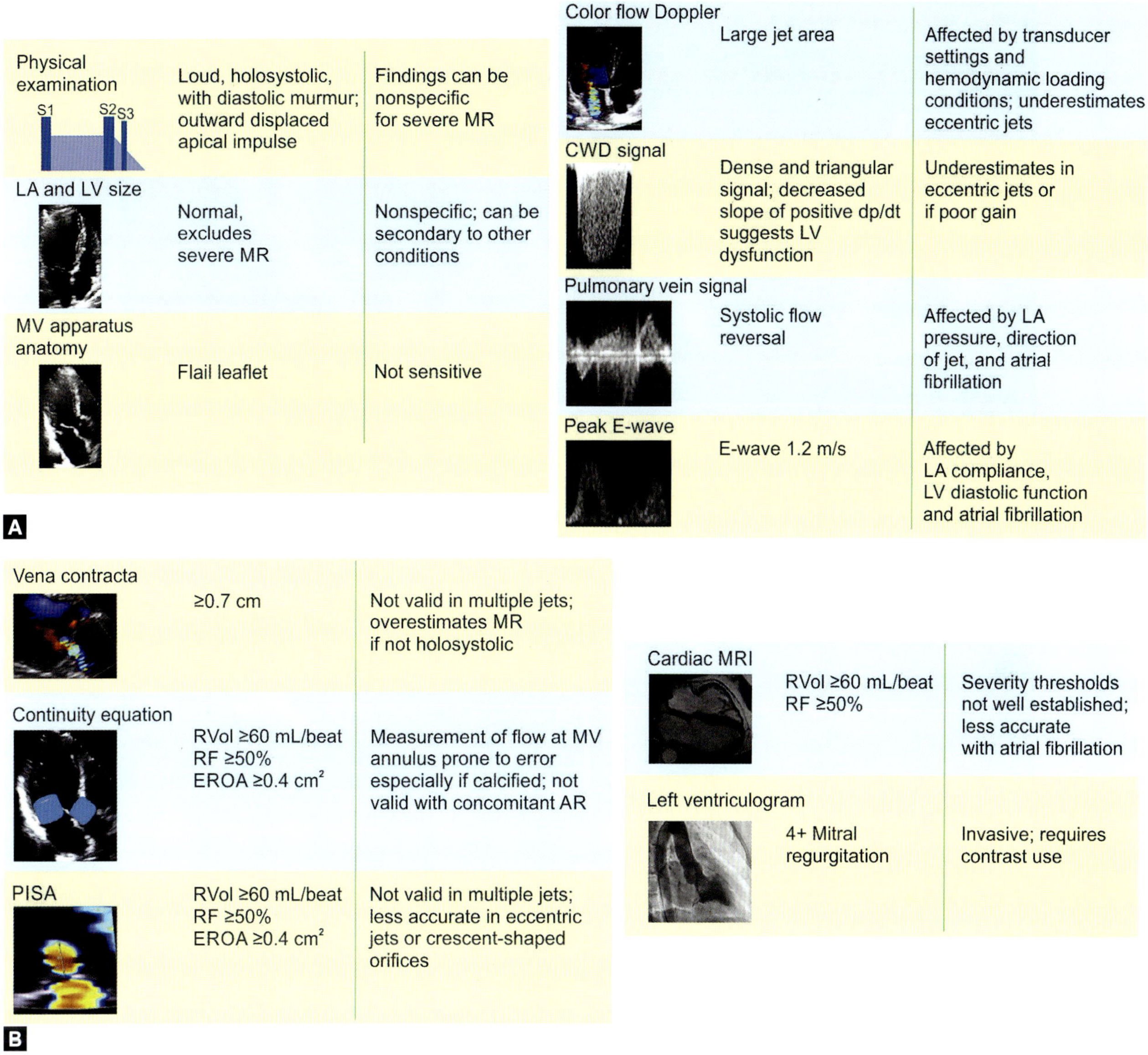

FIGS. 7A AND B: (A) Qualitative parameters and (B) Quantitative parameters for assessment of mitral regurgitation.

- Flail width <15 mm (largest horizontal dimension of flail segment measured on en face view of MV using 3D TEE) **(Figs. 10A to D)**
- Coaptation depth <11 mm (vertical depth of first point of mitral leaflet coaptation during mid-systole, measured from the plane of MV annulus in LA to LV direction on four-chamber view)
- Coaptation length >2 mm (vertical length of contact of mitral leaflets in mid systole, measured in LA to LV direction on four-chamber view)
- Absence of calcium in the leaflet grasping zone
- Absence of significant cleft of A2 or P2 scallops
- Absence of bileaflet flail/prolapse
- Presence of both primary and secondary chordal support
- Mitral valve orifice area **(Fig. 11)** >4.0 cm^2
- Posterior mitral leaflet length ≥10 mm
- Normal leaflet thickness
- Normal leaflet mobility (exclusion of rheumatic/endocarditic valve)
- Absence of severe mitral annular calcification (MAC)
- Absence of a patent foramen ovale (PFO)/atrial septal aneurysm (ASA), which can interfere with adequate atrial septal puncture

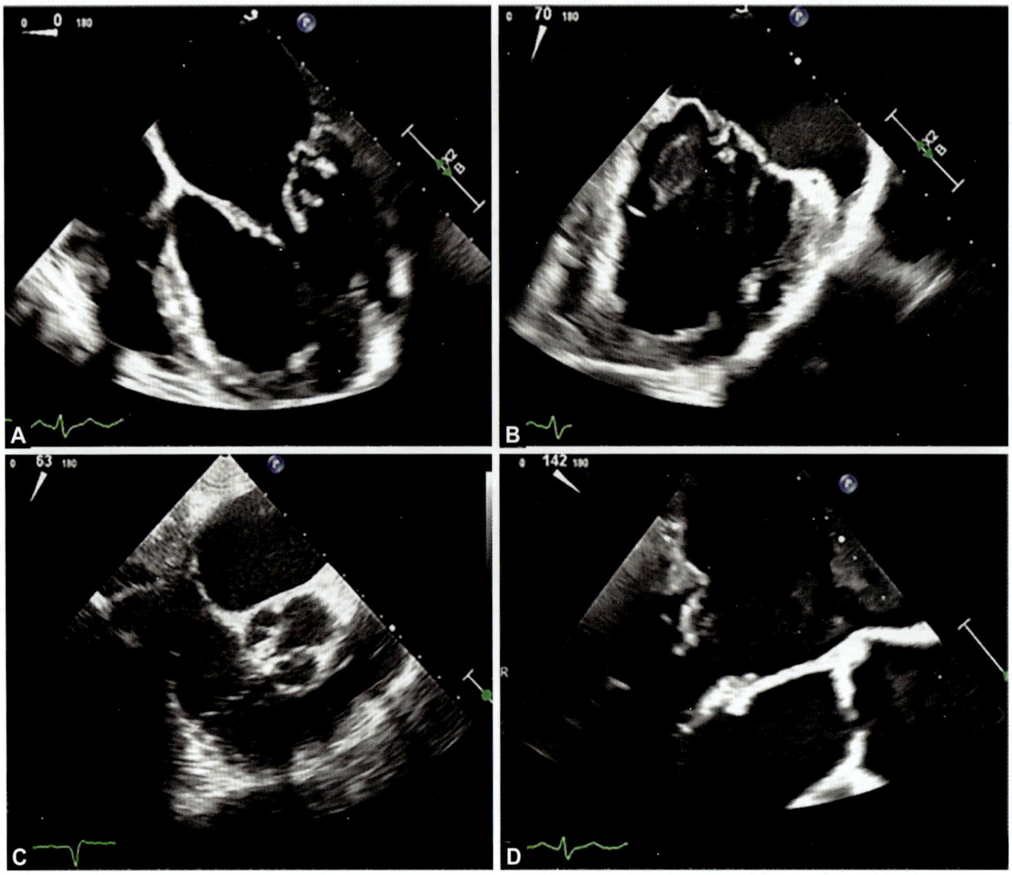

FIGS. 8A TO D: Mitral valve view TEE at (A) 0°; (B) bicommisure view; (C) short-axis view; and (D) long-axis view.

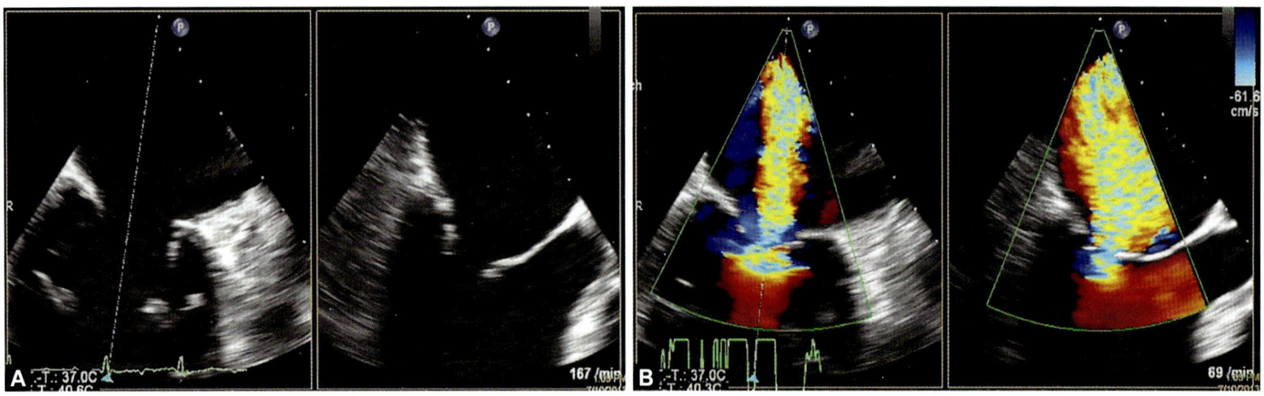

FIGS. 9A AND B: Commissure view showing mitral valve in orthogonal plane without colour and in second image with colour demonstrating the severity of mitral regurgitation.

Intraprocedural Transesophageal Echocardiography Guidance

The various steps during TEER when TEE guidance is paramount include:

- *Atrial septal puncture:* This is one of the most important steps during the procedure. The puncture site must be such that once the device catheter is introduced into the LA, enough maneuverability is possible along the lateral-to-medial axis (along MV coaptation line). The site must be at a posterior and superior location along the IAS. Adequate height of the puncture site from the plane of mitral annulus is also necessary for optimum device implantation (ideally 4–5 cm in primary MR and around 3.5 cm in secondary MR).[8] Any other puncture site or guide catheter introduction through PFO/atrial

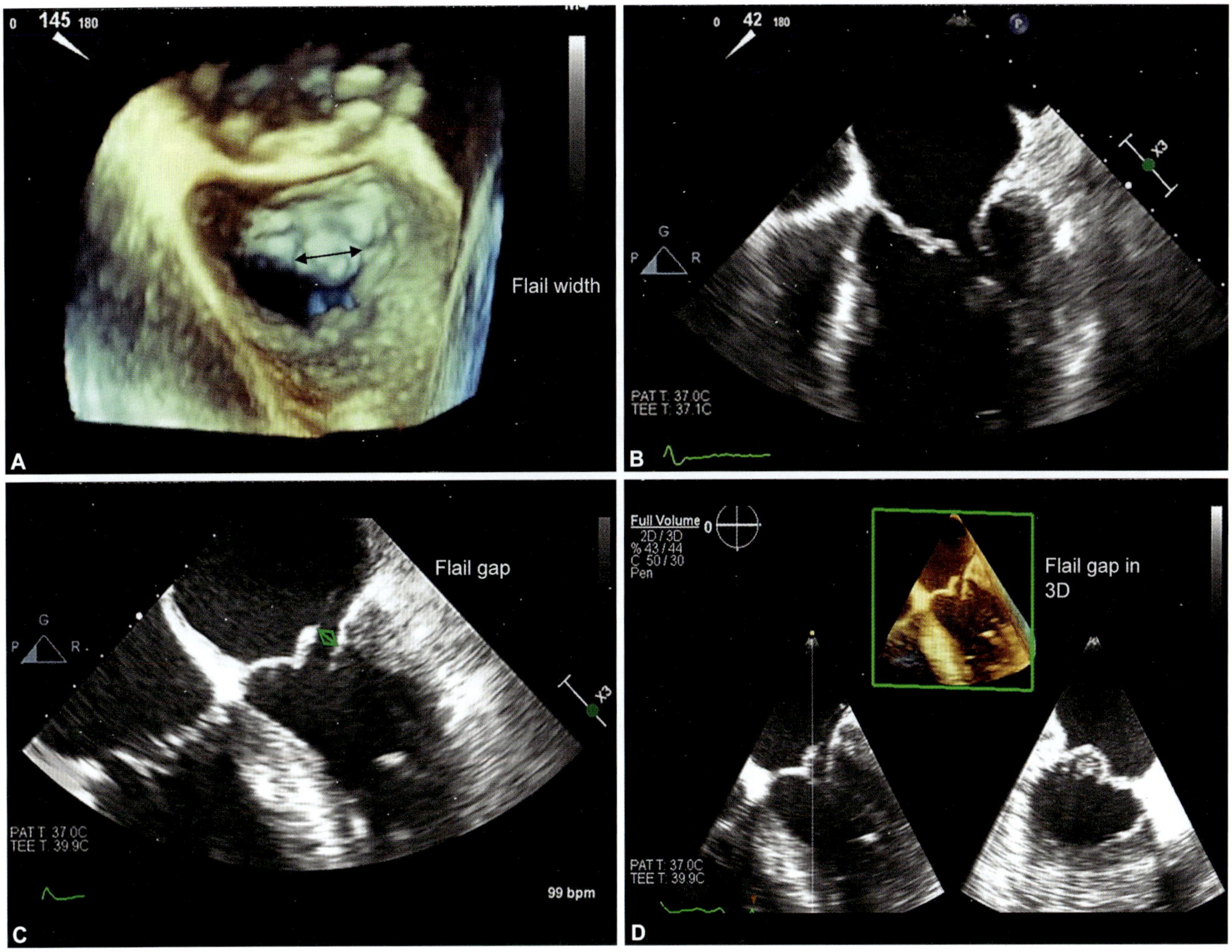

FIGS. 10A TO D: Flail gap and flail width highlighted in various views, 2D and 3D imaging.

septal defect (ASD) must be avoided to prevent device instability/malposition or IAS rupture. The TEE views required are **(Figs. 12 A and B):**
  - *Bicaval view (90–110°):* Superior–inferior orientation of IAS
  - *Short-axis view (40–60°):* Anteroposterior orientation of IAS
  - *Four-chamber view (0°):* Assessment of height of puncture site from mitral annular plane
- *Introduction of steerable guide catheter:* Following successful puncture and insertion of guidewire across the IAS, the guide catheter is introduced with the dilator under TEE and fluoroscopic guidance. Care must be taken that during the introduction of hardware, injury to lateral wall of LA should be avoided. Whenever possible, 3D TEE imaging should be performed at each step. Though adequate anticoagulation with heparin is ensured, attention must be paid toward any de-novo thrombus forming in the bulky hardware introduced during the procedure **(Figs. 13A and B)**.
- *Advancing the clip delivery system:* Subsequently, the clip device within the delivery catheter is advanced under fluoroscopic and TEE guidance. Care must be taken to avoid injury to LA wall with continuous echocardiographic imaging using orthogonal (X-plane) and 3D views. The guide catheter must always be in the LA across the IAS and not retracted backward during device propagation **(Figs. 14A to D)**.
- *Positioning the clip device over MV and advancement into LV:* These crucial steps are performed almost exclusively using TEE and 3D imaging support. The device must be oriented perpendicular to MV coaptation line. In contrast to the en face (surgeon's view) orientation of the valve on 3D, a "cardiologist's view" with aortic valve at 6 o'clock position and LAA orifice pointing to the right side is preferred, to assess adequacy of device positioning and medial-lateral movement of the device system.[10] Clockwise/anticlockwise and medial/lateral manipulation of the clip delivery system is needed to achieve optimum positioning. If implantation of more

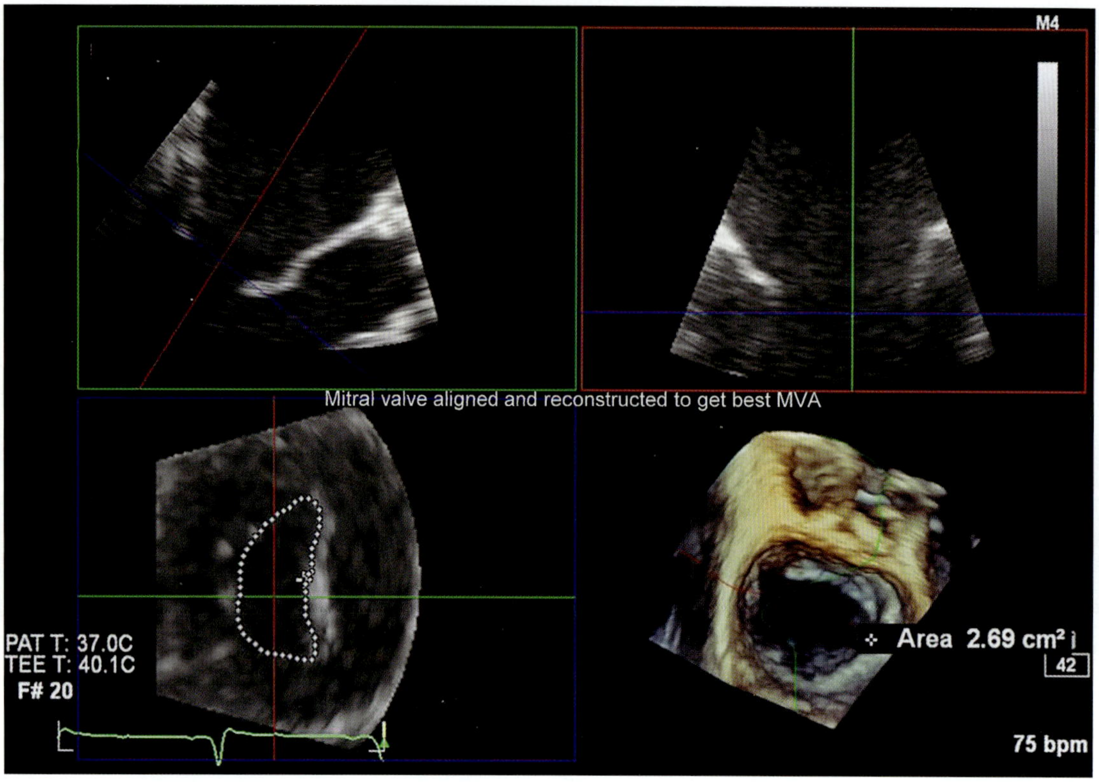

FIG. 11: Mitral valve area calculated by multiplanar reconstruction.

than one device is contemplated, then the first device must be implanted medially as medial deployment of device is of greater complexity in this procedure. Once a suitable orientation of the device is achieved, then the clips are partially opened and gradually crossed across the MV into LV under bicommissural and long-axis (120–140°) TEE views. On successful completion of this maneuver, the perpendicular device orientation must again be confirmed, and the clip arms are opened fully **(Figs. 15A and B)**.

- *MV leaflet capture and clip deployment:* Under TEE (2D and 3D) and fluoroscopic guidance, the leaflets are captured by deploying the grippers and the clip maneuvered into a semiclosed position (up to 60° closure). The bicommissural view should not show any of the clip arms separately, while on long-axis view, the arms must be visible perpendicular and grasping the leaflets, ensuring proper positioning. The leaflet flaps must bisect both the clip arms, which should be seen on long-axis view. Also, color Doppler imaging should confirm that the clip is positioned exactly on the MR jet origin point with splaying of jet by the clip. Once the correct positioning has been confirmed, then the clip is closed completely in a slow maneuver **(Figs. 16A and B)**.
- *Assessment of residual MR severity and final release of device*: Residual MR severity assessment echocardiographically is challenging as the jet is modified by the device and there may be more than one jet orifices with elliptical openings. Proximal isovelocity surface area (PISA) method of MR estimation is inaccurate in such circumstances. Hence, the MR jet must be carefully assessed in all the TEE views for severity and eccentricity. Quantitative MR assessment using 3D volumetric analysis (in absence of intracardiac shunts and significant aortic regurgitation) is contributory. Semiquantitative assessment using 3D vena contracta area and pulmonary vein flow patterns can be of help in identifying significant residual MR. However, definite consensus guidelines are needed in this regard. Assessment of mean transmitral pressure gradient (ideally <4 mm Hg) and MV planimetered area (>1.5 cm^2 using 3D planimetry) is mandatory to prevent iatrogenic mitral stenosis (MS).[8] If so, then clip repositioning may be required. Once these goals are adequately achieved, the clip is released and the MV morphology and MR are again assessed **(Figs. 17A and B)**.
- *Assessment for any complications and need for additional clip implantation*: Throughout the procedure, cautious monitoring must be ensured for the development of possible complications such as pericardial effusion/tamponade, thrombus formation, distortion/damage to MV leaflets, and subvalvular apparatus or clip dislodgement. IAS puncture site and shunt severity must be checked. If additional clips need to be implanted, then

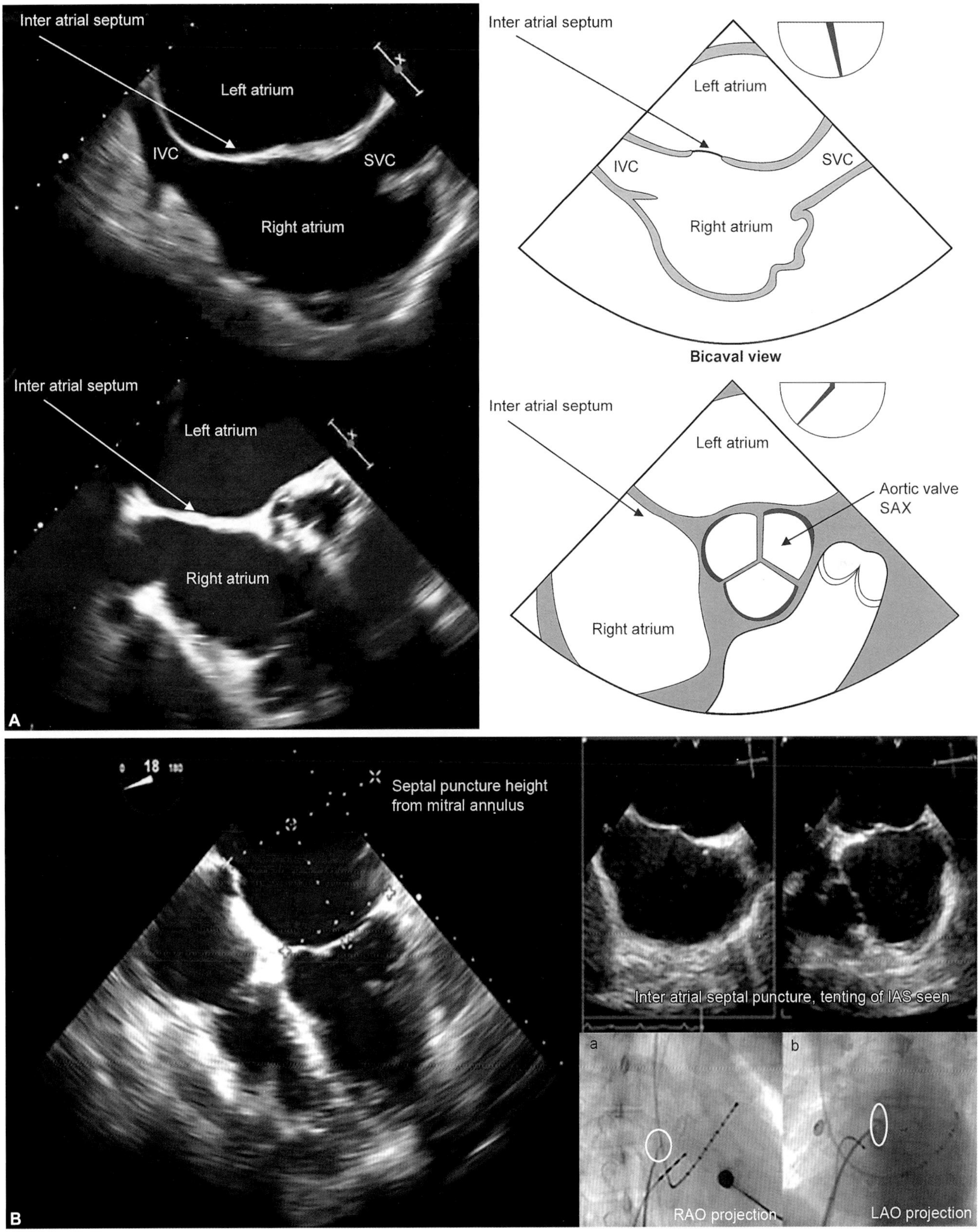

FIGS. 12A AND B: (A) Interatrial septum in long and short axis to select appropriate site for septal puncture and (B) showing height of septal puncture, one of the very essential steps, second image shows tenting of IAS in orthogonal planes.

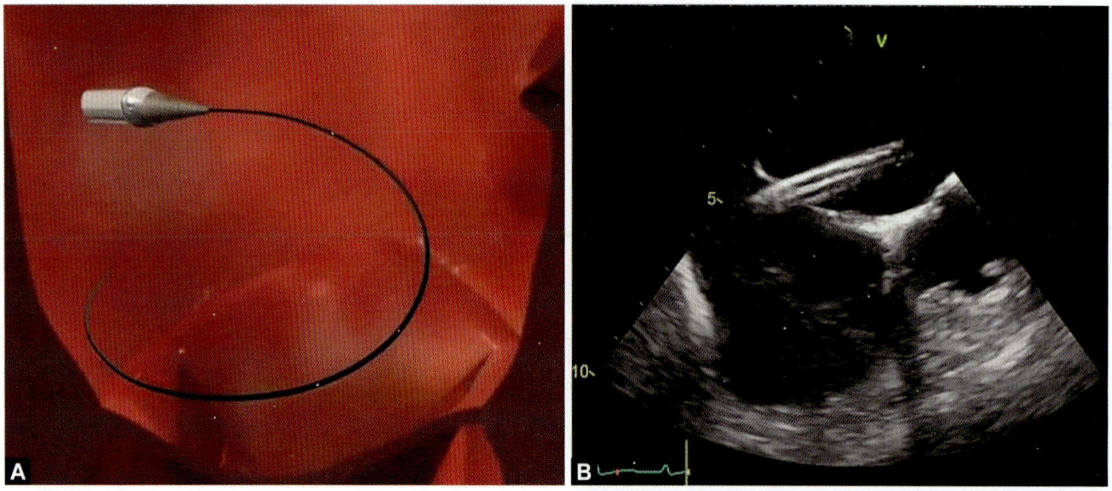

FIGS. 13A AND B: Introduction of steerable guide catheter across interatrial septum should be carried out in good visualization, with 2D and 3D imaging.

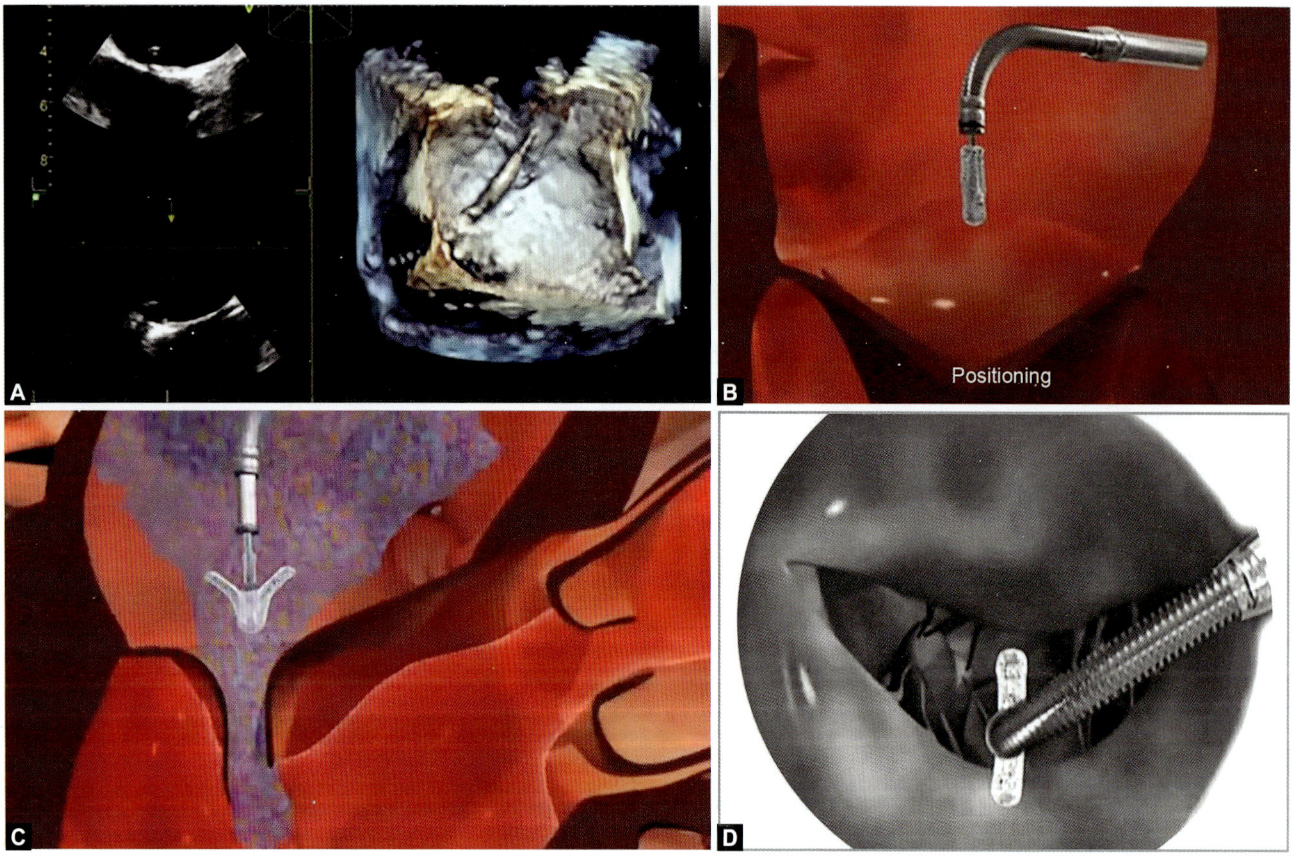

FIGS. 14A TO D: Advancing the clip delivery system is another key step. Full visualization of the whole during advancement is essential to avoid injury to adjoining structures.

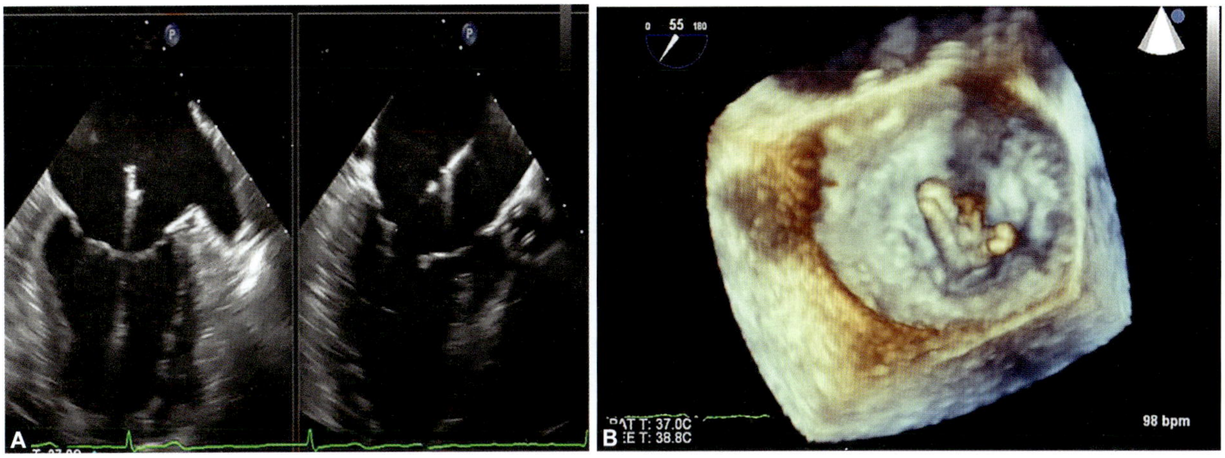

FIGS. 15A AND B: Positioning the clip device over MV and advancement into LV showing (A) bicommissural view X plane and (B) 3D en face view.

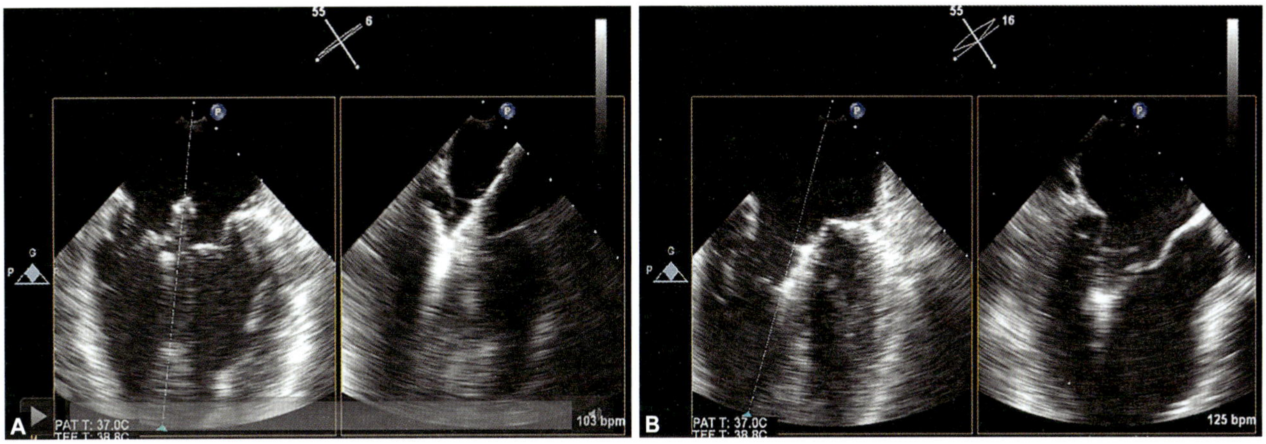

FIGS. 16A AND B: MV leaflet capture and clip deployment.

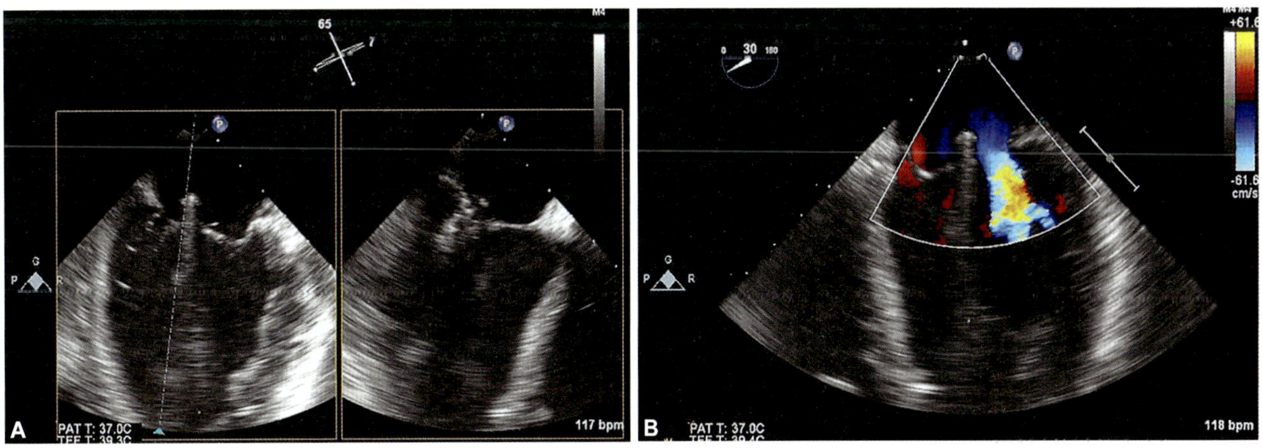

FIGS. 17A AND B: Assessment of residual MR severity and final release of device.

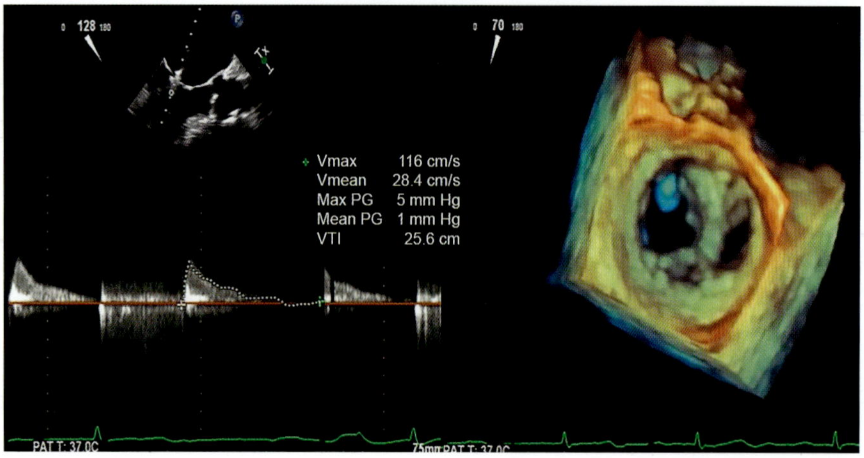

FIG. 18: 3D mitral valve image post MitraClip implantation along with the gradient across mitral valve.

fluoroscopy in addition to echocardiographic guidance aids in the correct positioning of subsequent clips parallel to the first clip **(Fig. 18)**.

PERIPROCEDURAL ECHOCARDIOGRAPHIC GUIDANCE FOR TRANSCATHETER MITRAL VALVE REPLACEMENT

The main indications of the procedure include: Valve in native valve, valve in prosthetic valve (degenerative bioprosthesis), valve in ring (in failed preexisting mitral annuloplasty ring), and valve in MAC situations. Available devices include *Tendyne®*, *Intrepid®*, *Tiara®*, *Evoque®*, *Sapien M3®* and *HighLife®*.

The assessment of MV apparatus and mechanism, and severity of MR are performed as outlined in guidelines.[6,7,11] A transapical or a transseptal approach is used. Due to the complexity and associated morbidity with the former, a transseptal approach is preferred whenever possible.[12] The TEE views are similar to those outlined in case of TEER. The desired transseptal puncture site is different, with a central location in bicaval view (90–110°) and a posterior location in short-axis view (40–60°). Also, an optimum puncture height 3–4 cm above mitral annular plane is ensured.[12]

Due to proximity of the MV to left ventricular outflow tract (LVOT), transcatheter mitral valve replacement (TMVR) risks the possibility of left ventricular outflow tract obstruction (LVOTO). Multidetector computed tomography scan (MDCT) is used preprocedurally to calculate the native LVOT area and the possible resulting neo-LVOT area following TMVR.[13] Recently, TEE-guided imaging algorithms have been devised that can be utilized in a similar way to calculate the neo-LVOT area.

A neo-LVOT area <2.0 cm^2 has been associated with significant LVOTO (LVOT pressure gradient >30 mm Hg).[12] In addition, an elongated AML, a small LV cavity, aortomitral angle <110°, small LVOT diameter, septal bulge, and redundant chordae are some other preprocedural morphological characteristics predisposing to LVOTO. To prevent such a possibility, catheter-based approaches such as LAMPOON procedure (mitral leaflet laceration) or alcohol septal ablation are performed. The reader is referred to excellent reviews discussing the indications and various methods for performing the LAMPOON procedure.[14] Catheter guidance and coaxial orientation of the valve delivery system are achieved using TEE, orthogonal imaging (x-plane), and 3D guidance.

Following valve implantation, TEE imaging is used to assess adequate deployment, valve gradients, paravalvular leak, and LVOTO. Complications of the procedure such as pericardial effusion/tamponade, encroachment of adjoining structures (particularly aortic annulus), new wall motion abnormalities due to left circumflex coronary artery compression and hemodynamically significant (post septal puncture) residual shunts must also be assessed.

CONCLUSION

Transcatheter mitral intervention is a viable option for patients with degenerative and secondary MR. Echocardiographic imaging is crucial at each stage of management in such patients. Selection of the ideal valve for intervention and imaging guidance at each step with 3D support ensures an optimum result with lower risk of complications.

ONLINE REFERENCES

Please scan the QR code provided at the end of the table of contents for References of this chapter.

CHAPTER

13

Atrial Functional Mitral Regurgitation: Diagnosis and Therapy Implications

Pankaj Harkut, Sunita Kumbhalkar, Seenu Prasanth A

ABSTRACT

"Atrial functional mitral regurgitation" (AF-MR) is a newly recognized condition where mitral regurgitation occurs due to left atrial disease, without left ventricular dilatation and intrinsic mitral valve disease. It is typically associated with long-standing atrial fibrillation and/or heart failure with preserved ejection fraction. This condition is characterized by a large left atrium, mitral annular enlargement, and normal left ventricular size and function. This should be differentiated from the conventional type of functional mitral regurgitation. The chapter reviews the diagnosis and therapy implications of atrial functional mitral regurgitation.

Keywords: Atrial functional mitral regurgitation (AF-MR), atrial fibrillation (AFib), heart failure with preserved ejection fraction (HFpEF)

INTRODUCTION

Mitral regurgitation (MR) is among the most common heart valve disorders.[1] Organic MR implies the presence of structural abnormalities of the mitral valve, whereas functional MR occurs in the setting of structurally normal leaflet tissue. The functional MR is caused by a restriction of leaflet motion resulting from the displacement of the papillary muscle-bearing segments of the left ventricle (LV). The displaced papillary muscles tether the mitral valve leaflets into the LV cavity such that adequate coaptation is no longer possible (as seen in ischemic MR and dilated cardiomyopathy).[2,3]

Gertz et al. demonstrated that functional MR is not only limited to patients with LV remodeling but that it can also occur in patients with left atrial (LA) and mitral annular enlargement caused by atrial fibrillation (AFib).[4] They retrospectively studied 53 patients with AFib, normal LV size, ejection fraction (EF) of ≥50%, and significant (moderate to severe) MR with structurally normal leaflets who were referred for catheter ablation. Follow-up echocardiography performed around 1 year after catheter ablation showed those with recurrent AFib had significantly larger LA volume and annular size as well as a >3 times higher rate of significant MR (82% vs. 24%; $p = 0.005$) compared with patients with sustained sinus rhythm. Gertz et al. used the term atrial functional MR (AF-MR) to distinguish MR in these patients from that which occurs in patients with LV remodeling, i.e., ventricular functional MR (VF-MR).[4]

EPIDEMIOLOGY AND NATURAL HISTORY

The prevalence of AF-MR varies between studies due to different definitions, diagnostic methods, study designs, and populations. In one study, referred for transthoracic echocardiography, significant AF-MR was found in 7% of patients.[4] A similar study showed that 3% of patients with AFib for ≤1 year had significant MR, compared to 28% with AFib for >10 years.[5] In a cohort with severe MR and preserved LV systolic function undergoing transesophageal echocardiography, AF-MR was found in almost 8% of patients.[5] In a community-based study, among individuals with significant MR, 27% had AF-MR, 38% had VF-MR, 32% had primary MR, and 2% had mixed etiology MR.[6]

The natural history of moderate/severe AF-MR was studied by Naser et al.[7] A total of 635 patients (median age 75 years, 51% female, 96% mild-moderate/moderate AF-MR, and 4% severe AF-MR) were included. Over a median of 2.2 years, incidence rates per 100 person-years were 3.2 for left ventricular systolic dysfunction ($p = 0.52$ vs. patients with no/mild AF-MR), 1.9 for progression of AF-MR, and 3.9 for regression. Female sex and larger LA volume index were independently associated with progression, whereas younger age, male sex, absent AFib, and higher LA emptying fraction were independently associated with regression. Neither AF-MR progression nor regression was independently associated with mortality. Instead, independent risk factors for mortality included older age, concentric LV geometry, and higher estimated LV filling and pulmonary pressures.[7]

PATHOPHYSIOLOGY

The pathophysiology of AF-MR include:

- Atriogenic leaflet tethering
- Abnormalities of mitral annular structure and dynamics
- Adaptive leaflet growth

Atriogenic leaflet tethering: The LA base and the posterior mitral annulus are situated within the LV inlet.[8] When these structures enlarge, the annulus becomes displaced onto the crest of the LV free wall. This displaced annulus tethers the posterior mitral leaflet (PML), thereby hamstringing it, a condition known as asatriogenic leaflet tethering.[9,10] Additionally, there may be evidence of anterior mitral leaflet (AML) pseudoprolapse **(Fig. 1)**.

Abnormalities of mitral annular structure and dynamics: The mitral annulus is a nonplanar fibrous structure that changes shape during the cardiac cycle. It undergoes a folding motion across its intercommissural axis during systole (saddle deepening).[11,12] This folding motion helps to reduce stress on the mitral leaflets. In patients with AFib, this folding is reduced and it is believed to be involved in the development of AFib and MR.[13]

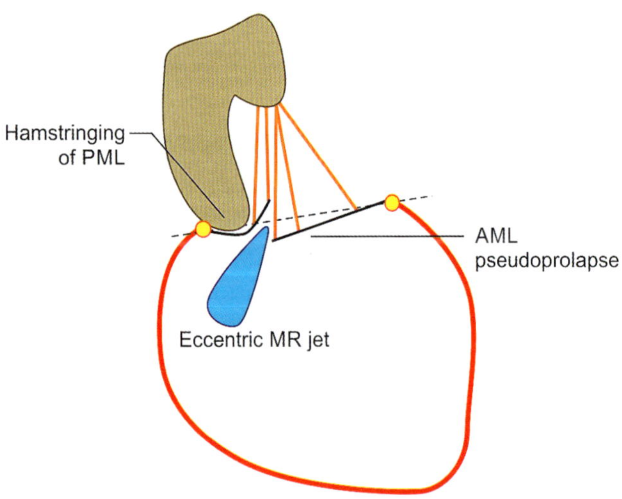

FIG. 1: Atrial functional mitral regurgitation example—giant left atrium with eccentric mitral regurgitant jet with preserved left ventricular size. Also, note hamstringing of PML (atriogenic leaflet tethering) and AML pseudoprolapse.

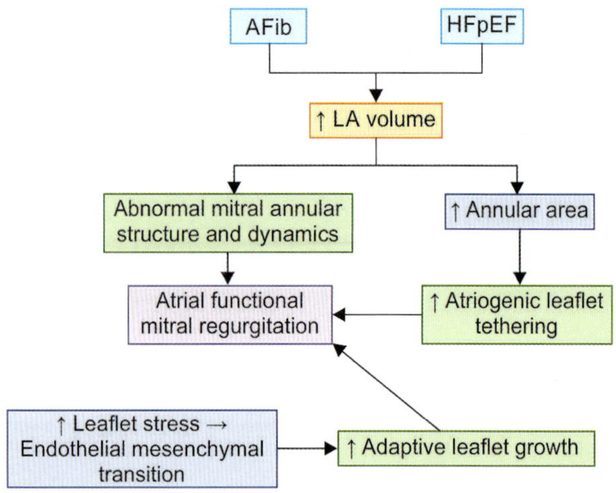

FLOWCHART 1: Pathophysiology of atrial functional mitral regurgitation.

Adaptive leaflet growth: In AF-MR, endothelial-mesenchymal transition, triggered by factors such as transforming growth factor-beta,[14] leads to migration of pluripotent endothelial cells into the valve, where they transform into fibroblasts and other mesenchymal cell lines, causing leaflet growth observed on echocardiography.[15] **Flowchart 1** summarizes the pathophysiology of AF-MR.

DIAGNOSIS

Echocardiography

Atrial functional MR should be assessed using the integrated approach. This should include color Doppler parameters and careful quantitative measurements of EROA and regurgitant volume, as well as qualitative supportive signs such as density, profile, and duration of the MR jet on continuous wave Doppler, pulmonary vein flow pattern, and mitral in flow E-wave velocity.

Echocardiographically, LV size and EF are more or less preserved in AF-MR. However, significant MR may lead to volume overload, causing left ventricular enlargement and a reduction in EF. Papillary muscle displacement that accompanies increased LV size tethers the mitral leaflets into the LV cavity, resulting in a picture of mixed AF-MR/VF-MR. Although not a diagnostic criterion, LV hypertrophy is commonly seen in AF-MR, particularly when HFpEF or hypertension coexist.[16] **Table 1** lists the differentiation between AF-MR and VF-MR.

The timing of the echocardiography assessment is crucial. When patients present with acute onset of AF and rapid ventricular response, moderate or severe MR can significantly improve after cardioversion.[17] Restoration of sinus rhythm with ablation can dramatically improve MR severity in AF-MR.[4] Assessment of MR severity is confounded by AF, especially in rapid or irregular rhythms. It is best

TABLE 1: Differentiation between AF-MR and VF-MR.

Criteria	Isolated AF-MR	Isolated VF-MR
LV size and geometry	• Normal by definition[22] (LV size may dilate secondarily in later stages of significant AF-MR)	• Often dilated[23] • Often increased LV sphericity[23]
LV systolic function	• Preserved regional and global function[22] • Peak LV GLS preserved (16–18%) or mildly reduced[22]	• Either global LV systolic dysfunction or focal wall motion abnormalities[23] • Peak LV GLS typically reduced (≤16%)[23]
LA size	• Dilated by definition[22] • LAVI usually moderately or severely enlarged (≥40 mL/m^2)	Often dilated[22]
Annular size	• Dilated by definition[22] • Sys D_{AP} > 35 mm in PLAX[24] or, sys D ≥ 36 mm in 4-chamber[25] or 3D mid-sys AA > 7.0 cm^2/m^2[26] • Annular flattening[22]	• Often dilated in response to LA dilation[22] • Annular flattening[23]
Leaflet morphology	• Macroscopically normal appearance[22] • At most, mild leaflet thickening[22]	• Macroscopically normal appearance[23] • Variable leaflet thickening[23]
Leaflet motion	Usually normal (Carpentier type 1 MR)[22]	Restrictive (Carpentier type IIIb MR)[23]
Leaflet coaptation point	At annular level or mildly displaced apically[22]	Displaced apically (subvalvular tethering)[23]
MR jet direction	Usually central but may be eccentric[22,27]	Eccentric or central[23]

(3D: three-dimensional; AA: annular area; AF-MR: atrial functional mitral regurgitation; AML: anterior mitral leaflet; D_{AP}: anteroposterior diameter; GLS: global longitudinal strain; LA: left atrium; LAVI: left atrial volume index; LV: left ventricle; LVEF: left ventricular ejection fraction; MR: mitral regurgitation; PLAX: parasternal long axis view; VF-MR: ventriculogenic functional mitral regurgitation)

to measure MR severity in sinus rhythm or AF when the ventricular rate is well controlled. It is recommended to use the indexed beat method by selecting a beat with similar preceding and following R-R intervals.[18]

Even in the best circumstances, AFib makes it challenging to measure MR using standard methods due to heart rate variability and beat-to-beat variation in LV stroke volume by 16–28%.[19,20] The proximal convergence method is also challenging in AF-MR due to variation in regurgitant orifice area, with the elliptical orifice shape commonly seen in AF-MR, leading to underestimation of MR. Some indirect markers of regurgitant severity, such as pulmonary venous Doppler, are also less reliable in AF. Advances in three-dimensional (3D) color Doppler technology may assist in refining this approach in the future. Some indirect markers of regurgitant severity are even less reliable, for example, pulmonary venous Doppler will show blunted systolic flow due to AF or high LA pressure even without any MR.

When quantifying AF-MR severity, it is important to consider the normal size and function of the LV. Studies **(Table 2)** show that LV end-diastolic volume averages in the normal range for AF-MR. AF-MR is associated with large LA volumes, which may accommodate the regurgitant volume if the LA is compliant. However, a "stiff" LA after extensive ablation could lead to elevated LA pressures even with lower regurgitant volumes.[21]

Role of Cardiac Magnetic Resonance and Cardiac Computed Tomography

While echocardiography is the first choice for evaluating mitral valvular morphology and hemodynamics because of its informativeness and accessibility, cardiac magnetic resonance (CMR) and computed tomography (CT) may contribute to the assessment of AF-MR even when echocardiography is suboptimal or when additional information is needed **(Table 3 and Figs. 2A to D)**. CMR and CT are limited by inadequate imaging windows or body habitus. However, they can accurately measure LV size and function and LA size.

However, CMR and CT require cardiac gating and may face some loss in image quality and challenge in quantitation of LVEF when cardiac rhythm is irregular in patients with AFib.

Cine imaging in CMR can assess mitral apparatus morphology and hemodynamics by quantifying MR severity. CMR may be more effective than CT at detecting annular distortion or abnormal leaflet motion. CMR phase contrast imaging accurately measures aortic systolic blood flow, which is then used to calculate mitral regurgitant volume and regurgitant fraction. Quantitation of MR regurgitant volume and fraction using CMR has been reported to be more reproducible than echocardiography.[33] In addition, CMR offers a more comprehensive assessment of LV remodeling by

TABLE 2: Quantitative echocardiographic studies in patients with AF-MR.

Reference	*n*	Age (years)	BSA (m²)	MR severity	EROA (cm²)	LAVi or LAV (mL or mL/m²)	LV size (end-diastole)	LVEF (%)	Persistent AF (%)
Cong et al.[28]	25	66	1.9 ± 0.2	Mod/Sev	0.47 ± 0.07	98 ± 22 mL	EDVi 89 ± 12 mL/m²	64 ± 2	70
Ito et al.[29]	16	72 ± 7	1.6 ± 0.2	Mod/Sev		95 ± 41 mL	EDD 55 ± 8 mm	66 ± 4	100
Kagiyama et al.[30]	28	75.9 ± 6.4	1.6 ± 0.2	Mod	0.26 ± 0.05	50.5± 19.5 mL/m²	EDD 49 ± 6 mm	62.5 ± 6.6	52
Kihara et al.[31]	12	69 ± 9		Mod/Sev			EDVi 79 ± 15 mL/m²	63 ± 6	100
Kim et al.[27]	23	68 ± 9	1.6 ± 0.2	Mod/Sev		69.7 ± 28.4 mL/m²	EDVi 57.2 ± 12.6 mL/m²	59 ± 6	100
Machino-Ohtsuka et al.[10]	25	66 ± 9	1.7 ± 0.2	Mod/Sev	0.41 ± 0.14	128 ± 105 mL	EDVi 54 ± 10 mL/m²	61 ± 9	100
Tang et al.[13]	21	71 ± 11	1.7 ± 0.1	Mod/Sev	0.27 ± 0.06	52 ± 10 mL/m²	EDVi 48 ± 10 mL/m²	59 ± 4	90
Uno et al.[32]	56	77 ± 10	1.8 ± 0.2	Mild/Mod/Sev	0.30 ± 0.11	83 ± 43 mL	EDVi 54 ± 18 mL/m²	60 ± 6	100

(AF: atrial fibrillation; BSA: body surface area; EDD: end-diastolic dimension; EDV: end-diastolic volume; EDVi: end-diastolic volume index; EROA: effective regurgitant orifice area; LAV: left atrial volume; LAVi: left atrial volume index; LV: left ventricle; Mod: moderate; MR: mitral regurgitation; Sev: severe)

TABLE 3: Role of cardiac CT and CMR in AF-MR.

	Cardiac CT	CMR
In suboptimal echocardiography	• Precisely measures of mitral leaflet morphology, mitral annular size across the cardiac cycle, tethering of leaflet motion, and orifice opening. CMR has advantages over CT due to higher temporal resolution and also the ability to quantify AF-MR severity • Quantify LV size and systolic function and LA size	
Other information		
Assessment of cardiomyopathy as underlying cause of MR	• Can rule out coronary artery disease and identify occult infarction • Assess the calcification of mitral valve apparatus • Can assess perivalvular anatomy in detail	• Identify myocardial infarction (including any involvement of the papillary muscles) • Assess myocardial fibrosis • Assess the severity of HFpEF
Quantify severity of MR	Does not quantify blood flow volume	Quantify regurgitant volume and regurgitant fraction (although accuracy reduced in AF)
Cardiac remodeling and preprocedural planning	Predict risk of LV outflow obstruction from percutaneous mitral valve replacement and characterize the landing zone of therapeutic devices	Predict recovery of adverse cardiac remodeling after mitral repair/replacement
Limitations	• Arrhythmias reduce image quality and accuracy of LVEF quantitation • Radiation exposure and iodinated contrast • Limited hemodynamic information	• Arrhythmias and cardiac devices lead to reduced image quality • Irregular rhythm leads to inaccuracy in the quantification of LVEF and MR • More operator dependent • Claustrophobia

(AF: atrial fibrillation; CMR: cardiac magnetic resonance; CT: computed tomography; HFpEF: heart failure with preserved ejection fraction)

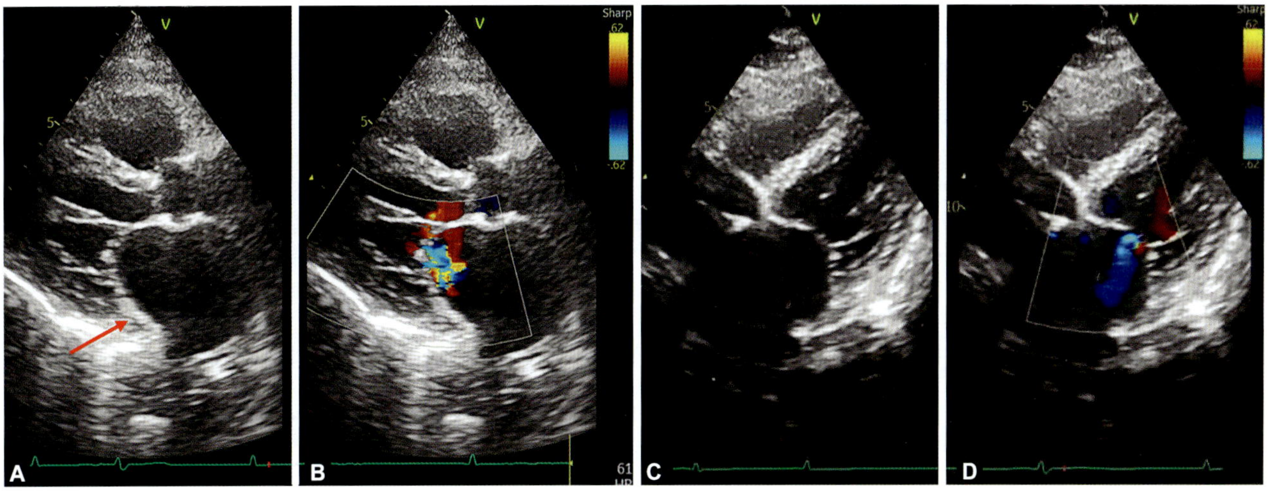

FIGS. 2A TO D: AF-MR—examples with echocardiographic images with color Doppler: (A and C) Systolic frame showing dilated LA and dilated mitral annulus with typically preserved LV size and function and concentric LV hypertrophy. (B and D) A central grade-II MR jet. Also, notice the tethering of the mitral valve (red arrow) and the underlying rhythm is AFib.

quantifying chamber size, LV function, and tissue fibrosis.[34] In patients in normal sinus rhythm, CT angiography accurately evaluates annular geometry, ventricular and atrial volumes and helps assess patients undergoing percutaneous mitral intervention. However, CT angiography lacks hemodynamic information and does not help adjudicate MR severity.[35]

In patients with multiple risk factors for HFpEF or prior chest radiation and evidence of impaired diastolic LV filling, CMR can provide insights on myocardial scar and fibrosis, aiding in understanding the severity and cause of cardiomyopathy. Additionally, CT allows for the identification and characterization of calcification of mitral apparatus that contributes to MR.

Strain Imaging

Patients with AF-MR have reduced LA (reservoir) strain,[5] which is associated with atrial fibrosis and increased likelihood of recurrent AFib when the LA reservoir strain is <15%.[36] Additionally, reduced LA strain is linked to higher mean LA and pulmonary artery systolic pressures, possibly due to poor LA compliance.[37]

TREATMENT

Medical Therapy and Rhythm Control

The 2020 Japanese Circulation Society heart valve disease management guidelines **(Box 1)** recommend (Class I recommendation) standard heart failure therapy for symptomatic patients with AF-MR,[38] including diuretics, which may reduce LA size. Rhythm control has been proposed as a means of reducing AF-MR by promoting atrial/annular reverse remodeling and restoring atriogenic and ventriculogenic contributions to annular contraction. Several small studies support this practice. Gertz et al.[4] findings had been previously discussed. Deferm et al.[39] observed a decrease in mean effective regurgitant orifice area from 0.27 to 0.15 cm^2 following electrical cardioversion in 15 patients with persistent AFib. Soulat-Dufour et al.[40] found that mean vena contracta width decreased from 0.40 to 0.21 cm in 47 patients with paroxysmal or persistent AFib following catheter ablation and/or electrical cardioversion. Finally, Masuda et al.[41] observed that more than three-fourths of patients with moderate AF-MR experienced improvement by one or more MR grades following catheter ablation. One study[42] demonstrated that catheter ablation significantly reduced the combined endpoint of heart failure hospitalization and stroke compared to patients treated with beta-blockers, calcium-channel blockers, digoxin, and/or antiarrhythmic drugs over a 3-year period.

In addition to reducing MR, rhythm control also leads to an increase in LVEF and also decreases brain natriuretic peptide levels.[41] The 2020 Japanese Circulation Society heart valve disease management guidelines **(Box 1)** consider catheter ablation reasonable (Class IIa recommendation) for symptomatic patients with persistent AFib and severe MR, if maintaining sinus rhythm is likely.

Surgery

The 2020 Japanese Circulation Society recommends surgical intervention is reasonable (Class IIa recommendation) for symptomatic patients with severe MR after failed standard heart failure therapy. In contrast, the 2020 American College of Cardiology/American Heart Association guidelines provide a Class IIb recommendation for surgery in similar patients **(Box 1)**.[43] Both recommendations are based on consensus (Level of Evidence: C). The 2021 European Society of Cardiology valvular heart disease management guidelines do not provide formal recommendations for the treatment of AF-MR. However, they mention that surgery and catheter ablation have been used to effectively treat AF-MR, although limited evidence supports this.

BOX 1 Treatment guidelines for AF-MR.[38,43]

2020 American College of Cardiology/American Heart Association Guidelines for the management of patients with valvular heart disease

In patients with chronic severe secondary MR from annular dilatation with preserved LV systolic function (LVEF of >50%) who have severe persistent symptoms (New York Heart Association functional Class III or IV) despite therapy for heart failure and therapy for associated atrial fibrillation and other comorbidities (Stage D), mitral valve surgery may be considered (COR: IIb; LOE: C)

2020 Japanese Circulation Society Heart Valve Disease Management Guidelines

- Standard medical therapy for heart failure, including diuretics, should be performed for symptomatic patients with AF-MR (COR: I; LOE: C)
- AFib catheter ablation is reasonable for symptomatic patients with persistent AFib and severe functional MR if successful ablation and maintenance of sinus rhythm can be expected from the duration of AFib and the LA size (COR: IIa; LOE: C)
- Mitral valve surgery is reasonable for patients with severe AF-MR who are consistently symptomatic despite standard medical therapy for heart failure (COR: IIa; LOE: C)[a,b]

[a] This recommendation can also be applied to patients with moderate AF-MR if MR worsens with heart failure exacerbations or during exercise stress testing.

[b] AF-MR is likely to accompany secondary atrial functional tricuspid regurgitation, and concomitant tricuspid surgery should be performed in patients with both AF-MR and tricuspid regurgitation.

(COR: class of recommendation; LOE: level of evidence)

Mitral valve surgery most often involves restrictive ring annuloplasty.[44] The presence of a large annular area may preclude coaptation unless significant ring undersizing is performed. This, however, increases the risks of dehiscence and mitral stenosis. In such cases, mitral valve replacement may be a suitable alternative. Patch augmentation of the PML using autologous pericardium has also been advocated, but the durability of this repair may be limited by leaflet shrinkage and stiffening.[45] Pseudoprolapse of the AML can typically be corrected with restrictive annuloplasty.[46]

The role of restoring sinus rhythm during mitral valve repair for AF-MR is not well-defined. One study found that patients who underwent Cox maze IV procedures had a 94% freedom from recurrent MR at 3 years, compared to 44% among those who did not.[47] However, only half of the patients undergoing mitral valve repair had Cox maze or CryoMAZE procedures.[44] Consideration of AFib duration and LA size is important when contemplating surgical intervention. Restoration of sinus rhythm becomes less likely when LA diameter exceeds 6.0 cm.[48]

Atrial functional TR caused by tricuspid annular enlargement frequently coexists with AF-MR.[49] The 2020 Japanese AF-MR guidelines recommend tricuspid valve repair in patients with combined AF-MR and AF-TR[38] (Class IIa recommendation). While surgery may improve symptoms, there is a lack of available data on the outcomes.

Percutaneous Interventions

The available percutaneous mitral valve interventions for patients with AF-MR include edge-to-edge repair (MitraClip, Abbott Vascular; PASCAL Mitral Valve Repair System, Edwards Life sciences), direct annuloplasty (Cardioband Mitral System, Edwards Life sciences; Millipede IRIS Ring, Boston Scientific), and indirect annuloplasty (Carillon Mitral Contour System, Cardiac Dimensions). Notably, transcatheter heart valves designed for the mitral position have not been studied in patients with AF-MR.

The multicenter Spanish MitraClip registry reported that 94% of patients experienced an acute reduction in MR from 3 to 4+ down to ≤2+.[50] Before the procedures, 90% of patients were in NYHA functional class III–IV; 12 months after the procedures, 20% were in class 3, and none were in class 4. Recurrent MR of >2+ developed in 20% by 12 months. In comparison, the Italian MITRA-TUNE registry reported a midterm MR recurrence rate of 11%.[51] The MITRA-TUNE registry also showed a reduction in annular dimensions that persisted for a median follow-up period of 1 year related to fibrosis caused by Mitraclip.[51,52] The long-term effect of this structural alteration on MR severity is not known.

The European Registry of Transcatheter Repair for Secondary Mitral Regurgitation includes a record of 126 patients, making it the largest cohort of symptomatic AF-MR patients reported. Procedural success, defined as MR of ≤2+, was achieved in 87% of registrants. The 2-year survival was 70%. Before repair, approximately 90% of patients were classified as NYHA functional class III/IV compared to about 40% after repair. NYHA functional class IV, right ventricular dysfunction, defined as reduced right ventricular–pulmonary artery coupling [(tricuspid annular plane systolic excursion) ÷ (pulmonary artery systolic pressure) < 0.34 mm/mm Hg], was a strong independent predictor of 2-year survival.[53]

A wide posterior leaflet angle, short residual PML, significant annular enlargement, pseudoprolapse, and jet eccentricity may predict worse outcomes after transcatheter edge-to-edge repair. The Italian MITRA-TUNE registry reported worse outcomes when preprocedural intercommissural annular diameter exceeds 34 mm.[51] Periodic echocardiographic surveillance for recurrent MR after transcatheter edge-to-edge repair seems prudent, particularly in patients with "high-risk" mitral valve geometry and/or jet eccentricity. Whether addressing annular enlargement by restoring sinus rhythm further reduces MR is uncertain, and randomized trials are needed to determine the efficacy of this combined approach.

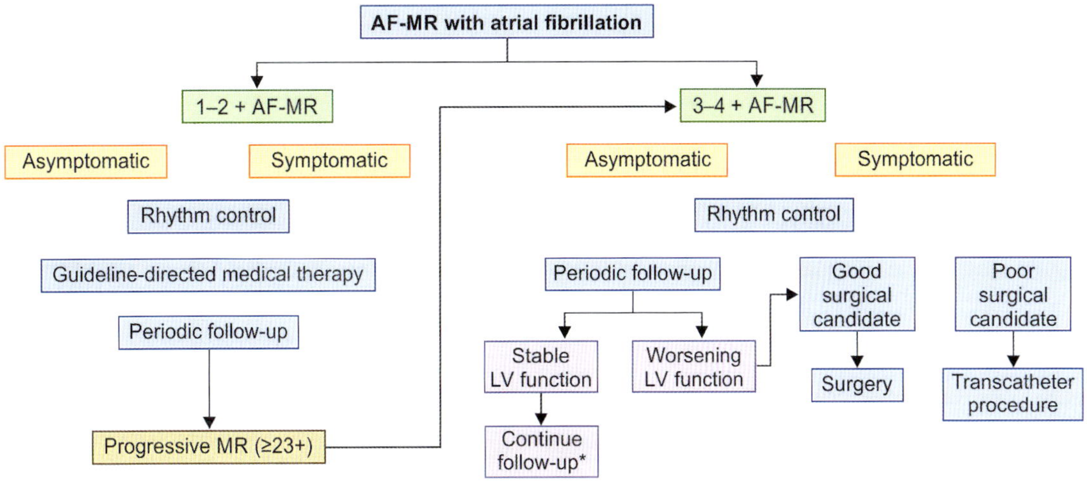

*Follow-up: Echocardiographic assessment of left ventricular size and function.

FLOWCHART 2: An integrated approach to the treatment of AF-MR.

Transcatheter annuloplasty devices could be an option for AF-MR patients at high surgical risk or with unfavorable anatomy for transcatheter edge-to-edge repair. In a series of 15 patients with moderate–severe AF-MR, the Carillon device led to a significant reduction in annular anteroposterior diameter and effective regurgitant orifice area at 3 months.[54] Another study comparing the Carillon device to the MitraClip in patients with AF-MR caused by HFpEF found no significant difference in functional status at 12 months.[55]

Integrated Approach to Treatment of Atrial Functional Mitral Regurgitation

Due to limited data, there is no consensus on treating patients with AFib and AF-MR. The integrated approach to the treatment of AF-MR is shown in **Flowchart 2**. However, according to the EAST AF-NET trial, restoring sinus rhythm within 1 year of AFib onset has been shown to decrease cardiovascular death, stroke, and other complications.[56] Therefore, rhythm control strategies should be pursued regardless of MR severity or symptom status. Symptomatic patients with advanced MR (3–4+) should be referred for surgery or transcatheter intervention. Asymptomatic patients with moderate to severe MR (3–4+) need regular follow-up to monitor for any deterioration in LV function, development of pulmonary hypertension, or signs of heart failure, which should trigger further intervention.

CONCLUSION

- AF-MR occurs in the setting of long-standing AFib and/or HFpEF.
- The pathophysiology includes atriogenic mitral leaflet tethering, abnormalities of mitral annular structure and dynamics, and variable adaptive leaflet growth.
- Echocardiographic features are large LA, mitral annular enlargement, and a normal left ventricular size and function. There may be variable leaflet restriction, variable anterior leaflet pseudoprolapse, and central or eccentric MR jets.
- Imaging modalities other than echocardiography, CT for anatomic detail, and mitral annular measurements in the context of transcatheter procedures, CMR imaging for assessment of LA fibrosis, and strain imaging for LA (reservoir) strain.
- There is no consensus on the medical management of patients with AF-MR. Standard heart failure therapy including a diuretic can be used, and some studies show an effect of rhythm management on MR reduction among these patients. However, outcomes data are lacking.
- There is no consensus on the role of surgical intervention in treating AF-MR. If pursued, surgery typically involves reduction annuloplasty, patch augmentation of the PML, or surgical mitral valve replacement could be considered.
- Transcatheter options to treat AF-MR include edge-to-edge repair and direct or indirect annuloplasty, albeit with limited available outcomes data. Transcatheter heart valve replacement has not been studied among patients with AF-MR.
- AF-MR due to AFib commonly is accompanied by atrial functional tricuspid regurgitation. Diuretic therapy can be considered, although surgery might be associated with improved symptoms; outcomes data are lacking.

ONLINE REFERENCES

Please scan the QR code provided at the end of the table of contents for References of this chapter.

CHAPTER

14

Left Atrial Strain: Clinical Applications and Limitations

Jacob Jose, Jesu Krupa

ABSTRACT

The left atrium (LA) modulates left ventricular filling by its reservoir function in systole, as a conduit during diastole, and pump function during atrial contraction. LA strain analysis using speckle tracking can be used for the assessment of this phasic LA function. The normal value for LA reservoir strain (LARS) is >24%. It is usually determined in a LA-focused apical four-chamber view or in combination with an apical two-chamber view, keeping the zero reference as the R wave on ECG and tracking the LA endocardium. LARS may be helpful in assessing diastolic dysfunction and LA pressure, especially when it is indeterminate by the existing algorithms. It is useful in predicting the risk of recurrence of atrial fibrillation and stroke. It also correlates with outcomes in chronic kidney disease (CKD), hypertrophic cardiomyopathy (HCM), and cardiac amyloidosis. It has been studied to a limited extent in a variety of other cardiac conditions including valvular heart diseases such as mitral regurgitation and aortic stenosis. It is also found to be low in diabetic patients compared to controls. Patients with hypertension show improvement in LARS with better blood pressure control. Hence, this simple tool is likely to be of great clinical value in the days ahead.

Keywords: Left atrium reservoir strain, hypertrophic cardiomyopathy, chronic kidney disease

INTRODUCTION

The left atrium (LA) modulates the left ventricular (LV) filling by its reservoir function in systole, as a conduit during diastole, and pump function during atrial contraction. LA dysfunction is a major contributing factor for elevated LA pressure (LAP). Usually, LA function is assessed by volumetric methods such as LA volume and LA expansion index, or by Doppler methods using mitral flow pattern. More recently, LA strain analysis has been used for the assessment of LA function. LA strain measurements can be done using tissue Doppler, velocity vector imaging, or 2D speckle tracking echocardiography (STE). With the speckle tracking method, LA phasic function can be easily assessed. The reservoir strain component is easy to obtain, and it is the single index that we can use for the estimation of LAP as well. In this chapter, we summarize the methodology and clinical applications.

METHODOLOGY

Though LA strain can be studied using tissue Doppler or STE, the latter method has now become the most acceptable measurement of LA strain. LA strain is quantified as global longitudinal strain (GLS) of the entire LA wall. Segmental LA strain is not measured or clinically relevant. Given the limited thickness of the LA wall and the minimum thickness of any region of interest, a distinction of endocardial strain and full wall strain is not done.

Our zero reference is end diastole which can be marked by the ECG trigger for R wave or nadir of the atrial strain if the QRS is wide. Some studies have used zero reference at the beginning of atrial contraction. This causes confusion by giving a different curve and is hence not recommended.

The morphology of the strain curve is characterized by a monophasic systolic part where the LA fills and stretches prior to opening of the mitral valve. When the mitral valve opens, LA emptying starts and there is a decline in the strain, and it reaches a plateau. With atrial contraction, there is another dip.

The European Association of Cardiovascular Imaging/American Society of Echocardiography[1] recommends LA strain analysis by tracing the LA endocardial border, starting at the medial mitral annulus excluding the pulmonary veins and going up to the lateral mitral annulus, using the *apical four-chamber view*. Biplane LA strain (from four- and two-chamber views) could also be considered as an option. The LA appendage (LAA) orifice is excluded in the apical two-chamber view. The myocardial region of interest of the LA is defined by the endocardial border and the epicardial border, like LV strain measurement. If the tracking software requires the definition of the region of interest, a default width of 3 mm is recommended. The region of interest size and shape should be adjusted in order to include the thickness of LA wall and to avoid including the pericardium. If the tracking software uses endocardial tracking only, the *endocardial contour* is delineated. The user should visually assess the tracking to the motion of the underlying LA wall in order to judge the accuracy of the LA strain estimate.

LEFT ATRIUM STRAIN WAVEFORMS

There are three strain values that can be obtained, but the one that is clinically most useful is the reservoir strain **(Fig. 1)**. *LA reservoir strain* (LARS) is the peak atrial longitudinal strain which is positive and occurs due to atrial filling during ventricular systole against a closed mitral valve. *Conduit strain* is calculated as the strain value at the onset of atrial contraction minus the peak atrial longitudinal strain and it is always negative. *LA contraction strain* (LASc) is calculated as the difference of the strain value at end diastole and the value at the onset of atrial contraction. This is always a negative value since it occurs during late diastole as a result of atrial contraction and emptying. In short, the value is positive during LA filling and negative during emptying.

NORMAL STRAIN VALUES

The strain values differ based on age and gender. In the study by Morris et al. of 393 normal persons, the LARS was 45.5 + 11.4% and the lowest expected value was 23%.[2] In the study by Singh et al., they used a vendor-independent software and did include individuals from several countries. The normal value for LARS is >24%.

HEMODYNAMIC DETERMINANTS OF LARS

As the LARS in systole, it should reflect the systolic function of the ventricle. Mitral annulus descent that occurs in systole is directly related to LV systolic function. LARS is also affected

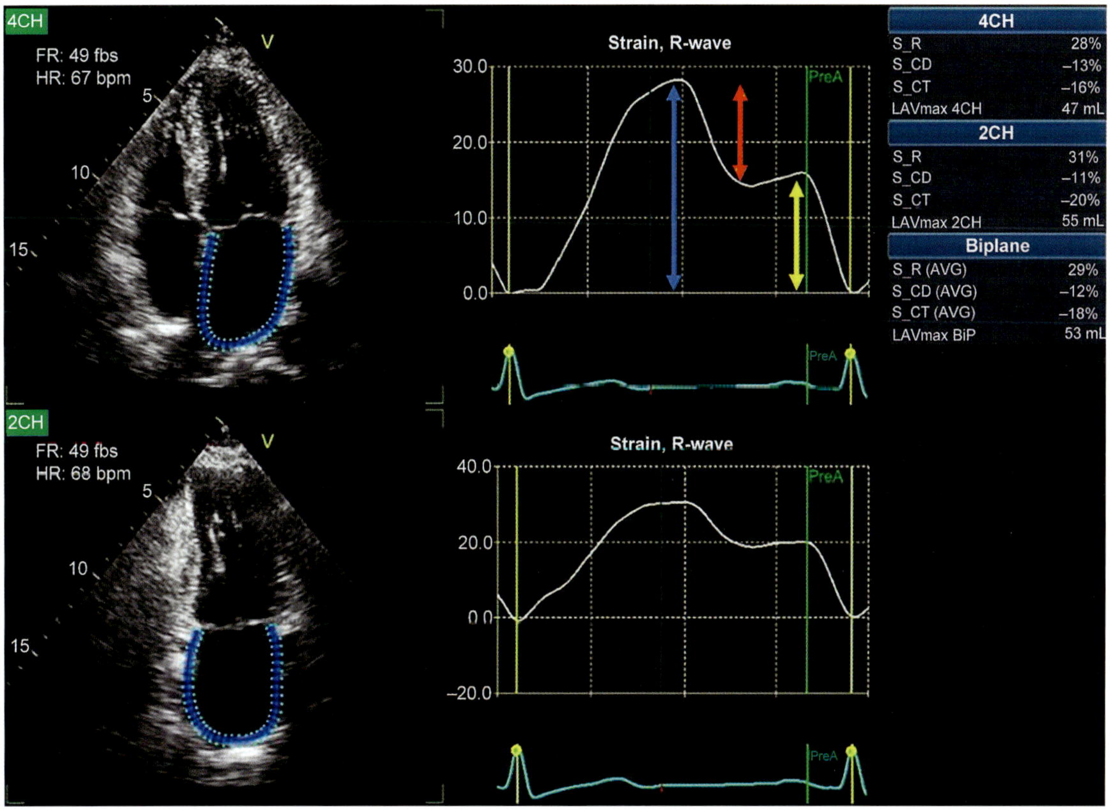

FIG. 1: A 53-year-old, asymptomatic diabetic and hypertensive with normal LVEF, abnormal LV GLS of –15.3%, grade 1 LV diastolic dysfunction with normal LV filling pressure at rest. LA strain in four-chamber and two-chamber views showing reduction in LARS but still >20–24%. The blue arrow shows the peak LA strain or reservoir strain, the red arrow shows the conduit strain, and the yellow arrow shows the atrial booster pump strain.

by LA chamber stiffness. The stiffer the LA, the lower will be the pressure gradient between the pulmonary veins and the LA and hence LARS will be reduced. The main determinants of LARS as invasively studied in patients undergoing transcatheter mitral valve edge-to-edge repair were LV relaxation, LV GLS, and LA chamber stiffness.[3]

LARS FOR DIASTOLIC DYSFUNCTION

Five parameters have been suggested for the assessment of diastolic dysfunction.[4] Of the five, *E/e′* ratio is the one that correlates reasonably well with the LAP. In the study by Singh et al., when *E/e′* ratio is compared with LARS with simultaneous pulmonary artery wedge pressure, LARS was better than the *E/e* ratio. Hence, many authors have tried to use LARS in the diagnosis of diastolic dysfunction. As per the diastolic dysfunction algorithm, a subset will be called indeterminate. It is in this group of patients we can use LARS. In the study by Potter et al.,[5] they used LARS instead of LA volume (LAVI), and they could reduce the indeterminate cases by 75%. In another study, they looked at this intermediate group with exercise. LARS has been used for the assessment of LAP with exercise in patients with heart failure with preserved ejection fraction (HFpEF). The addition of LARS improved the diagnostic value of HFpEF score with area under the curve from 0.7 to 0.8.[6]

Left atrium reservoir strain has been the most accurate for the estimation of LAP in patients with depressed LVEF, rather than with preserved ejection fraction. In patients with preserved EF, a LARS <18% has a high specificity for increased LV filling pressure.[7]

A comparison of LARS and LAVI is given in **Table 1**, adapted from the editorial of Cho and Hwang.[8]

LEFT ATRIUM STRAIN FOR PROGNOSIS

The addition of LARS can be useful for not only identifying patients with diastolic dysfunction but also prognostication. Risk of heart failure hospitalization was increased at an odds ratio of 6.6 (CI 2.6–16.6) in a group of patients with normal LAVI, but abnormal LA strain. The absolute increase in the prognostic value was 9.9% when LARS was added to LAVI.[9]

TABLE 1: LA volume versus LA strain.

	LAVI	LARS
Abnormal cutoff	>34 mL/m^2	<23%
Feasibility	90–93%	89–97%
Correlation with wedge pressure	Mild	Modest
Reflection of diastolic function	Chronicity	Early
Marker of LA fibrosis	May not be	May be
Prognostic value	Weak	Strong

LEFT ATRIUM STRAIN AND HEART FAILURE WITH PRESERVED EJECTION FRACTION PHENOTYPES

It has been proposed to phenotype HFpEF to those with reduced LV GLS and those with preserved LV GLS. Those HFpEF patients with reduced LV GLS may have reduced LARS which is likely to be secondary to LV myocardial disease and consequently elevated LAP. However, in those HFpEF patients with preserved GLS who have reduced LARS, the mechanism of LA dysfunction is believed to be due to *LA myopathy* which is disproportionate to the extent of LV disease. This subgroup of patients has a worse hemodynamic profile with chronotropic incompetence and higher pulmonary artery pressure and pulmonary vascular resistance, along with a lower stroke volume. **Figure 2** illustrates this new concept of disproportionate LA myopathy which emphasizes the pivotal role of the LA in heart failure.[10]

PREDICTION OF ATRIAL FIBRILLATION

Left atrium strain parameters have been shown to predict atrial fibrillation (AFib) in many studies. In the fifth Copenhagen City Heart Study which had 4,466 participants who were followed up for a median of 5.3 years, 4.3% developed AFib. For patients with LA strain of <23%, there was a 6.8-fold increased risk of developing AFib. Thus, integrating LA strain into an echo study for the general population will be useful for risk stratification.[11]

Left atrium strain has been useful for predicting recurrence of AFib following AFib ablation. In a study of 172 patients undergoing cryoablation, 50 of them had recurrence. A LARS of <17% is the highest incremental predictive value for AF recurrence (HR 9.45; 95% CI 3.17–28.13; $p < 0.001$). Even in patients with nondilated LA, the predictive value for recurrence was HR 5.39; 95% CI 1.66–17.52.[12]

RISK OF STROKE AND LEFT ATRIUM STRAIN

In a study, a cohort of 806 adults without stroke or AFib was followed for 10.9 years. New-onset stroke occurred in 53 participants (7%). Reduced LA strain was independently associated with new stroke even after control of other factors such as LA volume, AFib, and LV strain. Thus, in the elderly population, adding the LA strain may risk stratify patients who may develop stroke in the future.[13] A recent large study by Zhang et al. showed that after adjustment for LARS, AFib was not significantly associated with the risk of stroke or dementia.[14] However, the ARCADIA trial which randomized patients with cryptogenic stroke and LA myopathy but no AFib to apixaban versus aspirin failed to show any difference

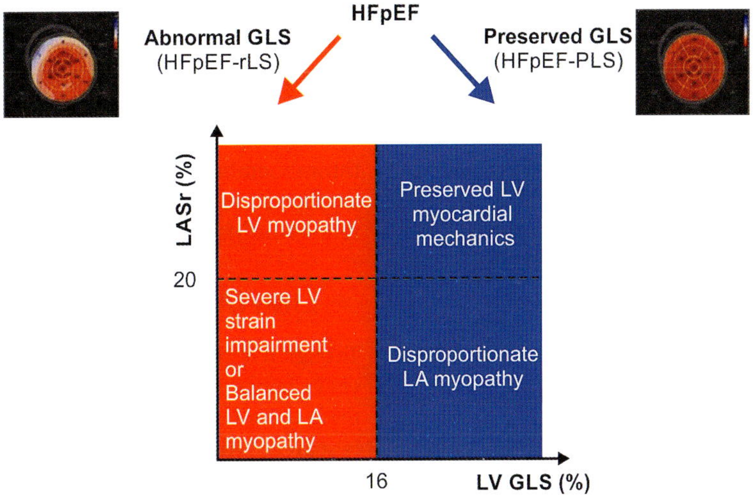

FIG. 2: Heart failure with preserved ejection fraction (HFpEF) phenotypes and disproportionate LA myopathy.

in stroke events in the two groups [hazard ratio 1.00 (95% CI 0.64–1.55)].[15]

Role of Left Atrium Strain in Post-myocardial infarction Patients

Left atrium reservoir strain is noted to be a good predictor for AFib in patients following myocardial infarction (MI). In a study of 392 patients of ST-elevation MI treated with primary angioplasty who were followed for 5.6 years, 6.3% of patients were noted to have AFib. The LA strain was 24.1% or less in patients with incident AFib.[16]

Role of Left Atrium Strain in Chronic Kidney Disease Patients

Chronic kidney disease (CKD) patients are known to have a higher cardiovascular risk. In a study of 243 patients with CKD and no previous heart disease who were followed up over 5 years, LA peak strain was the only predictor for the primary end point for death.[17] In another study of 280 patients with CKD stage 3 or 4, reduced LARS was associated with a 2.5-fold higher risk of composite outcomes (HR 2.51; 95% CI 1.19–5.30; $p = 0.02$) and was the only echocardiographic parameter that predicted progressive renal failure independent of established clinical risk factors for end-stage renal failure.[18] In a systematic review of LA strain in CKD patients that included six studies, it was noted that this is a promising marker for cardiovascular events.[19]

Left Atrium Strain in Hypertrophic Cardiomyopathy

Hypertrophic cardiomyopathy (HCM) is expected to have diastolic dysfunction. LA strain has been studied in this group as a prognostic marker for the development of heart failure, stroke, and death in a small study. In this study, there was lower event-free survival in patients with reservoir strain ≤23.8% or conduit strain ≤10.2%.[20]

Left Atrium Strain in Hypertension

In hypertensives, LA strain was abnormal despite normal volumetric measures of LA, suggesting that LA strain becomes abnormal earlier than LA dilatation.[21] It has also been shown that strain improves with blood pressure control. This improvement is not dependent on the class of drugs but on the level of blood pressure control. In a study of 160 patients of mild to moderate hypertension, nebivolol was compared with irbesartan and there was no significant difference between these two drugs for LA strain reduction.[22]

Left Atrium Strain in Diabetes

Diabetes is usually associated with strain abnormalities of the LV, and diabetic patients also have diastolic dysfunction. Impairment of LA reservoir and conduit function by STE strain has been shown even in the absence of LV hypertrophy or hypertension. In a systematic review of and meta-analysis of 41 studies with 6,668 asymptomatic patients with DM compared to 7,218 healthy controls, it was shown that LARS was significantly lower in individuals with diabetes compared to healthy controls [28.0% (23.9, 32.1) vs. 36.5 (34.2, 38.9)] with a large mean difference of –8.41 (–11.5, –5.33).[23]

Left Atrium Strain in Other Diseases

Left atrium strain has been studied in a variety of other cardiac conditions and the practical utilities of this need to be studied further. In a study of 65 patients with *mitral regurgitation* who were followed up after surgery for the development of heart failure and mortality, it was noted that a peak atrial strain <21% was the best discriminator for the development of these end points.[24] LA strain has been shown to be a better marker than natriuretic peptides in patients with *aortic stenosis* and preserved ejection fraction to identify patients who are likely to worsen their NYHA class or hospitalization heart failure. In this study of 173 patients, LARS of <20% was the best cutoff.[25] LA function has been shown to be abnormal in *obese* individuals and LA strain in obese individuals between the age of 35 and 55 years was studied in the Asklepios Study. As the BMI increased, the LARS decreased significantly from 35% in those with BMI <25 kg/m^2 to 30% in those with BMI of 30 kg/m^2 or more. This suggests that with increasing obesity, LA function is important for diastolic function and loss of this compensatory function may contribute to the AFib and heart failure in these patients.[26] LA strain has been studied in patients with *cardiac amyloidosis* and it has been shown that LARS <13.2% was associated with less survival **(Figs. 3A to D)**.[27] In a recent study of 448 patients with AL and ATTR cardiac amyloidosis, there were 64 patients (14.3%) who had a thromboembolic event. Of these, 75% of patients were in sinus rhythm and never had AF. It was also shown that it further refines the Mayo prognostic staging in this group of patients.[28]

LIMITATIONS

Though it is attractive, data are still emerging and LA strain is yet to become part of most clinical guidelines. Evidence for therapy for heart failure or stroke prevention based on LARS is scarce. LARS does not independently reflect LA function and may depend on LV longitudinal function.

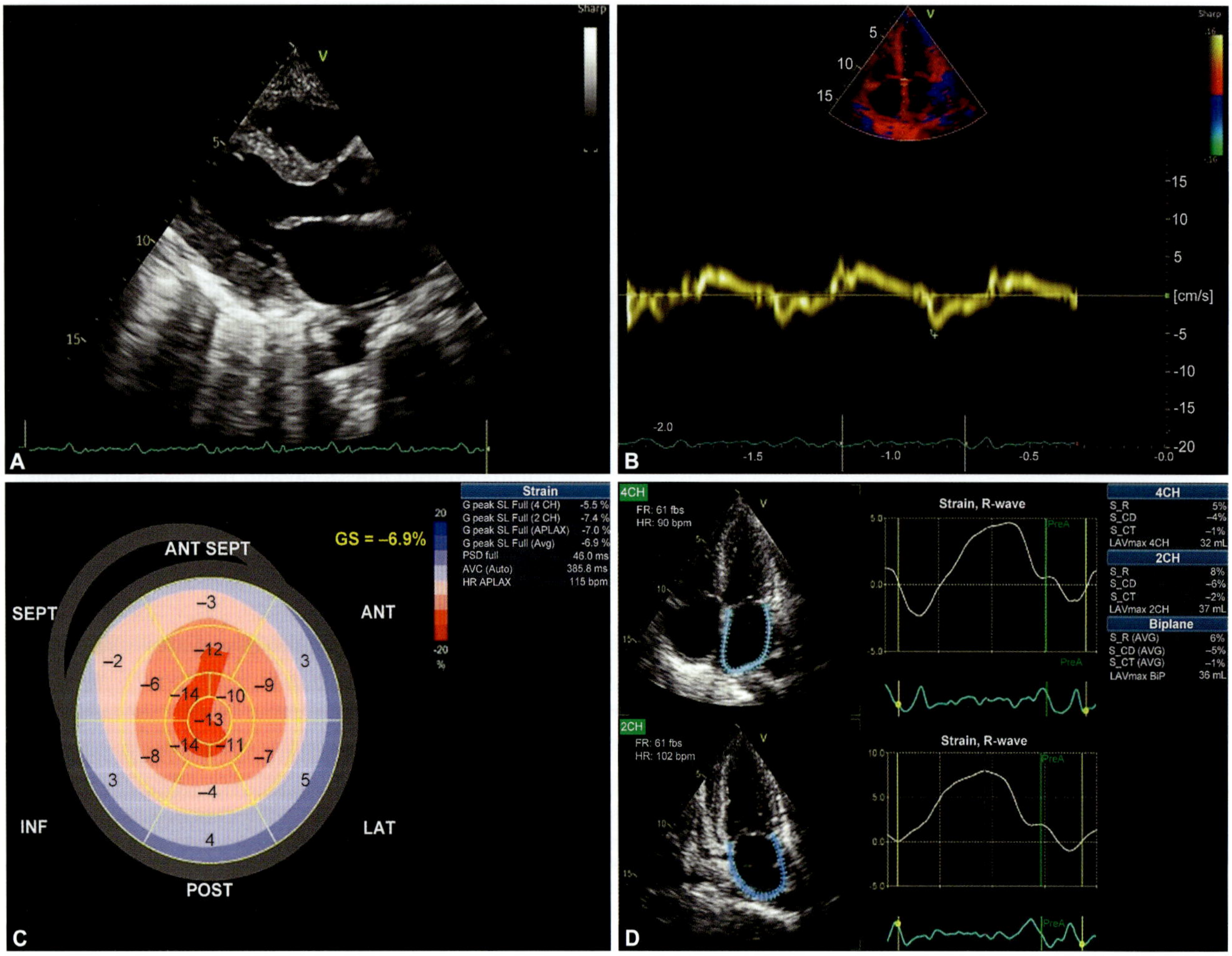

FIGS. 3A TO D: A 43-year-old female with heart failure symptoms and low-voltage QRS complexes on ECG. (A) LV with thick walls and a dilated LA; (B) Reduced mitral annular tissue Doppler velocities, medial *e′* = 5 cm/s; (C) "Cherry on top" appearance of LV GLS; and (D) Markedly reduced four-chamber and two-chamber LA strain, biplane LARS = 6%. These findings are typical of cardiac amyloidosis. The markedly reduced LA strain is indicative of severe LA dysfunction and could predispose to LA clot and thromboembolic phenomena even though the patient is in sinus rhythm.

CONCLUSION

Left atrium strain has become easy to measure with the newer echo machines due to built-in software for speckle tracking. Many of the machines have automatic measurement of the same. LARS may be particularly useful in the large group of patients with indeterminate diastolic function assessment. In addition, it plays a major role in the risk stratification of various patients and in the prediction of AFib. In the coming years, this will be another robust measure in our echo armamentarium.

ONLINE REFERENCES

Please scan the QR code provided at the end of the table of contents for References of this chapter.

CHAPTER

15

Coronary CT Angiography: Principles, Techniques, and Clinical Application

Priya Jagia, Sreelal Thazhathu Veettil

ABSTRACT

Coronary CT angiography (CCTA) is a noninvasive modality for assessment of coronary arteries. With excellent sensitivity, it is now a key step in the evaluation of both acute and chronic coronary artery disease. Optimum enhancement of the coronary arteries postinjection of contrast agent needs precise acquisition techniques. Different methods can be used depending on the indication and patient characteristics. In this brief chapter, we focus on the principles, modes of acquisition, and clinical applications of CCTA.

Keywords: CCTA, CT, techniques, principles, sensitivity

INTRODUCTION

Computed tomographic angiography (CTA) has come up as a crucial modality in the evaluation of coronary arteries. It is a fast and noninvasive modality that gives an excellent anatomic visualization of the coronary arteries, the cardiac chambers, and surrounding structures. Precise use of contrast agent dose and injection parameters tailored to the scanner is needed for optimal enhancement of the coronary arteries. Interpretation of the images needs an understanding of the anatomy and pathology of coronary artery disease and the potential artifacts in scans. Functional evaluation of lesions and cardiac structures remain a challenge, though tackled to an extent with the recent innovations in technology. Technological advancements have also dealt with the age-old issue of radiation.

Improved sensitivity to detect coronary artery disease helps in ruling out the disease in specific target populations. *It has found a niche in the evaluation of both acute and chronic coronary artery diseases. It has helped in reducing the number of unwarranted invasive coronary angiographies.*

PRINCIPLE

Administration of iodine-containing contrast agents results in selective enhancement of the contrast containing structures, which are the arteries in this case. An HU value of 250–300 is ideal for visualizing the coronary arteries.[1] The technique of acquisition mainly focuses on imaging the coronary arteries at this peak enhancement. Another issue with visualizing the coronary arteries is their movement during the cardiac cycle. Even with the modern scanners, the time taken for scan completion is more than the duration of a single cardiac cycle, which could result in blurring of the coronary artery. By gating the scan, we can map the entire cardiac cycle from one R wave to the next. Within this, areas of minimal cardiac motion during the diastole and systole are identified and focus is given to them to prevent motion artifacts.

ACQUISITION AND INTERPRETATION

Patient Preparation

Considering the possible risk of contrast allergy which may lead to aspiration, patients are usually requested to avoid solids for a minimum of 3 hours prior to the scan. They can continue to take clear fluids and are even encouraged to do so. A renal function test and subsequent calculation of estimated glomerular filtration rates is done in patients at risk for kidney disease. Heart rate-lowering medications targeting a heart rate of 60–70 become necessary in older generation of scanners with poor temporal resolution. Nitroglycerine (NTG) may be administered to dilate the coronary arteries prior to the scan. Patients should be screened for comorbidities prior to the administration of these agents. Screening is also done for pregnancy and conditions which may prevent them from holding breath for 5–10 seconds.

Intravenous Access

Contrast Volume

Typically, volumes of 1 mL/kg suffice in the modern scanners.[2] Postprocessing, using artificial intelligence-based software help in reducing the noise and enhancing the signals, making it possible to evaluate the coronary arteries using lesser amounts of contrast.

Region of Interest

Modern scanners can be set to automatically start the scan (trigger) once a predetermined enhancement level is reached at a specified region—the region of interest (ROI). Another method of acquisition is using a test bolus of contrast to obtain the enhancement curve of the artery and thus, predetermining the ideal time for acquisition.

Scan Delay

Scan delay is the time taken for acquisition to complete after intravenous administration of contrast agent. This includes the time it takes for the monitoring to start at the carinal level (monitoring delay), time taken to reach the threshold value in the ROI, and time taken for the scanner to move from the position of ROI to the intended starting point of the scan and the actual scan duration.

Rate of Administration

After fixing the contrast volume, the rate is determined so that the completion of contrast injection occurs prior to the acquisition of scan. A saline chase is also administered to clear the veins and right sided heart of any residual contrast.

ECG Gating

The mapping of the cardiac cycle using the ECG tracing can be done in two ways:

1. *Retrospective gating*: Scanning is done for the entire cardiac cycle and mapping is done after acquisition of the scan. Areas of least cardiac motion within the acquired scan range are identified and labeled. In patients with irregular heart rates, this method is more reliable. This scanning mode also allows for functional evaluation of the heart. As the entire cardiac cycle is scanned, the radiation dose is higher.
2. *Prospective gating*: The ECG tracing is read by the system and selective acquisition of a particular portion of the cardiac cycle is done where the cardiac motion is expected to be minimal. In patients with regular heart rate and rhythm, the machine can accurately acquire the scan. Radiation dose is significantly lower, and this method of acquisition should be considered as the default. Post-acquisition, cardiac phases outside of the target cannot be evaluated, which makes this mode more at risk of being noninterpretable and precludes functional evaluation.

These methods are compared in **Table 1**.

Postprocessing: In the machine, ECG editing can be done to remove unwanted cardiac cycles, which creates artifacts. In the console, multiplanar reconstructions of the images are possible. Apart from these curved reconstructions make it possible to visualize the coronary arteries in their entire extent.

Virtual reconstructions and 3D reformations of the coronary arteries help in demonstrating the anatomy better and identification of anomalies easier.

CT-derived fractional flow reserve: The Achilles heel of CCTA is its relative lack of specificity. Lesions that appear significant on CCTA may not have a hemodynamic significance and even some lesions that are having <50% stenosis may be significant hemodynamically. CT-derived fractional flow reserve (CT-FFR) is a recent modality that creates a physiological simulation data from routine CCTA which can provide the flow, pressure, and resistance across coronary artery segments using computational fluid dynamics.[3] A value of <0.75 is indicative of a significant lesion and warrants invasive catheter angiography. Addition of CT-FFR to routine CCTA reduces the downstream invasive coronary angiographies and the overall cost of healthcare.[4] However, majority of the trials have failed to demonstrate differences in outcomes of major adverse cardiovascular events and all-cause mortality.

TABLE 1: Comparison of commonly used methods of acquisition in CCTA.

	Retrospective	Prospective	Prospective helical
Phases acquired	All cardiac phases	Limited to 1–6 phases	Single phase
Radiation dose	4–10 mSv	2–4 mSv	~1 mSv
Functional evaluation	Possible	Not possible	Not possible
Artefacts	Less	Step/stitch artefacts, artefacts with higher heart rates	More artefacts at higher heart rates
Acquisition	4–8 seconds	2–4 seconds	<3 seconds

CT Perfusion

The attenuation of tissues after contrast administration is proportional to the blood flow in that territory. By measuring the changes in attenuation prior to contrast administration and in phases following contrast administration, qualitative or quantitative evaluation of the perfusion can be done. This principle is used in CT perfusion (CTP), which gives hemodynamic information about a stenotic lesion by assessing myocardial perfusion.[5] Stress perfusion images can be obtained after administering appropriate medications. The additional acquisition of images, especially in dynamic CTP, leads to higher radiation doses.[6]

CLINICAL APPLICATIONS

Acute Coronary Syndrome

The initial evaluation of patients with suspected acute coronary syndrome is aimed at classifying the patients based on risk. Following initial history, examination, ECG, enzyme levels and cardiovascular risk assessment, various risk assessment methods can be used to do this. Patients with a <1% risk of myocardial infarction (MI) in the next 30 days is considered low risk. According to the latest ACC/AHA guidelines, these patients can be safely discharged without further testing.[7]

Intermediate-risk Patients

In patients with no ST elevation on ECG and having intermediate-risk probability of acute coronary syndrome with normal or equivocal troponin levels or a high sensitivity troponin value of <99th percentile and normal functional testing in the past 1 year, a coronary CTA is appropriate investigation as shown in **Figure 1**. The role of CCTA has been questioned in the era of high-sensitivity troponin assays.[8] In the RAPID-CCTA trial, early coronary CTA was able to reduce the number of invasive coronary angiographies with no effect on subsequent myocardial ischemia (MI), revascularization or preventive treatment.[9] A combination of high-sensitivity troponin assay level of <99th percentile and high-risk plaque features on CCTA may be a better predictor of severity, as demonstrated in the PRECISE-CTA trial.[10] The high-risk plaques are an important consideration in patients with ACS, as a high number of these lesions are nonobstructive. High-risk plaque features include positive remodeling, low attenuation, napkin ring sign, and spotty calcification **(Fig. 2)**. In patients with features of high-risk plaque, further functional evaluation may be done with CT-FFR or CTP. CT-FFR helps in downgrading lesions found to be severe on CCTA and may also find out hemodynamically significant lesions with only mild-to-moderate stenosis on CCTA.[11] CTP can also stratify patients based on rest perfusion. A strategy of combined CCTA and CTP was both cost-saving and also reduced the duration of hospital stay in patients at intermediate probability of ACS when compared with nuclear perfusion study.[12] Thus, a strategy utilizing CCTA

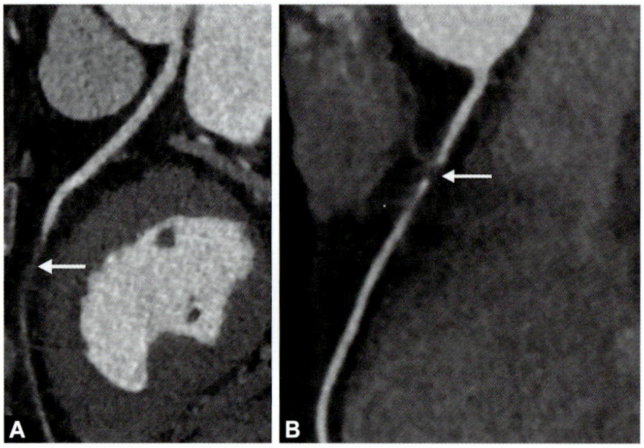

FIG. 1A AND B: Curved reformatted images of two patients who presented to the emergency room with complaints of acute-onset chest pain and atypical ECG changes. (A) Noncalcified plaque in the left anterior descending artery (LAD) causing long segment occlusion (white arrow) and poor distal opacification. (B) Noncalcified focal plaque causing significant stenosis (~90%) of the LAD.

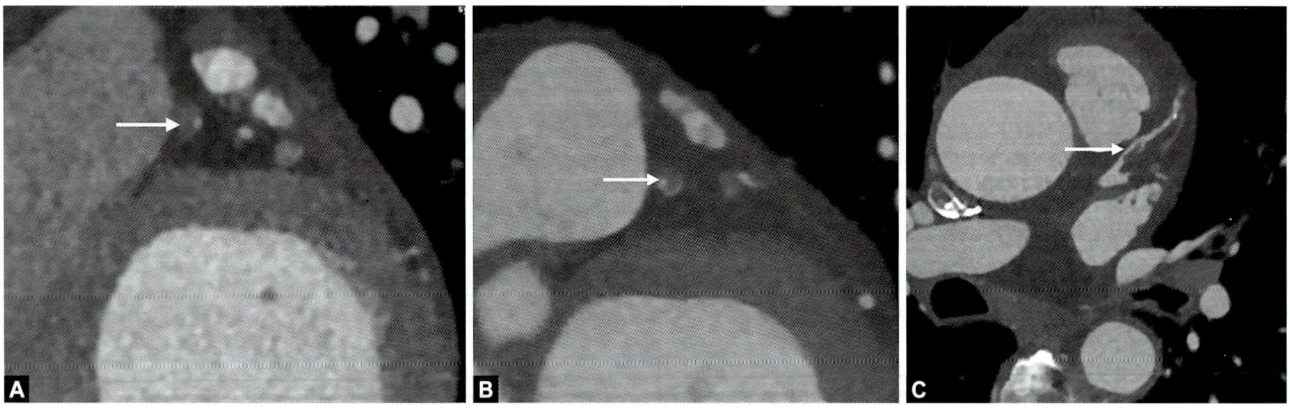

FIGS. 2A TO F: *Continued*

Continued

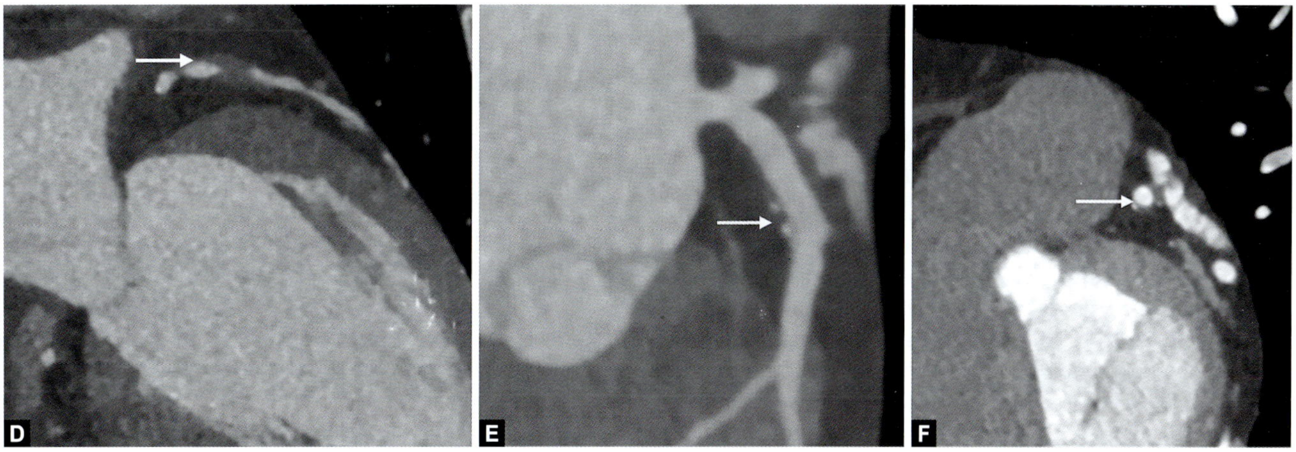

FIGS. 2A TO F: High-risk plaque features. (A) Low-attenuation plaque (white arrow) causing significant stenosis of the left anterior descending artery (LAD). (B and C) Short axis and four-chamber views of the LAD with an eccentric plaque (white arrows) causing significant stenosis. Note the short-axis view showing central hypodensity and rim of hyperdensity. (D) Positive remodeling caused by a plaque in the LAD causing significant stenosis. (E and F) Eccentric plaques with spotty calcifications causing mild stenosis of the LAD.

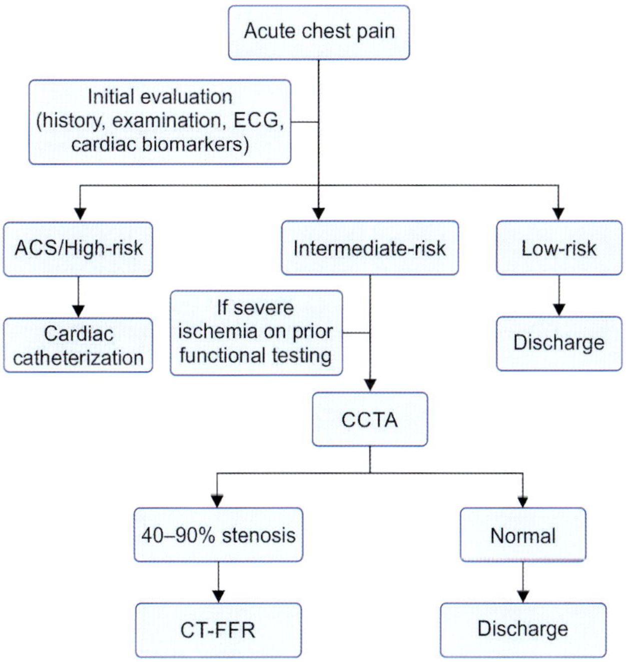

FLOWCHART 1: A prospective algorithm for the evaluation of patients presenting with acute coronary symptoms.

(CCTA: coronary CT angiography; CT-FFR: CT derived fractional flow reserve; ACS: acute coronary syndrome)

Source: Adapted from the 2021 ACC/AHA guidelines on chest pain.[7]

with additional use of CT-FFR or CTP when available in the presence of high-risk plaque features or moderate-to-severe stenosis may be utilized in this patient group. A flowchart showing a prospective algorithm for evaluation of patients with acute chest pain is as shown in **Flowchart 1**.

High-risk Patients

This includes patients with a high pretest probability of CAD, but with no features of ACS on ECG and normal troponins. Functional testing or invasive angiography is usually the preferred modality of investigation in these patients. CCTA may be appropriate in this setting in patients with no chest pain to rule out obstructive lesions.[13]

Non-ST Elevation MI

In patients with acute coronary syndrome with Non-ST elevation MI (NSTEMI), an invasive coronary angiography within 24 hours is considered the preferred investigative modality. However, a CCTA can be used in the intervening period to confirm the need for invasive angiography or as a triage for more urgent angiography.

Chronic Coronary Artery Disease

Risk Stratification

In patients with stable symptoms of CAD, CCTA can help in identifying patients more at risk for major adverse cardiovascular events (MACE). The recent CONFIRM registry findings show the findings of CCTA to be a better predictor of MACE compared with traditional risk factors. In patients with nonobstructive CAD, the extent of atherosclerosis on CCTA performed better than presence of diabetes or hypertension.[14] While diabetes and hypertension predicted MACE in patients with nonobstructive CAD, they were unable to do so in patients with a normal CCTA. The burden of noncalcified plaque was the strongest predictor of fatal or not fatal MI in the SCOT-HEART sub-hoc analysis, performing better than coronary artery calcium score and the severity of stenosis.[15] It becomes important to identify patients with any atherosclerosis, especially noncalcified plaque, on CCTA and to start preventive therapy based on the same.

CCTA versus Functional Testing in Suspected Patients with Coronary Artery Disease

CCTA has emerged as a first-line investigation in patients with stable CAD symptoms. This approach prevents unwanted invasive catheter angiographies and has a favorable cost-benefit analysis. A testing strategy that employed CCTA with selective FFR-CT in patients with 30–90% stenosis was compared with usual functional testing strategy in patients with stable CAD in a prospective multicenter randomized controlled trial, the PRECISE trial.[16] In the patients in CCTA arm, lower rates of angiographies without obstructive coronaries were seen without significant differences in the safety outcomes (all cause death and MI) at 1 year. An initial risk stratification using traditional risk factors was used to defer testing in patients who had a low risk in the CCTA group, which prevented excessive testing. Need for additional investigations was previously found as a shortcoming in the trials that evaluated CCTA as a first-line investigation. *CCTA first strategy has an equivalent efficacy in preventing major cardiovascular events and may present a better alternative in both financial and feasibility point of views.*[17] In patients with a nondiagnostic functional test, CCTA provides an alternate test for selecting patients for further investigations. A prospective algorithm for evaluating patients with stable coronary symptoms is shown in the **Flowchart 2**.

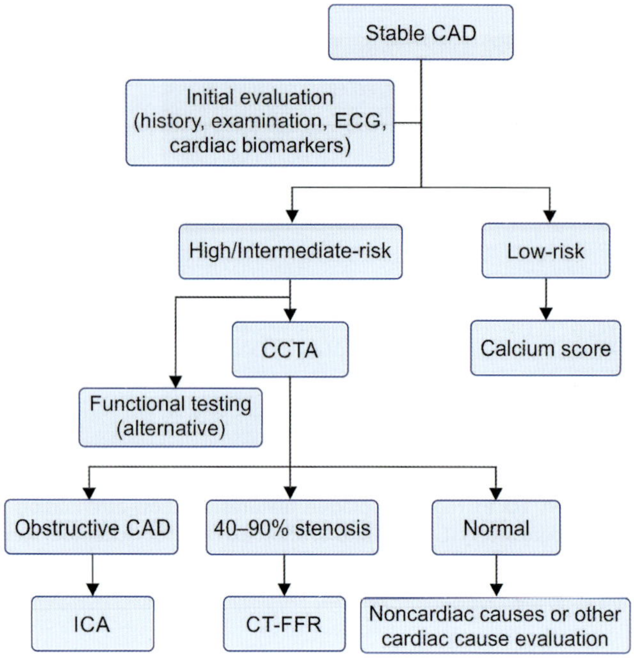

FLOWCHART 2: An algorithm for the evaluation of patients with stable coronary symptoms.

(CCTA: cardiac CT angiography; CT-FFR: CT derived fractional flow reserve; ICA: invasive catheter angiography)

Source: Adapted from the 2021 ACC/AHA guidelines on chest pain.[7]

Patients with Prior Revascularization

CCTA can be used for the evaluation of patency in stents > 3 mm. A recent meta-analysis showed sensitivity of 90 % and specificity of 94% in evaluation postpercutaneous stenting. It is also a reasonable modality for investigating stents <3 mm with thin struts in proximal nonbifurcation regions **(Fig. 3)**.[18] CCTA is a first-line investigation in the imaging of patients postcoronary artery bypass grafting (CABG). Graft patency can be evaluated accurately. The native vessel evaluation may be limited in view of excessive calcified plaques.[18]

Tables 2 and **3** summarize the latest ACC/AHA guidelines on chest pain, chronic coronary syndromes, and acute chest pain regarding the indications for CCTA.[7,19,20]

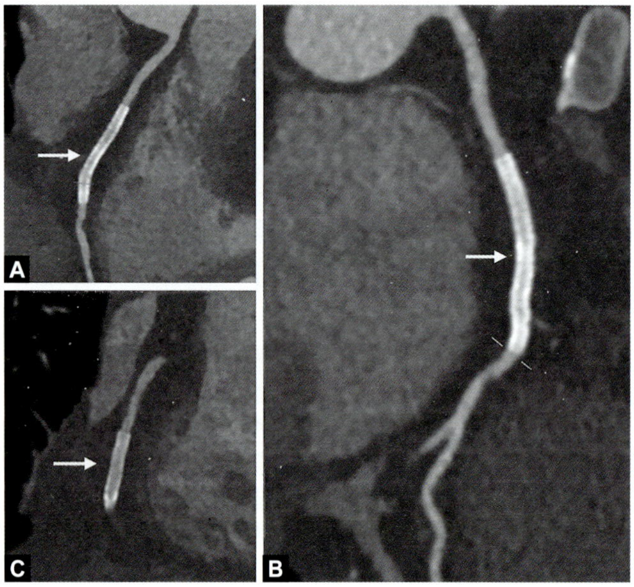

FIGS. 3A TO C: Coronary artery evaluation postpercutaneous angioplasty and stenting of coronary arteries. (A to C) Curved reformatted images of stented coronary arteries with no significant in-stent restenosis.

PREPROCEDURAL EVALUATION

CCTA is an appropriate investigation to rule out significant coronary artery disease in patients planned for noncoronary cardiac surgeries **(Fig. 4)**.[21,22] In patients undergoing noncardiac surgeries, coronary risk assessment may be needed in patients with intermediate or high cardiovascular risk. CCTA is an alternative modality to functional testing or invasive angiography in these situations. It can be useful in the preprocedural planning of patients undergoing

TABLE 2: Indications for coronary CT angiography in patients with chest pain/suspected coronary artery disease.

Recommended	May be considered	Not recommended
Nonacute chest pain/stable coronary symptoms		
• Likely anginal symptoms with no known CAD and no prior testing • Abnormal ECG, inconclusive or equivocal enzymes, inconclusive or mildly positive functional testing results or calcium score between 100 and 300	• Calcium score <100 or >300 • Less likely anginal chest pain, age above 50 years and two or more cardiovascular risk factors • Moderately or severely positive functional testing	Less likely anginal chest pain with age less than 50 years and one or fewer cardiovascular risk factors
Acute chest pain (ACP) patients suspected of acute coronary syndrome (ACS)		
• For intermediate pretest probability patients and no known CAD, if eligible for cardiac testing after initial evaluation • Intermediate probability patients with inconclusive/mildly abnormal functional testing within 1 year	• Triple rule-out • Intermediate probability patients with known nonobstructive (<50% stenosis) CAD • *High-risk pretest probability*: Alternative to functional testing or invasive coronary angiography • Non-STEMI with equivocal ECG and cardiac troponins for assessing need for invasive testing	Definite STEMI
Patients suspected of ischemic chest pain after coronary revascularization		
• Graft patency evaluation after coronary artery bypass graft (CABG) • Stents > 3 mm in diameter with normal or equivocal ECG and cardiac troponins	Stents < 3 mm in proximal coronary segments/ nonbifurcation region	• Stents < 3 mm in distal coronary segments/at bifurcation sites • Prior incomplete revascularization

TABLE 3: Asymptomatic patients with prior revascularization.

Recommended	May be considered	Not recommended
For isolated evaluation of bypass graft patency	• Asymptomatic patients in whom CABG was performed >5 years ago • Asymptomatic patient with PCI performed >2 years ago • Incomplete revascularization	• Asymptomatic patients in whom CABG was performed <5 years ago • Asymptomatic patient with PCI performed within 2 years

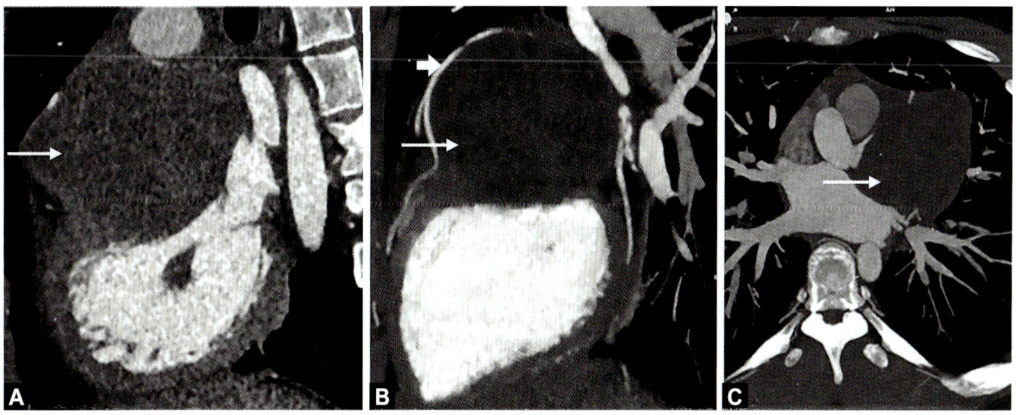

FIGS. 4A TO E: *Continued*

Continued

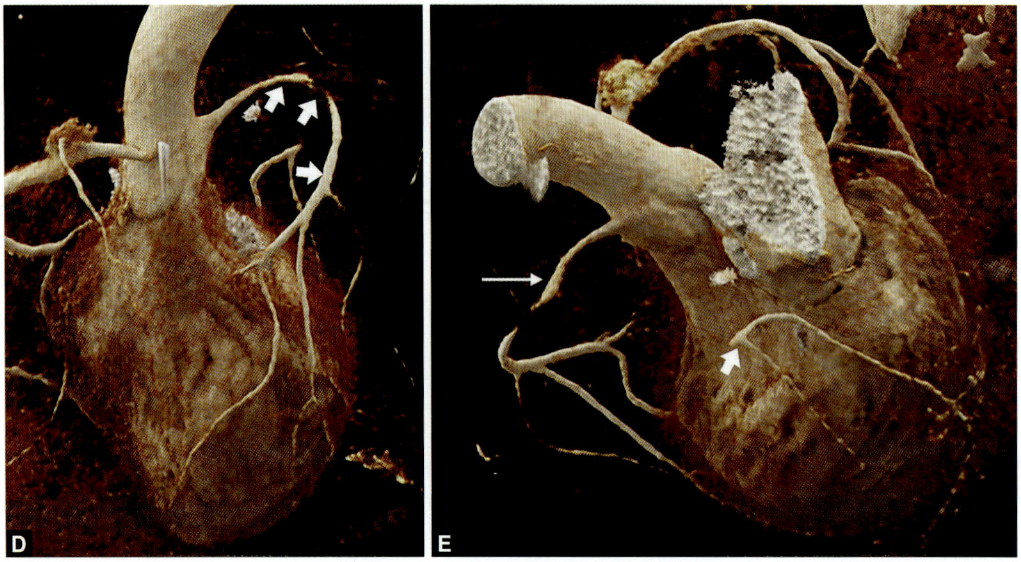

FIGS. 4A TO E: A young male diagnosed to have cardiac hydatid cyst. (A to C) Coronary artery evaluation was done using CCTA showing the hydatid cyst in short axis and axial reformats (white arrow). The left anterior descending artery (LAD) was seen to be compressed by the hydatid cyst (white arrowhead in B) and left circumflex artery (LCx) was not visualized. (D) The virtual reconstructed (VRT) image of the left anterior descending artery with significant compression (white arrowheads). (E) LCx getting reformed distally (white arrowhead) and not visualized proximally (white arrow) from the left main coronary artery.

TABLE 4: CTCA for surgical risk assessment.

Recommended	May be considered	Not recommended
Coronary artery assessment prior to noncoronary cardiac surgery		
• Patients with low-to-intermediate risk • Younger patients with nondegenerative valvular conditions		In high-risk patients
Risk assessment in patients undergoing noncardiac surgery		
	Alternative to functional testing in patients with intermediate ASCVD risk	For risk assessment prior to low-risk noncardiac surgeries

transcutaneous aortic valve implantation (TAVI), where accurate sizing and planning can be done based on CT measurements **(Table 4)**.

EVALUATION OF CARDIOMYOPATHIES AND ARRHYTHMIAS

Coronary artery disease may be a causative or contributing factor toward heart failure in a proportion of patients with cardiomyopathy. Detection and treatment for patients with significant coronary artery disease are protective.[23] CCTA is a noninvasive alternative to catheter angiography for evaluation of coronary arteries in these patients. In addition to evaluating the coronary arteries, the cardiomyopathy phenotype can also be assessed **(Fig. 5)**. In patients who have a contraindication for MRI, basic and objective functional evaluation is possible. Changes in the lung parenchyma and presence of enlarged mediastinal lymph nodes could also aid in narrowing the differential diagnoses **(Table 5)**.

CTA in Pediatric Population for Coronaries

Although the role of CTA in the evaluation of congenital heart disease is being redefined, there are several generally accepted clinical indications for which the benefits of imaging outweigh the risks. CCTA is especially useful in small children and infants, where breath holding is a problem, due to very fast acquisition time of multislice CT. It is extremely helpful in excluding coronary anomalies, which may cause the coronary artery to course anterior to right ventricular outflow tract. Prior knowledge of anomalous coronary artery can help prevent injury to it when the chest is opened. It is useful in diagnosis and follow-up of patients with Kawasaki disease where it shows exact morphology of coronary aneurysms and the associated findings **(Table 6)**.

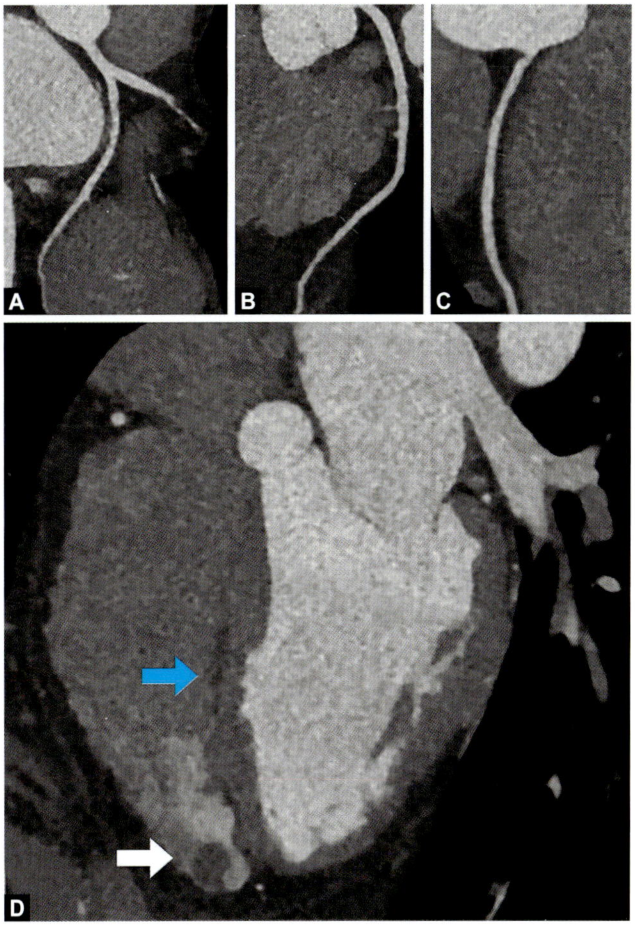

FIGS. 5A TO D: A young male aged 27 years presented with complaints of exertional palpitations. (A to C) Curved reformatted images of the coronary arteries (left circumflex, left anterior descending and right coronary arteries, respectively) which do not show any significant disease. (D) The four-chamber reconstructed image of the patient shows dilated right ventricle (RV) with fat infiltration in the RV side of the interventricular septum (blue arrowhead) and thrombus at the RV apex (white arrowhead). Note also the trabeculated RV-free wall. A cardiac MRI confirmed the diagnosis of arrhythmogenic cardiomyopathy.

RADIATION CONSIDERATIONS AND SAFETY

The radiation doses associated with routine CCTA scans have shown a significant reduction in the past decade, with average radiation doses reducing by as much as 78%.[24] *With the use of modern technology, average effective dose for CCTA have come under 3 mSv.*

Some of the methods of radiation dose reduction are as discussed in the following text.

Low tube potential (kVp): By reducing the tube potential from 120 kVp to 90–100 kVp, radiation dose can be reduced by ~50% and up to 68% when using 80 kVp.[25] Modern scanners use specialized applications to reduce the tube potential according to the patient's body habitus. In scanners without such protocols, BMI-based tube potential selection may suffice. In patients with <25 kg/m^2, a tube potential of 80 kVp is suggested and in patients with 25–30 kg/m^2, 100 kVp can be used.

Automated tube current modulation: Phases of the cardiac cycle with least motion are considered ideal. The tube current during the scan can be tailored to use optimum tube current during these "best" phases and minimize the tube currents during rest of the cycle.

Iterative image reconstruction: This is a computational method employed by majority of the modern scanners that help in reducing the noise (unwanted signal) after acquisition of the scan. Use of these methods obviates the need for higher tube potentials to improve contrast between different tissues and to reduce noise. A 33% reduction in radiation dose can be achieved using iterative reconstruction methods when compared to the classic image reconstruction.[25] Further reductions in radiation doses can be achieved with the use of deep learning-based software that continuously improve their noise reduction capabilities by feedback mechanisms.[26]

High-pitch helical scans: Increasing the pitch also helps in reducing the radiation dose—this principle is used in these protocols, which also enhances the speed of acquisition.

TABLE 5: CCTA in the evaluation of cardiomyopathies and arrhythmias.

Recommended	May be considered	Not recommended
• Patients with *newly diagnosed heart failure* with preserved or reduced ejection fraction and no known CAD • Evaluation of *transplant vasculopathy* • Exercise induced ventricular tachycardias (VT) • In sustained VT and in ventricular fibrillations	• Frequent ventricular premature contractions (VPCs) or nonsustained ventricular tachycardias • In patients with *syncope*, without ischemic equivalent when cardiovascular abnormality is suspected	• Infrequent VPCs • New-onset atrial fibrillation/flutter • Paroxysmal supraventricular tachycardia

TABLE 6: CCTA in pediatric population.

Congenital heart disease		
Recommended	**May be considered**	**Not recommended**
• Anomalous coronary artery • Complex congenital heart disease • Postoperative evaluation in congenital heart diseases		
Coronary CT angiography in Kawasaki disease patients		
• Symptomatic Kawasaki heart disease patients with no prior testing • For follow-up of patients with Kawasaki disease	Asymptomatic Kawasaki disease patients with no prior testing	

Prospective acquisition using high-pitch helical scans can reduce the radiation doses by ~50%.[27]

CONCLUSION

CCTA relies on precise acquisition parameters to ensure adequate enhancement of the coronary arteries post-iodinated contrast injection. With optimal enhancement, excellent sensitivity for coronary artery assessment is obtained. Other cardiac structures, lung parenchyma and the adjacent mediastinum, can also be evaluated. There has been significant reduction in the radiation doses with current generation of scanners and tailored acquisition can further this trend.

ONLINE REFERENCES

Please scan the QR code provided at the end of the table of contents for References of this chapter.

CHAPTER

16

Cardiac Magnetic Resonance Imaging for Cardiologists

Mona Bhatia, Amit Garg, Prasit Maity, Sachin Raiya

ABSTRACT

Cardiac MRI is an advanced imaging modality with broad clinical applications in diagnosing and managing cardiovascular diseases. Its primary strengths include the detailed assessment of ischemic heart disease, where it excels in evaluating myocardial function, infarct detection, and viability assessment. MRI effectively distinguishes between different types of myocardial compromises, such as hibernating and stunned myocardium, and identifies myocardial infarctions through delayed hyperenhancement. It also provides critical insights into nonischemic conditions like hypertrophic, dilated, and restrictive cardiomyopathies, as well as myocarditis and pericardial diseases. The modality's ability to evaluate cardiac masses, thrombi, and valvular diseases further highlights its utility. While MRI is less dependent on operator skill compared to echocardiography and avoids ionizing radiation, it faces challenges such as long scan times and high costs. Future developments, including advancements in contrast agents and real-time imaging techniques, promise to enhance MRI's role in cardiac interventions and regenerative therapies.

Keywords: Cardiac MRI, ischemic heart disease, cardiac masses, nonischemic cardiomyopathy, myocarditis, pericardial disease, coronary magnetic resonance angiography, atherosclerotic plaque evaluation, valvular disease

INTRODUCTION

Magnetic resonance imaging (MRI) is noninvasive, nonionizing, and provides exceptional resolution and soft-tissue contrast; its role in cardiac assessment has historically been limited.[1,2] Recent advancements in cardiac magnetic resonance have addressed previous limitations, which enables precise and reliable evaluation of cardiac anatomy and function, including myocardial viability, cardiomyopathies, pericardial disease, cardiac masses, congenital and valvular heart conditions, and aortic and pulmonary vessel assessment.[1,2] Emerging applications are expanding into myocardial perfusion, ischemia, atherosclerotic plaque evaluation, coronary artery and vessel wall analysis, and even therapeutic uses such as electrophysiology and interventional procedures.[1]

TECHNICAL ASPECTS OF CARDIAC MAGNETIC RESONANCE IMAGING

Magnetic resonance imaging employs a range of scanning protocols, generally categorized as either dark blood or bright blood methods. Dark blood techniques are primarily used to examine the anatomical structure of the heart and major blood vessels. In contrast, gradient-echo sequences are employed for assessing cardiac function. These include end-diastolic and end-systolic volumes, stroke volume, ejection fraction (EF), cardiac output, and myocardial mass[3,4] **(Table 1)**. Additionally, MRI enables flow quantification through phase contrast imaging. This capability proves invaluable when evaluating stenosis, regurgitation, and cardiac shunts. Furthermore, pressure differences across

TABLE 1: Left ventricular functional analysis.

End-diastolic volume	77.4 mL
End-systolic volume	29.8 mL
Ejection fraction	61.5%
Stroke volume	47.6 mL
Stroke index	23.3 mL/beat/m^2
Cardiac output	6.3 L/min
Cardiac index	3.1 L/min/m^2

cardiac abnormalities can be determined by analyzing blood flow velocities.[3]

Another valuable technique for assessing heart muscle function is myocardial tagging using a dark grid pattern to enable a three-dimensional (3D) examination of how the heart rotates, stretches, moves, and changes shape throughout its beating cycle. It allows to study the behavior of different layers of heart muscles: The inner (subendocardial), middle, and outer (subepicardial) sections, providing insights into localized heart function.[1,5]

Inversion recovery protocols are employed to suppress specific signals in MRI images. For instance, they can be used to cancel out signals from healthy heart tissue, making abnormal areas more visible. Alternatively, they can eliminate signals from fat when needed for certain diagnostic purposes.

After administering gadolinium contrast, enhanced imaging techniques become possible. These are useful for several cardiac assessments:

- Evaluating blood flow to the heart muscle
- Detecting areas of heart attack damage
- Identifying infiltrative diseases affecting the heart
- Distinguishing between masses and blood clots within the heart

These advanced MRI methods provide a wealth of information about heart structure and function, aiding in accurate diagnosis and treatment planning for various cardiac conditions.[3]

IMAGE ACQUISITION

Capturing clear images of the heart presents unique challenges due to motion from breathing and heartbeats. These movements can degrade image quality. To address these issues, specific techniques are employed:

- *Respiratory motion:* Patients are often asked to hold their breath during image acquisition.
- *Cardiac motion:* Electrocardiography (ECG) gating is used to synchronize image capture with specific phases of the heartbeat.
- *Advanced gating method:* In some cases, vector cardiogram gating is preferred over standard ECG gating.
- *Cine imaging:* This method uses ECG-triggered segmentation to capture multiple images throughout the cardiac cycle.

IMAGING PLANES

Magnetic resonance imaging offers versatile imaging capabilities, allowing for image acquisition in multiple orientations. While standard MRI scans can be performed in axial, coronal, and sagittal planes, cardiac MRI employs additional specialized views to capture the heart's unique structure and function:

- Vertical long-axis view
- Horizontal long-axis view (four-chamber view) **(Fig. 1)**

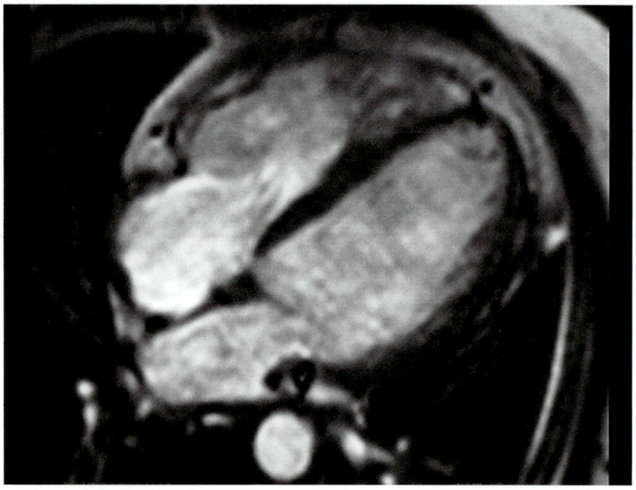

FIG. 1: Cardiac MRI—four-chamber view.

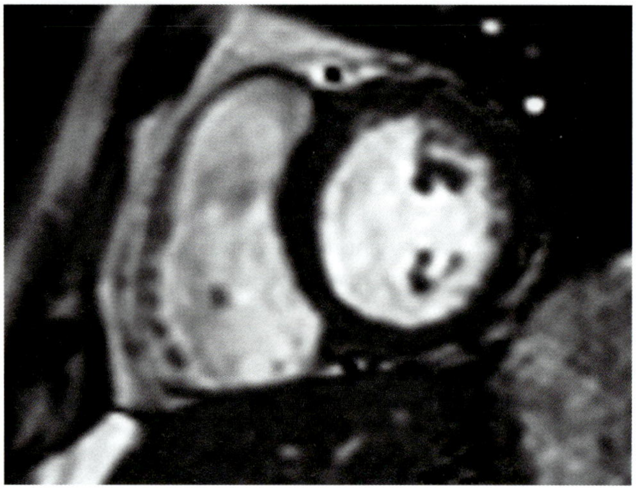

FIG. 2: Cardiac MRI—short-axis view.

- Short-axis view **(Fig. 2)**
- Three-chamber view **(Fig. 3)**

INDICATIONS AND APPLICATIONS

Cardiac MRI has the following common clinical applications.

Ischemic Heart Disease

In the context of ischemic heart disease, MRI serves as a powerful diagnostic tool, offering a comprehensive evaluation of heart function and structure. Here is a breakdown of its capabilities:

- *Functional assessment:*
    - MRI can evaluate both regional (specific areas) and global (overall) myocardial function.
    - It is considered the gold standard for analyzing ventricular volumes.

- Quantitative measurements
- *Wall function analysis:*
    - As shown in **Figure 4**, MRI can assess myocardial function and wall thickening.
- *Infarct and ischemia detection:*
    - MRI can identify both acute (recent) and chronic (long-standing) heart attacks.
    - It can detect areas of ischemia (reduced blood flow) that have not yet resulted in infarction.
- *Myocardial viability assessment:*
    - MRI can distinguish between different states of compromised heart muscle:
        - Hibernating myocardium (alive but dysfunctional due to chronic low blood flow)
        - Stunned myocardium (temporarily dysfunctional after an ischemic event)
        - Infarcted myocardium (dead heart tissue)

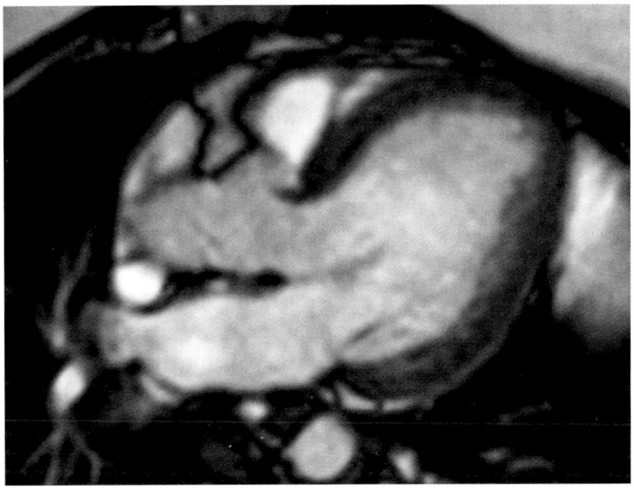

FIG. 3: Cardiac MRI—three-chamber view.

    - This ability to determine tissue viability is crucial for treatment planning, as it helps identify areas that might recover with improved blood flow.[2,3]

Delayed hyperenhancement (DHE) is linked to myocyte necrosis, making it a more dependable marker for infarction **(Fig. 5)**. By combining first-pass and delayed imaging, enhancement patterns have been investigated to evaluate tissue viability and forecast functional recovery. A significant perfusion deficit or DHE observed in early-phase MRI studies is a strong indicator of subsequent scar formation.[6]

Both acute and chronic myocardial infarctions exhibit regional wall motion abnormalities. In the case of acute infarctions, T2-weighted imaging may reveal increased signal due to edema. Severe acute infarctions might show a nonenhancing subendocardial region surrounded by an area of enhancement, indicative of microvascular obstruction (MVO). Typically, this MVO pattern resolves within 2 weeks, leaving behind only DHE. The presence of MVO on delayed enhanced images is associated with a poorer clinical prognosis.[3]

The prognostic significance of delayed enhancement in myocardial infarction is closely linked to its extent and transmurality **(Fig. 6 and Table 2)**.[2] Generally, a larger area of transmural enhancement—such as hyperenhancement affecting >50% of the myocardial wall thickness—correlates with a lower likelihood of functional recovery following acute myocardial infarction. This means that patients with extensive transmural infarctions are less likely to experience improvement in cardiac function after undergoing revascularization or receiving beta-blocker treatment **(Fig. 7)**.

Myocardial infarction can lead to several changes, including myocardial thinning (<6 mm) **(Fig. 4)**, hypertrophy of the noninfarcted myocardium, ventricular dilation, and aneurysmal transformations. Following an infarction, intraventricular thrombus formation may occur adjacent to

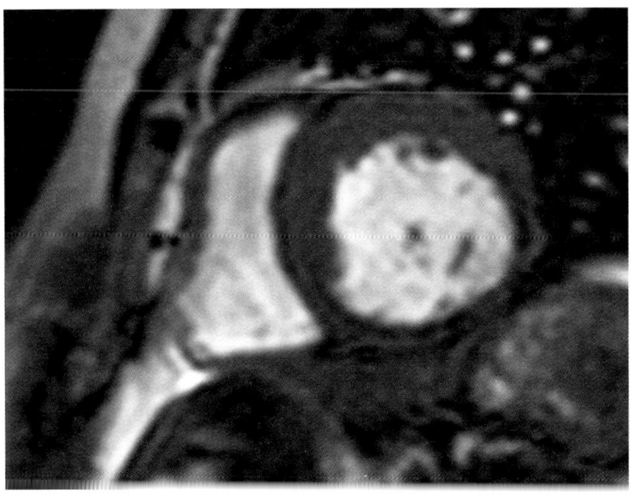

FIG. 4: Cardiac MRI—wall thinning in ischemic heart disease.

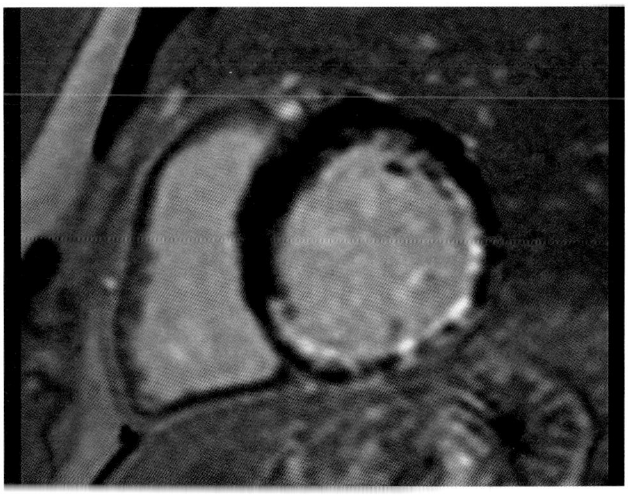

FIG. 5: Cardiac MRI—myocardial infarction.

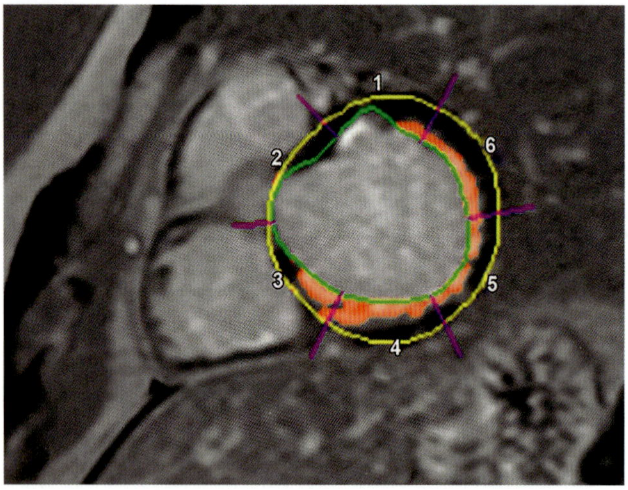

FIG. 6: Cardiac MRI—quantification of myocardial infarction.

TABLE 2: Cardiac MRI—percentage quantification of the infarcted myocardium.

Enhanced volume	15,277 mm^3
Myocardial volume	92,201 mm^3
Percentage enhanced	16%

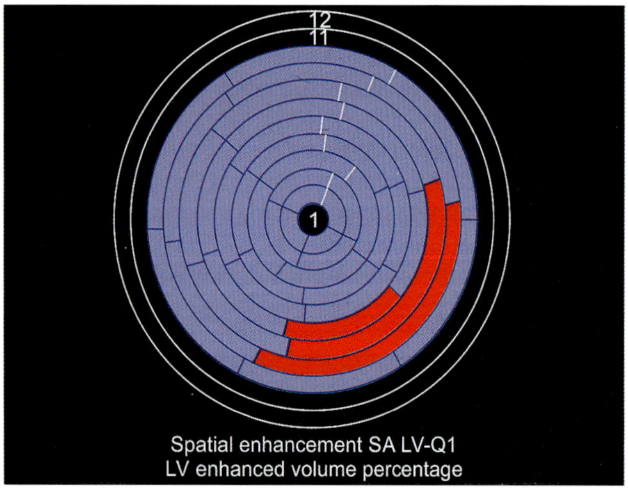

FIG. 7: Cardiac MRI—bull's eye view depicting enhanced scar tissue.

akinetic myocardium **(Fig. 8)**. Viability of myocardial tissue can be assessed using cine MRI without contrast during a low-dose infusion of dobutamine (5–10 µg/kg/min) or after administering adenosine. An increase in left ventricular wall thickening during stress in a segment that is dysfunctional at rest indicates tissue viability.[2] Dobutamine stress MRI is also effective in detecting ischemic myocardium.[2] It is important to note that DHE can also be observed in conditions other than acute or chronic infarcts, such as myocarditis, cardiomyopathy, sarcoidosis, amyloidosis, and

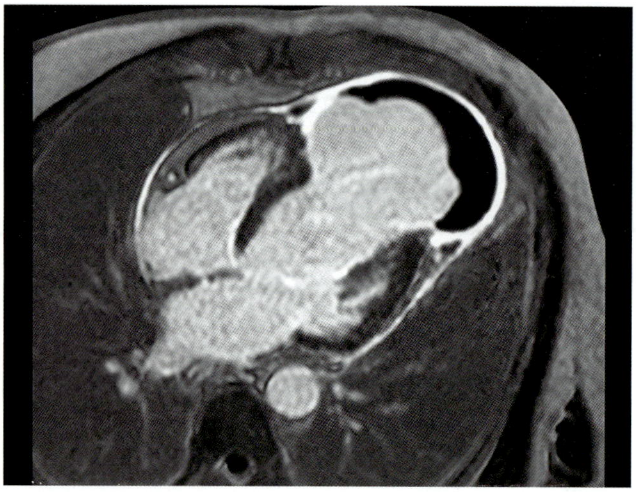

FIG. 8: Cardiac MRI—postinfarction left ventricular aneurysm with intraventricular thrombus.

arrhythmogenic right ventricular dysplasia. The pattern and distribution of hyperenhancement in these conditions—whether mid-wall, epicardial, or global endocardial—differ from the subendocardial or transmural patterns seen in infarcts.[2,4]

Comparison with Other Imaging Modalities

Perfusion MRI, both at rest and following pharmacologic stimulation with agents such as adenosine and dipyridamole, has been compared with traditional diagnostic methods like angiography and radionuclide scintigraphy. It has shown moderate sensitivity (67–83%) and specificity (75–100%).[1]

Myocardial delayed-enhancement MRI results align well with dobutamine stress echocardiography[2] and exhibit excellent correlation with positron emission tomography (PET), achieving 96% sensitivity and 84% specificity when compared with 18F-fluorodeoxyglucose PET.[7,8] However, a study found that while SPECT detected almost all nearly transmural infarctions, it missed 47% of subendocardial infarctions that were identified using myocardial delayed-enhancement MRI.[9]

Cardiac Masses, Thrombi, and Infections

Magnetic resonance imaging provides detailed insights into their morphological and histological characteristics, including extent, origin, hemorrhage, vascularity, and calcification.[2,1] One of MRI's notable advantages is its ability to differentiate between thrombi and tumors. On spin-echo images, both thrombi and tumors may appear with intermediate signal intensity. However, thrombi typically exhibit low signal intensity on gradient-echo images due to the presence of deoxyhemoglobin, unlike tumors.[4,10]

Myxomas, the most prevalent type of benign cardiac tumor, generally originate from the interatrial septum and can present as pedunculated or sessile with smooth edges.[4] Myxomas may also prolapse through the mitral valve, as seen on cine imaging. When a myxoma appears hypointense due to calcification or hemorrhage, postcontrast imaging can easily differentiate it from a thrombus, as tumors enhance while thrombi do not **(Fig. 9)**.[4]

Magnetic resonance imaging is also valuable for evaluating other cardiac tumors, such as metastases, fibromas, rhabdomyomas, hemangiomas, pheochromocytomas, lymphomas, malignant fibrous histiocytomas, and angiosarcomas **(Fig. 10)**.

Nonischemic Cardiomyopathy and Myocarditis

Magnetic resonance imaging provides precise evaluations of ventricular morphology, function, myocardial wall enhancement patterns, and wall motion abnormalities. These capabilities are crucial for the accurate characterization of conditions such as cardiomyopathy and myocarditis.[1]

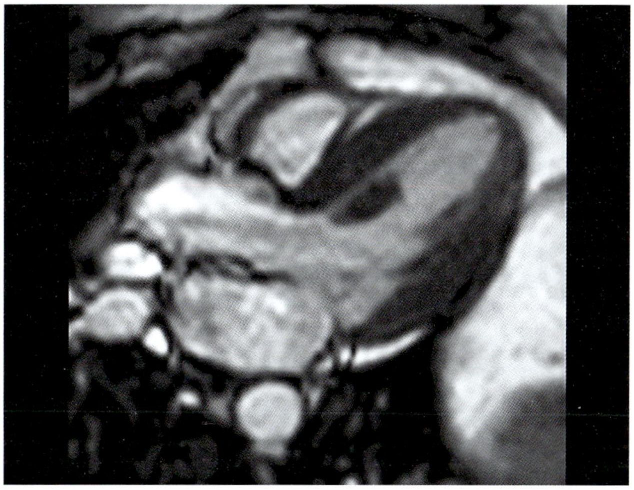

FIG. 9: Cardiac MRI—intraventricular thrombus.

Hypertrophic Cardiomyopathy

Cardiac MRI is highly effective in assessing the extent of hypertrophy in hypertrophic cardiomyopathy (HCM), particularly at the ventricular apex. HCM leads to hypertrophied myocardium and diastolic dysfunction. The condition can present in various forms, including asymmetric, concentric, or papillary muscle hypertrophy **(Fig. 11)**. The most common form is asymmetric hypertrophy, often affecting the interventricular septum, and it may involve the left ventricular outflow tract (LVOT), known as hypertrophic obstructive cardiomyopathy.[3]

Magnetic resonance imaging excels in visualizing apical HCM, LVOT obstruction, and systolic anterior motion of the mitral valve. Myocardial tagging is valuable for detecting regional function abnormalities, including asymmetric septal, symmetrical, and apical HCM.[11] It also quantifies turbulent flow and velocity in LVOT obstruction and evaluates mitral regurgitation. DHE is useful for identifying scar tissue within the hypertrophied myocardium, which can be a focus for potentially life-threatening arrhythmias. Additionally, cardiac MRI plays a crucial role in monitoring patients following ventricular septal resection or percutaneous ablation.[1,3]

Dilated Cardiomyopathy

In dilated cardiomyopathy, MRI is adept at evaluating various parameters, including wall thickness, impaired fiber shortening, end-systolic wall stress, and dilated heart chambers, as well as delayed-enhancement patterns.[1] Although subendocardial enhancement may be similar to that seen in infarction, mid-wall myocardial enhancement helps differentiate it from an ischemic cause **(Fig. 12)**. The extent of

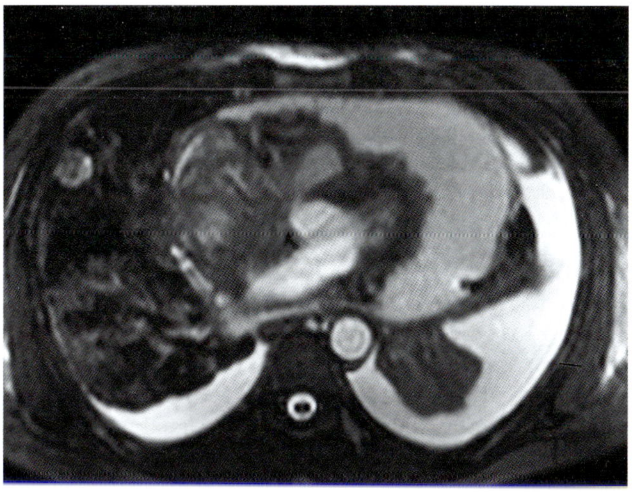

FIG. 10: Cardiac MRI—angiosarcoma with intra- and extracardiac mass with pulmonary metastasis.

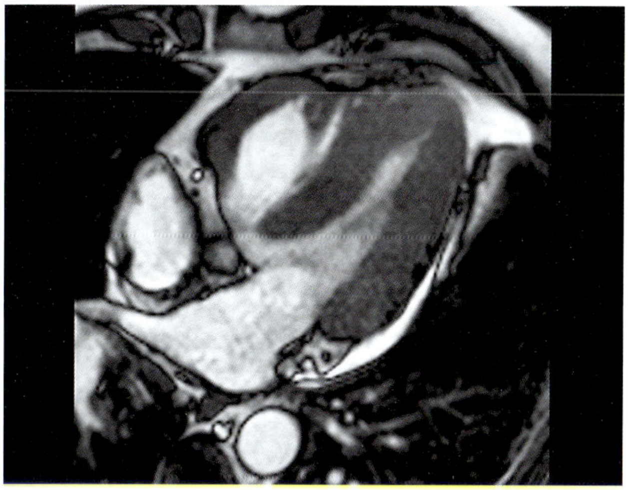

FIG. 11: Cardiac MRI—hypertrophic cardiomyopathy.

myocardial enhancement on MRI correlates with the severity of functional impairment.[2]

Restrictive Cardiomyopathy

Restrictive cardiomyopathy, caused by myocardial infiltration with fibrosis or other tissues, is characterized by normal left ventricular size and systolic function but severe diastolic dysfunction and biatrial enlargement. MRI is effective in evaluating various restrictive diseases.[1,3,11]

- *Sarcoidosis:* MRI can identify lesions with variable signal characteristics depending on the disease stage. These lesions may appear high intensity on T2-weighted images and exhibit central low intensity on T1- and T2-weighted images, often surrounded by a high-signal ring. Postgadolinium contrast enhancement typically shows a patchy mid-wall and epicardial pattern **(Fig. 13)**. Advanced cases may also reveal septal thinning, systolic and diastolic left ventricular dysfunction, and pericardial involvement.[2]
- *Hemochromatosis:* MRI detects extensive signal loss in native T1- and T2-weighted images, especially in the context of a notably "dark" liver, which confirms iron deposition and systemic hemochromatosis.[1] Iron deposition is primarily subepicardial.
- *Amyloidosis:* MRI may show ventricular wall thickening with DHE and thickening of the atrial septum. Septal thickness of 6 mm or more in the atrial septum or the right atrial posterior wall is fairly specific for amyloid infiltration.[1,12]
- *Endomyocardial fibrosis:* Also known as Loeffler endocarditis, this condition features extensive subendocardial fibrosis, apical thrombus formation, and progressive diastolic dysfunction.[11] MRI provides detailed quantification of both the morphological and functional aspects of endomyocardial fibrosis.

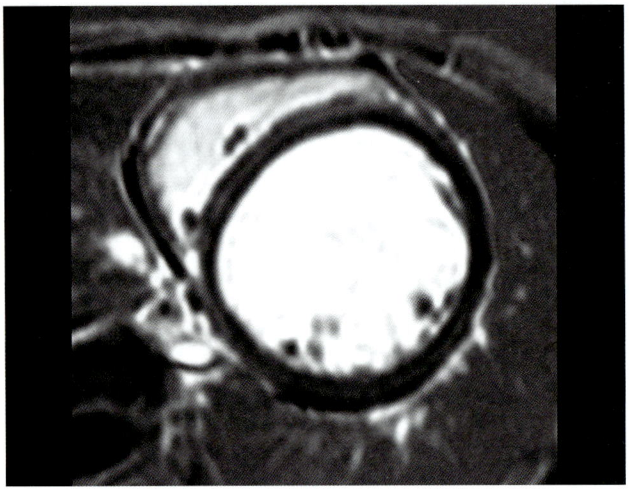

FIG. 12: Cardiac MRI—dilated cardiomyopathy with mid-wall enhancement.

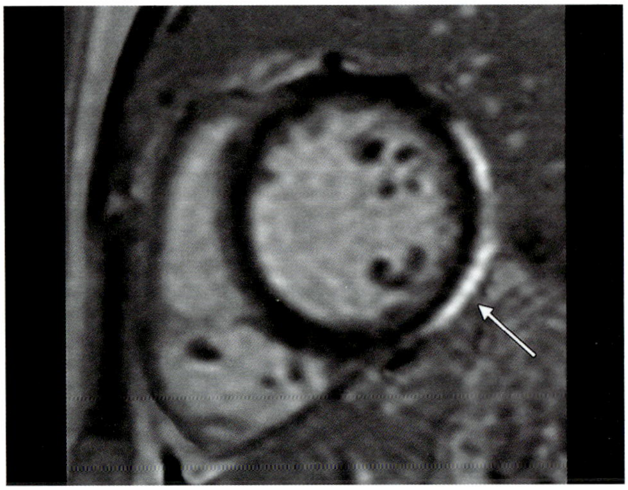

FIG. 13: Cardiac MRI—subepicardial scar.

Arrhythmogenic Right Ventricular Dysplasia

Magnetic resonance imaging is the preferred method for diagnosing arrhythmogenic right ventricular dysplasia (ARVD). Key indicators on MRI include fatty infiltration, thinning of the ventricular wall, abnormal regional wall motion, and dysplastic trabecular formations.[11] Additional findings may include localized bulging during early diastole and saccular aneurysmal outpouchings.[1] Delayed enhancement of the right ventricular myocardium can also aid in the diagnosis.[2,3]

Myocarditis

Viral or other forms of myocarditis typically begin with focal mid-wall enhancement and wall motion abnormalities, which can progress to more diffuse, transmural enhancement in both ventricles, sometimes accompanied by right ventricular pseudoaneurysm formation.[13]

In hypereosinophilic syndrome, myocardial involvement often presents with ventricular thrombi.[2] MRI is also useful in identifying inflamed regions, which can help guide the selection of biopsy sites during endomyocardial biopsy.[1] After transcatheter septal ablation, delayed enhancement indicates successful myocardial tissue destruction.[2]

Pericardial Disease

Pericardial disease is primarily assessed using echocardiography. However, echocardiography has limitations when no effusion is present or when the effusion is complex.[4] T1-weighted spin-echo MRI imaging shows the normal pericardium as a thin, low-signal band (about 2 mm), bordered by epicardial and pericardial fat. Unlike echocardiography, MRI is effective in detecting pericardial thickening, and a thickness greater than 2 mm may indicate inflammation, especially if effusion is present. A pericardial thickness of 4 mm or more is considered abnormal and indicative of fibrous pericarditis.[1]

Magnetic resonance imaging is also valuable in identifying effusions complicated by adhesions or loculations and in distinguishing between effusions based on signal characteristics and contrast enhancement.[1] On spin-echo imaging, simple effusions appear with low-signal intensity on T1-weighted images and high-signal intensity on T2-weighted images, while chylous and hemorrhagic effusions show higher signals on T1-weighted images.[3]

Cine MRI can reveal associated findings in the ventricles and cardiac valves,[1] such as a small right ventricular chamber, restricted diastolic filling, biatrial dilation, and septal or ventricular alterations like septal bounce. Tagged images may detect adhesions between the pericardium and epicardium,[1] and diastolic chamber collapse suggests tamponade. MRI is highly sensitive in differentiating constrictive pericarditis from restrictive cardiomyopathy, with pericardial thickening of 4 mm or more having an accuracy of 93%.[4]

Coronary Magnetic Resonance Angiography

Coronary artery angiography presents several challenges, primarily due to the small size of the coronary arteries, their tortuous paths, constant cardiac and respiratory motion, and the surrounding bright epicardial fat on MRI.[14]

Advancements in imaging sequences and contrast agents are bringing the possibility of routine noninvasive magnetic resonance coronary angiography closer to reality.[1,2] Contrast-enhanced magnetic resonance angiography can also assess the patency of coronary artery bypass grafts,[15] although its accuracy currently lags behind CT imaging.[16,17] MRI is capable of evaluating both saphenous vein and internal mammary bypass grafts,[15] including detecting saphenous vein graft aneurysms that may require surgical intervention. However, local artifacts caused by metallic clips, graft markers, and sternal wires remain a limitation in MRI imaging **(Fig. 14)**.[1]

Atherosclerotic Plaque Evaluation

Advanced pulse sequences and 3T magnetic resonance systems have the potential to become valuable tools for evaluating the regression and characterizing the tissue composition of atherosclerotic coronary plaques.[1]

Valvular Disease

Cardiac MRI is an effective tool for identifying and quantifying stenotic or regurgitant lesions, as well as directly visualizing abnormal valvular anatomy. It excels in measuring myocardial hypertrophy, ventricular dilation, and ventricular function, which are key factors in determining the timing of valve replacement surgery.[3] MRI has a high sensitivity (98%), specificity (95%), and accuracy (97%) for diagnosing both aortic and mitral regurgitation.[18] Phase contrast MRI can assess valvular stenosis severity by measuring peak jet velocity, calculating valve orifice area, and determining the transvalvular pressure gradient.[19]

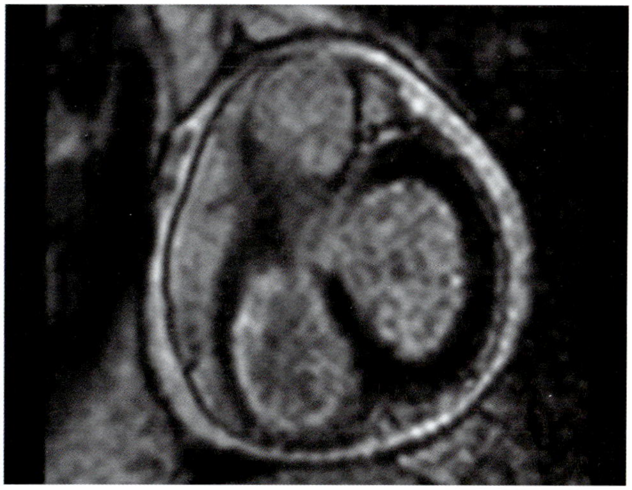

FIG. 14: Cardiac MRI—constrictive pericarditis.

FUTURE DEVELOPMENTS

In the future, contrast-enhanced MRI may play a role in guiding cardiac interventions, such as real-time monitoring of electromagnetic catheter-directed radiofrequency (RF) ablations enabling more precise positioning of the RF ablation site within the heart.[20] Emerging treatments for heart failure involve transplanting primitive cells, like stem cells or myoblasts, into damaged cardiac tissue, where they can differentiate into functional tissue.[21] Stem cells labeled with iron-based contrast agents have been used to track their myocardial localization after implantation,[22,23] enabling in vivo evaluation of their retention, engraftment, and migration.

CONCLUSION

Magnetic resonance imaging (MRI) is rapidly becoming a leading noninvasive tool for assessing cardiovascular diseases. Its nonionizing nature makes it safe for use in children and pregnant women. In addition to offering high-resolution, 3D imaging of cardiovascular structures, MRI provides significant advantages in evaluating blood flow, pressure gradients, and ventricular volumes, as well as analyzing ventricular contractile function, including for the right ventricle. Unlike echocardiography, MRI is less dependent on the operator and is not hindered by nearby bones or air.[3]

However, cardiac MRI also has drawbacks, including long scan times, which can make it unsuitable for unstable or uncooperative patients, higher costs, limited availability, and incompatibility with devices like pacemakers and cochlear implants.[1,3] Gadolinium-based contrast agents have also been linked to rare conditions like nephrogenic systemic fibrosis.[4]

Despite these challenges, advancements in MRI technology, such as MRI-compatible catheters for electrophysiology and ablation procedures, and its role in interventional cardiology and cell-based therapies for heart failure, signal a promising future for cardiac MRI. As these innovations continue to evolve, MRI is poised to significantly transform cardiology practices, with expected exponential growth in its applications.[1]

ONLINE REFERENCES

Please scan the QR code provided at the end of the table of contents for References of this chapter.

SECTION 3

Artificial Intelligence in Cardiology

Section Outline

CHAPTER

17

Artificial Intelligence in Echocardiography: Where are We and Where are We Going

Ramdas G Pai, Ajit D Pai, Vinutha Rajesh

ABSTRACT

Artificial intelligence (AI) is a rapidly evolving field with major current and potential applications in cardiovascular imaging including echocardiography. The AI tools can aid in image acquisition, improve image acquisition skills of the imager, help to process images and do measurements, and help with image interpretation. This can improve the speed and accuracy of image acquisition, interpretation, and reporting. Ability of AI to extract structured and unstructured data from the electronic medical records will help in understanding the context in which the echocardiogram is performed and add data from the echocardiogram and other sources to fine-tune clinical diagnosis, prognostication, and patient management.

Keywords: AI, echocardiography, images, interpretation, echocardiogram

INTRODUCTION

The use of artificial intelligence (AI) in cardiology is not new. Automated interpretation of electrocardiogram (ECG) has been performed since the 1990s. Stress nuclear images are segmented and analyzed by AI making its reporting easy for physicians. AI has been applied to perform multiple tasks in echocardiography, cardiac computed tomography (CCT), and magnetic resonance imaging (CMR). AI can assist in patient interviews, chart abstraction, assist in diagnosis and in patient management. AI tools are well suited for analysis of big data, finding nonlinear patterns and producing predictive models superior to traditional statistical models. In this chapter, we aim to summarize current applications of AI in the field of echocardiography and make a bold prediction where it is likely to go.

EVOLUTION OF THE ROLE OF AI IN ECHOCARDIOGRAPHY

Echocardiography is a commonly utilized imaging technique in the diagnosis, treatment, and monitoring of patients with cardiovascular disease (CVD).[1] Echocardiogram offers valuable information on the etiologies of CVD and effectiveness of various treatments. It is a critical noninvasive tool in tracking the progress toward treatment goals. Echocardiography accounts for 50% of all cardiac imaging studies performed among Medicare beneficiaries.[2]

Echocardiography protocol typically includes M-mode, 2D imaging, Doppler imaging including color and spectral Doppler, 3D images, left ventricular (LV) strain, LV volume, left atrial (LA) volume assessment, right ventricular (RV) volume, RV function, cardiac hemodynamics, and heart valves assessments. Echocardiographic scanning of the patient typically takes 40–60 minutes. It also takes 20–30 minutes to read these studies by an experienced echocardiographer depending on the pathology and image quality.

Obtaining optimal images in echocardiography is challenging due to various factors, including the sonographer skills, the patient's medical conditions, body habitus, echocardiographic equipment used, and the reader's experience. These challenges often result in timing issues, missed diagnoses, and inefficiencies in the imaging process that must be addressed.[3] There is a significant need for specialized medical training in the area of echocardiography due to the existing limitations.

In the last two decades, the use of AI in echocardiography for diagnosis and treatment of cardiac disorders has demonstrated the ability to solve these issues. In 1978, Fourier used M-mode to evaluate anterior mitral leaflet.[4] Convoluted neural network (CNN), a branch of deep learning (DL) is an essential tool used to recognize various views of the heart in

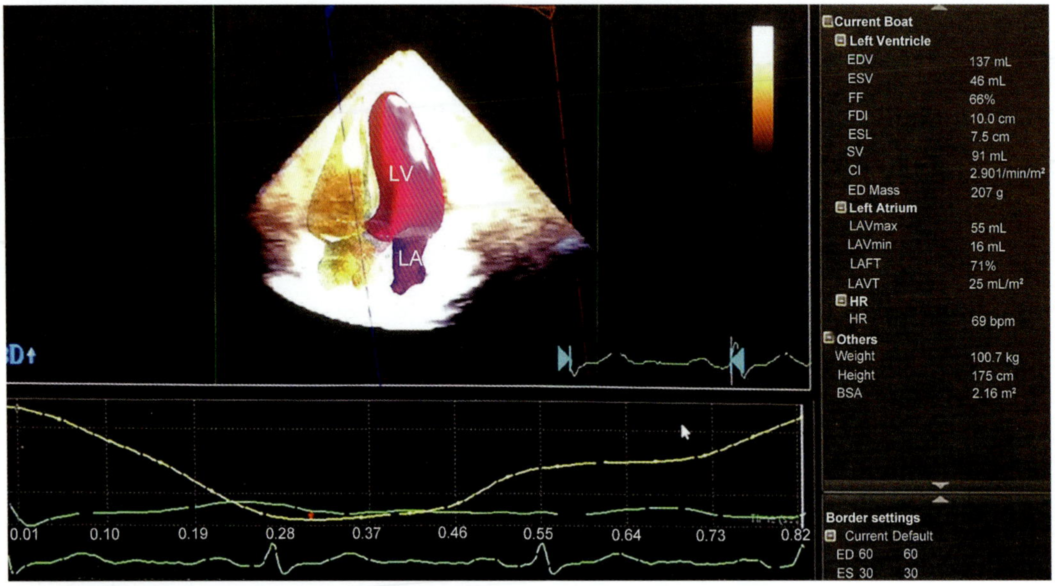

FIG. 1: 3D echocardiographic imaging of the left ventricle (LV) and left atrium (LA) from transthoracic apical window using Philips system. The system automatically tracks to endocardium to yield LV and LA volumes throughout the cardiac cycle and ejection fractions.

machine learning (ML) to accurately identify basic views of the LV.[5]

There are a large number of studies using AI in echocardiography to facilitate image acquisition, quantification, segmentation, analysis, and reporting. In addition, application of AI to selected dynamic images can also help make cardiac diagnosis with precision and prognosticate. This review discusses the current and evolving applications of AI in echocardiography **(Fig. 1)**.

CLINICAL DATA ABSTRACTION IN PREPARATION FOR ECHOCARDIOGRAPHY

Echocardiography is not performed in a clinical vacuum and its value is additive to clinical diagnosis or differential diagnosis. Adequate clinical and laboratory data should be abstracted before performing an echocardiogram. A clear indication and clinical question should be known. Recording of rhythm and blood pressure are important as well. These are generally deficient in the requests and are somewhat hard for the sonographers to capture adequately and accurately. In addition, the process is time-consuming. The AI tools can help abstract both structured and unstructured data from electronic medical records (EMRs) to make echocardiographic examination and data more meaningful. Potentially, the order management tool in the EMR can prefetch and export relevant data to the echocardiographic systems without much of human interface. This would save time, avoid errors, and operations more efficient.

AI-ASSISTED ECHOCARDIOGRAPHIC IMAGE ACQUISITION

Echocardiographic image acquisition requires in-depth training of cardiac anatomy, function, various abnormalities, and technical skills to acquire comprehensive set of images from multiple acoustic windows. This is generally performed by trained cardiologists or sonographers. There is a shortage of trained sonographers globally. In addition, such expertise to image the heart is not available at points of care such as intensive care unit, the emergency room, and patient's home, nursing home or remote areas of the world where the value of getting reliable images and accurate interpretation is of immense value. AI-assisted tools interfaced with echocardiographic equipment have been developed to address these unmet needs. Mor-Avi et al. used real-time AI-guided image acquisition tool, UltraSight Ltd, interfaced with Philips echocardiographic system to test the hypothesis that this can help echocardiographic novices to perform at a very high level after minimal training.[6] These novices performed 240 echocardiographic studies and these approached the quality of expert sonographers. A similar study performed by Narang et al. using Caption Health Echo GPS tool yielded similar results.[7] These tools are being incorporated into major echocardiographic equipment from different vendors. And these will level the echocardiographic playing field and democratize availability of echocardiography at points of care and in remote areas where expertise in image acquisition may not be available. These techniques are based on DL and are rapidly evolving and are being adopted into mainstream echocardiography.

IDENTIFICATION OF VIEWS AND IMAGE CLASSIFICATION

Automated chamber and view classification is the key for both AI-guided image acquisition and quantitation. DL and CNNs have been able accomplish this after adequate training. Madani et al. used these tools in 267 echocardiograms and achieved near perfect accuracy.[5] Zhu et al. achieved 99% accuracy in 895 patients with several thousand images.[8] Hence, labeling and tracking chambers and structures during real time imaging are very possible. This will also help sonographers to help identify and optimize structures with or without AI-guided image acquisition. This can also help novices to get self-taught through AI-assisted image classification and labeling to achieve higher levels of performance.[7-9]

CARDIAC CHAMBER QUANTIFICATION

Techniques of automatic quantification (AQ) and automatic border detection (ABD) are not new. Using AI, vendors were able to do these in the 1990s. Philips came up with AI assisted, operator facilitated automatic LV endocardial border detection and tracking throughout the cardiac cycle using AQ. This yielded LV volumes, EF, and dynamic volume changes over time from 2D images. Philips also created a tool called color kinesis (CK) for endocardial tracking and wall motion analysis.

Transthoracic 2D and 3D left heart chamber quantification using an automated adaptive analytics algorithm using heart model was developed by Philips and other vendors.[10-14] TomTech was one of the first vendors to generate dynamic 3D data sets of the heart using a TEE "Echo CT" technique with ECG and respiratory gating. This was developed in the 1990s and the technique has been extended to many echocardiographic equipment. The processes for generation of various nonorthodox tomographic planes were developed from the dynamic 3D data set. The concepts of electronic vivisection to simulate surgical or other views were developed along with image segmentation to extract the structures of interest such as the mitral or aortic valves or various chambers or atrial septum or atrial appendage, etc.

Liu et al. developed a DL algorithm based on U-Net (DPS-Net),[10] good performance was obtained for LV segmentation. DPS-Net was associated with high correlations and good agreements for the LVEF measurement with ROC > 0.94 for both normal and abnormal hearts in 340 subjects. This new strategy of feature extraction and fusion could enhance the accuracy of automatic LVEF assessment based on multiview 2D echocardiographic sequences. High diagnostic performance for the determination of heart failure was obtained by using DPS-Net in cases with different phenotypes of heart diseases.

The same EchoNet dynamic algorithm Liu et al. used has been extended to automate LV strain measurement and chamber segmentation. It has also been used in very large data sets of LV four-chamber views to even detect anemia, elevated serum BNP and troponin levels, and presence of liver disease. The DL training was based on 70,000 training four-chamber views.

The FAST-EFs multicenter study was performed using TomTec software to obtain automated EF and LV longitudinal strain in 255 patients.[15] The average calculation time was 8 seconds and both were performed with a very high degree of accuracy saving both time and effort.

Using the AI tools, one can easily segment the LV and obtain its volumes and EF by both 2D and 3D techniques and these tools are commercially available.[16] These tools, not only save time, but are more accurate than sonographer derived EFs and volumes and more reproducible. In addition, one can get LA and RV volumes as well by AI algorithms. The 3D RV volume by echocardiographic approximates to that derived by cardiac MRI, the cardiac MRI being the gold standard.

Calculating the LV strain in a fully automated fashion is by AI is available in most of echocardiographic equipment. This uses speckle tracking, a feature in the myocardium identified by AI and tracked to follow the movement of that piece of the myocardium. For the left ventricle, one can obtain both regional and global longitudinal strain, radial strain, circumferential strain and torsion, or angular strain. Abnormal strain is an early sign of myocardial dysfunction and its measurement automation has great value in a variety of cardiovascular disorders. AI algorithms also allow strain measurements from the LA and RV walls by speckle tracking technology **(Fig. 2)**.

The RV segmentation to evaluate the anatomy and function is more challenging compared to LV because of its more complex anatomy. The implementation of a multi-chamber model can facilitate a comprehensive evaluation of various clinical conditions that affect the cardiac chambers.

DETECTION OF CAD AND WALL MOTION ANALYSIS

There is considerable inter-reader variability in the interpretation of wall motion analysis, even among experienced readers. The variability seems to be more than for the evaluation of LV ejection fraction. To assess wall motion, one looks at endocardial excursion in relation to the center line as well as regional wall thickening during systole and its exact timing to decide if there is adequate thickening, whether it is delayed (tardikinesis) or there is thinning during systole with paradoxical thickening during early diastole. The interpreter's retinal refreshment rate may not be as high as the rates of these changes. AI-powered tools have been developed to automatically interpret resting and stress wall motion abnormalities. EchoGo Pro by Ultromics is one such tool that is available and has been trialed to interpret stress echocardiograms both in US and UK's NHS hospitals.[17] The EVEREST study enrolled 8,000 patients undergoing stress

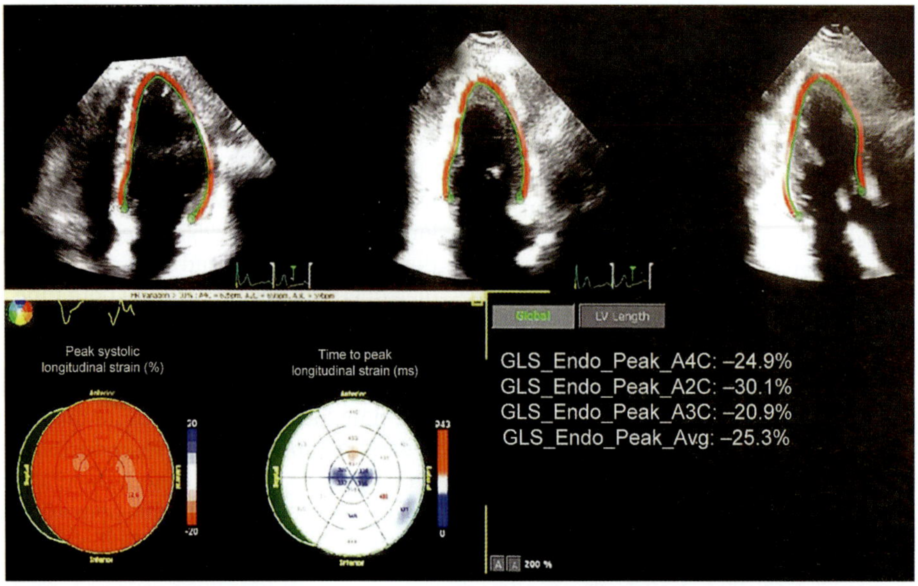

FIG. 2: Technique of using the speckle tracking to track LV wall motion and shortening in the longitudinal plane to obtain regional and global longitudinal strain of the LV. The same tool can be used to evaluate right ventricular and left atrial strains as well.
(GLS: global longitudinal strain)

echocardiograms and preliminary results were recently presented at ESC meeting.[18] The performance seemed to be similar to expert human interpretation. Despite that, the tool will empower institutions where advanced expertise is not readily available and will increase the adoption of stress echo in such places. The tool was cleared by FDA in 2021. The PROTEUS trial has enrolled 2,500 patients undergoing stress echocardiography in NHS hospitals; results are awaited.[19,20]

AUTOMATED DOPPLER ANALYSIS

Major advances have been made since the early introduction of Doppler technology into echocardiography in the 1980s when the output was Doppler shift. From this one had to factor in Doppler frequency and calculate the velocity of blood flow. Automated display of velocity was a major advancement. Now most of the echocardiographic equipment can automatically trace the Doppler spectral signals to give peak and mean velocities, velocity time integrals, and peak and mean gradients. There are also tools available to factor in the size of the area through which the flow occurs along with the flow velocity quantitation to obtain flow such as stroke volume from the LV outflow tract. There tools that have been developed to automatically quantitate mitral regurgitation (MR) color Doppler signal as well.

Mitral Valve Quantitation

Mitral apparatus is a complex structure and consists of not only the mitral annulus, leaflets, chordae tendineae, and papillary muscles, but the left atrium and left ventricle as well. Abnormalities in any of these structures can produce MR and multiple abnormalities may exist in a given patient. Customizing repair to abnormal dynamic anatomy of this complex apparatus is important for adequate and durable repair. Also, it is important to quantitate MR accurately when the jets are complex or multiple.

AI technology on aortic and mitral valvular heart disease is helpful in evaluating regurgitation severity using PISA method.[21] Automated measurements of morphological mitral valve parameters, such as 3D ring length and height, 2D area, commissural width, and overlap width, 3D leaflet area can be used to analyze valve morphology. These are similar to human expert measurement.

Munafo et al. used 3D TEE data sets from patients undergoing mitral clip procedure using Philips ultrasound system and developed automatic AI-generated mitral anatomy maps and measurements.[22] The automated displays were excellent and measurements were within 1–2 mm of expert measurements in terms of annulus size and shape and various mitral leaflet measurements **(Flowchart 1)**. These tools are very promising to enhance the repairability of mitral valves both during surgery and percutaneous repairs, but to improve the outcome as well by better fitting the repair technique to the anatomic defect. In a similar fashion, Jegannathan et al. performed automated 3D analysis of mitral valve anatomy with a Siemens ultrasound system with a similar degree of accuracy.[23]

Aortic Valve Quantitation

The aortic valve apparatus consists of the LV outflow tract, the aortic annulus, the leaflets, sinus of Valsalva, and the sinotubular junction from which the leaflets are suspended.

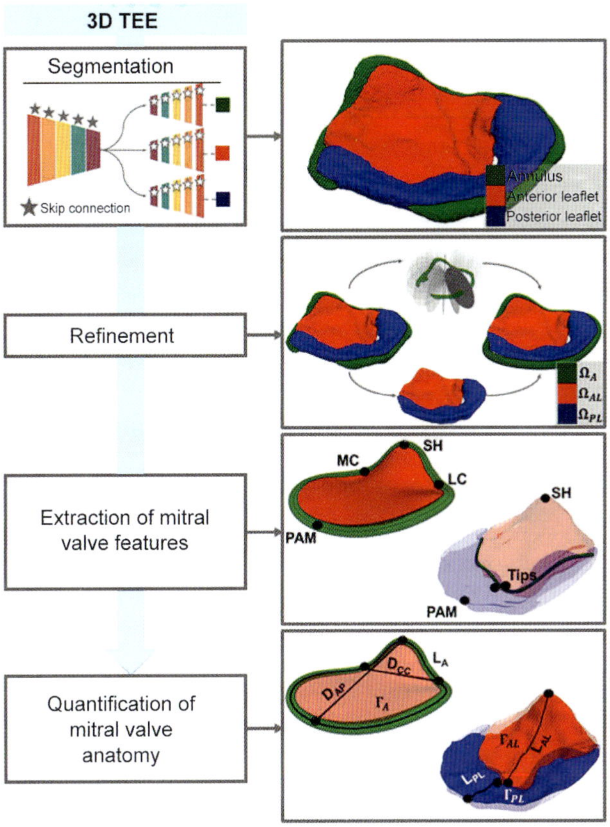

FLOWCHART 1: Schematic representation of the implemented automatic pipeline for mitral valve anatomy assessment through the four steps of segmentation, refinement, extraction, and quantification of mitral valve data from 3D TEE data set.

(D_{AP}: anteroposterior diameter; D_{CC}: inter-commissural diameter; L_A: annulus length; L_{AL}: anterior leaflet length; LC: lateral commissure; L_{PL}: posterior leaflet length; MC: medial commissure; PAM: posterior annulus mid-point; SH: saddle horn; Tips: leaflets tips; Ω_A: annulus surface; Ω_{AL}: anterior leaflet surface, Ω_{PL}: posterior leaflet surface)

Source: Reproduced through creative common agreement from Munafo R, Saitta S, Ingallina G, et al. (2023). A Deep Learning-based Fully Automated Pipeline for Regurgitant Mitral Valve Anatomy Analysis From 3D Echocardiography. [online] Available from https://iris.unisr.it/retrieve/13cdb1bb-1431-4cae-8fef-eb7611b4f224/ [Last accessed October, 2024].

In addition, in TAVR planning, one needs to know the coronary artery heights and sinus size so that the prosthetic valve and native leaflets do occlude the coronary ostia. Delineation of this anatomy is also important in aortic regurgitation patients undergoing potential repair.

Though most of these data have been obtained by CCT examinations, 3D TEE-obtained images with AI-guided or automatically performed measurements have been fairly accurate for clinical decision making. Various major vendors (e.g., Philips, Siemens, TomTec, etc.), have these capabilities and analysis and measurements can be performed with a few seconds of image acquisition.[24] In addition, AI driven, automated tools for assessment of aortic stenosis have become robust.[25] These tools developed using nearly half a million patients with aortic stenosis were not only able to predict severe aortic stenosis with about 75% agreement with the current guidelines, but were able to risk stratify and predict survival **(Flowchart 2 and Fig. 3)**.[25]

DISEASE DETECTION, PHENOTYPING AND PROGNOSTICATION

AI has been able to extract and use features that are not apparent to the human eye or mind. For example, AI, adequately trained, can predict a person's biological age, chronological age, gender, and even survival or sudden death risk from a simple ECG alone. If this is combined with the vast amount of structured and unstructured electronic health record data, the potential is simply mind-boggling.

AI tools have been developed to make a diagnosis of cardiac amyloidosis, coronary artery disease, hypertrophic cardiomyopathy, severe aortic stenosis, restrictive cardiomyopathy, constrictive pericarditis, heart failure with preserved EF, etc.[26-32] The list is expanding and this is all based on echocardiographic feature extraction. The potential is huge when other patient data are mined and used to arrive at the diagnosis and prognostication instead of just echocardiographic data.

Cardiac amyloidosis is not that infrequent and is grossly underdiagnosed. Both AL and ATTR amyloidosis are amenable to treatment, especially when diagnosed early. Otherwise, prognosis is grim. Using AI-extracted data from ECG and echocardiographic images, researchers have been able to diagnose cardiac amyloid with a high degree of certainty, with C-statistic in the range of 0.85–1.000.[26] The certainty should be higher if clinical data are added.

HFpEF is frequently missed leading to excess morbidity, HF hospitalization and mortality and a missed opportunity to treat early. Akerman et al. developed an AI-based tool to diagnose HFpEF from just a four-chamber view resulting in an area under ROC of 0.95.[27] Nearly, 3,000 patients and similar number of controls were used to develop the AI tool. Such an AI tool also predicted hospitalization and mortality with precision.[29]

Sengupta et al. developed an AI tool to diagnose severe aortic stenosis and predict survival.[30] The diagnostic accuracy approached that of expert reviewers using current ACC/AHA guidelines. AI tools can also predict rate of AS progression which tends to be highly variable in patients with AS.[31] One of the most rewarding area is the detection of rheumatic heart disease by AI algorithms.[32] This has vast implications in global health by making the tool available in remote underserved areas of the world to make a diagnosis and offer rheumatic fever prophylaxis.

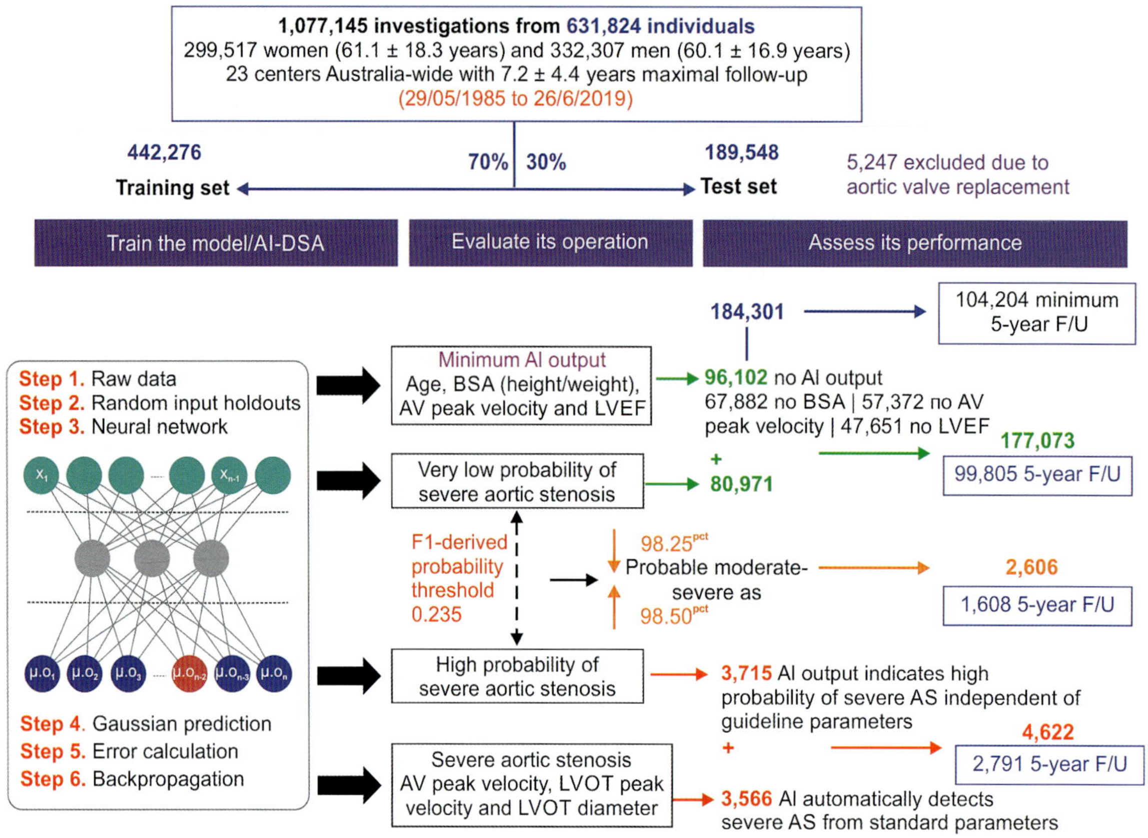

FLOWCHART 2: The training, evaluation, and testing of the AI-DSA to detect severe forms of AS. This schema shows the distribution of cases/investigations from the NEDA cohort used to train and evaluate the AI-DSA (investigation-based, no mortality data) and then test/assess its performance in accurately detecting the severe form of aortic stenosis associated with high 5-year mortality (individual-based). The highest F1 score was chosen as the probability at the peak of the precision/recall relationship, corresponding to a probability of 0.235. The moderate-to-severe aortic stenosis group corresponds to a probability output of >0.0625 (98.25–98.5 percentile of probability spectrum below the f1-derived threshold).

(AI-DSA: artificial intelligence decision support algorithm; AS: aortic stenosis; AV: aortic valve; BSA: body surface area; F/U: follow-up; LVEF: left ventricular ejection fraction; LVOT: left ventricular outflow tract; NEDA: National Echo Database of Australia; pct: percentile)

Source: Reproduced through creative common agreement from Strange G, Stewart S, Watts A, Playford D et al. Enhanced detection of severe aortic stenosis via artificial intelligence: a clinical cohort study. Open Heart. 2023;10(2):e002265d.

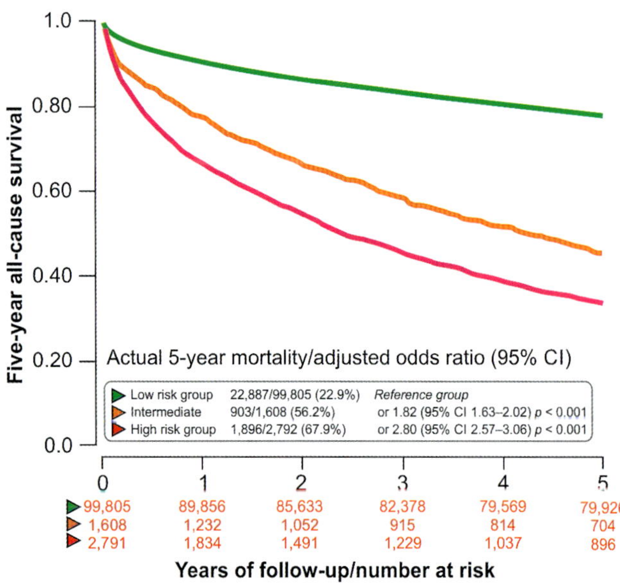

FIG. 3: Actual 5-year all-cause mortality according to three main outputs from the AI-DSA. This graph shows the 5-year actual mortality curves (all-cause and with no censoring of cases) for the three main output groups from the AI-DSA—with low probability individuals being the reference group). The ORs for age and sex were 1.08 (95% CI 1.08 to 1.08 per annum) and 1.50 (95% CI 1.46–1.55 for men vs. women).

(AI-DSA: artificial intelligence decision support algorithm)

Source: Reproduced through creative common agreement from Strange G, Stewart S, Watts A, et al. Enhanced detection of severe aortic stenosis via artificial intelligence: a clinical cohort study. Open Heart. 2023;10(2):e002265.

MINING UNSTRUCTURED DATA FROM ECHOCARDIOGRAPHIC REPORTS

Echocardiogram report has abundant nonstructural data which gets challenging in data mining.[33] Previous research on extracting echocardiographic data through natural language processing (NLP) from unstructured sources had limitations in terms of automation, and accuracy. Nath and colleagues showcased an NLP software named Echoinfer. This program can extract echocardiographic elements and values from structured, semistructured, and unstructured data found in echocardiography reports and organize them in a structured format. Echoinfer was able to extract eighty data elements including ventricular size, atrial size and their function, stenosis and regurgitation parameters of the valves, and hemodynamics accurately from large data base.[34]

To quote Bose et al., "To bridge this gap, we developed a specialized echocardiographic data engineering pipeline, leveraging extraction, transformation, and load (ETL) processes with NLP and ML techniques. Emphasizing its relevance to institutions and national registries in imaging, this approach transforms semistructured echocardiographic data into a structured, accessible format. Enhancing EMR integration and potentially establishing a comprehensive, population-based echocardiographic clinical data warehouse registry are pivotal".[35]

CONCLUSION

To make a bold prediction, AI will make echocardiography easier, faster, more reliable, and more powerful. The process of performing the echocardiogram will be better and faster with less sonographer work-related musculoskeletal injuries. The images will be better, measurements will be more accurate, reports will be autogenerated and integrated with clinical, laboratory, and other imaging data to offer robust clinical diagnosis. This amazing clinical imaging tool will be available globally, even where the expertise does not exist, to offer the same level of service as in a quaternary care hospital. The highest level of expertise, either through artificial or human intelligence will be available to every patient around the globe, rich and poor, thus leveling the playing field and democratizing healthcare.

ONLINE REFERENCES

Please scan the QR code provided at the end of the table of contents for References of this chapter.

CHAPTER

18

Artificial Intelligence and Heart Failure

Arijit Kumar Ghosh

ABSTRACT

Heart failure (HF) is a heterogeneous syndrome prevalent globally. It is a dynamic disease with varying definitions and classifications due to multiple pathophysiologies and etiologies. Artificial intelligence (AI) can play a pivotal role in the management of HF with its ability to integrate and synthesize large amounts of data with multidimensional interactions offering early detection and precise diagnoses. AI will improve the physicians' ability to make timely and better decisions. However, its challenges include data access, model interpretability, ethical concerns, and generalizability across diverse populations. Despite these ongoing efforts to refine AI models, it suggests a promising future for HF management.

Keywords: Heart failure, artificial intelligence, machine learning, application

INTRODUCTION

Heart failure (HF) is a clinical syndrome with symptoms and/or signs caused by a structural and/or functional cardiac abnormality and corroborated by elevated natriuretic peptide levels and/or objective evidence of pulmonary or systemic congestion.[1] HF is a long-term, advancing condition where the cardiac muscle debilitates due to various factors, leading to an insufficient supply of blood to meet the body's oxygen demands. HF is a common cause of hospitalization and poses challenges in diagnosis and management.[2]

Patients receive numerous diagnostic tests, invasive procedures, and therapies over the course of their illness, generating large amounts of data, which pose challenges for traditional analytical methods to make sense of them. To address this, big data approaches and artificial intelligence (AI) have been developed that can effectively predict future observations and outcomes, enabling precise diagnoses and management of patients with HF.

These AI-driven approaches have made significant strides in various aspects of HF research, including diagnosis, outcome prediction, classification of HF phenotypes, and optimization of treatment strategies. AI can play an important role in bridging these gaps in HF and has important advantages over traditional human-derived models.

ARTIFICIAL INTELLIGENCE

Artificial intelligence is a term that depicts machines to simulate human intelligence. AI focuses on equipping machines with human intelligence and decision-making capabilities to offer forms of support to individuals. It revolves around training machines to make decisions independently through various algorithms and mathematical calculations without actual human involvement. AI utilizes technology to provide personalized treatment plans for patients and excels at handling tasks that may be too complex or demanding for humans.[3]

Machine Learning

Machine learning (ML) is a subfield of AI that allows computers to analyze data, find patterns, and make predictions without explicit instructions. ML, or AI, involves the process of learning, where it familiarizes itself with a large set of data and identifies and interprets patterns better than a human brain.[4] ML encompasses computational techniques that can extract patterns from data, acquire knowledge, and apply this knowledge to tasks. ML methods can handle temporal, large-volume, and multimodality data. ML contributes to a significant chunk of AI today.

There are five categories within ML:

1. Supervised learning predicts known outcomes from labeled datasets, suitable for classification and regression, but demanding substantial data and time. In supervised ML, human-labeled datasets guide algorithms to accurately categorize information or forecast outcomes. This approach has successfully diagnosed HF using electrocardiography time series data.
2. Unsupervised learning uncovers hidden patterns without human guidance but may face challenges with biased training datasets and difficulty in identifying initial cluster patterns, leading to potential inaccuracies. Unsupervised ML involves grouping and analyzing unlabeled datasets to uncover hidden patterns without human intervention.
3. Semisupervised learning combines elements of both supervised and unsupervised approaches using labeled and unlabeled datasets. Unlabeled data are grouped based on similarities with labeled data to enhance the learning process.
4. Reinforcement learning, often used in robotics and gaming scenarios, relies on negative feedback to improve models. Machines with sensors, cameras, and GPS systems interact with their environment to better understand their surroundings.
5. Active learning algorithms.

Deep Learning

Machine learning has one of the advanced stages within techniques called deep learning (DL). Deep learning is a subset of ML that differentiates itself by the way it solves problems. ML involves training algorithms to learn from data and make predictions or decisions without being explicitly programmed for specific tasks. It uses neural networks to read, analyze, and interpret large and complex data collections.[5] DL techniques utilize artificial neural networks with multiple layers to find complex patterns to classify data and produce more precise predictions.[6] DL within AI/ML excels at handling intricate datasets derived from images or videos used in medical contexts. DL algorithms have been widely utilized in medicine for supervised and unsupervised training to automate the analysis of images.[7]

Artificial Intelligence-based Clinical Decision Support System

An artificial intelligence-based clinical decision support system (AI-CDSS) could aid in detecting HF in high-risk patients through AI algorithms. AI-CDSS offers an adaptable medical assistant platform for medical conditions. Choi et al. created the AI-CDSS and applied it in the diagnosis of HF among patients presenting with dyspnea in the outpatient clinic. They used a hybrid system where ML was integrated with knowledge acquired by expert-driven acquisition. AI-CDSS demonstrated a higher diagnostic accuracy compared to non-HF specialists.

- *Machine learning applications in HF*:
  - Prediction of incident HF[8,9]
  - Diagnosis of HF[10,11]
  - Classification of HF phenotypes[12-14]
  - Prediction of outcomes following HF diagnosis[15-17]
- *Optimization of medical and device therap*ies:
  - Medical therapy
  - Device therapy—patient selection and care

ARTIFICIAL INTELLIGENCE AND HEART FAILURE DIAGNOSIS

Traditional methods of diagnosing HF are a composite process involving clinical history and examinations, along with the evaluation of imaging techniques and laboratory parameters. HF can be challenging because it is a complex syndrome caused by both structural and functional cardiac disorders rather than a single disease entity.

The vast number of variables and quantity of data required to process and diagnose a complex syndrome like HF is a challenge for the human brain.[18] Thus, the ability of AI to identify and interlink subtle findings is an asset in efficient and effective decision-making. Gladding et al. incorporated AI with multiple sources of information from patients suffering from HF which included sources such as DNA sequencing, genomics, metabolites, data from wearables, digital ECG findings, and echocardiography. These data were used to substratify HF patients and show AI's potential to diagnose HF compared to conventional techniques.[19]

Rather than using traditional methods of analysis using human brains, it is far more feasible to use AI to do the job and help cut expenses by reducing the diagnosis time, leading to early diagnosis and early initiation of treatment. AI-based models to improve the diagnosis of HF have encompassed various data sources such as electrocardiograms (ECG), echocardiography, X-rays, and electronic health record (EHR) data.[20-23]

Early detection, diagnosis, and treatment are significant for HF, slowing its progression to the advanced stage and improving overall outcomes. ML models such as random forests, decision trees, logistic regression, and support vector machines help interpret complex healthcare data and accurately track primary modalities associated with HFs, such as heart rate, blood pressure, ECG signals, cholesterol levels, classification and severity of HF, predicting adverse events such as destabilization, rehospitalization, and mortality.[24]

Artificial intelligence serves as an essential tool to help physicians improve their clinical judgment and achieve precise diagnoses of diseases such as HF. To detect and diagnose HF, multiple data sources are integrated, and further AI algorithms are developed to improve the diagnostic accuracy.

Artificial intelligence algorithms could help physicians identify HF in at-risk patients early and develop an AI-CDSS. AI-CDSS is a scalable and flexible medical assistant platform for different types of diseases.[25]

Artificial Intelligence in Reading Electrocardiograms and Left Ventricular Dysfunctions

Attia et al. showed that the application of AI to ECG can be a powerful screening tool to identify left ventricular dysfunction in asymptomatic individuals. To achieve high accuracy, Kwon et al. analyzed 55,163 ECGs of 22,765 patients and developed a deep-learning algorithm for ECG-based HF identification. In addition, the DL model applied to ECG was shown to have a high performance in the detection of HF with preserved ejection fraction (HFpEF).[20,21]

There are also more specific risk markers that can be derived from ECGs, with models developed to identify the cross-sectional presence of LVSD that are also able to identify those at three- to fourfold higher risk of developing LVSD in the future and those at risk of developing clinical HF. These risks may have therapeutic implications.

In a study conducted by Bachtiger et al., an ECG-enabled stethoscope and a DL system called AI-ECG were used, and it was found that the single-lead ECGs could be used to detect HFrEF with a left ventricular ejection fraction (LVEF) of 40% or lower.[26]

Leveraging Artificial Intelligence and Cardiac Biomarkers

Integrating ML algorithms and biomarker analysis can help healthcare professionals gain valuable insights into the underlying mechanisms of HF, identify high-risk individuals, and develop targeted early intervention strategies to prevent the progression of HF and potentially reduce mortality rates.

Use of Artificial Intelligence in Automated Analysis of Imaging

AI has been used to interpret chest X-rays for detecting HFpEF, which helps reduce the dependence on more expensive imaging modalities such as echocardiography and cardiac MRI. Early diagnosis of HF will lead to early treatment initiation and fewer admissions or rehospitalization of patients, enabling better prognosis, lower cost-bearing, and better resource prioritization.

Artificial Intelligence in Wearables

The combination of wearable devices and AI can be used for cardiovascular (CV) monitoring at a fraction of the cost of expensive medical-grade devices. This results in more cost-efficient prevention and early detection of HF. Moreover, having a large number of data for AI to assess is beneficial since it provides more examples for the learning process. A study by Arman et al. involves monitoring CV biomarkers, including heart rate and step count. It was achieved using consumer-grade smartwatches, cloud technology to store big data, and applying self-supervised and multiple-instance learning techniques with AI to detect HF and AF.[27] This demonstrates AI's potential to help facilitate cost-effective CV monitoring of outpatients and prevent exacerbations in HF patients.

Enhancement of Cardiopulmonary Exercise Stress Testing in Heart Failure

SVM, an ML tool, was used by Inbar et al. to identify patients with chronic HF using cardiopulmonary exercise (CPX) test.[28] Furthermore, because CPX testing involves rigorous testing, research is actively underway to develop ML-based methods for estimating patient response to exercise in the early stages, as well as for estimating the dynamics of oxygen consumption from heart rate and inputs from the treadmill, cycle, and accelerometer. These methods will be integrated into smart devices.

Artificial Intelligence and Advanced Cardiac Imaging in Heart Failure

Multiple data sources, such as the ECG, EHRs, and imaging data [like echocardiography and cardiac magnetic resonance (CMR) imaging], are combined to detect and diagnose HF. Newer AI algorithms are being developed to improve diagnostic accuracy further. Research includes echocardiography image analysis, natural language processing for EHR data mining, and ECG analysis. Cho et al. demonstrated that HF with a reduced ejection fraction could be screened by a wearable device that used AI algorithms and a single-lead ECG instead of a standard 12-lead ECG. By incorporating such algorithms, AI can significantly aid in analyzing raw imaging data from cardiac imaging methods. AI methods may improve the effectiveness of auxiliary tools such as MRI, CT, and echocardiography. LVEF is crucial in determining the prognosis of HF, resynchronization therapy, and defibrillator. An ML method that can reliably and automatically quantify LVEF was proposed by Asch et al.[29] The accuracy of the ML in extracting LVEF was comparable to that of physicians.

In CV imaging, CMR imaging has become a vital tool over the last few years. Significant technological advancements have improved CMR's capacity for risk assessment and diagnosis. For noninvasive left ventricular volume and ejection fraction evaluation, CMR is considered superior. It also makes tissue characterization possible to determine medical management. Strain is a newly discovered biomarker that, like echocardiography, can aid in the ascent of CMR. However, several CMR procedures, such as volume measurement and contour tracing, require significant time. By integrating ML architectures, CMR can reach new heights and explore uncharted territory in CV imaging.

ARTIFICIAL INTELLIGENCE AND CLASSIFICATION OF HEART FAILURE PHENOTYPES AND TREATMENT

The present HF classification may be enhanced using ML. Phenotype mapping was performed in a prospective trial with 397 ambulatory patients with HFpEF using ML algorithms and data from EHRs. A novel classification method for HFpEF was created using this technique, which grouped study participants into phenotypes based on their clinical traits, echocardiographic parameters, ECG, invasive hemodynamics, and outcomes.

Another unsupervised ML analysis of 1,693 hospitalized patients with HF across the LVEF spectrum identified six distinct phenogroups based on the common comorbidities: Coronary artery disease, valvular heart disease, atrial fibrillation, chronic obstructive pulmonary disease, obstructive sleep apnea, or a few comorbidities. This grouping stratified the CV risk more effectively than LVEF. ML algorithms can be used to improve HF treatment by assessing the heterogeneity of the response to HF therapies. Ahmad et al. studied 44,886 patients with HF in the Swedish HF registry and utilized ML to classify patients into four subgroups based on their response to therapeutics and 1-year survival rates. This stratification allowed the identification of those most likely to benefit from guideline-directed medical therapy. ML can be used to prioritize patients who are most likely to benefit from interventions to optimize evidence-based therapies. Moreover, ML algorithms can assist clinicians in determining optimal sequencing and dosing of evidence-based therapies.

ARTIFICIAL INTELLIGENCE AND PREDICTION OF HEART FAILURE OUTCOMES

Heart failure is the leading cause of hospitalization in people aged 65 years and older. Moreover, patients with HF have a high risk of readmission, especially immediately after discharge. Therefore, risk stratification is important for HF, and ML can be particularly valuable in predicting readmission for these patients. Golas et al. showed that DL techniques outperformed traditional techniques in predicting 30-day readmission in patients with HF. Furthermore, Kwon et al. showed that a DL-based algorithm predicted in-hospital mortality and long-term mortality more accurately than the existing scores, including the Get with the Guidelines-Heart Failure Score (GWTG) and Meta-Analysis Global Group for Heart Failure (MAGGIC) score. This might be because DL algorithms do not restrict the number of input or features without limiting to those with established associations or biologically plausible rationales. Cardiac monitoring data can be used to develop risk prediction algorithms. In a cohort study of 900 patients, data from implanted cardiac resynchronization therapy (CRT) were collected. The alert algorithm used heart sounds, respiratory rate, tidal volume, heart rate, and patient activity to provide a sensitive and timely predictor of impending HF decompensation.[15]

MACHINE LEARNING-BASED PREDICTION OF RESPONSE TO CARDIAC RESYNCHRONIZATION THERAPY

The prognosticating role of AI may also extend to enabling high-value care practices and individualizing how therapies may affect outcomes. For instance, despite the heterogeneous risk, primary prevention implantable cardioverter defibrillators (ICDs) are recommended in a large subset of patients with HF. Through multimodal integration of imaging phenotypes and tabular characteristics, AI tools may provide actionable risk discrimination for arrhythmic versus nonarrhythmic mortality, guiding personalized risk–benefit discussions. AI models are also improving upon traditional rule-based approaches in discriminating underlying rhythm, thus preventing inappropriate shocks. Further insights into personalized disease trajectories may be provided by "digital twin" approaches that model the effects of varying population features and their simulated effects on outcomes. In patients with HF with poor left ventricular function with conduction abnormalities, CRT is recommended. But about one-third of the patients are nonresponders. AI and ML-based models can be used to predict response to CRT. A post-hoc analysis of the Multicenter Automatic Defibrillator Implantation Trial with CRT demonstrated that ML algorithms, by integrating clinical parameters and cardiac cycle imaging data, could classify a phenotypically heterogeneous HF cohort into distinct phenotypes, thus potentially optimizing the response rate to CRT. ICDs reduce the risk of sudden cardiac death in patients with HF. One study showed that unsupervised ML-based phenomapping could identify distinct phenotype subgroups in patients with clinically heterogeneous HF receiving secondary prophylactic ICD therapy, thus aiding the implementation of personalized medicine for these patients. Shakibfar et al. revealed that ML using daily summaries of ICD measurements in the absence of clinical information could predict the short-term risk of electrical storms.[30] In addition, a DL model can assist in selecting patients with HF who are eligible for subcutaneous ICD. The potential of ML to select patients for medical and device therapies needs to be harnessed through prospective testing and validation in clinical studies.[16,17]

IMAGING HEART FAILURE WITH ARTIFICIAL INTELLIGENCE

- Image obtaining and identification
- Image segmentation
- AI-based echocardiography

Artificial intelligence has been incorporated into echocardiographic evaluations as a means of getting more accurate echocardiographic images and sparing valuable time for clinical practices and aids in the correct diagnosis, treatment resulting in better healthcare for the patients, and reducing the need for repeated hospitalizations.

He et al. designed a trial including 3,495 echocardiographic reports in order to assess an LVEF evaluation based on AI. They found that the initial assessment of LVEF by AI was noninferior, but even superior to the assessment by sonographers, suggesting that AI can ameliorate efficacy and efficiency in assessing cardiac function.[31]

In a prospective study mainly targeting the robustness of an AI-based diagnosis, Chen et al. evaluated 80 hospitalized patients with acute left HF.[32] A deep convolutional neural network (DCNN) algorithm model was created in order to set up the image processing. AI-based assessment demonstrated higher diagnostic accuracy and was related to lower rehospitalization and mortality rates.

Artificial intelligence-assisted echocardiographic evaluation could help address the unmet need for an accurate diagnosis in the large, heterogeneous group of patients with HFpEF. AI-assisted echocardiographic interpretations can be applied retrospectively on an echocardiographic data basis in order to enhance our surveillance for undetected cases of relatively infrequent findings or early findings of dysfunction which may escape the attention of human interpreters. Measurements can be completely automated without lacking the reliability of the diagnosis at the same time. An automated approach for interpreting echocardiograms has the potential to promote accessibility to echocardiography, transferring heart assessments to primary care facilities and remote rural regions, thereby making it more widely available.

Cardiac Magnetic Resonance Imaging

Cardiac magnetic resonance is acknowledged as the superior method for evaluating the cardiac structure and overall systolic function and is achieved by measuring precise blood and myocardial volumes. The process of acquiring images is standardized and can be completed quickly. However, the analysis of these images is both time-consuming and reliant on the operator, leading to inherent variability between different observers and even within the same observer. DL can offer a solution by automating this task with high levels of accuracy and precision. AI algorithms play a crucial role in cardiac imaging, particularly in ventricular segmentation using techniques like cardiac MRI. ML can accurately segment heart chambers from cardiac MRIs, providing imaging biomarkers for predicting congestive heart failure (CHF).[33]

In a cohort study, AI-generated contours for feature tracking and strain analysis in CMR produce results that are on par with manual segmentations.

Artificial intelligence has also demonstrated potential in the field of CMR tissue characterization. Late gadolinium enhancement imaging is a crucial biomarker for assessing left ventricular scar volume, essential for risk assessment and procedure planning. DL convolutional neural networks (CNNs) can differentiate between left ventricular scar tissue and normal myocardium based on image-based characteristics. This capability allows for the precise measurement of scar volume in patients with ischemic and hypertrophic cardiomyopathies.

Cardiac magnetic resonance indicators can also be integrated into ML models to improve the accuracy of risk prediction. Ambale-Venkatesh and colleagues, as described in their study, utilized a random forest algorithm to demonstrate that among 725 clinical and imaging factors, the left ventricular structure and function derived from CMR imaging were identified as significant predictors of the onset of HF in a cohort of 6,814 participants from the MultiEthnic Study of Atherosclerosis.[34,35]

TECHNOLOGY IN THE DEVELOPMENT FOR EARLY DETECTION OF HEART FAILURE DECOMPENSATION

ZOLL μCor™

A clinical trial for predicting HF decompensation is now being conducted to test the ZOLL μCor™, which is a patch that has been approved by the FDA and is equipped with an ECG monitor, a radiofrequency sensor, and a transmitter. The patch is designed to quantify the amount of fluid in the pulmonary system.[36]

HeartLogic™ Algorithm

Multisensor Chronic Evaluation in Ambulatory Heart Failure Patients (MultiSENSE) was the source of the data utilized in developing the HeartLogic algorithm. Lung impedance, activity, respiratory rate, volume, and heart sounds (S1, S3) were all elements that were incorporated into the sensor measurements. According to a retrospective review, the HeartLogic algorithm may also help detect the gradual worsening of HF and stratify the risk of HF decompensation. Several trials have established the efficacy of remote telemedicine management in improving life expectancy, quality of life, and reducing HF rehospitalizations.[36]

ONGOING RESEARCH

Ongoing research is focused on areas such as ECG analysis, natural language processing for EHR data mining, and echocardiography image analysis. AI can be of great assistance in analyzing raw imaging data from cardiac imaging techniques. With the increasing amount of data from remote monitoring and wearable devices, the role of AI is expanding. Kwon et al. showed that an AI-enabled smartwatch with a 2-lead ECG detected HF with reduced ejection fraction with acceptable performance.

LIMITATIONS AND CHALLENGES OF ARTIFICIAL INTELLIGENCE AND HEART FAILURE

Major challenge to current AI/ML-based monitoring systems is the lack of rigorous prospective evaluation. Moreover, few studies have been shown to affect clinical end points such as mortality or make predictions that could directly inform clinical decision-making. AI/ML tools may also be limited in practice by the lack of standardized platforms to report predictions to clinicians and noise in ambulatory data, with some studies reporting that valid data are present for as little as half of the monitoring time. Solutions may involve deriving more informative time-varying metrics for longer periods of time.

An example of perpetuation or even augmentation of diagnostic uncertainties with ML. The two currently used algorithms for HFpEF diagnosis are HFA-PEFF and HF2FPEF. These two algorithms disagree in approximately 40% of the cases. Thus, the HFpEF clusters obtained with the use of unsupervised ML will strongly depend on which algorithm was used and the diagnostic uncertainty will culminate in cluster definition uncertainty.

Limitation of Artificial Intelligence in Heart Failure Diagnosis

There are two published algorithms for HFpEF diagnosis: H2FPEF and the European Society of Cardiology HFA-PEFF. The ESC HFA-PEFF score shares certain variables with the H2FPEF score but incorporates additional parameters leading to the anticipation of variations in the prevalence of HFpEF depending on the scoring system employed. Given the above discrepancies, disagreements may be present regarding which score should be utilized by the ML system in order to diagnose HFpEF.

Limitation of Artificial Intelligence Left Ventricular Ejection Fraction-based Heart Failure Classification

Several factors, including loading conditions and structural changes in the left ventricle, influence LVEF. Hence, even though LVEF does not directly contribute to myocardial contractility, it is misinterpreted as such. Therefore, the reliance on LVEF in the existing AI models for HF classification is another example of the challenges in the availability of accurate and high-quality data. Inconsistencies in data quality and biases in the datasets when using diverse data sources can result in skewed AI models that eventually become unreliable tools for diagnosing HF.

Artificial intelligence applications that have been trained impeccably can generate incorrect results when provided with inaccurate input. AI and ML models face several limitations including lack of external validation, limited generalizability, opaque decision-making, logistical challenges in implementation due to reliance on digital infrastructure, error propagation between iterations, and dataset shift. It would be rather unrealistic to assume that we could avoid providing the system with faulty importation regarding HF diagnosis and treatment, since there is abundant evidence advocating that our level of established knowledge is still inadequate. Issues that remain unresolved concern diagnosis, classification, and treatment; consequently, AI outcomes should always be interpreted with caution.

The effectiveness of ML models of HF in improving outcomes at the point of care needs to be tested prospectively in randomized controlled trials. There is an increasing need for prospective AI validation studies.[37]

ETHICAL CONSIDERATIONS

Ethical concerns frequently impose restrictions on ML-based models. Systemic biases have impeded the inclusion of under-represented minority groups in ML algorithms.[38]

LEGAL IMPLICATIONS

AI systems often require vast amounts of data, raising concerns about user consent, data protection, and privacy. Bias in AI systems can lead to discriminatory outcomes, making it the biggest legal issue in the AI landscape. Patients' informed consent regarding the utilization of their personal data the question of legal and ethical consequences also arises from the fact that there are chances of misdiagnoses.[39]

CONCLUSION

Even though advancements in medicine over the last few decades have resulted in a decrease in the morbidity and mortality associated with almost all CV diseases, HF remains an exception. Therefore, more advanced diagnostic modalities have become the need of the hour for early detection and treatment of HF.[6]

The utilization of AI in the diagnosis, classification, and prognosis of HF is expanding and has showcased promising outcomes. ML improves early diagnosis of HF, classification of HF, device selection, medication titration, risk prognostication, and clinical trial enrolment and retention. Various data, including ECG, echocardiography, and EHRs, are used in AI. In addition, the integration of data from remote monitoring and wearable devices has expanded the potential applications of AI in HF.

However, challenges such as access to high-quality data, validation, model interpretability, ethical concerns, and generalizability across diverse populations remain. Ongoing efforts to refine AI models indicate a promising future for diagnosing HF with AI technology. ML is a rapidly growing field that may improve HF care; however, further work on validation and interpretability is needed before it is incorporated in routine care. The incorporation of AI tools is expected to revolutionize HF management and significantly impact patient outcomes, thereby enabling more precise and personalized care of patients with HF.

With the advent of modern technologies, we now live in the "big data" era where we have enormous data in eHealth records, genomics, pathological results, imaging results, data from telemonitoring using implantables, wearable devices, and various mobile applications. Cardiologists need to assimilate these different data for early diagnosis and risk stratification, thus improving the quality of care in patients with HF.

ONLINE REFERENCES

Please scan the QR code provided at the end of the table of contents for References of this chapter.

CHAPTER

19

Artificial Intelligence in Transcatheter Aortic Valve Replacement

Preetish Rath, Pradeep Kumar Mustepally, PC Rath

ABSTRACT

Transcatheter aortic valve replacement (TAVR) has become treatment of choice and alternative option to surgical aortic valve replacement (SAVR) in elderly patients above 75 years of age. With recent real world evidence and clinical trials, TAVR is now indicated in low-risk patients apart from high risk. Artificial intelligence involves the development of algorithms that enable computers to learn from and make decisions based on data. Machine learning (ML) is a subset of artificial intelligence. These algorithms have made significant inroads across various fields, including healthcare, where it has demonstrated tremendous potential in enhancing diagnostic accuracy,[1,2] personalizing treatment plans,[3,4] and improving patient outcomes.[5,6]

Keywords: TAVR, artificial intelligence, machine learning

INTRODUCTION

Transcatheter aortic valve replacement (TAVR), revolutionized the management of severe aortic valve stenosis. The expanding indications for TAVR now include intermediate and low-risk patients, indicating its proven benefits and increasing acceptance across different subset of patients. Based on numerous registries and large-scale studies, number of TAVR procedures performed has increased globally, outnumbering surgical aortic valve replacement.[7,8]

The TAVR is a complex procedure, for successful intervention and recovery, precise planning and execution have to be done. In order to assist cardiologists, artificial intelligence (AI) could play a critical role in various stages of the TAVR process, from patient selection and preoperative planning to intraoperative guidance and postoperative care.[9,10] AI involves the development of algorithms that enable computers to learn from and make decisions based on data. AI provides automated analysis and deeper interpretation of data. Additionally, AI enhances the interpretation of cardiac imaging, leading to more accurate diagnosis and better-informed treatment decisions.[8]

AI algorithms assist in identifying the most suitable candidates for TAVR by analyzing extensive clinical data and predicting potential risks and outcomes.[11] In preoperative planning, ML enhances the accuracy of imaging interpretation, providing detailed anatomical models that help in selecting and sizing the appropriate valve prosthesis.[12] During the procedure, real-time ML-driven monitoring and decision support systems guide cardiologists, improving precision and reducing complications.

Artificial intelligence automated software may have several benefits:

- Increase the precision of measurements by removing bias, subjectivity, and intraobserver variability.
- Provide a "second opinion" to assist the decision-making process in patients with borderline anatomies.
- Reduce the time required for preprocedural planning.

AUTOMATED DETECTION OF AORTIC STENOSIS USING ARTIFICIAL INTELLIGENCE

The automated detection of aortic stenosis (AS) using machine learning (ML) is a significant advancement in the early identification and management of valvular heart disease. AS is often underdiagnosed and undertreated, but early detection is critical for timely intervention. Two studies highlight the effectiveness of ML in detecting AS using echocardiographic data. A recent study developed a convolutional neural network (CNN) model for the automated detection of AS using limited 2D echocardiographic datasets.[13] This approach utilizes CNNs trained on transthoracic echocardiograms (TTEs) to identify view types and diagnose AS severity, achieving a high area under the receiver operator curve (AUROC) of 0.96 for distinguishing AS from non-AS cases. The model can differentiate between mild, moderate, and severe AS with significant accuracy, making it a powerful tool for screening and diagnosing AS in clinical settings. Another study explored the use of deep learning algorithms to enhance the diagnosis of severe AS.[14] The study employed a large dataset of echocardiograms and demonstrated that ML could accurately identify severe AS with a sensitivity of 92% and a specificity of 88%. This study highlights the potential of ML to augment clinical decision-making by providing reliable, automated assessments of AS severity.

TRANSCATHETER AORTIC VALVE IMPLANTATION RISK PREDICTION AND PATIENT SELECTION

Machine learning plays a crucial role in enhancing risk prediction and patient selection for Transcatheter Aortic Valve Implantation (TAVI). Traditional risk scores, such as the Society of Thoracic Surgeons (STS) score and Euro SCORE II, provide useful benchmarks but have limitations in accurately predicting outcomes for all patient subsets. To address these limitations, ML models such as the TAVI Risk Machine (TRIM) scores[12] have been developed, leveraging large datasets to improve the accuracy and interpretability of risk predictions. The TRIM scores utilize random algorithms to predict 30-day survival and assist in decision-making for treatment and postprocedural care. TRIM scores have shown to outperform traditional risk scores in predicting outcomes. For example, the TRIM postscore achieved a C-statistics value of 0.79, significantly higher than the STS score's C-statistics value of 0.69.[15] This higher predictive accuracy is critical in selecting appropriate candidates for TAVI, ensuring that high-risk patients are identified accurately and receive optimal care. Furthermore, ML models incorporate a wide range of heterogeneous variables, including demographic data, comorbidities, and procedural specifics. For instance, a study integrating these variables into a neural network model achieved an area under the curve (AUC) of 0.82 for predicting 30-day mortality, compared to an AUC of 0.76 in the absence of these variables.[15] By providing a more nuanced risk assessment, these models support clinicians in making better-informed decisions, ultimately improving patient outcomes.

PREDICTING LONG-TERM MORTALITY

Predicting long-term mortality in TAVI patients is another area where ML models have shown significant promise. Researchers have developed models using support vector machines, neural networks, and random forests to predict 1-year survival rates. These models integrate a variety of clinical, laboratory, and imaging variables to provide accurate prognostic assessments. A recent study utilized a genetic variable selection algorithm followed by a random forest model, to achieve a negative predictive value (NPV) of 96% and a positive predictive value (PPV) of 92% for 1-year mortality.[16] Such high accuracy levels are crucial for optimizing patient follow-up and resource allocation, ensuring that patients receive the appropriate level of care based on their long-term risk profiles. Additionally, survival analysis models, which incorporate time-to-event data, have also been employed to predict long-term outcomes for patients with calcific aortic valve disease. A recent study compares traditional cox proportional hazard (CPH) with ML methods, finding that ML models, using variables such as albumin, age, BMI, glucose, hypertension, and clonal hemopoiesis of indeterminate potential (CHIP), predict 1-year mortality with a C-index of 80%, demonstrating superior prediction capabilities to identify patients at high risk of mortality.[17]

PHENOGROUPING FOR IMPROVED RISK STRATIFICATION

Semisupervised learning techniques for phenogrouping represent another innovative application of ML in TAVI. Semisupervised learning is a ML approach that combines a small amount of precisely labeled data with a large pool of unlabeled data to improve predictive accuracy and model performance. A recent semisupervised approach involved clustering patients into phenogroups based on their clinical characteristics, which can then be used to refine risk predictions and tailor treatments.[18] By combining topological data analysis (TDA) with supervised learning, researchers have created models that identify unique patient phenotypes and predict their outcomes more accurately than traditional methods. Integrating phenogroups with the STS score significantly enhanced the prediction of 30-day cardiovascular mortality compared to using the STS score alone. This integration yielded an AUC of 0.96 versus 0.80 when using the STS score alone.[18] This improvement in predictive accuracy is essential for better risk stratification. Moreover, by identifying distinct phenogroups, ML models enable clinicians to develop tailored treatment plans that address the specific needs of each patient group. For example, patients in a high-risk phenogroup may benefit from more intensive monitoring and follow-up care, while those in lower-risk groups can be managed with less aggressive interventions.

PROCEDURAL PLANNING AND GUIDANCE

Machine learning also plays a critical role in procedural planning and real-time guidance during TAVI. Advanced imaging analysis powered by ML algorithms can provide detailed anatomical assessments, identify optimal implantation sites, and predict potential complications. This enhances the precision and safety of the procedure, leading to better outcomes for patients. ML-driven imaging analysis has been used to evaluate coronary calcium and epicardial adipose tissue, which are important factors in procedural planning.[15,18] These analyses help in selecting the appropriate valve size and placement strategy, thereby reducing the risk of complications such as paravalvular leak and valve malposition. For example, a study using ML to analyze preoperative CT scans achieved a valve sizing accuracy of 94%, significantly reducing the incidence of paravalvular leaks. During the TAVI procedure, ML algorithms can provide real-time guidance by analyzing intraoperative imaging data. These algorithms assist in the precise positioning of the valve, ensuring optimal deployment, and minimizing the risk of complications. In one study, the use of ML-based real-time guidance reduced the incidence of major complications by 15%, highlighting the potential of these technologies to improve procedural outcomes.[15]

EARLY DISCHARGE STRATEGIES

The ML models are valuable in developing and validating early discharge strategies for TAVI patients. By predicting the likelihood of adverse events within the first 30 days post-TAVI, these models help clinicians identify patients who can be safely discharged early. This not only reduces hospital-related infections but also reduces healthcare costs and optimizes resource utilization. A recent study[12] developed ML-based TRIM scores and showed that their TRIM postmodel demonstrated a significant advantage in predicting early discharge candidates for patients undergoing TAVI. They identified 72.2% of patients as eligible for early discharge with a 1% risk of 30-day mortality, compared to only 31% identified by the STS score. Furthermore, among those predicted as dischargeable by TRIM post, only 7.3% experienced serious complications, a significantly lower rate than the 7.8% among those identified by the STS score, where the difference was not statistically significant. This highlights the TRIM postmodel's superior ability to accurately identify patients suitable for early discharge while maintaining a low risk of postprocedural complications.

CONCLUSION

The integration of AI in TAVI not only enhances the safety and effectiveness of the procedure but also contributes to personalized medicine, offering tailored treatment plans that cater to individual patient needs. As the technology continues to evolve, the scope and impact of AI in TAVI and broader cardiology are poised to expand, ushering in a new era of advanced, data-driven healthcare solutions. AI-driven software, allows fully automated segmentation and measurements of planning CTs. It yields precise and highly accurate measurements, saves time, and thus improves time efficiencies, costs.

ONLINE REFERENCES

Please scan the QR code provided at the end of the table of contents for References of this chapter.

Use of Artificial Intelligence Including Multimodal Systems to Improve the Management of Cardiovascular Disease

CHAPTER 20

Biyanka Jaltotage, Juan Lu, Girish Dwivedi

ABSTRACT

Cardiovascular disease (CVD) is the leading cause of death globally, with its burden expected to increase in the coming years. This has put pressure on healthcare systems and led to an overwhelming influx of complex data, causing information overload. Artificial intelligence (AI) has emerged as a potential solution to manage CVD on a large scale. AI, a computational algorithm capable of learning, reasoning, problem-solving, and understanding natural language, can analyze massive, dynamic, and diverse datasets, providing accurate and efficient decision support. AI-based multimodal analysis methods have emerged in select settings, synthesizing information from various modalities. However, ethical challenges, diversity within the training population, and the "black box problem" need to be addressed before widespread implementation. Groups are providing developers and governing bodies with tools to navigate these challenges.

Keywords: CVD, AI, systems, management, data

INTRODUCTION

Cardiovascular disease (CVD) stands as the predominant global cause of death, with current estimates suggesting that the burden of CVD is set to continue to surge over the coming years.[1] The escalating prevalence of CVD places growing demands on healthcare systems, and events like the COVID-19 pandemic have highlighted the strain on current resources. Moreover, the surge in CVD has also resulted in an overwhelming influx of complex data, leading to a state of information overload. Consequently, there is a pressing need for a solution capable of efficiently processing vast amounts of data with accuracy and speed.

In recent years, artificial intelligence (AI) has emerged as a viable solution to improve the management of CVD on a large scale. AI belongs to the field of computer science describing computational algorithms capable of performing advanced tasks such as learning, reasoning, problem-solving, and understanding natural language.[2] An AI system that can analyze massive, dynamic, and diverse datasets, that provide accurate and efficient decision support would be invaluable in healthcare, and groups are investigating how these systems could be implemented to improve the management of CVD.[2,3] The diagnosis and monitoring of CVD necessitate utilizing a diverse array of tests, offering rich datasets for training AI systems. These systems have remained largely purpose-built for specific clinical settings and applications, but with recent significant improvements in computing power AI-based multimodal analysis methods have emerged in some select settings that can synthesize information from a multitude of modalities, including images, text, video, audio, and language.[4] This chapter aims to overview the current and future applications of AI, with a review of both single-modal and multimodal techniques, in the management of CVD.

ARTIFICIAL INTELLIGENCE

Artificial intelligence is a comprehensive term describing algorithms designed to simulate human intellect. Machine learning (ML) is a large subset of AI which at its core is based on algorithms identifying relationships between data points in order to accurately make predictions with new input data.[5] On the other hand, deep learning (DL) is a subset of ML and is typically built on a framework consisting of a network of nodes arranged in layers.[5] Other architectures also exist, such as those consisting of a series of transformer blocks that utilize self-attention allowing the model to focus on the most vital aspects of an image and filter out less relevant details.[6]

Despite the possible widespread benefits of AI in the management of CVD, many clinicians remain wary. The technology brings with it unique challenges that need to be considered and addressed prior to widespread implementation. These include ethical challenges surrounding confidentiality, diversity within the training population, and the "black box problem". Groups have delved into these challenges in great detail and are providing developers and governing bodies with tools to navigate them.[2]

APPLICATIONS FOR ARTIFICIAL INTELLIGENCE IN CARDIOVASCULAR DISEASE

Modern clinical cardiology has witnessed numerous advancements over the years, spanning the introduction of antiplatelet agents and prognostic heart failure medications to the development of percutaneous coronary intervention (PCI) or transcatheter aortic valve replacement.[2] Many of these notable progressions stem from the cumulative insights gained through the utilization of multiple modalities. The strength of AI is the ability to identify patterns across a vast number of data points with short processing times. Integrating AI into the workflow can aid in standardizing the level of care delivered to patients by improving quality control. An understanding of the emerging technology provides insights into the prospective role of AI in routine clinical practice **(Fig. 1)**. While not exhaustive, this section will provide an overview of the current state of the technology.

Electrophysiology

The electrocardiogram (ECG) functions as a fundamental diagnostic tool employed by clinicians, yet interpretation can pose a challenge. The application of AI to ECG interpretation is therefore high yield.[7] Zhu et al. formulated an algorithm with DL for arrhythmia detection, and the resulting model was found to be superior to senior cardiology clinicians.[8] The authors also postulated that with high accuracy, the algorithm in the future could be integrated with wearable technology to provide real-time analysis. DL models that have been applied to smartwatches by Bumgarner et al. detected atrial fibrillation with excellent results; the sensitivity and specificity were 93 and 84%, respectively.[9] Similarly, DL has been applied to implantable

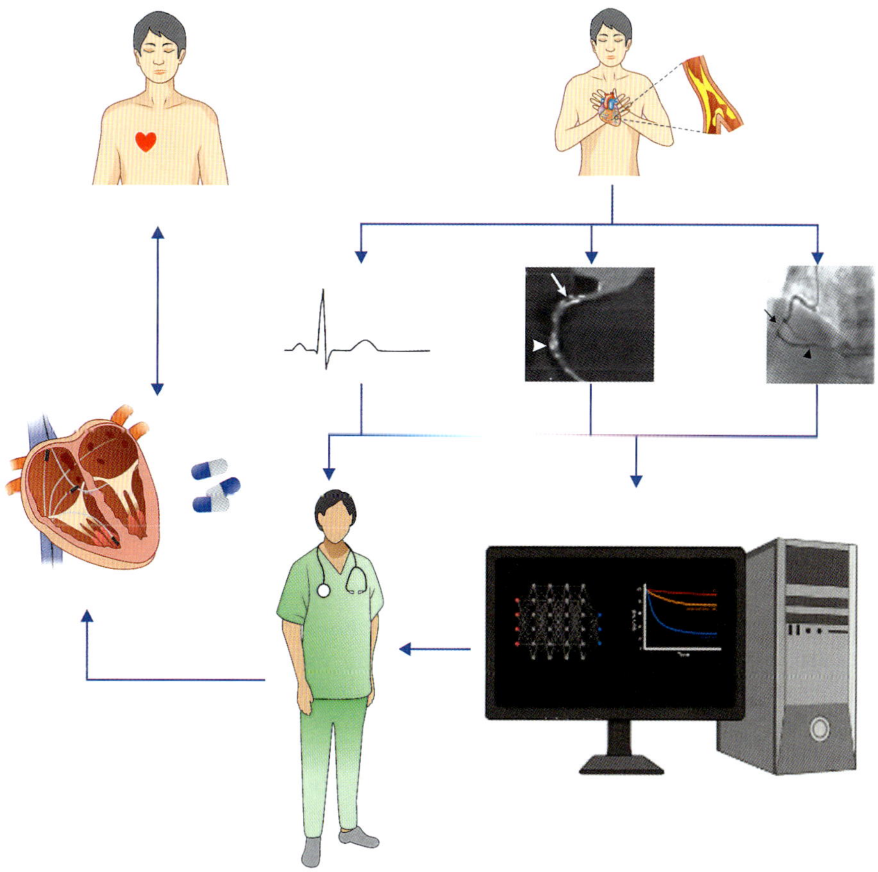

FIG. 1: Hypothetical artificial intelligence-based analysis of a presentation with chest pain. In the future patients presenting with common cardiac complaints such as chest pain could expect multimodality AI to analyze various aspects of their care such as the ECG, computed tomography scans, and coronary angiogram. Analysis of each modality can then be integrated and input into a system to guide clinical decisions.

loop recorders with a significant improvement in the positive predictive value from 53.9 to 74.5%.[10] Attia et al. have taken further steps with AI and analysis of ECGs in sinus rhythm to predict the presence of underlying paroxysmal atrial fibrillation with an impressive accuracy of almost 80%.[11] Further novel work in catheter ablation by You et al. investigated if robotic manipulation of catheters was possible; they employed reinforcement learning a subtype of ML that trains through trial and error.[12] The challenge for robotic systems with such tasks is the ability to compensate for external forces due to blood flow and respiration, yet success rates were impressive at up to 87%.

Interventional Cardiology

The field of interventional cardiology has expanded significantly in recent years, marked by the routine incorporation of intravascular imaging and coronary physiology, and is complemented by innovations in structural procedures. This expansion in the field has generated additional data points, which are increasingly conducive to AI involvement.

Invasive coronary angiography employs fluoroscopic imaging to evaluate the coronary arteries and image interpretation requires extensive training. In an attempt to assist clinicians with image analysis, Du et al. investigated a DL-based algorithm.[13] The algorithm demonstrated excellent accuracy for diameter stenosis at 88.2%, but also for advanced vessel characteristics including calcification, thrombus, and dissection with recall rates between 82.6 and 85.8%. With regards to interventional cardiology, there has also been an increasing shift, especially in complex lesions, in the routine use of intravascular imaging to improve lesion assessment and stent deployment.[14,15] Automation has proven to be feasible in intravascular ultrasound and optical coherence tomography, streamlining tasks such as vessel segmentation, plaque subtype analysis, and the detection of vulnerable plaque.[16]

Guidelines now endorse the use of coronary pressure wire-derived fractional flow reserve (FFR) (and instantaneous wave-free ratio) for ischemia-guided revascularization.[17] The uptake of FFR into routine revascularization decision-making has remained incompletely utilized, largely due to challenges surrounding time constraints, cost, invasiveness, and the need for hyperemia.[18] Furthermore, the interpretation of FFR is more nuanced than just using established cutoff values. FFR is a risk continuum, and lower values suggest more severe ischemia which correlates with more adverse events.[19] In addition, the pattern of coronary artery disease is also of importance with PCI of focal coronary disease more likely to improve symptoms and reduce ischemia; in contrast, percutaneous revascularization of extensive diffuse vessel plaque frequently fails to relieve ischemia and increases complication rates.[20] In an attempt to make FFR more accessible, Fearon et al. developed an algorithm with 92% accuracy for deriving FFR from analysis of conventional coronary angiographic images alone, eliminating the need for coronary pressure wire placement or hyperemia and reducing procedural time.[21] Davies et al. took an alternative approach and explored the development of an ML-based clinical decision support system to guide revascularization strategies based on the computational analysis of pressure wire pullback patterns, determining the disease pattern.[22] The software was compared to consensus by a team of multinational interventional cardiologists and was found to be noninferior in determining the appropriateness of PCI and the revascularization strategy. These advancements are examples of promising avenues for AI to be integrated into the complex landscape of interventional cardiology.

The field of structural cardiology has seen many advancements in recent years. The procedures are now growing in complexity, which is best highlighted by the recent developments in transcatheter valve interventions. Increasing procedural complexity leveraging virtual and augmented reality platforms, with AI support, offers substantial benefits. These platforms allow for improvements in both pre- and periprocedural planning and can improve the spatial awareness of the proceduralist.[23] The potential of these approaches has already been highlighted with reductions in procedural times and radiation exposure.[24]

Cardiac Imaging

Artificial intelligence is most advantaged in scenarios with large and complex data with a need for rapid and accurate analysis. Furthermore, DL algorithms such as convolutional neural networks excel with data in a visual format. The combination of these factors results in cardiac imaging being particularly well suited to the implementation of AI. Developers have therefore explored the applications of AI in a variety of imaging modalities including echocardiography, computed tomography (CT), and cardiovascular magnetic resonance (CMR) imaging. These techniques now allow for the assessment of cardiac structure, function, and hemodynamics, as well as the evaluation of coronary anatomy and characterization of myocardial edema and inflammation. This breadth of abilities limits the need for invasive procedures and limits patient exposure to unnecessary risks. Continued growth in this field is being propelled forward now with the help of AI technology.

Echocardiography is the most established cardiac imaging modality and remains a staple of first-line cardiac assessment due to its versatility and accessibility. The challenges surrounding echocardiography, however, are that image acquisition is technically difficult. In an attempt to obviate the need for specialized skillsets for image acquisition, Narang et al. developed DL-based software to guide novice scanners.[25] Images were deemed to be diagnostic in quality for basic cardiac parameters such as cardiac chamber size, myocardial function, and pericardial effusion characterization in up to 98.8% of cases. Similarly, Zhang et al. aimed to automate many of the manual measurements required for comprehensive assessment.[26] Early work has already demonstrated that algorithms employing DL techniques can now even extract hidden patterns revealing underlying pathogenic processes such as amyloidosis or hypertrophic cardiomyopathy.[5] Several other groups have focused on automating the assessment of valvular function.[27-29] Guidelines have moved away from more subjective assessment to the use of objective quantification with parameters such as proximal isovelocity area and regurgitant volume to grade the severity of valvular lesions.[30] These groups were able to demonstrate that AI-based quantification of valvular severity is viable with a high level of accuracy. In addition to valvular function, AI systems also have been shown to be effective in determining valve morphology.[31] Ongoing advancements are expected with AI and echocardiography over the coming years.

Computed tomography serves as the first-line test recommended for patients presenting with low- to intermediate-risk chest pain.[32] Given the routine use of CT, developers have strived to apply AI to expand its useability and overall utility.[3] One of the drawbacks of CT is the need for radiation and suboptimal imaging due to factors such as motion artifacts which can reduce diagnostic accuracy. Although the need for radiation cannot be completely eradicated, postprocessing by DL algorithms has shown that radiation exposure can be reduced by as much as 56% without compromising image quality.[33] Gong et al. were also able to develop AI software to minimize motion artifacts to improve image quality.[34]

Coinciding with developments in image acquisition, AI has also shown potential to assist CT image analysis. Ihdayhid et al. engineered a fully automated end-to-end system for calcium scoring that had an excellent correlation with manual measurements and an analysis time of only 13 seconds.[35] Other models have explored the application of AI to contrast studies. Lin et al. showed that their system had excellent correlation with expert readers for stenosis; outcome data also confirmed that their system was predictive of adverse cardiovascular events.[36] The same system was also able to accurately evaluate total plaque volume. Advanced CT markers of cardiovascular risk, including total plaque volume, are established predictors of cardiovascular risk, but their detection slows workflow which has hindered routine reporting.[3] An AI-based solution would promote the use of these valuable CT markers. Vulnerable plaques are another such marker. Kolossváry et al. formulated a model to improve the detection of vulnerable plaques with the use of radiomics, a subtype of AI extracting complex patterns from medical images.[37]

Until recently, CT has been limited in its ability to provide functional assessments to complement the detailed anatomical evaluation of coronary plaque. Traditionally, FFR has only been able to be measured invasively, but proprietary AI software utilizing advanced computational fluid dynamics has made noninvasive FFR_{CT} viable.[38] This FFR_{CT} has been shown to correlate well with invasive FFR and has resulted in a reduction in the rates of invasive angiography.[39,40] The software was approved by the Food and Drug Administration in 2014 and then in 2017 it was supported for routine clinical use in the United Kingdom by the National Institute for Health and Care Excellence.[41]

Pericoronary adipose tissue (PCAT), on the other hand, is a specific marker of coronary inflammation; elevated levels of inflammation are known to accelerate atherosclerosis and precipitate plaque rupture.[42] Before the application of AI, abnormalities in PCAT were detected using a Hounsfield units cutoff value. However, with the assistance of AI analysis, it is now understood that the relationship is not so binary. There are underlying complex patterns of inflammation that correlate with vascularity and fibrosis within PCAT that can improve precision in detecting those at the highest cardiovascular risk.[42] Although early work has been promising, the field of CT still has untapped potential when coupled with AI technology.

Similarly, early AI work has delved into the potential applications for CMR. In terms of cardiac volume and biventricular function assessments, CMR is the gold standard due to its high spatial resolution and the ability to perform multiplanar imaging, but measurements require manual inputs.[43] Both Bai et al. and Wang et al. demonstrated that this process can be successfully automated with the use of DL.[44,45] While CMR offers the advantage of being radiation-free compared to CT, a notable drawback is the relatively long acquisition times due to the need for multiple sequences to be performed, the need for contrast, and cardiac and respiratory motion-related artifact. With the use of DL algorithms, it is possible to image sequences in parallel, perform complex image reconstructions, and compensate for motion artifact reducing scan time by approximately five times.[46] Another advantage of CMR in comparison to other imaging modalities is that it is the gold standard for myocardial tissue characterization. This is largely due to the application of gadolinium contrast and resulting patterns of late gadolinium enhancement (LGE), but it is limited by the need for intravenous access and renal impairment. Zhang et al. utilized a DL model to reconstruct virtual LGE-equivalent images without the need for gadolinium to be administered.[47] The virtual images demonstrated excellent agreement with traditional LGE images, and readers even rated the virtual images to be of significantly superior quality. CMR guides diagnostic and therapeutic decision-making, and AI shows promise in extending its utility even further.

MULTIMODALITY ARTIFICIAL INTELLIGENCE IN CARDIOVASCULAR DISEASE

From a technical perspective, multimodality AI requires the incorporation of data in multiple forms such as image, text, video, audio, and language **(Fig. 2)**.[4] Analysis can

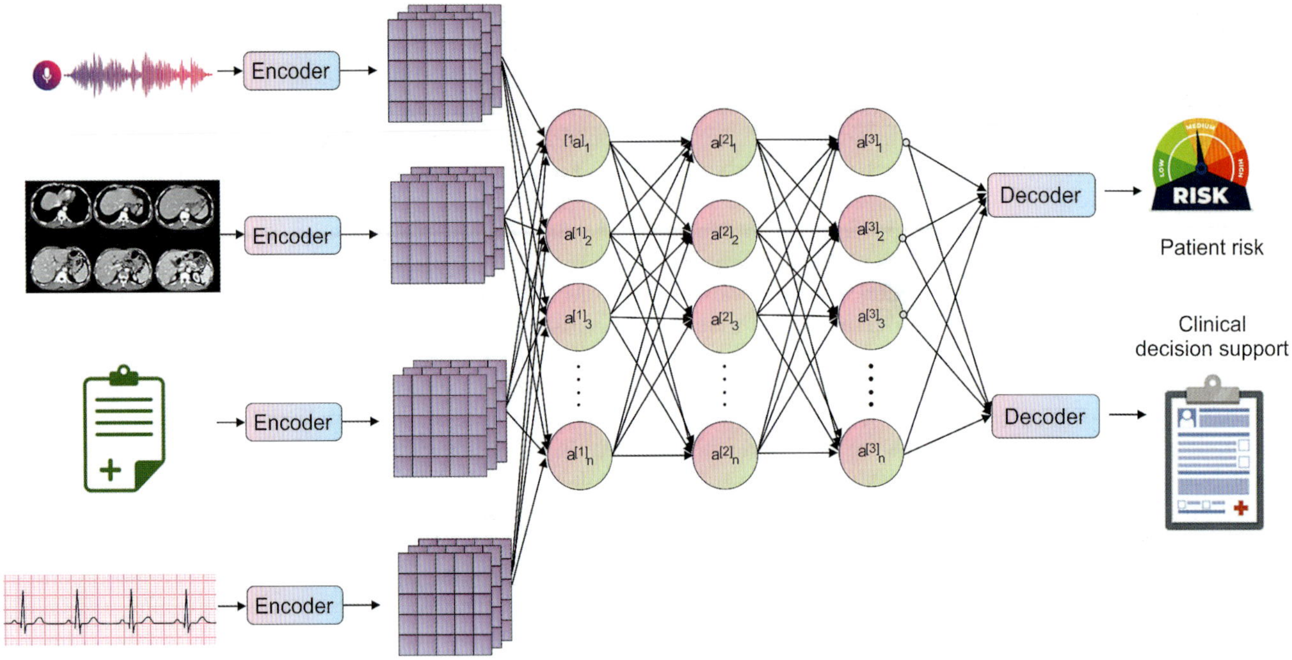

FIG. 2: Multimodal artificial intelligence system. A multimodal artificial intelligence system, utilizing data from audio, imaging, clinical reports, and bedside testing, to produce outputs to estimate individual patient risk and provide clinicians with clinical decision support.

then be performed using a range of AI techniques tailored to optimize each input data type. The theory is to provide algorithms with data from a diverse dataset to allow for precise predictions of clinical scenarios. In many ways, this is not dissimilar to how clinicians including cardiologists or humans in general utilize all their senses to guide decision-making. Each additional modality provides incremental crucial clinical information allowing for more precise outputs. Despite the presence of multimodal AI systems in other fields, medical systems have lagged behind.[48] This delay is likely attributed to the complexity and extensive array of data points needed to ensure accuracy across a wide range of populations, particularly in assisting clinical decisions that could have life-altering consequences.

Despite the scarcity of truly multimodal AI systems in health care, some do exist. Soto et al. created one such model to differentiate causes of left ventricular hypertrophy by the combination of ECG and echocardiography data.[49] The resulting fusion system was found to have superior sensitivity and specificity when compared to human experts. Another multimodal system by Puyol-Antón et al. analyzed both echocardiography and CMR imaging to predict responses to cardiac resynchronization therapy.[50] Inspiration for further multimodal algorithms can be gleaned from exploring other disciplines. In oncology, a comprehensive system integrating electronic medical records, histopathology, genomics, and radiology findings has been proposed to uncover latent patterns that refine cancer diagnosis and management while guiding the discovery of novel biomarkers and therapeutic targets.[51] On the other hand, in psychiatry, ongoing research is investigating emotion detection based on video data, audio signals, and motion detection through sensors and wearable technology.[52] Similarly, there is potential for multimodal AI in cardiology.

As evidenced by the AI systems discussed in this paper, most systems for CVD detection currently do not employ multimodality AI techniques. This renders existing systems impractical to implement into existing workflows, as analysis of each modality requires a multitude of AI applications. In addition, licensing for all these programs individually adds complexity and costs and likely necessitates an overhaul of current hardware. Healthcare AI systems are still lagging behind those in other industries. Inspiration can be drawn from autonomous driving vehicles, which seamlessly interpret objects, maps, and text through a single interface. The current lack of available multimodal AI in CVD acts as a barrier preventing further uptake of AI-based technology into more routine clinical care. The development of comprehensive complex multimodal AI algorithms will counterintuitively have the potential to simplify the experience for users.

In the future, there is a consensus that AI will play a pivotal role in the management of CVD, influencing numerous stages of patient care. With an increasing array of touch points during a patient's journey, AI developers should prioritize software consolidation to eliminate the need for a multitude of applications. In addition, there is a need for general refinement and seamless integration into existing workflows. Successful optimization of systems into current workplace systems is challenging and will hinge on close collaboration with end users, a key factor in achieving widespread adoption and the ultimate success of AI in CVD. It is likely that multimodal AI algorithms are the future and will be commonplace in clinical practice, as clinicians increasingly favor these integrated systems over their nonmultimodal counterparts.

CONCLUSION

In every realm of cardiology, there is now evidence of the benefits that AI can bring. There are, however, further benefits still to come with the exploration of proficient AI software across modalities. The advent of multimodality AI not only holds promise for enhancing algorithmic performance, but also streamlines the integration of AI into existing workflows. The field of cardiology is positioned at the forefront leading the design of multimodality AI services due to the already large AI-related research base available. Currently, only isolated examples of multimodal systems exist, but this is likely to change. The journey into the future of CVD management holds exciting prospects for improving patient care and reshaping traditional clinical care.

ONLINE REFERENCES

Please scan the QR code provided at the end of the table of contents for References of this chapter.

CHAPTER

21

Effects of Air Pollution on Cardiovascular Diseases: AI-based Analysis of Pollutant–Disease Relationships from PubMed Articles

Sudeshna Jana, Manjira Sinha, Tirthankar Dasgupta

ABSTRACT

In recent decades, environmental pollution has emerged as a significant global health concern. World Health Organization (WHO) data reveal that a significant part of the population is exposed to air containing elevated pollutant levels beyond the safety guidelines. Among the health impacts of pollution, cardiovascular diseases (CVDs) stand out. CVDs such as coronary artery disease, heart attacks, strokes, and hypertension contribute significantly to morbidity and mortality worldwide. Recent studies highlight the adverse effects of pollutants such as fine particulate matter ($PM_{2.5}$, PM_{10}), heavy metals, and toxic gases on cardiac health. Exposure to increased $PM_{2.5}$ concentrations over prolonged hours can trigger heart attacks and mortality; its long-term exposure raises cardiovascular mortality risk and reduces life expectancy. Epidemiological data demonstrate strong correlations between air pollutants and CVDs, supported by animal studies linking pollutants to thrombosis and atherosclerosis. However, gaps remain in understanding cumulative exposure's impact over decades, causal pathways, vulnerable populations, and emerging contaminants. Our work addresses these gaps by utilizing generative AI to construct a knowledge graph visualizing pollutant–cardiovascular relationships, aiding effective strategies to mitigate their impact on public health.

Keywords: Large language model (LLM), generative AI, knowledge graph, air pollution, cardiovascular diseases

INTRODUCTION

In recent decades, the increasing level of environmental pollution has become a major health concern worldwide. World Health Organization (WHO) data show that almost all of the global population (99%) breathes air that exceeds WHO guideline limits and contains high levels of pollutants, with low- and middle-income countries suffering from the highest exposures.[1] Among the numerous health effects of pollution, its impact on cardiovascular diseases (CVDs) is particularly alarming. CVDs, which include conditions such as coronary artery disease, heart attacks, strokes, and hypertension, are a leading cause of morbidity and mortality worldwide.[2]

Recent studies indicate that pollutants such as fine particulate matter (like $PM_{2.5}$, PM_{10}), heavy metals, and toxic gases significantly impact cardiac health.[3-6] Research by US Environmental Protection Agency (EPA) has found that exposure to increased concentrations of $PM_{2.5}$ over a few hours to weeks can trigger CVD-related heart attacks and death. Longer-term exposure can lead to increased risk of cardiovascular mortality and decreases in life expectancy. There are several epidemiological data that show a strong correlation between air pollutants and increased rates of CVDs and heart failure. Additionally, animal studies support these findings, demonstrating that pollutants can increase the chances of thrombosis and atherosclerosis.[7]

However, the findings do not demonstrate how cumulative exposure impacts cardiovascular health over decades, and the precise causal pathways by which these pollutants lead to cardiovascular damage. Also, it needs to identify which populations are most vulnerable to specific pollutants and why, due to genetic, environmental, and preexisting health and lifestyle factors. Furthermore, it is noticed that new pollutants and emerging contaminants, such as microplastics and various chemicals from industrial processes, are not yet well studied. Motivated by these above facts, our work aims to address several of these gaps by constructing a comprehensive knowledge graph that visualizes the causal relationships between pollutants and CVDs based on a large number of scientific literatures. We have also explored how varying concentrations of pollutants impact cardiovascular health differently across different populations. This knowledge will help deepen our understanding on how pollutants contribute to CVDs and develop more effective strategies to mitigate their impact on public health.

RELATED WORKS

Empirical Experiments on the Effect of Pollutants on Cardiovascular Diseases

Several empirical studies offer valuable insights into how pollutants impact CVDs. In 2012, Feng and Yang[8] demonstrated that there is an increased risk associated with $PM_{2.5}$ and PM_{10} exposure and CVDs. Subsequently, in 2020, Miller et al.[9] showed that cardiovascular risks like coronary artery disease, hypertension, and arrhythmias can happen from particulate matter, especially ultrafine particles from diesel emissions. Recently, in 2021, Lederer et al.[10] highlighted the significant role of pollutants such as $PM_{2.5}$ and nitrogen dioxide (NO_2) in increasing cardiovascular morbidity and mortality. They also found $PM_{2.5}$ associated with oxidative stress and thrombosis, while NO_2 is linked to systemic inflammation and autonomic dysfunction.

Computational Models on the Effect of Pollutants on Cardiovascular Diseases

In this era of artificial intelligence, various machine learning and deep learning techniques are increasingly used by many researchers to understand and predict the effects of pollutants on cardiovascular health. In 2017, Park et al.[11] developed an Environmental Risk Score (ERS) to estimate the health effects of pollutant mixtures and demonstrated the cumulative risk from pollutants such as cadmium, arsenic compounds, cobalt, and barium on gamma-glutamyl transferase and hypertension. Recently, in 2022, Lee et al.[12] predicted nonaccidental cardiovascular and respiratory mortality with the help of meteorological and air pollution data using several machine learning models.

Most of the studies have focused on how air pollution affects the cardiovascular system based on location-specific pollution data. In our research, however, we take a broader approach by examining the comprehensive effects of pollutants on CVDs across various locations and populations. In our work, we analyze a wide range of pollution-related scientific literature to understand these effects more thoroughly. Additionally, we explore new and emerging pollutants and their adverse effects on cardiovascular health in recent years.

PROPOSED METHODOLOGY

Downloading PubMed Abstracts

For our research work, we have collected 4,716 PubMed abstracts* using keywords "cardiovascular disease" and "pollution." Each abstract is associated with a unique identifier, "PMID." Additionally, we have also extracted the year of the study, which enables us to perform a temporal analysis to explore how the impact of pollutants on cardiovascular health has evolved over time. **Figure 1** shows a sample PubMed abstract with different portions of text color-coded, to highlight the different entities such as pollutant name, pollutant concentration, disease name, location, and target population that an abstract may contain.

Entity Identification and Relation Extraction

From these PubMed abstracts, we have extracted the following entities and relations:

- *Pollutant names (P)*: Name of pollutants mentioned in the abstract

Air pollution is associated with elevated cardiovascular mortality and an increase in cardiovascular risk factors. However, the literature data on associations between air pollution and cardiovascular risk factors are contradictory. To explore the relationship between residential exposure to atmospheric pollutants and cardiovascular risk factors (lipid biomarker and blood pressure levels). We studied a sample of 2339 adult participants in the ELISABET study from the Dunkirk and Lille urban areas of France. The mean annual exposure to atmospheric pollutants (PM10, NO2 and SO2) at the home address was estimated via an air dispersion model. The associations were probed in multivariate linear regression models. The mean NO2 level was 26.05 µg/m3 in Lille and 19.96 µg/m3 in Dunkirk. The mean PM10 level was 27.02 µg/m3 in Lille and 26.53 µg/m3 in Dunkirk. We detected a significant association between exposure to air pollutants and the high-density lipoprotein (HDL) (which is a protective factor against cardiovascular diseases) level: for a 2 µg/m3 increment in PM10, the HDL level decreased by 1.72% (p = 0.0037). None of the associations with other lipid variables or with blood pressure were significant. We didn't find evidence significant associations for most of the risk factors but, long-term exposure of adults to moderate levels of ambient air pollution was associated with a decrement in HDL.

Pollutant | Disease/Abnormality/Effect | Concentration | Location | Demography (Age, Gender)

FIG. 1: Example of an abstract with highlighted entities.

*https://pubmed.ncbi.nlm.nih.gov/

- *Pollutant level (C):* Concentration level of each pollutant
- *Disease name (D):* Diseases or abnormalities caused by the pollutants
- *Study location (Loc):* Location where the study was conducted
- *Population details (S):* Age group, gender of the affected population
- *Relation (R):* How a pollutant is related to a disease—"causes," "may cause," or "does not cause"

For the entity extraction, we have utilized a large language model (LLM), trained on extensive amounts of textual data, to learn the intricacies of language, enabling it to perform tasks such as answering questions, text generation, summarization, and translation.[14] With prompt-based learning, LLM model is adapted for various tasks by using natural language prompts to guide its responses.[15] In our work, GPT-3.5 turbo was used for the purpose of entity identification and relation extraction using the prompt, depicted in **Figure 2**.

Entity Standardization

All the entities extracted from the LLM are not always in the standard form. For instance, the pollutant "ultrafine particles" may be referred to as "ufp", "pm < 0.01 µm aerodynamic diameter" in different articles. Same thing happened with disease names, e.g., "hypertension" may be referred to as "high blood pressure," "arterial hypertension," or "hypertensive disorder" by different researchers. Therefore, all the extracted entities were standardized using the Unified Medical Language System (UMLS) Metathesaurus,[16] which contains an exhaustive list of such situations and assigns a "Concept Unique Identifier (CUI)" to each. After standardization, we got the final list of around 300 different pollutants, and around 936 disease names.

GPT User Prompt

```
gpt_user_prompt = f""" You have been provided with an PubMed abstract. You
    need to perform the following tasks:

    1. Identify all the pollutant names along with any disease/abnormality
        names mentioned in the abstract.
    2. Find whether there exists any causal relationship between the
        POLLUTANTs and disease/abnormalities mentioned in the abstract.
    3. If any causal relationship exists, your task is to identify specific
        POLLUTANT NAMEs and their relationship (cause/may cause/does not cause
        )
       with DISEASES or ABNORMALITIES from the given abstract.
    4. Capture the level of CONCENTRATION of that pollutant and level of
        EFFECT on the disease/abnormality if specified in the abstract
       or else "N/A".
    5. Capture demographical information of the subjects (LOCATION, AGE GROUP,
         GENDER) for whom the experiment
       was conducted if mentioned in the abstract or else "N/A".
    6. Give the output in the following JSON structure in text:
       [{"causality": "<Causal or not(True/False)>", "pollutant_name": "<
           POLLUTANT NAME>", "pollutant_concentration": "<CONCENTRATION>",
       "disease_or_abnormality": "<DISEASE OR ABNORMALITY it is causing>", "
           relation": "<how the pollutant is related with the
       disease/abnormality(causes/may cause/does not cause)>", "effect": "<
           level of EFFECT on the disease/abnormality>",
       "location": "<DEMOGRAPHICAL REGION where the experiment was conducted
           >", "age_group": "<Age information if provided in abstract>",
       "gender": "<gender information if provided in abstract>"}]
       Use "N/A" for ANY MISSING INFORMATION in any fields.
       If there is no causal relationship existing between the pollutants and
           disease/abnormalities in the abstract,
       put "False" in causality field and "N/A" in other fields.
    Now here is the PubMed abstract:
    "{abstract}"
    """
```

FIG. 2: Our prompts to LLM for identifying entities and relation extraction.

Constructing Knowledge Graph

After all the pollutant names and disease names were standardized, we have constructed a knowledge graph to provide a structured representation of complex relations, easier to understand and navigate relationships between different entities. In this knowledge graph, we have defined pollutants along with their concentration levels and diseases as nodes, and relation between pollutant and disease is indicated as a directed edge from pollutant to disease.

This graph helps us to understand how individual pollutants are linked to specific diseases and helps to explore the broader relationships between different pollutants and diseases. Additionally, it can reveal how diseases might be related through common pollutants and highlights the most prominent pollutants and diseases (refer to **Fig. 9**).

RESULTS AND DISCUSSIONS

This research offers a thorough understanding of how pollutants relate to various CVDs and abnormalities through the knowledge graph. The detailed analysis and outcomes are explored in the subsequent subsections.

Temporal Analysis

In this study, we have done a trend analysis on the variation of each pollutant, disease, and their interrelations over time. We use the study year of each abstract as the time variable for this analysis. This analysis helps us to understand how pollutants and disease rates change over time and to also identify long-term trends and patterns, and also any unusual or unexpected changes in pollutant levels or disease rate. Furthermore, through this analysis, we can evaluate the effectiveness of interventions or policy changes aimed at reducing pollution or mitigating disease.

Pollutant Trends

Figure 3 depicts the trends of occurrence of top five pollutants identified in the PubMed abstracts over the years 2012–2024. The data are suggestive of the fact that the $PM_{2.5}$ exposer has shown a clearly rising trend which was at its peak in 2022 and then decreased slightly. NO_2 has also experienced a steady increase, particularly after 2020. In contrast, ozone, carbon monoxide, and sulfur dioxide have exhibited more stable trends with slight fluctuations.

Furthermore, **Figure 4** illustrates the trends of some pollutants that were previously of little significance but have gained attention in recent years. Specifically, PM_1 has shown a dramatic increase in mentions starting from 2019, reaching its peak in 2023 and maintaining high levels in 2024. Ammonium and cadmium, which predominantly appeared in the discussion of those years, also showed a substantial increase, with ammonium escalating after 2016, and cadmium remarkably increasing, for instance, from 2020 to 2024.

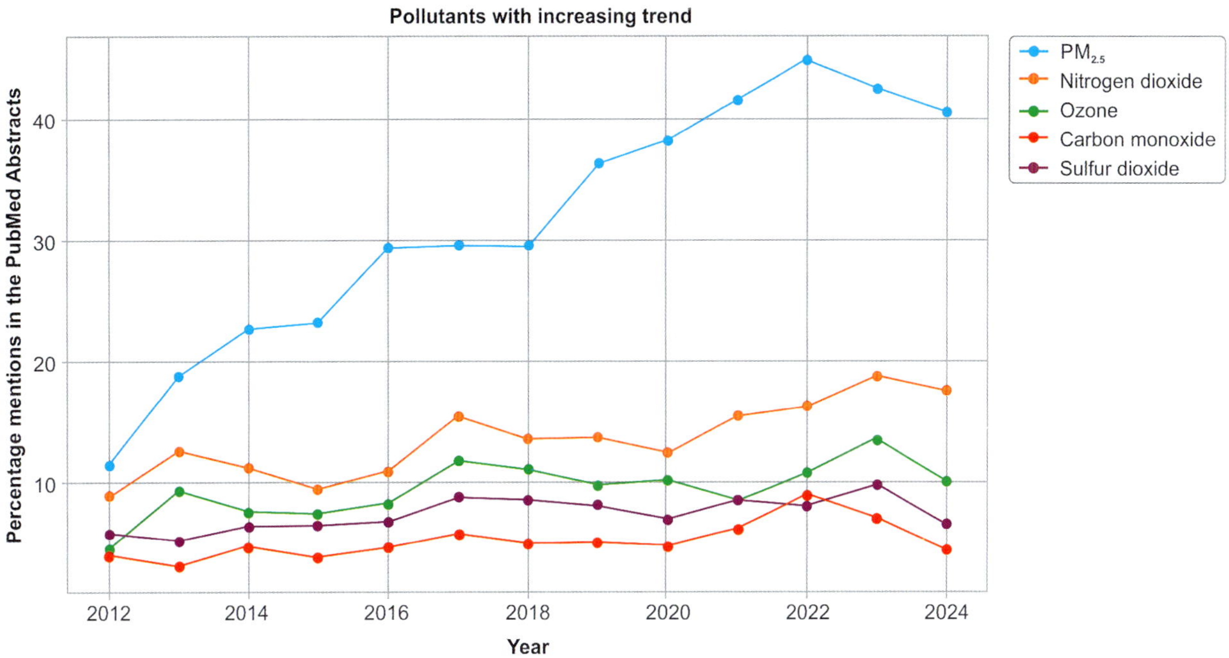

FIG. 3: Trends of top five pollutants over the years 2012–2024.

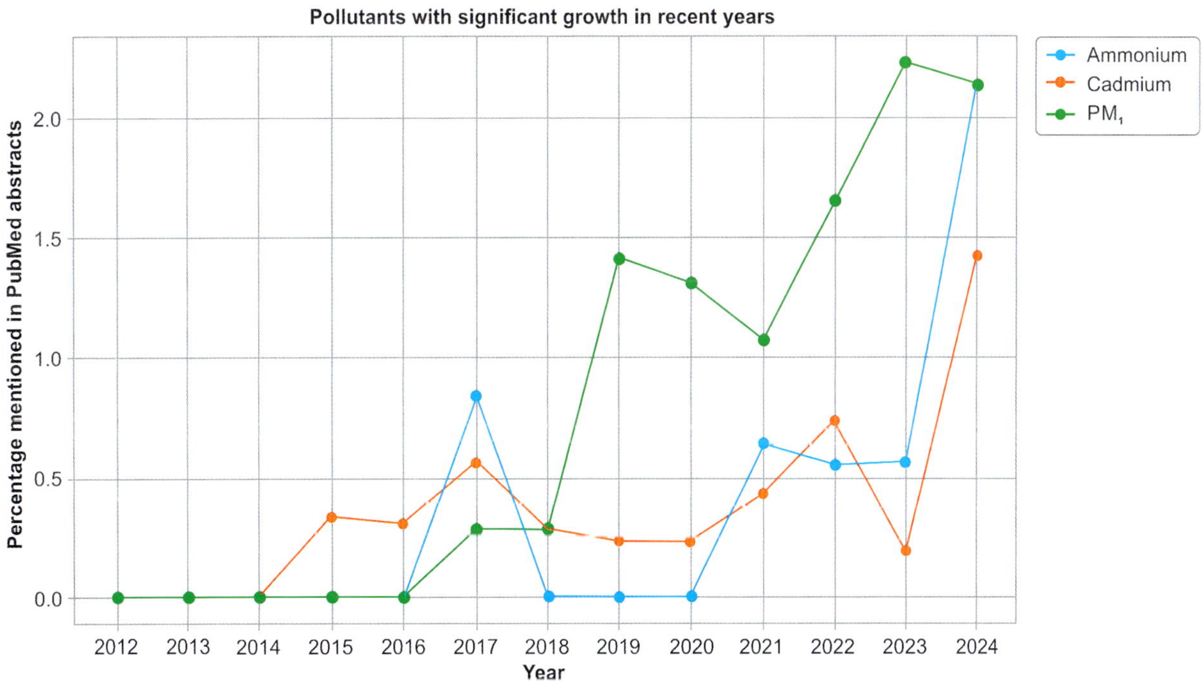

FIG. 4: Some emerging pollutants in recent years have.

Disease Trends

Figure 5 showcases the trends of top five diseases mentioned in PubMed abstracts from 2012 to 2024, highlighting their increasing trends over time. Hypertensive disease shows a remarkable upward trend, peaking around 2018 and maintaining high mentions >6% through 2024. Other diseases, such as ischemic stroke and atrial fibrillation, exhibit more gradual increases with slight fluctuations. Cardiometabolic syndrome and diabetes display a steady, though less pronounced, rise in mentions.

Moreover, **Figure 6** illustrates the occurrence of three diseases or abnormalities—dyslipidemias, metabolic diseases, and ST-segment elevation myocardial infarction (STEMI)—in PubMed abstracts from 2012 to 2024. It high-

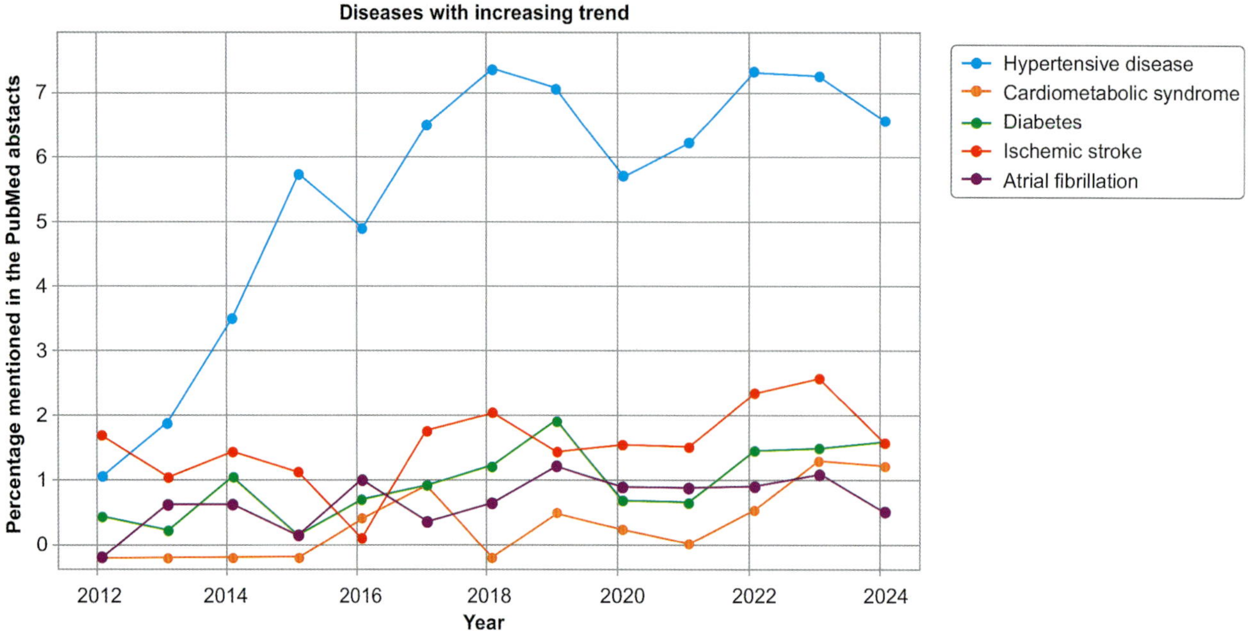

FIG. 5: Trends of top five diseases over the years 2012–2024.

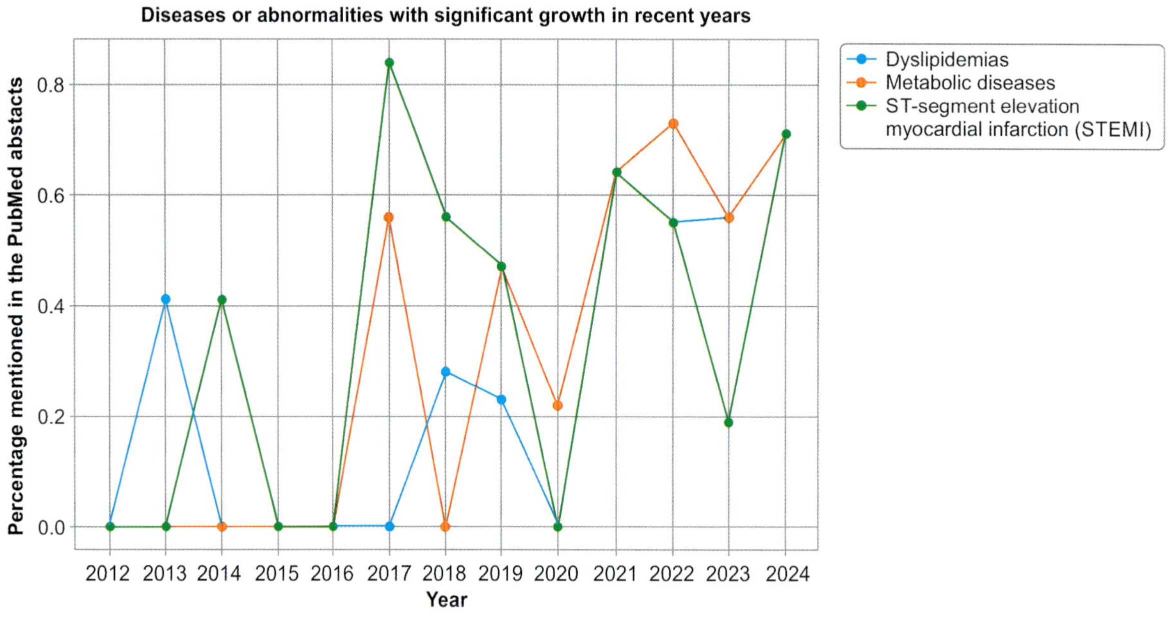

FIG. 6: Some emerging diseases in recent years.

lights periods of significant growth for each condition. Notably, STEMI experienced substantial peaks in 2017 and 2020, with the highest reaching in 2017. Metabolic diseases saw the most important increases around 2017 and 2020, and a consistent upward trend from 2021 to 2024. Dyslipidemias had more irregular proliferation, with peak points in 2013, 2017, and 2019, and a small spike in 2020.

Trends of Pollutant Disease Correlation

Figure 7 illustrates the increasing trend of $PM_{2.5}$ and PM_{10}, most occurring pollutants, causing various diseases over time, as reflected in PubMed abstracts from 2012 to 2024. $PM_{2.5}$ and PM_{10} register a remarkable rise in their relationship with certain disorders such as hypertensive disease, cerebrovascular accidents, myocardial ischemia, and atherosclerosis. $PM_{2.5}$ is the only name to be specifically related to hypertensive disease and cerebrovascular accidents, dominant after 2018.

Figure 8 displays the percentage of the most common pollutant–disease correlations. In this heatmap, a higher intensity of color indicates a stronger correlation, while a lower intensity reflects weaker correlations. Notably,

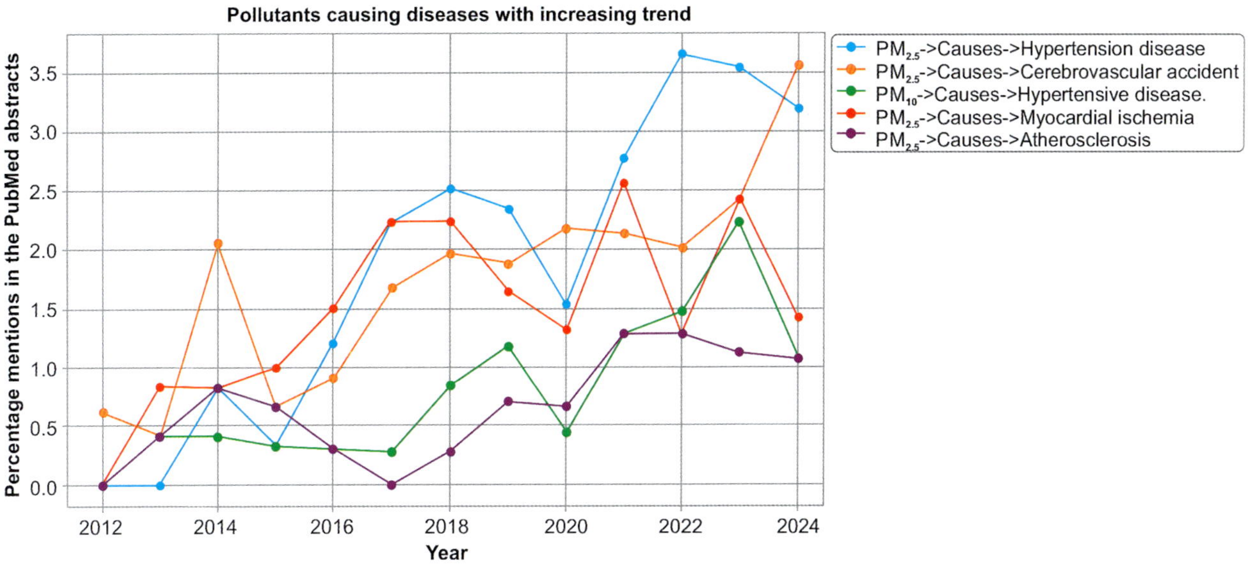

FIG. 7: Most occurring diseases caused by $PM_{2.5}$ and PM_{10}.

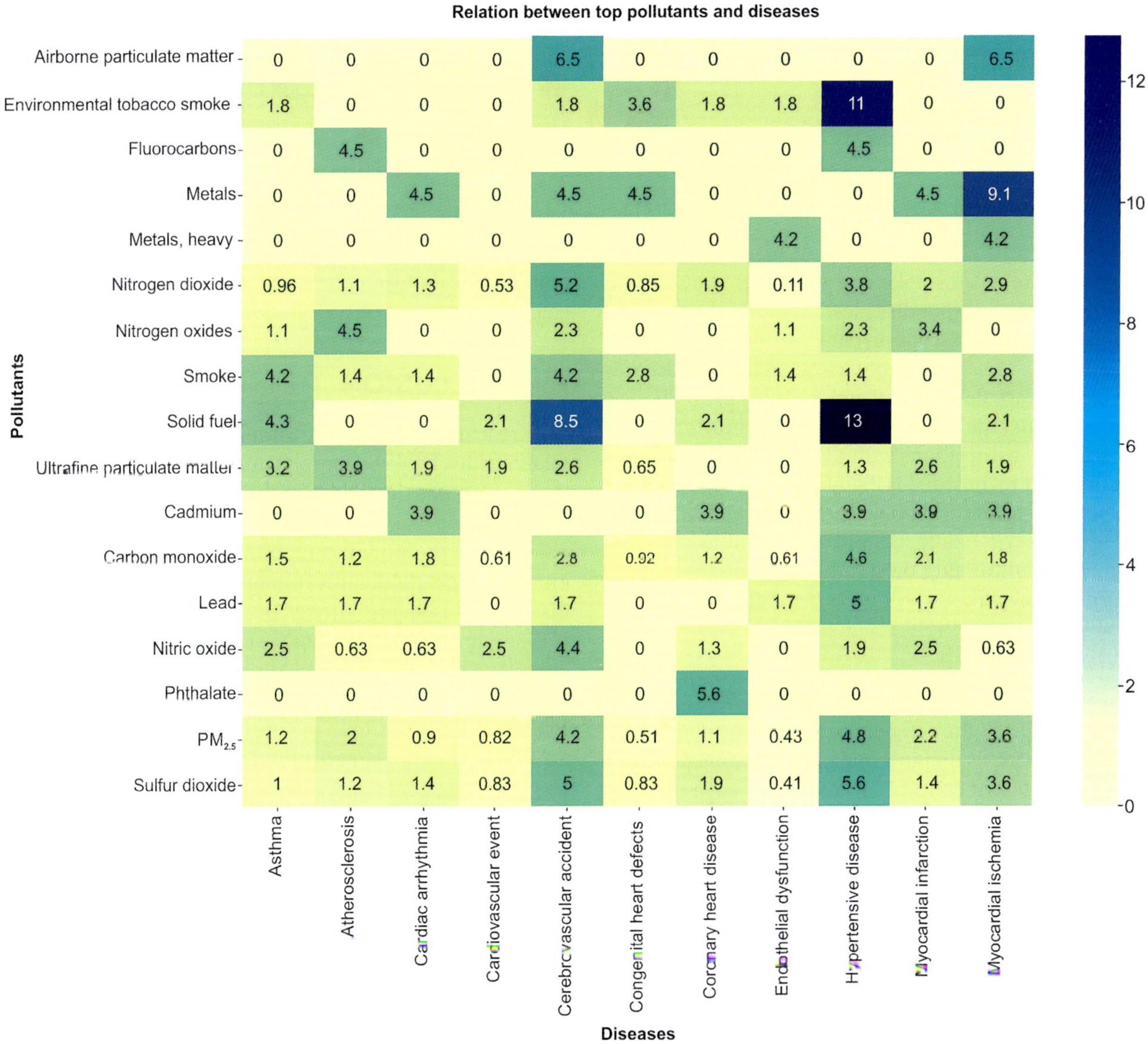

FIG. 8: Heatmap showing correlation between major pollutants and diseases.

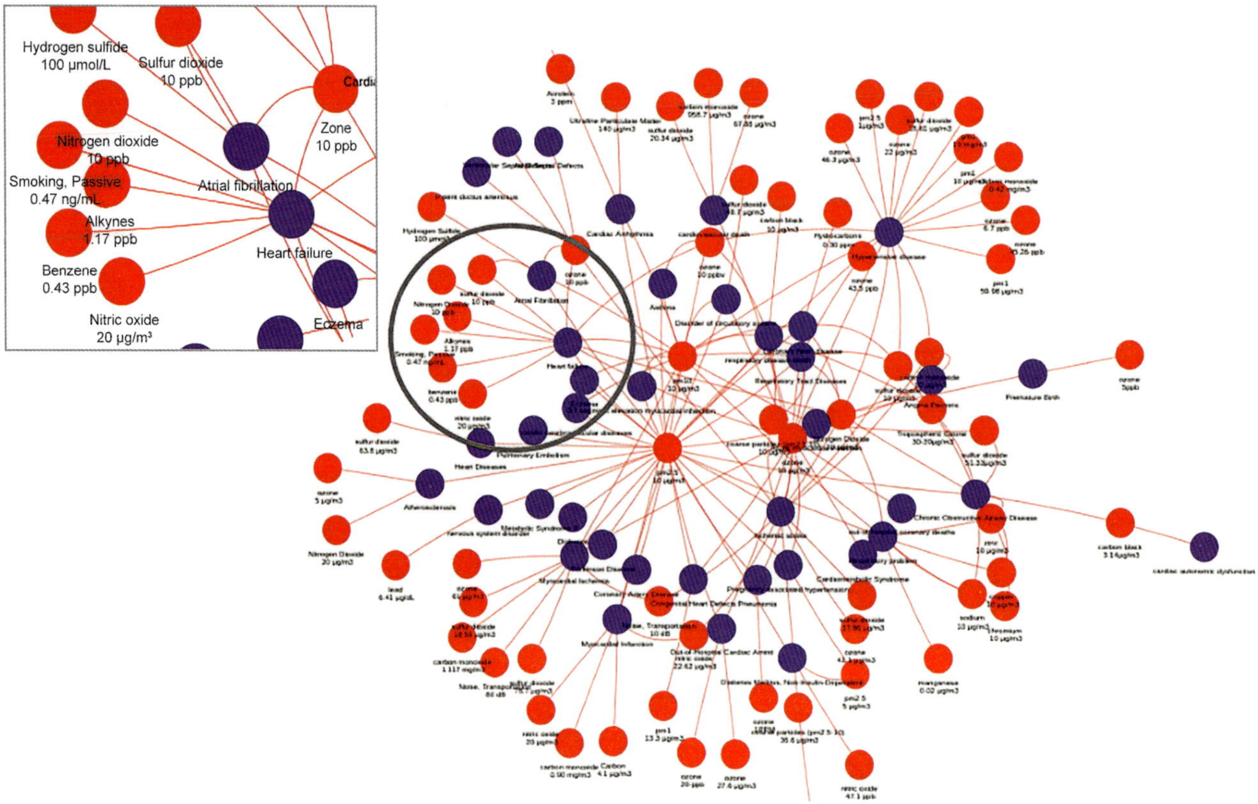

FIG. 9: Pollutant–disease knowledge graph. Pollutants are in red and diseases are in blue; edge indicate "cause."

environmental tobacco smoke and solid fuel show strong correlations with multiple diseases, including myocardial infarction and cardiovascular events. Airborne particulate matter and NO_2 are significantly associated with diseases such as cerebrovascular accident and coronary heart disease. Additionally, specific pollutants like cadmium and lead exhibit selective associations with diseases like endothelial dysfunction and myocardial ischemia. This comprehensive heatmap highlights critical pollutants that have the highest impact on various health conditions, emphasizing the importance of addressing these environmental factors to improve public health.

Knowledge Graph

Our knowledge graph includes a total of 1,907 nodes, comprising 1,029 pollutant nodes and 878 disease nodes, with 5,618 edges. It features multiple nodes for the same pollutant to represent different concentrations, where such data are available. **Figure 9** depicts a snippet of the knowledge graph; pollutant nodes are colored in red, and disease nodes are colored in blue.

CONCLUSION

This research is aimed at understanding intricate causal relationships between various pollutants and CVDs through the creation of a detailed knowledge graph. By standardizing and analyzing data from over 4,700 PubMed abstracts, we are able to find prominent pollutants, such as $PM_{2.5}$ and NO_2, and their specific health impacts, including hypertensive disease and ischemic stroke. The knowledge graph not only clarifies direct pollutant–disease connections but also reveals complex interrelations, providing a comprehensive tool for understanding and mitigating the cardiovascular health effects of air pollution. In future, we aim to incorporate multimodal data on pollution from other data sources to analyze the indirect effects of air pollution and to enrich the knowledge graph.

ONLINE REFERENCES

Please scan the QR code provided at the end of the table of contents for References of this chapter.

CHAPTER 22

Essentials for Artificial Intelligence Research in Cardiology: Challenges and Mitigations

Biyanka Jaltotage, Girish Dwivedi

ABSTRACT

Artificial intelligence (AI) is a computational process that simulates human intellect for problem-solving. It has made significant advancements in recent years, allowing algorithms to analyze vast amounts of data quickly and accurately. This makes AI attractive for data-heavy, repetitive tasks. However, caution is needed in high-stakes healthcare environments like managing cardiovascular disease (CVD). The COVID-19 pandemic has highlighted the strain on health services, and the ongoing metabolic syndrome epidemic is likely to intensify this burden. This chapter aims to improve the understanding of AI studies in cardiology.

Keywords: AI, human, data, CVD, COVID-19

INTRODUCTION

Artificial intelligence (AI) describes computational processes that simulate human intellect with the purpose of problem-solving.[1] The concept was initially described by Alan Turing as early as the 1950s.[2] Propelled by the processing power afforded by modern computing, these concepts have now been transformed to reality, and the field of AI has experienced substantial advancements in recent years. These algorithms are now capable of analyzing vast amounts of data in only seconds with exceptional accuracy, and they are not vulnerable to the fatigue that is experienced by humans.[3] Naturally, this makes AI attractive for data-heavy or repetitive tasks that are time-consuming. Recently, it has become evident that current health services are struggling to cope with the escalating demands of managing cardiovascular disease (CVD). The COVID-19 pandemic has underscored the strain on current health services in the management of CVD, a burden likely to intensify with the ongoing metabolic syndrome epidemic.[4,5]

Despite the excitement surrounding AI systems, a degree of caution is still needed. This is especially crucial in high-stakes healthcare environments like the management of CVD. Over the last few years, there has been an explosion in the number of AI-related studies, with researchers developing algorithms to assist clinicians in improving both speed and accuracy for a variety of tasks.[6] Despite these benefits, it cannot be forgotten that AI brings with it unique challenges that need to be carefully considered and extensively critiqued prior to implementation into everyday clinical practice. Further understanding is therefore needed on how to analyze AI studies in cardiology. This chapter aims to improve the understanding of what constitutes the essentials of an AI study across healthcare, with a specific focus on the field of cardiology.

ARTIFICIAL INTELLIGENCE

Artificial intelligence is an encompassing term referring to the development of systems or algorithms capable of advanced tasks such as learning, problem-solving, language understanding, and visual perception.[7] In cardiology, AI systems already exist that are being studied to improve arrhythmia detection, automate cardiac imaging analysis, and even to support clinicians in decision-making to guide coronary intervention.[7] With such a breadth of systems in the pipeline, an understanding of AI is necessary to appreciate how to evaluate these studies. Therefore, this section, although not comprehensive, will aim to provide a brief overview of the topic.

Machine learning (ML) lies at the core of AI identifying relationships between training data points not visible to

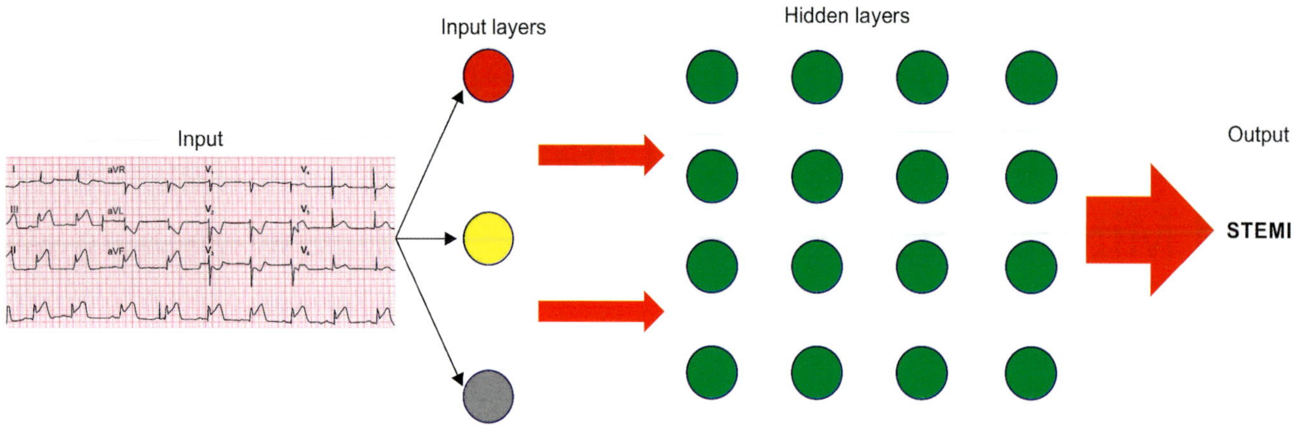

FIG. 1: The framework of deep learning: An input such as an electrocardiogram is analyzed by a deep learning algorithm through a network of notes. Each node requires a sufficient trigger to activate and then to trigger the subsequent nodes (hidden layers). This process concludes at the output layer which is then processed to provide an outcome to the end user.
(STEMI: ST elevation myocardial infarction)

humans, and with appropriate training, accurate predictions based on new previously unseen data is possible.[8] Despite the effectiveness of ML, some tasks are better suited to deep learning (DL), a specialized subset of ML. The framework for DL consists of networks of nodes arranged in layers, the first layer also called the input layer when provided with a sufficient trigger is directed to a further layer called the hidden layer of which there may be multiple, and ultimately ending in the output layer **(Fig. 1)**.[9] DL excels in the areas of image analysis, natural language processing, and speech recognition. Convolutional neural networks (CNNs) are the most frequently utilized DL models in healthcare. These CNNs predominantly process image-based data into layers of learnable weights and biases.[7] The field of cardiology is dense with visual data and CNNs excel in these environments.

With the use of these AI techniques, systems are now capable of performing rapid analyses with the potential to enhance productivity to manage increasing workloads while preserving accuracy, and ultimately improving outcomes for patients. Groups have been working on these algorithms for years and many are already in existence covering all aspects of cardiology. For example, automated ECG analysis tools using DL now have the potential to be more accurate than senior cardiologists.[10] Systems used in cardiac imaging have also demonstrated competency in automating assessments of echocardiography, computed tomography, and magnetic resonance imaging.[7] Furthermore, clinical decision support systems utilizing ML have been shown to be effective in determining appropriate revascularization strategies using percutaneous coronary intervention.[11] Considering this encouraging data, the increasing adoption of AI by various groups to address challenges is not unexpected.

CONSIDERATIONS AND CHALLENGES FOR AN ARTIFICIAL INTELLIGENCE STUDY

With the potential for AI to revolutionize healthcare, a degree of caution with the uptake of technology is rational. It is crucial to recognize that AI introduces its own set of challenges, which need to be carefully considered in all AI-related work to prevent negatively impacting patient care. Outlining these challenges will ensure that algorithms are designed from the ground up to be effective, but also safe.

Privacy and Confidentiality

Systems utilizing AI require access to a variety of data to produce accurate predictions. Frequently the data processing is performed in a cloud-based setting, creating the potential for data breaches which could compromise confidentiality.[7] It is essential that extensive measures are taken by developers to maintain end-to-end data confidentiality, prior to even being contemplated for use in clinical practice. Approaches such as the use of generative AI models have potential by generating synthetic datasets that resemble actual datasets, thereby nullifying the need for the system to hold sensitive data.[12] Another proposed approach includes training AI systems from encrypted patient data such that the system is never exposed to patient data directly.[12] Federated learning is another viable option to preserve data confidentiality. The fundamentals of federated learning involve a local copy of the relevant ML algorithm for users to utilize on their device.[13] The local algorithm learns, and these newly updated parameters are sent to a pooled centralized cloud server to improve the overall model. In this process, the raw data is not exposed and remains on the local device. If systems are allowed that lack confidentiality, patients and clinicians will lose confidence in the technology, impeding future developments.

Algorithm Bias

Cardiovascular disease is common worldwide and affects individuals from all walks of life, regardless of culture or ethnicity. AI systems are entirely dependent on their training population for precision and training populations lacking diversity are at high risk of underperforming with minority groups.[14] If there is widespread adoption of these AI systems, suboptimal training populations could legitimately risk widening already existing health inequalities. Software bias against minority groups is already being seen; one such example is that of an AI-assisted model to automate segmentation of the ventricles and myocardium on cardiac magnetic resonance imaging. Accuracy was found to be significantly different depending on the patient's race.[15] Mitigating bias within AI systems entails implementing various strategies **(Table 1)**. Incorporating built-in alarms that alert users when the system detects a high risk of bias could be a highly effective tool.[16] Additionally, ensuring diversity within the training population helps counteract biases inherent in datasets, and subsequently minority subpopulation testing could be performed. Furthermore, given the dynamic nature of local populations due to global migration, there will be a need for AI systems to remain up to date to sustain future accuracy and relevance. Lastly, in some situations, bias can be insidious and inherent to the design of the system. Obermeyer et al. discovered this by investigating a widely used algorithm used to estimate patient risk to target patients for "high-risk management programs."[17] The authors found that compared to White individuals, those who were Black had their risk significantly underestimated. Despite the richness and diversity of the dataset, it was found that the bias stemmed from training data reliance on health costs as a surrogate for health needs. This error failed to recognize that Black individuals often faced barriers to access to healthcare, so despite lower healthcare costs, the level of health among the Black population was poorer. Understanding the intricacies of bias in such circumstances requires transparent algorithm design.

TABLE 1: Checklist for developers to address system bias.

Checklist	Description
Training population diversity	Algorithms need to be trained using diverse populations. A lack of diversity increases the risk of poor performance in minority groups
Subgroup performance testing	Specific testing of the algorithm should be performed in minority groups to ensure accuracy remains high in these populations
Built-in alarms	Developers should design alarm systems for users in scenarios at high risk of bias
Adaptations to changing demographics	A process needs to be established for system updates to incorporate factors such as changing demographics over time, ensuring the algorithm's accuracy in the future
Transparency in algorithm design	Bias can be insidious and inherent to the algorithm. Therefore, transparent software design provides a deeper understanding allowing for the detection of design flaws at earlier stages

Overfitting

A further challenge faced by AI studies relating to the training population is the concept of overfitting. As described earlier, the algorithms learn from the training data by identifying patterns, but this creates the risk of variations in the data being detected and extracted that are only specific to the training dataset. Models that suffer from overfitting, lack external applicability to the general population.[18] The issue of overfitting needs to be suspected when a model performs increasingly well on the training data, but the same accuracy is not seen with the validation dataset. Overfitting is most problematic with smaller training populations, but simply increasing the population may not always be feasible. However, techniques do exist to overcome overfitting without having to increase the training cohort. With data augmentation, it is possible to artificially enrich the existing dataset by introducing minor alterations to the original dataset. For instance, with a set of images, this could include cropping, flipping, rotation, or skewing to improve the diversity of the existing training data.[18] On the other hand, another strategy is transfer learning. This consists of utilizing a model that has already been optimized from a large training dataset which is then redirected to a new task. Transfer learning works on the concept that some tasks may have similar processing requirements and that using an already existing system improves efficiency while reducing the risk of overfitting.[19] With the use of similar techniques, all good AI studies need to take purposeful steps to address overfitting and improve the generalizability of their algorithms.

The Black Box Problem

All AI technology faces the challenges of the "black box problem," and no simple solution exists. Explainability refers to the ability to grasp the general workings of a model's decision-making process without examination of intricate details in a model.[20] Frequently, explainability can be poor for AI systems as they are capable of connecting complex patterns in a way that no human ever could.[21] Ethically, the concept of the black box is challenging. In medical decision-making, the "black box problem" becomes particularly sensitive, as many feel transparency and understanding are crucial to maintaining patient safety. This sensitivity is heightened in high-acuity areas fields like cardiology.

As previously mentioned, AI technology also holds the potential to exacerbate health disparities, with some of these disparities potentially obscured within the opaque nature of the black box. The algorithm could create outputs based on confounding factors such as gender and race, which could be detrimental to overall population health. Gichoya et al. proved this concept by developing a DL model that was able to accurately predict race based on medical images alone.[22] Therefore, it is likely a degree of explainability is required in any AI study and may help to detect similar scenarios.

A number of techniques are now accepted to improve algorithm explainability. For example, saliency maps are an attractive visual solution; images such as a chest X-ray demonstrating heart failure could be color-graded, depending on regions that are most critical to the system's ultimate output **(Figs. 2A and B)**.[23] The drawbacks of saliency maps are the risk of oversimplification of complex models, which could result in inaccuracies and the inherent limitations of this technique to only visual data. An alternative option is feature visualization; with this technique the model's internal patterns are highlighted to better understand how a variety of inputs are influencing the outcome of the algorithm's decision-making **(Figs. 3A and B)**.[24] The challenges with this method include the complexity in interpreting the outputs, difficulties with scalability for large datasets, and a lack of flexibility with feature visualization which performs best with visual data and CNNs. There are post-hoc methods that are frequently utilized and two of the

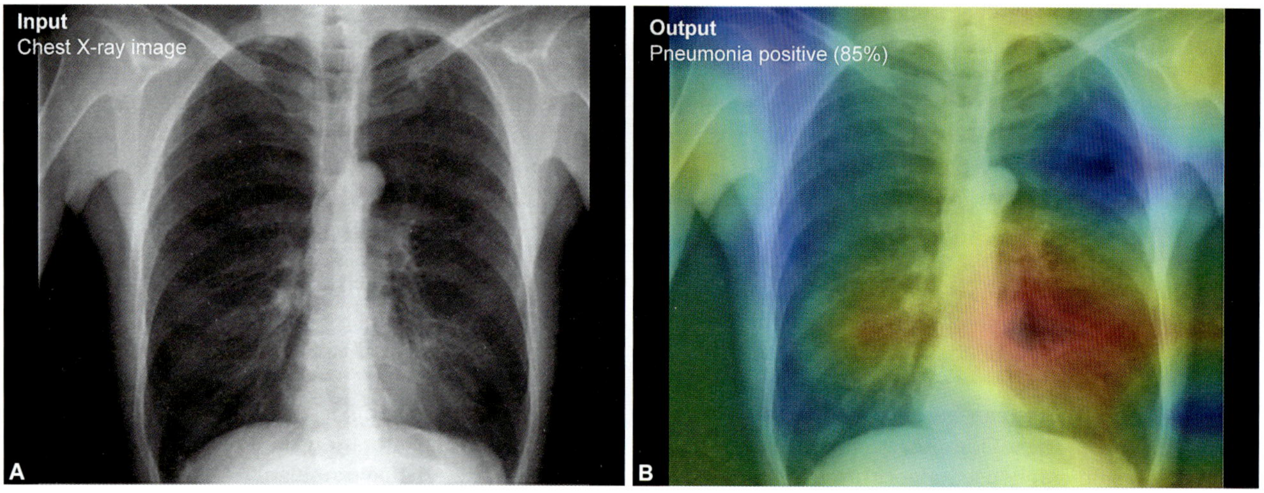

FIGS. 2A AND B: Explainable artificial intelligence with saliency maps: A chest X-ray is evaluated by an AI system, and a heat map is utilized to improve explainability. In this case, the system has produced an output with a likely diagnosis of pneumonia. The saliency map on the right image highlights in red the region of the image most critical to the final diagnosis.

Source: Adapted with permission from Ghassemi et al. (2021).[23]

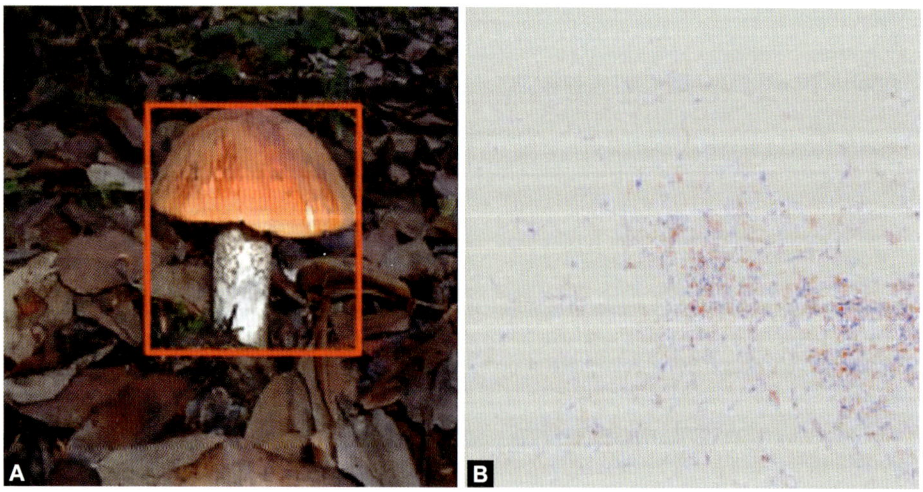

FIGS. 3A AND B: Feature visualization: This technique identifying internal data patterns that were employed by an algorithm to detect a mushroom in this image.

Source: Adapted with permission from Mohamed et al. (2022).[24]

most established techniques are locally interpretable model-agnostic explanations and Shapley values. When applying locally interpretable model-agnostic explanations, precise adjustments are made to specified inputs to discern which inputs are changing outputs most significantly.[23] Likewise, Shapley values provide a standardized method to ascertain the fractional contributions of a wide range of inputs.[25] The shortcomings of these post-hoc methods are the complexity, computational intensiveness for large datasets, and a lack of generalizability across the entire dataset as they provide local explanations only.

Despite the recent advancements made in the field of explainability, it is likely that shifting the focus to interpretable AI rather than explainability will yield the greatest benefits. Interpretable systems are transparent in design without the need to apply further tools or analysis to improve comprehension. On the other hand, explainability requires additional analysis and techniques to be applied to algorithms. A fixation on explainability can also prove to be detrimental as explainable models are not entirely faithful to the original models which may lead to errors with potentially significant consequences.[26] An interpretable approach has been supported by the Food and Drug Administration (FDA) in their 2021 action plan as part of the good ML practices.[27] Interpretability is seen best in cases that are designed from the ground up by developers with this idea in mind. However, interpretable models will not be necessary in all scenarios. Lower risk decisions such as a system used to create patient appointments would not require a high level of interpretability. Similarly, the need for interpretability is less stringent if clinicians can verify and modify a system output; an example could be an ML model that quantifies the severity of valvular lesions on echocardiography which is then subsequently reviewed by an imaging specialist.[28]

Ethical Considerations

Despite the widespread opportunities for benefits with the implementation of AI in cardiology, clinicians still have their reservations. The concepts of privacy and confidentiality, algorithm bias, and the black box problem detailed above all raise ethical concerns. In addition, there are further ethical concerns to be considered. For example, with the volumes of data being input into these systems, data ownership rights become unclear. Furthermore, with the use of AI-assisted decision-making, questions arise regarding liability. If and when medical errors occur, will the liability be with the user or software manufacturer, or would there be a concept of "shared liability?"[29] Lastly, there are societal concerns that need to be tempered surrounding automated systems. Most surveys of the general public have shown that automated decision-making without any human input is not supported in healthcare environments.[30] This highlights the importance of ongoing clinician involvement despite the availability of AI algorithms.

IMPLEMENTATION OF ARTIFICIAL INTELLIGENCE

The underpinnings of AI technology can be complex, and only individuals with specialist knowledge in the field will have a comprehensive understanding. Therefore, if these algorithms were to be incorporated into everyday clinical practice, the majority of users would lack this specialized knowledge. Moreover, it would be unreasonable to expect all users to have intimate knowledge of AI. Consequently, good AI systems will therefore need to focus on ease of use. A large aspect of this will be the development of an approachable user interface without a significant learning curve. Interfaces that are easily learnable will encourage the uptake of the technology, while also minimizing the opportunity for user error which could adversely affect patients. The technology should also aim to seamlessly integrate into existing workflows, which likely improves the success rates of end users utilizing the software in routine practice. Another consideration for smooth integration is the minimum hardware requirements. AI-based systems frequently demand substantial processing power, potentially limiting overall usability. Hence, it is essential that AI studies should also emphasize accessibility, by optimizing system efficiency and reducing the need for major overhauls of existing hardware.

Ensuring the appropriate use of AI models as intended is paramount. There may be a temptation for users to extend the application of such systems beyond their original scope, posing a risk to patients. To address this concern the concept of "model facts" was introduced.[31] It aims to inform users of the appropriate circumstances for utilizing an AI system in clinical decision-making, as well as when not to do so. It has been proposed that "model facts" should accompany the release of any AI software intended for clinical use as standard practice. Educating users through such methods will maximize the potential benefits of each system while minimizing the risks.

Artificial intelligence developers also encounter a myriad of challenges when crafting AI systems for healthcare applications. Similarly, governing bodies shoulder immense responsibility in scrutinizing such software to guarantee its safety and suitability for deployment. Consequently, several expert panels have contributed their insights to aid successful AI integration.[32-34] In line with these efforts, our group has pioneered a traffic light system, striving to provide further clarity in this complex landscape **(Box 1)**. Furthermore, updates have been made to both the CONSORT and SPIRIT guidelines which provide evidence-based recommendations to improve the reporting of randomized controlled trials and clinical trial protocols, respectively. The updates have focused on addressing AI and have culminated in the establishment of the CONSORT-AI and SPIRIT-AI guidelines.[35,36] With more accessible resources, developers and reviewers of novel

BOX 1 Proposed traffic light system checklist for an artificial intelligence (AI) algorithm.

Purpose:

- Describe the objective of the algorithm and why an approach with AI is needed
- Clearly define the task of the algorithm and its scope

Design:

- Describe the datasets used in detail, with explanations on why they were chosen and specifically the diversity of the dataset. This includes the validation dataset
- Detail how the data was prepared to preserve confidentiality but also to remain clean and consistent. Include if data augmentation or similar techniques were used
- What data records and inputs were required to develop the algorithm?
- Outline the completeness of the original dataset and the values that were missing and how these were managed. Include any techniques to manage outliers
- Describe the AI techniques used to develop the algorithm and why
- Who were the team members involved in the development of the algorithm and did they have a wide range of expertise and backgrounds?
- Detail the steps taken to ensure the technology can be integrated into existing healthcare systems. What is the expected workflow?
- How has the usability of the AI system and its interface been optimized and assessed?

Robustness:

- Describe the accuracy of the system and any outcome data. How does it compare to systems that are currently in place?
- Has the intraobserver and interobserver variability been described?
- What steps have been taken to optimize the performance of the algorithm?
- Are there alerts built to warn users when levels of certainty fall below the threshold? How was certainty defined and how was the threshold chosen?
- Describe the mechanisms in place to monitor performance, and for the system to adapt over time to ensure accuracy does not wane
- What considerations and techniques have been used to prevent overfitting?

Ethical considerations:

- Outline the techniques utilized to provide explainability. How has the degree of explainability of the algorithm been assessed?
- What steps have been taken to identify and address bias?
- How has patient data been secured to maintain confidentiality?
- How transparent is the algorithm code in order to allow for reproducibility?

Note: Each point should be assessed by an independent body, and if appropriate considerations have been made a green light is given. If considerations do not pass, then a red light is given, and the system is not passed into clinical use. A yellow light can be given if with modifications the system could be approved.

Source: With permission from Jaltotage et al. (2023).[7]

AI solutions have more guidance to optimize safety and performance.

Overall, the regulatory landscape for AI in healthcare is unique to other regimes and still remains underdeveloped.[37] A stepwise approach such as the traffic light checklist could provide the blueprint for the necessary structure for developers and regulators **(Box 1)**. Similarly, the FDA, Health Canada, and the United Kingdom's Medicine and Healthcare Products Regulatory Agency jointly established 10 guiding principles for developers to navigate good ML practices.[38] The principles highlight areas such as workflow integration, data quality assurance, robust cybersecurity, and generalizable results to the population of interest in real-world settings. Together these 10 principles currently form the basis to evaluate healthcare-related AI technology. As the field continues to evolve, further updates are inevitable, and regulatory bodies have shown a commitment to openness by encouraging discussion and actively seeking feedback from stakeholders.[39] The FDA offers publicly available lists of AI-enabled medical devices that have successfully met all premarket requirements, and at the time of writing 171 devices have made the published list.[40] A review in 2021 of this list revealed that despite FDA approval most medical AI devices had only undergone retrospective study at a small number of sites. Furthermore, almost half of all published reports did not include sample sizes, and of those that did the median sample size was modest at approximately 300.[41] Since that time, the 10 guiding principles have been introduced which do highlight and address these shortcomings. However, this underscores the ongoing need for regulatory innovation in parallel to advancements in AI-related technology, to optimize overall performance and patient safety.

CONCLUSION

The field of AI has made substantial advancements in recent years. It seems inevitable now that this technology will impact everyday life, including healthcare. The specialty of cardiology, in particular, stands to gain significantly given it is data heavy, can be repetitive, and consists of an array of image-based tests where AI can excel. Despite the potential benefits, AI brings with it unique challenges that need to be addressed for it to be successful in the healthcare space. There is also no current consensus on the key components of a good AI study to guide designers of these algorithms. Given the current state of the knowledge base, further work is still needed to establish a universal understanding of the essential elements constituting a robust AI study.

ONLINE REFERENCES

Please scan the QR code provided at the end of the table of contents for References of this chapter.

CHAPTER

23

Wearable Technology in Cardiovascular Disease

Satyavan Sharma, Akash Shah

ABSTRACT

A new era of wearable digital health technology driven by consumer market has emerged in healthcare with potential benefits in diagnosis, prevention, and management of cardiovascular disorders. The data generated from common wearables like smartwatches, wrist-worn devices, skin patches, and electrocardiographic devices will be available for patient management. At this stage, randomized data and clearcut recommendations about choice of wearable, the benefits, and their limitations are unclear. The technologies are evolving, and wearable technology will soon acquire a valuable place in cardiac care.

Keywords: Wearable technology, digital health technology, wearable devices, smartwatches

INTRODUCTION

Cardiovascular diseases (CVDs) continue to be the leading cause of morbidity and mortality globally.[1] There have been remarkable advances in treatment and prevention; however, a lot needs to be done to reduce the burden. Wearable technology has the potential to revolutionize the way we monitor and predict cardiovascular (CV) events in high-risk individuals. The field of cardiology has long used wearable medical devices to monitor heart rate and rhythm. In 1949, Norman J Holter reported the transmission of "radio-electrograph" employing an 85-pound wearable backpack.[2]

Wearable digital health technology (DHT) has emerged as a promising tool for monitoring and predicting CV events by tracking physiologic data, day-to-day activity, and sleep. The consumer (public) is eager to adopt these devices into everyday life with the hope to quickly identify and monitor CVD. The integration of this technology accelerated during the COVID-19 pandemic with the explosive growth of telehealth. According to evolving data, approximately 45% of Americans use smartwatches with a huge majority of the users reporting effective utilization of device for health surveillance. The overall market for the wearable DHT is estimated to grow to $70 billion by year 2025.[3,4]

The following topics will be discussed in this chapter.

- Growth of wearable technology
- Engineering principles
- Wearables in cardiac care
- Challenges and future directions

GROWTH OF WEARABLE TECHNOLOGY

The future of CV care will no doubt integrate wearable devices, remote monitoring, machine learning, artificial intelligence (AI), and algorithms to risk stratify individuals. The last decade has seen the emergence of many commercially available devices adopted by professionals and consumers. These devices can be worn on body as an accessory or embedded into clothing. Common wearables include smartwatches, wristbands, wrist-worn devices, skin surface patches, electrocardiograms (ECG), recording devices, and electrodes **(Fig. 1)**. Many of these wearables are not approved by FDA or other regulatory bodies and the reliability of the data can be questioned.

Ambulatory devices are becoming increasingly popular for continuous monitoring of cardiac diseases. They provide early detection of important physiological events, leading to timely alerts for seeking medical advice. **Box 1** shows parameters that can be monitored using wearable devices. Rhythm, activity, physiological, biochemical, and other variables can be tracked on daily basis. Pedometers, accelerometers, and wrist straps are commonly used to monitor daily activities and heart rate (HR) by athletes, sportspersons, and public. Heart-healthy wearables can be

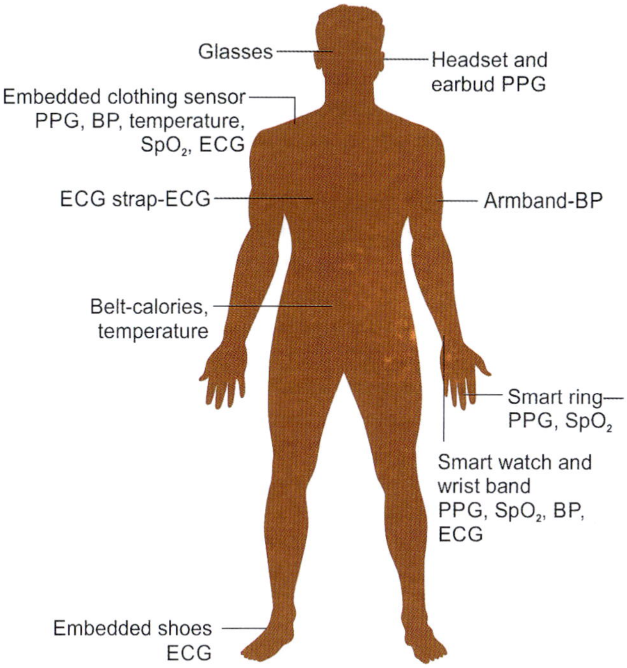

FIG. 1: Wearable devices.

(BP: blood pressure; ECG: electrocardiogram; PPG: photoplethysmography; SpO_2: oxygen saturation)

BOX 1 Parameters that can be monitored by WHT.

- Daily activity
- ECG monitoring and arrhythmia detection
- Physiological monitoring, (HR, RR, SPO_2, HR variability, BP, skin temperature, and sleep)
- Blood glucose and other biochemical parameters
- Hemodynamics parameters (intravascular volume)

(HR: heart rate, RR: respiratory rate, SpO_2: oxygen saturation; BP: blood pressure; WHT: wearable hemodynamic technologies)

used to assess and monitor user physiology, CV fitness, and can be a good way to provide motivation and achieve goals. Activity trackers are already a part of day-to-day monitoring by certain individuals.

Most exciting development is use of wearables for the diagnosis of arrhythmias, hypertension (HTN), coronary artery disease (CAD), valvular heart disease (VHD), congestive heart failure (CHF), and pulmonary hypertension (PH). The proper use of these devices may improve healthcare. Consumer-grade smartphone-based devices and smartwatches have been found to have high sensitivity and specificity for detection of atrial fibrillation (AF). The most useful advancement in DHT has been in recording of ECG and diagnosing rhythm disorders **(Box 2)**.

There is a virtual epidemic of CHF, and it has necessitated research and development of technologies that can help identify patients with early signs of decompensation. Clinical signs of heart failure are often preceded by asymptomatic increase in left ventricular end-diastolic pressure (LVEDP) and pulmonary capillary wedge pressure (PCWP). Emerging wearable hemodynamic technologies (WHTs) that measure dielectric sensing and bioimpedance may detect preclinical changes in intravascular volume.

BOX 2 Electrocardiogram (ECG) monitoring devices.

- Smartwatches (Apple watch, smartphone apps, and Fitbit)
- Handheld ECGs
- Ambulatory cardiac monitoring devices:
  - Holter monitoring (24–49 hours)
  - Long-term continuous (3–14 days)
  - External loop and event recorder (up to 30 days)
  - Mobile cardiac telemetry (up to 30 days)
  - Implantable cardiac monitor (up to 5 years)

ENGINEERING PRINCIPLES

Wearable ambulatory sensors have the potential to provide critical monitoring and diagnostic insights to prevent and treat health problems.[5] Being small in size and comfortable, they are suitable for long-term use. Some of the devices work in a standalone fashion, whereas others work in conjunction with other compact and portable equipment such as smartphone. The sensors utilized in wearables measure either activity, heart rate and rhythm, blood pressure (BP), or others. depending on the function. Wearable DHT can capture continuous or semicontinuous data measurements that can often be captured without patient initiation. The passively collected wearable biosensor data is instantaneously collected, analyzed, and then fed back to patient/physician for appropriate management. **Table 1** predicts different type of sensors, measurement undertaken, and their clinical utility.

Activity Sensors

Physical activity is inversely related to adverse CV outcomes and almost all professionals recommend appropriate exercise to patients and general public.[6] The wearables and smartphones can accurately assess physical activity and energy expenditure through various sensors. Triaxial accelerometer with differential capacitance is commonly used in currently used wearables due to excellent performance. The placement site on human body determines the accuracy and a centrally-located sensor on the torso is best suited for detecting posture, acceleration, and body movement. An ankle-mounted sensor is better suited to measure steps and energy expenditure; however, wrist-worn devices are preferred due to convenience. Global positioning system (GPS) and barometers have also been utilized as wearables to assess physical activity. GPS utilizes a system of 24 or more satellites that continuously emit signals to identify position.

TABLE 1: Sensors in wearable devices.

Sensors	Measurements	Clinical utility
Activity		
Accelerometer	Step count, speed, exercise, etc.	• Risk assessment • Primary and secondary prevention • Rehabilitation management
Barometer	Stair count	• ACS diagnosis • Hyperkalemia and long QT diagnosis • HF management • Therapy titration
GPS	Distance traveled and calorie burnt	• Risk prediction • HTN screening • Rehabilitation
Biometric		
ECG	Single and multiple ECG, arrhythmia detection, and interval (QTc) monitoring	Diabetes and HF management
PPG	HR, HRV, BP, rhythm, sleep, SV, CO, and SaO_2	
Oscillometric	Wrist cuff BP	
Others		
Biochemical sensors	Glucose and electrolytes monitoring	
Biomechanical sensors	CO, SV, and lung fluid volume	

(ACS: acute coronary syndrome; BP: blood pressure; CO: cardiac output; GPS: global positioning system; HF: heart failure; HR: heart rate; HTN: hypertension; HRV: heart rate variability; SV: stroke volume; SaO_2: oxygen saturation)

Heart Rate and Rhythm Sensors

The relationship between HR and CV risk is well established with long-term studies showing an association between a higher resting rate and CV disease and adverse clinical outcomes. HR monitors using chest-strap electrodes have been used in sports for decades. High resting HR in normal population has been associated with increased risk of CVD and all-cause mortality. Elevated HR strongly correlates with adverse events in CHF. Impaired HR recovery after exercise portends adverse CV events. Heart rate variability (HRV) has been linked to unfavorable outcomes in healthy population and in those with heart failure and reduced ejection fraction (HFrEF).

Wearable medical devices such as Holter ECG monitors have been used in healthcare for decades. Nowadays, devices purchased by public **(Fig. 1)** including smartphones, wristbands, watches, scales, shirts, rings, and eyeglasses are equipped with this type of functionality. There are a number of wearables **(Box 2)** that record ECG and measure HR and HRV. ECG sensors come in various forms and are the gold standard for HR and rhythm monitoring. Commercially available wearables measure HR and rhythm using ECG or photoplethysmography (PPG) by calculating beat-to-beat intervals and using algorithms to classify heart rhythm. Most consumer-grade devices (Apple and Fitbit) for detecting arrhythmias use PPG technology, which measures volumetric changes in blood flow that translate into pulse waves and tachogram recordings. Smartwatches and Fitbit (a wrist-worn device) can record a single-lead ECG as needed by placing a contralateral finger on the crown. The single-lead ECG can be useful for diagnosis of simple arrhythmias like AF but is insufficient for diagnosis of complex arrhythmias, myocardial infarction (MI), and QT and QRS interval abnormalities.

Blood Pressure Sensors

Hypertension is a major global health problem. Incorporating BP measurement with wearables has potential to improve screening for HTN and identify exercise-induced and nocturnal HTN. BP can be measured without a cuff, increasing the feasibility and ease of monitoring BP throughout the day. This technology combines ECG and PPG measurements to estimate BP by calculating the pulse transit time (time taken by arterial pulse to travel from the heart to a distal vessel). Another proposed wearable is based on flexible pressure sensor, which consists of a noninvasive, ultra-flexible, and transparent device that can be worn on a continuous basis. Pulse wave velocity-based measurements are also being investigated. There are wristwatches being developed with built-in cuff.

Other Sensors

Biochemical sensors can measure body fluid and electrolytes with the use of electromechanical transducers offering valuable information about volume status. Biomechanical sensors are used to measure cardiac output, stroke volume, and other hemodynamic variables.

WEARABLES IN CARDIAC CARE

A great deal of evidence has accumulated in the literature supporting use of WHT in healthcare and research.[3,7] The relevant areas are discussed here briefly.

Risk Assessment and Lifestyle Alterations

The CV disease assessment is traditionally based on clinical risk scores that estimate 10-year risk. Moderate-to-vigorous exercise (MVPA) measured with the use of triaxial accelerometers was associated with a lower mortality when compared with light physical activity or sedentary behavior in several Swedish and US population cohorts. Frequent wearables-generated HR measurements (HR, HRV, and HR recovery) can be incorporated unto CV risk scores. HR-guided training is gaining popularity; however, clinical trials need to document the benefits of this practice.

Cardiorespiratory Fitness

The 6 minutes walk test (6MWT) is widely used for evaluating cardiopulmonary fitness of an individual. A wearable, wireless multiparameter device has been developed with features to monitor SpO_2, HR, and 6MWT. The wearable and wireless sensor can detect the dynamic changes during the 6MWT and has potential for use as an ambulatory monitoring system.

Stress Diagnosis

Stress is well known to trigger/cause cardiac events. A stress-monitoring patch capable of monitoring the arterial pulse wave, conductance, and skin temperature is user-friendly and provides estimates of RR variability.

Arrhythmia Detection

The diagnosis of arrhythmias has also moved from burdensome strategies, such as ambulatory monitors, to more convenient wearables. The Holter can be worn for short periods and might miss paroxysmal arrhythmias. On the other hand, the loop recorders are invasive devices and require special training to insert and analyze. Wearables can provide continuous single-lead ECG monitoring, such as Zio patch or continuous PPG heart rhythm monitoring (Apple watch). PPG sensors can detect AF, the most common significant arrhythmia with a high sensitivity and specificity of 91–100% as compared with ECG. The Zio patch is an FDA-approved adhesive waterproof patch, which provides a relatively long-term monitoring of cardiac rhythms. The patch is applied to left pectoral region and can be kept up to 14 days without the need of battery recharge or replacement. The Zio patch is superior to Holter for detecting arrhythmias.[3] The Zio patch is recommended in patients with palpitations, syncope, or dizziness and has a good yield for detecting AF, ventricular tachycardia (VT), and bradyarrhythmia. The wearables have also been used to see progression of paroxysmal AF to permanent and optimize ventricular rate during rest and activity.

The Apple Heart Study investigated the use of smartwatch-based arrhythmia detection in 419,297 participants.[8] This is a remarkable trial that brought Apple technology into the domain of public healthcare. The technology-driven trial has its strengths of being a large-scale passive screening trial for a common disease—AF. Over 400,000 participants (mean age 41 years) were involved in their self-care study. The watch utilized optical sensors to intermittently generate "tachograms", which were interpreted as regular or not regular. The participant was asked to come for a telehealth check if an arrhythmia was suspected. The yield from the study was low and only 0.25% of participants received irregular pulse notifications. Another disappointment was that only 20.8% of notified individuals presented for further investigations and AF was confirmed in only 1/3. Nonetheless, this study is a landmark for integration of WHT in clinical care.

Hypertension Detection

Initiating HTN screening in population (particularly young) is widely recommended for preventing CVD. Oscillometric or cuff-less BP monitoring devices that can be worn continuously on the wrist might prove more convenient than traditional methods for screening purposes. Certain manufacturers from USA and Japan have developed and validated devices that can provide reliable measurements of BP from the wrist. These devices have been commercially available and have compared well with office-based sphygmomanometer readings but less closely with simultaneously performed ambulatory monitoring.[7] The use of these WHT is going to increase and it will be beneficial if international organizations provide validation and standard guidelines to physicians to incorporate these devices in practice.

Management of Ischemic Heart Disease

Wearable devices are likely to have enormous impact in management of patients following acute coronary syndrome (ACS) and in chronic coronary syndrome (CCS). Strategies for secondary prevention of CAD can be achieved by better control of modifiable risk factors through WHT. The use of Apple watch and Bluetooth-guided applications in post-ACS patients in a small study revealed better implementation of guideline directed medical therapy (GDMT) and reduced adverse events. Wearables can also be used to titrate beta-blocker therapy and screen for arrhythmias.

The UP-STEP ACS study will be the first randomized study utilizing Fitbit (Fitbit, San Francisco, USA) in post-ACS patients to study the effect of the wearable on improving the effort tolerance and secondary prevention.[7]

Heart Failure

Several randomized controlled trials (RCTs) have assessed the role of invasive and noninvasive telemonitors in management of CCF with mixed results.

In the management of CHF, wearables can be used to assess physical activity, HR, and HRV and accordingly, risk stratify. Wearable actigraphy devices have been validated with patient's symptoms and activity during rehabilitation. A review of wearable monitoring in these patients revealed reduced physical activity to be associated with poor clinical outcomes, mortality, and morbidity.[7] There are devices that can be integrated into clothes to measure and detect changes in intrathoracic impedance and guide diuretic management. Remote dielectric sensing (ReDS) and electromagnetic signals across the chest are used in home-monitoring wearables and applications designed to detect pulmonary congestion. Early data shows promising results and reduction in CHF admissions using these appliances.

Pulmonary Hypertension

Pulmonary HTN is a serious condition with progressive symptoms, reduced exercise capacity, and high morbidity and mortality. Activity monitoring using WHT has been incorporated in several drugs and devices outcome trials. The FIT-PH study is aimed to study the patient's activity and quality of life (QOL) data using Fitbit put on the wrist. The QOL data is to be correlated with implanted pulmonary artery monitoring pressure devices.

QT Measurement

A prolonged QT interval can predispose patients to life-threatening arrhythmias. The use of a single-lead ECG available in most wearables does not provide an accurate assessment of QTc. However, accurate measurement may be possible in future using innovative techniques like device manipulation and AI algorithms that enable multilead recordings.

Hyperkalemia Diagnosis

Hyperkalemia is a common cause of life-threatening rhythm disturbances in patients with CAD and associated renal dysfunction. Elevation of potassium is also a threat in patients who are on CHF therapies. ECG recording techniques have the potential to recognize the electrical changes like peaked tall T waves, QRS widening, PR shortening, and bradyarrhythmias. The clinical data at present is limited and conflicting with false positives and negatives.

Peripheral Vascular Disease

The first line of treatment in patients with peripheral vascular disease and intermittent claudication is a supervised program of gradually increasing exercise. WHT has tremendous potential in management of these patients.

CHALLENGES AND FUTURE DIRECTIONS

There is no doubt that future belongs to wearable technology; however, several challenges can hinder their widespread use. The consumers fueled by media hype/information of trendy but often evolving technologies are pushing for rapid adoption of WHT in clinical practice. The scientific community needs to trend with caution. Incorporating data from wearables into clinical decision-making is feasible but not straightforward. Patients are already coming to the physicians with a lot of data acquired by their smart devices. The data may create a lot of anxiety, especially in healthy individuals. At this stage, doctors need to be extremely cautious about the source of the device and whether the use is off-label. It is also important to know that currently, there is dearth of studies that have shown improvement in outcomes.

Moving into future, we need the following:

- Information about device accuracy (actionable data versus noise), regulatory approvals, patient privacy issues, and cost.
- Develop comprehensive evaluation frameworks in close collaboration between technical and medical personnel, regulatory tract, and RCT data. A position paper by European Society of Cardiology is a major step in formulating policies and directing further research strategies.[9]
- Cardiologists and physicians will need to assimilate these data sources and learn to utilize the data for patient management. Physicians need training in WHT and telehealth.
- An extremely important study[10] reported significantly lower use of WHT amongst those with CVD with only 18% reporting the wearable use. Surprisingly, the population who need to benefit the most utilize it least due to lower socioeconomical and educational status. Unfortunately, cost is a barrier to its use in elderly. This raises another important and unanswered question about who should be medically prescribed WHT and which one.

CONCLUSION

The WHT has shown promising applications in certain CVDs; however, the integration and application of this data into clinical practice is still in infancy.

ONLINE REFERENCES

Please scan the QR code provided at the end of the table of contents for References of this chapter.

SECTION 4

Dyslipidemia Management

Section Outline

CHAPTER

24

CSI Clinical Practice Guidelines for Dyslipidemia Management

JPS Sawhney

ABSTRACT

Dyslipidemias are the most important coronary artery disease (CAD) risk factor. Proper management of dyslipidemia is crucial to control the epidemic of premature CAD in India. The *Cardiological Society of India* developed consensus-based guidelines for better lipid management for CAD prevention and treatment.

The focus of these guidelines is on management of specific dyslipidemias relevant to India-raised low-density lipoprotein (LDL) cholesterol, non-high-density lipoprotein cholesterol (non-HDL-C), apolipoproteins, triglycerides, and lipoprotein(a). In these guidelines, management of dyslipidemias in the elderly, young and children, and patients with comorbidities-stroke, peripheral arterial disease, kidney failure, posttransplant, human immunodeficiency virus (HIV), and familial hypercholesterolemia is also presented. The CSI guidelines for dyslipidemia management are based on data from Indian population wherever available, major international guidelines (mainly European) and expert opinion of lipid management leaders from India with focus on the dictum: *earlier the better, lower the better, longer the better and together the better*. In the present chapter salient points from the CSI Dyslipidemia Guidelines are summarized.

Keywords: Dyslipidemia, guidelines, cardiovascular disease, statins, nonstatins, cholesterol

INTRODUCTION

India has the dubious distinction of having the highest number of coronary artery disease (CAD) patients in the world. Case-control and prospective studies in India have reported that lipid abnormalities, especially raised total, low-density lipoprotein (LDL), and non-high-density lipoprotein-cholesterol (non-HDL-C), triglycerides and apolipoprotein B (ApoB) are the most important risk factors. Lipid management based on LDL-C and non-HDL-C target is crucial to reduce the incidence of CAD in both primary and secondary prevention settings. A number of challenges exist which include premature occurrence of major CAD risk factors; large burden of premature CAD; high prevalence of raised total, LDL and non-HDL-C, familial hypercholesterolemia (FH), hypertriglyceridemia (in association with diabetes and metabolic syndrome); and elevated lipoprotein(a) [Lp(a)]. Low status of population-level and individual-level awareness and treatment of dyslipidemias and extremely low status of guideline recommended control in the community and the clinic is also a barrier for optimal lipid management. There is also lack of large randomized controlled studies of various pharmacological and clinical interventions in India to develop context specific evidence based guidelines. The current consensus document for management of various dyslipidemias, has been developed through a review of major international guidelines on lipid management and local evidence (data for prevalence of dyslipidemia in India), clinical trials of statin and nonstatin where Indian population participated, genetic studies of our country [FH and Lp(a) and small studies on responses of statin in our population], and reflects opinions of the leaders in lipid management in the country. This chapter highlights specific focus areas of CSI clinical practice guidelines for dyslipidemia management.[1]

EPIDEMIOLOGY OF DYSLIPIDEMIAS IN INDIA

- Atherogenic dyslipidemia is prevalent in our country.
- Raised triglycerides are an important and unique feature of dyslipidemias in India.

- HDL cholesterol has recently been relegated as a risk marker and not a risk factor.
- The 2023 ICMR-INDIAB study has also reported the prevalence of various dyslipidemias in all the states of the country **(Figs. 1A to D)**. The prevalence of total cholesterol ≥ 200 mg/dL ranges from 4.6–7.9% to 45.6–50.3%; LDL cholesterol ≥ 130 mg/dL from 4.6–6.2% to 46.8–52.1%; triglycerides ≥ 150 mg/dL from 21.2–22.7% to 43.4–47.9%; and low HDL cholesterol ranges from 51.8 to 83.1%.
- This study has reported higher prevalence of hypercholesterolemia in few Northern and Southern states, more in urban than rural areas with interstate and inter regional variability, whereas the prevalence of high triglycerides and low HDL cholesterol is similar throughout the country.

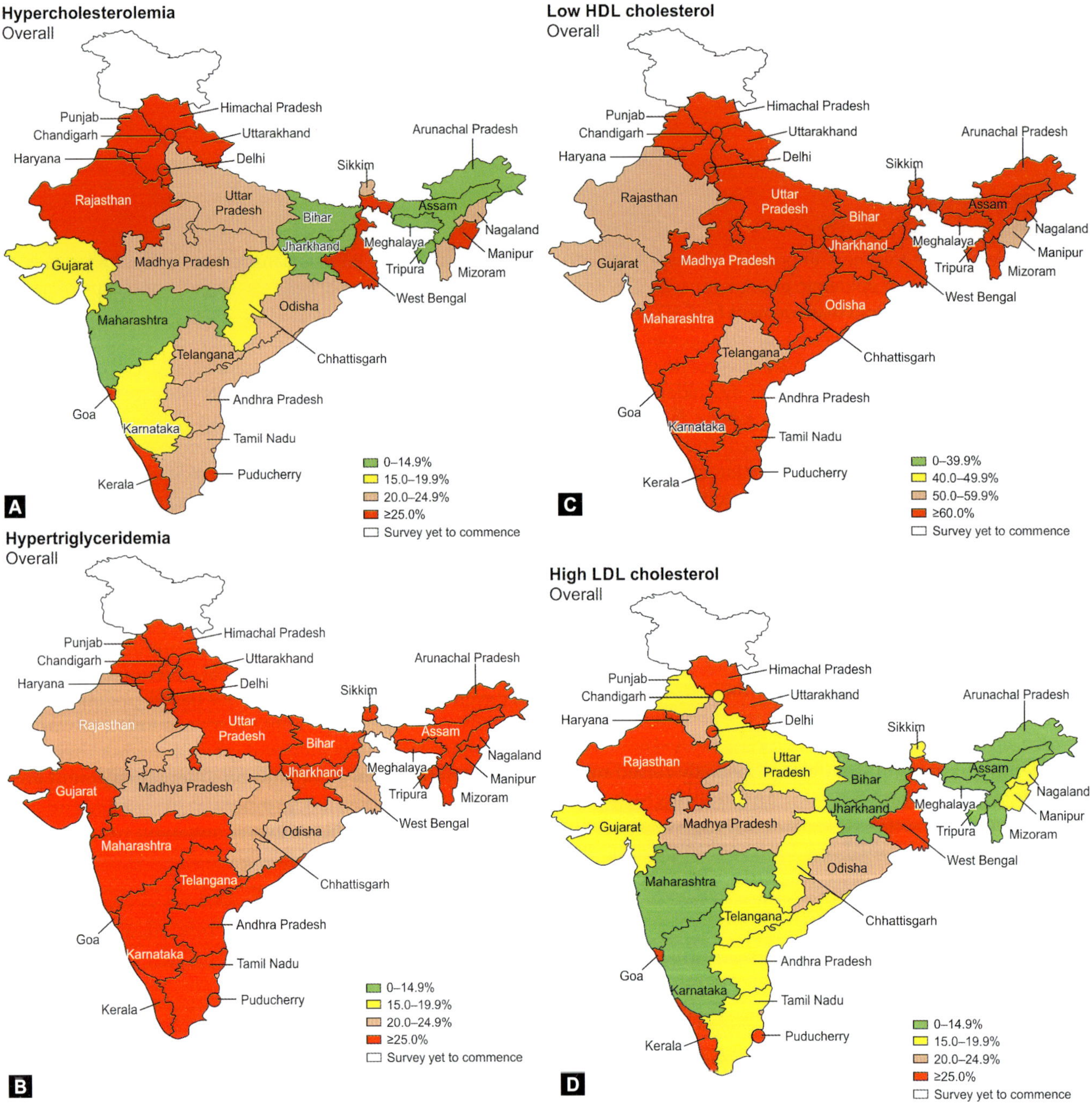

FIGS. 1A TO D: State level prevalence of various dyslipidemias in ICMR-INDIAB study.

Source: Anjana RM, Unnikrishnan R, Deepa M, et al.; ICMR-INDIAB Collaborative Study Group. Metabolic noncommunicable disease health report of India: the ICMR-INDIAB national cross-sectional study (ICMR-INDIAB-17). Lancet Diabetes Endocrinol. 2023;11(7):474-89.

- Few other epidemiological studies have reported variable prevalence rates of important dyslipidemias in urban India. The prevalence of total cholesterol ≥ 200 mg/dL ranges from 25 to 30%, non-HDL cholesterol ≥ 130 mg/dL: 50–55%, LDL cholesterol > 100 mg/dL: 50–55%, triglycerides > 150 mg/dL: 30–40% and low HDL cholesterol: 60–70%.
- Studies have also reported low status of population-level and individual-level awareness and treatment of various dyslipidemias.

EVALUATION OF LIPID PARAMETERS

- Measurement of nonfasting levels of total cholesterol, LDL cholesterol, HDL cholesterol, non-HDL cholesterol, and triglycerides for risk estimation and guiding treatment is recommended.
- Measurement of lipid profile in clinics and emergency departments can lead to early estimation of CAD risk and rapid initiation of lipid lowering lipid lowering therapies.
- CAD risk and baseline levels of LDL cholesterol guide intensity of lipid lowering therapies **(Table 1)**.
- There is an urgent need for standardization of lipid estimation in medical laboratories across the country so that every eligible individual can receive evidence-based lipid lowering interventions.

CARDIOVASCULAR RISK CLASSIFICATION AND SUGGESTED TARGETS

- Risk stratification is important to guide lipid lowering therapy and to identify goals **(Flowchart 1)**.
- *Five categories are recommended*: Low risk, moderate risk, high risk, very high risk, and extremely high-risk groups. Goals for various dyslipidemias are summarized in **Table 1**.

ACUTE CORONARY SYNDROME (FLOWCHART 2)

- In acute coronary syndrome (ACS) patients, a nonfasting lipid profile is acceptable as the goal is to achieve LDL cholesterol below 55 mg/dL as early as possible.
- A proven concept in LDL cholesterol management in ACS hit hard and hit early with combination lipid-lowering therapy.
- High dose of statins alone may not be able to attain the LDL cholesterol goal in a significant number of patients. Therefore, addition of ezetimibe at initiation of treatment is recommended.
- It is recommended to add another nonstatin drug if LDL cholesterol target of <55 mg/dL is not achieved at 4 weeks: Choices are bempedoic acid, PCSK9 inhibitors or inclisiran. Maximum effect of statin comes at 4 weeks. Beyond 4 weeks there is no further reduction of LDL-C.
- Down titrate the dose if this is SAMs, or rising trend of HbA1c in prediabetic patient (metabolic syndrome).

STABLE ATHEROSCLEROTIC CARDIOVASCULAR DISEASE (FLOWCHART 3)

- Chronic coronary syndrome (CCS) and other ASCVDs are common in clinical practice.

TABLE 1: Standard lipid testing panels and targets for various risk groups (all values in mg/dL).

	Desirable levels of various lipid fractions			
Lipid parameter	**Low risk**	**Moderate risk**	**High risk**	**Very high risk**
LDL cholesterol	<100	<100	<70	<55
Non-HDL cholesterol	<130	<130	<100	<85
HDL cholesterol	>40 M, >50 W	>40 M, >50 W	>40 M, >50 W	>40 M, >50 W
Triglycerides	<150	<150	<150	<150
Lipoprotein(a)	<50	<50	<50	<50

Note:
- Calculate non-HDL if TGY > 150 mg/dL. Non-HDL = Total cholesterol–HDL-C.
- Low risk—no cardiovascular risk factor.
- Moderate risk—any one of major CVD risk factors (smoking/tobacco, hypertension, diabetes, dyslipidemia, family history of young heart attack, central obesity).
- High risk—diabetes with one or more risk factor, hypertension with one or more risk factor, chronic kidney disease, familial hypercholesterolemia.
- Very high risk—clinical evidence of blockage in arteries (angina, heart attack, stroke, and limb vessel disease), diabetes > 20 years/diabetes with complications, familial hypercholesterolemia with CVD.
- CVD—cardiovascular disease (disease of arteries of heart, brain, and limb).
- Elevated Lp(a) above 50 mg/dL is associated with high risk of CVD, heart failure, and aortic valve disease.

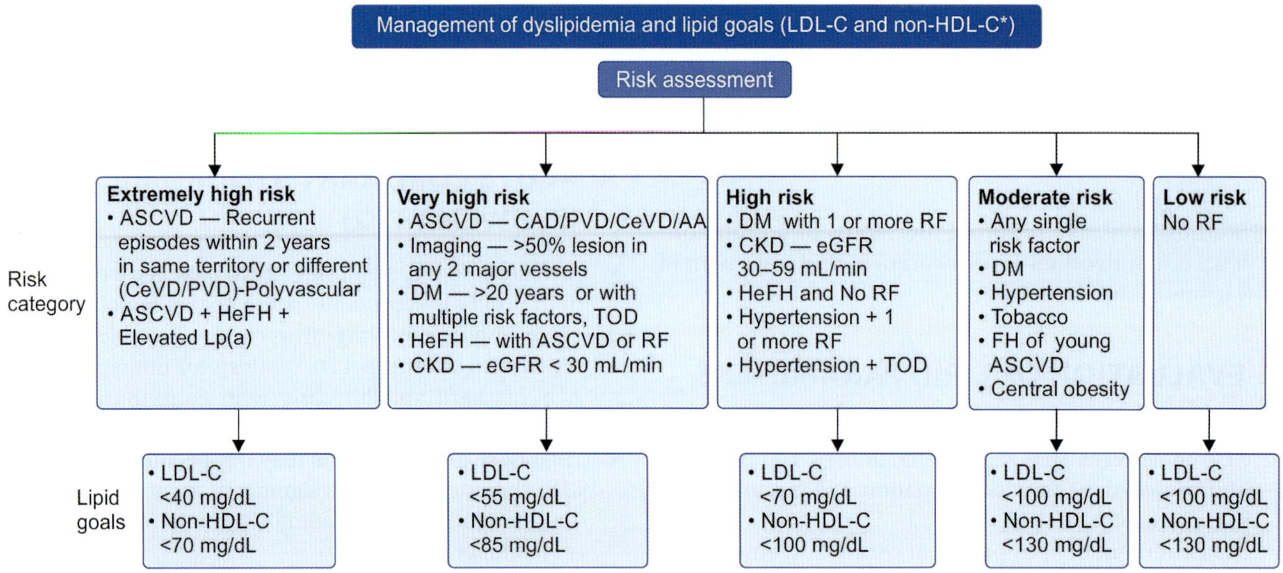

In the absence of our own risk score calculator, only risk factors are used for risk assessment.

*Non-HDL-C as coprimary goal because of increase prevalence of atherogenic dyslipidemia in our country.

FLOWCHART 1: Cardiovascular risk estimation and lipid management goals.

(AA: aortic aneurysm; ASCVD: atherosclerotic cardiovascular disease; CAD: coronary artery disease; CeVD: cerebrovascular disease; CKD: chronic kidney disease; DM: diabetes mellitus; FH: family history; HDL-C: high-density lipoprotein cholesterol; HeFH: heterozygous familial hypercholesterolemia; LDL-C: low-density lipoprotein cholesterol; PVD: peripheral vascular disease; RF: risk factor; TOD: target organ damage)

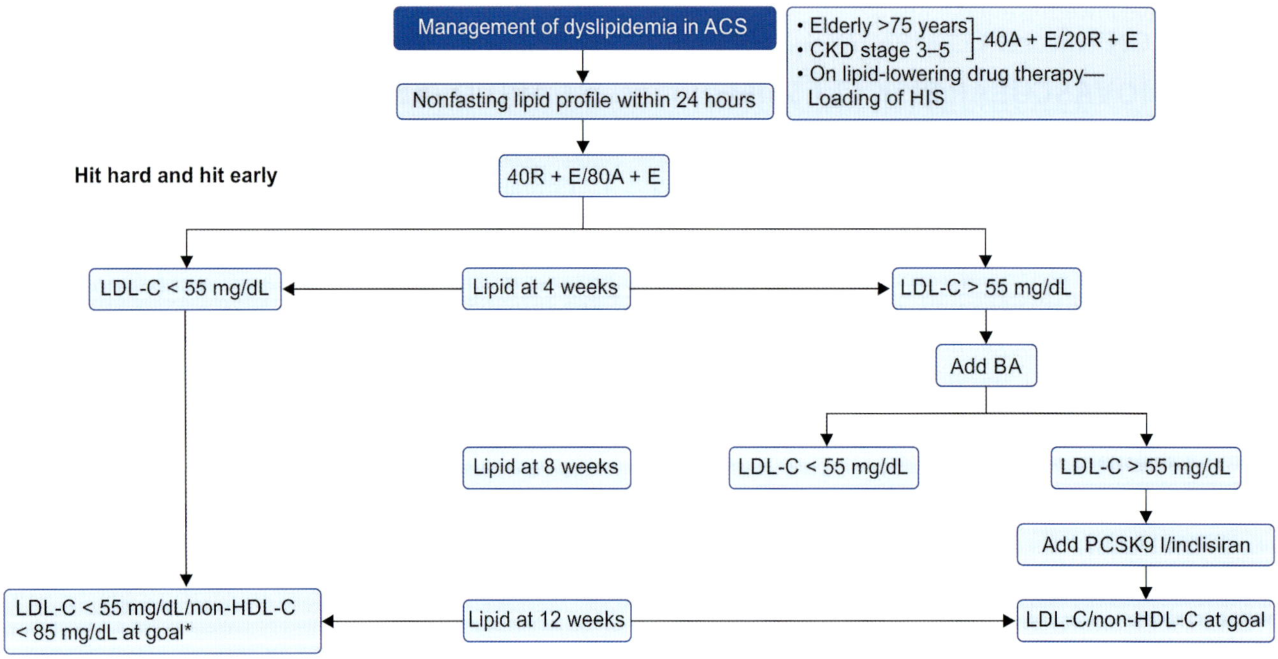

*Look for non-HDl target if TG is ≥ 150 mg/dL;

If non-HDL-C not at goal—add bempedoic acid;

If recurrent ACS, goal should be LDL-C < 40 mg/dL/non-HDL-C < 70 mg/dL;

If patient has statin-associated muscle symptoms (SAMS), new-onset diabetes or worsening HbA1c—down titrate statin followed by lipid profile (R 40 to R 20 or A 80 to A 40).

FLOWCHART 2: Lipid management in the setting of acute coronary syndromes.

[ACS: acute coronary syndrome; FU: follow-up; HIS: high intensity statin (R 20–40 mg, A 40–80 mg); BA: bempedoic acid; A: atorvastatin; R: rosuvastatin; E: ezetimibe]

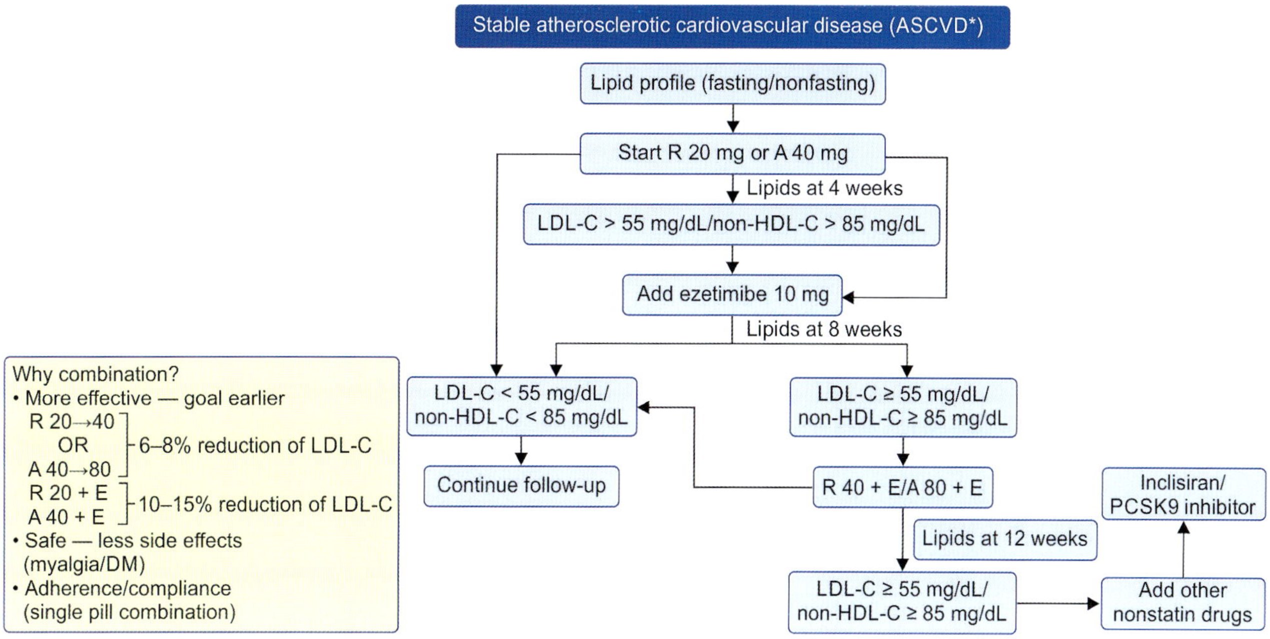

* ASCVD includes CAD/CeVD/PVD

FLOWCHART 3: Lipid management in chronic coronary syndromes.

- In these patients, the goal is to achieve LDL cholesterol <55 mg/dL and non-HDL cholesterol <85 mg/dL **(Table 1)**.
- A significant proportion of Indian population suffers from atherogenic dyslipidemia (raised small dense LDL cholesterol and triglycerides with low-HDL cholesterol). In such patients, it is recommended to initiate high intensity statin therapy **(Table 2)**. A significant proportion shall also require additional ezetimibe.
- Instead of doubling the dosage it is recommended to add ezetimibe which can reduce LDL-C by 15% and help to achieve the goal early with safety (less myalgia and new-onset diabetes).

DRUG THERAPY

Statins in Dyslipidemia Management

Triglycerides, Non-HDL Cholesterol, and low-HDL Cholesterol

- Non-HDL cholesterol is comprised of all proatherogenic lipoproteins containing ApoB which include VLDL, IDL, LDL, chylomicron remnants, and Lp(a).
- Target non-HDL-C if TGy is >150 mg/dL.
- Hypertriglyceridemia is managed by treatment of underlying causes and ASCVD risk factors, lifestyle modifications, statins and nonstatin drugs to lower non-HDL-C, control of diabetes, and pharmacotherapy **(Flowchart 4)**.

TABLE 2: Commonly available statins in India and daily dose according to intensity of treatment.

Drug	High intensity	Moderate intensity	Low intensity
Atorvastatin	40–80 mg	10–20 mg	5 mg
Rosuvastatin	20–40 mg	5–10 mg	-
Pitavastatin	-	2–4 mg	1 mg

- Though omega-3 fatty acids can bring down triglyceride levels, only icosapent ethyl has been shown to reduce cardiovascular (CV) events.
- Fibric acid derivatives can lower triglyceride levels by 30–50%, but have not been shown to reduce CV events when used without background statin therapy.
- In patients with mild to moderate hypertriglyceridemia (TG 150–499 mg/dL), there is no role for fibric acid derivatives. In those with diabetes or ASCVD, IPE may be considered if TG remains high after lifestyle measures and control of diabetes.
- Measurement of non-HDL cholesterol is simpler, more convenient and more predictive of ASCVD than LDL-C, but less often used because LDL-C is more widely used in randomized controlled trials and international guidelines but we have included non-HDL-C as coprimary goal in our guidelines. If TGY > 500 mg/dL, give fenofibrate and EPA, saroglitazar if high TGY is associated with DM or patient has MAFLD.

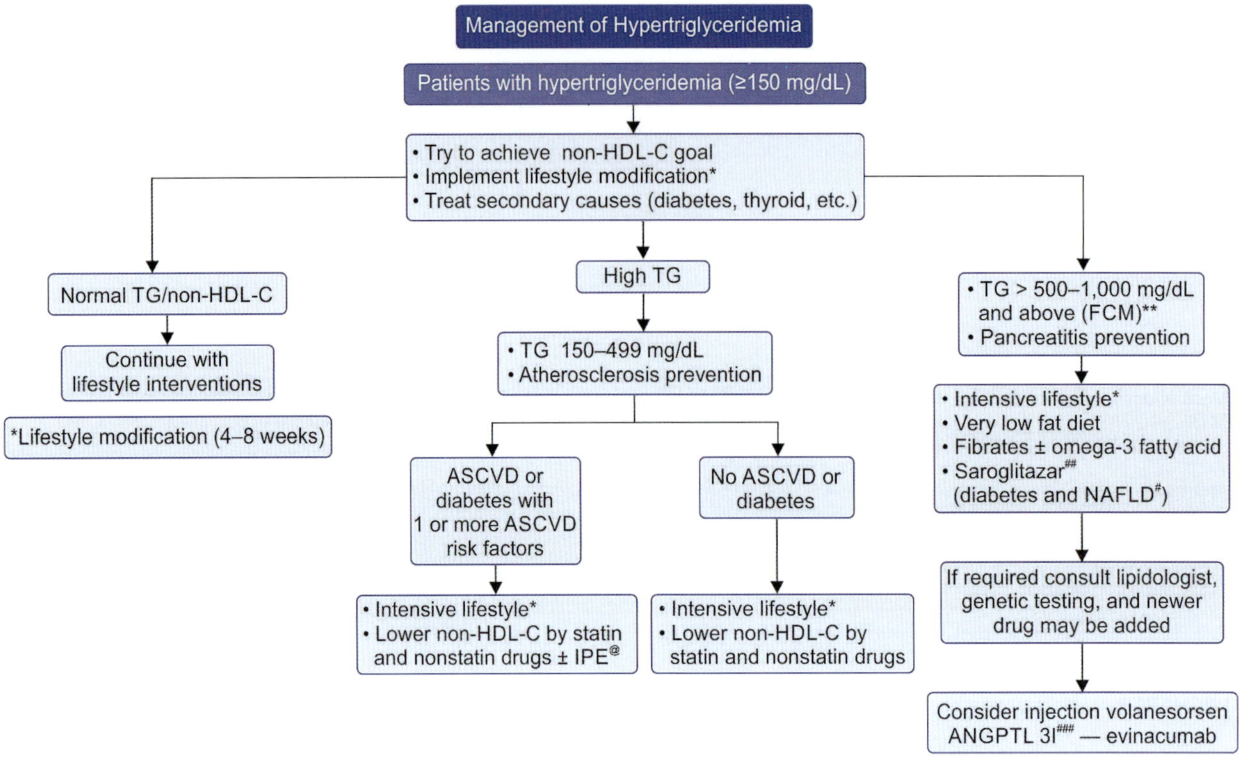

*Reducing carbohydrates, TFA, SFA; Alcohol abstinence; Tobacco cessation; Increasing physical activity; Weight reduction

**FCM: Familial chylomicronemia syndrome.

@IPE Icosapent ethyl.

#NAFLD: Nonalcoholic fatty liver disease.

##Saroglitazor: No endpoint data, no long term safety data.

###ANGPTL 3I: Angiopoietin-like protein 3 inhibitor.

FLOWCHART 4: Management of hypertriglyceridemia.

LIFESTYLE MANAGEMENT

Issues in Dietary Management

- Food patterns, choices, and preparation influence health, rather than rigid counting of calories or proportion of macronutrients.
- Weight management is best achieved using healthy dietary patterns combined with regular exercise.
- Severe restriction on total fats in diet is not supported by evidence. Increased intake of combination unsaturated fats as in Mediterranean diets is recommended. Omega-3 polyunsaturated fatty acid (PUFA) supplementation may be useful in reducing ASCVD events in moderate to high-risk individuals with high triglycerides.
- Plasma saturated fats correlate better with dietary refined carbohydrates. LDL cholesterol slightly increases with higher intake of saturated fats but restriction has no discernible effect on ASCVD incidence or mortality in randomized trials.
- Atherogenic dyslipidemia is best managed by restriction of excess calories, sugars, refined carbohydrates, fried foods, and trans fats while maintaining ideal body weight.
- Isolated elevation of LDL cholesterol is managed by restriction of trans fats and saturated fats.
- The healthiest oils appear to be those high in monounsaturated fatty acid (MUFA) and PUFA with a high N-3/N-6 ratio. The combination of MUFA- and PUFA-containing oils is a good option.
- Trans fats should be totally avoided. Trans fats are present in fried foods and are influenced by cooking practices.
- Minimize deep frying in refined oils because refined oils degrade easily. Traditional Indian oils with a high smoking point may be considered for frying, while reinforcing that fried foods are harmful. Palm oils should be avoided.
- Refined carbohydrates, sugar-sweetened beverages, and processed foods should be strongly restricted and replaced with healthy grains and fiber.
- Dairy fats are controversial; due to recent data suggesting a neutral association with CVD, these may be advocated to replace unhealthy foods like refined carbohydrates or processed foods.

- Healthy diets are plant-based, but an omnivorous diet with eggs, dairy, and occasional intake of unprocessed meats is acceptable. In ASCVD patients, egg yolk and red meat should be restricted. The emphasis is on intake of fruits, vegetables, whole grains, legumes, poultry, fish, and nuts.
- Modest consumption of nuts reduces cardiometabolic risk.
- Alcohol intake should be restricted as much as possible and is not recommended for preventing heart disease.
- Moderate consumption of tea (three to five cups of day) and coffee (one to three cups per day) is acceptable.

SPECIFIC COMORBIDITIES

Stroke

- Dyslipidemias, especially raised LDL cholesterol, are important risk factors for atherothrombotic ischemic stroke.
- Treatment targets for LDL cholesterol (<55 mg/dL) in stroke survivors leads to a lower risk for additional CV events.
- If the LDL cholesterol goal (<55 mg/dL) is not achieved or in statin-intolerant patients, a combination of ezetimibe and/or bempedoic acid along with the maximum tolerated dose of statin may be considered. Evolocumab treatment decreases CVD and ischemic stroke risk.

Peripheral Arterial Disease

- Prevalence of CAD in PAD is 65%. PAD is considered as very high risk and the LDL cholesterol goal is <55 mg/dL.
- High-intensity lipid-lowering therapy is the mainstay of treatment.
- Ezetimibe when added to statin leads to significant reduction of major adverse CV events in PAD.
- PCSK9 inhibitors have been reported to significantly reduce adverse events in PAD versus non-PAD patients.

Congestive Heart Failure

- Routine statin administration is not recommended in nonischemic congestive heart failure (CHF).
- Statins should be continued in CHF with CAD.
- Lipophilic statins (simvastatin, pitavastatin, or atorvastatin) may have beneficial effects on CV outcomes irrespective of the etiology and left ventricular function.
- PCSK9 inhibition appears to have no benefit in HF without ASCVD.

Diabetes

- Dyslipidemia is common in diabetes and is characterized by low-HDL cholesterol, raised triglycerides, and small dense LDL cholesterol.
- Persons with diabetes are risk-stratified according to the duration of their disease, risk factor burden, and presence or absence of target organ damage.
- LDL cholesterol goal is <55 mg/dL for diabetes with ASCVD and diabetes >20 years or with multiple risk factors. Diabetes with any risk factor should have LDL cholesterol <70 mg/dL. Diabetes without risk factors or new-onset diabetes could have LDL cholesterol <100 mg/dL.
- Good glycemic control helps in reducing serum triglycerides in a person with poorly controlled diabetes. Noninsulin glucose-lowering drugs may have a beneficial impact on lipid profile.
- The risk-benefit ratio of statin therapy is beneficial in persons with diabetes, and this should be clearly communicated to all stakeholders.
- While statins remain the first choice of therapy, in intensive or moderate dosage, bempedoic acid, ezetimibe, PCSK9 inhibitors, or fenofibrate can be used to intensify treatment if targets are not met.

Chronic Kidney Disease

- Large clinical studies have reported that statins reduce all-cause mortality and CV events in people with CKD.
- Lipid-lowering therapy with a statin with or without ezetimibe is recommended in patients with eGFR < 60 mL/min/1.73 m^2 and also in those with a preserved GFR but who have an increased urinary albumin-to-creatinine ratio (2.3 mg/mmol) for at least 3 months.
- Statin treatment should not be started for the majority of hemodialysis patients without evidence of ASCVD.
- Patients who were already taking statins, ezetimibe, or a statin/ezetimibe combination at the time of dialysis should consider continuing these medications, especially if they have ASCVD.
- Fibrates should not be used in conjunction with statins in patients with CKD, and ezetimibe monotherapy is not recommended.
- PCSK9 inhibitors are effective in lowering LDL cholesterol in CKD patients without affecting renal outcomes, although more data is awaited.
- Bempedoic acid is safe in patients with mild or moderate renal impairment.

Solid-organ Transplant Patients

- Patients of organ transplant are at a significantly higher risk of developing ASCVD, triggered largely by the dyslipidemia associated with immunosuppressants.
- Drug interactions with ongoing immunosuppressant therapy remain a major challenge in managing these patients with dyslipidemia.
- Before initiating drug therapy for dyslipidemia, lifestyle measures such as physical activity, a Mediterranean diet, feasibility of replacing cyclosporine and mTOR inhibitors should be implemented.

- Various lipid-lowering drugs particularly statins may be given, but there are no large studies available in this subset of patients. There is evidence of benefit for statins in patients undergoing transplant.
- Statins intolerance or dyslipidemia despite on maximally tolerated dose, alternative or additional ezetimibe therapy may be considered. Ezetimibe should be avoided in patients who are on cyclosporine.

Pregnancy

- Serum triglycerides and total cholesterol levels are often elevated in pregnancy.
- Dietary interventions are the mainstay of the management in pregnant women.
- Omega-3 fatty acids and bile acid sequestrants are safe but only moderately effective.
- Statins are contraindicated in pregnancy due to the risk of teratogenicity and should also be avoided during lactation.
- Statins are not recommended in premenopausal women considering pregnancy and not using adequate contraception.
- Ezetimibe and bempedoic acid are not recommended in pregnancy.

Liver Disease

- Statins are the first-line treatment for dyslipidemia in metabolic dysfunction-associated steatotic liver disease (MASLD).
- Mild elevation (up to threefold) of liver transaminases is not a contraindication for statins.
- Statins are contraindicated in decompensated cirrhosis or acute liver failure.
- Drug interactions must be considered when prescribing statins to these patients particularly when given with antiviral drugs for hepatitis B and C.
- Combination of ezetimibe with rosuvastatin may be more effective in reducing liver fat.
- Both fibrates and omega-3 fatty acids reduce triglyceride levels but not liver fat.
- Saroglitazar is approved to treat NAFLD and being evaluated for benefits in MASLD.

Inflammatory Diseases

- Autoimmune connective disorders and inflammatory conditions such as rheumatoid arthritis (RA) and systemic lupus erythematosus (SLE) increase the risk of CVD.
- The most common derangements are high triglycerides, small dense LDL and Lp(a) and low-HDL cholesterol. There is direct correlation of C-reactive protein (CRP) with HDL cholesterol.
- Hydroxychloroquine has been shown to reduce total and LDL cholesterol.
- Cyclophosphamide reduces levels of LDL and VLDL cholesterol.
- Statins are the first-choice drugs to reduce LDL cholesterol and choice depends on magnitude of lowering required and drug interactions.
- Treatment of underlying condition can reduce dyslipidemia while anti-inflammatory drugs such as steroids and calcineurin inhibitors can aggravate it.

SPECIFIC PHENOTYPES

Dyslipidemia in the Elderly

- Initiation of drug therapy for dyslipidemia for primary prevention in the elderly should be individualized considering comorbidities, drug interactions, and patient preferences.
- All elderly patients must be counseled for lifestyle measures and medication adherence.
- Statin use as primary prevention for the elderly is supported by meta-analysis and statins are recommended in elderly with high risk of CVD or CAD.
- Statins should be started at a low dose with monitoring for adverse effects. The dose should be titrated to achieve LDL cholesterol goals **(Table 1)**.
- Among very elderly (>80 years) there is inadequate evidence for drug treatment of dyslipidemia for primary prevention and clinical judgment and patient preferences should guide decisions.
- In the elderly, the goals for LDL cholesterol are similar to the nonelderly **(Table 1)**.
- In the elderly with high and very high CAD risk, the addition of ezetimibe is likely to be beneficial.
- Evolocumab is safe and effective in the elderly and could be an alternative in high and very high CAD risk.

Dyslipidemia in the Young

- Myocardial infarction (MI) and sudden cardiac deaths in young adults (<40 years) are common in India. Dyslipidemia and tobacco are one of the primary drivers.
- All individuals should have their lipid profile evaluated by the age of 18 years. Screening may be of particular benefit in identifying young adults with elevated LDL cholesterol due to unrecognized HeFH. Young adults (18–40 years) having ASCVD should be on intensive lipid-lowering therapy to keep LDL-C below 55 mg/dL.
- If a young adult has LDL cholesterol of ≥190 mg/dL on repeated evaluation, statin therapy should be initiated.
- Young adults with hypertension and diabetes should receive mild to moderate-intensity statin therapy to achieve the LDL-C goal **(Table 2)**.
- Additionally, all individuals should be advised to lead a healthy lifestyle, increase physical activity, adhere to dietary restrictions, and refrain from smoking and tobacco use.
- Young adults who are carrier of *HeFH* gene should be on healthy lifestyle and small to moderate dose of statin.

Pediatric Hyperlipidemia

- Identifying dyslipidemia in childhood is an opportunity for preventing adult CAD.
- Encouraging a healthy lifestyle with high levels of physical activity, tobacco avoidance, and intake of a healthy diet is necessary.
- Secondary dyslipidemia due to drugs, metabolic, renal, and hepatic causes should be excluded.
- Dyslipidemia due to genetic defects in lipid metabolism should also be considered.
- In children, drug therapy is indicated only with very high LDL cholesterol levels or in children with risk factors following failure of lifestyle changes.
- Pharmacotherapy is best avoided in children <10 years of age except in the presence of severe primary hyperlipidemia and children who are carrier of FH.
- Statins and fibrates, respectively, are first-line drugs for hypercholesterolemia and hypertriglyceridemia. Monitoring of liver functions, creatine kinase, and lipid profile should be performed following 1 month of therapy and every 3–6 months thereafter.
- Ezetimibe can be given to children above the age of 10 years.
- A phase 4 study in India, which included children 12–18 years, reported that PCSK9 inhibitor-evolocumab was safe and well-tolerated.

GENETIC DYSLIPIDEMIA

Familial Hypercholesterolemia

- FH is caused by genetic defects in LDL cholesterol pathways. It is associated with elevated LDL cholesterol and a risk of premature CAD.
- Studies have reported an FH prevalence of 15–20% in premature CAD in India. FH is more common in younger patients with higher LDL levels and with lower incidence of other risk factors such as diabetes, hypertension, and smoking.
- Dutch Lipid Clinic Network (DLCN) criteria are simple clinical tools for FH diagnosis. DLCN is based on a scoring system. A score > 8 suggests definite HF, a while score 6–8 is probable FH.
- DLCN criteria could also be used after applying correction factors in patients already on statins. Genetic testing is confirmatory.
- Statins are used to treat adult HeFH with a LDL cholesterol goal of <70 mg/dL for primary prevention and <55 mg/dL for secondary prevention. High-intensity statin with ezetimibe is recommended as initial therapy. If targets are not achieved, other nonstatin drugs (bempedoic acid, PCSK9 inhibitors, and inclisiran) should be considered **(Flowchart 5)**.

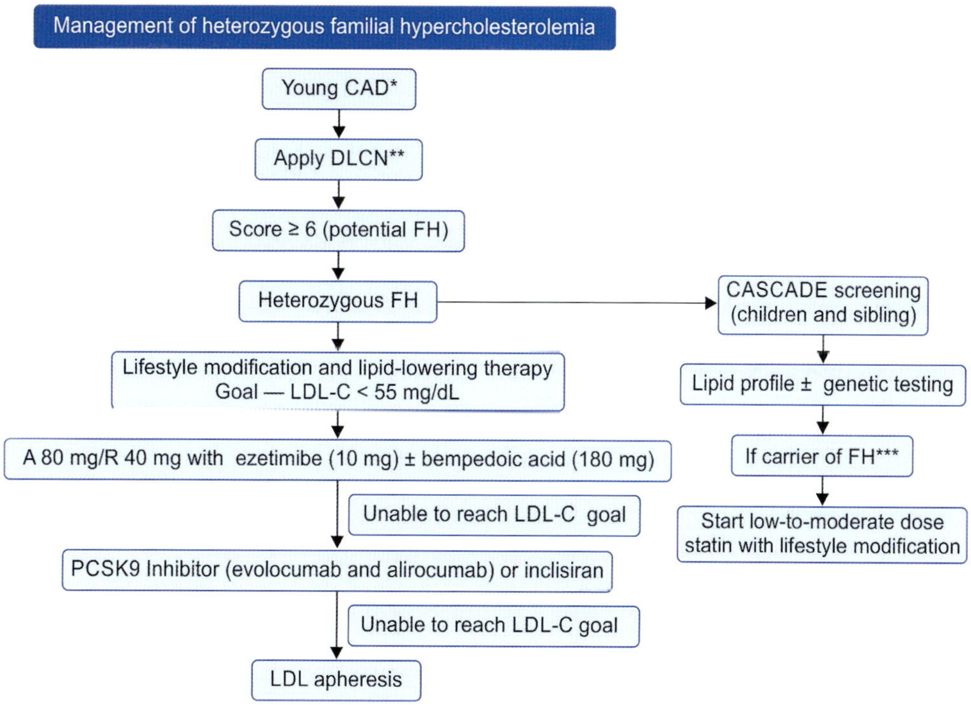

*Young CAD < 55 years male, <65 years female.

**DLCN: Dutch Lipid Clinical Network;
Potential–Definite + Probable FH;
DLCN score 3–5 possible FH (genetic testing is preferred).

***Carrier of FH: Adults—LDL-C >160 mg/dL;
Children >150 mg/dL or genetic positive.

FLOWCHART 5: Familial hypercholesterolemia diagnosis and management.
(A: atorvastatin; R: rosuvastatin)

- Cascade screening of family members is recommended following diagnosis of FH in an individual. HeFH detected children should be managed with statins to achieve an LDL cholesterol target of <130 mg/dL.
- Patients with HoFH high-LDL cholesterol > 500 mg/dL and require combination therapy with high-intensity statins, ezetimibe, and PCSK9 inhibitors. Mipomersen, lomitapide, and plasmapheresis are approved for HoFH treatment.

Elevated Lipoprotein(a)

- Lp(a) is inherited, independent, and causal risk factor for CAD and other ASCVD. Epidemiological, genome-wide association, and Mendelian randomization studies have demonstrated an association between increased Lp(a) levels incidence of MI, aortic stenosis, ischemic stroke, heart failure, and CV and all-cause deaths.
- Elevated Lp(a) is not uncommon and one in five individuals worldwide have elevated Lp(a) (>50 mg/dL or >125 nmol/L). In South Asians, the prevalence is one in four.
- The Lp(a)-mediated CVD risk is mediated by proinflammatory, prothrombotic, and proatherogenic processes.
- Elevated Lp(a) is genetically determined, not influenced by diet and exercise, and remains stable over time. The levels may increase in thyroid diseases, CKD, inflammation, and sepsis. It also increases in pregnancy and menopause. It should be measured at least once in a lifetime.
- An Indian study reported association of Lp(a) > 50 mg/dL with severe angiographic CAD. Elevated Lp(a) in 43 % of FHeH patients and higher levels in young CAD patients compared to the elderly.
- Presently there are no approved therapies but many are in pipeline. Comprehensive lifestyle and aggressive risk factor control is recommended.
- Novel antisense oligonucleotide and small interfering RNA treatments that target apo(a) in hepatocytes reduce Lp(a). Some drugs being evaluated for outcomes are pelacarsen, olpasiran, and other antisense oligonucleotides.

CONCLUSION

Lipid management is crucial for ASCVD prevention and management. Dyslipidemias are widely prevalent in the general population and CAD patients. There is humongous evidence that lowering LDL cholesterol using statins and other nonstatin drugs can reduce the incidence of primary CAD events, and also prevent recurrent events in established ASCVD patients. The Cardiological Society Clinical Practice Guidelines have given simplified algorithm to manage dyslipidemia based on risk estimation.

This guideline has uniquely discussed lipid management in specific comorbidities and patient phenotypes. These issues are especially relevant in India. Adherence to lifelong therapy is a challenge and we believe that better health literacy, financial support, and the use of algorithm-based therapies can improve initiation and continuation.[1]

ACKNOWLEDGMENTS

We would like to express our sincere gratitude to the co-authors for their invaluable contributions to "Indian Clinical Practice Guidelines for Dyslipidemia management". All the authors (JPS Sawhney, Sivasubramanian Ramakrishnan, Kushal Madan, Saumitra Ray, P Balagopalan Jayagopal, Dorairaj Prabhakaran, Tiny Nair, Geevar Zachariah, Peeyush Jain, Jamshed Dalal, Sitaraman Radhakrishnan, Arun Chopra, Sanjay Kalra, Ashwani Mehta, Arvind K Pancholia, Nitin K Kabra, Dhiman Kahali, Tapan Ghose, Satyavir Yadav, Prafulla Kerkar, Ajay Yadav, Debabrata Roy, Mrinal Kanti Das, Vijay H Bang, Pratap Chandra Rath, Dhurjati Prasad Sinha, PS Banerjee, Rakesh Yadav, and Rajeev Gupta) provided critical insights and contributed significantly for enriching the chapter. Their dedication and collaborative efforts have been instrumental in shaping the final outcome of these guidelines.

ONLINE REFERENCES

Please scan the QR code provided at the end of the table of contents for References of this chapter.

CHAPTER

25

Lipid Metabolism: Insights into Regulation and Dysregulation

Subrat Kumar Muduli

ABSTRACT

Lipids are a group of hydrophobic compounds transported in the blood in the form of lipoproteins to various organs of the body to be used for cell growth, energy generation, storage, and utilization. Fatty acids (FAs) are the building blocks of every lipid. The exogenous pathway of lipid metabolism starts with the absorption of dietary fat and their transport in lymphatics as chylomicrons, whereas the endogenous pathway starts with the production and secretion of very low-density lipoproteins into circulation to be finally degraded into fatty acids and other forms. Hepatic lipases convert intermediate-density lipoproteins produced from very low-density lipoproteins, into low-density lipoproteins. Cholesterol is transported to tissues through low-density lipoproteins; whereas, their removal from tissues is mediated through high-density lipoproteins, a process called reverse cholesterol transport. These steps are tightly regulated by hormone-sensitive lipases. Fasting stimulates glucagon, epinephrine, and cortisol release which activate these lipases and lead to lipolysis. Insulin promotes lipogenesis. Genetic mutations in any of the enzymes involved in lipid metabolism or receptors involved in clearance of the lipoproteins lead to the accumulation of lipids in various parts of the body, such as the cornea, skin, liver, and various arteries. Atherosclerotic cardiovascular diseases are the final expression of such derangement. Drugs such as statins and fibrates exploit these pathways to produce their clinical benefits.

Keywords: Lipid, hormonal regulation, lipoprotein disorder, statin

INTRODUCTION

Lipid metabolism comprises the whole spectrum of absorption, transport, catabolism, synthesis, and utilization of various lipid molecules inside the human body. Lipid molecules are hydrophobic and hence insoluble in blood. After absorption, they are packaged into lipoproteins for their transport to distant peripheral cells. Lipids are essential for membrane integrity, signal transduction, cellular proliferation, and energy production essential for human survival. Dysregulation of this pathway has been implicated in a myriad of disorders, such as obesity, diabetes, fatty liver, atherosclerosis, and even cancers.

The five classes of lipids are (1) fatty acids, (2) free sterol, (3) sterol esters, (4) triacyl glycerol, and (5) phospholipids. Fatty acids are the primary building blocks of any lipid molecule. Its uptake and catabolism contribute to energy generation, cell growth, and membrane synthesis. Toxic lipid derivatives such as acylcarnitine and ceramides are also a byproduct of such metabolism and can lead to individual cell death.[1]

Primarily two pathways exist that mediate lipid metabolism; one is the exogenous path for the consumed dietary fats in the intestine and the other one is the endogenous pathway which starts from the liver.[2] The two pathways with the liver sitting at the convergence of two are depicted in **Figure 1**.

LIPID METABOLISM PATHWAYS

Exogenous Pathway

It refers to the transport of absorbed dietary fat into blood circulation and finally liver. Dietary free fatty acids react with glycerol to form triglycerides (TGs) in intestinal cells, and they are packaged into chylomicrons after interacting with Apo B48. This process is mediated by microsomal triglyceride transfer protein (MTP).[3] In the absence of MTP there occurs a

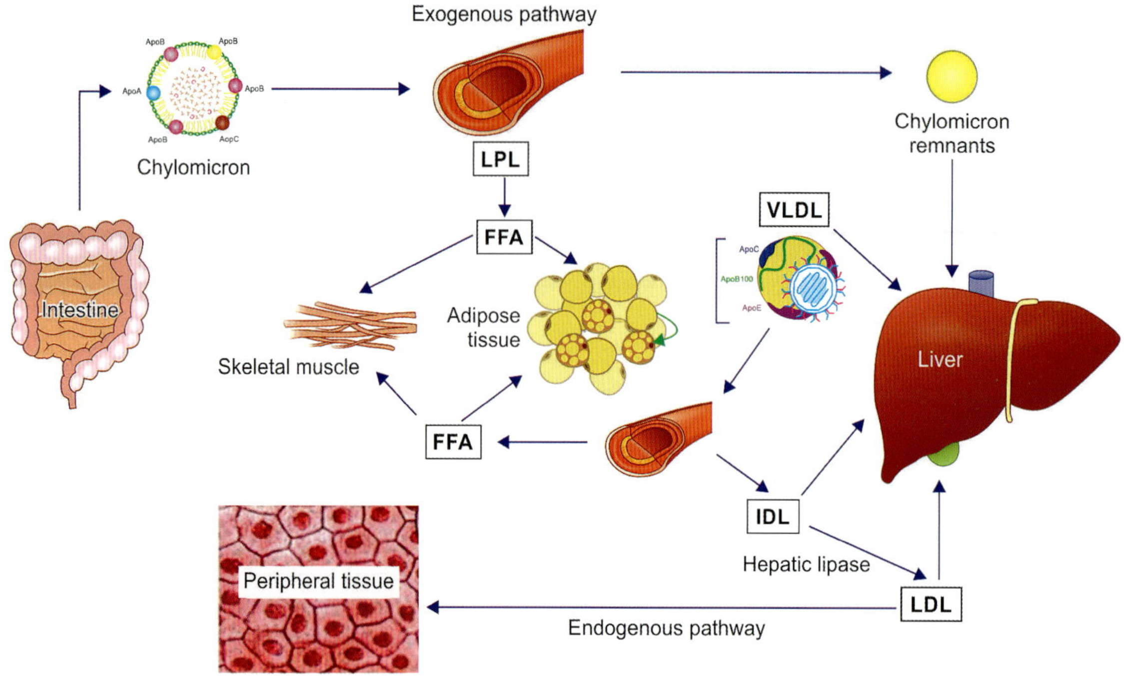

FIG. 1: Exogenous and endogenous pathway of lipid metabolism.

Note: The exogenous pathway starts with dietary fat absorption in the intestine whereas the endogenous pathway starts in the liver with the production and secretion of VLDL. The liver sits at the convergence of two pathways.

(FFA: free fatty acid; IDL: intermediate density lipoproteins; LDL: low-density lipoprotein; LPL: lipoprotein lipase; VLDL: very low-density lipoprotein)

severe decrease in ApoB containing lipoproteins.[4] Esterified cholesterol is also similarly packaged into such chylomicron lipoproteins. Then the chylomicrons circulate through lymphatic channels and the left subclavian vein to peripheral tissues such as adipose tissue, and cardiac, and skeletal muscle for further use. Lipoprotein lipase in peripheral cell capillaries readily hydrolyzes these chylomicrons and releases free fatty acids. As the chylomicrons lose fatty acids their size progressively decreases into remnant forms which helps them cross the fenestrated endothelial barrier of the liver. Remnant forms are taken up by hepatic cells though ApoE. ApoE is acquired in the circulation from HDL particles.

Endogenous Pathway

It starts from the secretion of lipoprotein particles from the liver and finally ends with their utilization in peripheral cells for energy generation. Chylomicron remnants taken up by the liver are left with few TGs and cholesterol. Cholesterol is also synthesized de novo in hepatic cells through the mevalonate pathway.[5] Statins act on this de novo cholesterol synthesis pathway from mevalonate to reduce cholesterol levels in the body. The degraded chylomicron remnants with cholesterol combine with ApoB100 to form the VLDL. Cholesterol components are higher in VLDLs compared to Chylomicrons. Packaging of TGs, cholesterol esters, vitamin E, and ApoB100 is mediated by MTP similar to that in enterocytes. VLDL after getting secreted into circulation acquires a lot of ApoC and ApoE from HDL. It gets degraded in circulation by lipoprotein lipase, an enzyme present in vascular endothelial cells, into IDL. Hydrolysis of VLDL, similar to chylomicrons, releases fatty acids and glycerol. ApoCII is essential for LPL activation and this ApoCII can be found in chylomicrons, VLDL, and IDL. IDL can be retaken up by hepatic cells through LDL receptors or can be further degraded by hepatic lipase. 40–60% of IDLs are retaken up by liver cells. IDL sheds ApoE and TGs to form LDL particles. LDL particles transport the cholesterol to tissues and eventually are taken up by the liver or extrahepatic cells through LDL receptors mediated by ApoB100. Around 70% of LDL is cleared by endocytosis into hepatic cells. LDL particles in liver cells can acquire Apo synthesized in the liver and form Lp(a). Excess levels of LDL cholesterol can result in cholesterol accumulation in various arteries. LDL cholesterol and Lp(a) levels are independently associated with atherosclerotic cardiovascular diseases.

Reverse Cholesterol Transport

Nascent HDL is formed by phospho-lipidation of ApoA1 by adenosine triphosphate (ATP)-binding cassettes protein transporter A1 (ABCA1) protein in intestinal cells as well as liver cells. It also contains cholesterol. More mature HDL particles are produced by acquiring more cholesterol from macrophages and other extrahepatic sites. Cholesterol gets esterified into cholesterol esters by lecithin cholesterol acyl transferase (LCAT) and these cholesterol esters internalize into its core making HDL more spherical and denser. HDL particles transfer this cholesterol either to hepatic cells or apo B containing lipoproteins in exchange for TGs. This process is mediated by cholesteryl ester transfer protein (CETP). This process of cholesterol removal through HDL is known as reverse cholesterol transport.[6] HDL can also directly bind to liver cells through scavenger receptor class B1 receptors and gets internalized. Due to this role of HDL as the remover of tissue cholesterol, HDL is considered good cholesterol and plays a protective role in atherosclerosis. CETP inhibitors have also been tested in clinical trials for cardiovascular risk reduction by raising HDL levels.

After CETP-mediated exchange, HDL becomes rich in TGs which are hydrolyzed by the liver. Endothelial lipase also plays a role in the hydrolysis of HDL phospholipids so that they can be catabolized faster.

The Ultimate Endpoints: Fatty Acid Synthesis and Beta-oxidation

During conditions of excess energy, particularly glucose-repleted state de novo lipid synthesis occurs using acetyl-CoA and NADPH.[7] Acetyl-CoA is generated from ingested glucose or carbohydrate through the glycolysis process. Acetyl-CoA gets converted to malonyl-CoA by acetyl-CoA Carboxylase beta. Malonyl-CoA is the definitive precursor for fatty acid synthesis as well as a regulator for beta-oxidation of fatty acids. Most of the required fatty acids are synthesized in the human body by fatty acid synthetase enzymes from various precursors in adipose tissue and are stored there.

Adenosine triphosphate is the major energy source for the survival of tissue cells in the body. ATP is generated through beta-oxidation of free fatty acids in mitochondria during conditions when glucose availability is in sparse.[8] Heart, skeletal muscles, and liver primarily use FFA for energy generation. In the liver, the incomplete beta oxidation leads to the formation of ketone bodies which are used by the brain in fasting states for energy generation. Beta oxidation leads to the formation of acetyl-CoA which is a substrate for the TCA/Krebbs cycle to be finally broken down to CO_2 and H_2O. This FFA oxidation is regulated by peroxisome proliferator activator receptor alpha (PPAR-α).[9] Alpha oxidation and omega oxidation occur in peroxisomes and endoplasmic reticulum, respectively. Omega oxidation removes the long chain of toxic fatty acids. Alpha oxidation helps in the breakdown of long-chain fatty acids but the enzymes are different.

HORMONAL REGULATION OF LIPID METABOLISM

Lipid pathways are primarily involved in energy generation, storage, and utilization. Adipocytes play a central role in energy use and expenditure during large variations in energy intake. These are one of the largest human cells containing TGs and cholesterol esters in central vacuoles. Fasting stimulates TG breakdown and the release of nonesterified fatty acids and glycerol into the blood through the activation of hormone-sensitive lipase.[10] It also reduces the uptake and storage of TGs. These actions are largely mediated through hormones. Most of the hormones act on the metabolic pathways directly except leptin and norepinephrine. In a fasting state, levels of glucagon, cortisol, growth hormone, and epinephrine are raised combined with low insulin and leptin levels.[11,12] Leptins play a limited role and their levels are affected during conditions of prolonged fasting. Hormone-sensitive lipase is stimulated by these elevated hormones directly or in an indirect manner. Glucagon and epinephrine directly activate the membrane-bound cAMP-CREB-CPT 1 pathway. Cortisol acts through the GR alpha-ANGPTL4 pathway and GH activates the PLC pathway. All these pathways finally lead to phosphorylation of HSL which leads to DGA, monoacyl glycerol formation, and fatty acid oxidation. Insulin plays a central role by promoting lipid synthesis, inhibiting breakdown, and facilitating the conversion of glucose to fatty acids. It acts through the PI3 Akt pathway. The downstream regulatory pathway includes the sterol regulatory element-binding protein 1c (SREBP1c) and the carbohydrate response element-binding-protein (ChREBP), which belong to lipogenic transcription factors activating lipogenic genes, such as *Fasn*, *ACC*, *Scd1*, and *Elovl6*. Insulin reduces LDL release. Epinephrine promotes lipid synthesis and storage in adipose tissue. Thyroid hormones enhance TG synthesis as well as lipid beta-oxidation. Estrogen potentiates fatty acid oxidation and decreases TG synthesis while the opposite is done by testosterone. During periods of stress, sepsis, organ failure, aging, and cancers these hormones play a major role in regulating lipid pathways. The role played by various hormones with their mechanism of action is described in **Table 1**.

MOLECULAR MEDIATORS OF LIPID METABOLISM

Peroxisome Proliferator-activated Receptor Alpha

Peroxisome proliferator activator receptor alpha is a transcription factor activated by ligand binding, such as free fatty acids. Its role comes during conditions of energy deprivation. PPAR-α is abundantly expressed in the liver, skeletal muscle, and heart. It promotes fatty acid uptake and mitochondrial as well as peroxisomal beta-oxidation by binding with retinoic acid receptors and targeting genes in a peroxisome proliferator response elements (PPREs) dependent manner.[13] It inhibits glycolysis and promotes gluconeogenesis and glycogenesis. In macrophages, it inhibits LDL uptake. Fibrates activate PPAR-α, upregulate LPL, and increase HDL and ApoC. They ultimately lead to

TABLE 1: Hormonal regulation of lipid metabolism and the molecular pathways involved in regulation.

Hormone	Molecular pathway	Effect on lipid
Insulin	SREBP↑, ChREBP↑, Fox O1↓	Promotion of synthesis
Glucagon	SREBP↓, ChREBP↓, ACC↓	Inhibition of synthesis
	PPAR-α, Aox, CTP1, Ctp1a↑, HSL in adipocytes↑	Promotion of catabolism
Thyroid hormone	• SREBP↑, ChREBP↑, ACC↑ • HMG CoA reductase↑ • PPAR-γ↓	Promotion of synthesis
	HSL ↑, ATGL↑, PPAR-α↑, Lipophagy↑	Promotion of catabolism
Estrogen	PPAR-γ↓, ACC↓	Inhibition of synthesis
Progesterone	SREBP↑	Promotion of synthesis
Androgen	SERBP↑, ChERB↑, ACC↑, Fasn↑	Promotion of synthesis
	Not known clearly	Promotion of catabolism
Growth hormone	• PPAR-γ↓ • Reducing insulin sensitivity	Inhibition of synthesis
	• WAT lipolysis↑ • HSL↑	Promotion of catabolism

Note: Fasting suppresses insulin levels and increases levels of glucagon, cortisol, and norepinephrine. This activates hormone-sensitive lipase which induces lipid breakdown and fatty acid release. Insulin promotes lipogenesis.

(ACC: acetyl CoA carboxylase; Aox: acyl CoA oxidase; ATGL: adipose triglycerol lipase; ChREBP: carbohydrate response element binding protein; CTP: carnitine acyl transferase 1; Fasn: fatty acid synthase; Fox: forkhead box; HSL: hormone-sensitive lipase; PPAR: peroxisome proliferator-activated receptor; SREBP: sterol regulatory element-binding proteins; WAT: white adipose tissue)

the clearance of TG-containing lipoproteins and reduce TG levels.[14]

Angiopoietin-like Proteins

Angiopoietin like 4 (ANGPLT4) is widely distributed in the human body. It serves as an autocrine regulator of LPL activity during fasting. In a fasting state, its levels are upregulated which increases the degradation of LPL and hence decreases the hydrolysis of TGs. This upregulation of ANGPLT4 is brought in by a combined action of decreased insulin levels, raised glucocorticoids, and free fatty acids.[15] During cold its levels are decreased in brown adipose tissue (BAT) but elevated in white adipose tissue (WAT). Most of the actions of ANGPLT4 occur at the posttranslational level. Its actions are antagonized by ANPLT 8.

Hypoxia-induced Lipid Droplet Association Proteins

Hypoxia-inducible factors (HIFs) are another group of heterodimeric transcription factors. Hypoxia enhances lipogenesis by HIF-dependent modulation of proteins involved in fatty acid (FA) uptake, synthesis, storage, and usage. Uptake of extracellular fatty acid and TAG synthesis are promoted under hypoxia by transcription factor *PPAR-γ*, the gene of which is directly activated by HIF-1.[16] Extracellular fatty acid influx and lipogenesis under hypoxia are also enhanced via HIF-1-mediated induction of the expression of fatty acid-binding protein (FABP) 3 and 7 in cancer cells.[17] In addition, HIF-1 can promote the endocytosis of lipoproteins, by upregulating the expression of low-density lipoprotein receptor-related protein (LRP1), the receptor that internalizes LDL in vascular smooth muscle cells, as well as the expression of VLDL receptor in cardiomyocytes.[18]

Hypoxia-inducible factor activation induces obesity. Hypoxia and obesity are also linked to liver diseases, such as nonalcoholic fatty liver disease (NAFLD), characterized by inflammation, fibrosis, and steatosis. Although the causality and molecular mechanisms that underlie NAFLD are not completely understood, the development of hypoxia in the liver is implicated in the pathogenesis of the disease.

STATES OF DYSREGULATION

A deregulatory state involving lipid metabolic pathways can cause the elevation of unwanted or bad lipids which finally lead to their accumulation in various arteries and precipitate ischemic events. They can arise from various genetic mutations or from acquired diseases. Familial forms of such lipid disorders are classified into five categories of hyperlipidemia by Fredriksons depending on the pathways involved and their health effects.[19]

Lipid Disorders with Elevated Triglycerides

Familial chylomicronemia syndrome (FCS, Fredriksons Type I), familial hypertriglyceridemia (FHTG, Fredriksons

Type IV, V), and familial dysbetalipoproteinemia (FDBL, Fredriksons Type III) are characterized by severe elevations of TGs.[19] Patients suffering from FDBL usually have a lower TG:Cholesterol ratio. Since chylomicrons and VLDL share a common metabolic pathway accumulation of either of two can result in TG elevation. FHTG and FCS are not associated with any major atherosclerotic cardiovascular disease (ASCVD) events, but the risk of pancreatitis is there when TG levels are above 500 mg/dL. DP1HBP1 homozygous mutations, LPL deficiency, and Apo CII deficiency result in hyperchylomicronemia. Hepatic lipase deficiency results in the accumulation of remnant lipoproteins.

Secondary causes of TG elevation are much more common than the familial forms. Obesity, insulin resistance, alcohol intake, estrogen treatment, and even excessive carbohydrate intake can cause an elevation of TGs. Drug therapy with beta-blockers, thiazide diuretics, and steroid therapy also leads to TG elevations.

Lipid Disorder with Elevated Cholesterol

Familial hypercholesterolemia (FH, Fredriksons Type IIa) causes an elevation in cholesterol levels with normal TG.[19] Familial hypercholesterolemia results from an absent LDL receptor function or a defective receptor function. LDL cholesterol levels are elevated due to decreased clearance of LDL itself and also from an increased conversion from IDL. FH is characterized by tendon xanthomas and premature CAD. ATP binding cassette gene mutations can lead to sitosterolemia characterized by the elevation in both plant sterols and cholesterol.[20] It results from increased intestinal absorption and decreased excretion of sterols. Hemolysis due to the incorporation of plant sterols into cell membrane is a characteristic feature of this disease. Gain of function mutation in the *PCSK9* gene results in an autosomal dominant form of hypercholesterolemia because of increased degradation of LDL receptors in lysosomes. Hypothyroidism, nephrotic syndrome, cholestasis, acute intermittent porphyria, and drug therapy are the usually encountered secondary causes.

Abnormal High-density Lipoprotein Metabolism Defects

Inherited deficiency of ApoA1 and LCAT enzyme causes low levels of HDL cholesterol.[21] ApoA1 is required for LCAT activity, so ApoA1 deficiency causes secondary LACT deficiency which results in increased levels of free cholesterol. This hinders the formation of mature HDL particles. Unlike Complete ApoA1 deficiency missense or nonsense mutation in *ApoA1* genes or LACT deficiency are not associated with premature ASCVD. Tangiers disease is characterized by ABCA1 deficiency that results in decreased efflux of cholesterol from cells to nascent ApoA1. This results in rapid removal of ApoA1 producing a clinical picture similar to LCAT deficiency. LDL cholesterol levels are also reduced in this disease.

Many inherited conditions can cause a rise in HDL cholesterol levels. Loss of function mutation in the *CETP* gene allele can increase their levels to >150 mg/dL.[22] LDL cholesterol levels are reduced. Though studies suggest that CETP deficiency protects against ASCVD pharmacological inhibition of CETP with torcetrapib gave disappointing results in clinical trials in reducing CV risk. **Table 2** summarizes the

TABLE 2: Familial lipid metabolism disorders and their clinical features.

Molecular defects (familial syndrome)	Lipoprotein levels	Clinical features
LPL and ApoCII deficiency (familial chylomicronemia syndrome)	Elevated chylomicrons	Eruptive xanthoma, hepatosplenomegaly, pancreatitis
LDL R, ApoB100, PCSK9 deficiency (familial hypercholesterolemia)	Elevated LDL	Tendon xanthomas, premature ASCVD
ABCG5, ABCG8 defects (sitosterolemia)	Elevated LDL	Tendon xanthomas, premature ASCVD
ApoE defects (familial dysbetalipoproteinemia)	Elevated chylomicron and VLDL remnants	Palmar and tuberoeruptive xanthoma, premature ASCVD
ApoA-V deficiency (familial hypertriglyceridemia)	• VLDL • VLDL and chylomicrons	Eruptive xanthoma, hepatosplenomegaly, and pancreatitis
Hepatic lipase deficiency	VLDL remnants	Pancreatitis, premature ASCVD
ABCA1 deficiency (Tangier's disease)	Low HDL levels	Hepatosplenomegaly, orange tonsils, neuropathy, premature ASCVD
LCAT deficiency	Low HDL level	Corneal opacification, renal disease, and hemolytic anemia
CETP deficiency	High HDL levels	Deceased ASCVD risk (uncertain)

(ABC: ATP-binding cassette transporter; ASCVD: atherosclerotic cardiovascular disease; CETP: cholesterol ester transfer protein; HDL: high-density lipoprotein; LCAT: lecithin cholesterol acyl transferase; LDL: low-density lipoprotein; LDL R: low-density lipoprotein receptor; LPL: lipoprotein lipase; PCSK9: proprotein convertase subtilisin/kexin 9; VLDL: very low-density lipoprotein) familial forms and the secondary forms of dyslipidemia, and their clinical picture.

Secondary Forms of Lipid Metabolic Disorder

Obesity, diabetes, hormone therapy, thyroid disease, nephrotic syndrome, and cholestasis are commonly encountered clinical disorders associated with dyslipidemia. Obesity is characterized by insulin resistance. This enhances fatty acid synthesis in the liver. Expanded adipose tissue mass delivers excess of free fatty acids liver. In the liver esterification of fatty acids occurs leading to increased formation of TGs. VLDL secretions are increasing. Some LDL elevation can be there. HDL levels are low due to reduced lipolysis. Obesity increases the risk of NAFLD characterized by the accumulation of fat in the liver. Adipocytes secrete various proinflammatory cytokines such as leptin, hepatocyte growth factor, TNF-α, IL-1β, and IL-6 which increase the risk of metabolic syndrome progression, steatohepatitis, and development of diabetes. Similarly high insulin levels in DM are associated with a decrease in LPL activity resulting in reduced clearance of chylomicrons and VLDL. VLDL synthesis is also increased; though, LDL levels are usually normal increased levels of dense LDL are seen. Estrogen therapy characteristically causes an elevation in both TGs as well as HDL cholesterol, a diametrically opposite phenomenon, due to an increase in synthesis rates of both. A similar pattern might also be seen with prolonged alcohol use. However, Alcohol consumption primarily causes raised TGs which can be severely elevated in the presence of an underlying primary lipoprotein disorder. Hyperlipidemia in nephrotic syndrome is due to a rise in synthesis as well as decreased clearance of VLDL and increased synthesis of LDL. Renal failure leads to mildly elevated VLDL and remnant lipoproteins. Cholestatic conditions result in hypercholesterolemia and skin lesions, such as FDBL (palmar and eruptive xanthomas). Lamellar particles LP-X which are found in the plasma of cholestatic patients which are formed from cholesterol combined with phospholipid.[23]

CONCLUSION

Lipid metabolism is the prime pathway of energy generation, storage, and utilization in the human body. Dietary sources and lipoprotein particles secreted from the liver are the starting points of the exogenous and endogenous pathways of lipid metabolism respectively. Steps in the pathways are tightly regulated by hormones secreted during fasting and energy repleted states. Both genetic mutations and acquired conditions can lead to derangement in these pathways and hence accumulation or even deficiency of particular kinds of lipids which ultimately lead to atherosclerotic cardiovascular events. Beneficial effects of drugs such as statins, fibrates, and CETP inhibitors are observed by modulating these pathways. Drugs such as PCSK9 inhibitors are the recent drugs to be added to such classes and many more are being tested in recent clinical trials exploiting these pathways.

ONLINE REFERENCES

Please scan the QR code provided at the end of the table of contents for References of this chapter.

Intensive Lipid-lowering Therapy for Early Achievement of Low-density Lipoprotein-C Targets in Cardiovascular Disease

CHAPTER 26

Saumitra Ray, Somnath Mukhopadhay, Srina Ray

ABSTRACT

Blood lipids are the most important risk factor for atherosclerotic cardiovascular disease. Of the different lipoproteins, low-density lipoprotein (LDL) has emerged as the primary culprit. Different patient populations have different targets for the LDL levels, as very clearly depicted by various guidelines. However, the ideal time frames to attain these goals remain rather elusive. An immediate and intense regimen of multiple LDL-lowering drug combinations can achieve these targets much faster than a stepwise approach. But how much they translate into clinical advantages remains to be fully addressed. There are some conflicting evidences for either approach. But with the advent of effective and safe options, the early intensive lowering of LDL is gaining momentum of late.

Keywords: Lipid-lowering therapy, LDL-C targets, intensive early regimen

INTRODUCTION

The world has witnessed an evolving era of lipid-lowering therapy (LLT) where different drugs of different classes have been used to modify our lipid values with the support of ever-changing guidelines to direct our journey. Till date, the most coveted goal is low-density lipoprotein (LDL) lowering. Studies revealed reduction of major adverse cardiovascular events (MACE) by 40–50% with each LDL-C reduction of 30 mg/dL.[1] Despite significant improvements in cardiovascular (CV) outcome with statin, around 40% of patients still suffer from CV events with ongoing statin therapy.[1]

LDL-C AS A PREDICTOR OF CARDIOVASCULAR DISEASE

Globally, an association between CV disease and cholesterol was seen as early as the mid-twentieth century.[2] Carl Muller observed high plaque deposition in familial hypercholesterolemia (FH) in 1939 and these patients faced a very high risk for CV death.[2-4] In 1952, John Gofman found high LDL in patients having myocardial infarction (MI) compared to healthy individuals.[2,5] The Framingham Heart Study established serum LDL-C as an independent risk factor for atherosclerotic cardiovascular disease (ASCVD) in 1977.[2,6]

LOW LDL-C AND DEMOGRAPHIC INSIGHT

Different studies showed that LDL-C of an average American is far from optimal values. The hunter-gatherer population of Hadza of Tanzania and Pacific Islanders of Pukapuka and Tokelau had lower serum cholesterol and a lower prevalence of CVD than the US population.[7-9] A survey of the Tsimane of Bolivia, a population with the lowest documented prevalence of atherosclerosis, revealed that they had an average LDL-C of 72 mg/dL.[10,11]

CURRENT RECOMMENDATION

Dyslipidemia management should be done according to the most recent guidelines with a combination of pharmacotherapy and lifestyle modification. Recent trials have shown consistent benefit of lowering LDL-C after acute coronary syndrome (ACS) in reducing CV events. There are numerous studies which already have shown benefit of LLT in CCS also. LLT remains one of the most meaningful therapies for primary and secondary prevention.

Over the last decade, LDL-C target has become consistently lowered. The American College of Cardiology/American Heart Association (ACC/AHA) in 2013 recognized that most clinicians used LDL-C targets of <100 and

<70 mg/dL for the primary and secondary prevention of ASCVD, respectively; the guidelines did not give specific targets due to the lack of clinical trials testing specific LDL-C targets. But they recommended high-intensity statin (HIS) to reduce LDL-C by 50% in high-risk patients and moderate-intensity statin to lower LDL-C 30–49% in intermediate-risk group.

In 2017, the American Association of Clinical Endocrinologists (AACE) and American College of Endocrinology (ACE) advised LDL-C goal of <55 mg/dL at an extreme risk for ASCVD.[12]

According to the latest European Society of Cardiology (ESC) guidelines, the current treatment goal is to lower LDL-C to <55 mg/dL and to achieve ≥50% reduction from baseline (Class I) **(Flowchart 1)**. For patients who experienced a second CV event within 2 years, not necessarily of the same type as the first event, an LDL-C goal < 40 mg/dL appears to confer more benefit (Class IIb).[13]

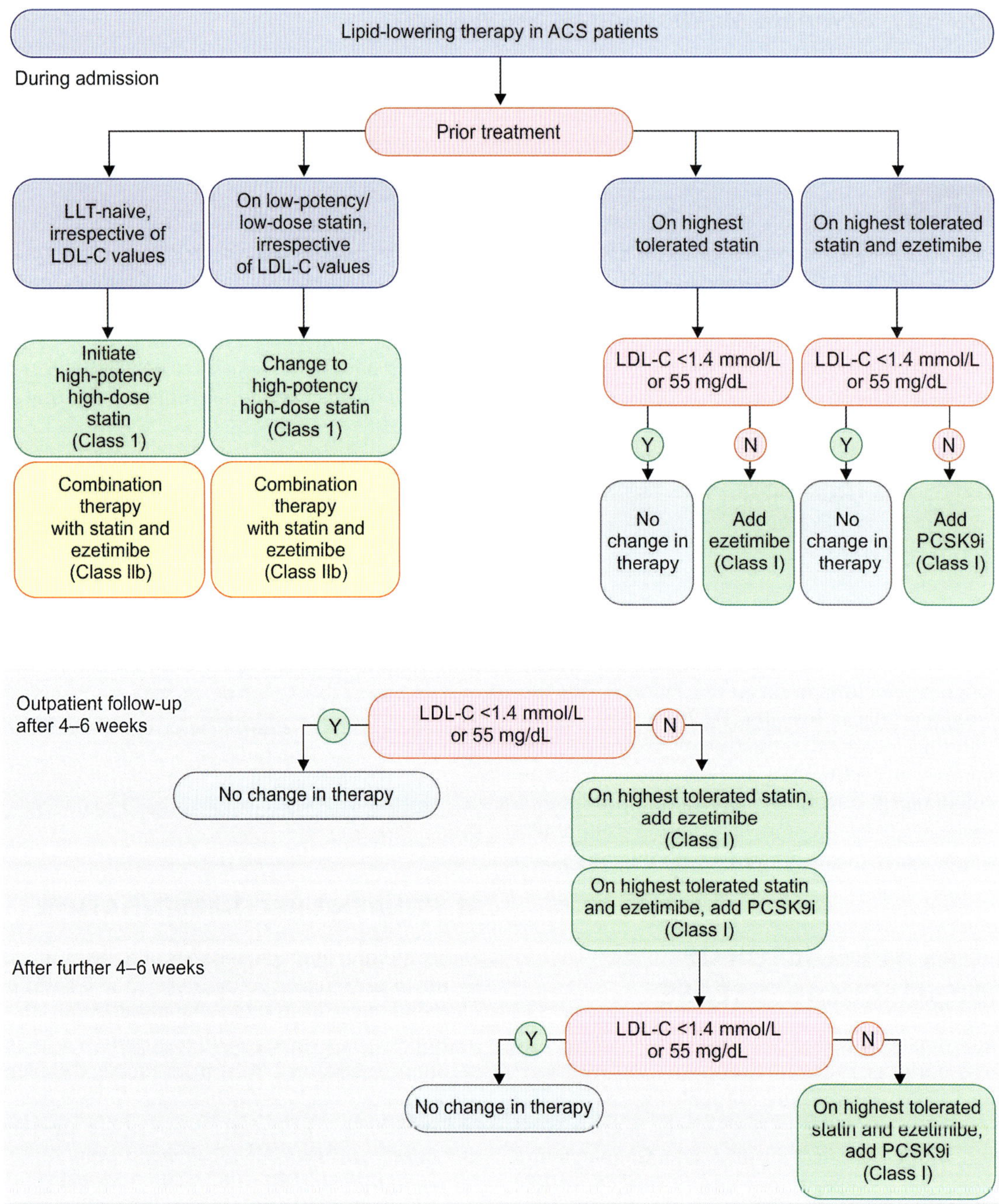

FLOWCHART 1: Guideline-directed LLT in ACS.

The 2020 LAI guidelines recommended treatment target 100 mg/dL for low or intermediate risk, 70 mg/dL for high risk, and 50 mg/dL for very high risk, defined as preexisting ASCVD, DM with ≥2 risk factors/target organ damage or homozygous FH. For extreme-risk patients—those with CAD and one or more feature of high-risk group [i.e., DM with zero to one other major ASCVD risk factor, CKD stage 3B or 4, coronary calcium score > 300 HU, Lp(a) > 50 mg/dL, etc.]—a treatment target of 50 mg/dL was recommended with an optional goal of 30 mg/dL. Individuals at an extreme risk with recurrent ACS, polyvascular disease, or an additional "very high risk" factor were recommended a more intensive treatment target of 30 mg/dL.[14]

After an ACS event, an intensive early regimen with LLT should be initiated as early as possible for prognostic benefit and for better patient adherence.[15] HIS should be given in maximum tolerated dose to achieve LDL-C goal. After the IMPROVE-IT trial, add-on therapy of ezetimibe with statin appeared safe and provided long-term benefit for CV outcomes. After the ODYSSEY OUTCOMES trial, treatment with proprotein convertase subtilisin/kexin type 9 (PCSK9) inhibitor alirocumab appeared safe and effective in reducing LDL-C after hospitalization with ACS. Recent data also showed improvements in plaque phenotype and plaque regression in ACS treated with PCSK9 inhibitor. In all scenarios, lipid profile should be re-evaluated 4–6 weeks after each treatment or dose adjustment to find out treatment goal achievement and safety issues. The therapeutic regimen can then be decided accordingly.

INDIAN PERSPECTIVE OF RECENT GUIDELINES

Recently, the Cardiological Society of India elaborated these managements in a simplified and acceptable fashion. They have stratified the risk and given algorithms for the management of dyslipidemias in different scenarios **(Flowcharts 2 to 4)**.

Lipid-Lowering Pharmacotherapy

See **Table 1**.

The Lower the Better

There are numerous trials which showed benefits of statin in primary prevention as well as in secondary prevention. The Scandinavian Simvastatin Survival Study (4S) showed not only CV event reduction but also survival benefit with a 30% relative risk reduction in all-cause mortality with simvastatin.[17] In the MIRACL study, atorvastatin, shortly initiated after MI, showed 16% relative risk reduction of the primary end point.[18] In the TNT study, atorvastatin 80 mg showed 22% major CV outcome reduction in stable CHD patients compared to atorvastatin 10 mg.[19] Moreover, a meta-analysis comprising 26 RCTs manifested around 10% reduction in all-cause mortality with each 1.0 mmol/L LDL-C reduction by more intensive statin therapy **(Flowchart 5)**.[20]

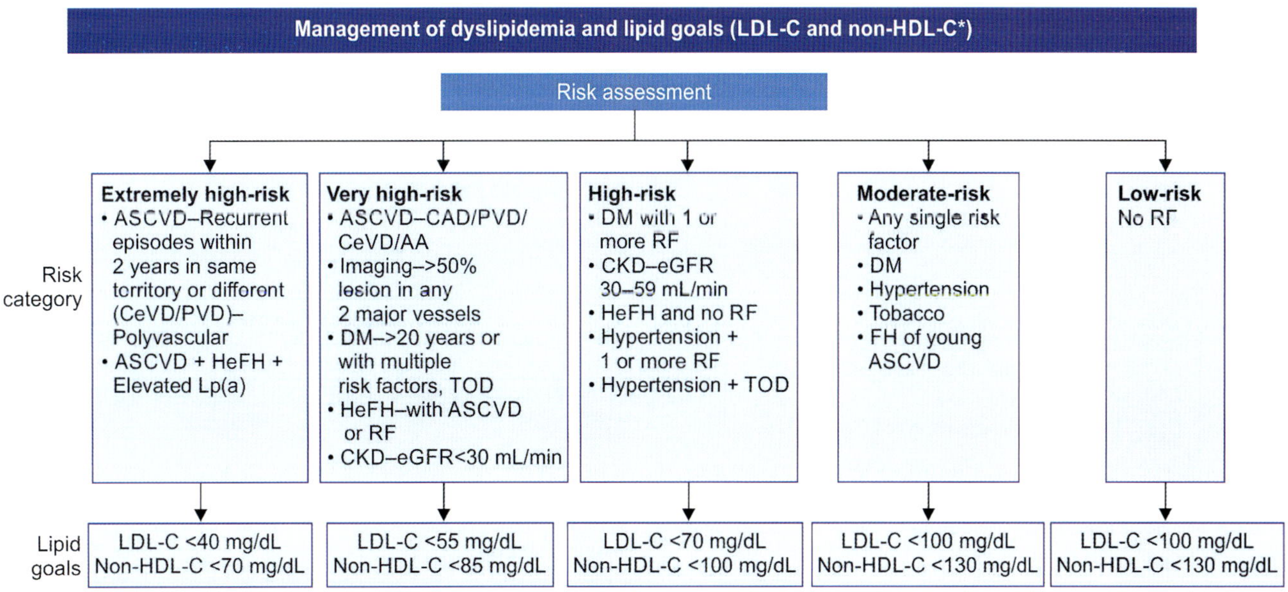

*Non-HDL-C as coprimary goal because of increased prevalence of atherogenic dyslipidemia in our country.

FLOWCHART 2: Management of dyslipidemia and lipid goal.[16]

Note: In the absence of our own risk score calculator, only risk factors are used for risk assessment.

(AA: arotic aneurysm; ASCVD: atherosclerotic cardiovascular disease; CAD: coronary artery disease CeVD: verebrovascular disease; CKD: chronic kidney disease; DM: diabetes mellitus; FH: family history; LDL-C: low-density lipoprotein cholesterol; HDL-C: high-density lipoprotein cholesterol; HeFH: heterozygous familial hyperchloesterolemia; PVD: peripheral vascular disease; RF: risk factor; TOD: target organ damage)

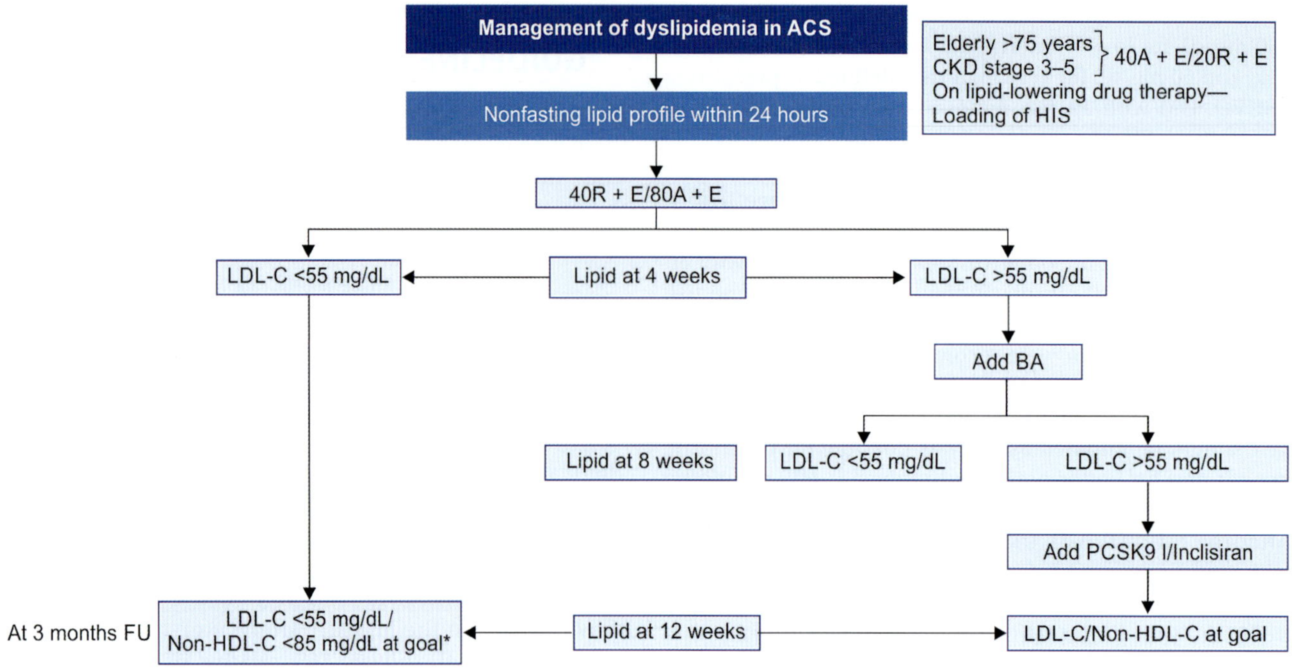

*Look for Non-HDL target if TG is ≥ 150 mg/dL, If Non-HDL not at goal—add bempedoic acid, If extreme high riskm goal should be LDL-C <40 mg/dL/non-HDL <70 mg/dL.

FLOWCHART 3: Management of dyslipidemia in ACS.[16]

Note: If patient has statin-associated muscle symptoms (SAMS), new-onset diabetes or worsening HbA1c in prediabetic patient—downtitrate statin (R40 to R20 or A80 to A40) followed by lipid profile at 4 weeks.

[A: atovastatin; ACS: acute coronary syndrome; BA: bempedoic acid; E: ezetimibe; FU: follow-up; HIS: high intensity statin (R-20-40 mg, A-40-80 mg); R: rosuvastatin]

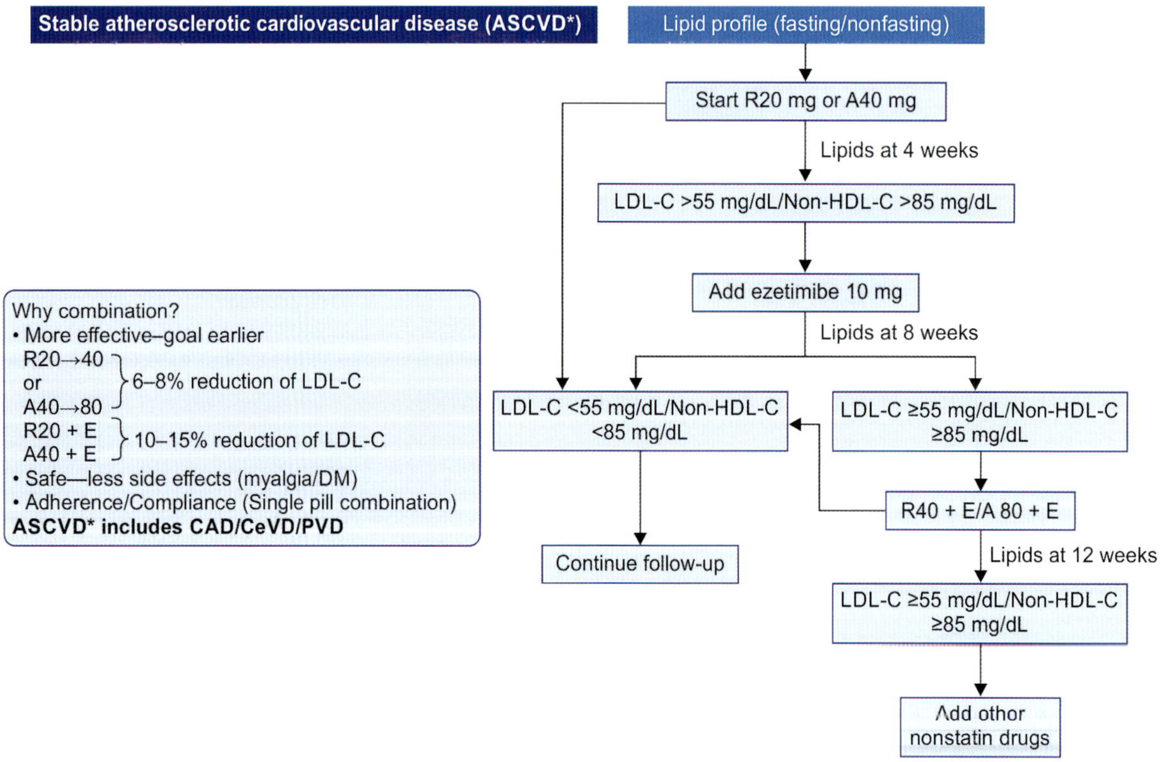

FLOWCHART 4: Management of dyslipidemia in ASCVD.[16]

(A: atorvastatin; E: ezetimibe; R: rosuvastatin)

TABLE 1: Drugs for dyslipidemia and their details.

Drug	Year of FDA approval	Mechanism of action	Major trial	Comments
Nicotinic acid (niacin)	1950	Not well-defined	(a) Coronary Drug Project (b) AIM-HIGH (c) HPS2-THRIVE	(a) 11% lower mortality with h/o MI compared to placebo (b) and (c) did not demonstrate vascular event reduction compared to statin monotherapy
Bile acid sequestrants (cholestyramine, colesevelam, colestipol)	1970	Increased cholesterol metabolism via bile excretion	LRC-CPPT	Colestipol reduced risk of CHD mortality by 24% in middle-aged men with primary hypercholesterolemia
Fibrates (gemfibrozil, fenofibrate)	1970	Promote receptor-mediated LDL-C clearance and increased catabolism of LDL-C	• Helsinki Heart Study • FIELD • ACCORD	34% reduction in incidence of CHD in middle aged men with dyslipidemia in the HHS study, but not supported by the other two
Lovastatin	1987	Competitive inhibitor of HMG-CoA reductase	AFCAPS/TEXCAPS	Reduced risk of major coronary events by 37% in patients with moderately elevated cholesterol
Pravastatin	1991	Competitive inhibitor of HMG-CoA reductase	CARE	Reduced incidence of fatal coronary events or nonfatal MI by 24% in patients with MI who had cholesterol level <240 mg/dL
Atorvastatin	1996	Competitive inhibitor of HMG-CoA reductase	Treating to New Targets (TNT)	22% relative risk reduction in CV events with 80 mg/day over 10 mg/day in stable CHD
Simvastatin	1998	Competitive inhibitor of HMG-CoA reductase	Scandinavian Simvastatin Survival Study (4S)	30% reduction in mortality in CHD
Rosuvastatin	2003	Competitive inhibitor of HMG-CoA reductase	Justification for the use of Statins in Prevention Trial Evaluating Rosuvastatin (JUPITER)	Rosuvastatin decreased CV events by 44% in patients with LDL-C <130 mg/dL but elevated CRP
Ezetimibe	2004	Inhibitor of NPC1L1 cholesterol transporter	Improved Reduction of Outcomes: Vytorin Efficacy International Trial (IMPROVE-IT)	Ezetimibe–simvastatin therapy provided reduction in LDL-C levels with 6% relative risk reduction in adverse CV outcome compared to statin monotherapy
Lomitapide	2012	Microsomal triglyceride transfer protein inhibitor	Phase III Trials	50% reduction in LDL-C at 26 weeks in homozygous FH
Mipomersen	2013	Small interfering RNA inhibitor of apolipoprotein B	RCT with FH on Lipid-lowering Therapy	36% reduction in LDL-C and significant reductions in apolipoprotein B
Alirocumab	2015	Monoclonal antibody inhibitor of PCSK9	Evaluation of Cardiovascular Outcomes after an Acute Coronary Syndrome during Treatment with Alirocumab (ODYSSEY OUTCOMES)	15% relative risk reduction for ASCVD events in ACS already on statin
Evolocumab	2015	Monoclonal antibody inhibitor of PCSK9	Further Cardiovascular Outcomes Research with PCSK9 Inhibition in Subjects with Elevated Risk (FOURIER)	15% relative risk reduction for ASCVD events in ASCVD patients on statin therapy

Continued

Continued

Drug	Year of FDA approval	Mechanism of action	Major trial	Comments
Bempedoic acid	2020	Adenosine triphosphate citrate lyase inhibitor	Cholesterol Lowering via Bempedoic Acid, an ACL-Inhibiting Regimen (CLEAR OUTCOMES)	Bempedoic acid compared to placebo given to patients with statin intolerance demonstrated a reduction in primary end point of CV mortality, nonfatal MI, nonfatal stroke, or coronary revascularization of 13%
Evinacumab	2021	Monoclonal antibody inhibitor of angiopoietin-like protein 3	Evinacumab for Homozygous Familial Hypercholesterolemia (ELIPSE HoFH)	49% reduction in LDL-C
Inclisiran	2021	Small interfering RNA inhibitor of PCSK9	Inclisiran for Participants with Atherosclerotic Cardiovascular Disease and Elevated Low-density Lipoprotein Cholesterol (ORION-10 and -11)	50% reduction in LDL-C in ASCVD patients on maximally tolerated statin; CV outcome trials are ongoing

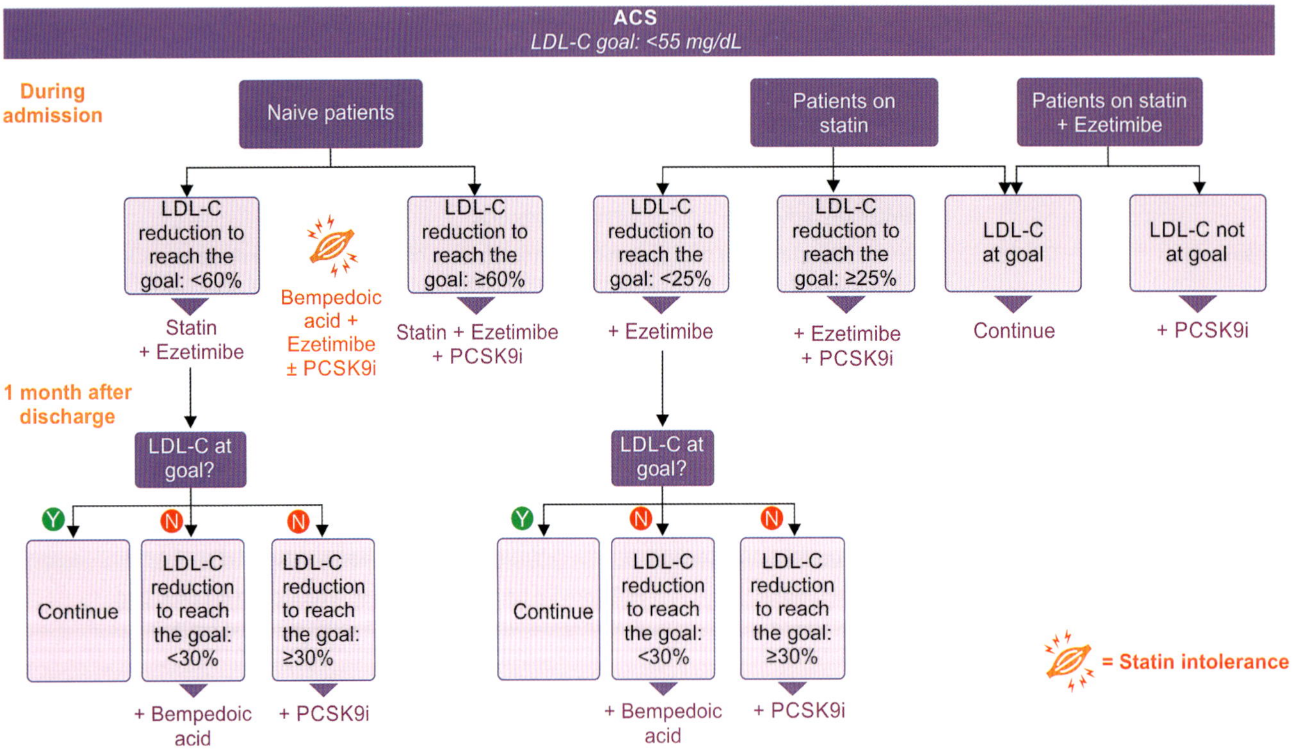

FLOWCHART 5: Proposed algorithm to manage LDL-C after ACS.[1]

The IMPROVE-IT trial showed that adding ezetimibe to statin further reduced LDL-C from 70 to 54 mg/dL with a relative risk reduction in CV outcome of 6.7% over 7 years in ACS setting.[21] In the FOURIER trial, the PCSK9 inhibitor evolocumab had been tested in stable CHD patients over a median follow-up of 2.2 years. It lowered LDL-C by 59% to a median of 30 mg/dL, which led to a 15% relative risk reduction of the primary end point—a composite of CV death, MI, stroke, hospitalization for unstable angina, or coronary revascularization.[22] This benefit was extended with evolocumab over 8 years with persistent low rates of adverse CV events compared to delayed initiation as suggested by the FOURIER-OLE study.[23] The ODYSSEY study echoed similar findings with alirocumab after ACS with a median follow-up of 2.8 years. LDL-C reduction was around 63% and relative risk reduction was 15% for primary end point—composed of death from coronary heart disease, nonfatal MI, fatal or nonfatal ischemic stroke, or unstable angina requiring hospitalization.[24] Aggressive LDL-C lowering was associated with reduction of CV events and recurrence which was approximately double that of the first occurrence of an ASCVD primary end point, indicating that the benefits of profound LDL-C lowering extend beyond the prevention of the first ASCVD events.[25,26]

In the FOURIER trial, we found that patients achieving LDL-C levels < 20 mg/dL after 4 weeks of evolocumab had the lowest risk for ischemic events in the entire study population without a rise in adverse events.[27] Similarly, the ODYSSEY Outcomes study reported that LDL-C of <25 mg/dL had a particularly low risk of MACE similar to that of patients who achieved LDL-C levels of 25–50 mg/dL (0.65–1.3 mmol/L) without excess risk of hemorrhagic stroke or dementia.[28] These findings were further supported by a meta-analysis, including 10 RCTs and >38,000 subjects, which showed that very low LDL-C levels on intensive LLT were not associated with any adverse event and maintained a persistent reduction in CV events.[29] The GLAGOV study substantiated the potential benefit of PCSK9 inhibitor evolocumab, which when added to statin resulted in atherosclerotic plaque regression in CAD picked up by IVUS.[30]

Our new weapon is inclisiran. This is a small interfering ribonucleic acid (siRNA)-based technology which can degrade PCSK9 mRNA in the liver to inhibit its translation, and thus eliminates the source of PCSK9 in the circulation. Different studies showed that it can reduce LDL-C by up to 52% in a well-tolerated manner.[31] Phase III trials are there to show the potential benefit of inclisiran in reduction of MACE. However, larger studies are needed to validate this with longer follow-ups.[32]

In our current practice, an achievable LDL-C value can be predicted with a drug alone or in combination: An average reduction in LDL-C levels of 60% is with PCSK9 inhibitor therapy alone, 75% in combination with HIS, and even 85% in combination with statin and ezetimibe.[17] If we double the statin dose, a further 6% reduction can be done. Hence, there is a paradigm shift toward "high-intensity LLT" as the first line, especially in very high-risk patients. This may be a rational and effective approach. In the case of statin intolerance, the combination can be ezetimibe plus bempedoic acid or PCSK9i, according to the baseline values. A more intensive regimen comprising the statin, ezetimibe, and PCSK9 inhibitors should be prescribed to ACS patients who are already on a statin and ezetimibe, as well as those ACS-naïve patients whose LDL-C level should decrease ~80% to reach the LDL-C-recommended level. Triple therapy can also be given to the extremely high-risk patients.

REAL-WORLD EVIDENCE

In the real-world scenario, the achievements of LDL-C goal are much less considering the available guidelines. This gap in treatment has been shown in numerous studies. The Da Vinci study is an important study which reported that HIS monotherapy was used by 20% of the very high-risk patients for primary prevention and 38% of patients for secondary prevention. Higher use was mainly seen in CAD (51%) than in PVD (39%) or cerebral (40%) diseases. In a study called the Santorini study, 21.0% of very high-risk patients and 23.5% of high-risk patients did not have any LLT at all. Moreover, physicians frequently underestimated the very high risk in patients, leading to false risk stratification. According to physicians, 29.2% were classified as high CV risk and 70.8% as very high risk. But when the CV risk was assessed properly, only 6.5% of patients were at high risk and 91.0% of patients were in the very high-risk group. In an Indian study, it was seen that out of 575 study population, only around 21% managed to achieve a target LDL-C of <55 mg/dL after 1 year, despite being on HIS.

CONTROVERSIES

The *Journal of the American Heart Association* recently published a study where more than 14,000 participants were examined in the National Health and Nutrition Examination Survey (NHANES). This study found an increased risk of all-cause mortality (HR 1.45, 95% CI 1.10–1.93) in those with LDL-C < 70 mg/dL compared to those with LDL-C of 100–129.9 mg/dL (controlling for demographic factors and comorbidities) over around 20 years.[33] But there might have been some confounding factors like subclinical comorbidities which may not be adjusted for. Moreover, other clinical trials have not corroborated these results during achieving low LDL-C levels. Some association was there who had elevated high-sensitivity CRP levels > 2 mg/dL.[34,35] There was another warning of potential association between LDL-C < 70 mg/dL and the incidence of intracranial hemorrhage (ICH) stroke;[36] this association persisted during using LDL-C 70–99.9 mg/dL or LDL-C 100–129.9 mg/dL as the reference mark.[37,38] The IMPROVE-IT trial demonstrated a nonsignificant trend toward rise in hemorrhagic stroke treated to a relatively lower LDL-C goal with ezetimibe and simvastatin. But a subsequent 2017 analysis showed significant reductions in MACE when LDL-C was <30 mg/dL compared to ≥70 mg/dL, without a concomitant rise in rates of neurocognitive events, hemorrhagic stroke, or non-CVD deaths.[39] Contemporary clinical trials did not corroborate association between very low LDL-C and higher rate of adverse events. The EBBINGHAUS study demonstrated no difference in the effects on cognitive function with excess lipid lowering using evolocumab.[38,39] But definitely longer-term follow-up data is needed. Till date, competing data suggested that further CV and mortality benefits are there with aggressive LDL-C reduction. The AHA recently published a scientific statement on this perspective of LDL-C lowering and the risk for hemorrhagic CVA and dementia. They stated that achieving very low LDL-C did not increase the risk for hemorrhagic CVA and that the risk of a hemorrhagic CVA associated with statin therapy in patients without a history of CVD is small and consistently nonsignificant.[39]

FUTURE DIRECTION

Studies have not yet established whether inclisiran will result in reduction in clinical events as has been shown with other PCSK9 inhibitors. Inclisiran is being tested in the ongoing ORION-4 (NCT03705234) and VICTORION-2 Prevent (NCT05030428) trials in this respect. EVOLVE-MI will test the effect of adding evolocumab to the standard care on major CV events in 4,000 post-AMI hospitalized patients. Another study named VICTORION-INCEPTION in a post-ACS setting will assess the effectiveness of inclisiran with persistently high LDL-C despite statin. The AMUNDSEN trial is aiming to study LDL-C reduction at 12 months with tertiary clinical end points after randomizing patients to receive evolocumab with the first dose given before PCI. Current cutting-edge research in the field of LLT is gene editing. VERVE-101 is a CRISP-Cas 9-based genome editing medication prepared to permanently inactivate PCSK9 gene expression. It showed efficacy in reducing PCSK9 level and circulating LDL-C in nonhuman primates and mouse models.[39] The ongoing Heart-1 trial is the first-in-human study investigating a single intravenous infusion of VERVE-101 in patients with heterozygous FH and established ASCVD on maximally tolerated oral LLT. Early results demonstrate efficacy in PCSK9 downexpression, with a mean reduction of 69% in LDL-C levels without safety concerns in the short term, providing proof of concept for in vivo DNA base editing in a human body.

VACCINE

Though the vaccination to manage atherosclerosis is an attractive strategy, the development of an ideal vaccine is challenging. It can disrupt the body's tolerance to self-antigens without triggering an immune response from autoreactive T cells that could attack healthy cells. Thus, in spite of the promising initial results, the vaccine has never gone beyond animal models.

CONCLUSION

In recent days, intensive LLT is largely dominated by the PCSK9 inhibition beyond HIS and ezetimibe.[40,41] Efficacy and safety are making this path more acceptable, whereas cost remains the main barrier in our country. One important aspect is development of resistance by the formation of neutralizing antibodies against these anti-PCSK9 mAbs. Another important thing to mention is a physician's inertia toward high-intensity LLT. Despite substantial improvements in understanding, the LDL-C goal is often underachieved. But this exploratory science is always searching for the solution. Ever-advancing lipidology and pharmacotherapy are continuously raising hope to overcome the dynamic nature of lipid control and to promote good CV health.

ONLINE REFERENCES

Please scan the QR code provided at the end of the table of contents for References of this chapter.

New Low-density Lipoprotein Cholesterol—Lowering Agents: Update on PCSK9 Inhibitor Monoclonal Antibodies, Inclisiran, and Bempedoic Acid

CHAPTER 27

Vimal Mehta, Pratishtha Mehra, Jamal Yusuf

ABSTRACT

There is an epidemic of atherosclerotic cardiovascular disease (ASCVD) in India which is due to poor cardiovascular (CV) risk factor control, especially dyslipidemia. The incidence of ASCVD and associated mortality is decreasing in Western countries, whereas it continues to rise in India. Dyslipidemia is highly prevalent in our country and has maximum population-attributable risk for CV events. Although statins are the first line to control low-density lipoprotein cholesterol (LDL-C) levels, many patients are unable to tolerate them because of perceived or real side effects. Also, statin therapy has relatively limited efficacy, especially in patients with high baseline LDL-C levels; hence, newer therapies are required to attain ever-decreasing LDL-C targets. Therefore, introduction of newer treatment options will not only make possible the attainment of LDL-C goals but also help control the epidemic of ASCVD. This chapter describes the efficacy and safety of three novel treatment options like proprotein convertase subtilisin/kexin type 9 inhibitor monoclonal antibodies (PCSK9i mabs)—alirocumab/evolocumab, a small interfering ribonucleic acid (siRNA) targeting proprotein convertase subtilisin/kexin type 9 (PCSK9)—inclisiran, and adenosine triphosphate (ATP) citrate lyase inhibitor—bempedoic acid.

Keywords: Bempedoic acid, dyslipidemia management, extreme-risk group, inclisiran, low-density lipoprotein cholesterol, PCSK9 inhibitor monoclonal antibodies

INTRODUCTION

Indians develop atherosclerotic cardiovascular disease (ASCVD) about a decade earlier than the Western populations, despite having lower levels of low-density lipoprotein cholesterol (LDL-C).[1] Dyslipidemia is highly prevalent with the ICMR-INDIAB-17 study reporting low high-density lipoprotein cholesterol (HDL-C) levels along with hypertriglyceridemia as the most common lipid abnormalities.[2]

There is a huge gap between guideline-directed goals and LDL-C targets achieved in the real world, especially with ever-decreasing guideline-recommended LDL-C goals. Furthermore, there is no lower LDL-C threshold below which benefits cease to exist.[3] Recent trials/post hoc analyses have shown further significant reduction in cardiovascular (CV) events with very low LDL-C levels (≤30 mg/dL).[4,5] Accordingly, the Lipid Association of India (LAI) recommendations have given LDL-C targets of <50 mg/dL in very high-risk group, and <50, ≤30, and 10–15 mg/dL in extreme-risk group, categories A, B, and C, respectively, according to the LAI risk stratification algorithm.[6-8]

Several newer lipid-lowering agents with different mechanisms have become available recently, including proprotein convertase subtilisin/kexin type 9 inhibitor monoclonal antibodies (PCSK9i mabs)—alirocumab/evolocumab, a small interfering ribonucleic acid (siRNA) targeting PCSK9—inclisiran, and adenosine triphosphate (ATP) citrate lyase inhibitor—bempedoic acid **(Table 1)**.

PROPROTEIN CONVERTASE SUBTILISIN/KEXIN TYPE 9

Proprotein convertase subtilisin/kexin type 9 (PCSK9) is expressed predominantly in the hepatocytes and regulates the activity of LDL receptor (LDLR). PCSK9 binds to the LDLR resulting in lysosomal degradation of the LDLR after internalization of the receptor along with LDL particle inside the liver. If PCSK9 is absent during internalization of the LDLR to deliver LDL particle, the LDLR recycles

TABLE 1: Expected average percent reduction in blood LDL-C levels with various lipid-lowering regimens in patients without familial homozygous hypercholesterolemia.

Lipid lowering therapy	LDL-C lowering (%)
Moderate intensity statin	30–40%
High intensity statin	50–55%
Ezetimibe	18–20%
High intensity statin + ezetimibe	60–65%
Bempedoic acid with statins	≈15%
Bempedoic acid without statins	≈25%
Ezetimibe + bempedoic acid	≈36%
High intensity statin + ezetimibe + bempedoic acid	≈75%
PCSK9 inhibitor monoclonal antibodies	55–60%
PCSK9 inhibitor monoclonal antibodies + high intensity statin	75–80%
PCSK9 inhibitor monoclonal antibodies + high intensity statin + ezetimibe	80–85%
Inclisiran	45–50%

back to the hepatocyte surface to catch more LDL particles from the circulation. Thus, PCSK9 inhibitors prevent LDLR degradation, thereby increasing the concentration of LDLRs on the hepatocyte surface resulting in increased clearance of LDL-C from the circulation.[7]

PCSK9 Inhibitor Monoclonal Antibodies

Two fully human monoclonal antibodies targeting PCSK9 are available, alirocumab and evolocumab. In India, only evolocumab is marketed. The dose of alirocumab is 75 mg/150 mg administered subcutaneously every 2 weeks or 300 mg monthly. The evolocumab dose is 140 mg subcutaneously every 2 weeks or 420 mg monthly. The LDL-C levels should be checked about 2 weeks after third biweekly injection to determine the LDL-C-lowering response. Both decrease LDL-C levels by about 55–60%, triglycerides decrease by about 15%, lipoprotein(a) [Lp(a)] decreases by 25–30%, and HDL-C increases by 5–10%, but have no effect on high-sensitivity C-reactive protein (hsCRP) levels.[7,9,10]

Evolocumab Randomized Clinical Trials

The FOURIER (Further Cardiovascular Outcomes Research with PCSK9 Inhibition in Subjects with Elevated Risk) study randomized 27,564 patients who had prior MI, stroke, or symptomatic peripheral arterial disease (PAD) and LDL-C ≥ 70 mg/dL/non-HDL-C ≥ 100 mg/dL on maximal statins to evolocumab or placebo.[11] Evolocumab reduced median LDL-C levels from 92 to 30 mg/dL (59% decrease), non-HDL-C by 52%, and ApoB by 49% ($p < 0.001$). The 5-point primary end point (HR 0.85; $p < 0.001$) and secondary end point (CV death, MI, or stroke) (HR 0.80; $p < 0.001$) decreased significantly at a median follow-up of 2.2 years, mostly by ischemic endpoint reduction **(Table 2)**. The serious adverse events were similar, except minor injection-site reactions with evolocumab.[11] The CV events progressively decreased with further LDL-C lowering, with an adjusted HR of 0.69 with LDL-C < 10 mg/dL for primary end point and 0.59 for secondary end point compared with LDL-C ≥ 100 mg/dL. The high-risk subgroups like recent MI, multivessel disease, or PAD had more event rates and derived additional benefit.[12,13]

FOURIER-OLE was an open-label extension (OLE) study from the original FOURIER study enrolling 6,635 patients receiving evolocumab for a median of 5 years, with maximum duration on evolocumab for patients initially randomized to evolocumab being 8.4 years.[14] The median achieved LDL-C was 30 mg/dL at 12 weeks. Those who continued on evolocumab from the FOURIER study had 15% reduction in 5-point major adverse CV events (MACE) (HR 0.85; $p = 0.008$), 20% reduction in MI, stroke, and CV death (HR 0.80; $p = 0.003$), and 23% reduction in CV death (HR 0.77; $p = 0.04$) compared to those assigned placebo in the FOURIER study and who later received evolocumab. There were no safety concerns.[14] The above suggests that attaining very low LDL-C levels is not only safe but also associated with additional benefits especially when started early.

Alirocumab Clinical Trials

Alirocumab has been evaluated in many clinical studies. The ODYSSEY OUTCOMES trial enrolled 18,924 patients with a history of an acute coronary syndrome (ACS) in the past 12 months and LDL-C ≥ 70 mg/dL/non-HDL ≥ 100 mg/dL/ApoB ≥ 80 mg/dL despite statins. The patients were randomized to alirocumab (n = 9,462) or placebo (n = 9,462). At 2.8-year median follow-up, alirocumab decreased LDL-C levels by 54.7%. The 4-point primary end point significantly decreased with alirocumab versus placebo (HR 0.85; $p < 0.0003$) mainly due to decrease in ischemic events of nonfatal MI by 14%, stroke by 27%, and unstable angina by 39% **(Table 2)**. There were only minor injection-site reactions with alirocumab.[15] Interestingly, in patients with baseline LDL-C ≥ 100 mg/dL (30% of total cohort), the MACE reduced by 24%, with all end points showing significant reduction, including CAD and CV death reduction by 28% and 31% respectively, signifying the benefit of additional LDL-C lowering beyond stains, especially in patients at higher risk with high baseline LDL-C values.

PCSK9 Inhibitor Monoclonal Antibodies in Acute Coronary Syndrome

The risk of adverse CV events is the highest immediately after ACS. Therefore, it is plausible that very early LDL-C lowering to ultralow levels will be beneficial in reducing MACE.

TABLE 2: Baseline characteristics and cardiovascular outcomes in FOURIER and ODYSSEY OUTCOMES trials.

	FOURIER trial	ODYSSEY OUTCOMES trial
Total number of patients	27,564	18,924
Patient population	*Stable ASCVD*: History of myocardial infarction, nonhemorrhagic stroke, symptomatic peripheral artery disease	*Recent acute coronary syndrome (ACS)*: Hospitalization for ACS (myocardial infarction or unstable angina) 1–12 months before randomization
Age (mean, years)	63	58.5
Qualifying LDL-C (mg/dL)	≥70	≥70
Baseline LDL-C (mg/dL)	92 (median)	92 ± 31 (mean ± SD)
Follow-up (months)	26	34
Primary end point	*5-Point MACE*: Cardiovascular death, myocardial infarction, stroke, hospitalization for unstable angina, or coronary revascularization	*4-Point MACE*: Coronary heart disease death, nonfatal myocardial infarction, fatal or nonfatal ischemic stroke, or unstable angina requiring hospitalization
Secondary end point	Composite of cardiovascular death, myocardial infarction, or stroke	Composite of death from any cause, nonfatal myocardial infarction, or nonfatal ischemic stroke
High-intensity statin use (%)	69.5	89
Achieved LDL-C (mg/dL)	30 mg/dL at 12 weeks (median)	38 mg/dL at 4 months (mean, on-treatment analysis)
Cardiovascular outcomes (relative risk reduction)		
Primary end point (%)	15	15
Secondary end point (%)	20	14
Myocardial infarction (%)	27	14
Stroke (%)	21	27
Coronary revascularization (%)	22	12

The Evolocumab for Early Reduction of LDL-Cholesterol Levels in Patients with Acute Coronary Syndromes (EVOPACS) study randomized 308 ACS patients to evolocumab 420 mg or placebo, administered in-hospital and at 4 weeks plus atorvastatin 40 mg. The LDL-C <70 mg/dL was attained in 95.7% of patients given evolocumab compared with 37.6% on placebo at 8 weeks.[16]

The Evolocumab in Acute Coronary Syndrome (EVACS) trial randomized 57 patients with non-ST-elevation MI (NSTEMI) to a single evolocumab 420-mg injection or placebo within 24 hours of the index event. The LDL-C levels significantly decreased with evolocumab compared with placebo by day 3 demonstrating the efficacy of PCSK9i mabs in promptly attaining LDL-C goals. The LDL-C levels of <70 and <55 mg/dL at hospital discharge were attained in 80.8% and 65.4% of patients, respectively, compared with 38.1% and 23.8% on placebo.[17]

The PACMAN-AMI trial randomized 300 acute MI patients undergoing primary angioplasty to either biweekly 150 mg alirocumab ($n = 148$) or placebo ($n = 152$). Alirocumab decreased LDL-C level to 33.8 mg/dL resulting in placebo-controlled percent atheroma volume decrease of 1.21%, and increase in minimal fibrous cap thickness of 29.65 μm, assessed in two non-infarct-related coronaries at 52 weeks suggesting coronary plaque regression.[18]

Thus, initiation of evolocumab during index hospitalization results in marked LDL-C reduction with guideline-directed LDL-C goals achieved in majority as well as plaque regression. However, CV outcomes study of early PCSK9 inhibitors use is lacking and is needed to confirm the clinical benefit of intensive early LDL-C reduction after ACS.[19]

Regulatory Approval

The Central Drugs Standard Control Organization (CDSCO) in India permitted use of evolocumab in subjects with HoFH on February 21, 2017, and for clinical ASCVD on March 27, 2018.[20] Alirocumab is not yet approved in India.

INCLISIRAN

Inclisiran is a long-acting synthetic siRNA targeting PCSK9 mRNA that inhibits the translation of the PCSK9 protein in hepatocytes.[21,22] Therapies based on siRNA require less frequent dosing compared with other RNA-based therapies like antisense oligonucleotides. siRNA molecules (21–23 nucleotides) are double-stranded RNA molecules consisting of a guide (antisense) strand and a passenger (sense) strand.[21,22] In order to achieve the targeted uptake by the liver to avoid off-target effects, inclisiran is conjugated to the carbohydrate moiety triantennary *N*-acetylgalactosamine (GalNAc), which binds specifically to asialoglycoprotein receptors on hepatocytes.[21,22] The PCSK9 synthesis inhibition increases the recycling and expression of LDL-C receptors resulting in increased uptake of LDL particles, thereby reducing LDL-C levels.

Dosing and Administration

Inclisiran sodium is given as 300-mg subcutaneous injection (equivalent to 284 mg inclisiran) in the abdomen, thigh, or upper arm, with the first dose administered on the first day, followed by a second injection on day 90, and then every 6 months. This dosing schedule is based on the ORION-1 trial, which reported approximately 50% reduction in LDL-C levels at 180 and 240 days after two doses (days 1 and 90).[23] This schedule has been validated in the Phase 3 trials.[24,25] Inclisiran is available as 1.5-mL solution packaged in a prefilled glass syringe. Unlike the PCSK9i mAbs which are self-administered injections, inclisiran is recommended to be administered by a healthcare professional.

Pharmacokinetics

The peak plasma levels of inclisiran occur approximately 4 hours after dosing and are not detectable in plasma after 24–48 hours. Inclisiran is 87% protein bound with volume of distribution of about 500 L and is mostly metabolized by nonspecific nucleases into inactive shorter nucleotides with excretion partly through the kidneys. The terminal elimination half-life is approximately 9 hours with no accumulation occurring with multiple dosing.[26] Since inclisiran does not induce or inhibit cytochrome P450 enzymes or other common drug transporters, clinically significant drug–drug interactions are unlikely. It is not indicated in pregnant or breast-feeding women.[21]

If a planned dose is missed by <3 months, inclisiran should be administered and dosing continued according to the patient's original schedule. If a planned dose is missed by >3 months, a new dosing schedule should be started as in a new patient. In transitioning from PCSK9i mabs, inclisiran can be administered immediately after the last dose of PCSK9i mab or within 2 weeks after the last dose of PCSK9i mab.[21,22,26]

In patients with mild/moderate (Child–Pugh class A/B) hepatic disease or mild/moderate renal impairment, no dose adjustment is required. There are no data in patients with severe hepatic disease (Child–Pugh class C) or with severe renal impairment.[26] The safety and efficacy of inclisiran in children < 18 years and in solid organ transplant recipients is not established.

Clinical Efficacy and Safety

The efficacy of inclisiran has been tested in various trials under the ORION program. The phase II ORION-1 trial which evaluated different dosing schedules reported the highest LDL-C reduction with two 300-mg doses (days 1 and 90) of 52.6% at 180 days. At day 240, LDL-C was 47.2% lower and at 1 year, LDL-C was 31.4% lower compared to baseline. The PCSK9 levels decreased by 69.1 ± 12.1% at day 180, with sustained reduction of 40% at day 240. The non-HDL-C decreased by 46 ± 14.6%, ApoB by 40.9 ± 14.8%, triglycerides by 14.2%, VLDL-C by 16%, and Lp(a) by 25.6% at day 180. The HDL-C increased by 8.6 ± 14.9% at day 180.[23]

ORION-9 randomized 482 adult heterozygous familial hypercholesterolemia (HeFH) patients on maximal statins ± ezetimibe with a baseline LDL-C ≥ 100 mg/dL to inclisiran on days 1, 90, 270, and 450 or placebo. The mean LDL-C reduction was 39.7% at day 510. The PCSK9 levels decreased by 60.7%. There was significant LDL-C reduction across the genetic variants (LDLR, ApoB, and PCSK9).[24]

The ORION-10 and ORION-11 trials assessed the efficacy of inclisiran in secondary prevention and high-risk primary prevention patients with LDL-C ≥ 70 mg/dL and ASCVD (ORION-10 and ORION-11) or LDL-C ≥ 100 mg/dL and ASCVD risk equivalent such as diabetes, familial hypercholesterolemia, or 10-year ASCVD risk ≥ 20% (ORION-11).[25] The LDL-C levels reduced by 52.3% in the ORION-10 trial and by 49.9% in the ORION-11 trial ($p < 0.001$). The placebo-corrected reduction in Lp(a) was 26% in the ORION-10 trial and 19% in the ORION-11 trial.[25] A pooled analysis of ORION-9, 10, 11 studies described mean placebo-corrected decrease in LDL-C of 50.7% at day 510 with inclisiran.[27]

In ORION-3, an open label 4-year extension study, patients receiving inclisiran in ORION-1 were given twice-yearly inclisiran (inclisiran-only arm), whereas patients receiving placebo in ORION-1 first received evolocumab 140 mg every 2 weeks until day 360 and then twice-yearly inclisiran (switching arm). In the inclisiran-only arm, the mean sustained LDL-C reduction was 44.2% over nine injections. In the switching arm, evolocumab resulted in 61% LDL-C reduction. After switching to inclisiran, the 3-year time-averaged LDL-C reduction was 45.3% over seven injections. This suggests that evolocumab is more effective in reducing LDL-C.[28]

Clinical Use

Inclisiran has effectively lowered LDL-C but cardiovascular outcome data are lacking. It may improve adherence by a twice-yearly maintenance dosing schedule. The high cost imposes selective use in patients who are not at LDL-C goal despite being on statins along with ezetimibe and bempedoic acid.

Adverse Effects

The adverse-event profile of inclisiran was similar to that of placebo except for transient, minor injection-site reactions.[23-25] Mild elevations of serum hepatic transaminases ≤3 times upper limit of normal were more common with inclisiran than with placebo. Inclisiran has not been shown to be carcinogenic in experimental animals.[26]

Regulatory Approval

Inclisiran was approved in the European Union in December 2020 and by the US FDA in December 2021 as an adjunct to diet and maximal statin therapy for adult patients with HeFH or ASCVD.[26,29] Inclisiran was approved in India by the CDSCO in July 2023.[30]

Ongoing Trials

ORION-8 (NCT03814187) is an extension trial of ORION-9, 10, 11 and includes patients with homozygous FH. The TIMI 65/ORION-4 trial (NCT03705234) aims to compare clinical outcomes for 5 years among 15,000 adults with established ASCVD. VICTORION-1 PREVENT aims to evaluate patients at high risk of developing ASCVD by assessing the incidence of 4-point MACE. VICTORION-2 PREVENT is studying patients with established ASCVD and LDL-C ≥70 mg/dL on stable lipid-lowering therapy. The VICTORION-PLAQUE (NCT05360446) is evaluating inclisiran efficacy on atherosclerotic plaque progression in subjects with nonobstructive CAD.

BEMPEDOIC ACID

Bempedoic acid is a prodrug that is converted to its active component, bempedoyl-coenzyme A, by the enzyme very long-chain acyl-CoA synthetase-1 expressed in the liver.[31] A cytosolic enzyme called ATP-citrate lyase, which is upstream of HMG-CoA reductase in the cholesterol biosynthesis pathway, is competitively inhibited by bempedoyl-coenzyme A. The inhibition of cholesterol synthesis in the liver increases the hepatic expression of LDLRs, thereby decreasing the circulating LDL-C levels. The absence of acyl-CoA synthetase 1 in skeletal muscle, the activating enzyme of bempedoic acid, prevents muscle toxicity.[31-33]

Pharmacokinetics

The half-life of bempedoic acid, an oral, once-daily, small molecule, is 15–24 hours with median time to maximum concentration (T_{max}) of 3.5 hours. It is available as a 180-mg tablet, which is absorbed in the small intestine, and food has no impact on oral bioavailability. The pharmacokinetic properties are not affected by age, sex, race, or weight. The steady state is reached after 7 days of treatment. The drug is about 99% protein bound in plasma.[32,33]

The major metabolites of bempedoic acid are glucuronides of bempedoic acid and bempedoyl-CoA. With 70% of excretion occurring in urine and 30% in feces, the kidneys are the primary route of elimination. The exposure rises by 1.4 and 1.9 times with mild and moderate renal impairment, respectively. Patients who have mild/moderate hepatic impairment have 22% lower plasma levels. Patients with Child–Pugh class C hepatic cirrhosis and end-stage renal disease have not been studied. Being mild organic anion transporter 2 (OAT2) inhibitor, competition between uric acid and bempedoic acid glucuronide metabolite for the same renal OAT2 transporter results in minor increases in plasma uric acid and creatinine.[31-33]

Drug–Drug Interactions

There are few significant drug interactions with bempedoic acid. The cytochrome P450 enzymes CYP3A4/CYP2C9, which are involved in metabolism of statins, do not metabolize bempedoic acid or bempedoyl-CoA. Hence, cytochrome P450-mediated medication interactions do not exist. Warfarin does not interact with bempedoic acid. Simvastatin and pravastatin concentrations increase by about 2- and 1.5-fold, respectively, in combination with bempedoic acid.[31-33]

Clinical Studies

The CLEAR (Cholesterol Lowering through Bempedoic acid, an ACL-Inhibiting Regimen) program tested bempedoic acid in five randomized clinical trials in different patient populations. CLEAR Tranquility and CLEAR Serenity evaluated patients with hypercholesterolemia and statin intolerance, whereas CLEAR Harmony and CLEAR Wisdom explored bempedoic acid in patients with ASCVD or high risk of ASCVD and HeFH. CLEAR Outcomes was a large study evaluating impact on clinical end points.

In the CLEAR Serenity trial, 345 subjects with hypercholesterolemia (mean LDL-C 157.6 mg/dL) and statin intolerance were randomized 2:1 to bempedoic acid or placebo for 24 weeks. At week 12, LDL-C decreased significantly in the bempedoic acid group (placebo-corrected decrease 21.4%; $p < 0.001$). The non-HDL-C decreased by 17.9%, total cholesterol by 14.8%, ApoB by 15.0%, hsCRP by 24.3% (all $p < 0.001$), and HDL-C by 4.5% ($p = 0.003$). The new-onset diabetes or diabetes worsening was lower with bempedoic acid (2.1% vs. 4.5%).[34]

The CLEAR Tranquility trial randomized (2:1) 269 participants with statin intolerance and LDL-C ≥100 mg/dL to bempedoic acid or placebo in addition to ezetimibe 10 mg/day for 12 weeks. Bempedoic acid + ezetimibe group had 28.5% placebo-corrected LDL-C reduction ($p < 0.001$). The efficacy of bempedoic acid in decreasing LDL-C was more without background statins versus with statins (–34.7% vs. –20.5%), since both drugs act on the identical pathway.[35]

The CLEAR Harmony study randomized (2:1) 2,230 patients with ASCVD, HeFH, or both, on maximal statins with LDL-C ≥70 mg/dL to bempedoic acid or placebo. The mean LDL-C levels reduced by 16.5%, $p < 0.001$, at 12 weeks.[36] In the CLEAR Harmony 78-week, OLE study (overall 130 weeks), bempedoic acid was given to all patients. The mean LDL-C decreased by about 15%, non-HDL-C by 11%, ApoB by 7%, total cholesterol by 10%, and hsCRP by

17% at 78 weeks, showing sustained LDL-C-lowering efficacy over 2.5 years without any safety concerns.[37]

In the CLEAR Wisdom trial, 779 patients with ASCVD, HeFH, or both were randomized to receive bempedoic acid or placebo for 52 weeks on top of optimal statin therapy. The baseline LDL-C of 120.4 ± 37.9 mg/dL decreased by 15.1% at 12 weeks in the bempedoic acid group.[38]

The combined analysis of 4 trials which included 3,623 patients showed a mean initial LDL-C level in patients with either ASCVD or HeFH or together decreased from 107.6 mg/dL by 16% with bempedoic acid, whereas in patients with statin intolerance, it decreased from 144.4 mg/dL by 23% at 12 weeks, with sustained LDL-C lowering at 52 weeks, confirming better efficacy of bempedoic acid in the absence of statins.[39]

The CLEAR OUTCOMES trial randomized 13,970 patients to bempedoic acid or placebo group with a median follow-up of 40.6 months. There were 22.7% of patients on statin and 11.5% on ezetimibe. The mean baseline LDL-C level of 139 mg/dL showed placebo-corrected reduction of 21.1% in the bempedoic acid group at 6 months. The primary endpoint incidence reduced significantly with bempedoic acid versus placebo (11.7% vs. 13.3%; HR 0.87; $p = 0.004$) as did the incidence of composite of CV death, nonfatal MI, or nonfatal stroke (8.2% vs. 9.5%; HR 0.85; $p = 0.006$). The endpoint reduction was due to significant reduction in ischemic events of MI and coronary revascularization with no effect on CV or all-cause death.[40]

Bempedoic acid significantly lowered LDL-C as well as hsCRP, with no significant effect on fibrinogen and IL-6 levels.[41] In a real-world open-label study, 122 patients with ACS received concurrent triple therapy with rosuvastatin 40 mg/day, ezetimibe 10 mg/day, and bempedoic acid 180 mg/day that resulted in 57.7, 61.7, 61.9, and 60.6% reductions in LDL-C at week 1, 2, 4, and 6, respectively ($p < 0.001$).[42]

Clinical Use

Bempedoic acid is a third-line drug after statins and ezetimibe **(Flowchart 1)**. Patients with a history of gout may have exacerbation during treatment with bempedoic acid, and uricosuric drugs may be required. The monitoring of uric acid levels may be needed in patients with hyperuricemia.

Adverse Events

In phase III studies, the minor side effects occurred equally commonly in bempedoic acid and placebo groups. Muscle symptoms were seen when bempedoic acid was given with statins; however, no increased frequency was seen when given alone. Bempedoic acid reversibly increases mean uric acid levels by about 0.80 mg/dL which can exacerbate gout. Few cases of tendon rupture have been reported; however, there was the presence of confounding factors like older age and corticosteroids use. There can be a clinically insignificant increase in blood urea nitrogen and serum creatinine. The incidence of cholelithiasis was higher with bempedoic acid in the CLEAR OUTCOMES trial.[37-40]

Regulatory Approval

In India, the CDSCO granted permission to manufacture/market bempedoic acid 180-mg tablets on April 6, 2022.[43]

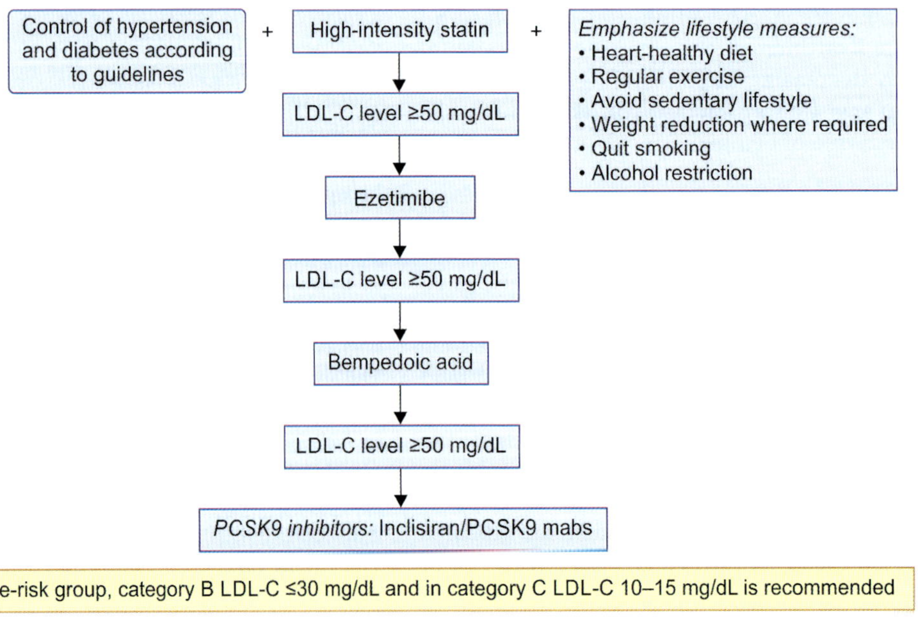

FLOWCHART 1: Treatment algorithm to achieve LDL-C goals in secondary prevention according to the Lipid Association of India.

CONCLUSION

As emphasized by LAI, LDL-C targets are to be attained in all patients as per the LAI risk stratification algorithm. High-intensity statin therapy (atorvastatin 40–80 mg or rosuvastatin 20–40 mg OD) is the backbone of lipid lowering followed by ezetimibe 10 mg OD and bempedoic acid 180 mg OD in patients with established ASCVD and HeFH.[8] In patients with true statin intolerance, ezetimibe 10 mg OD alone or in combination with bempedoic acid is recommended.[31] PCSK9 inhibitors are required when targets are still not achieved **(Flowchart 1)**.[7] Physician's decision is paramount along with a detailed discussion with the patient (shared decision) before initiating intensive lipid-lowering therapy.

ONLINE REFERENCES

Please scan the QR code provided at the end of the table of contents for References of this chapter.

CHAPTER

28

Lipoprotein(a) in Clinical Practice: A Guide for Clinicians

Arvind Kumar, Vipin Kumar

ABSTRACT

Residual risk remains in many patients despite aggressive lipid lowering and risk factor management. Lipoprotein(a) [Lp(a)] is another novel risk marker, which has independent effect on atherosclerotic cardiovascular disease (ASCVD) risk and calcific aortic valve stenosis (CAVS). It is genetically determined by *LPA* gene and its level remains stable throughout life. Hence, Lp(a) measurement is recommended at least once in a lifetime to assess ASCVD risk. Management includes lifestyle modification, aggressive low-density lipoprotein (LDL)-C reduction by statins, and other antilipid therapies. Proprotein convertase subtilisin/kexin type 9 (PCSK9) inhibitors can be added in patients with high LDL-C and LP(a) with high-dose statins and they reduce Lp(a) also by 20–30%. Lipoprotein apheresis is the only approved specific therapy to target high Lp(a) and recommended for high-risk patients with familial hypercholesteremia (FH) and ASCVD, whose Lp(a) level remains ≥60 mg/dL (~150 nmol/L) and LDL-C ≥100 mg/dL on maximally tolerated lipid-lowering therapy. Various targeted Lp(a) therapies are in development, such as antisense oligonucleotide and small interfering RNA (siRNA), which can reduce Lp(a) by 80–100%.

Keywords: Lipoprotein(a) [Lp(a)], atherosclerotic cardiovascular disease (ASCVD), ASCVD risk, calcific aortic stenosis, novel biomarker

INTRODUCTION

Assessment and management of atherosclerotic cardiovascular disease (ASCVD) risk include lipid measurements and its reduction with high-dose statin therapy and other targeted antilipid therapies like ezetimibe, bempedoic acid, proprotein convertase subtilisin/kexin type 9 (PCSK9) inhibitors, and novel synthetic small interfering RNA (siRNA), inclisiran. Significant residual risk remains in many patients, even with targeting these and other traditional cardiovascular risk factors. Lipoprotein(a) [Lp(a)] is another promising biomarker, the elevated levels of which have been found to be associated with an increased risk of ASCVD as well as calcific aortic stenosis.[1,2] Lp(a) is a type of low-density lipoprotein (LDL) that contains apolipoprotein(a) [Apo(a)] attached to its surface in addition to apolipoprotein B100.[3] About 20–30% of the world's population has been estimated to have high levels of Lp(a),[4] although there is high variation observed in different racial groups. Clinical implications of Lp(a), its pathogenic mechanism, and current management strategies are reviewed here.

WHAT IS LIPOPROTEIN(a)?

Lipoprotein(a) is a type of LDL particle, which contains additional Apo(a) linked to the apolipoprotein(B) [ApoB] component of the LDL particle by a disulfide bond.[5] Risks associated with Lp(a) are attributed to both its components Apo(a) and ApoB, which have an adverse impact on atherosclerosis, thrombosis, and inflammation.[3,6]

PATHOGENESIS OF LIPOPROTEIN(a)

Apolipoprotein(a) moiety of Lp(a) contains oxidized phospholipids, which increase production of proinflammatory cytokines, induce arterial wall inflammation, and promote atherogenesis, while ApoB contributes to atherogenesis through entry into the vessel wall and subsequent oxidation to highly inflammatory oxidized LDL (oxLDL), as with other LDL and ApoB100 particles.[7] Apo(a) also has structural similarity to plasminogen, which may also pose a procoagulant effect[8] and leads to Lp(a) binding to plasminogen receptors on vascular endothelial cells, causing inhibition of plasmin generation and fibrinolysis.[9] Apo(a) also binds to exposed vascular endothelium, which leads to endothelial uptake and accumulation of Lp(a) within atherosclerotic lesions and endothelial dysfunction.[10]

Lipoprotein(a) binding to valvular endothelium via Apo(a) and its deposition into valvular cells has been attributed to the development of calcific aortic valve disease.[11] Proinflammatory activity associated with oxidized phospholipids found in the Lp(a) molecule promotes differentiation of vascular cells into osteoblasts leading to calcification of valves.[12-15] Further calcification is promoted by autotaxin and lysophosphatidylcholine distributed with Lp(a) in aortic valvular interstitial cells.[16]

METABOLISM

LPA gene primarily determines Lp(a) concentration in serum in an autosomal-dominant fashion, and the number of kringle domains in it determines Apo(a) size.[6,17,18] *LPA* gene completely expresses itself by 1–2 years of age and its peak level is achieved at age 5 years. Although there is considerable heterogeneity in terms of Apo(a) size, present evidence suggests that atherogenesis related to Lp(a) appears to be mediated by the concentration of Lp(a) only.[19] Plasma Lp(a) concentration varies reversely with the size of Apo(a) particles and is not greatly influenced by dietary factors.[6] It can also be affected by several other single-nucleotide polymorphisms within the *LPA* gene.[20,21] These variations and polymorphisms in the *LPA* gene contribute to individual heterogeneity.[5] Lp(a) clearance is likely to be mediated by hepatic scavenger receptors and plasminogen receptors, and it remains in plasma longer than LDL.[6]

EVIDENCE OF ASSOCIATION WITH ATHEROSCLEROTIC CARDIOVASCULAR DISEASE/CALCIFIC AORTIC VALVE STENOSIS/MORTALITY

Elevated Lp(a) levels have been found to be associated with a high risk of cardiovascular events, most consistent with myocardial infarction (MI) and calcific aortic valve stenosis (CAVS).[20,22-25] It is also associated with an increase in the risk of peripheral artery disease, abdominal aortic aneurysms, and major adverse limb events,[26] while no association has been found for venous thromboembolism.[20,27] A higher Lp(a) level is required to see a similar increase in the risk of heart failure,[20,23] ischemic stroke,[20,22,23,25] and cardiovascular mortality.[23,25,28,29] For example, in European ancestry in the Copenhagen General Population Study, the Lp(a) level associated with HR of 1.5 for MI was 193 nmol/L (89.5 mg/dL) and for CAVS was 154 nmol/L (71.3 mg/dL), whereas the levels were higher for ischemic stroke [323 nmol/L (150 mg/dL)] and heart failure [261 nmol/L (121 mg/dL)].[20]

A continuous, log-linear relationship between baseline Lp(a) and risk for ASCVD events was observed in two analyses of the UK Biobank, with a small increase in risk even at low levels of Lp(a) (25–50 nmol/L).[22,23] Hence, clinical risk assessment and decision-making should involve the degree of Lp(a) elevation and presence of other risk factors, not merely by elevation of Lp(a) alone above a threshold of 125 nmol/L or 50 mg/dL. Also no impact of race on Lp(a)-attributable risk was found despite observed differences in median Lp(a) levels between different racial/ethnic groups.[22,23] Analysis of a large multiethnic US pooled cohort of five prospective studies showed consistent increases in ASCVD risk associated with higher Lp(a) levels by sex and race/ethnicity.[30] Hence, race-based definitions of elevated Lp(a) are not recommended.[31]

Studies by both Cowell et al. (SALTIRE investigators) and Zheng et al. found that the greatest tertile of Lp(a) level (>35 mg/dL) is associated with a higher degree of aortic valve calcification.[15,32] A specific single-nucleotide variation located within the *LPA* gene (rs10455872) was significantly linked to the existence of aortic valve calcification (OR per allele, 2.05) in a study involving 6,942 participants from the CHARGE cohort.[33] Similarly, Lp(a) levels >30 mg/dL were linked to increased calcification activity, as measured by ^{18}Fsodium fluoride on PET scans, and a higher rate of progression of the disease, as seen on CT scans and echocardiography.[15]

Also in a study, Lp(a) levels have been found to provide incremental and independent prognostic information to C-reactive protein levels for risk estimates of ASCVD, MI, and CAVS.[34]

Prevalence of elevated Lp(a) levels in Indians and south Asians is approximately 25% and considering more prevalent malignant and premature CAD in Indians, the role of Lp(a) as a risk factor becomes more important.[35] In an observational cohort study of Indian participants, Lp(a) >30 mg/dL was associated with higher incidences of cardiac death, major adverse cardiovascular events (MACE), MI, and revascularization.[36] Similarly in an smaller case-control study involving south Indian participants, elevated Lp(a) levels were found to be associated with more severe coronary artery disease.[37]

LABORATORY MEASUREMENT OF LIPOPROTEIN(a)

Lipoprotein(a) levels remain stable throughout a person's lifetime, as >90% of its values are determined by genetics related to the *LPA* gene, not being significantly affected by diet or environment.[7,38] Hence, Lp(a) measurement needs to be done only once in a lifetime.[13] On the basis of genetic and epidemiological evidence, current consensus statement from the ESC recommends measuring Lp(a) once in a lifetime for all adults to determine individuals at high CVD risk.[20]

Lipoprotein(a) measurement is not done in routine lipid measurement assays. Total Lp(a) mass in milligrams per deciliter, as measured in older-generation assays, used measurement of Apo(a) and was dependent on the isoform size.[14,39] Hence, use of particle concentration units (nmol/L) rather than mass units is preferred because of this isoform size heterogeneity. Although if correctly measured, both were found to be similarly predictive of cardiovascular event risk,[40] the National Lipid Association (NLA) recommends Lp(a) measurement in nmol/L.

Lipoprotein(a) genetic risk scores incorporating genetic variants at or near LPA locus can identify higher-risk individuals,[25,41,42] but have no incremental value for CVD risk classification compared with Lp(a) concentrations alone.[25] Therefore, Lp(a) measurement alone is preferable for risk stratification.

CURRENT GUIDELINE-BASED RECOMMENDATIONS ON SCREENING FOR LIPOPROTEIN(a)

Elevated Lp(a) remains a risk factor for ASCVD even with aggressive LDL-C lowering by statins and other antilipid therapies.[43-45] As risks associated with elevated LDL-C and non-high-density lipoprotein cholesterol (non-HDL-C) levels along with elevated Lp(a) levels are increased manifold, more intensive therapy is required in these patients.[20]

The 2018 American College of Cardiology/American Heart Association (ACC/AHA) Task Force guideline for the management of blood cholesterol and the 2019 ACC/AHA guideline on the primary prevention of cardiovascular disease recommended measurement of Lp(a) in patients with a family history of premature ASCVD and provided a threshold of Lp(a) ≥ 50 mg/dL or ≥125 nmol/L as a risk-enhancing factor for CVD to help guide preventive intervention.[46,47] The 2019 ESC/European Atherosclerosis Society guideline for management of dyslipidemias and most recently NLA[31] recommend measurement of Lp(a) at least once in an adult's lifetime, for selected patients with a family history of premature ASCVD (similar to ACC/AHA) and suspected familial hypercholesterolemia, and for reclassification in people between moderate and high risk.[8] Lp(a) measurement can be used in individuals with first-degree relatives with premature ASCVD, personal history of premature ASCVD, and primary severe hypercholesterolemia, to clarify ASCVD risk.[48] The NLA recommends values of Lp(a) ≥ 125 nmol/L (≥50 mg/dL) to be considered high risk, levels < 75 nmol/L (<30 mg/dL) as low risk, and intermediate values as intermediate risk.[31] The Lipid Association of India (LAI) defines Lp(a) > 50 mg/dL as high-risk criteria and between 20 and 49 mg/dL as a risk modifier for risk stratification of ASCVD risk.[49]

CURRENT MANAGEMENT STRATEGIES IN PATIENTS WITH ELEVATED LIPOPROTEIN(a)

Managing individuals with elevated Lp(a) levels should involve a multipronged approach, identification, and aggressive risk factor management. They should optimize the therapy of other modifiable risk factors such as hypertension, smoking, diabetes, weight, and physical inactivity. They should achieve a LDL-C goal of <70 mg/dL (the lower the better), through lifestyle modifications either alone or with various medications. First-degree relatives of individuals with high Lp(a) should be screened to identify familial risk. Individuals with elevated Lp(a) (≳125 nmol/L) with optimal cardiovascular health scores had a lower risk of incident CVD compared with individuals with lower Lp(a) levels with poor cardiovascular health in a large prospective observational study.[50]

Aspirin for primary prevention is not well established with some trials suggesting more harm than benefit. The 2019 ACC/AHA guideline on the primary prevention of CVD recommends aspirin in adults with an elevated ASCVD risk but at a low risk of bleeding (Class IIb recommendation).[47] However, individuals with elevated Lp(a) levels may have beneficial effects with aspirin therapy, which is seen in analyses of Women's Health Study[51] and the Aspirin in Reducing Events in the Elderly (ASPREE) trial.[52] As Lp(a) has prothrombotic effects, aspirin may be beneficial in patients with elevated Lp(a), with no increased risk of bleeding.[52] Therefore, aspirin is recommended for primary prevention in patients with elevated Lp(a), after assessing risks and benefits.[31]

Despite the inability to decrease and mild propensity to increase Lp(a),[53] statins remain the mainstay therapy for LDL-C reduction and clearly showed reduction in ASCVD risk and MACE.[54,55] Hence, statins should not be discontinued because of this small Lp(a) elevation.

Lipoprotein(a) levels are not found to be significantly reduced by either ezetimibe or bempedoic acid.[56,57]

Lipoprotein(a) levels show about 20–30% reduction with PCSK9 inhibitors (evolocumab and alirocumab) and siRNAs (inclisiran).[45,58,59] In the Further Cardiovascular Outcomes Research with PCSK9 Inhibition in Subjects with Elevated Risk (FOURIER) trial in stable ASCVD patients, evolocumab, individuals with elevated Lp(a) had a greater relative risk reduction than those without elevated Lp(a). Patients with baseline Lp(a) above the median (120 nmol/L; HR 0.75) achieved 25% reduction in MACE as compared to 11% in those with baseline Lp(a) at or below the median (HR 0.89). This data points that higher-risk patients get more benefit from intensive LDL-C- and Lp(a)-lowering therapy.[45] Similar findings were observed in ODYSSEY outcomes, in which reduction in MACE was higher among patients with higher baseline Lp(a).[60] Therefore, in higher-risk patients with elevated LDL-C and Lp(a) with maximally tolerated statin therapy, a PCSK9 inhibitor may be added to further reduce risk, though PCSK9 inhibitors are not approved for use only to reduce Lp(a) levels.

Niacin therapy lowers Lp(a) levels by about 23% by decreasing Apo(a) production rate.[61] Combination therapy of niacin and statins did not show clinical benefit despite ~20% reductions in Lp(a) level in two recent trials, AIM HIGH and HPS2 THRIVE.[61,62] A higher risk of diabetes, myopathy, and infection was noted in these trials. Therefore, niacin is not recommended for Lp(a) lowering.

Lipoprotein apheresis (LA) is the only FDA-approved therapy to lower Lp(a) levels, which can be used in patients with uncontrolled Lp(a) levels > 160 mg/dL and with a history of CVD or >300 mg/dL without CVD.[63-65] It is now approved for use in high-risk patients with familial hypercholesteremia (FH) and ASCVD whose Lp(a) level remains ≥ 60 mg/dL (~150 nmol/L) and LDL-C ≥ 100 mg/dL on maximally tolerated lipid-lowering therapy. Both LDL-C and Lp(a) values reduce after LA, but decrease is not persistent and levels return back to previous levels.

While Lp(a) lowering may be beneficial in reducing ASCVD risk, it has no effect on the treatment of valvular aortic stenosis (VAS), as with other available lipid-lowering drugs.[13]

LIPOPROTEIN(a) TARGETED THERAPIES IN DEVELOPMENT

Various targeted therapies to reduce Lp(a) levels are in different stages of trials. Pelacarsen is an antisense oligonucleotide, which targets the *LPA* gene transcribing mRNA and can reduce Lp(a) levels by >80%.[66] Olpasiran is an siRNA that prevents the translation of the Apo(a) protein and reduces circulating Lp(a) levels up to ~100%.[67] Large cardiovascular outcome trials in secondary prevention patients with elevated Lp(a) levels are ongoing, which will establish the impact of these therapies on MACE: HORIZON[68] and OCEAN(a)—Outcomes Trial.[69] Phase 2 trials are underway for other siRNA therapies targeting Lp(a), zerlasiran,[70] and lepodisiran.[71,72] Additionally, an oral agent (muvalaplin), which interferes with the Apo(a) and ApoB interaction and disrupts the formation of Lp(a), is being tested in early phase trials.[73]

CONCLUSION

Lipoprotein(a) level measurement is important for risk assessment and leads to actionable strategies even though specific Lp(a)-lowering therapies are not currently available.[74] Hence, it should be measured at least once in lifetime for all adults to identify high-risk individuals. Since the relation between Lp(a) and ASCVD risk is continuous and log-linear, no specific single threshold can be defined to identify patients at risk; rather, it should be used as continuum of cardiovascular risk. Individuals with Lp(a) levels < 75 nmol/L should be identified as low risk and with values ≥125 nmol/L as high risk. These risk categories apply for all races and ethnicities with no specific race-based definition applied. Individuals with Lp(a) levels between 75 and 125 nmol/L should be considered as intermediate risk. This should be used to guide advice on lifestyle modification and aggressive lipid-lowering therapy with statin and other drugs including PCSK9 inhibitors, if LDL-C and Lp(a) remain high. It should also be used to identify family at risk, and high value mandates screening in first-degree family members. At present, LA is the only FDA-approved therapy for high-risk individuals, while many Lp(a) targeted therapies are in development.

ONLINE REFERENCES

Please scan the QR code provided at the end of the table of contents for References of this chapter.

CHAPTER 29

Lipoprotein(a): Why Measure and What to Do

Tanmoy Majee, Sidhartha Chattopadhyay, Arup Dasbiswas

ABSTRACT

Lipoprotein(a), a cholesterol-rich lipoprotein, is found in the blood and is linked to cardiovascular diseases such as coronary artery disease, heart attack, and stroke. High levels of Lp(a) contribute to plaque buildup and blood clot formation. Genetics determine Lp(a) levels, which can be challenging to modify through lifestyle changes or medications.

Keywords: Lipoprotein, cardiovascular, coronary artery disease, heart attack, stroke, challenges

INTRODUCTION

Lipoprotein(a), often abbreviated as Lp(a), is a type of lipoprotein found in the blood. It consists of a cholesterol-rich core surrounded by a protein shell, including a specific protein called apolipoprotein(a) [Apo(a)], which is attached to apolipoprotein B-100.[1]

The Lp(a) is similar to low-density lipoprotein (LDL) but with an additional protein component. High levels of Lp(a) in the blood are associated with an increased risk of cardiovascular diseases, such as coronary artery disease (CAD), heart attack, and stroke. This is because Lp(a) can contribute to the buildup of plaque in the arteries and promote blood clot formation.[2]

Genetics play a significant role in determining Lp(a) levels, and these levels can be difficult to modify through lifestyle changes or standard medications. However, some newer treatments, and experimental therapies targeting Lp(a) specifically, are being investigated for their potential to lower Lp(a) levels and reduce cardiovascular risk.[3]

ETIOLOGY

The etiology of Lp(a) involves a combination of genetic and potentially some environmental factors. Here is a breakdown of its primary causes.

Genetic Factors

- *Genetic variations*: Lp(a) levels are predominantly influenced by genetic factors. The gene encoding *Apo(a)*, which is a component of Lp(a), is highly polymorphic. Variations in this gene can lead to different Lp(a) levels in the blood. The size of the Apo(a) isoforms, which varies due to genetic differences, is a key determinant of Lp(a) levels. Larger isoforms are generally associated with higher Lp(a) concentrations. Adult levels are reached in childhood typically by the age of 5 years.
- *Inheritance pattern*: Lp(a) levels are largely inherited in an autosomal codominant manner, meaning that the level of Lp(a) is influenced by the genetic contributions from both parents. This inheritance pattern is responsible for the variability in Lp(a) levels among individuals.

Environmental Factors

- *Diet and lifestyle*: Unlike LDL cholesterol, Lp(a) levels are less likely to be affected by diet and lifestyle changes. However, some studies suggest that factors such as obesity, smoking, and physical inactivity might have a modest impact on Lp(a) levels.
- *Hormonal influences*: Hormonal changes, such as those related to pregnancy or menopause, might influence Lp(a) levels, although the impact is generally smaller compared to genetic factors.

EPIDEMIOLOGY

The epidemiology of Lp(a) focuses on the distribution, prevalence, and impact of elevated Lp(a) levels in different populations. Here is an overview.

Prevalence

- *General population*: Lp(a) levels vary widely among individuals, but elevated levels are common. Approximately 20–30% of people have Lp(a) levels that are considered high, with thresholds often defined as greater than 30 mg/dL or the 90th percentile for the population.[4]
- *Ethnic variability*: The prevalence of elevated Lp(a) levels varies by ethnicity:
    - *African populations*: Tend to have higher average Lp(a) levels and a higher prevalence of high Lp(a) compared to other ethnic groups.
    - *European and Asian populations*: Also have a significant proportion with elevated Lp(a) levels, though the average levels and prevalence can be lower compared to African populations.
    - *North American populations*: Display a diverse range of Lp(a) levels depending on genetic background, but generally follow similar patterns to other populations.
    - *Indian and southeast Asian population*: Approximately 25% of Indians have elevated Lp(a) levels (>50 mg), rendering Lp(a) a risk factor of great importance similar to diabetes.

Cardiovascular Risk

- *Association with cardiovascular disease*: Elevated Lp(a) levels are associated with an increased risk of cardiovascular diseases, including premature CAD, stroke, and peripheral artery disease. The risk appears to be independent of other lipid markers like LDL cholesterol.
- *Risk assessment*: Lp(a) is increasingly recognized as an important marker for cardiovascular risk assessment. Elevated Lp(a) levels can help identify individuals at higher risk who might benefit from more intensive monitoring or specific therapeutic interventions.

Gender and Age

- *Gender differences*: There is some evidence suggesting that Lp(a) levels may be higher in men compared to women, although the differences are generally modest. The impact of Lp(a) on cardiovascular risk might also differ by gender.
- *Age*: Lp(a) levels are relatively stable throughout life but can slightly increase with age. However, elevated Lp(a) levels in younger individuals are particularly concerning due to their potential long-term cardiovascular risk.

PATHOPHYSIOLOGICAL MECHANISMS

- *Atherosclerosis*:
    - *Plaque formation*: Lp(a) is considered proathero sclerotic, proinflammatory, prothrombotic, and anti-fibrinolytic. It increases the expression of vascular cell adhesion molecule (VCAM 1) and E selectin, thereby promoting the adhesion of monocytes to the endothelium and initiating the process of atherosclerotic plaque formation. Lp(a) exhibits a higher affinity for vascular walls, proteoglycans, and fibronectin on the endothelial surface compared to LDL cholesterol and other ApoB-containing lipoproteins. This leads to accumulation of Lp(a) in the arterial intima. Macrophages can take up Lp(a) leading to the formation of foam cells which is the hall mark of early atherosclerosis.
- *Thrombosis*:
    - *Prothrombotic effects*: Apo(a) has structural similarities to plasminogen, which plays a crucial role in breaking down blood clots. Elevated Lp(a) levels can inhibit plasminogen's ability to dissolve clots by competing with it for its specific binding sites on fibrin leading to reduced fibrinolysis. Thrombogenesis is also stimulated by Lp(a) as it leads to increased plasminogen activator inhibitor 1.
    - *Increased clot stability*: Lp(a) may contribute to the persistence and stability of blood clots, making it harder for the body to dissolve them. This can lead to a higher risk of thrombotic events.
- *Inflammation*:
    - *Endothelial dysfunction*: The accumulation of Lp(a) in arterial walls can induce inflammation and oxidative stress. Inflammatory cytokines and oxidative products can further damage endothelial cells, leading to increased plaque formation and progression.
    - *Inflammatory markers*: Elevated Lp(a) levels are associated with increased levels of inflammatory markers, which contribute to the overall inflammatory state and cardiovascular risk.

SCREENING FOR LP(a)

The primary reason for screening patients for Lp(a) is to help identify those at high risk for heart disease, especially in the absence of other major risk factors. It also helps to identify patients who need more intensive lipid lowering therapy. Today there is a variability in opinion on when to screen and whom to screen for Lp(a).

The National Lipid Association recommends considering Lp(a) testing in cases with a significant family history of premature atherosclerotic cardiovascular disease among first-degree relatives, personal history of premature atherosclerotic cardiovascular disease and severe primary hyperlipidemia. Canadian Cardiovascular Society guidelines recommend universal screening for Lp(a). The European Atherosclerosis Society has established guidelines for screening for Lp(a) in patients with history of premature cardiovascular disease, those experiencing recurrent cardiac events despite on statins therapy.

European Society of Cardiology recommends universal screening for Lp(a) at least once in individual s lifetime.

There is no generalized consensus on Lp(a) risk thresholds:

- >50 mg/dL is an accepted target in ACC/AHA, Canadian guidelines.
- <30 mg/dL is considered normal, 30–50 mg/dL intermediate, and >50 mg/dL abnormal in the European Atherosclerotic Society consensus statement.
- >50 mg/dL is accepted as a risk enhancing cut off in the National Lipid Association scientific statement.

CLINICAL SIGNIFICANCE AND TREATMENT

Hormonal drugs may improve Lp(a) levels but are not necessarily associated with improved cardiovascular outcomes. Estrogens may improve Lp(a) levels and has been thought of improving potential cardiac risk profiles but is not currently in use for the same. In fact, it carriers potential risk s in certain patient population. Similarly testosterone has also been thought to reduced Lp(a) levels but needs further research to be useful for this purpose. Testosterone may also decrease HDL concentration thereby can lead to increased atherosclerosis. Levocarnitine has potential to reduce Lp(a) but has been associated with increased levels of trimethylamine N-oxide which in turn is associated with increased atherosclerosis. Many candidate medications are in pipeline which actually reduce or have the potential to reduce Lp(a) but whether they will improve overall cardiovascular morbidity and mortality is the big question. Some dietary and lifestyle changes reduce the risk associated with high Lp(a) levels. Consuming more vegetables, fruits, and flaxseed may reduce Lp(a) levels in varying amount in different studies. Contrary to mild-to-moderate exercise, severe intensity in long term can increase Lp(a) levels.

Patients with significantly higher levels of Lp(a) should generally be treated to achieve a target of <50 mg/dL. Treatment with niacin can lower Lp(a) levels by 20–30%, but it has not been associated with improved cardiac outcomes.[5]

CONCLUSION

Though statins are primary treatment options for dyslipidemia, they have not shown consistent effects on Lp(a) levels. Nonetheless high levels of Lp(a) indicate the need for more intense statin therapy. PCSK9 inhibitors are also an option for reducing Lp(a). Promising results from the ODYSSEY OUTCOMES trial of alirocumab and the FOURIER trial of evolocumab have been achieved. A meta-analysis showed PCSK9 inhibitors to reduce Lp(a) levels to around 26% in addition to improved cardiac outcomes.

The guidelines set by the European Atherosclerosis Society recommend screening for Lp(a) in individuals with a history of premature cardiovascular disease. Patients who experience recurring cardiac events despite being on statin therapy should undergo testing at least once in their adult life. The purpose is to identify individuals with very high inherited Lp(a) levels exceeding 180 mg/dL (> 430 nmol/L). These individuals may have a heightened lifetime risk of atherosclerotic cardiovascular disease (ASCVD), equivalent to the risk associated with heterozygous familial hypercholesterolemia.[6]

Several novel therapies targeting the *LPA* gene transcription rate using small interfering RNA and gene translation with antisense oligonucleotides are in phase 2 and phase 3 trials. Initial results of Lp(a) HORIZON with pelacarsen have shown almost 35–80% reduction of Lp(a) level depending on dose . OCEAN (a) preliminary results with olpasiran showing 70–110% reduction at 36 weeks. ORION 11 with inclisiran showing almost 28.5% reduction of Lp(a) in preliminary results. However, these minor therapies need further evaluation of long-term follow-up to be considered in reducing Lp(a) in patients.

ONLINE REFERENCES

Please scan the QR code provided at the end of the table of contents for References of this chapter.

CHAPTER

30

Elevated Triglyceride: Current Concepts

Manoranjan Mandal, Anindya Mukherjee, Mainak Mandal

ABSTRACT

Hypertriglyceridemia is multifactorial and a common clinical problem. Impaired clearance or increased production of triglyceride-rich lipoproteins (TRL) along with genetic factors have come up as important contributors to hypertriglyceridemia and atherosclerotic cardiovascular disease (ASCVD). Low-density lipoprotein is targeted for lipid lowering therapy. Targets reflecting the contribution of TRL such as Apo-B and non-HDL-C are emerging as recommendations. This chapter summarizes the present epidemiology, recent concepts of genetics, and the newer treatment strategies for elevated triglycerides.

Keywords: Triglycerides, triglyceride rich lipoproteins (TRL), hypertriglyceridemia (HTG)

INTRODUCTION

The triglyceride-rich lipoproteins (TRL) has come up as important contributors of atherosclerotic cardiovascular disease (ASCVD) in recent past. The concern of pancreatitis and ASCVD has led to further research and advent of newer treatment modalities for increased triglycerides (TG).

DEFINITION

The American guidelines classify hypertriglyceridemia (HTG) as moderate HTG when fasting or nonfasting TG is 2.0–5.6 mmol/L (175–499 mg/dL). Severe HTG is defined as fasting TG ≥5.6 mmol/L (≥500 mg/dL).[1] An elevated TG of >10 mmol/L (>885 mg/dL) is associated with increased risk of acute pancreatitis.[2]

EPIDEMIOLOGY

The prevalence of HTG is about 10–25% in adult population and it varies widely from region to region.[3-7] Mild-to-moderate HTG is on the rise over the past few decades contributed by obesity and diabetes. Prevalence of severe (>885 mg/dL) and very severe (>1,770 mg/dL) HTG ranges from 0.1 to 0.2% and 0.01 to 0.02%, respectively.[3]

ETIOLOGY

Both genetic and acquired HTG are prevalent. Monogenic causes are relatively rare compared to polygenic among the genetic causes.[3,4] The genetic causes are often known as the primary causes and acquired causes are stated a secondary causes. **Boxes 1 and 2** depict the primary and secondary etiologies of HTG.[3,8,9]

BOX 1 Primary causes of hypertriglyceridemia.

- *Monogenic chylomicronemia (hyperlipoproteinemia type 1 or familial chylomicronemia syndrome):* Mutation in one of five genes—LPL (80% cases), APOC2, APOA5, LMF1, and GPIHBP1
- *Multifactorial or polygenic chylomicronemia (hyperlipoproteinemia type 5 or mixed hyperlipidemia):* Accumulated genetic defect of TG raising polymorphism in APOA1-C3-A5; FADS1-2-3, NCAN, APOB, and ANGPTL3 genes
- Multifactorial or polygenic hypertriglyceridemia (hyperlipoproteinemia type 4 or familial hypertriglyceridemia)
- *Dysbetalipoproteinemia (hyperlipoproteinemia type 3):* APOE E2/E2 homozygosity or APOE dominant rare variant heterozygosity
- *Combined hyperlipoproteinemia (hyperlipoproteinemia type 2B or familial combined hyperlipidemia):* Accumulation of common small effect LDL-C raising polymorphisms

PATHOPHYSIOLOGY

Chylomicrons secreted by the intestine transport dietary TG, while liver secretes very low-density lipoproteins (VLDL) and this transports TG of endogenous origin. Chylomicrons and VLDLs are the two main types of lipoproteins which help in TG transport. These lipoproteins also contain a lipid core found by TG and cholesterol esters, surface apolipoprotein, phospholipids, and free cholesterol.[3,4] VLDL and chylomicron are metabolized by lipoprotein lipase (LPL). The remnants are taken up by liver. Some VLDL remnants undergo further metabolism by hepatic lipase to form low density lipoproteins (LDL).[4] The efficiency of LPL mediated lipolysis and subsequent uptake of the remnants determine the level of circulating TG. These mechanisms can get saturated, therefore when plasma TG levels rise beyond a certain limit, lipolysis decreases.[10,11] TRL starts accumulating in blood when acquired or genetic causes lead to reduced LPL activity resulting in impaired clearance of exogenous and/or endogenous TRL.[3] Alcohol consumption, diets high in saturated fats or high glycemic index, obesity causes increased chylomicron and VLDL production which in turn causes HTG.[3] Nonhigh density lipoprotein (non-HDL) contains VLDL and remnants as important components and therefore increase in non-HDL would also lead to HTG.[12,13] Apolipoprotein B-100 forms a key component of both VLDL and its remnants and therefore the levels of apolipoprotein B (Apo-B) are raised in HTG.[12] Highly atherogenic small, dense LDL particle levels are also increased in patients with HTG. Decreased activities of cholesterol ester transfer protein (CETP) and LPL leads to reduced production and alteration of HDL composition, this leads to HDL catabolism resulting in reduced HDL levels in patients with HTG.[14] **Figure 1** gives an overview of the pathophysiology.

BOX 2 Secondary causes of hypertriglyceridemia.

- *Medical conditions*: Diabetes mellitus, metabolic syndrome, insulin resistance, obesity, chronic kidney disease, nephrotic syndrome, hypothyroidism, third trimester of pregnancy, myeloma, systemic lupus erythematosis, liver disease, HIV infection, Cushing syndrome, and sarcoidosis
- *Lifestyle factors*: Excessive alcoholism, saturated fats and high glycemic index diet, and sedentary lifestyle
- *Medications:* Glucocorticoids, anabolic steroids, estrogens, thiazide and loop diuretics, noncardioselective β-blockers, isotretinoin, bexarotene, propofol, bile acid sequestrants, cyclophosphamide, asparaginase, capecitabine, interferon, tacrolimus, sirolimus, cyclosporin, protease-inhibitors, second-generation antipsychotics such as clozapine and olanzapine

CLASSIFICATION

The present classifications are streamlined based simply on the TG level as demonstrated in **Box 3**.[9,15]

PRESENTATION

The HTG can clinically present as various forms of ischemic heart disease but the most concerning presentation probably is acute pancreatitis or acute coronary syndrome. Typically, it is silent and often detected on screening for dyslipidemia.[3] Early management averts the development of clinical signs.[8] Eruptive xanthoma, lipemia retinalis, and hepatosplenomegaly are the characteristic features of chylomicronemia. Infants can present with abdominal pain and failure to thrive.

APPROACH

- *History*: Family history, medical history such as diabetes, obesity, hypothyroid, lifestyle factors such as sedentary habits, high fat intake, medication history such as antipsychotics, anabolic steroids are the important bits

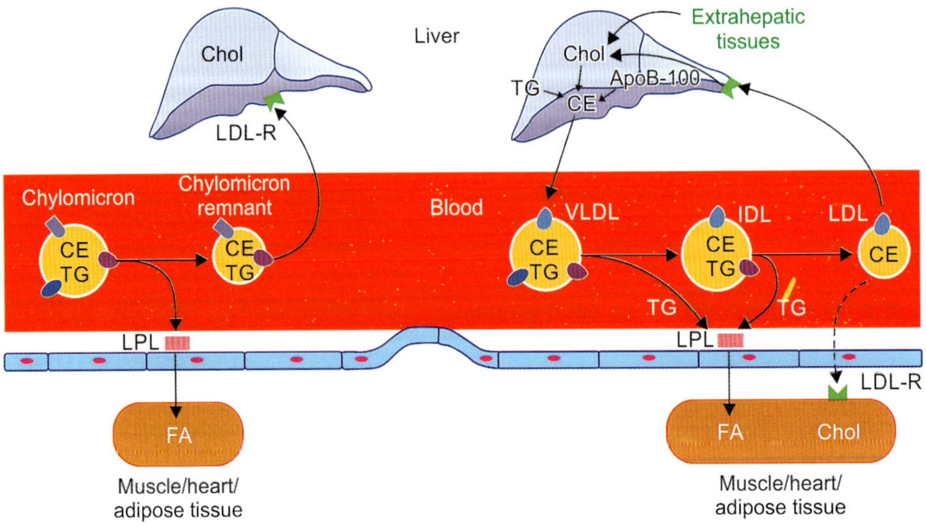

FIG. 1: Triglyceride metabolism.

BOX 3 Classification of hypertriglyceridemia.

- *American Heart Association/American College of Cardiology:*
  - *Moderate HTG*: 2.0–5.6 mmol/L (175–499 mg/dL)
  - *Severe HTG*: ≥5.6 mmol/L (≥500 mg/dL)
- *European Society of Cardiology/European Atherosclerosis Society*:
  - *Mild-to-moderate HTG*: 2–10 mmol/L (175–885 mg/dL)
  - *Severe HTG:* >10 mmol/L (>885 mg/dL)

Note: The 2021 American College of Cardiology expert consensus defines fasting TG ≥1.7 mmol/L (≥150 mg/dL) or nonfasting TG ≥2.0 mmol/L (≥175 mg/dL) and TG <5.6 mmol/L (<500 mg/dL) as moderate HTG.

BOX 4 Risk factors for hypertriglyceridemia.

Strong:
- Family history of hyperlipidemia
- High saturated fat in diet
- Food with high glycemic index
- Excess alcohol consumption
- Family/personal history of obesity
- Family or personal history of diabetes
- Insulin resistance
- Nonalcoholic fatty liver or nonalcoholic steatohepatitis
- Nephrotic syndrome
- HIV infection
- Medications as discussed in **Box 2**

Weak:
- Cushing syndrome
- Inflammatory/immune disorders such as sarcoidosis, systemic lupus erythematosus, and myeloma
- Organ transplant (possibly related to use of immunosuppression)
- Hypothyroidism
- Pregnancy

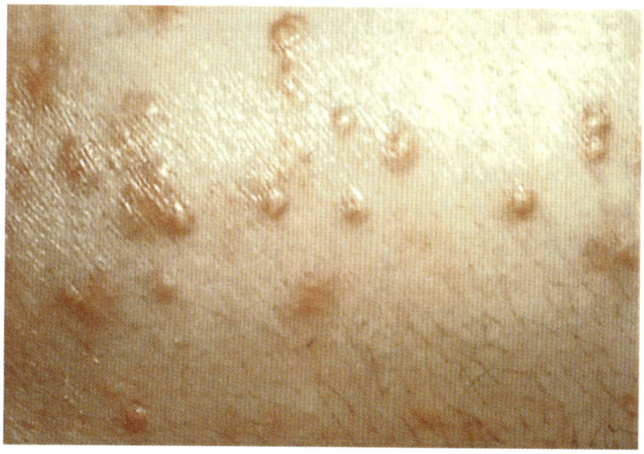

FIG. 2: Eruptive xanthoma.

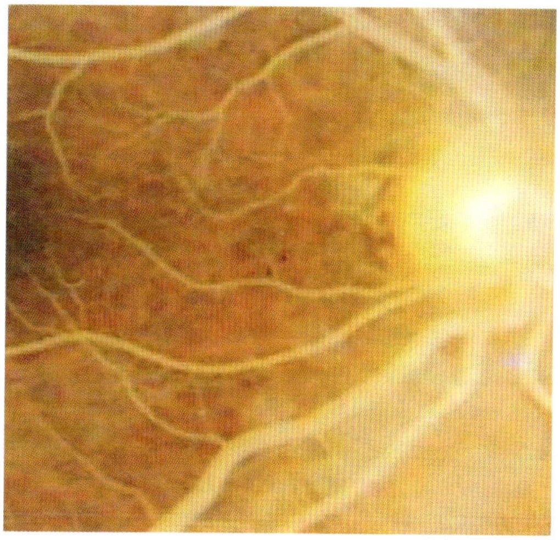

FIG. 3: Lipemia retinalis.

in history taking.[3,9] Risk factors can be classified as strong and weak as depicted in **Box 4**.

- *Clinical features*: Severe HTG and chylomicronemia lead to characteristic features, such as eruptive xanthomas (raised crops of small yellowish papules encircled by erythematous halos on extensor surfaces of the extremities, the buttocks, and the shoulders) **(Fig. 2)** and lipemia retinalis (whitish-pink appearance of retinal vessels and retinal pallor with pinkish hue seen on fundoscopy) **(Fig. 3)**.[10] Other less common features could be quite generic in the form of abdominal pain, pallor, diarrhea, etc.
- *Investigations*: A full lipid profile usually includes TG. Calculated LDL is not accurate when TG is above 4.6 mmol/L (400 mg/dL). 12 hour fasting TG is usually the recommended way to test for HTG but nonfasting TG has been demonstrated to be associated with risk of atherosclerosis.[16] Apo-B is being used increasingly but the standards need to be set universally to make it a proper tool.[13] Fasting or nonfasting states do not affect its value.

Secondary causes such as diabetes, hypothyroidism, and liver dysfunction should be investigated. Coronary imaging, myocardial perfusion scan, and liver ultrasounds can be useful accessory investigations.[16] The investigations to be considered are listed in **Box 5**. Significant HTG can be identified just from a peripheral blood sample as shown in **Figure 4**.

SCREENING

Dyslipidemia is an established risk factor for ASCVD. While in the UK and Europe lipid screening starts at 40 years age, in the USA, guidelines suggest 5 yearly screening from 20 years of age.[15,17] Diabetes, family history may expedite the screening process.

TREATMENT

Two main objectives of treatment are:
1. Prevention of ASCVD
2. Prevention of acute pancreatitis

BOX 5 Tests in suspected hypertriglyceridemia.

First test to order:
- Twelve hour fasting triglycerides

Other tests to consider:
- Apolipoprotein B
- Fasting plasma glucose
- Renal function test
- Urinary albumin
- Thyroid function study
- Liver function test
- C-reactive protein

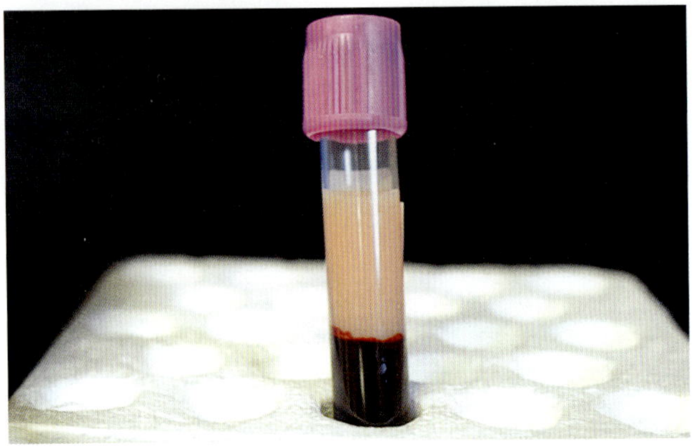

FIG. 4: Blood sample showing a milky white upper layer of triglycerides in a patient with severe hypertriglyceridemia.

The TG levels <1.7 mmol/L (<150 mg/dL) poses lower risk of ASCVD as per the recent European guidelines.[15] TG ≥5.6 mmol/L (≥500 mg/dL) prompts reduction of the levels to prevent acute pancreatitis.[9]

Nonpharmacological Treatment

This is mainly used in mild-to-moderate HTG and also as an adjunct in severe HTG. This includes alcohol limitation, low fat diet, avoiding foods with high glycemic index, prevention and management of secondary causes such as diabetes, hypothyroid, etc.[9] Referral to a registered nutritionist might be helpful.

Patients with familial chylomicronemia syndrome have severe genetic deficiency of lipolysis. A stringent low-fat diet is recommended (<15% of daily caloric intake from fat).[3,11] Medium chain fatty acids get directly absorbed into the portal circulation and therefore are good alternatives.[11] Supplemental essential fatty acids, fat soluble vitamins, and referral to lipid specialist could be considered.[11]

Pharmacological Management of Mild-to-moderate Hypertriglyceridemia

Fasting TG ≥1.7 mmol/L (≥150 mg/dL) following 4–12 weeks of lifestyle intervention, a stable dose of maximally tolerated statin therapy when indicated, and evaluation and management of secondary causes has been defined as persistent HTG.[9] Persistent HTG and 10-year ASCVD risk 5–<7.5% should lead to patient-clinician discussion regarding the initiation of moderate-intensity statin therapy.[9] Ezetimibe, proprotein convertase subtilisin/kexin type 9 (PCSK9) inhibitors, or bempedoic acid have been used as an adjunct to reduce LDL but has minimal effect on TG, therefore not advised for HTG.[18] Addition of icosapent ethyl led to a significant reduction in the risk of ASCVD and cardiovascular mortality in patients with HTG.[19] Addition of icosapent ethyl may be considered in patients with persistent TG ≥1.7 mmol/L (≥150 mg/dL) despite maximally tolerated statin therapy and consideration of lifestyle factors according to the USA guidelines. Those with ASCVD and either LDL-cholesterol <1.8 mmol/L (<70 mg/dL) or LDL-cholesterol 1.8–2.6 mmol/L (70–99 mg/dL), or those age >50 years without ASCVD, but with diabetes and one or more high-risk factors for ASCVD can be considered for icosapent ethyl if they have moderate HTG.[9,20] High-risk patients with TG levels between 1.5 and 5.6 mmol/L (135–499 mg/dL) despite statin treatment should be considered for icosapent ethyl in combination with a statin as per European recommendations.[15,19] The European guidelines also recommend that in patients who are at LDL-cholesterol goal but still have TG levels >2.3 mmol/L (>200 mg/dL), fenofibrate may be considered in combination with a statin. This is contrary to the USA guidelines.[15]

Pharmacological Management of Severe Hypertriglyceridemia

Statins alone can neither reduce such high levels of TG nor can reduce the risk of acute pancreatitis. Fibrates and possibly omega-3 fatty acids can achieve this most efficiently.[21]

If statin and fibrate need co-prescription, fenofibrate is the safer fibrate option with a lower risk of muscle related complications when combined with statins.

For those with a 10-year ASCVD risk 5–<7.5% and persistent HTG, patient-clinician discussion is recommended regarding the initiation of moderate-intensity statin therapy.[2,9]

Adults with TG ≥5.6 mmol/L (≥500 mg/dL), and especially fasting TG ≥11.3 mmol/L (≥1,000 mg/dL), should have a very low-fat diet, avoiding refined carbohydrates and alcohol, taking prescription omega-3 fatty acids, and, if necessary, fibrate therapy.[9] In individuals with, a ≥30% reduction in TG is possible with omega-3 fatty acids in patients with TG ≥5.6 mmol/L (≥500 mg/dL).[20] Management of pancreatitis is out of scope of this text. But prophylactic fibrate therapy is recommended after stabilization to prevent further episodes of pancreatitis.[9]

PROMINENT, an ongoing trial evaluates Pemafibrate (K-877, Kowa), a selective PPAR modulator, lowers TG levels by 35–45% in patients with T2DM and HTG.[22] STRENGTH trial evaluates ASCVD outcomes of 4 g daily omega-3 carboxylic acids containing eicosapentanoic acid and docosahexanoic acid.[23] Usual dose of icosapent ethyl is 2 g orally twice daily while the usual dose of omega-3-acid ethyl esters is 4 g/day orally given in 1–2 divided doses.

EMERGING THERAPIES

Reduction of Apolipoprotein C-III

Apolipoprotein C-III (Apo C-III) circulates with TRL and is associated with higher ASCVD. Volanesorsen, impairs translation of Apo C-III mRNA. It is an antisense oligonucleotide designed to inhibit the formation of Apo C-III. Olezarsen (also known as AKCEA-APOCIII-LRx) and ARO-APOC3, are in development. These are also antisense oligonucleotide targeting Apo C-III. European Medicines Agency (EMA) have approved volanesorsen in genetically confirmed familial chylomicronemia syndrome not responding to usual therapies. The US Food and Drug Administration (USFDA) has not approved volanesorsen due to the risk of thrombocytopenia.[24-29]

Reduction of Angiopoietin-like Protein 3

The monoclonal antibody evinacumab and the antisense therapies IONIS-angiopoietin-like protein 3 (ANGPTL3)-LRx and ARO-ANG3 reduce ANGPTL3 which is a genetically validated target for HTG. These have shown reductions of TG of 50–80%.[25,28,30]

Novel Krill-derived Omega-3 Phospholipid/Free Fatty Acid

Pooled data from the TRILOGY 1 and 2 phase 3 randomized controlled trials investigated omega-3 phospholipid/free fatty acid (omega-3-PL/FFA) derived from krill oil and demonstrated that in patients with severe HTG (fasting TG levels from 500 to 1,500 mg/dL), omega-3-PL/FFA reduced blood TG levels at 12 weeks (26.0% compared with 15.1% with placebo), with reductions persisting even at 26 weeks. Omega-3-PL/FFA was well-tolerated.[31]

PRIMARY PREVENTION

Primary prevention involves identification and treatment of modifiable risk factors as discussed before.

SECONDARY PREVENTION

This involves physical activity, reduction of fat intake, and improved lifestyle. As per the US Preventive Services Task Force (USPSTF) recommendation, adults between 40 and 75 years with estimated 10 year ASCVD risk of ≥10% should start a statin and those with a risk of 7.5–10% may be offered a statin selectively.[32]

MONITORING

Six weekly monitoring of TG levels is recommended while initiation and optimization of therapy. Half yearly to 1 yearly lipid profile check is recommended when the values are stable. Liver function should be done at baseline, during a drug or dose change and then 6–12 monthly when the individual is on statins or fibrates.

PROGNOSIS

Prognosis has improved and is improving with proper detection and management of HTG. Proper follow-up improves the prognosis even further.[33]

CONCLUSION

Epidemiologic and genetic studies have shown that TRL and their remnants significantly contribute to ASCVD. Besides LDL-C, current guidelines recommend targeting Apo-B and non-HDL-C. The initial step in treatment involves lifestyle changes, followed by LDL-C reduction with statins to lower vascular risk, independent of TRL reduction. Previous trials with fibrates, niacin, and CETP inhibitors did not conclusively show ASCVD risk reduction in patients with optimal cholesterol levels. However, recent studies highlight role of TRL in residual risk for ASCVD patients on statins. Emerging therapies, such as high dose omega 3 fatty acids (icosapent ethyl) and selective PPAR modulator (Pemafibrate), may benefit patients through TRL reduction. New treatment targets based on TRL molecular pathways, including Apo C-III antisense oligonucleotide (volanesorsen), ANGPTL3 inhibitors (evinacumab; ASO IONIS-ANGPTL3-LRx), and therapies targeting Apo C-II, A-V, and ANGPTL4, are in clinical testing. TRLs have emerged as crucial markers of residual risk and treatment targets. Ongoing trials will assess novel strategies to lower serum TG, potentially making TRL treatment a key aspect of lipid management alongside LDL-C reduction.

ONLINE REFERENCES

Please scan the QR code provided at the end of the table of contents for References of this chapter.

CHAPTER

31

Dyslipidemia in Asymptomatic Young Indians

Sunandan Sikdar, Rathindra Nath Karmakar

ABSTRACT

Dyslipidemia in young is an important public health problem in a populous country like India. Diet, lifestyle, comorbidities and genetic causes contribute to it. Recent guidelines have stressed on therapy based on risk stratification and achieving targets. Though statins are the mainstay of therapy, the emergence ezetimibe, bempedoic acid, and biological therapies have revolutionized the field.

Keywords: Asymptomatic, dyslipidemia, South Asian phenotype, statins

INTRODUCTION

India has one of the highest numbers of persons in the age-group of 18–40 years because of its demographic dividend. The prevalence of hypercholesterolemia in India varies from 10 to 15% in rural to 25 to 30% in urban populations in various studies.[1] The Indian dyslipidemia is of different phenotype (South Asian phenotype) from that observed in western populations. This phenotype has low high-density lipoprotein cholesterol (HDL-C) (<40 mg/dL in males and <50 mg/dL in females), low apolipoprotein A1, and higher triglycerides (TG), lipoprotein (a) and apolipoprotein B along with visceral adiposity. The total levels of low-density lipoprotein cholesterol (LDL-C) in South Asians are comparable to those of Caucasians, but there is an increased small-dense atherogenic component. Asian Indians have been found to develop CVD at a younger age than other populations.[2] In India 25% of all myocardial infarctions (MI) occur before age of 40 years—in INTERHEART study, the median age of MI among Indians was 53.0 years compared to 58.1 years in other countries.[3]

An important implication of asymptomatic dyslipidemia is that a significant number of subjects are exposed LDL-C for a prolonged period of time. Results from Mendelian studies have clearly shown than even a small reduction in LDL-C achieved at an early age and maintained over decades leads to several fold greater reductions in ASCVD risk compared to more aggressive LDL-C lowering initiated later in life.[4] Further, in case of population of South Asian ancestry like Indians, ASCVD risk estimators may be giving us a false sense of security due to age being an important parameter (most tools begin with age including that of Lipid Association of India where age > 45 years in males and > 55 years in females are major risk factor).[5] A dedicated risk prediction score derived from the Indian population is needed, although QRISK 3 score is better for risk assessment in Indians.

EPIDEMIOLOGY

The ICMR INDIAB study was done in 2,000 rural and urban participants from four states of India. The prevalence of dyslipidemia was around 79%. The most common lipid abnormality was low HDL-C in 72.3%, with 44.9% of the patients having it as an isolated abnormality.[6] It was found that 4.8% of the population had all four lipid abnormalities (hypercholesterolemia + hypertriglyceridemia + low HDL-C + high LDL-C). In The Center for Cardiometabolic Risk Reduction in South Asia Cohort Study, females had a higher prevalence of low HDL-C and males had high TG.[7]

INDIAN DIET AND ITS IMPLICATIONS

We are exposed to a particular type of diet from our childhood in India. Indian diets contain lower fat as well as saturated fatty acids (SFA), both in urban as well as rural surveys. In India, of total energy 19–24% come from fat compared to 36% in the western diets. On the other hand, 71% of rural and 63% of urban energy intake come from carbohydrate compared to 51% in high-income economies. In India n-3 polyunsaturated fatty acid consumption (PUFA) is very low except in coastal areas as it comes from marine fish. Though recommended amount of n-3 PUFA is 200 mg/day, Indian consumption is one-tenth. Further due to increased awareness, increased use of safflower oil has increased n-6 oil consumption and the recommended balance of n-6/n-3 ratio has been skewed.[8] The role of Indian diet as a causal factor in promoting the South Asian phenotype of dyslipidemia is yet to be determined.

CAUSAL FACTORS

Dyslipidemia is a lifestyle disease. Diet, lack of exercise, obesity, and metabolic disorders (like diabetes, hypothyroidism) are implicated. However, polygenic and monogenic factors are also associated with it. Among monogenic diseases, homozygous familial hypercholesterolemia (HoFH) and heterozygous familial hypercholesterolemia (HeFH) must be excluded. Three main genes are associated with FH—*LDL receptor*, *PCSK9*, and *Apo B* gene.

Familial hypercholesterolemia: Indian study on the general population ($n = 4{,}000$) patients showed a prevalence of 1 in 1,000 (0.1%) was found for definite FH.[9] A subanalysis showed that out of the enrolled 90 patients with high LDL cholesterol, about 20% (definite + probable) were FH. The data regarding asymptomatic FH (mostly HeFH) with only dyslipidemia is scarce. Diagnosis is established by genetic test or by criteria like Dutch Lipid Clinic Network (DLCN).

There are some monogenic disorders causing dyslipidemia in young as described in **Table 1**.

There are some less discussed conditions, which are more important as a cause of dyslipidemia in young individuals in our country:

Pregnancy-induced hypertension and eclampsia are both associated with increased risk of development of ASCVD.

Polycystic ovarian disease affects nearly 4–22% reproductive age women and have associated metabolic syndrome, visceral adiposity and dyslipidemia—high total cholesterol, low HDL, and high TG.[10]

Viral infection: Immune activation caused by human immunodeficiency virus (HIV) and the treatment with antiretroviral therapy (ART), which induces dyslipidemia, jointly contribute to development of atherosclerotic heart disease. Studies with pitavastatin showed significantly reduced the risk of major adverse cardiovascular events by 35% over a mean follow-up of 5 years.[11]

Diagnosis and time of screening: At the age of 18 years all individuals should be screened for dyslipidemia. Individuals with family history of lipid disorders should be screened earlier.[12]

Risk stratification: Family history of premature ASCVD (defined as occurrence of an ASCVD event in a male first-degree relative < 55 years of age and in a female first-degree relative < 65 years of age or before menopause) identifies individuals at an elevated ASCVD risk. Unlike other risk factors, it truly reflects the net consequences of various known and unknown genetic factors as well as environmental and epigenetic risk factors that may be prevalent in a family.[5]

Because all risk assessment tools lack accuracy when predicting the presence of subclinical atherosclerosis in asymptomatic subjects, widely available screening tests are required that can predict at an individual level.

Guidelines have been published by Cardiological Society of India. The patients have been divided into five categories. However, only low risk (no risk factor) or moderate risk (single risk factor: Diabetes, hypertension, tobacco, FH) may have asymptomatic dyslipidemia in usual circumstances and thus shall be under purview of this chapter.[13]

Though as mentioned before, QRISK 3 score is better for risk assessment in Indians compared to the pooled cohort equations, a dedicated risk prediction score derived from the Indian population is needed.[5] Four parameters may be considered under this heading as an addendum to the already established parameters:

1. *Coronary Artery Calcification Score (CACS) and its use in risk stratification*: Patients with CACS > 100 but no conventional risk factors had higher event rates than those with 3 or more risk factors but no coronary artery calcification (i.e., zero CACS). On the other hand, CACS 0 has nearly zero 5-year mortality risk provided they have no risk factors. Patients with risk factors may have noncalcified coronary plaque as 50% of plaques may not have calcium. CACS 1-99 may be more difficult to stratify as they do have higher risk of ASCVD. In the Coronary Artery Risk Development in Young Adults (CARDIA) study, 3043 subjects underwent CACS measurement at a mean age of 40.3 ± 3.6 years. Among 58 individuals (1.9%) with CACS ≥ 100, the absolute all-cause mortality rate was 22.4% over a follow-up of 12.5 years, a strikingly high mortality rate for young participants.[14] LAI has classified CACS values into four groups: (i) CACS 0, (ii) CACS

TABLE 1: Monogenic disorders causing dyslipidemia.

Disease	Gene	Lipid component	Manifestation	Transmission
Familial hypercholesterolemia	*LDL R, Apo B, PCSK9*	LDL	Tendon xanthoma, CAD, raised LDL	AD
Familial dysbetalipoproteinemia	*Apo E*	Chylomicron, VLDL remnants	Palmar and tuberoeruptive xanthomas, CAD, PAD	AR, AD
Familial hepatic lipase deficiency	*Hepatic lipase*	VLDL remnant	CAD, pancreatitis	AR
Sitosterolemia	*ABCG 5, ABCG 8*	LDL	Tendon xanthoma, CAD	AR

(AD: autosomal dominant; AR: autosomal recessive; CAD: coronary artery disease; PAD: peripheral artery disease)

1-99, (iii) CACS 100-299, and (iv) CACS > 300 for risk stratification in subjects of 30 years and above.

2. *Nonalcoholic fatty liver disease*: In recognition that ASCVD is the leading cause of death in patients with NAFLD, the LAI designates NAFLD with fibrosis grade 2 or 3 as a high-risk feature. The presence of NAFLD would require an LDL-C goal < 50-70 mg/dL, depending on the overall risk profile of the patient. Statins substantially reduce the ASCVD risk in NAFLD and the benefit is much greater than that seen in patients without NAFLD.[5]
3. *Polygenic Risk Score (PRS)*: Though validated for subjects of European ancestry may help in risk stratification. Individuals with high PRS (overall score in the top 5 percentile) have more than threefold increased odds of early-onset MI, a risk which is equivalent to that seen in individuals with genetically confirmed FH. Since a high PRS has a much higher prevalence (10-20% higher) than FH mutations, the former may have a much greater relevance for ASCVD risk assessment.[15,16]
4. *Carotid and femoral ultrasonography for risk stratification*: The Carotid And FEmoral ultrasound morphology Screening and CArdioVascular Events in low-risk subjects study (CAFES-CAVE) recruited 14,300 healthy, asymptomatic individuals from Italy and followed for 10 years. Among subjects with nonobstructive carotid or femoral plaque (defined as wall thickening ≥1 mm in association with irregular, increased echogenicity involving all the ultrasonic layers), the 10-year event rate was 39.1%. Both carotid and femoral arteries had comparable predictive value, but their combination was associated with an almost 15% higher rate of events.[17]

TREATMENT

Asymptomatic Young Individuals, Raised LDL without Risk Factors

They must undergo lifestyle modification if LDL > 100 mg/dL. If these measures do not improve LDL, a low-dose statin—atorvastatin 10 mg, rosuvastatin 5 mg, or pitavastatin 1-2 mg may be tried.[12]

Lifestyle modification starts with a healthy diet. The components of a heart healthy diet is given in brief in **Table 2**. Target to be achieved are for low-risk and moderate-risk patients: LDL-C < 100 mg/dL; non-HDL-C < 130 mg/dL; HDL > 40 mg/dL (male), >50 mg/dL (female); TG < 150 mg/dL; and Lp(a) < 50 mg/dL **(Table 3)**.[13]

TABLE 2: Recommended diet in brief.

Carbohydrate	Protein	Fat
Fresh fruits and vegetable	Fish (>300 g/week)	Vegetable oil—3 tsf/day
Whole grains (brown rice/chapati)	Lean meat/one egg/day	Avoid deep fried food
Legumes	1 cup milk/day	

Source: Adapted from Sawhney et al.[13]

TABLE 3: Targets for dyslipidemia.

Parameter (mg/dL)	Low-risk	Moderate-risk	High-risk
LDL	<100	<100	<70
Non-HDL	<130	<130	<100
HDL	>40 males, >50 females	>40 males, >50 females	>40 males, >50 females
TG	<150	<150	<150
Lp(a)	<50	<50	<50

Asymptomatic Young Individuals, High Triglyceride with Normal LDL

Individuals with TG > 150 mg/dL have predisposition to atherosclerotic heart disease, especially if they have concomitantly low HDL. LAI has kept fasting TG > 150 mg/dL and nonfasting TG > 175 mg/dL as risk modifier. For asymptomatic patients, lifestyle modification—including low refined carbohydrate, low-fat diet, exercise, and other weight reduction measures, avoiding drugs (e.g., betablockers, thiazides) that raise TG and treating underlying conditions like hypothyroidism and hyperglycemic state. Statin treatment is recommended as the first drug of choice for reducing CVD risk in high-risk individuals with hypertriglyceridemia [TG > 2.3 mmol/L (200 mg/dL)].[18] TG > 500 mg/dL warrants therapy in all cases. In high-risk (or above) patients with TG between 135 and 499 mg/dL, despite statin treatment, n-3 PUFAs (*icosapent ethyl* 2 × 2 g/day) should be considered in combination with statins **(Table 4)**. Fenofibrate, omega-3 fatty acid are other drugs in the armamentarium. As per recent CSI guideline Fenofibrate can be given if TG > 500 mg/dL. Saroglitazar, a novel dual PPAR α/γ agonist, with predominant PPARα effect and moderate PPARγ effect, developed in India, is indicated in diabetics with hypertriglyceridemia and also in often associated fatty liver disease. If non-HDL cholesterol > 130 mg/dL then statins should be added.

Asymptomatic Familial Hypercholesterolemia

Statins are used to treat adult HeFH patients. To achieve the LDL goal of <70 mg/dL for primary prevention, 55 mg/dL for secondary prevention, and <40 for FH with elevated Lp(a), statin doses can be increased to the maximum tolerated dose. These goals are difficult to achieve in homozygous variety with statins alone **(Table 5)**. In primary prevention, for individuals with FH at very high risk, an LDL-C reduction of ≥50% from baseline and an LDL-C goal of <55 mg/dL should be considered. Many patients are unable to achieve recommended LDL-C target levels despite intensive statin therapy, with or without ezetimibe.

Proprotein convertase subtilisin/kexin type 9 (PCSK9) inhibitors can be used to treat these patients. PCSK9 inhibitors have been shown to reduce Lp(a) by 25–30% in addition to LDL-C. Because they are used in patients with HoFH, knowledge of the underlying genetic defect is useful. Patients with receptor-negative status may not respond to PCSK9 inhibitors as well as patients with receptor-defective status. The Tesla B study found that patients with one or two defective LDL receptor mutations had a 40.8% mean reduction in LDL-C, compared to no reduction in patients with two negative mutations.

Other newer agents available: Patients with HoFH have high LDL-C > 500 mg/dL and require a high dose of statins, ezetimibe, and PCSK9 inhibitors. *Mipomersen* and *lomitapide* (not available in India) are FDA-approved drugs for the treatment of HoFH patients, but they have toxic side effects. For HoFH, LDL apheresis may be a reasonable and effective option in our country.

Inclisiran is a small interfering RNA (SiRNA) molecule that reduces hepatic PCSK9 production and significantly lowers LDL-C levels. In a randomized trial of FH patients already on maximally tolerated statins (ORION-9), inclisiran demonstrated both safety and efficacy in lowering LDL-C by 45%. It is given as a subcutaneous injection twice a year.

Evinacumab is a monoclonal antibody against angiopoietin-like 3 (ANGPTL3) that can be given subcutaneously or intravenously in patients with homozygous hypercholesterolemia as well as in patients with or without HoFH who have refractory hypercholesterolemia. ANGPTL3 is a secreted protein expressed primarily in the liver. It inhibits the activity of LPL and endothelial lipase (EL), and retards clearance of TRLs upstream of LDL production. At the maximum dose, evinacumab-reduced LDL-C by >50% in patients with refractory hypercholesterolemia. In phase III clinical trial (ELIPSE) in 65 patients with HoFH a significant 47% decrease in LDL-C levels was observed in patients receiving evinacumab together with maximum doses of lipid-lowering therapy compared to baseline levels, and a 49% difference from the placebo group receiving maximum doses of lipid-lowering therapy alone.

TABLE 4: Asymptomatic hypertriglyceridemia.

TG level (mg/dL)	Subjects	Management
<150	Any	Lifestyle modification
150–499	Diabetic/ASCVD risk factors	Statins + Icosapent ethyl
150–499	Nondiabetic or risk factors	Statin + Nonstatin drugs
>500	Familial hyperchylomicronemia	Low-fat diet Fibrates + Omega 3 FA + Saroglitazar

Source: Adapted from Sawhney et al.[13]

TABLE 5: Management of genetic hypercholesterolemia.

Condition	Diagnosis	Treatment (increasing intensity if not on target—recommended target is LDL < 55 mg/dL)
HeFH	DLCN score > 6	*Level 1*: High-dose statin + Ezetimibe
HoFH		*Level 2*: Add PCSK9i/Inclisiran
		Level 3: Evinacumab (yet to be launched in India)
		Level 4: LDL apheresis

(DLCN: Dutch Lipid Clinic Network)

Statin-intolerant Patients with Asymptomatic Hypercholesterolemia

Statin intolerance occurs due to its side effects: (1) Statin-associated muscle symptoms (SAMS)—10–15% in observational studies and even less in blinded studies; (2) statin-associated rhabdomyolysis very rare (1–3 cases/100,000 patient years); (3) raised transaminases 0.5–2% and usually mild; (4) statin-induced diabetes (highest with rosuvastatin) is very mild and rare—one case in 255 statin-treated patient in 4 years. It is less common in young.

In case of SAMS the options are based on risk stratification: Low risk (5-year MACE < 5%)—no treatment, moderate risk (5-year MACE 5–15%)—ezetimibe, and high risk (5-year MACE 15–20%) and very high risk (5-year MACE > 20%)—ezetimibe + PCSK9 inhibitor. Inclisiran is an alternative.[19] Recent CSI guideline has emphasized that if SAMS occur with more than four times creatinine phosphokinase, statin should be stopped and rechallenged after 4 weeks at lower alternate day dosing.[13]

Bempedoic acid is available as a nonstatin treatment option in statin-intolerant patients. Combination of bempedoic acid and ezetimibe can be used if LDL target is not met by single nonstatin drug.

CONCLUSION

Dyslipidemia in asymptomatic Indians is a problem that requires urgent attention due to long-term implications on atherosclerotic disease burden. Large-scale screening is needed to uncover this population as effective therapies exist.

ONLINE REFERENCES

Please scan the QR code provided at the end of the table of contents for References of this chapter.

CHAPTER

32

Ten Commandments of Lipidology

Arpita Katheria, Rakesh Maurya, Aditya Kapoor, Rajeev Agarwal

ABSTRACT

Atherosclerotic cardiovascular disease (ASCVD) is the leading cause of mortality worldwide, particularly in India, where it develops earlier than the western population. Deranged lipid profiles are a risk factor, with lowering LDL-C being the main therapy target. Despite ongoing research, understanding lipidology is crucial for clinicians.

Keywords: ASCVD, mortality, India, lipid profiles, LDL-C

INTRODUCTION

Atherosclerotic cardiovascular disease (ASCVD) is the most common cause of mortality world-wide, and its prevalence continues to increase with time.[1] The problem is even more worrisome in India, as Indians tend to develop ASCVD a decade earlier than western population, and thus require early and more aggressive primary and secondary preventive strategies.[2] Deranged lipid profile has been an established risk factor for ASCVD. Although studies have shown Apo-B, lipoprotein(a) [Lp(a)], and triglycerides as causally related to ASCVD, lowering of LDL-C has shown definitive benefit, and remains the main target of therapy.[1] There is a lot of ongoing research targeting different components of lipid profile, and it may be challenging to keep up with the same. Here the salient features of lipidology are highlighted as ten commandments of lipidology for clinicians' usage.

COMMANDMENT 1

Atherosclerosis is a childhood disease that matures in adulthood and is aggravated by social determinants: Coronary artery disease is commonly encountered during adulthood and is, therefore, considered a disease of adults. But atherogenesis starts early in life, often, during childhood. A study conducted on human fetal aortas in 82 spontaneously aborted fetuses and premature newborns, who died within 12 hours of birth, showed that fatty streak formation had started during fetal development and was worse in fetuses with maternal hypercholesterolemia.[3] Many other studies have shown that atherosclerosis starts during childhood and progresses into adulthood.[4] It has also been shown that risk factors during childhood predict clinical cardiovascular events during mid-life.[5] Studies have also shown favorable, kind environments, leading to lesser incidence of atherosclerosis despite cholesterol-rich diet, in experimental animals.[6] Thus, it is imminent that steps such as healthy diet, lifestyle changes, positive emotional environments are taken from childhood itself so as to prevent coronary events later in life.[7]

COMMANDMENT 2

LDL-C is the main driver for atherosclerosis: There are four compelling lines of evidence that prove that LDL-C is the main driving force for atherosclerosis **(Fig. 1)**. These include *epidemiological data* which shows that increased LDL-C is directly related to increased risk of atherosclerosis,[8] *genetic association* of familial hypercholesterolemia with higher risk of premature atherosclerotic cardiovascular disease,[9] *experimental evidence* of increased coronary events in animals with induced hypercholesterolemia,[10] and *evidence of therapy* with statins, PCSK9 inhibitors which decrease LDL-C and also reduce MACE. In the CTT collaborators meta analysis, more intensive lipid-lowering therapy produced a 15% further reduction in major vascular events, with significantly lower coronary death or nonfatal MI, coronary revascularization, and ischemic stroke.[11]

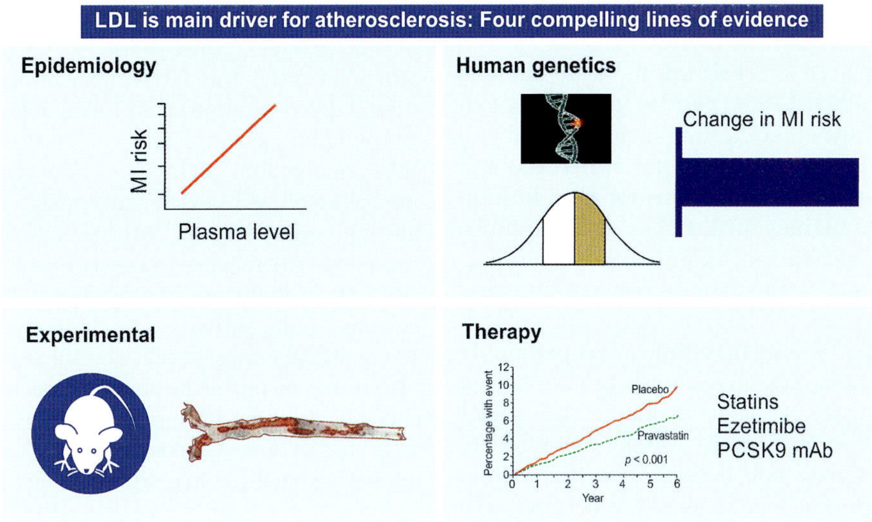

FIG. 1: Lines of evidence suggesting LDL-C as the main driver for atherosclerosis.

COMMANDMENT 3

Lower LDL-C is better: The invention of statins marked the beginning of a new era in the management of atherosclerosis. PROVE-IT trial was the first to show that high-intensity statin (atorvastatin 80 mg/day) was associated with lower rates of MACE in ACS patients compared to moderate-intensity statin (pravastatin 40 mg/day). The median LDL-C achieved was 62 and 95 mg/dL, respectively. This study showed that achieving lower levels of LDL-C levels resulted in greater protection against major cardiovascular events or death.[12] This was further substantiated by the IMPROVE-IT trial, in which, simvastatin and ezetimibe combination therapy (median LDL-C 53.7 mg/dL) led to improved cardiovascular outcomes in ACS patients, compared to simvastatin monotherapy (median LDL-C 69.5 mg/dL).[13] The trials of PCSK9 inhibitors have shown that LDL-C can be safely lowered to 30 mg/dL or lower, with incremental reduction in risk of cardiovascular events.[14,15] LAI guidelines have recommended aggressive lowering of LDL-C, with the target LDL-C of 30 mg/dL in extreme risk patients, with consideration for further reduction to 10–15 mg/dL if recurrent ASCVD events occur at LDL-C of 30 mg/dL.[2]

COMMANDMENT 4

Combination therapy should be standard of care: A meta-analysis done on individual patient data of eight large RCTs on statins studied over 38,000 patients and found large interindividual variation in LDL-C reduction, with > 40% patients not achieving target LDL-C of 70 mg/dL with high-intensity statin therapy, and having higher risk of MACE.[16] This study highlights the fact that statin may not be enough in achieving target LDL-C levels, and there is need for combination therapy with ezetimibe, PCSK9 inhibitors, bempedoic acid etc. to reach target LDL-C levels. The benefit of combination therapy is that it uses synergistic action of these drugs in cholesterol synthesis and absorption, and receptor recycling, also it helps with dose-dependent side effects of certain drugs, such as statins.[17] LDL-C reduction with moderate-intensity statin is 30–50% and 50% with high-intensity statin therapy, 20% with ezetimibe, and 60% with PCSK9 inhibitors. The maximum theoretical LDL-C reduction achieved by combination of high-intensity statin with ezetimibe is 60%, with HI statin + PCSK9 inhibitors is 80%, and with HI statin + PCSK9 inhibitors + ezetimibe is 84%.[17] Recent studies have also shown the superiority of combination therapy of statin with ezetimibe compared to statin monotherapy in reducing MACE. The Racing trial in patients with established ASCVD compared MI statin combined with ezetimibe with HI statin monotherapy and showed that the combination therapy was noninferior to HI statin monotherapy ($p = 0.48$) in terms of composite primary end-point of cardiovascular death, major cardiovascular events, or nonfatal stroke with better LDL-C control in combination therapy (LDL-C < 70 mg/dL in 72% patients in combination therapy and 58% with statin monotherapy).[18] A cohort study in Korean population showed that combination of MI statin with ezetimibe was superior to HI statin monotherapy in reducing the composite outcome of myocardial infarction, stroke, and death in primary prevention population with dyslipidemia.[19] LAI (2023) guidelines recommend to calculate % reduction in LDL-C required to achieve target levels of LDL-C at week zero and start therapy accordingly: MI statin for 30%, HI statin for 50%, HI statin + ezetimibe for 65% reduction in LDL-C, add Bile acid sequestrant or bempedoic acid for additional 20% reduction, and PCSK9 inhibitors for >20% reduction.[2]

COMMANDMENT 5

It does not matter how LDL-C is lowered: There are multiple pathways through which LDL-C can be lowered. It can be done through lifestyle modification including diet and exercise, pharmacological therapy, lipid apheresis, and intestinal bypass surgery. Diet and lifestyle modification has been shown to reduce LDL-C by 10–15%.[20] The CTT meta-analysis has shown that 1 mmol/L (39 mg/dL) reduction in LDL-C led to 10% decrease in all-cause mortality and 24% decrease in both major coronary events and revascularization.[11] Studies have shown that per mg/dL reduction of LDL-C, cholestyramine and ezetimibe showed similar cardiovascular risk reduction as statin.[20] This shows that cardiovascular benefits of lipid-lowering therapies are proportional to LDL-C reduction; it does not matter whether it is done using a single drug, or a combination of drugs, with or without lifestyle modification. This is in contrast to diabetes treatment, where some drugs such as SGLT-2 inhibitors have proven cardiovascular benefits, over and above blood glucose lowering **(Fig. 2)**.

COMMANDMENT 6

Intensive lipid lowering causes plaque stabilization and regression: It has been established previously that intensive lipid lowering with statin as well as other agents decreases LDL-C levels, and in turn lower LDL-C levels lead to lower rates of MACE. Recent studies using intravascular imaging have also shown that better lipid control may also lead to plaque stabilization and even regression. A case report by Nishihira et al. showed that intensive lipid lowering with a combination of statin and ezetimibe leads to plaque stabilization on near-infrared spectroscopy (NIRS) with a marked decline in maximum lipid core burden index (LCBI) of 701 to 237 at 1 month of follow-up.[21] The GLAGOV trial also showed that addition of evolocumab to statin led to significant decline in percentage atheroma volume (PAV) as well as total atheroma volume (TAV) on IVUS.[22] A post-hoc analysis of this trial also showed plaque regression with LDL-C levels of <50 mg/dL. More recently, the HUYGENS study **(Fig. 3)** demonstrated that in patients of NSTEMI, with raised LDL-C levels, combination of statin and evolocumab caused favorable changes in plaque phenotype (improved minimum fibrous cap thickness, reduced maximum lipid arc and macrophage index).[23] Similarly, in PACMAN AMI trial, alirocumab caused plaque regression (decreased PAV, decreased LCBI, and improved fibrous cap thickness) in noninfarct-related arteries among patients with acute myocardial infarction.[24] These studies suggest that stabilization and regression of plaque may be one of the potential mechanisms for improved clinical outcomes with very low levels of LDL-C. Further large-scale studies are required to definitively determine the role of lipid-lowering drugs in plaque stabilization and regression.

COMMANDMENT 7

LDL-C 30 is the new LDL-C 50: The concept that a human being can thrive on low values of LDL-C was originally postulated by Brown and Goldstein in their Nobel lecture in 1985. They suggested that LDL-C of 25 mg/dL would be sufficient to nourish body cells, and that plasma LDL-C of 25–60 mg/dL might be physiological for human beings.[25] Results of trials of PCSK9 inhibitors in which LDL-C levels were very low (median achieved LDL-C of 30 mg/dL in Fourier trial) found that these low levels of LDL-C were safe and effective.[14,15] There were initial concerns over long-term safety of these drugs, but the FOURIER OLE trial showed that evolocumab did not show more serious adverse events, neurocognitive events, or hemorrhagic stroke compared to placebo.[26] LAI (2023) guidelines have divided patients into five groups: Low risk, moderate risk, high risk, very high risk, and extreme risk. The last category is further subdivided into category A, B, and C. They recommend the target LDL-C of <100 mg/dL in low and moderate risk, <70 mg/dL in high-risk group, <50 mg/dL in very high-risk group, and extreme risk-category A, a target

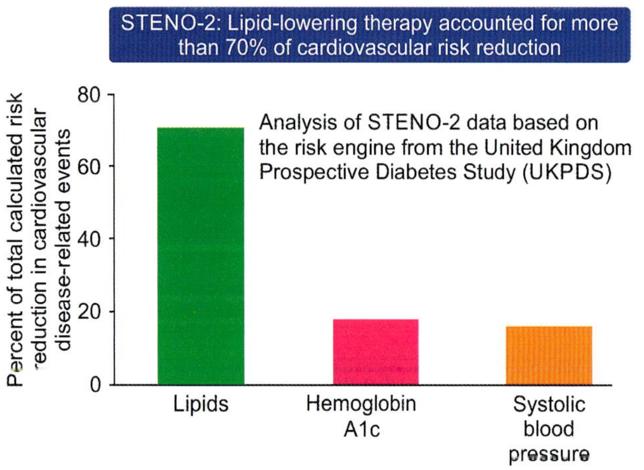

FIG. 2: Lipid-lowering therapy accounted for greater than 70% of total cardiovascular risk reduction in STENO-2 trial.

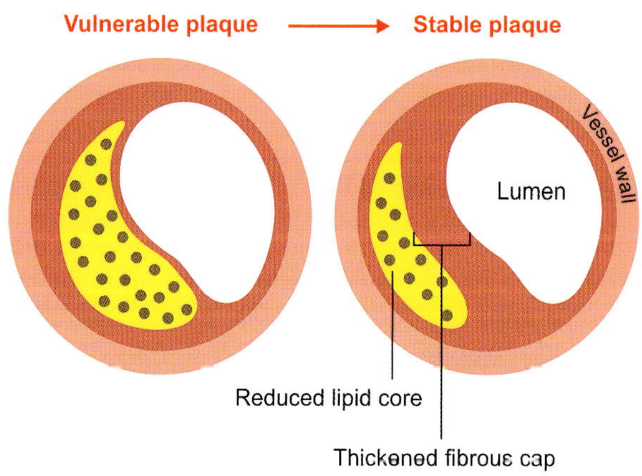

FIG. 3: Addition of evolocumab to statin caused plaque stabilization in HUYGENS trial.

LDL-C of <30 mg/dL is optional in extreme risk category A, but mandatory in extreme risk-category B patients, with target of 10–15 mg/dL in extreme risk-category C, where recurrent ASCVD events occur at LDL-C of 30 mg/dL.[2]

COMMANDMENT 8

Triglyceride is mere cosmetic correction: Mendelian randomization studies have shown a causal association between TRLs and ASCVD, though the extent of this association has been different in various studies and at times lost significance in multivariate analysis.[27] A recent randomized study has suggested that all lipoproteins containing Apo-B increase ASCVD risk, and that the ASCVD risk of TRLs is due to their Apo-B particles rather than TG content.[28] All LDL-C-lowering drugs also lower TG levels by 5–15%, while greater TG lowering (25–45%) is seen with fibrates, omega-3 fatty acids, and niacin. Fibrates, including the recently studied pemafibrate, have not shown any benefit over and above statin therapy in reducing MACE.[29] In the PROMINENT trial, diabetic patients with serum TG 200–499 mg/dL with HDL-C <40 mg/dL and LDL-C <100 mg/dL were taken. Pemafibrate 0.4 mg/day failed to reduce MACE, even after decreasing TG by 31%, rather, it increased LDL-C by 14% (likely due to conversion of TRL remnants to LDL-C).[30] Similarly, trials of niacin have also shown no benefit.[27]

Studies done on omega-3 fatty acids have shown contradictory results. The REDUCE-IT trial enrolled over 8,000 patients (70% established ASCVD and 30% DM with additional risk factors), with TG 135–499 mg/dL and LDL-C <100 mg/dL on statin therapy were given Icosapent ethyl (4 g/day) or placebo (mineral oil). The study showed much lower rates of MACE in EPA group compared to placebo (HR = 0.75; $p < 0.001$). At the end of study, triglycerides reduced by 21.6% with EPA, while LDL-C increased by 3.1%, while in the placebo group, TG decreased (–6.5%) and LDL-C increased (+10.2%).[31] The subsequent STRENGTH trial enrolled over 13,000 high risk patients on statin with low HDL-C, high TG (180–499 mg/dL), and LDL-C < 100 mg/dL were given omega 3 CA 4 g/day (EPA + DHA) or placebo (corn oil). There was no difference between the two groups in terms of MACE (HR = 0.99; $p = 0.84$).[32] The major differences between the two studies could be attributed to: (1) Mineral oil showed significant increase in inflammatory markers such as hs-CRP, IL-1B, IL-6, Lp(a), Apo-B, which were not shown by corn oil, which could have led to worse outcomes in placebo group in REDUCE-IT.[33] (2) The modest 20% decrease in TG levels cannot on its own explain the 25% reduction in MACE, as much better TG reduction with fibrates and niacin did not cause significant reduction in MACE in previous trials, and perhaps other properties of **Ω**3FA may have played major role in outcomes.[34] (3) EPA may have independent benefit in reducing CV outcomes, which are decreased by DHA.[29] This shows that TGs were enrollment criteria but not an outcome-based metric and perhaps, REDUCE IT is more a vascular trial than a TG-lowering trial. Current recommendations from LAI (2023) are that fasting TG > 150 mg/dL or nonfasting TG > 175 mg/dL is considered a risk modifier and have recommended addition of icosapent ethyl if persistent TG >150 mg/dL despite LDL-lowering therapy.[2]

COMMANDMENT 9

Intensive lipid lowering is safe: Neonates have LDL-C in the range of 30–70 mg/dL, with LDL-C values of <30 mg/dL reported in healthy neonates.[35] Genetic loss-of-function mutations in PCSK9 leading to low levels of LDL-C confers cardiovascular protection, lowering rates of cardiovascular events in these patients without any neurological damage. On the other hand, other genetic conditions such as abetalipoproteinemia, which is associated with undetectable levels of LDL-C secondary to absence of Apo-B containing lipoproteins, are characterized by severe neurological manifestations, although these have been found to be due to deficiency of fat-soluble vitamins, particularly vitamin E, which causes demyelination, and low LDL-C has not been found to be specific cause of the neurological manifestations.[36] Also, brain utilizes de-novo synthesized cholesterol and is not much affected by peripherally acting LDL-reducing agents. Many studies have shown increased risk of hemorrhagic stroke with lower levels of LDL-C, although this has not been shown with trials of PCSK9 inhibitors.[35] Long-term follow-up study, FOURIER-OLE which had follow-up of up to 8.4 years, showed that evolocumab did not show more serious adverse events, neurocognitive events, or hemorrhagic stroke compared to placebo, with median LDL-C of 29 mg/dL at the end of study and 15% lower risk of cardiovascular death, myocardial infarction, stroke, or hospitalization for unstable angina or coronary revascularization.[26] The increased risk of new onset diabetes seen with LDL-C lowering with statin use has not been seen with PCSK9 inhibitors. Also, there is no significant effect of low LDL-C on steroid hormones, which use cholesterol as a precursor.

COMMANDMENT 10

Lp(a)—a new pathway to target: Lp(a) has been causally associated with cardiovascular disease, although there are limited therapeutic options that target it, and treatment is directed at lowering LDL-C in such patients. It has been shown that elevated Lp(a) confers additional increased cardiovascular risk over and above the risk associated with raised LDL-C.[37] A genetic study found Lp(a) to be more atherogenic than LDL-C.[38] Among the existing therapy, statins, ezetimibe, and bempedoic acid have no or minimal effect on Lp(a), while PCSK9 inhibitors lowers Lp(a) by approximately 25%. Lipoprotein apheresis causes maximum 60% reduction in Lp(a) levels.[39] Three important drugs specifically targeting Lp(a) are in various stages of trials. These include pelacarsen, an antisense oligonucleotide, olpasiran and SLN360, both siRNA against Lp(a) mRNA.

The phase 3 HORIZONS outcome trial of pelacarsen is ongoing and will shed more light on cardiovascular outcomes of this new molecule.

CONCLUSION

Atherosclerosis is a metabolic curse for South Asians, particularly Indians, with earlier disease onset, and worse prognosis. The risk of ASCVD is directly proportional to LDL-C levels. Despite all the advancements in therapeutics, controlling dyslipidemias, and in turn ASCVD still remains a big challenge, particularly in developing countries such as India, where affordability and accessibility are important issues to consider. The ongoing research on therapies for molecules other than LDL-C such as Lp(a) may provide additional therapeutic targets to clinicians in future. To rephrase William Osler, the good physician treats stenosis, and the great physician treats atherosclerosis.

ONLINE REFERENCES

Please scan the QR code provided at the end of the table of contents for References of this chapter.

CHAPTER

33

Management of Pediatric Hyperlipidemia

Amit Malviya, Preethi Caleb Harris, Animesh Mishra

ABSTRACT

Diagnosis of pediatric lipid disorders is commonly missed in our day-to-day practice. Researchers in the past have highlighted that as many as 50% of the children with lipid abnormalities are missed because of lack of routine screening. Because atherosclerosis begins in childhood, there is an extended latent period, between the elevated risk and the actual occurrence of cardiovascular outcomes. This provides a window of time to explore early processes that contribute to the development of atherosclerotic cardiovascular disease (ASCVD) and to target intervention. This chapter highlights the importance of diagnosing hyperlipidemia in children and initiating treatment in childhood, which may reduce or prevent its progression into development of ASCVD. This chapter also highlights the causes of pediatric hyperlipidemia, screening recommendations, and treatment options available.

Keywords: Pediatric hyperlipidemia, screening for hyperlipidemia in children, lipid lowering therapy in children

INTRODUCTION

Lipids are an essential component of our daily diet. There are four major classes of plasma lipids which are clinically important, namely cholesterol, triglycerides, phospholipids, and free fatty acids. These are essential for cell membrane formation, energy transport, formation of hormones, synthesis of bile acids, etc. Excess of these triggers atherosclerosis. Hyperlipidemia has always been considered as a disorder among adults, and lipid levels in children are seldom measured and given importance. Evidences show that atherosclerotic changes start to begin in childhood, as early as by 2 years of age.[1] The introduction of electronic gadgets, emergence of fast foods, decreased outdoor activity, and the COVID pandemic have made all children globally at risk for childhood obesity, thereby leading to hyperlipidemia. There is evidence that early subclinical atherosclerosis during childhood leads to morbidity and mortality during adulthood.[2-5]

Dyslipidemias are abnormal amount of lipids (cholesterol or triglycerides) and/or lipoproteins (aggregate molecules made up of lipids and apolipoproteins that bind to lipids) in the blood.

IS HYPERLIPIDEMIA REALLY A PROBLEM IN CHILDREN AND ADOLESCENTS IN INDIA?

According to the Comprehensive National Nutrition Survey (CNNS, 2016–2018), the first and the largest nutrition assessment survey undertaken in children in India:[6]

- 2% of under-5 children were overweight or obese.
- 4% of school aged children (5–9 years) overweight or obese (BMI for age > +1 SD).
- 5% of adolescents (10–19 years) were overweight or obese (BMI for age > +1 SD).
- 2% of adolescents had abdominal obesity (waist circumference-for-age > +1 SD).
- The prevalence of high total cholesterol was 3% and 4% among school-age children (5–9 years) and adolescents (10–19 years), respectively.
- About 34% of children, 5–9 years, and 16% of adolescents had high triglycerides.
- The prevalence of low HDL cholesterol was 26% and 28% among school-age children and adolescents, respectively.
- 1 in 10 children was prediabetic and 1% of children were already diabetic.

A higher prevalence of low HDL cholesterol was observed among children and adolescents who resided in rural areas. These parameters indicate that the future working population is at an increased risk for atherosclerotic cardiovascular disease (ASCVD). This is a serious cause of concern and needs to be addressed.

These above statistics indicate that there is a paradigm shift in the nutritional status of children in India with the trend heading toward childhood obesity. So, it is indeed a necessity to identify children who are at risk of ASCVD.

Normal Values of Lipids in Children

Levels of lipids fluctuate at various stages of childhood and adolescence. They are influenced by various metabolic, hormonal, genetic and environmental factors, age, and sex.[7] Total cholesterol in umbilical cord blood is approximately 70 mg/dL. These levels increase significantly during infancy and then increase slowly thereafter up to 9–11 years, when they more closely reflect adult values. During puberty, secondary to hormonal changes, the total cholesterol and LDL cholesterol levels decrease and HDL and TG levels also fluctuate. The Dietary Intervention Study in Children (DISC) showed an average decrease of LDL of 23.3 mg/dL in boys and 10.6 mg/dL in girls in Tanner stage 4 or 5 compared to Tanner stage 1.[8] The plasma cholesterol levels tend to be higher in girls when compared to boys. Baseline values are attained around the second decade of life. Hence, screening is not recommended during the pubertal period due to high rates of false-negative results.

Historically, an overnight fast was deemed compulsory before lipid screening. Studies in children have shown that the difference between fasting and nonfasting lipid values was not statistically significant. Fasting is advisable only if nonfasting screening lipid profile shows derangement in triglyceride levels.[9] Lipid levels if abnormal should be repeated again and an average of both must be taken. Based on the NLHBI integrated guidelines for cardiovascular health and risk reduction in children and adolescents, the values are categorized into acceptable, borderline, and high **(Table 1)**.[10]

TABLE 1: Lipid values in children and adolescents.†

	Cutoff level category (mg/dL)*		
Lipid	**Acceptable**	**Borderline**	**High/low**
Total cholesterol	<170	170–199	≥200
LDL-C	<110	110–129	≥130
Non-HDL-C	<120	120–144	≥145
Apolipoprotein B	<90	90–109	≥110
Triglycerides			
Age 0–9 years	<75	75–99	≥100
Age 10–19 years	<90	90–129	≥130
HDL-C	>45	40–45	<40
Apolipoprotein A-1	>120	115–120	<115

*The cut points for high and borderline high represent approximately the 95th and 75th percentiles, respectively. Low cut points for HDL-C and ApoA-1 represent approximately the 10th percentile.

†For children, fasting refers to consuming nothing except water after midnight.

(HDL-C: high-density lipoprotein cholesterol; LDL-C: low-density lipoprotein cholesterol)

IS SCREENING THE NEED OF THE HOUR?

Given the evidence that the diagnosis of hyperlipidemia among children has been a rarity so far, the above evidence concludes that screening is an essential part for primary prevention of adult ASCVD.

Guidelines for screening for dyslipidemia in the pediatric population have evolved over the past 26 years. It remains controversial because it involves testing for a risk factor for atherosclerosis and not for the disease per se.[11] Screening for family history for cardiovascular disease (CVD) can be challenging because of limited time for history taking during patient encounters.[12] Before 2011, there were two major approaches to screening for hyperlipidemia in children: screening in selected populations and screening in the general population. Traditionally, screening of high-risk children with multiple risk factors, a family history of CVD, or the presence of hypercholesterolemia in the family members was the recommendation. The results of the Coronary Artery Risk Detection in Appalachian Communities project indicated that the targeted screening processes most likely resulted in missed opportunities, overlooked many with significant dyslipidemia, and failed to detect genetic dyslipidemias, which require early pharmacological treatment.[13] In 2011, the US National Institutes of Health National Heart, Lung, and Blood Institute (NHLBI) Expert Panel recommended additional "universal screening" for all children and adolescents.

GUIDELINE RECOMMENDATIONS REGARDING SCREENING

See **Table 2** and **Flowcharts 1 and 2**.

CLASSIFICATION OF HYPERLIPIDEMIAS

Hyperlipidemias can be classified as primary or secondary.

Primary hyperlipidemia is caused by genetic mutations resulting in abnormal levels of lipids and apolipoproteins **(Table 3)**.

The most common is FCH followed by FH. FH can be diagnosed with a personal or family history of hypercholesterolemia or premature ASCVD. The patients present

TABLE 2: Guideline recommendations for screening in children.

Organization	Universal screening recommendation	Target screening recommendation
AHA (2018)	In children and adolescents without cardiovascular risk factors or a family history of early CVD, it may be reasonable to measure a lipid profile once between the ages of 9 and 11 years and again between the ages of 17 and 21 years[11]	• In children and adolescents with: ○ A family history of either early CVD (MI, documented angina, or atherosclerosis by angiography in parents, siblings, grandparents, aunts, or uncles with age < 55 years for men and <65 years for women) or ○ Significant hypercholesterolemia (≥240 mg/dL, LDL-C ≥190 mg/dL, non-HDL-C ≥ 220 mg/dL, or known primary hypercholesterolemia) • It is reasonable to measure a fasting or nonfasting lipoprotein profile as early as age 2 years to detect FH or rare forms of hypercholesterolemia[11] • In children who have been found to have moderate or severe hypercholesterolemia, it is reasonable to do a reverse cascade screening • Lipid profile screening is done in first- and second-degree relatives, and if possible, third-degree relatives to detect familial lipid disorders
AAP (2017)[10]	Screen once (fasting or nonfasting) between 9 and 11 years of age and once between 17 and 21 years of age	Selective screening (fasting lipid profile) between 2 and 8 years of age if (1) parent, grandparent, aunt/uncle, or sibling with MI, angina, stroke, CABG/stent/angioplasty at <55 years in males and <65 years in females; (2) parent with TC ≥ 240 mg/dL or known dyslipidemia; (3) child has a moderate- or high-risk medical condition which includes any one of the following: • *High risk*: ○ Diabetes ○ Hypertension that requires pharmacological treatment ○ BMI ≥ 97th percentile ○ Chronic kidney disease ○ Postorthotopic heart transplant ○ Kawasaki's disease with current aneurysm ○ Smokes cigarettes • *Moderate risk*: ○ Exposed to secondhand smoke ○ Hypertension not requiring pharmacological treatment ○ Obesity, BMI > 95th percentile and overweight in adolescents ○ Nephrotic syndrome ○ Kawasaki's disease with regressed coronary aneurysms ○ Chronic inflammatory disease ○ HIV infection Selective screening (fasting lipid profile) between 12 and 16 years of age if there is new knowledge of one of the criteria above, but BMI cut point of ≥85th percentile

with ASCVD by the age of 20 years. Carotid intima-media thickness gives a clue to the burden of ASCVD. Diagnostic criteria include Simon Broome system, Dutch Lipid Clinic Network criteria, and MEDPED criteria.

Secondary hyperlipidemia is usually caused due to an underlying nonlipid disorder. Treatment of the causes usually resolves the lipid abnormalities **(Table 4)**.

MANAGEMENT

Lifestyle modification is the first line of treatment in the management of any pediatric hyperlipidemia. There is enough evidence to back up such an approach among pediatric population. Adopting healthy behaviors such as proper dietary approach, weight loss, daily physical activity, and appropriate sleep often results in favorable outcomes. Pharmacological treatment is recommended only when the trial of nonpharmacological measures fails and in hereditary hyperlipidemias.

Lifestyle Modification

Lifestyle modification plays an important role. It primarily focuses on dietary changes and physical activity. Parents play an important role in encouraging their children in this aspect.[14]

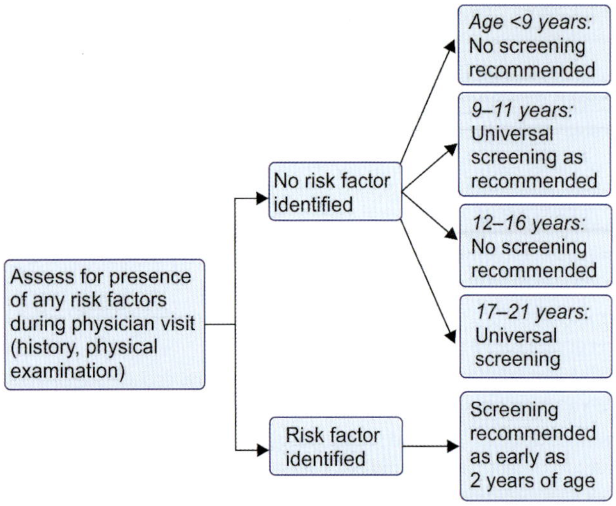

FLOWCHART 1: Screening for pediatric hyperlipidemia.

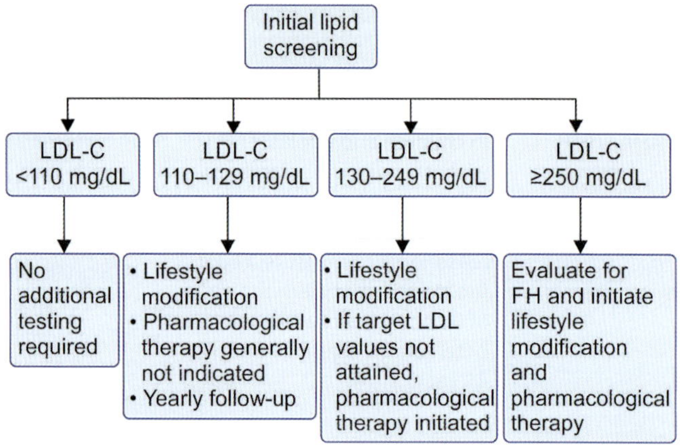

FLOWCHART 2: Interpretation of lipid profile results and management algorithm.

TABLE 3: Classification of genetic dyslipidemias and their clinical features.

Type	Genetic abnormality	Excess lipoproteins	Disease	CV risk	Risk of pancreatitis	Other clinical features
I	Absent lipoprotein lipase or apoC-II, apoA5, GPIHBP1, LMF1	Chylomicrons, triglycerides	Familial chylomicronemia syndrome	+	++	• 1–2/million children • Manifests in infancy; eruptive xanthoma, lipemia retinalis, hepatosplenomegaly
IIa	Absence or reduction of LDL receptors—most common *APOB, PCSK9, LDLRAP1* mutations	LDL	Familial hypercholesterolemia (FH)	++++	–	• Can be homozygous (1 in 1 million) or heterozygous (1 in 500) depending on the severity of lack of LDL receptor • Tendon and cutaneous xanthomas may be seen (rarely found before 10 years of age) • Aortic stenosis
IIb	ApoB100 overproduction	LDL, VLDL	Familial combined hyperlipidemia (FCH)	++	–	• 1 in 200–300 • Linked to T2DM, metabolic syndrome, and CKD
III	APOE mutation	Chylomicron, VLDL remnants	Familial dysbetalipoproteinemia	++	+	• Palmar xanthoma • Not usually seen in childhood
IV	Overproduction of VLDL	VLDL, TG+ *Low* HDL	Familial hypertriglyceridemia	+	++	Hepatomegaly, DM, lipemia retinalis, eruptive xanthomas
V	Overproduction of VLDL and decreased lipoprotein lipase	VLDL, TG++ *Low* HDL	Familial hypertriglyceridemia	+	++	

Daily Physical Activity

In the era of COVID pandemic where there has been an exponential surge of use of electronic gadgets by the children, it is essential to emphasize the importance of outdoor physical activity in order to improve the physical and mental health of the future generation. Recommendations are:[15]

- *3–5 years of age*: At least 180 minutes of physical activity per day. They should not be sedentary for >60 minutes at a time except during sleep.
- *6–17 years of age*: 60 minutes or more of moderate to vigorous physical activity every day.

Good Sleep Pattern

Adequate nighttime is important for the prevention of obesity. A positive dose-response relationship has been observed between total sleep hours and risk of development of obesity.[16] Educating parents regarding the importance of establishing a healthy sleep routine for themselves and their

TABLE 4: Secondary causes of dyslipidemia.

Dietary factors	• Diet rich in saturated fatty acids and carbohydrates • Sedentary lifestyle • Alcohol
Endocrine–metabolic disorders	• Diabetes mellitus • Hypothyroidism • Hypopituitarism • Cushing syndrome • Acromegaly • Polycystic ovarian syndrome • Obesity • Pregnancy • Lipodystrophy • Glycogen storage disorders
Kidney disease	• Nephrotic syndrome • Chronic kidney disease
Liver disease	• Alcoholic hepatitis • Biliary cirrhosis • Cholestasis (biliary atresia, Alagille syndrome, benign recurrent intrahepatic cholestasis)
Infections	• Acute viral or bacterial infections • Human immunodeficiency virus • Hepatitis
Inflammatory conditions	• Systemic lupus erythematosus • Juvenile rheumatoid arthritis
Drugs	• Thiazide diuretics • Beta-blockers • Immunosuppressants (cyclosporine, tacrolimus, l-asparaginase) • Corticosteroids • Oral contraceptives • Retinoids • Antiretroviral therapy
Miscellaneous	• Kawasaki disease • Congenital heart disease • Anorexia nervosa • Solid organ transplantation • Childhood cancer survivor

children is needed. The American Academy of Pediatrics recommends the following guidelines regarding sleeping hours per day for children:

- *1-2 years of age*: 11–14 hours
- *3-5 years of age*: 10–13 hours
- *6-12 years of age*: 9–12 hours
- *13-18 years of age*: 8–10 hours

Screen Time

Sedentary behaviors like excessive television viewing are associated with higher triglycerides and lower HDL levels. Limiting screen time promotes physical activity in children. It has been identified as an independent predictive factor of obesity.[17]

Dietary Modifications

One of the best ways to achieve a healthy lifestyle among children is to create a positive and healthy home environment. Often, children mimic the healthy behaviors adopted by their parents.

Studies have shown that preschool children who were exposed to three household routines of eating dinner regularly as a family, getting sufficient nighttime sleep, and limited screen time had lower obesity rates when compared to those who were not following these routines.[18,19]

Parents are the gatekeepers for food, snacks, and beverage availability at home. Studies have shown that the exposure to healthy snacks like fruits and vegetables at 2–4 years predict the child's food preferences at 8 years. Reducing unhealthy snack availability at home may be the first initiative to promote cardiovascular health.

Dietary modifications can have a significant impact on improvement in BMI and abnormal lipid levels in children. The modifications focus on reducing total and saturated fat and cholesterol. Increased intake of dietary fiber through fruits, vegetables, and whole grains is recommended (**Table 5**).

The first step would be to place the child on a CHILD-1 diet. If the child's fasting lipid levels after a 3-month trial intervention exceed the therapeutic target, the child must be placed on an even more restricted diet, the CHILD-2 diet. If lipid levels have not reached target levels even

TABLE 5: CHILD-1 and CHILD-2 dietary recommendations by the National Cholesterol Education Program (NCEP).[20]

Recommendations	CHILD-1	CHILD-2
Total fat consumption	20–30% of total caloric intake	20–30% of total caloric intake
Saturated fat	<10% of total calories	<7% of total calories
Average daily total cholesterol	<300 mg	<200 mg
Daily calories from MUFA	Should not exceed 10–15%	Should not exceed 10–15%
PUFA intake	Up to 10%	Up to 10%
Dietary fibers	5 or more times a day	5 or more times a day

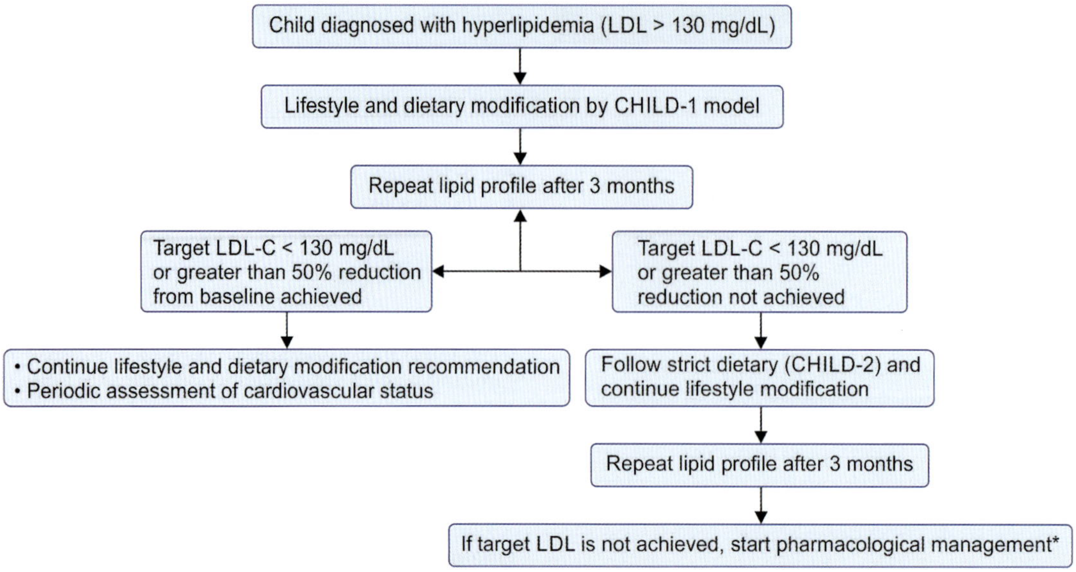

*If LDL-C levels > 190 mg/dL, initiate statin therapy depending on the age;
LDL 160–189 mg/dL—if features of familial hypercholesterolemia;
Or family history of premature CVD, initiate statin therapy;
If target level is not achieved, consider starting on other lipid-lowering agents.

FLOWCHART 3: Management of pediatric hyperlipidemia.

after a 3-month trial of even more stringent diet, then pharmacological therapy is recommended **(Flowchart 3)**.

The target LDL level recommended is <130 mg/dL or >50% reduction from baseline.

PHARMACOLOGICAL THERAPY

In a subgroup of patients, especially those with primary hyperlipidemias, lifestyle modifications may not be sufficient to mitigate the risks of ASCVD. When pharmacological therapy is initiated, it is important to continue the implementation of lifestyle modification. Both act synergistically and may attenuate the need for a higher dose of pharmacological therapy. According to the AHA guidelines, in children and adolescents 10 years or older who have LDL > 190 or >160 mg/dL with clinical features consistent with FH, who do not respond to lifestyle modification, statins are recommended.

Exception is children with homozygous familial hypercholesterolemia where treatment can be initiated as early as 2 years of age **(Table 6)**.

Statins

To date, statins are considered to be the first-line drugs in the management of pediatric hyperlipidemia, due to their safety, efficacy, and cost. Currently, seven of the commercially available statins are approved for their use in children and adolescents and multiple trials have been conducted and have proven the efficacy and safety profile of statins in children. Rosuvastatin is approved for use in children from the age of 7 years, pravastatin and pitavastatin from the age of 8 years, and simvastatin, atorvastatin, lovastatin, and fluvastatin may be used from the age of 10 years.[21] Statins act in a dose-dependent mechanism and reduce LDL levels up to 33%.

TABLE 6: Commonly used drugs and their doses for treatment of pediatric hyperlipidemia.

Drug	Age (years)	Dose	Expected LDL-C (% reduction)
Rosuvastatin	8–9	5–10 mg	44–52
	10–17	5–20 mg	44–63
Pravastatin	8–13	20 mg	30
	14–18	40 mg	36
Atorvastatin	10–17	10–20 mg	37–42
		10–80 mg (HoFH)	37–60
Fluvastatin	10–16	20–80 mg	20–36
Simvastatin	10–17	10–40 mg	30–40
Lovastatin	10–17	10–40 mg	20–30
Colesevelam	10–17	3.75 g	10–15
Cholestyramine	6–12	80 mg/kg TID, maximum dose 8 g/day	20
	10–17	4 g BD	
Ezetimibe		10 mg	20

They can be used in children with both FH and secondary hyperlipidemia. The choice of statins is a matter of provider preference and can be influenced by the amount of expected reduction in LDL. The primary goal is to achieve LDL levels < 130 mg/dL or ≥50% reduction. If reduction is not achieved with the initial dose, doubling the dose can be considered provided the maximal dose has not been reached. However, doubling the dose will cause an additional 6% reduction only.

The FDA has approved the use of statins for both heterozygous and homozygous FH.[22]

In heterozygous FH patients, where LDL level reduction with trial of lifestyle modification has not been satisfactory, statins can be initiated. In a 20-year follow-up of children with hypercholesterolemia treated with statins by Ilse et al., it was shown that statins slowed the progression of carotid intima-media thickness and reduced the risk of adulthood CVD. LDL levels should be maintained < 130 mg/dL.[23,24]

In homozygous FH patients, LDL levels should be maintained <100 mg/dL or ≥50% reduction from baseline. However, in practice, up to 80% of homozygous FH patients do not achieve target LDL values with statins alone.

Transaminase levels should be checked before starting statins. Liver enzymes, creatinine kinase, and pubertal growth development and growth monitoring need to be done on a periodic basis. They are contraindicated in breastfeeding and pregnancy due to their potential teratogenicity. There appear to be no available data till date on the risk of development of diabetes in children treated with statins.

Ezetimibe

Ezetimibe is a cholesterol absorption inhibitor, whose action is mediated through the Niemann–Pick C1-like 1 receptor present in GI tract epithelial cells. It is well tolerated by children. It can be used alone or in combination with a statin. In combination with statins, LDL levels are reduced by up to 15%. They can be initiated by 10 years of age.[25]

Bempedoic Acid

Bempedoic acid is an ATP citrate lyase inhibitor. However, its safety and effectiveness in children < 18 years of age have not been established.

Bile Acid Sequestrants

Before the introduction of statins, bile acid sequestrants were the first-line drugs in the management of hyperlipidemia in children. They bind to the bile salts in the gastrointestinal tract and prevent reuptake. This leads to increased conversion of cholesterol to bile in hepatic cells, upregulation of LDL receptor, and increased clearance of LDL from blood. But they can lead to elevation in TG levels; hence, they are not recommended in HoFH. As much as 15% reduction in LDL levels was achieved. But the main problem was tolerance to the drugs because of unpleasant taste, nausea, vomiting, diarrhea, and flatulence leading to low treatment adherence in children. In addition to bile acids, they may bind to vitamins and hence children receiving this group of drugs should be periodically examined for signs of fat-soluble vitamin deficiencies and folate deficiency. Colesevelam has shown to have better tolerability than cholestyramine and colestipol. It is approved for HeFH > 10 years of age.[26]

PCSK9 Inhibitors

PCSK9 inhibitors bind to the circulating proprotein convertase subtilisin/kexin type 9 (PCSK9) and decrease the LDL receptor catabolism in liver cells, leading to its increased expression and increased clearance. Evolocumab and alirocumab are the two available drugs. They reduce the LDL cholesterol levels by 55–60% and 20–25% in adult heterozygous FH and homozygous FH, respectively. Response to treatment in children with HoFH depends on the residual LDL receptor activity (defective or null).

Trials have demonstrated that evolocumab (TAUSSIG, HAUSER) can be used safely in children > 10 years of age. The FDA has approved its use in children with both HeFH and HoFH in addition to other lipid-lowering agents.[27]

Dose is 420 mg once monthly, subcutaneous route.

Based on a multicentric phase 3 RCT ODYSSEY KIDS, the FDA has recently approved the use of alirocumab in patients with heterozygous FH who had LDL levels 130 mg/dL or greater while on other lipid-lowering therapies.[28]

Both the drugs have a good safety profile and can be safely used in children > 10 years of age.

Inclisiran

Inclisiran is a small interfering RNA (siRNA) which inhibits PCSK9 synthesis in liver cells by binding to the RNA-induced silencing complex and cleaves the messenger RNA complex that is responsible for encoding of PCSK9. This unique mechanism brings about a reduction in intracellular and extracellular PCSK9 levels, resulting in extended reduction of LDL cholesterol.

ORION 16 and ORION 13 are two clinical trials evaluating the safety of inclisiran in adolescents who have not attained target LDL levels with lipid-lowering therapy in HeFH and HoFH, respectively.[29]

Lomitapide

Lomitapide is a microsomal triglyceride transfer protein inhibitor. Phase 2 trials have shown promising results, but it is not yet approved for its use in children.[30]

Evinacumab

Evinacumab is an ANGPLT-3 inhibitor.

TABLE 7: Drugs used in the treatment of hypertriglyceridemia.

Class of drug	Drug	MOA	Side effects	Approval status
Fibric acid derivatives	Gemfibrozil, fenofibrate	Increase LPL activity and decrease VLDL production	Diarrhea, mild elevation of transaminases	Not approved in adolescents < 18 years of age
Omega fatty acid	• EPA/DHA • Icosapent ethyl	Inhibits diacyl glycerol, reduces VLDL production, and increases rate of peroxisomal beta oxidation in liver	Headache, nausea, arthralgia, dysgeusia	Not evaluated in children
Apolipoprotein C-III synthesis inhibitor	Volanesorsen (antisense oligonucleotide)	Targets mRNA to reduce apolipoorotein C- III synthesis and activates LPL-mediated hydrolysis of TG	Thrombocytopenia	No pediatric data available

(DHA: docosahexaenoic acid; EPA: eicosapentaenoic acid)

In the ELIPSE trial among adults with HoFH who had high LDL levels despite the use of high-dose statins, ezetimibe, PCSK9 inhibitors, lomitapide or plasmapheresis, evinacumab showed a 49% reduction after 6 months of treatment. Adverse effects include headache, UTI, upper respiratory tract infection, arthralgia, myalgia, and transaminitis.[31]

In HoFH patients of age 12 years or more, evinacumab showed a 47% decrease in LDL. In March 2023, it was approved for use in children as young as 5 years of age with HoFH.[32]

Dose: For children aged 12 years or more, 15 mg/kg/dose IV every 4 weeks.

Plant sterols and stanols can be used in children >2 years of age. They inhibit cholesterol absorption and cause an 8–10% reduction of LDL when used as an additive to statins.

Plasmapheresis is advised for patients who are aged 10 years and older, not responding to lipid-lowering therapy.

Drugs for Hypertriglyceridemia

Drugs for hypertriglyceridemia depend on the severity. Currently, there are no FDA-approved medications for the treatment of hypertriglyceridemia **(Table 7)**.

- *TG 150–399 mg/dL*: Dietary and lifestyle changes. If still not reducing, statins can be used. The main treatment goal is non-HDL cholesterol < 130 mg/dL.
- *TG 400–999 mg/dL*: Fibrates can be tried but are not approved by FDA.

CONCLUSION

Numerous other medications, fibrates, niacin, DGAT inhibitors, and others are still being evaluated. Other emerging therapies include liver-directed gene transfer of the LDL receptor, vaccines targeting key proteins involved in cholesterol metabolism, and CRISPR-based gene editing of PCSK9 and ANGPTL3.

ONLINE REFERENCES

Please scan the QR code provided at the end of the table of contents for References of this chapter.

SECTION 5

Hypertension

Section Outline

CHAPTER

34

Ambulatory and Home Blood Pressure Monitoring: Update 2024

A Muruganathan

ABSTRACT

This topic provides a comprehensive overview of the importance of blood pressure (BP) monitoring in diagnosing and managing hypertension, highlighting the limitations of traditional office BP measurements. Hypertension diagnosis traditionally relies on office BP measurements, which, despite being widely used, present limitations such as variability in readings and a lack of comprehensive data on BP fluctuations throughout the day. Notably, office BP readings do not capture critical nocturnal BP levels or early morning surges, both of which are vital indicators of cardiovascular risk.

Given these limitations, the medical community has increasingly turned to out-of-office BP measurements, including home blood pressure monitoring (HBPM) and ambulatory blood pressure monitoring (ABPM), as recommended by recent guidelines. These methods provide more reliable and continuous data, identifying phenomena like white-coat and masked hypertension, and offering a clearer picture of a patient's BP profile over 24 hours. Such detailed monitoring is essential for accurate diagnosis, better risk stratification, and effective management of hypertension.

Home blood pressure monitoring, in particular, has gained popularity due to its convenience, cost-effectiveness, and ability to empower patients in managing their condition. However, it also presents challenges, such as potential inaccuracies in device readings, improper use, and the inability to capture nocturnal BP variations.

The text concludes that a prudent approach would be to judiciously decide which patients would benefit from ABPM and to review the advantages and disadvantages of HBPM and ABPM for both diagnosis and effective management of hypertension. It emphasizes the need for clinicians to carefully assess the benefits and limitations of each monitoring method to determine the most appropriate approach for each patient, and highlights the potential for integrating these tools with telemedicine to enhance treatment decisions and improve patient outcomes.

Keywords: Ambulatory blood pressure monitor (ABPM), home blood pressure monitor (HBPM), systolic blood pressure (SBP), diastolic blood pressure (DBP)

INTRODUCTION

Hypertension is the most common preventable and modifiable risk factor for cardiovascular disease (CVD). Proper measurement of blood pressure (BP) is essential to make a diagnosis of hypertension, grade of hypertension, and arrive at treatment decisions. Office BP measurement is the most commonly used method for the diagnosis of hypertension. But, office BP is associated with several disadvantage, such as large variability in office BP readings. BP is known to exhibit circadian variations. Several factors affect BP all through the day. Currently, nocturnal risk of BP or nondipper pattern of hypertension is an important aspect to be considered when treating hypertensive patients and predicting patients who would be at high risk of strokes or cardiovascular (CV) events. Early morning rise of BP is another risk factor for CV events.[1] The office BP readings only provide a snapshot of BP readings at a specific time point during the clinic visit. Office BP measurements do not give 24 hour BP reading, nocturnal BP readings, or BP readings in the early morning hours. Hence, if treatment decisions and risk of stroke or CV events is based only on office BP measurements, inappropriate treatment decisions may be taken, and the best treatment approach may be missed.

Two alternative and better methods of measuring BP called out of office BP measurements have been recommended by guidelines today.[1] These include home blood pressure monitoring (HBPM) and ambulatory blood pressure monitoring (ABPM). The recent trends based on clinical studies and guidelines have recommended use of home blood pressure measurements over office BP readings and have recommended ambulatory blood pressure measurements in selected groups of patients.[1] Out-of-office BP measurements (by patients at home or with 24-hour ABPM) are more reproducible than office measurements, more closely associated with hypertension-induced organ damage and the risk of CV events and identify the white-coat and masked hypertension phenomena.[1] In untreated or treated subjects with office BP classified as high-normal BP or grade 1 hypertension (systolic 130–159 mm Hg and/or diastolic 85–99 mm Hg), the BP level needs to be confirmed using home or ambulatory BP monitoring.[1]

A prudent approach for the clinicians would be to judiciously decide, which patients would benefit from ABPM. Reviewing the advantages and disadvantages of HBPM and ABPM is essential for both diagnosis and more effective management of hypertension in the real world setting.[2]

TABLE 1: Advantages and disadvantages of HBPM.[6]

Advantages	Disadvantages
Multiple readings can be taken over a period of time	Some devices may not be accurate
Avoids white-coat hypertension	Patients may not place the cuff properly
Reproducible	Patients may change dose of drugs without medical advice
Better predictor of CV mortality than office BP	No recording at night
Can diagnose white-coat hypertension and masked hypertension	
Can detect increased BP variability	
Increases patient awareness of BP control	

HOME BLOOD PRESSURE MONITORING[3]

Over the past decade, HBPM has emerged as an effective and convenient means of screening for hypertension. HBPM allows patients to monitor BP as often as they wish. Monitors that use the oscillometric method are accurate, reliable, easy to use, and relatively inexpensive.[4,5] Several advantages have been reported with use of HBPM **(Table 1)**. Office BP measurements overestimated BP response compared with HBPM.

The National Institute for Health and Care Excellence (NICE) guidelines for HBPM have made three recommendations when using HBPM to confirm a diagnosis of hypertension: (1) For each BP recording, two consecutive measurements must be taken, at least 1 minute apart with the person seated; (2) BP must be recorded twice daily, ideally in the morning and evening; and (3) BP recording should continue for at least 4 days, ideally for 7 days. Measurements taken on the first day should be excluded and the average value of the remaining days after day one is discarded can be used.[7]

Utility of Home Blood Pressure Monitoring in the Real World Setting[8]

- *Guide treatment decisions*: HBPM can be effectively used to guide treatment decisions for optimum CV outcomes.
- *Improve patient compliance and adherence to treatment:* Incorporation of HBPM into routine management of patients with uncontrolled hypertension may improve BP control. With HBPM, patients can regularly monitor their own progress in controlling BP. Increased involvement of patients in their own health may improve patients compliance to treatment.[9]
- *Partner with telemedicine:* HBPM is very effective when it is coupled with telemonitoring. If the BP readings from HBPM instantly relayed to a primary healthcare professional, he can immediately guide treatment changes or dose adjustments.[10]

Limitations of Home Blood Pressure Monitoring[11]

Home blood pressure monitoring may give systolic daytime BP readings in children lower when measured with than daytime ABPM, whereas no such difference exists in adults. HBPM does not provide nocturnal recordings and cannot give information regarding the diurnal patterns in BP. Caution should be exercised in the use of HBPM in the elderly. Accuracy of devices is a limiting factor associated with HBPM use. Although standard cuffs are appropriate for most patients, in patients with small (<24 cm) or large (>32 cm) arm circumference, only appropriately designed cuffs of the right size should be used. Another imitation of HBPM is inappropriate placing of the cuff by patients or caregivers. To measure BP accurately, the cuff must be wrapped correctly, and proper posture of the patient is essential during the measurement. Inexperienced users find it difficult to wrap the cuff in the correct position. An incorrectly wrapped cuff can lead to less accurate BP readings. In addition, irregular pulses due to arrhythmias lead to inaccurate BP readings.

The Latest Development in Home Blood Pressure Monitoring Technology[5]

The latest development in HPBM technology is Intelli wrap cuff technology. It has a longer inflatable area within the cuff that wraps all the way round the arm. This decreases pressure loss on the brachial artery, increases the "acceptable range" of placement and thus reduces the impact of cuff placement on BP measurement accuracy. It is also pre-formed, and hence the user can easily fit it with one hand.

Research and Development of Nighttime Home Blood Pressure Monitoring

Historically, ABPM has been the gold standard for measuring nighttime BP. However, advancements in HBPM have introduced the ability to measure nighttime BP during sleep using self-measured devices. This progress has been driven by collaborations such as the one between Jichi Medical University and Omron Healthcare Co., Ltd., which aims to develop new HBPM systems and clinically relevant BP profiles through projects at the SURGE (SUper ciRculation monitorinG with high TEchnology) R&D Center.[1]

Key Developments and Evidence[12]

- *Medinote (HEM-5041; Omron Healthcare)*:
    - Year: 2010
    - Source: Kario et al.
    - Function: Automatic BP monitoring during sleep with fixed intervals
    - ICT-based: Not available
    - Competing device: Coleman et al.; Watch BP Home N (microlife)
- *HEM-7252G-HP (Omron Healthcare)*:
    - Year: 2017
    - Source: Kario et al.
    - Function: Automatic BP monitoring during sleep with fixed intervals, timer function after going to bed, and built-in third-generation mobile communication.
    - ICT-based: Available
    - Competing device: Takahashi et al.; Watch BP Home N (microlife)
- *Triggered Nighttime Blood Pressure Monitoring (TNP)*:
    - Year: 2006
    - Source: Shirasaki et al.
    - Function: Automatic BP monitoring during sleep with fixed intervals and triggered BP function based on oxygen saturation and heart rate.
    - ICT-based: Not available
    - Competing device: Viera et al. (not for additional function but for HEM780REL itself)
- *ICT-based TNP (ITNP)*:
    - Year: 2014
    - Source: Kario et al.
    - Function: TNP with built-in third-generation mobile communication facility for night-by-night evaluation
    - ICT-based: Available
    - Competing device: None
- *Wearable Beat-by-Beat Surge BP Monitoring (WSP)*:
    - Year: 2016
    - Source: Kario
    - Function: Wrist-type continuous BP monitoring based on the tonometry method
    - ICT-based: Not available
    - Competing device: None

Key Studies and Findings[13]

- *J-HOP study*:
    - Using the Medinote device, the J-HOP (Japan Morning Surge Home Blood Pressure) study successfully measured nighttime home BP at fixed intervals (2:00 AM, 3:00 AM, and 4:00 AM) for 14 days in 2,562 participants.
    - Findings demonstrated that self-measurement of nighttime BP at home is feasible and comparable to ABPM measurements. Nighttime BP was significantly correlated with various CV risk markers.
- *J-TOP trial*: The J-TOP (Japan Target Organ Protection) trial used nighttime HBPM to assess BP in a clinical intervention trial, finding that reductions in nighttime home BP were more closely associated with regression of left ventricular hypertrophy than clinic BP.

Advanced Nighttime Home Blood Pressure Monitoring Devices[4]

- *Medinote with ICT-based telemonitoring*: The Medinote device has evolved into the HEM-7252G-HP, an ICT-based nighttime home BP telemonitoring system that transmits data directly from the patient's home.
- *Trigger Nighttime HBPM (TNP)*: This device includes hypoxia-trigger and low heart rate-trigger functions, allowing BP measurements during specific conditions such as hypoxic episodes and periods of low heart rate.
- *Wearable Beat-by-Beat Surge BP Monitoring*: Omron Healthcare has developed a prototype wearable wrist-type tonometry BP monitor, aimed at providing continuous BP monitoring during sleep. This device detected significant variations in BP during different sleep stages.

Clinical Implications and Future Research[14]

- *SPREAD study*: The ongoing SPREAD (Sleep Pressure and Disordered Breathing in Resistant Hypertension and Cardiovascular Disease) study is evaluating the clinical implications of nighttime BP surges in high-risk patients.
- *ICT-Based TNP (ITNP) system*: The ITNP system enables repeated, real-life assessments of nighttime BP and OSA-related surges, enhancing the sensitivity of OSA detection and the evaluation of CPAP therapy effectiveness.

- *CPAP therapy evaluation*: ITNP has shown that effective CPAP therapy can significantly reduce nighttime BP surges, although some patients may still experience CV events despite therapy.[15]

Management of Nocturnal Hypertension[16]

- *Guidelines and recommendations*: The 2017 AHA/ACC guidelines recommend a nighttime BP control goal of <110/65 mm Hg. Morning home BP-guided titration of antihypertensive drugs is the first step toward achieving 24-hour BP control.
- *Practical strategy*: Based on the HONEST study, a three-step strategy is recommended for controlling morning hypertension, progressing to the control of masked nocturnal hypertension with a target nighttime BP < 110/85 mm Hg.

Nighttime HBPM is emerging as a valuable tool for assessing and managing nocturnal hypertension, with accuracy comparable to ABPM and potential advantages in detecting and managing specific conditions, such as OSA. Continued research and technological advancements will likely enhance the clinical utility and patient outcomes associated with nighttime HBPM.

AMBULATORY BLOOD PRESSURE MONITORING[17]

Ambulatory blood pressure monitoring devices are worn by patients over a 24-hour period with multiple measurements and are considered the gold standard for BP measurement. Ambulatory blood pressure readings provide a profile of BP behavior over a 24-hour period.

The definition of hypertension by using ABPM criteria continues to evolve **(Table 2)**. In clinical practice, a satisfactory ABPM recording should have ≥70% of expected measurements. Unlike recommendations from guidelines, position papers have considered it reasonable to increase the minimum of daytime measurements to 20 while retaining a minimum 7 measurements at night based on measurements being performed every 30 minutes, or more frequently throughout the entire 24-hour period. The ABPM recordings may have to be repeated if certain criteria are not met **(Box 1)**.[8]

The indications for performing ABPM are given in **Box 2**. The indications for ABPM include suspected white-coat hypertension, masked hypertension, resistant hypertension, labile hypertension, and orthostatic hypotension, to study the nocturnal BP profile and to assess the 24-hour control of BP **(Box 3)**. Over the past few years, there has been increasing interest in BP patterns during sleep, and nocturnal BP is now considered to be superior to daytime BP in predicting CV risk.[22]

TABLE 2: Thresholds for hypertension diagnosis based on ABPM.[18]

Thresholds for hypertension diagnosis			
24-hour average	≥130/80 mm Hg		
Awake (daytime) average	≥135/85 mm Hg		
Asleep (nighttime) average	≥120/70 mm Hg		
Suggested values for upper limit of normal	**Optimal**	**Normal**	**Abnormal**
Daytime	<130/80	<135/85	>140/90
Nighttime	<115/65	<120/70	>125/75
24 hours	<125/75	<130/80	>135/85

Benefits of using ABPM in Therapeutics[23]

- *Identifying nocturnal hypertension or nondipper pattern:* ABPM gives a continuous BP recording of BP over 24 hours. This helps in picking up alterations in the normal circadian pattern of BP. BP is usually higher during the day (or periods of wakefulness) and lower at night (or periods of sleep). At night, the expected physiological fall in BP is >10% (dipping), whereas a reduction of < 10% in BP at night is defined as "nondipping"; patients with "a riser (or reverse dipping)" pattern show an increase in BP during sleeping hours to levels (BP fall is <0%) that may be higher than those during the day (i.e., nocturnal hypertension). "Extreme dipping" is seen in patients who show a marked (>20%) nocturnal

BOX 1 Criteria for repeating ABPM recording.[19]

- 24-hour recording with ≥70% of expected measurements
- 20 valid awake (0900–2100 h) measurements
- 7 valid asleep (0100–0600 h) measurements
- Blood pressure measurements at 30 minutes intervals throughout 24 hours
- For research purposes ≥2 valid daytime and 1 valid nighttime measurement per hour

BOX 2 Indications for ABPM.[20]

- Identify white-coat hypertension
- Identify masked hypertension
- Identify the 24 hour BP pattern
- Nocturnal hypertension
- Identify nondippers
- Morning hypertension and morning blood pressure surge
- Study BP variability
- Assess the response to treatment
- Assess 24 hour BP control
- Diagnose refractory hypertension
- Identify ambulatory hypotension
- Identifying blood pressure patterns in Parkinson disease
- Endocrine hypertension

BOX 3 Definition of white-coat and masked hypertension phenomena.[21]

White-coat hypertension:
- Untreated subjects with elevated office blood pressure ≥ 140/90 mm Hg
- 24-h ABPM < 130/80 mm Hg
- Awake ABPM < 135/85 mm Hg
- Sleep < 120/70 mm Hg
- Home blood pressure < 135/85 mm Hg

Masked hypertension:
- Untreated subjects with office blood pressure < 140/90 mm Hg
- 24-h ABPM ≥ 130/80 mm Hg
- Awake ABPM ≥ 135/85 mm Hg
- Sleep ≥ 120/70 mm Hg
- Home blood pressure ≥ 135/85 mm Hg

Masked uncontrolled hypertension:
- Treated subjects with office blood pressure < 140/90 mm Hg
- 24-h ABPM ≥ 130/80 mm Hg
- Awake ABPM ≥ 135/85 mm Hg
- Sleep ≥ 120/70 mm Hg
- Home blood pressure ≥ 135/85 mm Hg

fall in systolic BP (SBP) and or diastolic BP (DBP), or have a night/day SBP or DBP ratio of <0.8. Nocturnal BP as assessed by ABPM is the most reproducible and reliable parameter for risk stratification. Nocturnal hypertension (BP ≥ 120/70 mm Hg) indicates the presence of comorbidities, such as obstructive sleep apnea (OSA). The riser pattern of nighttime BP is associated with a poor prognosis and occurrence of stroke and cardiac events. The morning BP surge (the difference between the lowest nighttime BP and morning BP measured 2 hours after awakening) is associated with an increased risk of CV and cerebrovascular adverse events, especially hemorrhagic stroke. ABPM facilitates diagnosis of nondipper profile, the morning surge of BP, and BP variability.[24]

- *Guide drug treatment and monitor patients after initiation of drug treatment for hypertension*: ABPM is indicated in all patients before starting pharmacological therapy for hypertension. Several drugs such as diuretics and valsartan have been suggested to restore the normal dipper pattern in BP, but the benefit of conversion from nondipper pattern to dipper pattern needs further studies.

ABPM can also be used to monitor therapy in patients after treatment initiation.[2]

- *ABPM can predict outcomes in hypertensive patients.* Longitudinal studies conducted over a period of 12 months have demonstrated that ABPM has better predictive value than in clinic BP regarding antihypertensive treatment-induced regression of left ventricular hypertrophy. ABPM has distinct benefits in different patient population with hypertension in the real world setting **(Table 3)**.
- *ABPM in special patient populations:* ABPM may prevent misclassification of grade of hypertension in patients with chronic kidney disease (CKD). Nondipping pattern may be associated with decline in renal function, microalbuminuria, and death, independent of BP load in CKD patients.[26]

Ambulatory monitoring helps in evaluating the efficacy of antihypertensive treatment in transplants. Immediately after transplantation, many patients have nocturnal hypertension associated in up to 30% of patients. Ambulatory monitoring is also being used to assess for hypertension in potential organ donors.[27]

- *Assess blood pressure variability (BPV)*:[28] Greater variability in SBP is a significant independent predictor of mortality. ABPM data can be used to calculate a number of important indices of short-term BPV, such as the standard deviation (SD), coefficient of variation (CV), average real variability (ARV), variability independent of the mean (VIM) for daytime and nighttime BP, weighted SD of 24-hour BP values, and peak and trough values for daytime and nighttime BP.

Here are some ABPM monitors from 2023 and 2024:[29]
- *Custo Med GmbH*: This is the first ABPM recorder worldwide that has been successfully validated according to stringent requirements of the ESH-IP-2010 protocol.
- *Medaval Star-Rated ABPM monitors*: These monitors have been clinically validated.
- *BPro*: This is a small wrist-worn device that captures users' arterial pulse wave data and converts the data into 24-hour ABPM readings via a proprietary algorithm.
- *Oscar 2 ABP monitor*: This monitor is independently used and provides a patient-focused solution with unsurpassed comfort, data reliability and confidence.
- *Kenz BPM AM 300 CE*: This monitor uses a small body and can manage BP readings at any time of the day.
- *ABPM-05*: This is one of the smallest and lightest ambulatory monitors, weighing only 190 g.
- *SEIVA TonoTrack*: This ABPM records from 24 to 48 hours and uses the oscillometric measurement method.
- *TM-2441 ABPM*: This monitor features an all-in-one design and is equipped with advanced sensors and a large display to enable in-clinic spot checks.

Limitations of Ambulatory Blood Pressure Monitoring[30]

The limitations of ABPM include discomfort felt by the patient during nighttime periods, occasionally ABPM may not be able to detect genuine artefactual measurements, and finally the limited availability due to the high cost of ABPM in the real-world setting could limits its use. All HBPM devices require validation, but this may not be possible in the real-world setting and inaccurate readings have been found in a high proportion of monitors.

TABLE 3: Benefits of ABPM in different patient profiles.[25]

Patient profile	Use of ABPM	Comment
Untreated patients who have a clinical diagnosis of high blood pressure based on office readings	• ABPM can help to categorize patients into various levels of cardiovascular risk • *Low risk*: White-coat hypertension • *High risk*: Sustained hypertension	ABPM can help in diagnosis of white-coat hypertension
Patients who have started antihypertensive treatment	• ABPM can help individual tailoring of treatment regimens • Monitor response to treatment • Helpful in cases of apparent drug resistance • Corroborate the findings of excessive variability in multiple clinical readings • Detect hypotension in patients with symptoms, who have apparently normal clinic blood pressure readings	ABPM is indicated for patients suspected of having resistant hypertension before up titrating the doses of current medications or adding additional blood pressure-lowering medication

CONCLUSION

The escalating burden of hypertension and increased awareness among the general population has witnessed an increased acceptance of HBPM devices and ABPM devices. Office BP readings only give a snap shot of BP reading at a particular time point. They do not reflect the BP variability. HBPM gives useful and extensive BP information obtained under fixed time frames and conditions over a long period of time. These BP readings are stable and have a high degree of reproducibility. The availability of economical HBPM devices has increased the reach of this HBPM facility to a large proportion of the hypertensive population. HBPM aids in treatment decisions, helps to monitor response to treatment, helps to detect refractory hypertension, and has a good predictive value for future CV events and stroke. HBPM can help categorize patients into low or high CV risk and help initiate early treatment. A prudent use of HBPM and ABPM in the real-world setting would help clinicians treat their hypertensive patients more effectively, reduce CV morbidity and mortality, and help more patients reach target BP levels owing to appropriate treatment interventions.[31]

ONLINE REFERENCES

Please scan the QR code provided at the end of the table of contents for References of this chapter.

CHAPTER

35

Various Guidelines for Hypertension: Which One Best Suits for India

Abhishek Garg, Gautam Singal, Gurpreet S Wander

ABSTRACT

Hypertension, a leading modifiable risk for cardiovascular diseases, has seen significant guideline evolution in the past two decades. Initially lacking clear screening or treatment recommendations, guidelines are now provided to specific at-risk groups. Most of these guideline changes focused on establishing and adjusting thresholds for elderly subgroups and patients with diabetic kidney disease, and stroke. Treatment choice now considers disease stage, comorbidities, and other factors, rather than ethnicity. This chapter offers a brief overview of global and Indian hypertension guidelines.

Keywords: Hypertension, clinical practice guidelines, Indian guidelines

INTRODUCTION

Hypertension, affecting around 1.39 billion people globally and causing 10.4 million premature deaths annually, continues to rise worldwide.[1,2] Despite this trend, many cases remain undiagnosed or poorly managed. In a 2017 multinational study, 35% of participants were found to have hypertension, with 58% receiving antihypertensive treatment.[3] Among those treated, 46% did not achieve adequate blood pressure (BP) control.[3] Effective BP management is crucial, given its impact on other major health conditions.[4] Various organizations, such as the American Heart Association (AHA) and Joint National Committee (JNC), as well as Indian entities like the Ministry of Health and Welfare Society (MoHWS) and the Indian Guidelines on Hypertension (IGH), have developed guidelines to help healthcare providers and patients achieve optimal BP levels through lifestyle changes and medications. These guidelines have evolved over the years in response to advancing knowledge and understanding. This chapter will compare global and Indian hypertension guidelines.

EPIDEMIOLOGY

Globally

A 2015 Global Burden of Disease analysis found that the prevalence of elevated systolic BP (≥140 mm Hg) increased by 3.2% from 17.3% in 1990 to 20.5% in 2015.[5-8] During the same 10-year period, low- and middle-income countries experienced a significant rise in hypertension prevalence, increasing from 23.8% in 2000 to 31.5% in 2010.[8] In contrast, high-income countries saw a decline in hypertension prevalence from 31.1 to 28.5%.[8] This rise is primarily attributed to the high prevalence of risk factors such as hypertension, diabetes, and dyslipidemia.[9] Hypertension is linked to 12.8% of all deaths worldwide.[10]

India

India is witnessing an epidemic of cardiovascular diseases (CVD), largely driven by uncontrolled hypertension.[9] Hypertension, according to the INTERHEART and INTERSTROKE studies, contributes to 17.9% and 34.6% of the population's attributable risk for coronary artery disease and stroke, respectively.[11] Presently, hypertension prevalence is 33.8% in urban areas and 27.6% in rural areas, with an overall prevalence of 29.8%.[11] In Indian populations, recent studies indicate a progressive increase in mean arterial pressure across the general population over the past two decades.[11] However, the rates of awareness, treatment, and control of hypertension in India remain suboptimal.[9] Hypertension prevalence also varies regionally due to social, economic, and dietary differences, as reflected in human development and urbanization indices.[9]

REVIEW OF VARIOUS HYPERTENSION GUIDELINES

The American College of Cardiology/ American Heart Association Guidelines

The AHA/American College of Cardiology (ACC) began consolidating evidence and releasing guidelines specific to hypertension in 2013. Initially, these guidelines were developed in conjunction with the Centers for Disease Control and Prevention (CDC). In 2013, the AHA/ACC/CDC[12] established a BP threshold of 139/89 mm Hg for all adults. However, this was revised in 2014 to a screening threshold of 140/90 mm Hg for all adults.[4] Subsequently, in 2015, the AHA/ACC maintained the same screening threshold of 140/90 mm Hg for all adults, but there were variations in thresholds for certain demographic groups.[4] Specifically, for adults over 80 years old, the BP goal was set at <150/90 mm Hg.[4] For adults with CAD, the target was <140/90 mm Hg; for adults who had experienced a stroke, it was <130/80 mm Hg.[4]

The 2017 ACC/AHA[13] guideline introduced changes to the classification of hypertension, eliminating the category of prehypertension and dividing hypertension into three stages (as shown in **Table 1**). A significant change in the 2017 guideline was the revision of the hypertension definition from ≥140/90 to ≥130/80 mm Hg.[13] This guideline established a screening threshold of 130/80 mm Hg for diagnosing hypertension, regardless of age or comorbid conditions, aiming for stricter BP control.[13] This lower diagnostic threshold (≥130/80 mm Hg) was backed by evidence from the Systolic Blood Pressure Intervention Trial (SPRINT),[14] which revealed a reduction in cardiovascular (CV) events (5.2% vs. 6.8%, $p < 0.0001$) and all-cause mortality (3.3% vs. 4.5%, $p = 0.0003$) with a lower cutoff (120/80) compared to the previous guideline's threshold of 140/90 mm Hg.[14] Furthermore, the 2017 ACC/AHA guideline recommended a screening threshold of 130/80 mm Hg for ambulatory, noninstitutionalized, community-dwelling adults aged 65 years and older.[13] This recommendation was also backed by data from the SPRINT trial,[14] indicating improved outcomes with intensive BP management in patients aged 75 years and older. Additionally, the guideline set a screening threshold of 130/80 mm Hg for specific conditions such as heart failure, diabetes mellitus, chronic kidney disease, and poststroke.[13] Accurate BP measurement is emphasized in the ACC/AHA guidelines, advocating for standardized measurement conditions using properly sized cuffs and validated devices.[13] The guidelines also introduce new recommendations for out-of-office BP measurement to confirm the diagnosis of hypertension.[13] They also address critical topics including BP thresholds for initiating antihypertensive drug treatment, treatment goals, and strategies to enhance hypertension treatment and control.

Limitations to American College of Cardiology/ American Heart Association Considerations

The SPRINT[14] and ACCORD[15] clinical trials have significantly influenced the latest ACC/AHA guidelines. However, both studies have limitations that may have impacted their findings. First, the SPRINT trial demonstrated improved CV outcomes in the intensive treatment group (targeting systolic BP <120 mm Hg) compared to the standard treatment group (targeting systolic BP <140 mm Hg).[14] However, the trial excluded individuals with diabetes, end-stage chronic kidney disease, and those with dementia, limiting the external validity of its results.[14] Second, the ACCORD BP trial indicated that intensive BP control did not confer benefits over standard therapy.[15] Nonetheless, some scholars criticized the study for being "underpowered" due to its design limitations.[15]

European Society of Cardiology/European Society of Hypertension Guidelines

Initially, the European Society of Hypertension (ESH) and European Society of Cardiology (ESC) relied on the World Health Organization's (WHO) hypertension guidelines, rather than issuing their specific recommendations.[4] The 2003 recommendations prioritized a patient's CV risk profile over simple BP readings when deciding on medication.[4] Antihypertensives were to be started only for patients with high or very high CV risk if they had "high-normal" BP,[4] for grade 1 and 2 hypertension if patients had high or very high risk or moderate risk with sustained high BP for 3 months.[4] Grade 3 hypertension required immediate medication, while low-risk individuals with borderline high BP could consider treatment.[4] The guidelines aimed for a target BP of ≤140/90 mm Hg for all, with a stricter goal of <130/80 mm Hg for diabetics, though achieving this in elderly patients was acknowledged as challenging.[4] Combination therapies, such as diuretics with angiotensin-converting enzyme inhibitors (ACEi)/angiotensin II receptor blockers (ARBs), beta blockers, or calcium channel blockers (CCBs), were recommended.[4]

The significant updates in the 2007 guidelines and recommendations included the necessity of using peak and trough or ambulatory measurements to ensure 24-hour BP monitoring. Additionally, alongside CCBs and thiazide diuretics, ACEi and beta blockers were advised for treating hypertension in elderly patients. The ESC/ESH advocated for a stricter BP target of 130/80 mm Hg for patients with a history of stroke and renal dysfunction, recommending an even lower target for those with >1 g/day of protein in their urine.[4] They also suggested the use of fixed-dose combinations to promote adherence.[4]

In the 2013 guidelines,[16] the committee reversed some earlier decisions regarding the initiation of drugs and treatment targets for elderly patients and those with comorbidities such as diabetes mellitus and poststroke conditions. The committee recommended a systolic BP of <140 mm Hg for all patients, including elderly patients under 80 years of age.[16] For elderly patients over 80 years old, a systolic BP reduction to between 150 and 140 mm Hg was recommended. A diastolic BP of <90 mm Hg was adopted for all patients, except for those with diabetes, who were found to benefit from a diastolic BP reduction to between 85 and 80 mm Hg, but not below 80 mm Hg.[16] In terms of therapeutic strategies and drug choices, the committee largely reaffirmed the positions of the earlier guidelines, including the use of combination therapy, fixed-dose formulations, major classes of antihypertensives suitable for initiating treatment, and the selection of drugs for comorbid conditions.[16]

In 2018, the ESC/ESH committee[17] implemented significant changes based on new evidence from studies on when to initiate drug treatment, target BP, and manage hypertension in patients with comorbidities across different ages. For all nonfrail elderly patients, treatment should be initiated when systolic BP is ≥160 mm Hg.[17] Treatment should also be started for fit elderly patients with systolic BP of 140–149 mm Hg. The committee discouraged discontinuing therapy in fit patients based on age when the treatment is tolerated.[17] Treatment should also be initiated for patients with chronic kidney disease, diabetes mellitus, or a history of stroke if their office systolic BP is ≥140 mm Hg or diastolic BP is ≥90 mm Hg. The goal is to maintain their BP below 140/90 mm Hg, provided it is well tolerated.[17] The treatment objectives of the 2018 ESC guidelines are shown in **Table 1**. Therapeutic strategies, drug choices, and other related therapeutic guidelines remained unchanged.

The 2023 ESH guidelines[18] largely maintained their core recommendations but have been updated to more closely match the 2017 ACC/AHA guidelines as shown in **Table 2**. The primary recommendations focus on BP measurement and the diagnosis of hypertension.[18] Given the variety of automatic BP measurement instruments available in the market, the ESH stresses the importance of using clinically validated electronic, upper-arm devices. Hybrid manual auscultatory devices should be used only if automated devices are unavailable.[18] The diagnosis of hypertension is based on an office systolic BP value of ≥140 mm Hg or a diastolic BP value of ≥90 mm Hg, accurately measured during two or more separate visits.[18] Exceptions to this include patients with a BP ≥180/110 mm Hg, a history of CVD, organ damage, or "hypertension-related symptoms," in which case the diagnosis may be made based on readings from a single

TABLE 1: Globally various hypertension guidelines on blood pressure.

	Globally CPGs		
	2017 ACC/AHA[13]	**2018 ESC[17]**	**2020 ISH[25]**
Non-HTN	*Normal*: <120/<80 *Elevated*: 120–129 and <80	*Optimal*: <120 and <80 *Normal*: 120–129 and/or 80–84 *High normal*: 130–139 and/or 85–89	*Normal*: <130 and <85 *High normal*: 130–139 and/or 85–89
HTN	≥130 or ≥80 *Stage 1*: 130–139 or 80–89 *Stage 2*: ≥140 or ≥90	≥140 or ≥90 *Grade 1*: 140–159 and/or 90–99 *Grade 2*: 160–179 and/or 100–109 *Grade 3*: ≥180 and/or ≥110	≥140 or ≥90 *Grade 1*: 140–159 and/or 90–99 *Grade 2*: ≥160 and/or ≥100
BP threshold (mm Hg) for adding pharmacological therapy	≥140/90 ≥130/80 if high CVD risk	≥140/90 ≥160/90 if age ≥80 years Consider 130–139/85–89 if very high risk of CVD	≥140/90
BP target (mm Hg)	<130/80	*18–65 years*: 120–129/70–79 *≥65 years*: 130–139/70–79	*<65 years*: 120–130/70–80 *≥65 years*: <140/90

(CPG: Clinical Practice Guidelines; HTN: hypertension)

TABLE 2: Similarities between ACC/AHA and ESH guidelines on hypertension.

Guideline similarities	2017 ACC/AHA[13]	2023 ESH[18]
Accurate BP measurement	It is recommended to perform office blood pressure measurements using a validated, cuffed device, along with HBPM or ABPM, before diagnosing hypertension	
CV risk calculator for treatment thresholds	The pooled cohort equation and SCORE2/SCORE2-OP offer estimates for the 10-year risk of fatal and nonfatal CV events and should guide treatment decisions	
Initial pharmacotherapy	• Initial therapeutic choices include ACEi, ARBs, thiazide, and CCBs • Single-pill combination therapy is a first-line treatment strategy for many patients	

(CV: cardiovascular)

TABLE 3: Classification of hypertension according to 2023 ESC/ESH guidelines.[18]

Categories	Systolic (mm Hg)		Diastolic (mm Hg)
Optimal	<120	and	<80
Normal	120–129	and	80–84
High normal	130–139	and/or	85–89
Grade 1 hypertension	140–159	and/or	90–99
Grade 2 hypertension	160–179	and/or	100–109
Grade 3 hypertension	≥180	and/or	≥110

Stage 1: Uncomplicated hypertension (without any hypertension-mediated complications, CKD stage 1 or 2)
Stage 2: Presence of complication or CKD stage 3 or diabetes
Stage 3: Established CVD or CKD stage 4 or 5

visit.[18] Patients with hypertension are classified into grades and stages, as shown in **Table 3**. Based on the intersection of hypertension grade and stage, patients are categorized as having very low, low, moderately high, or high risk for CVD, following the risk stratification guidelines from the SCORE2 and SCORE2-OP charts.[18] Significant attention is given to home BP measurements (HBPM) and 24-hour ambulatory blood pressure monitoring (ABPM), which are recommended in addition to office BP measurements as class II recommendations.[18] The guidelines highlight that the primary benefits of antihypertensive drug treatment stem from BP reduction rather than drug-specific effects.[18] β-Blockers are included among the recommended first-line drugs.[18] They are particularly favored for patients with heart failure with reduced ejection fraction, chronic coronary syndromes, or atrial fibrillation requiring heart rate control.[18] The 2023 ESH guidelines' stance on β-blockers as first-line treatment differs from that of some other major Western guidelines.[18] Another key aspect of the 2023 ESH is the definition of BP targets for drug treatment, with the SBP/DBP target set at <130/80 mm Hg for patients aged 18–64 years.[18] These revised ESH guidelines now suggest renal denervation therapy as an alternative option for patients with uncontrolled resistant hypertension or those experiencing adverse effects from medications.[18]

Trials Considered in European Society of Cardiology/European Society of Hypertension Guidelines and Their Limitations

The Cardiovascular Health Study,[4] Atherosclerosis Risk in Communities Study,[4] HOT study,[4] Australian Blood Pressure Study,[4] ALLHAT,[19] and SPRINT[14] were the key trials informing these guidelines. These randomized trials, which were of short duration, generally lasted 4–5 years. Exclusion and selection criteria often targeted high-CV-risk patients, making extrapolation to other risk levels uncertain. Although meta-analyses are not the highest level of evidence, they offer greater statistical power than individual trials and provide useful average treatment effects.[4] However, they are post hoc analyses with nonhomogeneous trials, and most are not powered for secondary end points. Additionally, therapeutic programs and patient compliance in trials often differ from clinical practice.[4]

Indian Guidelines on Hypertension—Best Suits for the Indian Population

The Indian population has special features for early onset of hypertension, clustering of multiple CV risk factors, significant season variation of BP, low awareness, treatment and control rate, and early hypertension-mediated organ damage.[5] Guidelines for hypertension were first developed in 2001. Subsequent versions were released in 2007 and 2013, with the latest update (IGH-IV) published in 2019.[5] The main objective of these guidelines is to provide well-rounded information to aid clinicians, without imposing strict rules that might limit their professional judgment in patient management.[5]

The classification of BP for adults is presented in **Table 4**. This classification applies to individuals who are not on antihypertensive medication and have no acute illness.[5] It is based on the average of two or more BP readings taken on at least two separate occasions, 1–3 weeks apart.[5] These guidelines and the classification of hypertension are based on readings taken in a clinical setting by healthcare providers.[5] HBPM is recommended for follow-up and decision making in patients with hypertension.[5] Both white coat hypertension and masked hypertension are recognized through the use of both office and HBPM.[5]

This guideline emphasizes the importance of accurately measuring BP and includes recommendations for out-of-office measurements using HBPM. Another method for out-of-office BP measurement is ABPM, which involves using a portable monitor worn on a belt and connected to a standard cuff on the upper arm.[5] BP readings are taken every 15–20 minutes over a 24- to 48-hour period.[5] This technique helps identify white coat hypertension, masked hypertension, nocturnal hypertension, and resistant hypertension, as well as evaluate the effects of antihypertensive drugs.[5] The diagnostic threshold for HBPM mean and daytime ABPM is >135/85 mm Hg, while a 24-hour mean ABPM of >130/80 mm Hg is also indicative.[5]

For managing hypertension in the Indian population, drugs that block the angiotensin pathway, such as ACEIs and ARBs, are preferred for those under 60 years old.[5] CCBs and diuretics are recommended for individuals over 60 years of age.[5] Most patients require more than one medication to control BP, and combination therapy

TABLE 4: Indian major hypertension guidelines on blood pressure.

Categories	Indian CPGs	
	2016 MoHFW[20]	2019 IGH-IV[5]
Non-HTN (mm Hg)	*Optimal*: <120 and <80 *Normal*: 120–129 or 80–84 *High normal*: 130–139 and/or 85–89	*Optimal*: <120 and <80 *Normal*: <130 and <85 *High normal*: 130–139 or 85–89
HTN (mm Hg)	≥140 or ≥90 *Grade 1*: 140–159 and/or 90–99 *Grade 2*: 160–179 and/or 100–109 *Grade 3*: ≥180 and/or ≥110	≥140 or ≥90 *Grade 1*: 140–159 or 90–99 *Grade 2*: 160–179 or 100–109 *Grade 3*: ≥180 or ≥110
BP threshold (mm Hg) for adding pharmacological therapy	≥140/90	>140/90 >130/80 if CVD
BP target (mm Hg)	*<80 years*: <140/90 *≥80 years*: <150/90	*<60 years*: 120–130/70–80 *≥60 years*: 130–140/80–90

(CPG: Clinical Practice Guidelines; HTN: hypertension)

in a single pill is encouraged to improve compliance.[5] For stage 2 hypertension, treatment should begin with a two-drug combination, preferably in a single pill. Certain combinations are preferred, such as ACEIs/ARBs with CCBs as a first-line combination, with diuretics as the third agent.[5] Beta blockers are no longer first-line agents and are reserved for specific indications (heart failure and atrial fibrillation).[5] The threshold for initiating antihypertensive drugs is 140/90 mm Hg for most patients. However, for patients with CAD and HF, therapy may begin at 130/80 mm Hg. The target BP should be <130/80 mm Hg for those under 60 years old, while targets for the elderly should be individualized.[5]

2016 Ministry of Health and Welfare Society[20]

In these guidelines, hypertension is defined by major Clinical Practice Guidelines (CPGs), including those from the WHO and Indian CPGs. All CPGs recommend adding pharmacological treatment to lifestyle interventions for BP readings of 140/90 mm Hg or higher.[21] Among Indian CPGs, only IGH-IV follows this lower threshold for patients with CVD or CVD risk. All major CPGs suggest starting treatment with single-pill combinations (SPCs) unless unaffordable (ACC/AHA) or contraindicated (ESC/ESH).[4] The IGH-IV advises using SPCs only for patients needing combination therapy, while the MoHWS recommends SPCs only after stabilizing BP with two separate drugs.[21] The MoHFW recommends maintaining BP below 140/90 mm Hg for those under 80 years old and below 150/90 mm Hg for those 80 years or older (as shown in **Table 4**).[20] The IGH-IV sets BP targets below 130/80 mm Hg for those under 60 years old and 130–140/80–90 mm Hg for those 60 years or older.[5] Only three CPGs specify time targets for achieving target BP: the ESC/ESH[17] recommends 3–6 months, the International Society of Hypertension (ISH) recommends 3 months,[22] and the MoHWS[20] advises 6–8 weeks. The IGH-IV prefers ABPM and HBPM. However, the MoHWS does not advocate for out-of-office BP measurements because of practical challenges in India.[20]

Other Guidelines

In addition to the major CPGs mentioned earlier, there were various worldwide guidelines for hypertension, including the 2015 and 2021 United States Preventive Services Task Force (USPSTF),[23,24] JNC 8,[25] ISH,[22] and the National Kidney Foundation hypertension guidelines.[26]

CONCLUSION

Over the past 24 years, hypertension guidelines have evolved to include a broader at-risk population by adopting various BP cutoffs specific to different populations. The development of antihypertension medications has also achieved significant success, supported by numerous clinical trials. We anticipate that future, mainly Indian hypertension guidelines, will include BP control targets tailored to ethnicity, sex, body muscle mass, and geographical location, enhancing the individualization of their clinical application.

ONLINE REFERENCES

Please scan the QR code provided at the end of the table of contents for References of this chapter.

CHAPTER

36

Initiating Combination Therapy for Hypertension: Background and Rationale

Tiny Nair

ABSTRACT

Recent guidelines in the management of hypertension talk about initiating pharmacological treatment with a combination of two drugs from different classes in a single pill. This conclusion comes from the fact that most patients need more than two agents for blood pressure (BP) control, and a single pill combination at therapy initiation would increase compliance, which in long-term would help achieve better BP control and eventually lesser morbidity and mortality. This narrative review would go through the background and rationale of such a strategy, focusing on its usage and benefits of initiating hypertension treatment with combination therapy in India.

Keywords: Monotherapy, combination therapy, hypertension management

INTRODUCTION

It is estimated that only around 20% of hypertensives globally attain target blood pressure (BP) goal of <140/90 mm Hg. India has 220 million hypertensives with 1 in 3 hypertensives diagnosed to have the disease, 1 in 5 are treated, and just around 1 in 12 are controlled to goal. This points out the dismal picture of hypertension in India. Treatment of hypertension starts with lifestyle alteration consisting of salt restriction, regular exercise, weight optimization by a balanced diet, no smoking, and moderation of alcohol intake, and it forms the bedrock of treatment. But despite the best efforts, most patients need drug therapy, that too more than one pharmacologic agent. Large studies have shown that most patients need two or three, and some more than three drugs for control of hypertension and to reach goal BP.

Presently available drugs, when used in combination, are extremely effective in controlling hypertension; a true treatment-resistant hypertension is estimated to be around 5% of all hypertensives.

This is the reason why proper strategy planning is as important as the discovery and introduction of novel drugs in the treatment of hypertension. The drug therapy strategies could be either monotherapy (single drug) or combination (multidrug) therapy.[1,2]

EVOLUTION AND BACKGROUND OF STRATEGIES

Monotherapy

The traditional strategy of treatment of hypertension starts with lifestyle measures such as salt restriction, exercise, and weight management. If it fails or does not attain the goal BP, a pharmacological agent thought appropriate for the patient is started. Drug treatment is also chosen straight away if the initial BP is very high, where BP control is unlikely to happen with lifestyle alone. Also, being an asymptomatic condition, a very high BP left solely on lifestyle alteration may end up in a CV event, and such risk may be substantial. Traditionally, in monotherapy, one drug—a diuretic, an angiotensin-converting enzyme inhibitor (ACEI), angiotensin receptor blocker (ARB), a calcium channel blocker (CCB), or a beta-blocker (BB) is chosen as the first-line agent. Choice of agent is based on either patient profile (age, gender, and chance of pregnancy), presence or absence of risk factors (diabetes, obesity, dyslipidemia), or comorbidities [chronic obstructive pulmonary disease (COPD), chronic liver disease (CLD), and chronic kidney disease (CKD)]. The dose of the drug is dictated by therapeutic response and tolerability/side effects. The drug is started initially at a small stable dose and gradually increased until BP is controlled or the patient shows signs of intolerance or side effects to that drug (pedal edema with CCB, bradycardia with BB).

The advantage of monotherapy is that if the patient gets controlled on one drug, he need not be exposed unnecessarily to a second chemical. But unfortunately, this turns out to be untrue. Most patients need more than one drug (mostly two or more), and hence the logic fails.[1,2]

Monotherapy Strategies

Two distinct strategies have emerged regarding the application of monotherapy in hypertension.

Increase Dose Monotherapy

Here, the drug dosage is increased gradually depending on the BP level and patient tolerability. The dose escalation stops once the BP goal is achieved, or a side effect emerges, or the therapeutic ceiling of the drug is achieved.[3]

Switch in Sequence Monotherapy

Hypertension is caused by and driven by one or several deranged pathophysiological mechanisms: vasoconstriction, volume overload, and an overactive renin–angiotensin system (RAS) axis. If a drug fails to achieve BP control, it could mean that the drug is ineffective or poorly effective, because the pathophysiological pathway responsible for hypertension in that particular patient remains unaffected or nonresponsive to the drug, since the mechanism of action (MOA) of the drug could be different. Hence, one logical approach could be stopping that drug altogether and trying a different drug. If a diabetic hypertensive is not responding to a diuretic, it could mean that, in that patient, volume overload is not a major causative factor driving his BP. Addressing his RAS axis by ACEI or ARB could be a better strategy. Similarly, for a volume-dependent, salt-sensitive individual, a diuretic may be a better choice than CCB or BB.

The main logic against this approach is that most patients have activation of more than one pathophysiological axis in hypertension. An obese diabetic hypertensive could have an accelerated RAS axis, a sympathetic overdrive, and a volume overload, and all these could play a role in the genesis of hypertension in this patient. He needs a combination of multiple drugs from different classes to be combined for optimal effect. In case one pathway is left unattended, this pathway may overact and by compensatory mechanism null the beneficial effects of the other drugs too. A vasodilator drug could end up in reflex tachycardia negating its beneficial effects.[4]

Data show that overall, 40% patients respond to monotherapy (much less reach BP goal) while 80% respond to two-drug therapy, and 95% to three-drug regimen. This clearly tilts the balance in favor of multidrug regimen.[4]

EVOLUTION OF MULTIDRUG "COMBINATION" THERAPY

Step Care

The traditional multidrug approach to treat hypertension was the typical step-care approach, where patient was started on one drug, and the dose was up titrated to maximum. If BP was still uncontrolled, a drug from another class was added, initially at a low dose, and then the dose of the second drug was hiked too.

The concept held good logic but took a longer time for BP control. The emergence of the "time in range" concept dictated that longer the time patient had uncontrolled BP, determined his hypertension-mediated target organ damage (HMOD). A longer delay in BP control may end up in irreversible HMOD with long-term sequelae such as loss of vision, LV dysfunction, heart failure with preserved ejection fraction (HFpEF), and reduced glomerular filtration rate (GFR).

The other disadvantage was that, after started on monotherapy, and the resultant being asymptomatic, the patient often failed to come back, and continued for review, resulting in suboptimal BP control. Also, time to reach the BP goal, as discussed, tends to dictate target organ damage.[1,2,4-6]

Initial Combination Therapy

The ACC/AHA guideline 2003 and the ESC/ESH 2007 and their subsequent revisions clearly favor an initial dual-drug combination to start off as the initial regimen in pharmacological management of hypertension.

In initial combination strategy, the treatment is typically begun with a combination, a RAS inhibitor, added to a diuretic or a CCB. The initial recommendations directed at benefit of patients who had a BP goal >20/10 mm Hg at initial presentation (BP > 160/90 mm Hg). Subsequent editions indicate the benefit of this strategy in almost all newly detected hypertensives beyond a trial of lifestyle changes. The exceptions to initial combination therapy are those who are fence sitters (borderline BP values), frail, extremes of age, or with a limited expected lifespan because of extensive disease.[1,2]

The CCB plus ARB combination is particularly attractive, being safe, effective, metabolic friendly, and has few side effects. In a country like India, with extremes of weather, dry summer months deplete volume while, diametrically opposite, humid monsoon tends to retain sodium. The seasonal change alters diuretic potency and results in hyponatremia. Also, diuretic-induced change of blood sugar has been a concern in India, with high prevalence of IFG and type 2 diabetes mellitus (T2DM).

When two drugs fail to control BP, all three drugs (ACEI/ARB with CCB and a diuretic) are combined.

BOX 1 Benefits of initial combination therapy.

- Address multiple physiological pathways at the same time right from the start
- Greater BP reduction
- Faster response to "at goal" level
- Consistent BP reduction (less heterogeneity at population level)
- Very little or no increase in hypotension
- Better adherence
- Less therapeutic inertia
- Lesser HMOD (resulting from faster control and better adherence)

Initial use of combination therapy has shown to cause a prompter attainment of BP goal and a more homogeneous attainment of goal BP at the population level. The benefits are many, but the major ones are highlighted in **Box 1**.[1,4,7]

SUPPORTING DATA

Large data from multiple clinical trials also point to the benefit of initial combination therapy over initial monotherapy.

HOPE 3 trial showed that compared to placebo treatment of grade 1 hypertension (BP 140–159 mm Hg) resulted in 24% reduction of CV events when treated with an initial combination therapy with an ARB and diuretic.[1,8] ALLHAT trial, which enrolled 42,000 patients, showed that an earlier control of BP had a better outcome and lesser HMOD.[9] VALUE trial, which looked into the efficacy of valsartan, in a post-hoc analysis found that earlier goal attainment with an initial two-drug combination produced a better outcome compared to single-drug regimen.[1]

Gradman et al., in a study involving 1,700 patients with hypertension, showed that initial two-drug combination therapy led to better BP control compared to initial monotherapy at 2 years follow-up. Surprisingly, this difference translated to a significant benefit of 38% reduction in CV events, 36% reduction in new heart failure, and 21% reduction in stroke.[10]

Real-life information comes from a community database from Lombardy in Italy, with a population of 10 million that had around 2 million patients of hypertension on therapy. Those on initial combination therapy had a 20% reduction in hospitalization because of ischemic heart disease, stroke, and heart failure compared to those on combination therapy.[3]

Rea et al. looked at the retrospective data of 2,212 hypertensive patients on antihypertensive treatment, on follow-up for at least 1 year. On retrospective analysis, compared to initial monotherapy, those on combination had a 56% lesser CV event rate and a 71% reduction in heart failure hospitalization.[11]

FUTURE PERSPECTIVE

The future of combination therapy looks bright. With newer drugs that are more effective and protective for HMOD beyond BP lowering is likely to change the scenario of combination therapy initiation for hypertension, especially for those with subtle HMOD or borderline comorbidities.

Combination of SGLT-2 inhibitors with nonhormonal mineralocorticoid receptor antagonists (MRA) is one of such emerging strategies, especially in the background of impaired fasting glucose (IFG) or diabetes with microalbuminuria.[12]

INDIAN SCENARIO

In India, multiple drug combinations are available in the market and are quite popular and prescribed freely. These are prescribed more with compliance and pill burden reduction and hence generally not started at initiation. Being an asymptomatic disease and given the dismal control rates of hypertension (mere 1 in 12), a strong campaign to start combination therapy at treatment initiation would greatly benefit the Indian hypertensive population.

CONCLUSION

Initiation of pharmacological treatment with a single-pill combination therapy has many benefits, both in terms of compliance and logic of inhibiting multiple pathophysiological pathways right from the start.

ONLINE REFERENCES

Please scan the QR code provided at the end of the table of contents for References of this chapter.

CHAPTER 37

The Role of Calcium Channel Blockers in Modern Treatment of Hypertension in 2024: Beyond Cilnidipine

Nakul Sinha

ABSTRACT

Hypertension affects 1.28 billion adults worldwide, with most in low- and middle-income countries. Calcium channel blockers (CCBs) have been a cornerstone in hypertension management for over three decades. This chapter explores newer agents, their mechanisms, benefits, and emerging trends in hypertension management. In India, CCB use is nearly equivalent to ARBs.

Keywords: Hypertension, worldwide, CCBs, management, trends

INTRODUCTION

Hypertension continues to be an important health issue across the globe, significantly contributing to cardiovascular morbidity and mortality. An estimated 1.28 billion adults aged 30–79 years worldwide have hypertension,[1] most (two-thirds) living in low- and middle-income countries. The management of hypertension has evolved over the years, incorporating a variety of pharmacological approaches to control blood pressure (BP) and mitigate associated risks. Among these pharmacological agents, calcium channel blockers (CCBs) have been a cornerstone in hypertension management for more than the last three decades. In this chapter, we explore the role of CCBs in the present-day treatment of hypertension, with a focus beyond the widely used cilnidipine, discussing newer agents, their mechanisms, similarities and differences, direct and indirect benefits, and emerging trends in hypertension management. Proportion of use of CCBs as antihypertensive monotherapy in India is almost equivalent to angiotensin II receptor blockers (ARBs).

OVERVIEW OF CALCIUM CHANNEL BLOCKERS

Depending upon the types of α1 subunit present, six different types of calcium channels have been identified: L-, N-, T-, P-, Q- and R-types. Of these, only the T-type are low-voltage-operated channels, while the rest belong to the high-voltage category. CCBs are a class of medications that inhibit the influx of calcium ions through different types of calcium channels in the vascular smooth muscle and cardiac myocytes. This inhibition results in vasodilation, reduced myocardial contractility, and decreased heart rate, collectively contributing to lower BP. Therefore, CCBs are classified based on the type of calcium channel they predominantly inhibit, viz., L-type (e.g., amlodipine), L/T-type (e.g., cilnidipine/azelnidipine), and L/N-type (e.g., benidipine). CCBs are broadly classified into two categories: Dihydropyridines (DHP) (useful for hypertension) and nondihydropyridines **(Flowchart 1)**.

- *DHPs:* These primarily act on vascular smooth muscle, causing vasodilation and are predominantly used in the management of hypertension.
- *Nondihydropyridines:* These act on both the heart and blood vessels, affecting heart rate and contractility in addition to vasodilation. Examples include verapamil and diltiazem **(Flowchart 2)**.

BEYOND CILNIDIPINE: EMERGING CALCIUM CHANNEL BLOCKERS

Azelnidipine

Azelnidipine is a newer DHP CCB with distinct pharmacological properties. It has a longer duration of action and

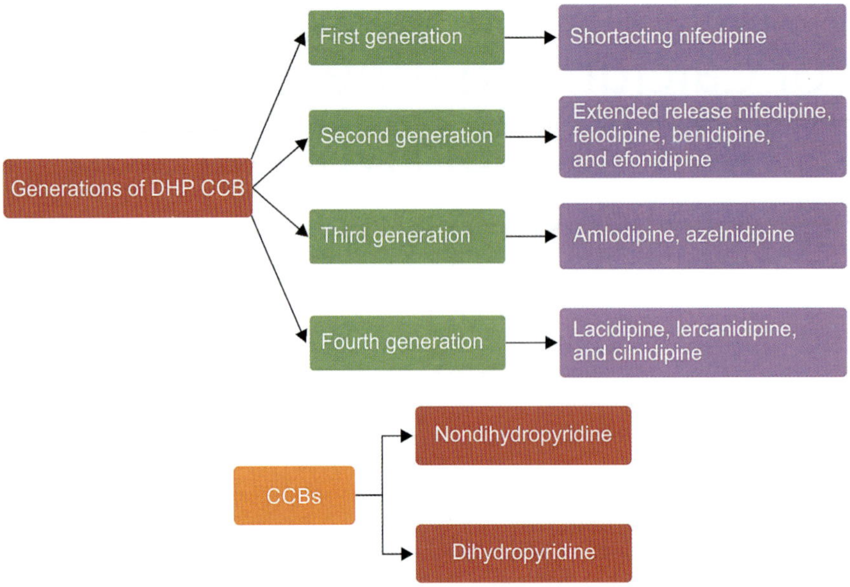

FLOWCHART 1: Classification of calcium channel blockers (CCBs).

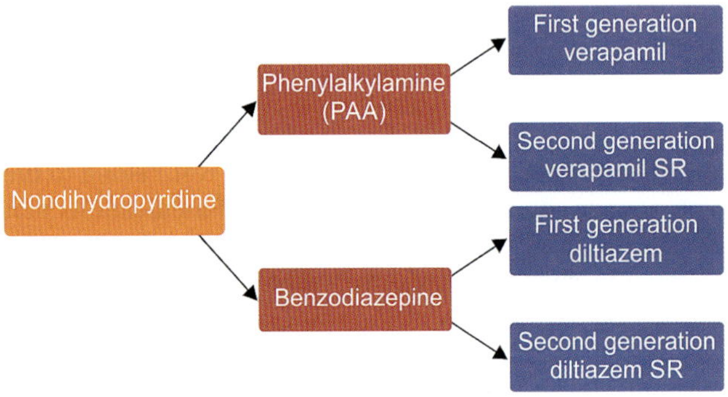

FLOWCHART 2: Division of nondihydropyridines.

provides gradual, sustained BP control. Azelnidipine mostly acts on L-type Ca^{2+} channels and has action on T-type Ca^{2+} channels also. Azelnidipine has strong lipophilicity and affinity to membranes of vascular smooth muscle cells.

Azelnidipine exhibits antioxidant properties, reducing oxidative stress and inflammation, which are critical in hypertensive patients with comorbid conditions like diabetes and chronic kidney disease (CKD). Clinical trials have demonstrated its efficacy in reducing BP without significant reflex tachycardia, making it a promising agent for hypertension management.

In At-HOME (Azelnidipine Treatment for Hypertension Open-label Monitoring in the Early morning) study, azelnidipine once daily in morning dose was given for 16 weeks. The morning and evening home BPs, clinic BPs, and pulse rates were all significantly ($p < 0.0001$) lowered.[2] Similarly in other studies azelnidipine, but not amlodipine, reduced urinary albumin excretion and carotid atherosclerosis in subjects with type 2 diabetes.[3] In a phase 3, double-blind, randomized, multicentric active control study in Indian patients comparing azelnidipine with amlodipine revealed that SBP and DBP reductions were similar.[4]

Barnidipine

Originally developed in Japan, Barnidipine is characterized by its highly lipophilic nature, allowing for enhanced vascular selectivity and prolonged action. It offers effective 24-hour BP control with once-daily dosing. Barnidipine has preferential effects on renal and mesenteric vasodilation, and it also significantly decreases both BP and plasma NE levels, indicating that it also lowers the BP by sympathoinhibition possibly via the central nervous system.[5] In two European multicenter randomized, double-blind studies, barnidipine was found to have antihypertensive efficacy comparable to that of amlodipine and nitrendipine, but with less adverse effects.[6]

Lacidipine

Lacidipine is a lipophilic DHP CCB with slow onset of action and potent antioxidant properties compared to other CCBs. It has been shown to improve endothelial function and reduce arterial stiffness, contributing to overall cardiovascular protection. Lacidipine's once-daily dosing regimen and minimal side effect profile enhances patient compliance and treatment adherence. In different RCTs, daily single dose of lacidipine (2–6 mg) has demonstrated similar antihypertensive efficacy to other long-acting CCBs, thiazides, enalapril, and atenolol.[7]

Efonidipine

Efonidipine hydrochloride is an L-/T-type DHP CCB with antihypertensive and antianginal properties with little/no reflex tachycardia. It is highly lipophilic and enters the cell membrane to reach binding site. It has slow onset and long duration of action. Efonidipine prolongs phase 4 depolarization of sinoatrial node, which contributes to its potent negative chronotropic effect and maintains cardiac output, a property beneficial in patients with angina. Efonidipine has an equipotent dilatory impact on both afferent and efferent arterioles, resulting in increased GFR without elevated intraglomerular pressure, thereby preventing hypertension-induced renal damage.[8]

Benidipine

It is an L-/T-type DHP CCB but has also been shown to inhibit N-type calcium channels. Benidipine has greater vasoselectivity due to "membrane approach" leading to high affinity for cell membranes from DHP binding site and is the key reason for its long-lasting activity. The renoprotective effects of benidipine are due to equivalent dilation of the glomerular afferent and efferent arterioles. By reducing activation of the aldosterone-induced mineralocorticoid receptor, benidipine also exerts a natriuretic effect. The COPE trial showed that the benidipine/thiazide diuretic combination reduced cardiovascular outcomes even in patients with poor BP control.[9] Different studies have shown anti-oxidative activity, stimulation of NO production, stimulation of osteoblast differentiation, suppression of adhesion molecules expression, and suppression of the proliferation of vascular smooth muscle cells and mesangial cells as well as myocardial protection.

Lercanidipine

Lercanidipine inhibits the influx of extracellular calcium across the myocardial and vascular smooth muscle cell membranes possibly by deforming the channel, inhibiting ion-control gating mechanisms, and/or interfering with the release of calcium from the sarcoplasmic reticulum. The decrease in intracellular calcium inhibits the contractile processes of the myocardial smooth muscle cells, causing dilation of the coronary and systemic arteries, increased oxygen delivery to the myocardial tissue, decreased total peripheral resistance, decreased systemic BP, and decreased afterload.[10]

Felodipine

Felodipine does not affect venous system; instead, it selectively dilates arterioles. According to in vitro investigations, Felodipine is more selective for vascular tissue than cardiac tissue when compared to other CCBs. Additionally, felodipine's clinical studies have not revealed any unfavorable inotropic effects. Both the diastolic and systolic BP levels decline in a dose-dependent manner after using felodipine.[11]

Isradipine

The strongest CCB in the DHP family is isradipine. It restricts the flow of calcium into heart and artery smooth muscle cells by binding to calcium channels with a high affinity and specificity. Because of alternate splicing of the channel's α1 subunit and a higher frequency of inactive channels in smooth muscle cells, it shows a higher degree of selectivity toward arterial smooth muscle cells.

Nicardipine

Nicardipine blocks the passage of extracellular calcium across the membranes of smooth muscle cells in the heart and blood vessels. This is achieved by channel deformation, blocking ion-control gating mechanisms, and/or obstructing the sarcoplasmic reticulum's ability to release calcium. The cardiac smooth muscle cells' contractile activities are inhibited by the reduction in intracellular calcium, which dilates the coronary and systemic arteries, increases oxygen delivery to the myocardial tissue, reduces total peripheral resistance, lowers systemic BP, and reduces afterload.[12]

Nitrendipine

Nitrendipine is a calcium entry blocker shown to inhibit the movement of calcium through the "slow channel" of cardiac and vascular smooth muscle, thus inducing peripheral vasodilation with consequent reductions in elevated BP. In individuals with mild-to-severe hypertension, nitrendipine quickly decreases BP and maintains this effect over time. Open trials of 1–12 months' duration have shown that nitrendipine (usually 10–40 mg daily) reduces systolic and diastolic pressures to within normal limits in 45–86% of patients with mild-to-moderate hypertension.[13]

MECHANISMS OF ACTION AND BENEFITS OF NEWER CALCIUM CHANNEL BLOCKERS

The newer generation of CCBs exhibit unique pharmacodynamic and pharmacokinetic profiles, enhancing their therapeutic efficacy and safety. Key mechanisms and benefits include:

- *Improved vascular selectivity:* Agents like barnidipine and azelnidipine exhibit high lipophilicity, allowing for targeted action on vascular smooth muscle without significant cardiac effects. This reduces the risk of reflex tachycardia and other cardiac side effects.
- *Antioxidant properties:* Oxidative stress plays a crucial role in the pathogenesis of hypertension and related

cardiovascular complications. Azelnidipine and lacidipine reduce oxidative damage and improve endothelial function.
- *Renal protection:* Barnidipine and cilnidipine, with their renoprotective effects, offer significant advantages for patients with hypertensive nephropathy.
- *Sustained BP control:* The newer CCBs provide prolonged action, ensuring stable and sustained BP control throughout the day. This minimizes BP variability, which is associated with better cardiovascular outcomes.

PLEOTROPIC EFFECTS

The pleotropic effects of CCBs include:
- Newer CCBs provide protective effects against hypertension-mediated organ damage (HMOD). In HF with preserved ejection fraction (HFpEF), the treatment of hypertension with all major antihypertensive drugs, including CCBs, is recommended by most guidelines. In HF with reduced ejection fraction (HFrEF), the initial recommendation is to combine drugs with sacubitril–valsartan/renin–angiotensin–aldosterone system (RAAS) blockers, β-blockers, aldosterone inhibitors, and SGLT-2 inhibitors. If BP control is still not achieved, a DHP-CCB can be added for BP control.
- *Atherosclerosis and vasospasm:* CCBs are highly effective in suppressing coronary vasospasm. Hypertension and LVH are often associated with myocardial ischemia and nonobstructive CAD. In such cases, treatment with CCBs can be beneficial.
- *Renal protection:* L-type CCBs increase glomerular pressure through dilation of the afferent artery and constriction of the efferent artery. In contrast, L/N-type and L/T-CCBs decrease glomerular pressure and improve glomerular microcirculation through vasodilatory activity on both afferent and efferent arterioles. Lercanidipine, an L/T-channel blocker, is highly lipophilic and directly dilates both the afferent and efferent glomerular arteries without altering intraglomerular capillary pressure. The combined treatment with RAS blockers and L/T-type CCBs reduces proteinuria without affecting kidney function and adverse effects. This finding is independent of BP and may be associated with decreased aldosterone also.
- *Prevention of cardiovascular events:* According to many studies, CCBs are beneficial in reducing cerebrovascular and cardiovascular events in hypertension. As a result, they are advised for use in both elderly individuals and ISH. Research has demonstrated that a quicker fall in BP leads to better outcomes and increased likelihood of protection. The ASCOT Legacy Study found that combination therapies with BP-lowering CCBs and lipid-lowering medicines are linked with long-term mortality benefits in patients with hypertension who have no history of CAD events.[14]
- *Antioxidative action:* CCBs are associated with mild antiatherosclerotic effects in patients with mild-to-moderate hypertension. This is thought to be due to their antioxidative action. In hypertensive patients scheduled for cardiac intervention, treatment with azelnidipine significantly reduced plaque volume 48 weeks after treatment initiation.[15]
- *Cerebral effects:* Studies have also looked at the effects of CCBs on cerebral circulation. A study by Kimura et al. showed that the treatment from azelnidipine maintained cerebral blood flow and cerebral vascular reserve.[16]
- *Anti-inflammatory activity:* Azelnidipine has anti-inflammatory activity that is independent of its hemodynamic effects suggested by in vitro and in vivo experiments.[17]

COMBINATION THERAPIES: ENHANCING EFFICACY

The management of hypertension often necessitates combination therapy to achieve optimal BP control. CCBs are frequently combined with other antihypertensive agents, enhancing their efficacy and reducing side effects.
- *CCB and angiotensin-converting enzyme (ACE) inhibitors/ARBs:* Combining CCBs with ACE inhibitors or ARBs offers synergistic effects. While CCBs provide vasodilation, ACE inhibitors/ARBs inhibit the RAAS, reducing vasoconstriction and fluid retention. This combination is effective in managing hypertension in patients with diabetes and CKD.
- *CCB and diuretics:* Diuretics enhance the antihypertensive effects of CCBs by promoting sodium and water excretion, reducing blood volume, and lowering BP. This combination is particularly useful in patients with salt-sensitive hypertension. Additionally, this also helps mitigate the ankle edema.
- *CCB and β-Blockers:* Combining CCBs with β-blockers is beneficial in patients with hypertension and concomitant coronary artery disease. CCBs provide vasodilation, while β-blockers reduce heart rate and myocardial oxygen demand, offering comprehensive cardiovascular protection.

SPECIAL POPULATIONS: TAILORING CALCIUM CHANNEL BLOCKER THERAPY

Elderly Patients

Hypertension is highly prevalent among the elderly, who often have multiple comorbidities and are at increased risk for adverse drug reactions. CCBs are particularly advantageous in this population due to their favorable side-effect profile and minimal impact on metabolic parameters. Long-acting agents provide sustained BP control with once-daily dosing, enhancing compliance in elderly patients.[18]

Patients with Diabetes

Diabetes is a common comorbidity in hypertensive patients, and managing both conditions simultaneously is crucial. CCBs, particularly those with renal-protective and antioxidant properties like azelnidipine, are effective in reducing BP without adversely affecting glycemic control.

Patients with Chronic Kidney Disease

Hypertension is a leading cause of CKD, and effective BP control is vital to slow disease progression. CCBs like cilnidipine and barnidipine, with their renal-protective effects, are beneficial in this population. These agents reduce glomerular pressure and proteinuria, offering dual benefits of BP control and renal protection.

Pregnant Women

Hypertension during pregnancy poses significant risks to both the mother and fetus. While some antihypertensive agents are contraindicated, CCBs like nifedipine are considered safe and effective for managing hypertension in pregnant women. Their rapid onset of action and ability to lower BP without compromising uteroplacental blood flow make them suitable for this special population.

FUTURE DIRECTIONS AND RESEARCH

The landscape of hypertension management continues to evolve, with ongoing research focused on improving the efficacy and safety of CCBs. Future directions include:

- *Development of novel CCBs:* Research is underway to develop newer CCBs with enhanced selectivity, longer duration of action, and additional organ protective effects. These agents aim to provide more comprehensive cardiovascular protection while further minimizing side effects.
- *Personalized medicine:* Advances in genetic research and pharmacogenomics hold promise for personalized hypertension treatment. Identifying genetic markers that predict responders to CCBs, can guide the selection of the most effective agents for individual patients, optimizing treatment outcomes.
- *Combination therapies:* Exploring novel combinations of CCBs with other antihypertensive agents continues to be an area of interest. Combining CCBs with newer classes of antihypertensives, SGLT-2 inhibitors, may offer synergistic effects and improve outcomes in patients with complex comorbidities.
- *Nonpharmacological interventions:* Integrating CCB therapy with lifestyle modifications and nonpharmacological interventions, such as dietary changes, physical activity, and stress management, can enhance overall hypertension management. Research into the effectiveness of these integrated approaches is being looked into to improve comprehensive care for hypertensive patients.

CONCLUSION

Traditional CCBs primarily block L-type calcium channels, while novel CCBs also block N-type and/or T-type channels, leading to organ-protective actions. Consequently, each CCB has unique pharmacokinetic profiles and side effects. A more potent BP-lowering effect and systolic BP variability was found to be lower in newer CCBs. CCBs have protective effects against HMOD both in HFrEF and HFpEF. CCBs when combined with RAS blockers, result in decreased proteinuria and improved kidney function and can effectively reduce CVD events in patients with ISH. CCBs are thus indicated for conditions including hypertension in the elderly, ISH, angina pectoris, and coronary vasospasm.

Calcium channel blockers continue to play a prominent role in the modern management of hypertension, with newer agents offering enhanced efficacy and safety profiles. Beyond cilnidipine, emerging CCBs like azelnidipine, barnidipine, and lacidipine provide additional benefits such as antioxidant properties, renal protection, and sustained BP control. The combination of CCBs with other antihypertensive agents further enhances their therapeutic potential. Tailoring CCB therapy to special populations and integrating nonpharmacological interventions are critical aspects of comprehensive hypertension management. As research advances, the development of novel CCBs and personalized treatment approaches will continue to shape the future of hypertension management, offering improved outcomes for patients worldwide.

ACKNOWLEDGEMENT

I'm grateful to Dr Nitish Tripathi for his help in preparing the manuscript.

ONLINE REFERENCES

Please scan the QR code provided at the end of the table of contents for References of this chapter.

CHAPTER

38

Diuretics for the Modern Management of Hypertension in 2024: Beyond Hydrochlorothiazide

Dipankar Ghosh Dastidar

ABSTRACT

All hypertension guidelines recommend diuretics as a first-line antihypertensive agent along with angiotensin-converting enzyme inhibitors (ACEI)/angiotensin receptor blockers (ARB) and calcium channel blockers (CACB). However, diuretics do not have class effect and efficacy differs significantly between agents. Thiazide-like diuretics like chlorthalidone and indapamide sustained release (SR) have an edge over conventional thiazide-type agents like hydrochlorothiazide (HCTZ). The improved efficacy of thiazide-like diuretics has been proven in terms of efficacy, pleiotropic benefits, and tolerability in large randomized controlled trials and their meta-analysis. Several novel diuretic molecules with improved efficacy and yet devoid of the deleterious side effects are in the pipeline. Hence, it is high time to look beyond thiazide diuretics.

Keywords: Diuretics, HCTZ, chlorthalidone, indapamide SR, pleiotropic benefits, novel diuretics

INTRODUCTION

Diuretics are first-line drugs in the management of systemic hypertension along with angiotensin-converting enzyme inhibitors (ACEI)/angiotensin receptor blockers (ARB) and calcium channel blockers (CACB). Salt retention is a key anomaly in the pathogenesis of hypertension. Diuretics are effective antihypertensive agents by causing increased natriuresis and diuresis. The role of diuretics as a first-line agent in the treatment of hypertension is established from the results of several landmark trials and their meta-analysis.[1-8] However, diuretic use has been plagued by issues of electrolyte imbalance like hyponatremia, hypokalemia, and unfavorable metabolic profiles like hyperuricemia, lipid abnormalities, and increased risk of developing type-2 diabetes mellitus.

DIURETICS AS FIRST-LINE AGENTS IN HYPERTENSION GUIDELINES

The role of diuretics as a first-line agent in the treatment of hypertension is established from the results of several landmark trials and their meta-analysis. The Antihypertensive and Lipid-Lowering Treatment to Prevent Heart Attack Trial (ALLHAT) was a randomized, double-blind, active-controlled clinical trial, recruiting patients from 1994 to 2002.[9,10] It clearly demonstrated that diuretics are just as effective as other drugs in preventing cardiovascular events and should be the first choice for treating high-risk hypertensive patients. This prompted all the major hypertension guidelines to give diuretics a class 1 indication in the first-line therapy for hypertension.

When compared for relative risk (RR) of stroke, heart failure, cardiovascular and all-cause mortality, diuretics, in fact, shared certain advantages over the other first-line antihypertensive agents in certain clinical scenarios. In the comparison between amlodipine and chlorthalidone, the 6-year RR of heart failure was higher with amlodipine than with chlorthalidone [RR 1.38; 95% confidence interval (CI) 1.25–1.52]. In the comparison between lisinopril and chlorthalidone, the RR of cardiovascular disease, stroke, and heart failure were significantly higher with lisinopril than with chlorthalidone (RR 1.10; 95% CI 1.05–1.16; RR 1.15; 95% CI 1.02–1.30; RR 1.20; 95% CI 1.09–1.34, respectively)[9,10] **(Fig. 1)** These data proves that diuretics apart from being potent antihypertensive agents, also have an edge over other first-line antihypertensives in certain other clinical scenarios like diabetes, elderly, stroke, patients of African origin, low renin, heart failure, and resistant hypertension.

All the major hypertension guidelines endorse diuretics as the first-line therapy along with ACEI/ARB and CACB[1-8] **(Fig. 2) (Tables 1 and 2)**.

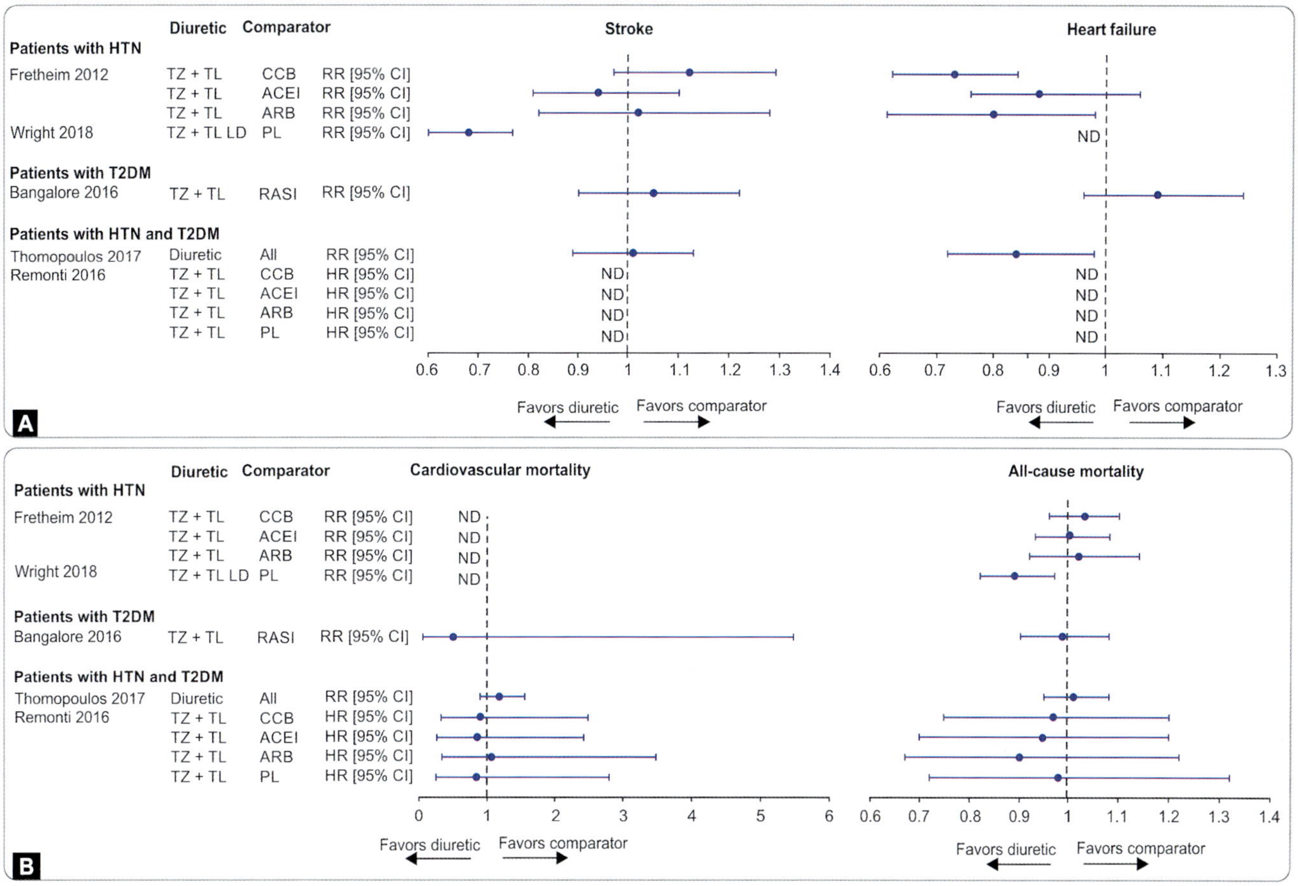

FIGS. 1A AND B: Diuretics compared with other first-line antihypertensives.[9,10]

MAJOR CLASSES OF DIURETICS

Major classes of diuretics include thiazide-type diuretics (containing benzothiadiazine ring) and thiazide-like diuretics (lacking the benzothiadiazine ring), loop diuretics, potassium-sparing diuretics, and mineralocorticoid receptor antagonists. Their classification is based on mechanism and site of action **(Fig. 3)**.

Different classes of diuretics have different mechanisms of action and target different regions of the nephron.

- *Proximal tubule*: Drugs like acetazolamide block carbonic anhydrase, thereby preventing the reabsorption of sodium, bicarbonate, and chloride and causing increased urinary loss of these substances. About 60–65% of filtered sodium is reabsorbed in the proximal convoluted tubule of the nephron.
- *Loop of Henle:* Loop diuretics act by inhibiting the sodium-potassium-chloride symporter in the thick ascending limb of the loop of Henle. Loop diuretics are highly protein-bound. So, they enter the urine through proximal tubular secretion via organic anion transporter 1 (OAT-1), OAT-2, and ABCC4 in the proximal tubule rather than through glomerular filtration. They are highly potent diuretics. About 20% of filtered sodium is reabsorbed in this part of the nephron.
- *Distal tubule:* Thiazides act by inhibiting the sodium chloride cotransporter in the distal convoluted tubules of the kidney. Thiazides are less potent than loop diuretics and are ineffective when the glomerular filtration rate falls below 30 mL/min. Thiazide diuretics are classified as thiazide-type diuretics (containing benzothiadiazine ring) and thiazide-like diuretics (lacking the benzothiadiazine ring).
- *Connecting tubule and collecting duct:*
    - *Blocking the epithelial sodium channel:* Some potassium-sparing diuretics, like amiloride and triamterene, bind to epithelial sodium channels (ENaCs) to prevent sodium reabsorption in the collecting tubule. This causes selective natriuresis and prevents potassium loss in urine.
    - *Aldosterone receptor antagonists:* Other potassium-sparing diuretics, like spironolactone and eplerenone, inhibit aldosterone receptors causing natriuresis and potassium retention.

This difference in mechanism of action of the different classes of diuretics can be used synergistically to overcome

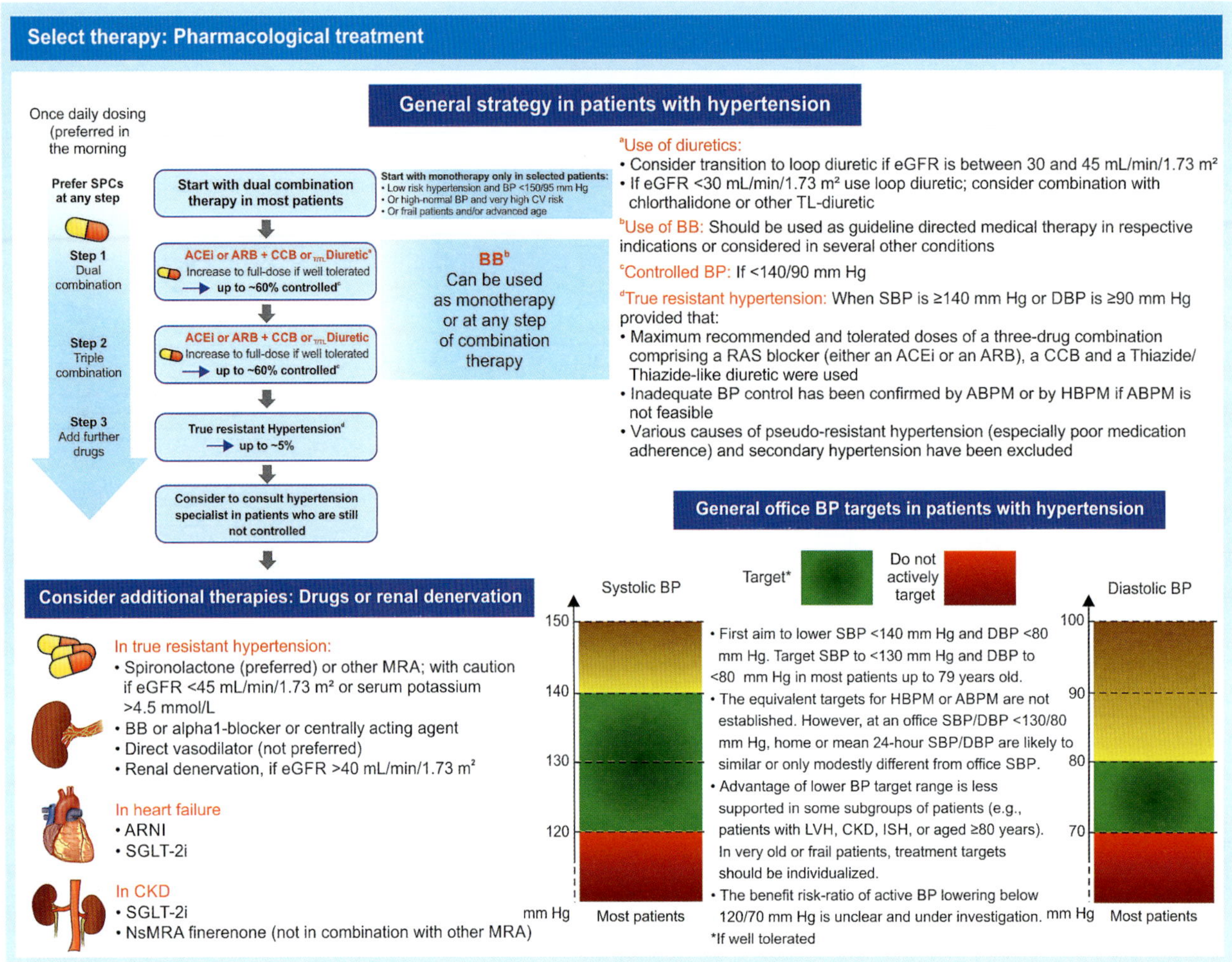

FIG. 2: 2024 European Society of Hypertension clinical practice guidelines for the management of arterial hypertension.[1]

TABLE 1: Major classes of oral antihypertensive drugs (Primary agents).[6,7]

Class	Drug	Usual dose, range (mg/day)	Daily frequency	Comments
Primary agents				
Thiazide or thiazide-type diuretics	Chlorthalidone	12.5–25	1	• Chlorthalidone is preferred based on prolonged half-life and proven trial reduction of CVD
	Hydrochlorothiazide	25–50	1	• Monitor for hyponatremia and hypokalemia, uric acid, and calcium levels
	Indapamide	1.25–2.5	1	
	Metolazone	2.5–5	1	• Use with caution in patients with history of acute gout unless patient is on uric acid-lowering therapy
ACEI	Benazepril	10–40	1 or 2	• Do not use in combination with ARBs or direct renin inhibitor
	Captopril	12.5–15.0	2 or 3	
	Enalapril	5–40	1 or 2	• Increased risk of hyperkalemia, especially in patients with CKD or in those on K^+ supplements or K^+-sparing drugs
	Fosinopril	10–40	1	• May cause acute renal failure in patients with severe bilateral renal artery stenosis
	Lisinopril	10–40	1	
	Moexipril	7.5–30	1 or 2	• Do not use if history of angioedema with ACEI
	Perindopril	4–16	1	• Avoid in pregnancy
	Quinapril	10–80	1 or 2	
	Ramipril	2.5–20	1 or 2	
	Trandolapril	1–4	1	

Continued

Continued

Class	Drug	Usual dose, range (mg/day)	Daily frequency	Comments
ARBs	Azilsartan	40–80	1	• Do not use in combination with ACEI or direct renin inhibitor • Increased risk of hyperkalemia in CKD or in those on K^+ supplements or K^+-sparing drugs • May cause acute renal failure in patients with severe bilateral renal artery stenosis • Do not use if history of angioedema with ARBs • Patients with a history of angioedema with an ACEI can receive an ARB beginning 6 weeks after ACEI is discontinued • Avoid in pregnancy
	Candesartan	8–32	1	
	Eprosartan	600–800	1 or 2	
	Irbesartan	150–300	1	
	Losartan	50–100	1 or 2	
	Olmesartan	20–40	1	
	Telmisartan	20–80	1	
	Valsartan	80–320	1	
CCB—dihydro-pyridines	Amlodipine	2.5–10	1	• Avoid use in patients with HFrEF; amlodipine or felodipine may be used if required • Associated with dose-related pedal edema, which is more common in women than men
	Felodipine	2.5–10	1	
	Isradipine	5–10	2	
	Nicardipine SR	60–120	2	
	Nifedipine LA	30–90	1	
	Nisoldipine	17–34	1	
CCB—nondihydro-pyridines	Diltiazem ER	120–360	1	• Avoid routine use with beta blockers because of increased risk of bradycardia and heart block • Do not use in patients with HFrEF • There are drug interactions with diltiazem and verapamil (*CYP3A4* major substrate and moderate inhibitor)
	Verapamil IR	120-360	3	
	Verapamil SR	120–360	1 or 2	
	Verapamil-delayed onset ER	100–300	1 (in the evening)	

TABLE 2: Major classes of oral antihypertensive drugs (Secondary agents).[6,7]

Class	Drug	Usual dose, range (mg/day)	Daily frequency	Comments
Secondary agents				
Diuretics—loop	Bumetanide	0.5–2	2	• Preferred diuretics in patients with symptomatic HF • Preferred over thiazides in patients with moderate-to-severe CKD (e.g., GFR <30 mL/min)
	Furosemide	20–80	2	
	Torsemide	5–10	1	
Diuretics—potassium sparing	Amiloride	5–10	1 or 2	• Monotherapy agents and minimally effective antihypertensive agents • Combination therapy of potassium-sparing diuretic with a thiazide can be considered in patients with hypokalemia on thiazide monotherapy • Avoid in patients with significant CKD (e.g., GFR <45 mL/min)
	Triamterene	50–100	1 or 2	
Diuretics—aldosterone antagonists	Eplerenone	50–100	1 or 2	• Preferred agents in primary aldosteronism and resistant hypertension • Spironolactone associated with greater risk of gynecomastia and impotence as compared with eplerenone • Common add-on therapy in resistant hypertension • Avoid use with K^+ supplements, other K^+-sparing diuretics, or significant renal dysfunction • Eplerenone often requires twice-daily dosing for adequate BP lowering
	Spironolactone	25–100	1	

Continued

Continued

Class	Drug	Usual dose, range (mg/day)	Daily frequency	Comments
Beta blockers—cardioselective	Atenolol	25–100	2	• Beta blockers are not recommended as first-line agents unless the patient has IHD or HF • Preferred in patients with bronchospastic airway disease requiring a beta blocker • Bisoprolol and metoprolol succinate are preferred in patients with HF*r*EF • Avoid abrupt cessation
	Betaxolol	5–20	1	
	Bisoprolol	2.5–10	1	
	Metoprolol tartrate	100–200	2	
	Metoprolol succinate	50–200	1	
Beta blockers—cardioselective and vasodilatory	Nebivolol	5–40	1	Induces nitric oxide-induced vasodilation. Avoid abrupt cessation
Beta blockers—noncardioselective	Nadolol	40–120	1	• Avoid in patients with reactive airways disease. • Avoid abrupt cessation
	Propranolol IR	80–160	2	
	Propranolol LA	80–160	1	
Beta blockers—intrinsic sympathomimetic activity	Acebutolol	200–800	2	• Generally avoid, especially in patients with IHD or HF • Avoid abrupt cessation
	Penbutolol	10–40	1	
	Pindolol	10–60	2	

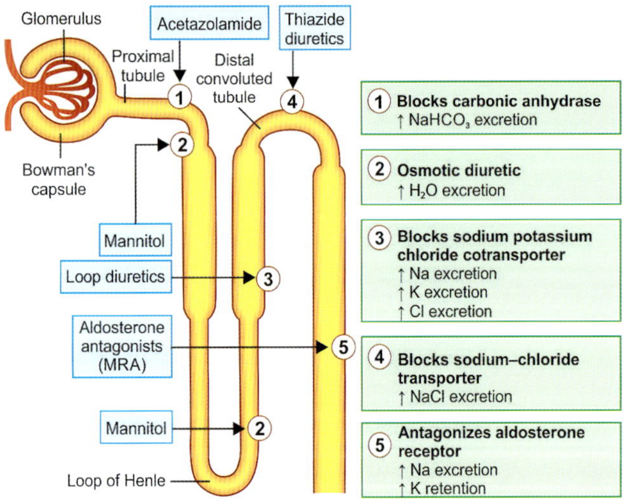

FIG. 3: Mechanism of action of various classes of diuretics.[11]

diuretic resistance or prevent dyselectrolytemia by combining a loop/thiazide diuretic with a potassium-sparing one. The magnitude of natriuresis declines over time. This is the so-called "braking phenomenon" and it is the result of both hemodynamic changes at the glomerulus as well as adaptive changes in the distal nephron.[12] These problems can be tackled by blocking different segments of the nephron by using two different classes of diuretics, a phenomenon called sequential nephron blockade.[12]

MECHANISM OF ANTIHYPERTENSIVE EFFECT OF DIURETICS

Diuresis

The initial phase of BP reduction is caused by natriuresis and diuresis. This effect lasts for the first 2 weeks. Later on, the resultant hypovolemia stimulates the renin-angiotensin mechanism, thereby offsetting the primary blood pressure (BP) reduction mechanism.

Vasodilatation

Vasodilation is the second phase, during which the diuretic treatment causes peripheral vasodilation that mediates the long-term BP reduction.[13-16] The vasodilating mechanism varies between cases of diuretics. Significant differences in vasodilating mechanism have been found between thiazide and thiazide-like diuretics in the form of calcium channel antagonism,[14] the opening of the KCA channel,[13] the inhibition of carbonic anhydrases,[16] and the inhibition of RhoA and Rho kinase expression **(Table 3)**.[14]

WHY LOOK BEYOND THIAZIDE-TYPE DIURETICS?

Initially, thiazide and thiazide-like diuretics were clubbed together as they both blocked the sodium-chloride

TABLE 3: How diuretics cause vasodilatation: Explaining the pleiotropic benefits of thiazide-like diuretics.[13-16]

	Hydrochlorothiazide	Chlorthalidone	Indapamide
Effect on KCA channels	+	ND	–
Desensitization to calcium via RhoA and Rho kinase	+	+	ND
Calcium channel antagonism	–	–	+
Carbonic anhydrase inhibition	+	+++	++
Increase in urinary prostaglandins PGE2 and PGF2α	ND	+	+
VEGF-C and TGF-β3 transcription decrease	ND	+	ND
Oxidative stress reduction	–	–	+
Platelet aggregation reduction	–	+	+

(KCA: potassium-activated calcium; ND: no data; PGE2: prostaglandin E2; PGF2α: prostaglandin F2alpha; TGF: transforming growth factor; VEGF: vascular endothelial growth factor)

transporter in the distal convoluted tubule. However, class differences among diuretics agents do exist. A number of recent hypertension management guidelines recommend the "preferred" use of thiazide-like diuretics rather than thiazide diuretics.[1-8]

Trial Results and their Meta-analysis

Meta-analysis of several trials of diuretics on hypertension has revealed better outcomes of thiazide-like diuretics like chlorthalidone and indapamide sustained release **(Fig. 4)**.

Thiazide-like Diuretics are more Potent, and the Efficacy is not Dose-dependent

Chlorthalidone and indapamide are more potent per milligram than hydrochlorothiazide (HCTZ) for BP reduction (HCTZ 50 mg is equipotent with chlorthalidone 12.5–25 mg). Moreover, indapamide and chlorthalidone have similar BP reductions in a non-dose-dependent manner over the 1–5 mg and the 12.5–75 mg ranges, while HCTZ treatment has BP reductions, which are dose-dependent **(Table 4)**.

Thiazide-like Diuretics are Longer Acting

Chlorthalidone and indapamide have longer durations of action than HCTZ. This results in better nighttime BP control and preventing early morning hypertension surges notorious for causing cardiovascular events. HCTZ, in contrast, had to be given in higher dosage for similar BP reductions and had daytime BP control only. These differences persisted in thiazide-like diuretic monotherapy or in combination with other antihypertensives. Chlorthalidone and azilsartan medoxomil combination provided better 24-hour BP control than HCTZ–azilsartan combination.[19]

In the Natrilix sustained release Versus Candesartan and Amlodipine in the Reduction of Systolic Blood Pressure in Hypertensive Patients Trial [(X-CELLENT); $n = 577$], 3 months of treatment with a regular 1.5 mg dose of indapamide sustained release was shown to reduce 24-hour, daytime, and

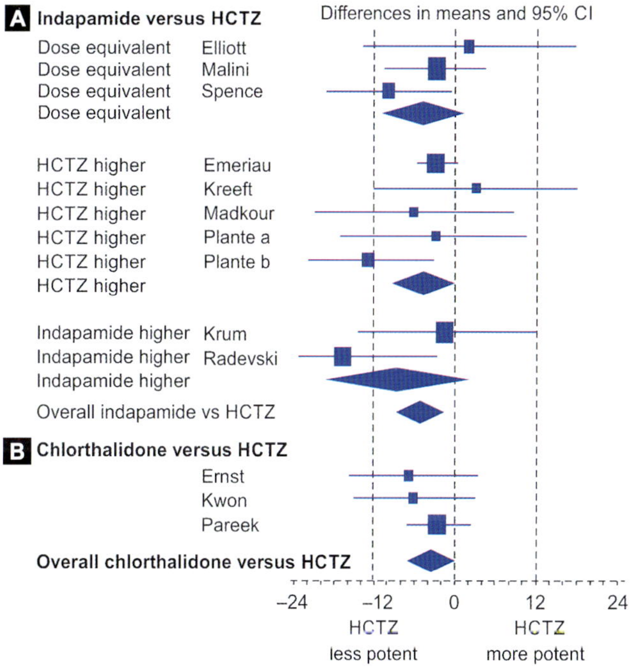

FIGS. 4A AND B: Meta-analysis for SBP reduction. (A) Indapamide versus HCTZ and (B) Chlorthalidone versus HCTZ.[17,18]

nighttime SBP.[20] BP variability, a marker of cardiovascular adverse events, was also less with long-acting thiazide-like diuretics.[21,22]

Tolerability and Side Effects

As stated before, thiazide-type diuretics need to be given in relatively higher dosage for effective BP control. This causes dyselectrolytemia and other metabolic derangements. Thiazide-like diuretics have improved BP reduction potency even at lower doses without any harmful side effects. A study of patients with mild-to-moderate hypertension (n = 690) when treated with indapamide

TABLE 4: Comparison between hydrochlorothiazide, chlorthalidone, and sustained release (SR).[17]

	Hydrochlorothiazide	Chlorthalidone	Indapamide SR
Half-life	6–15 hours	40–60 hours	14–24 hours
Duration of action	16–24 hours	48–72 hours	>24 hours
Equipotency for office SBP	25 mg	12.5 mg	1.5 mg
Dose effect for office SBP	Yes	Mixed data	No

TABLE 5: Comparison of laboratory parameters.[17]

Laboratory parameters	Hydrochlorothiazide	Chlorthalidone	Indapamide sustained release
Serum potassium	Decreased+	Decreased++	Decreased
Serum glucose	Increased	Increased	Neutral
Serum lipids	Increased	Mixed data	Neutral
Serum uric acid	Increased	Increased+	Increased+
Renal function	Decreased	Decreased	Neutral

Note: +,++ indicate the intensity of the variation from mild to moderate to intense.

sustained release 1.5 mg had equivalent BP reductions without hypokalemia and hyperuricemia than indapamide immediate release 2.5 mg.[23] Metabolic neutrality with sustained release indapamide has also been recorded in the elderly and in patients with type 2 diabetes mellitus in the NESTOR and HYVET studies.[24,25] However, both HCTZ and chlorthalidone cause hypokalemia and hyperuricemia. In the 2012 Peterzan meta-analysis, potassium decrease of 0.4 mmol/L was reached by a four times lower dose of chlorthalidone than of HCTZ (11.9 vs. 40.5 mg, respectively), and a urate increase of 36 µmol/L was found with a 12.3 mg dose of HCTZ and an 8.9 mg dose of chlorthalidone.[26] This might be a reason for drug discontinuation in a significant number of hypertensive patients. A rise in serum creatinine is expected with most short-acting diuretics like HCTZ because of reduction in renal perfusion pressure. This effect is more pronounced in hot, humid states, especially with concomitant use of other antihypertensives. Similarly, dyselectrolytemia and metabolic derangements like hypokalemia and hypocalcemia are more pronounced with HCTZ, especially in elderly females with low body weights **(Table 5)**.[27,28]

Effects on serum glucose, dysmetabolic effects, and increases in the probability of developing type 2 diabetes mellitus are typically considered to be similar for chlorthalidone and HCTZ. However, close analysis of the Elliott 2007 network meta-analysis (n = 143,153) suggests that new-onset diabetes was more common with HCTZ compared to chlorthalidone.[29] Indapamide is metabolically neutral, whereas HCTZ was associated with significant increases in triglycerides and glucose levels.[30-32] More than 10 years use of HCTZ is also associated with an increased risk of skin cancers due to its photosensitizing effect.[33,34]

Pleiotropic Benefits of Thiazide like Diuretics

Blood pressure-independent reduction of risk of cardiovascular events and heart failure, much like pleiotropic benefits occurred with thiazide-like, but not thiazide diuretics.[35-37]

Improvements in clinical endpoints are in large part attributable to decreases in BP. However, certain antihypertensives possess pleiotropic benefits in terms of cardiovascular and nephroprotection beyond BP reduction **(Table 6)**.

Indapamide was found to reduce left ventricular mass, an effect not seen with HCTZ.[38] A meta-analysis (12 trials, n = 1,005) showed that treatments with chlorthalidone, indapamide, and potassium-sparing diuretics reduced left ventricular mass, an effect not seen with HCTZ.[39] Indapamide use was associated with improved endothelial function and arterial compliance.[40] Strain imaging showed improved cardiac contraction. Increases in flow-mediated dilation were also observed with combination indapamide sustained release 1.5 mg, but not with HCTZ 25 mg.[40] Both indapamide and chlorthalidone have been shown to prevent platelet aggregation, an effect not seen with HCTZ. This had beneficial effects in onroke reduction.[41] Chlorthalidone, but not bendroflumethiazide, decreases vascular endothelial growth factor-C and transforming growth factor-β3 transcription, both of which are implicated in angiogenesis

TABLE 6: Pleiotropic benefits from recent meta-analyses in hypertensive patients.[35-38]

Study	Versus		BP adj	Cardio-vascular events	Coronary heart disease	Cerebro-vascular events/stroke	Heart failure	Cardio-vascular mortality	All-cause mortality
Olde Engberink et al., 2015									
Thiazide-like[b]	PL	RR (95% CI)	No	*0.67 (0.60–0.75)*[a]	—	*0.68 (0.57–0.80)*[a]	*0.47 (0.36–0.61)*[a]	—	*0.84 (0.74–0.96)*[a]
Thiazide[b]	PL	RR (95% CI)	No	*0.67 (0.56–0.81)*[a]	—	*0.52 (0.38–0.69)*[a]	*0.36 (0.16–0.84)*[a]	—	0.86 (0.75–1.00)
Thiazide-like[b]	PL	RR (95% CI)	Yes	*0.88 (0.79–0.98)*[a]	—	—	*0.71 (0.57–0.89)*[a]	—	—
Thiazide[b]	PL	RR (95% CI)	Yes	*1.00 (0.91–1.09)*	—	—	0.90 (0.68–1.21)	—	—
Chen et al., 2015[c]									
Thiazide-like[d] AC + PL OR (95% CI) No				*0.78 (0.68–0.90)*[a]	0.98 (0.91–1.05)	*0.82 (0.70–0.96)*[a]	*0.57 (0.41–0.76)*[a]	—	—
Thiazide[d]	AC + PL	OR (95% CI)	No	0.92 (0.79–1.07)	0.96 (0.78–1.19)	1.03 (0.67–1.56)	0.71 (0.44–1.15)	—	—
Thomopoulos et al., 2015									
Chlorthalidone	AC + PL	RR (95% CI)	Yes	—	*0.69 (0.49–0.97)*[a]	*0.63 (0.50–0.80)*[a]	0.48 (0.35–0.67)[a]	0.80 (0.61–1.04)	0.89 (0.75–1.06)
Indapamide	AC + PL	RR (95% CI)	Yes	—	1.02 (0.63–1.65)	0.73 (0.61–0.87)[a]	—	0.83 (0.69–1.01)	0.86 (0.75–0.99)[a]
Thiazide[e]	AC + PL	RR (95% CI)	Yes	—	0.80 (0.56–1.15)	0.59 (0.41–0.85)[a]	0.81 (0.45–1.46)	*0.79 (0.65–0.95)*[a]	0.92 (0.81–1.05)
United Kingdom National Clinical Guideline Centre									
Bendroflumethiazide	PL	HR (95% CI)	—	*0.78 (0.65–0.94)*[a]	1.00 (0.80–1.25)	*0.44 (0.30–0.63)*[a]			1.00 (0.81–1.24)
Chlorthalidone	PL	HR (95% CI)	—	4.31 (0.27–68.84)	2.0 (0.86–4.67)	*0.63 (0.49–0.80)*[a]	—	—	0.87 (0.73–1.04)
Indapamide	PL	HR (95% CI)	—	*0.77 (0.64–0.93)*[a]	*0.53 (0.36–0.77)*[a]	*0.72 (0.61–0.87)*[a]	—	—	*0.85 (0.74–0.99)*[a]

[a]Significant versus comparator

[b]Thiazide-like constitutes chlorthalidone and indapamide; thiazide constitutes chlorothiazide, hydrochlorothiazide, trichlormethiazide, bendroflumethiazide, and bendrofluazide.

[c]No adjustment for blood pressure

[d]Thiazide-like: Indapamide, chlorthalidone, metolazone; Thiazide: Chlorothiazide; HCTZ: Methyclothiazide, trichlormethiazide, polythiazide, and bendroflumethiazide

[e]Hydrochlorothiazide and Bendroflumethiazide,

Note: Significant values are indicated in italics.

(Ac: active; BP adj: blood pressure adjustment; CI: confidence interval; HR: hazard ratio; OR: odds ratio; PI: placebo; RR: risk reduction) and vascular permeability.[41] This could be the basis for heart failure reduction associated with chlorthalidone treatment. Indapamide selectively appears to reduce oxidative stress.

Amongst diuretics, markers of renal function respond differently to treatment with HCTZ, chlorthalidone, and indapamide.[24,42,43] Favorable changes in renal hemodynamics with improved urine albumin-creatinine ratio, urine neutrophil gelatinase-associated lipocalin, and renal resistive index were noted in the losartan/indapamide group rather than in the losartan/HCTZ group.[43]

Mortality

Diuretics were always known to have morbidity benefit without mortality benefit. However, meta-analysis by Olde Enberink et al. has shown that treatment with thiazide-like diuretics, but not thiazides, resulted in a significant reduction in all-cause mortality compared with placebo (RR 0.84; 95% CI 0.74–0.96). Similar observations were noted by the meta-analysis of Thomopoulos et al. (n = 195,267), where treatment with indapamide significantly reduced all-cause mortality (RR 0.86; 95% CI 0.75–0.99).[44] These mortality benefits of thiazide-like drugs were independent of BP reduction. Similarly, in placebo-controlled SHEP trial (n = 1,226), significant improvements in cardiovascular and all-cause mortality were noted after chlorthalidone treatment (adjusted hazard ratio 0.69; 95% CI 0.53–0.85 for cardiovascular mortality and 0.81; 95% CI 0.68–0.95 for total mortality).[44]

Thus, it appears that there exists a lot of differences in clinical outcomes between thiazide-type and thiazide-like diuretics though they have principally the same site of action on the nephrons. Guidelines are starting to appreciate differences between the different diuretic molecules. The Latin American Society of Hypertension guidelines prefer indapamide with a history of stroke or transient ischemic attack. The ACC/AHA hypertension guidelines recommend chlorthalidone. The Thomopoulos et al. 2015 meta-analysis highlights the important differences between chlorthalidone and indapamide.[37] Chlorthalidone trials showed benefits in coronary heart disease (RR 0.69; 95% CI 0.49–0.97). Indapamide data reached significance for all-cause mortality RR 0.86; (95% CI 0.75–0.99). Both treatments had significant effects on stroke and on the composite endpoint (stroke and coronary heart disease).

DIURETIC USE IN SPECIAL SITUATIONS IN HYPERTENSIVES

Type 2 Diabetes Mellitus

Type 2 diabetes mellitus is a frequent comorbidity in hypertensive subjects. Diabetic patients are prone to develop heart failure or renal impairment.[45] RAS inhibitors are the first-line treatment because of their efficacy in heart failure and renoprotection.[46] However, diuretics by causing natriuresis and venodilatation are equally potent in these clinical scenarios despite unfavorable profile on certain metabolic parameters.

In the Natrilix sustained release versus Enalapril Study in Hypertensive Type 2 Diabetics with Microalbuminuria (NESTOR; n = 565) trial of hypertensive patients with type 2 diabetes mellitus, natriuresis was more with indapamide sustained release 1.5 mg than enalapril 10 mg. Natriuresis is directly correlated with the degree of BP reduction and cardiovascular benefits. Even effects on microalbuminuria (urinary albumin: creatinine ratio) were equivalent suggesting that RASi were no superior than thiazide-like diuretics in nephroprotection.[24,47] However, hypokalemia (10.2% vs. 1.0%, respectively) was more with indapamide than enalapril.

Elderly

The elderly (≥65 years of age) group of population is a special substrate for choosing appropriate antihypertensive medications because of their multiple comorbidities and as they are at higher risk of having adverse events or electrolyte imbalances. Both Systolic Hypertension in the Elderly Program (SHEP; n = 4,736)[48-50] and ALLHAT substudy in elderly population showed significantly greater reduction in cardiovascular events with chlorthalidone.

Similar cardiovascular benefits have been observed with indapamide use in Hypertension in the Very Elderly Trial (HYVET; n = 3,845).[25]

History of Stroke

Metabolically neutral diuretics like indapamide have been shown to have positive role in stroke prevention. Both Post-Stroke Antihypertensive Treatment Study (PATS; n = 5665)[51] and Perindopril Protection Against Recurrent Stroke Study (PROGRESS; n = 6105)[52] showed significant reductions in stroke and other cardiovascular events with indapamide use.

Black Patients of African or Caribbean Descent

Several studies support the idea that diuretics are particularly efficacious in this patient population. In sub-analysis of ALLHAT in black patients (n = 11,792),[53] chlorthalidone treatment was superior to lisinopril treatment for stroke, heart failure, and combined endpoints of coronary heart disease and cardiovascular disease. Black populations have low renin hypertension, low nitric oxide bioavailability, and low aldosterone escape through non-ACE pathways, such as chymase and cathepsin. ACEI had inferior outcomes in terms of composite of mortality, myocardial infarction, and stroke: Hazard ratio 1.65; 95% CI 1.33–2.05; $p < 0.0001$, myocardial infarction (hazard ratio 4.00; 95% CI 1.34–11.96); $p = 0.01$, stroke (hazard ratio 1.97; 95% CI 1.34–2.92; $p = 0.001$], heart failure (hazard ratio 3.00; 95% CI 1.99–4.54); $p < 0.0001$], and all-cause mortality (hazard ratio 1.35; 95% CI 1.03–1.76), $p = 0.030$ compared with treatment with diuretics.[54]

SALT-SENSITIVE AND LOW-RENIN HYPERTENSION

This combination of salt-sensitive hypertension and/or low-renin hypertension is common in blacks, elderly, resistant hypertension, metabolic syndrome, diabetes mellitus, and chronic kidney disease.[55,56] These are mostly volume-overloaded states where diuretics work best.

NOVEL DIURETICS

The standard diuretics in clinical use today are however plagued by issues of long-term potency or efficacy because of development of diuretic resistance or braking phenomenon.[12] Issues of side effects limit their use. Hence, there is an utmost need to develop novel molecules, which are potent yet devoid of serious side effects. The promising diuretics are vasopressin receptor antagonists, sodium-glucose cotransporter-2 (SGLT-2) inhibitors, urea transporters inhibitors, aquaporin antagonists, adenosine receptor antagonists, natriuretic peptide receptor agonists, ROMK inhibitors, WNK-SPAK inhibitors, and pendrin inhibitors **(Fig. 5)**.[57]

Carbonic Anhydrase Inhibitors

Drugs like acetazolamide are used to treat glaucoma, idiopathic intracranial hypertension, altitude sickness, congestive heart failure, and epilepsy. Their effect on systemic hypertension is weak.[58] Thiazides and loop diuretics do possess some weak carbonic anhydrase inhibition activity, which may contribute to their antihypertensive efficacy beyond their inhibition of renal sodium transporters.[16]

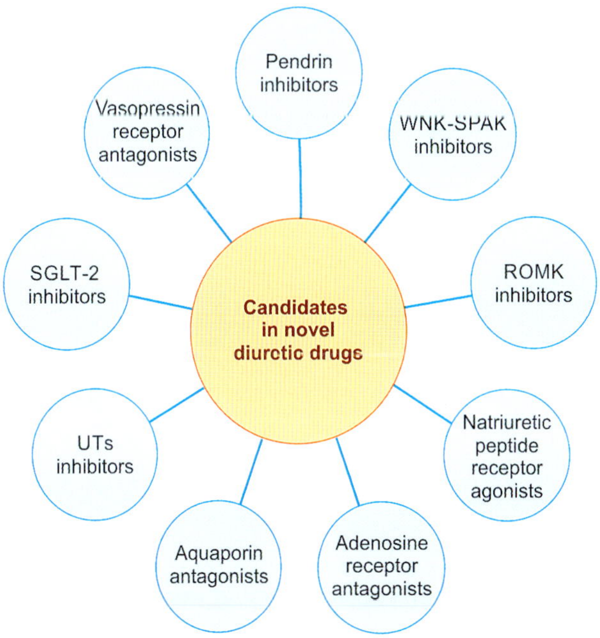

FIG 5: Novel diuretics in development.[57]

Osmotic Diuretics

Mannitol, glycerin, urea, and isosorbide are pharmacologically inert substances that increase the osmolarity of blood and renal filtrate, thereby causing diuresis. They are used to treat raised intracranial pressure and high intraocular pressure and are not preferred agents for systemic hypertension unless it is coexisting along with these disorders.[59]

Vasopressin Receptor Antagonists

Intravenous conivaptan and oral tolvaptan, lixivaptan, and satavaptan cause vasodilation (V_1) and inhibit water reabsorption (V_2). These drugs, popularly known as aquaretics are indicated in the management of hyponatremic hypervolemia [present in over 20% of patients with acute heart failure (AHF)].[60] Their current role as antihypertensive agents is limited.

Sodium-glucose Cotransporter-2 Inhibitors

Empagliflozin and dapagliflozin are a novel class of molecules causing reduction in the reabsorption of sodium and glucose in the kidney's proximal tubules, thereby causing natriuresis and diuresis. They act as antihypertensives, particularly in obese and type 2 diabetes mellitus patients.[61] They have pleiotropic benefits by which they offer cardiovascular protection, particularly against heart failure and nephroprotection.[61]

Urea Transporters Inhibitors

Agents like thiourea analogs, phloretin, and dimethylthiourea act by inhibiting urea transporters in the inner medullary collecting duct, thereby preventing urea recycling and countercurrent mechanisms.[62] They have fewer side effects on electrolytes than conventional diuretics. They are useful in hypertensives with edema.

Adenosine Receptor Antagonists

Adenosine type 1 receptor (A1-AR) antagonists like rolofylline induce diuresis and natriuresis in experimental animals and humans.[63] Much of this effect is due to inhibition of A1-ARs in the proximal tubule, which is responsible for 60–70% of the reabsorption of filtered Na^+ and fluid. However, seizures are an ominous side effect.

Natriuretic Peptide Receptor Agonists

The ANP-analogue MANP engages the guanyl cyclase- A receptor, thereby activating cGMP, reducing BP, enhancing sodium excretion, and suppressing aldosterone.[64] It has pleiotropic benefits in the form of preventing hypertrophy and having antifibrotic effects.

Renal Outer Medullary Potassium Inhibitors

Renal outer medullary potassium (ROMK) channel inhibitors like MK-7145 prevent salt and water reabsorption in the loop of Henle, facilitating natriuresis and diuresis.[58] They are longer acting than loop diuretics. They improve bone mineral density and plasma lipids.[65]

WNK–SPAK Inhibitors

Mutations within the with-no-K(Lys) (WNK) kinases cause Gordon's syndrome characterized by hypertension and hyperkalemia. There is activation of the STE20/SPS1-related proline/alanine-rich kinase (SPAK) protein kinase, which phosphorylates and stimulates the key Na^+:Cl^- cotransporter (NCC) and Na^+:K^+:$2Cl^-$ cotransporters (NKCC2) cotransporters that control salt reabsorption in the kidney and cause hypertension.[66] Rafoxanide and Closantel are examples of SPAK inhibitors with promising roles in salt-sensitive hypertension.

Pendrin Inhibitors

Concept of pendrin inhibition stems from findings of Pendred syndrome caused by mutations in pendrin (SLC26A4), where there is salt depletion, hypotension, and hypochloremic alkalosis apart from sensorineural deafness, hypothyroidism, and goiter.[67] PDSinh-C01, a small molecule acts as pendrin inhibitor causing diuresis in hypertension and edema.

CONCLUSION

There exists an overwhelming amount of data promoting thiazide-like diuretics over thiazide-type diuretics in terms of efficacy, pleiotropic benefits, diminished side effects, and improved tolerability. Certain hypertension guidelines also recommend thiazide-like diuretics. Most of them suggest a combination polypill taking advantage of the synergistic mechanism of action benefits to improve compliance and efficacy. It is now high time to look beyond hydrochlorothiazide in the management of hypertension.

ONLINE REFERENCES

Please scan the QR code provided at the end of the table of contents for References of this chapter.

CHAPTER

39

Inhibition of Angiotensinogen in the Treatment of Hypertension

Sudhir Chandra Sinha, G Venkateshwara Reddy

ABSTRACT

Systemic hypertension remains at the pandemic level at present. Even though it is a major contributor to adverse cardiovascular outcomes in terms of coronary artery disease, stroke, peripheral arterial disease, and kidney damage, still a reluctance exists in patients to use antihypertensive treatment as such and it seriously compromises the level of blood pressure control. The majority of adverse cardiovascular outcomes are noted in mild-to-moderate hypertensive, who form the major component of a cardiovascular pandemic. So, it has become important to find alternate antihypertensive pharmacotherapy that can help in improving compliance and adherence. Angiotensinogen is the only mother molecule of the renin–angiotensin system (RAS) cascade. So far inhibition of various steps in this cascade by angiotensin enzyme inhibitors, angiotensin receptor blockers, or direct renin inhibition has resulted in a paradoxical accumulation of angiotensinogen and renin and angiotensin II in plasma, what is now called the RAS escape phenomenon. Therefore, it becomes important to search for a therapeutic agent that can counter these limitations of present-day pharmacotherapy. Direct angiotensinogen inhibition by gene silencing is emerging as an important tool in managing hypertension in the future.

Keywords: Angiotensinogen, small interfering RNA, antisense oligonucleotides, CRISPR-Cas9, RAS escape

INTRODUCTION

Systemic hypertension, commonly abbreviated as hypertension, is a leading risk factor for cardiovascular disease, stroke, peripheral arterial disease, and renal failure. The pharmacotherapy of hypertension has evolved over the years with the regular addition of potent molecules such as diuretics, β-blockers, calcium channel blockers, α-blockers, centrally acting agents, angiotensin-converting enzyme (ACE) inhibitors, angiotensin receptor blockers, renin inhibitors, and direct arterial dilators. Despite such a big list of available pharmacotherapy, according to the World Health Organization (WHO), though >1.4 billion adult population in the world are affected with hypertension, <14% have adequate control.[1] It is responsible for more than three-quarters of cardiovascular deaths in low- and middle-income countries. Despite the availability of effective medications, approximately 10–20% of individuals are still labeled as resistant hypertension.[2]

Though blood pressure (BP) quantification in clinics became possible with the discovery of the sphygmomanometer cuff by Scipione Riva-Rocci in 1896 and the description of auscultatory sounds by Korotkoff in 1905, it was established as a risk factor in 1961 based on findings from the Framingham Heart Study. The pathophysiology of essential hypertension is still inadequately understood. The term "essential hypertension" was coined by Eberhard Frank in 1911 when a definite cause could not be ascertained. Despite scientific advancement, almost 85–90% of hypertension is still labeled as essential. It is recognized as a multifactorial disorder with a complex interplay of genetic, environmental, and lifestyle changes.

RENIN–ANGIOTENSIN SYSTEM

The first indirect BP measurement was performed on a kymograph by FA Mahomed in 1872. However, much earlier than that, Richard Bright in 1836, linked kidney disease to left ventricular hypertrophy. Later, Tigerstedt and Bergman 1898 reported the pressor effect of renal extracts and named it Renin based on its source. In 1936, researchers from Argentina and the USA were able to isolate a substance from renal extract that caused hypertension. They could also demonstrate that renin worked on a plasma protein to produce a new substance that had a pressor effect. The Argentine group called it hypertensin, and Americans called it angiotonin. Finally, in 1958, Irving H. Page (USA) and Eduardo Braun Menéndez (Argentina) agreed jointly to name it angiotensin. Page also described its origin from the liver. ACE was isolated by the group of scientists Leonard T Skeggs, Norman Shumway, and colleagues in 1956. Kevin KF Ng and John R. Vane in 1970 demonstrated that angiotensin I (Ang I) is converted to angiotensin II (Ang II) in the lungs.

Physiology of the Extended Renin–Angiotensin System[3]

Renin is produced by cleavage of prorenin present in the juxtaglomerular cells in afferent arterioles of the kidney by proconvertase 1 and cathepsin B. Mature renin is stored into the juxtaglomerular cells and released into the bloodstream if there is a decrease in renal perfusion or decrease in renal tubular sodium. The half-life of renin is 10–15 minutes.

Angiotensinogen (AGT) is alpha-2 globulin produced by the liver. It belongs to the serpin family and is called serpin 8. It is also known as the renin substrate. It has 485 amino acids. Renin cleaves ten peptides from it to form what is called angiotensin I. Conversion of AGT to Ang I by renin is the rate-limiting step in RAS. Ang I is further cleaved by removing two amino acids at the C-terminal by "classic" angiotensin converting enzyme (ACE) produced in the lungs to form Ang II. Chymase and cathepsin G can also convert Ang I to II. Ang II is the most potent vasoconstrictor substance. Ang II exerts its physiological effects by predominantly binding to Ang II type-1 receptors causing vasoconstriction, sodium, and water retention mainly by stimulating aldosterone release and fibrosis. Ang II is further cleaved by angiotensinases present in red blood cells and vascular smooth muscles into angiotensin III. It has 40% vasopressor activity as compared to Ang II. Further cleavage of angiotensin III produces a hexapeptide angiotensin IV.

Angiotensin II Type 1 Receptor

Angiotensin II binding to angiotensin II type 1 receptor (AT1R) produces vasoconstriction and sodium and water resorption. It is found in many organ tissues such as blood vessels, heart, kidney, adrenal gland, and the central nervous system. Its activation is also responsible for inflammatory response, oxidative stress, and hypertension.

Angiotensin II Type 2 Receptor

This receptor is present in the heart, brain, and kidney in adults but the concentration is very low. Activation of angiotensin II type 2 receptor (AT2R) causes vasodilation and prevents inflammation, a role just opposite to activation of AT1R. Activation of AT2R causes vasodilation and promotes anticell proliferation and apoptosis.

"Counterregulatory (Protective) Renin–Angiotensin System" Pathway

Recent research has extended RAS beyond Ang II. A counterregulatory pathway has been discovered. Similar to classic ACE, another enzyme, ACE-2 was discovered in 2000, which converts Ang I to angiotensin 1–9 (Ang 1–9) and it also converts Ang II to angiotensin 1-7 (Ang 1–7). This pathway and products had little attention in the past but now receiving significant attraction. ACE-2 thus plays a role in decreasing Ang II levels. Ang 1–7 acts through Mas receptors-1 to release nitric oxide synthase (NOS) and increases sodium excretion. Ang 1–9 acts on AT2R and bradykinin receptors to cause vasodilatation. In addition to all these, other components such as Ang (1–12), angiotensin A, and alamandine have been identified which may have important physiological effects. ACE-2 converts angiotensin A into alamandine (Ala). Alamandine is also produced by decarboxylation of Ang 1–7. It acts through MrgD and MasR receptors. Alamandine acts through MrgD receptors to cause antiproliferative, vasodilatory, and antinatriuretic effects. Thus, stimulation of AT1-R receptors produces hypertension and fibrosis whereas stimulation of AT2R, Mas-1, and MrgD receptors causes vasodilation. In healthy adults, there is a balance between ACE and ACE-2, whereas in hypertension ACE dominates.

Angiotensin-converting enzyme inhibitors were the first to be introduced for the treatment of hypertension and formed the backbone of hypertension management since 1981. Almost 10 ACE inhibitors were approved by the Food and Drug Administration (FDA) between 1981 and 1996. ACE inhibitor has certain important side effects such as cough and angioedema due to the accumulation of bradykinin and prostaglandins.

The development of ACE inhibitor was followed by the development of angiotensin II type-1 receptor blockers (ARB). Losartan was the first orally active ARB to be approved by the FDA in 1995.

Renin is the rate-limiting step of RAS physiology. Aliskiren was the first renin inhibitor to undergo a phase III trial and was approved by the FDA in 2007.

The focus has now shifted to either producing AGT inhibitors or analogs of ACE-2 end products.

ANGIOTENSINOGEN

Angiotensinogen is the only substrate and source of all other angiotensin peptides. Genetic manipulation causing depletion of AGT in experimental mice threatens viability. However, it is possible to inhibit AGT mRNA expression using antisense oligonucleotides (ASOs). ASOs are single-stranded, DNA-like synthetic nucleic acids. These hybridize specific base pairs of mRNA and so alter the production of a specific desired protein. AGT ASO was extensively studied in hypertensive rat models and it was found to effectively lower BP.[4] Targeting liver AGT in particular has a profound effect on BP. Another method of targeting liver AGT is by small interfering RNA (siRNA).

Renin–angiotensin System Escape Phenomenon

Renin acts on AGT to produce Ang I which degrades further into Ang II. Ang II has been demonstrated to control renin expression and release by a negative feedback loop. Therefore, inhibiting RAS with conventional agents such as direct renin inhibitors, ACE inhibitor, and ARB may suppress this negative feedback loop and increase renin levels and high plasma concentrations of AGT levels. This causes restoration in Ang II levels and concentration of Ang II at AT1R receptors. This may counteract RAS blockade and attenuate antihypertensive effects. This is known as the RAS escape phenomenon. Therefore, it becomes imperative to find a better molecule for RAS blockade.

Angiotensinogen Suppression: A New Tool to Manage Hypertension

Experimental studies have shown that liver AGT is the primary source of circulating, adipose tissue, and kidney AGT. Inhibition of liver AGT can suppress circulating and kidney AGT. Two approaches have been studied—one is the direct binding of N-acetyl galactosamine (GalNAc) to ASO that inhibits RNA translation, and another method is by siRNA that works via the RNA interference pathway. These two approaches have reached an advanced stage. A third approach is to utilize gene editing technology like clustered regularly interspaced short palindromic repeats/clustered regularly interspaced short palindromic repeat-associated protein 9 (CRISPR/Cas9). This causes permanent disruption of the target gene.

Antisense Oligonucleotides in Angiotensinogen Suppression

The ASO is single-stranded DNA. Hepatocytes are rich in asialoglycoprotein receptors. GalNAc binds to this receptor causing rapid endocytosis of the GalNAc-ASO complex. After endocytosis, it binds to the target mRNA. It is then cleaved by RNAse H1 in both cytoplasm and nucleus. This leads to the destruction of mRNA and the translation process of the target protein, AGT.[5]

IONIS-AGT-L_{RX} Phase I and Phase II Study

IONIS-AGT-L_{Rx} (Ionis Pharmaceuticals, Carlsbad, California), a hepatocyte-directed ASO molecule, was studied in two phase II trials (1) in patients with mild hypertension after washout of antihypertensive medications (AGT-ASO monotherapy study), and (2) in patients with uncontrolled BP who received antihypertensive background therapy with 2–3 antihypertensive medications[6] (add-on therapy study). In the monotherapy group, patients with mild hypertension, and systolic BP between 140 and 165 mm Hg were randomized into 2:1 fashion with 80 mg weekly subcutaneous injection of IONIS-AGT-L_{RX} versus placebo for 6 weeks then followed for 13 weeks. In the add-on strategy group, patients received 80 mg subcutaneous IONIS-AGT-L_{RX} for 8 weeks then 13 weeks follow-up period. It showed a very good safety and efficacy profile compared to placebo. In the phase II monotherapy group, there were 17 patients in the treatment arm. There was a mean BP reduction of –8/–1 mm Hg in the treatment arm but it did not reach statistical significance. However, IONIS-AGT-L_{RX} was well tolerated without any hypotension, renal dysfunction, or hyperkalemia. There were no significant changes in renin mass, aldosterone, or Ang II.

In the phase II add-on group, there were 18 patients in the treatment arm. Two-thirds of the patients were on two antihypertensive medications and one-third on three or more antihypertensive medications. There was a BP change of –12/–6 mm Hg but it did not reach statistical significance. However, a good safety profile was demonstrated.

Further trials are underway to assess the role of IONIS-AGT-L_{RX}: A study to assess the safety, tolerability, and efficacy of IONIS-AGT-L_{Rx} in ASTRAAS (ASO targeting the RAAS system). It will recruit 150 participants with uncontrolled BP who are on ≥3 antihypertensive medications and it will evaluate the effect of IONIS-AGT-L_{Rx} on in-office and 24-hours ambulatory SBP, DBP, and plasma AGT. A study to assess the safety, tolerability, pharmacokinetics, and pharmacodynamics of ION 904, a more potent ASO to AGT, is also underway.

Limitations of Antisense Oligonucleotides-angiotensinogen

The major limitation at the moment with ASO-AGT is the requirement of weekly injections. Also, larger studies and phase III trials are needed to study its impact on hard cardiovascular endpoints such as mortality, cardiovascular disease prevention, and target-organ damage.

Short Interfering Ribonucleic Acid as Angiotensinogen Inhibitor

In 1998, Fire A and colleagues[7] reported a novel way of silencing endogenous genes by injecting small nucleotide double-stranded RNA into the cells. It was used in the nematode *Caenorhabditis elegans* to alter gene expression. This post-transcriptional phenomenon was named *RNA interference (RNAi)*. It opened the door for gene silencing using double-stranded short interfering RNA (siRNA) which is capable of degrading a larger mRNA. These siRNAs exist in two forms—endogenous and exogenous. Endogenous siRNA is present in all animal cells, plant cells, bacteria, and viruses. It helps in cell division, differentiation, and growth. Exogenous siRNA are of special interest because they are medium-sized (14–16 KD), stable at room temperature, have long intracellular life (typically 3–6 months), easy to prepare, and easy to administer (subcutaneous), and can be self-administered.[8] The delivery is made by using lipid nanoparticles or conjugation with a ligand (GalNAc) leading to receptor-mediated endocytosis. Once inside the cell, it remains inactive until it combines with Argonaute, part of the RNA-induced silencing complex (RISC). There passenger strand is removed and the remaining antisense strand binds to the desired mRNA target. This prevents protein translation. GalNAc-siRNA is stable inside hepatic endosomes which causes long-life to it.

Zilebesiran (Alnylam Therapeutics in Cambridge, Massachusetts), also known as ALN-AGT, is the first-in-class GalNAc-AGT-siRNA that has undergone phase I human trials.[9] 107 patients were randomized to a single subcutaneous dose of Zilebesiran (10, 25, 50, 100, 200, 400, or 800 mg) or placebo in a 2:1 fashion and were followed for 24 weeks. In part B, the effects of an 800 mg subcutaneous dose of Zilebesiran on BP were assessed in high-low-salt diet conditions. In part E, it was coadministered with irbesartan. Pharmacodynamics, pharmacokinetics, safety, and efficacy in terms of reduction in systolic blood pressure (SBP) and diastolic blood pressure (DBP) as measured by ambulatory BP monitor were assessed. There was a dose-dependent decrease in SBP and DBP with dose ≥200 mg which persisted for 24 weeks. There were few injection site reactions.

Zilebesiran is now being evaluated in phase II trials in patients having mild-to-moderate hypertension without antihypertensive medications in KARDIA-1, KARDIA-2, and KARDIA-3 trials.

RNA Interference with Zilebesiran for Mild-to-moderate Hypertension. KARDIA-1 Randomized Clinical Trial[10]

The KARDIA-1 trial was a multicenter, randomized, double-blind, placebo-controlled in adults with mild-to-moderate hypertension evaluating subcutaneous zilebesiran doses of 150, 300, or 600 mg every 6 months or 300 mg every 3 months. It randomized 394 patients out of which 377 were eligible for analysis (302 zilebesiran and 75 placebo). There was a significant reduction of SBP –14.1 mm Hg, –16.7 mm Hg, and –15.7 mm Hg for zilebesiran 150 mg every 6 months, 300 mg once every 6 months, and 600 mg every 6 months, respectively. In terms of side-effects, 58%, 60%, 61%, and 64% reported at least one side-effect with zilebesiran 150 mg once every 6 months, 300 mg every 6 months, 300 mg every 3 months, and 600 mg every 6 months, respectively.

Zilebesiran in Combination with a Standard-of-care Antihypertensive in Patients with Inadequately Controlled Hypertension KARDIA-2 Trial

The KARDIA-2 trial evaluated patients with inadequately controlled BP with indapamide 2.5 mg, amlodipine 5 mg, or olmesartan 40 mg daily. Zilebesiran 600 mg subcutaneous single dose or placebo was added to standard therapy. Patients were followed for 6 months. The addition of an extra antihypertensive agent was permitted after 3 months if required to achieve target BP. The results were presented at the American College of Cardiology Annual Scientific Session[11] (ACC.24), Atlanta, GA, April 7, 2024. There was a significant reduction in SBP –18.5 mm Hg (indapamide/zilebesiran), –10.2 mm Hg (amlodipine/zilebesiran) and –7.0 mm Hg (olmesartan/zilebesiran as compared to placebo at 3 months. At 6 months, there was SBP reduction of –12.1 mm Hg (indapamide/zilebesiran), –9.7 mm Hg (amlodipine/zilebesiran) and –4.0 mm Hg (olmesartan/zilebesiran) as compared to placebo. This SBP reduction was sustained in indapamide and amlodipine over 6 months.

KARDIA-3 Trial

This is an ongoing phase II trial of zilebesiran in adult patients with uncontrolled hypertension with 2–4 antihypertensive agents and high cardiovascular risk. Cohort A will randomize approximately 270 patients with 300 or 600 mg zilebesiran or placebo in 1:1:1 fashion. In cohort B, approximately 120 patients will be randomized to 150, 300, or 600 mg of zilebesiran or a placebo in a 1:1:1:1 manner.

Advantages and Limitations of siRNA Therapy

The concept of siRNA-AGT looks attractive because of simplicity in dosing, longer duration of action, and positive outcomes in phase I and II studies. However, it has significant limitations. The initial studies have evaluated a very small number of patients. Phase 3 trials with larger enrollment probably will shed better light. Because it takes a longer time to act, this therapy is not suitable for severe hypertension or accelerated-malignant hypertension. The effects on cardiovascular outcome, mortality, and target organ damage have not been studied so far. Pharmacological interaction with other cardiovascular medicines and its role in complex cardiac patients with diabetes and renal failure need to be assessed. Finally, cost-effectiveness, especially in third-world countries where generic variants of original antihypertensive molecules are available at cheap rates, will play the most significant role in its adaptability. AGT remains an important physiological and humoral substance released during stress, sepsis, hypovolemia, and hypotension and it is linked with the patient's survival. AGT inhibition may theoretically compromise with patient's survival during emergencies.

CRISPR/CAS9 MEDIATED DELETION OF THE ANGIOTENSINOGEN GENE FOR HYPERTENSION

Another evolving approach to silence liver AGT is a gene editing technology known as clustered regularly interspaced short palindromic repeats/clustered regularly interspaced short palindromic repeat-associated protein 9 gene editing system proposed by Sun and colleagues.[12] The delivery of CRISPR-Cas9 into the liver reduced AGT expression by 40% and circulating AGT by 30% in spontaneously hypertensive rats. It reduced BP and also prevented the development of new BP in experimental models. Moreover, the BP-lowering effect was maintained for 1 year. The partial disruption of the hepatic *AGT* gene was sufficient to lower BP but did not affect the homeostatic response to cardiovascular stress. This is being viewed as a sustained, irreversible control of hypertension in humans if proven safe and effective in clinical studies.

ANGIOTENSIN II VACCINE[13]

Hironori Nakagami[14] and colleagues reported the first-ever phase I/IIa study of angiotensin II vaccine AGMG0201 in patients with mild to moderate hypertension. Twelve patients were enrolled to receive two doses of vaccine intramuscularly at 0 and 30 days and followed for 360 days. Vaccination resulted in high titers of antiangiotensin II antibody. Further studies are in progress to develop vaccines against various components of RAS such as renin, Ang I and II, and AT1R.

CONCLUSION

Angiotensinogen inhibition by genetic interference is being viewed as a promising pharmacotherapy for hypertension in the coming days. Technologies are still evolving. The trial data are still limited to experimental models or phase I/II human trials. If proven to be safe and effective, these agents may change the course of hypertension management in the future, especially for those who are unwilling to take daily pills. There is a chance that by using CRISPR–Cas9 like gene editing technology, hypertension may be cured at least in some individuals in the future. The angiotensin vaccine is also under evaluation. The products of the "protective" RAS pathway are also being evaluated in various phases for treatment of hypertension.

ONLINE REFERENCES

Please scan the QR code provided at the end of the table of contents for References of this chapter.

CHAPTER

40

Nocturnal Hypertension

Amal Khan, Anish Kumar Khan, Amartya Khan

ABSTRACT

Nocturnal hypertension is a clinical condition of elevated BP at night detected by ambulatory blood pressure monitoring. Guidelines defined mean BP as >120/70 mm Hg at nighttime.

Both nocturnal hypertension and nondipping status are associated with a higher cardiovascular risk and target organ damage, but debate remains over which is a better prognostic marker for CV outcomes. While current data remain inconclusive, many suggest that nocturnal hypertension is a more reliable and clinically significant marker of CV risk for nondipping status. Regarding management reducing nocturnal hypertension and nondipping HTN through chronotherapy specifically, evening-dosing antihypertensives have not been conclusively shown to provide long-term CV benefits.

Keywords: Ambulatory blood pressure monitoring (ABPM), home blood pressure monitoring (HBPM), hypertension-mediated organ damage (HMOD)

INTRODUCTION

Nocturnal hypertension is emerging as a residual cardiovascular risk.[1,2] There is much evidence that nocturnal hypertension is associated with target organ damages such as left ventricular hypertrophy, silent cerebral disease, and albuminuria, as well as with subsequent atherosclerosis, cardiovascular disease, and stroke.[3,4] A high prevalence of nocturnal hypertension is present in Chinese, Japanese, and other Asian populations rather than in Caucasians, which is probably associated with a high salt intake and salt sensitivity.[5-7] Nocturnal hypertension is considered to be a risk factor of target organ damage and cardiovascular and all-cause mortality, independent of daytime BP.[8,9] However, due to the disadvantages of routine home BP monitoring (HBPM) in daily practice, nocturnal hypertension has not been fully recognized and usually underdiagnosed.

DEFINITION AND EPIDEMIOLOGY

According to 2023 ESH guidelines for the management of hypertension, the nighttime hypertension is defined as an average BP 120/70 mm Hg recorded during the night hours with ambulatory blood pressure monitoring (ABPM). In recent years, dedicated home BP devices have emerged as a new method for obtaining BP values during sleep, and they could be a practical alternative to ABPM.[10] Two large studies have shown that having nocturnal hypertension in people with normal office BP and normal daytime BP, a condition called isolated nocturnal hypertension, is associated with a higher risk of hypertension-mediated organ damage (HMOD) and adverse outcomes.[10] Isolated nocturnal hypertension is a specific condition with mean nighttime BP ≥ 120/70 mm Hg while daytime BP < 135/85 mm Hg, which is more insidious and difficult to identify.[5,6] In a study conducted among the Chinese population, the authors demonstrated that isolated nocturnal hypertension is associated with increased arterial stiffness.[5] Mean nighttime BP ≥120/70 mm Hg while daytime BP < 135/85 mm Hg on antihypertensive medications is defined as uncontrolled nocturnal hypertension.[11] Isolated nocturnal hypertension has been found to be present in 9.2–12.9% of adults[12,13] and more prevalent in men with high-normal BP and high CV risk profile, Africo-American, older individuals, obese and diabetic patients, and patients with CKD.[14]

There are no large-scale epidemiological data on the prevalence of nocturnal hypertension. A cohort study done in China showed that the prevalence of isolated nocturnal hypertension was 10.9%.[5] The analysis of international ABPM databases disclosed that the prevalence of isolated nocturnal hypertension in Asian and South African populations was about 10%, while 6–7.9% in Europeans, indicating obvious regional and racial differences.[6]

PATHOPHYSIOLOGY

Various physiological and pathological factors associated with nocturnal hypertension are detailed in **Figure 1**.

- Within our Asian demographic, a significant factor contributing to nocturnal hypertension is the elevated consumption of salt or heightened sensitivity to salt, causing a rise in the requirement for renal sodium excretion during nighttime. This, in turn, leads to an escalation in renal perfusion pressure, ultimately resulting in the development of either nocturnal hypertension or a nondipping hypertension pattern.[15,16]
- Patients with chronic kidney disease or cardiac dysfunction may experience elevated circulatory volume, resulting in increased venous return while lying down, potentially causing a rise in blood pressure during nighttime hours.[1]
- Individuals suffering from diabetes, Parkinson's disease, sleep difficulties, or autonomic nerve dysfunction may exhibit elevated sympathetic activity during the night, which can disrupt their circadian rhythm and cause nocturnal hypertension.[1]
- Obstructive sleep apnea (OSA) has been extensively linked to nocturnal hypertension and nondipping as intermittent hypoxia and sleep fragmentation result in sympathetic excitation and subsequent vasoconstriction. Upregulation of the renin-angiotensin-aldosterone system, as well as increased oxidative stress and endothelial dysfunction, in OSA may also contribute to nocturnal hypertension and nondipping pattern.[17,18]
- Supine nocturnal hypertension may coexist with orthostatic hypotension in certain elderly people.[1,19] BP circadian rhythm disorders and nocturnal hypertension are common in elderly patients with reduced elasticity of large arteries, arterial stiffness or atherosclerosis, vascular endothelial dysfunction, or decreased BP autoregulation capacity resulting from reduced baroreceptor reflex sensitivity, among other factors.
- Certain secondary hypertensive conditions, including renovascular hypertension, renal parenchymal

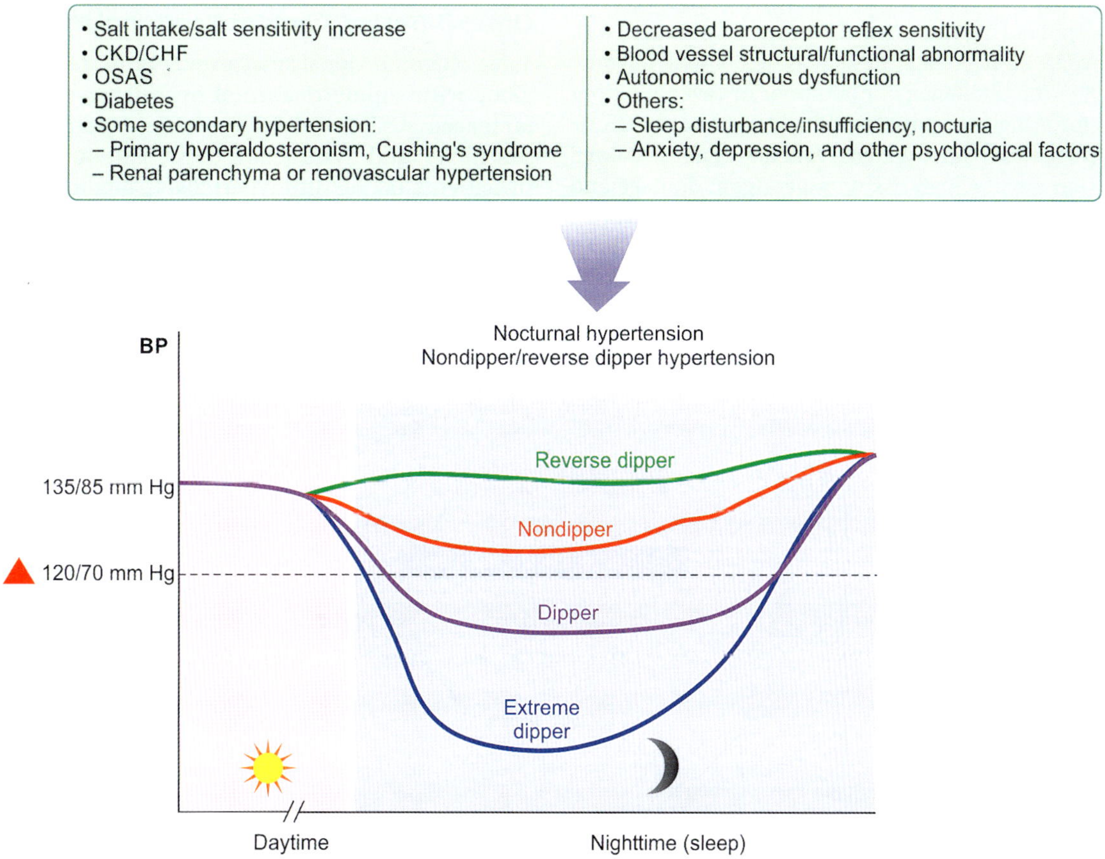

FIG. 1: Pathophysiology, definitions, and possible mechanisms of nocturnal hypertension. Extreme dipper: >20% reduction in nighttime BP; physiological dipping (dipper): >10% and <20% decrease in nighttime BP; nondipper: <10% reduction in nighttime BP; reverse dipper: rise in nighttime BP compared with daytime.

(CHF: chronic heart failure; CKD: chronic kidney disease; OSAS: obstructive sleep apnea syndrome) hypertension, Cushing syndrome, and primary hyperaldosteronism, typically result in nocturnal hypertension due to an increased volume load.[1]

- Elevated blood pressure at night can be attributed to various factors such as high environmental temperatures during sleep (during summer), inadequate sleep, frequent awakenings, anxiety, depression, cognitive impairment, and other psychological influences.

CLINICAL PHENOTYPES

As per the analysis of 24-hour ABPM, most of the patients having nocturnal hypertension demonstrated as having sustained hypertension during day and night, and some patients had isolated nocturnal hypertension.

Day–Night Sustained Hypertension

Day–night sustained hypertension refers to the situation in which ABPM shows the mean daytime BP ≥ 135/85 mm Hg and nighttime BP ≥ 120/70 mm Hg. According to the difference between mean daytime and nighttime BP, it can be divided into the following patterns: Dippers (nighttime BP drops by >10% to <20% on average compared with daytime BP), extreme dippers (≥22% fall), nondippers divided into reduced dippers (nighttime BP drops by <10–0% fall) and riser or reverse dippers (nighttime BP is higher than daytime BP), etc.[20-22] The incidence of nondipper or reverse dipper hypertension is higher in patients with old age, obesity, OSAS, CKD, and diabetes.[14] Since patients with day–night sustained hypertension are at a high risk of target organ damage and adverse cardiovascular events, it is necessary to evaluate circadian rhythm via ABPM and try to reach a goal of 24-hour BP control.[4] While both nondipping and reverse dipping are associated with abnormal LV mechanics, such as reduced LV longitudinal strain, only reverse dipping is associated with reduced circumferential strain and reduced right ventricular global longitudinal strain.[23-26]

Isolated Nocturnal Hypertension

Isolated nocturnal hypertension is characterized by an average nighttime BP of 120/70 mm Hg or higher in ABPM without the use of antihypertensive medications, while daytime BP remains below the diagnostic threshold for hypertension. This form of masked hypertension is typically detected and diagnosed through ABPM,[5] but it is often overlooked in clinical settings. Recent research suggests that individuals with isolated nocturnal hypertension are typically older, are male, have a higher BMI, consume more alcohol, have a faster nighttime pulse rate, and exhibit elevated levels of blood cholesterol or glucose. For men, smokers, obese individuals, and patients with metabolic syndrome, CKD, high-normal office BP, or evident target organ damage in the absence of other cardiovascular risk factors, a 24-hour ABPM is recommended to identify isolated nocturnal hypertension **(Flowchart 1)**.[27]

Other Different Types of Nocturnal Hypertension

Some older individuals may exhibit orthostatic hypotension along with supine nocturnal hypertension, often due to increased stiffness of large arteries, reduced baroreflex sensitivity, and dysfunction of the autonomic nerves.[28,29] In patients taking antihypertensive medications, uncontrolled nocturnal hypertension may arise if the drugs' effectiveness cannot be sustained throughout the day.

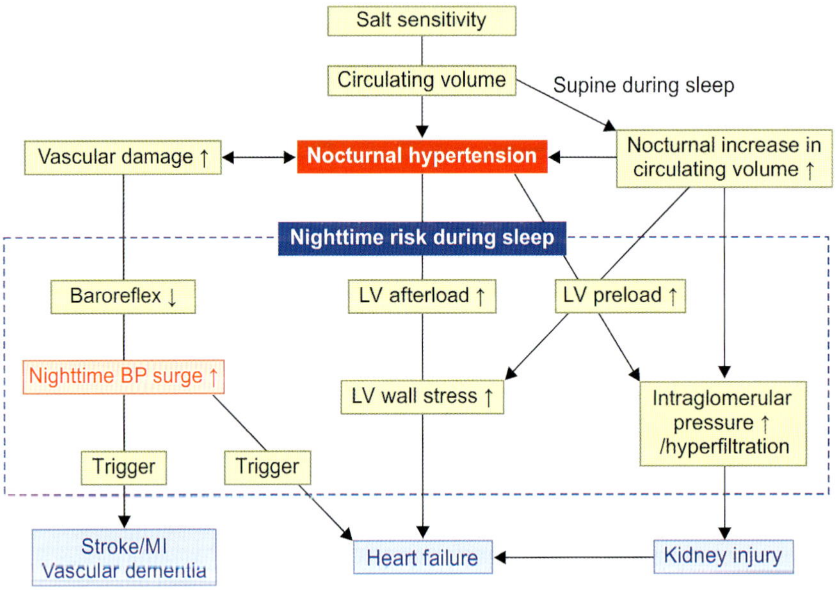

FLOWCHART 1: Possible mechanism of the effects of nocturnal hypertension leading to increased cardiovascular risk.
(BP: blood pressure; LV: left ventricular; MI: myocardial infarction)

Despite well-controlled daytime office or ambulatory blood pressure, nighttime blood pressure levels may remain elevated. Nocturnal hypertension can sometimes progress into morning hypertension during the early hours.[30] The nondipper or reverse dipper blood pressure pattern typically manifests in individuals with nocturnal hypertension, although it can also be observed in normotensive patients. Among hypertensive patients with diabetes, the prevalence of the nondipper pattern can reach 30%.[31] A meta-analysis has indicated that the nondipper pattern is linked to a higher risk of all-cause mortality and cardiovascular events,[32] but this conclusion is still subject to debate and requires further investigation.

Diagnosis and BP Monitoring

A 24-hour ABPM record is highly reproducible in the short term for detecting nocturnal hypertension, but its reproducibility is lower for identifying dipper and nondipper blood pressure patterns. Research indicates that 18% of untreated hypertensive patients had a change in their diagnosis of nocturnal hypertension, while 24% experienced a change in their blood pressure patterns (dipper or nondipper) after undergoing a repeated ABPM within 1 month.[25] Therefore, it is advisable to conduct a repeat 24-hour ABPM in 3–6 months to validate the diagnosis of nocturnal hypertension, particularly in patients who had poor sleep during the initial ABPM.[20] In specific situations, such as patients undergoing hemodialysis, a 44- to 48-hour ABPM is recommended.[26]

In recent times, there have been advancements in electronic arm or wrist-type BP monitors that can be utilized for HBPM at night to screen for nocturnal hypertension and for long-term follow-up. The reproducibility of nighttime HBPM is considered to be reliable. A validated HBPM should consist of a minimum of two consecutive nights with three readings taken per night.[33] A Japanese cohort study revealed that the nighttime BP levels measured by HBPM (they used an upper arm electronic sphygmomanometer, which automatically measures BP at 2:00, 3:00, and 4:00 AM in night) over a period of 14 consecutive days were slightly higher in systolic BP (by 2.6 mm Hg) and lower in diastolic BP (by 0.7 mm Hg) compared with nighttime BP levels measured by ABPM.[34] Meta-analysis results indicated that the nighttime BP levels obtained through HBPM and ABPM are similar, with a minor difference of 1.4/0.2 mm Hg,[35] suggesting a general agreement between nighttime home and ambulatory BP measurement. Therefore, the diagnostic BP threshold of ABPM can be applied to define nocturnal hypertension using HBPM, which is when the mean nighttime BP is ≥120/70 mm Hg. The consistency between HBPM and ABPM for diagnosing nocturnal hypertension was found to be 79% on the first night, 81% on the second night, and 80% for two nights of testing.[36]

Treatment

Lifestyle Modification

Lifestyle modifications for general hypertension population are also suitable for patients with nocturnal hypertension, including sodium intake restriction, healthy diet, sleep improvement, appropriate physical exercise, weight control, smoking cessation, mental stress relief, and moderate alcohol consumption.[21]

Strategy Based on Pressor Mechanisms

The elevation in the baseline blood pressure is influenced by the rise in circulating volume or the presence of advanced vascular disease, such as increased vascular stiffness and heightened vascular resistance due to small artery remodeling **(Flowchart 2)**.

Salt restriction, diuretics, aldosterone blockers, sacubitril/valsartan, and sodium-glucose cotransporter-2 inhibitors are recommended for patients with increased circulating volume, while calcium channel blocker monotherapy or combined therapy with a renin-angiotensin system inhibitor is preferred for patients with advanced vascular disease.[37,38] Recent clinical trials have shown that sacubitril/valsartan improves cardiovascular prognosis[39] and that sodium-glucose cotransporter-2 inhibitors reduce cardiovascular events, particularly in patients with heart failure, and prevent the decline of renal function.[40] Among the patients with OSA, sympatholytic treatment with β-/α-blockers and renal denervation are effective in reducing average and peak

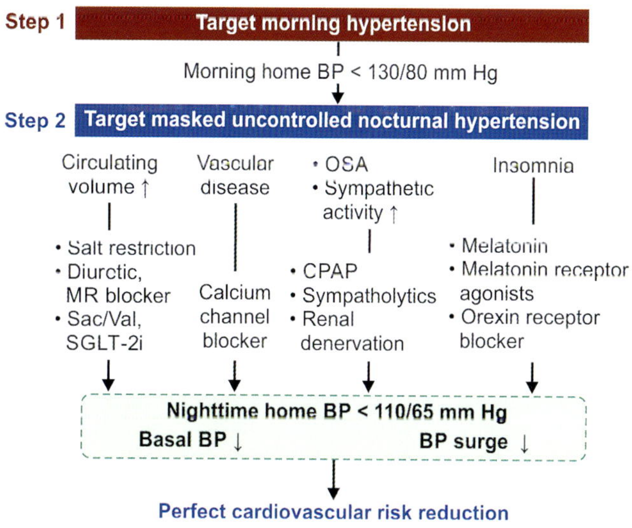

FLOWCHART 2: Pharmacological and other management strategies of nocturnal hypertension.

(BP: blood pressure; CPAP: continuous positive airway pressure; MR: mineral corticoid receptor; OSA: obstructive sleep apnea; Sac/Val: sacubitril/valsartan; SGLT-2i: sodium-glucose cotransporter-2 inhibitor)

TABLE 1: Recommendations for nighttime hypertension and BP phenotypes.[22]

Recommendations and statements	CoR	LoE
It is recommended to assess nighttime BP using ABPM because it is more predictive for outcomes than daytime BP, and because nocturnal hypertension, nondipping, and reverse dipping are associated with increased CV risk	I	B
For the identification of nighttime BP phenotypes, repeating ABPM is necessary, because of poor reproducibility	I	B
In isolated nocturnal hypertension, antihypertensive drugs may lower BP and may thus be considered	III	C
In general hypertensive population, morning dosing or bedtime dosing results in similar outcome	I	B

(ABPM: ambulatory blood pressure monitoring)

nighttime blood pressures.[41] Hypnotics, such as melatonin, melatonin receptor agonists, and orexin receptor antagonists, may help patients with sleep disorders.[42]

Chronotherapy

Chronotherapy is a therapeutic approach that involves administering drugs based on the circadian blood pressure rhythm of patients in order to achieve better blood pressure control, reduce adverse effects, and improve clinical outcomes.[43] Previous small-scale trials have explored the use of chronotherapy and combined controlled-release drug delivery technology for nighttime blood pressure control and nondipper hypertension, but the findings have been subject to debate **(Table 1)**.

CONCLUSION

There are still many issues to be solved for the management of nocturnal hypertension, especially for isolated nocturnal hypertension.

How can HBPM, especially smart wearable devices, as well as ABPM, play a part in the diagnosis of nocturnal hypertension?

What is the excellent treatment target and intervention approach for isolated nocturnal hypertension? Well-designed clinical trials should also be done in the future.

ONLINE REFERENCES

Please scan the QR code provided at the end of the table of contents for References of this chapter.

CHAPTER

41

Secondary Causes of Hypertension: A Quick Guide for Diagnosis

Vinod Sharma, Ruchi Sharma

ABSTRACT

Hypertension is a major noncommunicable disease responsible for high morbidity and mortality across the globe. Worldwide nearly 30% of adult population is suffering from hypertension. While in majority, the cause is unknown, in around 10% of patients, there is identifiable cause, and these patients fall under the category of secondary hypertension. The morbidity and mortality in this category of patient can be altered favorably by the treatment of underlying disorder, leading to secondary hypertension. This review aims to outline prevalence, diagnostic approach, and summary of therapeutic modalities of common causes of secondary hypertension.

Keywords: Secondary hypertension, pseudohypertension, pseudoresistance, renovascular hypertension, pregnancy-related hypertension

INTRODUCTION

Hypertension is one of the most common noncommunicable diseases, leading to high morbidity and mortality across the globe.

In India, hypertension is a major public health problem, both in a major adolescence and adults with a substantial burden on the healthcare system.

Recent epidemiological studies have reported that hypertension is increasing in India with a more rapid increase in rural and young populations.

The National Family Health Survey Study (NFHS-5) found that the prevalence of hypertension in the age group of 15–49 years was 22.80%.[1]

According to a recent survey, the prevalence of hypertension is 28–30% in adults older than 18 years, and nearly 2 in 3 remain undiagnosed across the country both in rural and in urban areas.[2]

A systematic review and meta-analysis found that the overall prevalence of hypertension is 29.8% but varies by region:

- North India : 14.6 % in rural and 28.8% in urban areas
- East India : 31.7% in rural and 34.5% in urban areas
- West India : 18.1% in rural and 34.8% in urban areas
- South India : 21.1% in rural and 31.8% in urban areas[3]

Primary hypertension, also referred to as essential hypertension, accounts for the majority (90–95%) of hypertension cases. The exact cause of primary or essential hypertension is often unknown, but it is a combination of genetic, lifestyle, and environmental facts, which plays crucial role in its causation.

Secondary hypertension defined as elevated blood pressure, secondary to an identifiable cause, is found in around 10% of patients. Because of the low prevalence and cost constraints, often routine evaluation are not performed in every case of hypertension. Identifying the cause of hypertension in select group of patients helps in guiding appropriate line of treatment. More, so it may result in complete cure of hypertension with complete elimination of antihypertensive therapy with resultant improvement in morbidity and mortality.

The prevalence of secondary hypertension varies with age, and it is most prevalent in extreme of age. It accounts for 70–80% of hypertension cases in children less than 12 years of age and approximately 17% of cases in adults aged 65 and older. The prevalence of secondary hypertension is lowest among hypertensive patients who are 19–39 years of age while its prevalence in adolescent (12–18 years) is 10–15%.[4]

ETIOLOGY OF SECONDARY HYPERTENSION

Renal Parenchymal Disease

- Diabetic nephropathy
- Glomerulonephritis
- Polycystic kidney disease
- Interstitial renal parenchymal disease
- Majority of patients with renal parenchymal disease are found to have hypertension.
- Incidence of hypertension increases with progressive deterioration of renal parenchymal disease.
- Emergency of hypertension carries a negative impact on renal parenchymal disease, and it further accentuates the worsening of renal function culminating into end-stage renal disease.

Renovascular Disorders

Hypertension due to stenosis of one or both renal arteries is not an uncommon cause of secondary hypertension. While fibromuscular dysplasia is a cause of renal artery stenosis, especially in female of young age, atherosclerosis is a common cause of renal artery stenosis in elderly population, leading to secondary hypertension.

Endocrine Disease

Increased secretion of hormones can lead to secondary hypertension. Common causes of secondary hypertension due to endocrinal causes are:

- *Primary aldosteronism*: It is responsible for majority of endocrine hypertension cases.
- Pheochromocytoma
- Cushing syndrome
- Rare endocrine disorders which may cause secondary hypertension are:
  - Acromegaly
  - Primary hyperparathyroidism
  - Thyroid disorders

Vascular Cases

- Coarctation of aorta, causing hypertension in young individuals
- Vascular of medium- or large-sized arteries and AV fistula

Drug-induced Secondary Hypertension—Common Offending Drugs

- Nonsteroidal anti-inflammatory drugs
- Systemic corticosteroids
- Mineralocorticoids such as ketoconazole, I alpha fludrocortisone, and carbenoxolone
- Estrogens, androgens, and oral contraceptives
- Decongestants such as phenylephrine or pseudoephedrine
- Drugs used for treatment of attention deficit hyperactivity disorder (ADHD)—amphetamine, methylphenidate, and dextroamphetamine
- Antidepressant such as monoamine oxidase inhibitors, tricyclic antidepressants, and serotonin-norepinephrine reuptake inhibitors
- *Miscellaneous drugs such as*:
  - Sodium-containing antacids
  - Appetite suppressants
  - Nicotine and alcohol

Miscellaneous Causes of Secondary Hypertension

- Obstructive sleep apnea
- Polycystic ovarian syndrome
- Preeclampsia

HOW TO SCREEN FOR SECONDARY HYPERTENSION?

Exclude Pseudohypertension and Pseudoresistance

Patients with resistant arterial hypertension should be screened for secondary dorms. However, before starting the screening, pseudohypertension and pseudoresistance should be excluded.

Pseudohypertension

Pseudohypertension is defined as cuff diastolic BP at least 15 mm Hg higher than simultaneously measured intra-arterial BP. It is found in elderly patients with calcified and rigid arteries who present with little or no target organ damage despite very high BP readings. In these patients, excessive cuff pressure is needed to compress the artery, resulting in falsely high readings. This entity may be identified using the Osler maneuver. However, this maneuver has a large intra- and interobserver variability. Assessment of brachial arterial stiffness by the measurement of carotid-radial pulse wave velocity may also help identify patients with this particular form of hypertension.[5,6]

Pseudoresistance: Inadequate Blood Pressure Measurement Techniques

There are two very common causes for pseudoresistance due to inaccurate BP measurement techniques: (1) BP measurement without letting the patient quietly sit for at least minute and (2) inadequate cuff size (too small cuff size may result in falsely increase BP >15 mm Hg).

Poor Treatment Control

Poor therapy control is sometimes related to physician's clinical inertia, i.e., they fail to up titrate therapy in order to reach target BP. Conversely, poor patient adherence to therapy is widespread reaching about 40% in patients with newly diagnosed hypertension.

White Coat Hypertension

White coat hypertension is a frequent cause of pseudo-resistance with a prevalence of about 20–30%. Twenty-four hour ABPM is valuable tool to assess the likelihood of secondary hypertension.

Drug-related Hypertension

Take a detailed history of drugs used by patients and rule out drug-induced hypertension.

Clues for Secondary Hypertension

In general, patients of hypertension with any of the following characteristics are pointers to secondary hypertension:

- Age of onset less than 40 years
- Abrupt onset of hypertension
- Abrupt worsening of hypertension despite previously good control
- Hypertensive urgency or emergency
- Resistant hypertension (blood pressure ≥140/90 mm Hg despite the consistent use of three antihypertensive drugs including a diuretic, or a need for four or more drugs to control the blood pressure)
- Target organ damage disproportionate to the degree of hypertension
- Family history of early-onset hypertension, stroke before the age of 40 years, or primary aldosteronism
- *Clinical clues*:
  - An excessive drop in potassium with a small dose of diuretic (primary aldosteronism or other endogenous or exogenous mineralocorticoid excess)
  - Excessive decrease in GFR with a small dose of an angiotensin-converting enzyme (ACE)-inhibitor (RAS, predominately when bilateral)
  - A remarkably resistant arterial hypertension
  - Paroxysmal hypertension or episodes suggestive of catecholamine excess (suggestive of pheochromocytoma)

STEPS IN ASSESSMENT OF SECONDARY HYPERTENSION

History and Physical Findings

The following history and physical examination findings point toward a specific cause of secondary hypertension:

- History of renal insufficiency, atherosclerotic cardiovascular disease, and edema may warrant further evaluation of chronic kidney disease (renal parenchymal disease).
- History of recurrent urinary tract infections, kidney stones, acute/chronic abdominal/flank pain, hematuria, and progressive renal failure may point toward autosomal dominant polycystic kidney disease (renal parenchymal disease).
- Snoring, obesity, and daytime sleepiness could be indicative of obstructive sleep apnea.
- Worsening renal function with ACE inhibitors and a systolic/diastolic abdominal bruit point toward the renovascular disease.
- Episodic hypertension, headache, and palpitation, associated with acute stress, in a perioperative setting, could be the signs of pheochromocytoma or paragangliomas.
- Decreased or delayed femoral pulses, radio femoral delay, and difference in the blood pressure into arms are seen in patient with coarctation with aorta and vasculitic causes of secondary hypertension.
- Weight gain, fatigue, weakness, hirsutism, amenorrhea, moon facies, dorsal hump, purple striae, and truncal obesity present in Cushing syndrome/disease.
- Fatigue, weight loss, hair loss, diastolic hypertension, and muscle weakness are seen in hypothyroidism.
- Heat intolerance, weight loss, palpitations, systolic hypertension, exophthalmos, tremor, and tachycardia will occur in hyperthyroidism.
- Kidney stones, osteoporosis, depression, lethargy, and muscle weakness present in hyperparathyroidism.
- Headache, fatigue, visual problems, enlargement of the hands, feet, and tongue are features of acromegaly.
- Heartburn, Raynaud phenomenon, and nail pitting on the examination may be suggestive of scleroderma.

Laboratory Evaluation

Confirmatory laboratory and radiology investigations are individualized and preceded by the screening test.

How to Screen?

Refer to **Table 1**.[7]

Renal Parenchymal Disease

- The initial screening tests for renal parenchymal diseases include serum creatinine with estimated glomerular filtration rate (eGFR), urine detailed report, urinary protein/protein to creatinine ratio, and renal ultrasound.
- A renal biopsy followed by histopathology is a gold-standard investigation, recommended for the diagnosis of specific conditions and pathophysiology of renal parenchymal disease.

Endocrine Disorder

Primary Aldosteronism

- Hypertension with hypokalemia is one of the characteristic features of primary aldosteronism, especially in those individuals with a family history of hypertension and cerebrovascular accidents at a young age.[8]

TABLE 1: Summary overview of the most common causes and screening method for secondary hypertension.

Secondary cause	Prevalence[a]	Prevalence[b]	History	Screening	Clinical findings	Laboratory findings
Obstructive sleep apnea	>5–15%	>30%	Snoring, daytime sleepiness, morning headache, and irritability	Screening questionnaire; polysomnography	↑ neck circumference, obesity, and peripheral edema	Not specific
Renal parenchymal disease	1.6–8.0%	2–10%	Loss of good BP control, diabetes, smoking, generalized atherosclerosis, previous renal failure, and nocturia	Creatinine, ultrasound of kidney	Peripheral edema; pallor, loss of muscle mass	↑ Creatinine, proteinuria; ↓ Ca^{2+}, ↑K^+, ↑ PO_4
Renal artery stenosis	1.0–8.0%	2.5–20%	Generalized atherosclerosis, diabetes, smoking, and recurrent flush pulmonary edema	Duplex, CT, MRI, or angiography (drive by)	Abdominal bruits and peripheral vascular disease	Secondary aldosteronism ARR →, ↓ K^+, ↓ Na^+
Primary aldosteronism	1.4–10%	6–23%	Fatigue, Constipation, polyuria, and polydipsia	Aldosterone-renin ratio (ARR)	Muscle weakness	↓ K^+ and ARR↑
Thyroid disease	1–2%	1–3%	Hyperthyroidism; palpitations, weight loss, anxiety, heat intolerance; hypothyroidism; Weight gain, fatigue, and obstipation	TSH	Hyperthyroidism: tachycardia, AF, accentuated heart sounds; exophthalmos; Hypothyroidism: bradycardia, muscle weakness; myxedema	Hyperthyroidism: TSH ↓; fT4 and/or fT3 ↑, Hypothyroidism: TSH ↑; fT4 ↓; Cholesterol↑
Cushing's syndrome	0.5%	<1.0%	Weight gain; impotence; fatigue, psychological changes, polydipsia, and polyuria	24-hour urinary cortisol; dexamethasone testing	Obesity, hirsutism, skin atrophy, striae rubrae, muscle weakness, and osteopenia	24-hour urinary; cortisol↑; glucose↑; cholesterol ↑; K^+↓
Pheochromocytoma	0.2–0.5%	<1%	Headaches, palpitations, flushing, and anxiety	Plasma-metanephrines; 24-hour urinary catecholamines	The "5 P's": *P*aroxysmal hypertension, *p*ounding headache, *p*erspiration, *p*alpitations, *p*allor	Metanephrines↑
Coarctation of the aorta	<1%	<1%	Headache, nosebleeding, leg weakness, or claudication	Cardiac ultrasound	Different BP (≥20/10 mm Hg) between upper-lower extremities and/or between right-left arm; ↓ and delayed femoral pulsations; interscapular ejection murmur; rib notching on chest X-ray	Not specific

[a]Prevalence in hypertensive patients.
[b]Prevalence in patients with resistant hypertension.[7]

(AF: atrial fibrillation; ARR: aldosterone-renin ratio; BP: blood pressure; Ca^{2+}: calcium; CT: computed tomography; fT3: free triiodothyronine; fT4: free thyroxine; K^+: potassium; NA^+: sodium; PO_4-: phosphate; TSH: thyroid-stimulating hormone)

The plasma aldosterone/renin ratio is the preferred screening test for primary aldosteronism, and it should be done at least 4 weeks after the withdrawal of aldosterone antagonists and after the correction of hypokalemia.

- The measurement of 24-hour urine aldosterone level after oral sodium loading and plasma aldosterone level after intravenous saline infusion are the diagnostic tests for primary aldosteronism, while renal vein sampling can be done for selected patients.
- Adrenal imaging is recommended for the localization of the lesion.

Pheochromocytoma

- Screening for pheochromocytoma/paraganglioma is recommended in the presence of episodic hypertension, along with palpitations, headache, postural hypotension, and stigmata of neurofibromatosis.[9]
- Measurement of urinary or plasma metanephrine is the recommended screening test for pheochromocytoma.
- Computed tomography or magnetic resonance imaging is recommended for the localization of the tumor.
- An overnight dexamethasone suppression test is the preferred screening investigation for Cushing syndrome.
- 24-hour urinary free cortisol and midnight salivary cortisol

Thyroid and Parathyroid Disorders

- Thyroid disorders are the rare causes of secondary hypertension, which can be diagnosed.
- Measuring the thyroid-stimulating hormone (TSH) and free T4/T3 levels.
- Ultrasonography and biopsy are recommended in selected patients with suspected thyroid malignancies.
- Serum calcium level is the best screening test for hyperparathyroidism, while the measurement of serum parathyroid hormone is recommended for the diagnosis of primary hyperparathyroidism.

Renovascular Hypertension

- Renal artery stenosis is suspected when patients present with uncontrolled hypertension and have renal bruit.
- Develop deterioration of renal function after taking ACE inhibiting drugs.
- Ultrasound renal Doppler is the initial recommended test for the screening and diagnosis of renal stenosis.
- Computed tomographic angiogram (CTA) and magnetic resonance angiogram (MRA) can be considered in a selected group of patients.
- The bilateral, selective renal artery angiogram is rarely required for the diagnosis of renal artery stenosis.[10]

Vascular and Other Causes of Hypertension

- Coarctation of the aorta is the major contributor to secondary hypertension in this group, and an echocardiogram is the best screening as well as a diagnostic test for the coarctation of the aorta.
- Computed tomographic aortogram (CTA) and MRA is recommended for the diagnosis and confirmation of coarctation of the aorta as well as vasculitis.
- Polysomnography (preferably in-laboratory polysomnography) is the diagnostic study of choice when there is a suspicion of obstructive sleep apnea.
- The clinical and laboratory findings consistent with scleroderma may include thrombotic microangiopathy, autoantibodies against RNA polymerase III, and positive antinuclear antibody (ANA).

Treatment/Strategy in Secondary Hypertension

Management of secondary hypertension comprises adequate control of blood pressure with a healthy lifestyle and appropriate antihypertensive drugs and addressing the secondary causes mentioned above.

Renal Parenchymal Disease

- Main focus of the management is to treat the reversible causes responsible for the progression to advanced kidney disease.
- Adequate blood pressure control is an essential component of management in CKD and contemporary guidelines recommend renin-angiotensin (RA) antagonists as the preferred drug therapy for the treatment of hypertension in CKD. The RA-blocking drugs not only control hypertension but also prevent the progression of CKD, especially in patients with proteinuria.[11]

Renovascular Hypertension

- Management of renovascular hypertension (renal artery stenosis) is divided into medical therapy and revascularization.
- Medical therapy involves the use of antihypertensive drugs to control blood pressure and in the case of atherosclerotic disease, the use of antiplatelets, statins, diet, and lifestyle changes.
- ACE inhibitors and ARBs are the antihypertensive drugs of choice in patients with unilateral renal artery stenosis; however, these drugs are contraindicated in bilateral renal artery stenosis due to the risk of rapid renal dysfunction.
- Other pharmacologic treatment options are calcium channel blockers and thiazide diuretics.
- Percutaneous revascularization is recommended along with medical therapy in selective patients, especially those with fibromuscular dysplasia.
- The combination of drug therapy and percutaneous revascularization has been reported to reduce blood pressure significantly, and this strategy has long-term

renoprotective effects in patients with fibromuscular dysplasia.

- Revascularization may be more beneficial than medical therapy alone in following subset of patients:
  - Patients with recurrent flash pulmonary edema
  - Failure or intolerance to optimal medical treatment
  - Refractory hypertension
  - Unexplained, progressive, a decline in renal function
  - Recent initiation of dialysis in a patient with suspected renal artery stenosis
  - An acute increase in creatinine after medical therapy and in patients with a renal resistive index of less than 80 mm Hg on Doppler.[12,13]

Endocrine Hypertension

- Unilateral primary aldosteronism (e.g., unilateral adrenal hyperplasia or aldosterone-producing adenoma) gets treated with unilateral laparoscopic adrenalectomy.
- If the patient is not a surgical candidate or a patient has the bilateral adrenal disease, then medical management with a mineralocorticoid receptor antagonist is recommended and spironolactone is the drug of choice for primary aldosteronism.
- Cushing syndrome or Cushing disease, an open surgical or laparoscopic resection of the lesion/tumor, is the treatment of choice
- The definite treatment of pheochromocytoma is surgical resection of the hormone-producing lesion; however, preoperative alpha and beta-adrenergic blocking drugs are an essential part of pheochromocytoma management.
- It is recommended to start alpha-adrenergic blocking drugs first and then add beta blockers for the treatment of tachyarrhythmias.
- Initiation of beta-adrenergic blocking drugs is not recommended alone/before the alpha-adrenergic blockade, as it results in hypertensive crisis due to the unopposed alpha-adrenergic effect.
- Pheochromocytoma crisis is treated with intravenous phentolamine followed by initiation of oral alpha-adrenergic blocking drugs.
- The specific treatment of patients with hypothyroidism included thyroid replacement therapy, while hyperthyroidism is treated with antithyroid drugs.
- The definite treatment of patients with hypertension due to acromegaly is transsphenoidal resection of the hormone-producing tumor.[12]

Vascular Hypertension

- Coarctation of the aorta is the major cause of vascular hypertension in the younger population.
- The choice of antihypertensive drugs for this population depends on the other coexisting conditions.
- The definite treatment is the percutaneous or surgical correction of the coarctation.
- Correction of coarctation at an early age provides better long-term outcomes, but one-third of the patients remain hypertensive even after surgical correction of the coarctation of the aorta.
- Vasculitides of the large vessels (e.g., Takayasu arteritis) may also lead to hypertension due to a significant rise in systemic vascular resistance.
- Corticosteroids or other immunosuppressant agents along with antihypertensive drugs are recommended for the treatment of secondary hypertension due to vasculitides.[14]

Obstructive Sleep Apnea

- Continuous positive airway pressure (CPAP) therapy is the mainstay of treatment for OSA.
- Lifestyle modifications, such as weight loss, along with the usage of CPAP have a synergistic effect on lowering blood pressure and are better than either intervention alone.
- An alternative to CPAP is oral appliances, used in mild-to-moderate OSA, which are noninferior to CPAP in the reduction of blood pressure and may even help with better compliance in patients.
- In patients refractory to the above treatment, few upper airway surgeries can be performed to help with symptoms and reduction in blood pressure, such as uvulopalatopharyngoplasty (UPPP) in adults and tonsillectomy and adenoidectomy in children.

Pregnancy-related Hypertension

- Interventions for hypertension in pregnancy are lifestyle modifications and antihypertensives.
- The antihypertensives commonly used in pregnancy are labetalol, nifedipine, and methyldopa.
- If an acute decrease in blood pressure is required, intravenous labetalol and intravenous hydralazine are options.
- Treatment/management of gestational and chronic hypertension in pregnancy is always indicated when blood pressures are in the severe range (>160/110 mm Hg) last at least 15 minutes apart. ACOG does not recommend treatment with antihypertensives for mild range pressures unless they were on the medication for pregestational hypertension (chronic hypertension) prior to pregnancy. The treatment indication for chronic hypertension is 140/90 mm Hg per ACOG. First-line therapies include labetolol, hydralazine, or nifedipine. Nifedipine is preferred if oral medication for acute oral treatment and nifedipine or oral labetalol preferred in the outpatient setting. Thiazide diuretics can be continued if used to treat chronic hypertension before pregnancy. Hydralazine and clonidine have been used in certain circumstances but are not commonly used in the longitudinal treatment of gestational or chronic

TABLE 2: Antihypertensive drugs that can be safely used in pregnancy.

Antihypertensive drug*	Class/action	Dose	Adverse effects
Labetalol	Beta blocker	100 mg twice a day to 400 mg three times a day	Bradycardia, bronchospasm, and headache
Nifedipine controlled release	Calcium channel antagonist	30 mg daily to 60 mg twice a day	Headache (fast-dose effect), flushing, tachycardia, peripheral, and edema
Methyldopa	Central action	250 mg twice a day to 750 mg three times a day	Depression, dry mouth, sedation, rarely hemolysis, and hepatitis
Hydralazine	Vasodilator	25 mg three times a day to 50 mg three times a day	Flushing, headache, and lupus-like syndrome
Prazosin	Alpha blocker	0.5 mg twice a day to 5 mg three times a day	Orthostatic hypotension

*Although oxprenolol is safe, it is no longer available in Australia.

TABLE 3: Antihypertensive drugs to avoid in pregnancy.

Antihypertensive class	Advice	Potential adverse effects	Recommendation
ACE inhibitors	Contraindicated	Teratogenic in the second and third trimester, resulting in fetal anuria, oligohydramnios Hypocalvaria, Intrauterine growth restriction and patent ductus artertosus, death	Stop drug ideally before conception or at diagnosis of pregnancy
Angiotensin receptor blockers	Contraindicated	Teratogenic in the second and third trimesters. Fetal anuda, lallgohydramnlos, and hypocalvaria. Intrauterine growth restriction, patent ductus artedosus, and death	Stop drug ideally before conception or at diagnosis of pregnancy
Diuretics	Avoid	Maternal hypovolemia, fetal hypoglycemia, thrombocytopenia, hyponatremia, and hypokalemia	Use an alternative antihypertensive
Beta blockers (other than labetalol)	Avoid	Fetal bradycardia and intrauterine growth restriction (atenolol)	Use an alternative antihypertensive
Calcium channel antagonists (other than nifedipine and diltiazem)	Avoid	Maternal hypotension and fetal hypoxia	Use an alternative antihypertensive

hypertension. ACE inhibitors, angiotensin receptor blockers, mineralocorticoid receptor antagonists, and nitroprusside are teratogenic and thus contraindicated in pregnancy. Nitroprusside can be used as a last resort in treatment-resistant hypertension. The treatment goal is to 140–150/90–100 mm Hg **(Tables 2 and 3)**.[15]

CONCLUSION

Hypertension, whether primary or secondary, is a major risk factor for cardiovascular events including cerebrovascular accidents and stroke, coronary artery disease, peripheral vascular disease, heart failure, and also for atrial fibrillation, especially in aged hypertension affects microvasculature of people two sensitive organs, i.e., kidney and eyes, leading to hypertensive retinopathy and chronic kidney disease. However, few complications are more common in secondary hypertension viz:

- Secondary hypertension is mostly a cause of resistant hypertension and often remains uncontrolled despite maximally tolerated dose of three antihypertensive drugs including a diuretic.
- Secondary hypertension accelerates end span damage with significant increase in premature cardiovascular events, especially if it remains undiagnosed and inadequately controlled.

ONLINE REFERENCES

Please scan the QR code provided at the end of the table of contents for References of this chapter.

CHAPTER

42

Resistant Hypertension: Latest Advances in Management

Satyendra Tewari, Harshit Khare

ABSTRACT

Resistant hypertension (RHT) is mainly a diagnosis of exclusion, defined as office systolic BP > 140 mm Hg and/or diastolic BP > 90 mm Hg despite the use of three or antihypertensives at maximum tolerated doses, one of which is diuretic. RHT carries much poor prognosis in terms of cardiovascular diseases as compared to the others. The prevalence is somewhere around 7.6% after excluding white coat hypertension. Workups for RHT include ambulatory BP monitoring to rule out white coat hypertension besides workups for other secondary causes of hypertension and excluding medication noncompliance.

The treatment strategies include altering lifestyle-related modifiable factors, pharmacotherapy-utilizing drugs targeting renin–angiotensin–aldosterone system, and advanced therapies based on renal denervation (RDN) and baroreceptor activation. The pharmacotherapy includes ACEis or ARBs in combination with CCB or beta-blockers along with diuretics, especially spironolactone. The RDN therapy and baroreceptor activation therapy can be offered as a last resort to those not responding to the pharmacotherapy.

Keywords: Resistant hypertension, antihypertensive therapies, renal denervation therapies, RAAS

INTRODUCTION

Resistant hypertension (RHT), as a disease entity, is often considered a deadlock situation in the medicine community due to limited therapeutic options and unfamiliarity with the nature of therapeutic response. The difficulty starts right from making the diagnosis. Wei et al. noted that "the diagnosis of resistant hypertension is actually a diagnosis of exclusion." They elaborated that RHT can be broadly defined as absence of ambulatory blood pressure control despite the use of guideline-directed medical therapy and maximum medication adherence on the part of patient. More specifically, it is defined as "the failure to achieve the office BP goal of systolic > 140 mm Hg or ambulatory BP goal of systolic < 135 mm Hg and/or diastolic office BP < 90 mm Hg or ambulatory diastolic BP < 85 mm Hg, respectively, despite use of three antihypertensive agents at maximum tolerated dosages (including one diuretic)." Further, some authors suggest including in this definition, even those with controlled BP if requiring more than four antihypertensives. A pseudo-RHT is defined as refractory hypertension that is either due to some other secondary cause or is being erroneously documented due to whitecoat hypertension.[1-3]

The AHA and ESC guidelines recommend that for diagnosing RHT, it is essential to exclude whitecoat hypertension with 24-hour ambulatory BP monitoring (ABPM) or home BP monitoring (HBPM) measurements in addition to ensuring adherence to antihypertensive medications and ruling out other potential causes of secondary forms of hypertension. Thus, true RHT is diagnosed by exclusion of pseudo-RHT.

Possible causes of pseudo-RHT include whitecoat hypertension, inadequate office BP measurements, and poor adherence to prescribed medications. Furthermore, many other factors can contribute to apparent RHT, such as excessive alcohol consumption, high intake of sodium, vasopressor or other sodium-retaining substances, including some herbal remedies, cocaine abuse, obesity, obstructive sleep apnea syndrome, and psychological stress. Even after considering all these factors, the prevalence of apparent or pseudo-RHT is relatively high in real-world practice.[1,2]

EPIDEMIOLOGY

There is a lack of prospective studies on hypertension that may have employed ABPM and followed up on patient adherence to medications, to enable diagnosis of RHT. That would be an ideal situation. Therefore, the reported prevalence of RHT is largely based on observational studies and few prespecified outcome trials. The prevalence of RHT varies widely in the reported literature, largely depending on the adopted diagnostic criteria, the number of antihypertensive drugs, the methods of BP measurements, and reference populations (e.g., general populations, hypertensive cohorts, treated uncontrolled hypertensive outpatients, and ethnic groups).

A meta-analysis, comprising a large population size of nearly 9.6 lakhs, reported a prevalence of 13.7% based on observational studies and 16.3% based on randomized trials when pseudo-RHT and poor medication compliance were not excluded.[4] Another large registry of around 68,000 patients from Spain reported RHT prevalence as 7.6% after excluding whitecoat hypertension.[5] Other good-sized studies have reported RHT prevalence of around 8% after excluding secondary causes of hypertension and nonadherence to medications.[6,7]

ASSOCIATION WITH CARDIOVASCULAR RISK

Resistant hypertension is associated with higher rates of diabetes mellitus (17.7%) as highlighted by US registry data and further has a higher risk for cardiovascular (CV) events, namely myocardial infarction, congestive heart failure, and stroke as evidenced by data from large trials such as ALLHAT.[8-10]

ASSOCIATED MODIFIABLE FACTORS

Resistant hypertension is linked to several comorbidities and risk factors, such as obesity, smoking, alcohol intake, the obstructive sleep apnea, and metabolic derangements such as hyperuricemia and hyperaldosteronism. Further studies show correlation between high salt intake and inadequate BP control.

A previous meta-analysis has shown that a significant weight loss results in modest reduction of 4.5 and 3.2 mm Hg in systolic BP (SBP) and diastolic BP (DBP), respectively. The evidence for specific dietary regimens for RHT is however limited. Moreover, reduced alcohol intake (<10 g suggested for women and <20 g for men), smoking cessation, and regular aerobic exercise spanning > 150 min/week may help attain BP goals better.[11]

PHARMACOLOGICAL TREATMENT

The various therapies for RHT evolved from the concept that systemic mean arterial pressure is the manifestation of constant interaction between sympathetic nervous system-efferent innervations and renal renin–angiotensin system with baroreceptors acting as a central control/brake. The prevalent pharmacotherapies are no different from this concept. The therapies targeting renin–angiotensin system, namely angiotensin-converting enzyme inhibitors (ACEis) or angiotensin receptor blockers (ARB), in combination with either calcium channel blockers or beta-blockers form the starting base of treating this ordeal. However, RHT is notorious in the sense that it is unlikely to be controlled by two or three classes of drugs. So the next step is to escalate doses of these medications to maximum tolerable dosages and using longer half-life medications for round-the-clock BP control. In the follow-up, monitoring with ABPM every 2–3 weeks is required, and failing to achieve target of <135 mm Hg systolic and <85 mm Hg diastolic BP calls for revision in treatment. In the next step, addition of diuretics is required. If however, ABPM continues falling short of target BP goals, then mineralocorticoid receptor antagonists need to be added. Not to mention, at this stage of treatment, we are definitely dealing with RHT. Trials of spironolactone, especially PATHWAY-2, have shown spironolactone to be most effective for lowering BP levels irrespective of plasma-renin levels, and the response is consistent in long-term as well. This has led to recommendations for adding spironolactone in treating RHT. Those who do not tolerate spironolactone, it is reasonable to add either eplerenone or amiloride. Further addition of vasodilatory therapeutics, namely potassium channel opener minoxidil and endothelin type A antagonist darusentan, hardly results in benefiting RHT patients because of limiting adverse effects with these drugs including fluid retention, edema, arrhythmia, and heart failure.[12,13]

ROLE OF RENAL DENERVATION

Recent enthusiasm in BP control with renal denervation (RDN) using catheter-directed radiofrequency or ultrasound ablation has met with limited success.

The initial studies, namely the SYMPLICITY HTN-1 (Renal Denervation in Patients With Refractory Hypertension HTN-1) and SYMPLICITY HTN-2 (Renal Denervation in Patients With Refractory Hypertension HTN-2) were remarkable in the sense that they showed SBP/DBP reduction of 14/10 and 32/12 mm Hg, respectively, with RDN. However, in SYMPLICITY HTN-3 (Renal Denervation in Patients With Uncontrolled Hypertension HTN-3), which was a sham-controlled single-blind study of 535 patients with RHT, the RDN procedure failed to show significant BP reduction. While there are various explanations available for the failure of SYMPLICITY HTN-3, the most important reason was probably nonadherence to medications. The study was not designed to assess medication adherence and lifestyle changes. Other explanations listed for failure of this study were broader patient selection, frequent changes in medication, limited experience with procedure, and inability to achieve complete circumferential ablation with first-generation catheters. More recent trials such as DENERHTN and INSPiRED, however, fared better due to more systematically followed-up medication adherence, more selective study population, and a standardized step-care antihypertensive treatment.[14-18]

The limited success with RDN trials shifted population selection to patients with untreated or milder hypertension. The SPYRAL HTN-OFF MED (Global Clinical Study of Renal Denervation With the Symplicity Spyral Multi-electrode Renal Denervation System in Patients With Uncontrolled Hypertension in the Absence of Antihypertensive Medications) did show BP control similar to monotherapy with antihypertensives, but due to invasive nature of this therapy, RDN could not be labeled as the first-line therapy. More recently, in SPYRAL HTN-ON MED (Global Clinical Study of Renal Denervation With the Symplicity Spyral Multi-electrode Renal Denervation System in Patients With Uncontrolled Hypertension on Standard Medical Therapy) RDN has performed better in achieving BP goals over both short-term (2–3 months) and medium-term (6 months). Similar results have been achieved with the use of ultrasound waves in RADIANCE-HTN SOLO study (A Study of the ReCor Medical Paradise System in Clinical Hypertension). It is again important to mention that all these recent studies had followed medication adherence throughout the study using biomarkers either in blood or urine samples. Furthermore, long-term follow-up from some of these studies (Global Symplicity Registry, SPYRAL HTN-ON MED, and RADIANCE-HTN SOLO) shows continued efficacy of the RDN procedure. While further studies are required to prove the efficacy of RDN better, it can be convincingly concluded from these studies that RDN can be offered to patients who are unable to achieve target BP goals despite adherence to best available medical therapies and incorporating possible lifestyle and dietary changes and have an adequate renal function.[19-21]

BAROREFLEX ACTIVATION THERAPY

Despite the novelty of concept, the evidence for stimulation of carotid baroreceptors as treatment for RHT is weak. Although initial nonrandomized studies (US Rheos Feasibility trial and DeBuT HT) showed safety and efficacy of baroreceptor stimulation, the double-blind RCT Rheos pivotal trial failed to achieve both its primary efficacy endpoint of reduction in office BP reading and procedure safety endpoint at 6 months. Perhaps, RCTs with better design, enrolling selective study population, and employing ABPM and medication adherence techniques will provide more insights into this developing science.[22-24]

ARTERIOVENOUS ANASTOMOSIS

A study employing ROX coupler (a self-expanding stent delivered under fluoroscopy to create a central arterio-venous anastomosis between the iliac artery and vein) has shown promising results in terms of office as well as 24-hour SBP and DBP reductions that were consistent at 12 months. However, the replication of this in RCTs is necessary before any recommendations can be made for the use of A-V anastomosis as the treatment for RHT. Moreover, long-term effects of such anastomosis remain to be seen.[25]

CONCLUSION

Lifestyle interventions along with stepwise escalation in pharmacotherapeutics hold the major ground against the battle with RHT. The RDN is a valid alternative when all measures have failed. The evidence for other device-based therapies is still limited and awaits further studies before they can be applied to clinical practice.

ONLINE REFERENCES

Please scan the QR code provided at the end of the table of contents for References of this chapter.

CHAPTER

43

Drugs for True Resistant Hypertension

SS Iyengar

ABSTRACT

True resistant hypertension (RH) is a high-risk clinical condition, and the concern is the heightened risk of cardiovascular disease, stroke, renal failure, and mortality in these patients. Mineralocorticoid hormone excess and volume overload are the underlying pathophysiologic mechanisms in most of these cases. There are safe and effective mineralocorticoid receptor antagonists and other drugs available for intensification of BP-lowering treatment. Identification of factors contributing to RH and stepwise management with antihypertensive drugs of differing mechanisms of action along with lifestyle intervention as an integral part of the management help in achieving the target BP in these patients. If the drug treatment fails, renal sympathetic denervation (RDN) is an option.

Keywords: Resistant hypertension, mineralocorticoid receptor antagonists, endothelin receptor antagonists, small interfering RNA

INTRODUCTION

True resistant hypertension (RH) is defined as blood pressure (BP) above goal [systolic BP (SBP) or diastolic BP that remains ≥140 or ≥90 mm Hg, respectively as per ESH guidelines[1] and ≥130 or ≥80 mm Hg, respectively as per ACC/AHA guidelines[2]] despite appropriate use of lifestyle intervention and optimal doses of three drugs comprising a renin-angiotensin-aldosterone (RAAS) blocker (either an angiotensin-converting enzyme inhibitor or an angiotensin receptor blocker), a calcium channel blocker, and a thiazide/thiazide-like diuretic.

Controlled RH that includes patients taking four or more drugs to maintain the goal BP and refractory hypertension, which is referred to as uncontrolled BP despite five or more drugs of different classes, including a diuretic are not a part of discussion in this paper.

Prevalence of RH varies, depending on the definition applied, centers, and the population studied. Taking all these factors into consideration, an estimate of RH prevalence has been projected as 5% of the hypertensive population.[1]

The pathophysiological mechanism implicated in true RH is an interplay between factors like raised levels of aldosterone, endothelin 1, and vasopressin and increased sympathetic activity.[1,3,4]

Resistant hypertension is associated with increased cardiovascular (CV) morbidity and mortality. A prospective observational study of 5,839 patients found that 7.2% patients had true RH. During a follow-up of 4.5 years, the adjusted risks of CV events and heart failure were significantly increased in patients with true RH compared to patients with controlled nonresistant hypertension.[5] Patients with RH necessarily need frequent assessment and may require hospitalization leading to enhanced healthcare costs. It is crucial to ensure appropriate assessment and adequate treatment for patients suspected of RH.[6]

DRUGS FOR TRUE RESISTANT HYPERTENSION

It is reasonable to adopt a stepwise approach to institute drugs for true RH.

Optimization of the existing treatment: It is important to emphasize and reinforce the lifestyle measures. Regular exercise, reduction in salt intake, and abstinence from smoking and alcohol contribute favorably. Weight reduction in obese patients has to be ensured. Use maximally tolerated recommended doses of the drugs. Use an appropriate diuretic. If eGFR is <30 mL/min/BSA, chlorthalidone is the preferred diuretic. In the CLICK trial, in patients with eGFR 15–29 mL/min/1.73 m^2 and true RH, chlorthalidone exhibited a better response (the adjusted change in the 24-hour ambulatory systolic BP from baseline to 12 weeks was –11.0 mm Hg in the chlorthalidone group as compared to –0.5 mm Hg in the placebo group) as compared to placebo.[7]

In end-stage renal disease (ESRD), loop diuretics need to be used.

- Add one or more of the following drugs to intensify the antihypertensive therapy so that BP should be reduced below 140/90 mm Hg and below 130/80 mmHg, if well tolerated.

Mineralocorticoid Receptor Antagonists

Spironolactone

Spironolactone is probably the most suitable fourth drug to be added to the three antihypertensive drugs in RH.

In PATHWAY-2 trial,[8] 335 patients of RH were randomly assigned to spironolactone, doxazosin, bisoprolol, and placebo. Spironolactone was clearly superior to placebo, doxazosin, and bisoprolol in reducing home SBP, and the treatment was well tolerated.

A meta-analysis of 12 trials of 1,655 patients assessed the antihypertensive effect of spironolactone compared with placebo, alternative drugs, RND, and no treatment. Spironolactone showed a significant reduction in office BP and ambulatory in patients with RH at 3 months.[9]

Spironolactone may have side effects like breast tenderness, gynecomastia and sexual impotence in men, and menstrual irregularities in women. eGFR and serum potassium should be closely monitored.

Eplerenone

Eplerenone is the other steroidal mineralocorticoid receptor antagonist (MRA). It interferes less with progesterone or androgen receptors, but it is less potent than spironolactone.[10]

Ameloride

Ameloride is another potassium-sparing diuretic and was found to be as effective as spironolactone in an open-label trial.[11]

Finerenone

Finerenone is a potent, selective, and nonsteroidal MRA. In a post hoc analysis, finerenone and spironolactone were compared in RH patients with moderate-to-advanced chronic kidney disease. Finerenone group had patients with an eGFR of 25–45 mL/min/1.73 m^2, serum potassium of 4.3–5.1 mmol/L, and an automated office SBP of 135–160 mm Hg at baseline. Spironolactone group with similar features of CKD and RH received patiromer, a potassium binder in addition. The authors concluded that in comparison to patients with true RH and chronic kidney disease treated with spironolactone with or without patiromer, finerenone was associated with a lower SBP reduction, lower risk of hyperkalemia, and lower treatment discontinuation, during 4 months of treatment.[12]

Sacubitril–Valsartan (ARNI)

The post hoc analysis of PARAGON-HF trial showed that 731 HFpEF patients (15.2%) had apparent RH and 135 (2.8%) had apparent MRA-RH. These patients had a poor outcome as compared to those with well-controlled hypertension. It was also noted that patients of RH on ARNI had greater reduction in SBP at 1 and 4 months than with valsartan. With ARNI, 47.9% of RH patients had controlled BP versus 34.3% who received valsartan.[13]

Other Commonly Used Drugs

Hydralazine and minoxidil are direct vasodilators that are not favored much in RH, as they are known to cause reflex sympathetic activation, tachycardia, and fluid retention.

Adrenergic Blockers

A small observational study involving 8,639 patients with RH received MRAs, beta-blockers (BBs), and alpha-1-blockers. The results showed that there was a nonsignificant benefit in favor of BBs and alpha-blockers. [14] These drugs, vasodilating BBs and alpha-blockers, are useful additions to achieve the goal BP in patients with true RH.

Aldosterone Synthase Inhibitors

Baxdrostat blocks aldosterone synthase, and thus reduces synthesis of aldosterone. It is highly selective and reduces plasma aldosterone levels but not cortisol levels. In a multicenter, placebo-controlled trial, 248 patients with RH received baxdrostat or placebo for 12 weeks. In these patients with RH, baxdrostat showed dose-related significant reductions in systolic and diastolic BP, without serious adverse events and instances of adrenocortical insufficiency. Hyperkalemia seen in two patients did not recur after withdrawal and reinitiation of the drug.[4]

Endothelin Receptor Antagonists

Aprocitentan: Endothelin-1 is a powerful vasoconstrictor that regulates vascular tone, remodeling, and BP. Aprocitentan is a dual endothelin-1 antagonist of ET-A and ET-B receptors. The “PRECISION” a multicenter, blinded, randomized, parallel-group, phase 3 study involved 730 patients of RH. At baseline, mean office BP was 153/88 mm Hg and mean 24-hour ambulatory BP was 138/83 mm Hg. Patients were randomized to receive daily oral aprocitentan or placebo, plus three drugs comprising amlodipine, valsartan, and hydrochlorothiazide. The study concluded that in patients with RH, aprocitentan was well tolerated and superior to placebo in lowering BP at week 4 with a sustained effect at week 40. Edema, a common side effect, was seen in about 10% of patients.[3]

In March 2024, the US Food and Drug Administration (FDA) approved aprocitentan as a new drug for treating patients with RH.

RNA Interference Therapeutics

Angiotensinogen, the precursor of angiotensin peptides, plays a key role in the pathogenesis of hypertension. Zilebesiran is an RNA interference therapeutic agent, has a prolonged duration of action, and interferes with angiotensinogen synthesis in liver. It is expected that zilebesiran will exert a sustained reduction of BP over a 24-hour period for months, with twice-yearly or quarterly subcutaneous administration.

In a phase 1 study, 107 patients with hypertension were enrolled. Single dose of zilebesiran (≥200 mg) showed a decrease in SBP (>10 mm Hg) and diastolic blood pressure (>5 mm Hg) by 8 weeks, the reduction being consistent throughout diurnal cycle and was sustained up to 24 weeks. It showed an augmented effect when irbesartan was coadministered. There were no adverse events like hypotension, hyperkalemia, or worsening of renal function, requiring intervention. Mild injection site reactions were reported.[15] Applicability of these results in a broader population with hypertension needs to be studied.

GUIDELINES

The recent guidelines of European Society of Hypertension[1] recommend the following BP targets and drugs for true RH.

- In patients with true RH, BP should be reduced below 140/90 mm Hg and below 130/80 mm Hg, if well tolerated.
- Drugs that can be considered as additional therapy in patients with true RH are spironolactone (or other MRA), BBs, alpha-1-blockers, centrally acting agents (clonidine), or amiloride.
- Thiazide/thiazide-like diuretics are recommended in true RH if estimated eGFR is ≥30 mL/min/1.73 m^2.
- Loop diuretics should be used if eGFR falls below 30 mL/min/1.73 m^2.
- Chlorthalidone can be used if eGFR is <30 mL/min/1.73 m^2.
- Patients with true RH should be followed up meticulously for BP control, target organ damage, and comorbidities.

MANAGING PATIENTS WITH TRUE RESISTANT HYPERTENSION

The approach to management of patients with true RH is given in **Flowchart 1**.

Patients with true RH are at a greater risk of developing target organ damage and thus are exposed to increased risk of morbidity and mortality.

The treatment they are already receiving should be rationalized and optimized, if there is a scope. Their lifestyle should be closely scrutinized and corrected, paying attention to diet, exercise, smoking, and alcohol. Comorbidities call for a closer look, like managing obesity, obstructive sleep apnea, diabetes, and cardiac and renal dysfunction.

Maximally tolerated doses of the antihypertensive drugs should be instituted. Single pill combinations are preferred, as they improve adherence. If eGFR is <30 mL/min/1,73 m^2, chlorthalidone is the diuretic to be used, and in ESRD, loop diuretics will be effective.

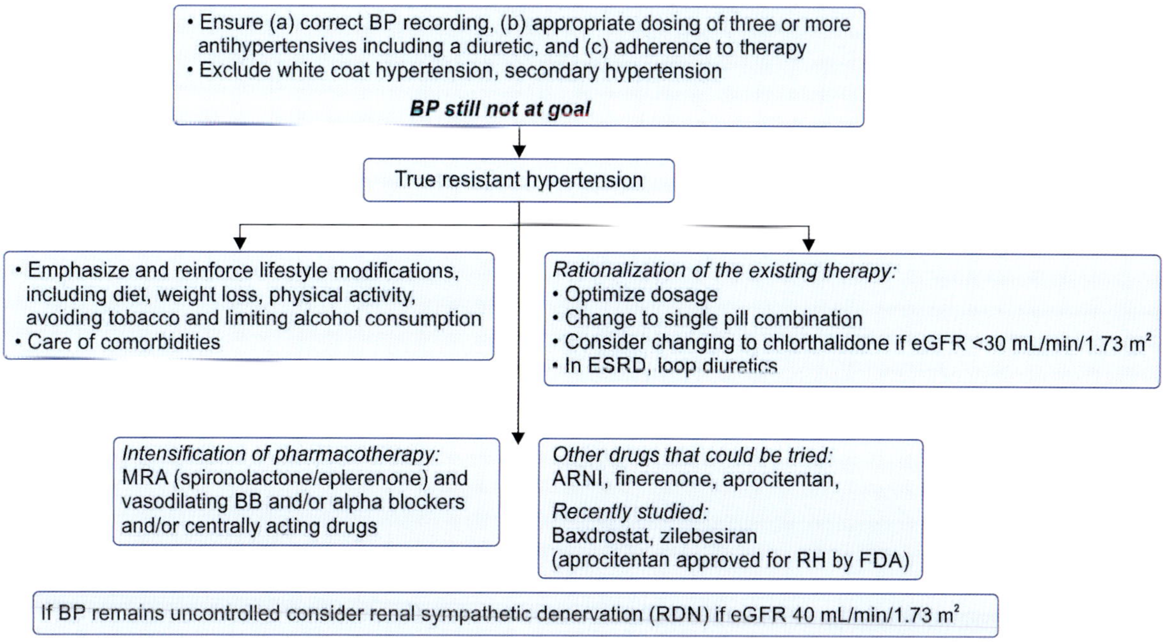

FLOWCHART 1: Management of true resistant hypertension.

The MRAs are clearly the choice as the fourth drug. Spironolactone and, if not tolerated, eplerenone are to be administered. To achieve a BP of 140/90 mm Hg or less (<130/90 mm Hg if tolerated), adding vasodilating BB and/or alpha-blockers and/or centrally-acting drugs sequentially will help. ACE-inhibitor or ARB may be replaced by ARNI with due precautions to derive additional benefit. Aprocitentan has been approved by FDA for RH. Baxdrostat and zilebesiran appear promising, awaiting clinical trials in RH.

The RDN can be considered as an additional treatment option in patients with true RH if eGFR is >40 mL/min/1.73 m^2.

CONCLUSION

Resistant hypertension remains a significant clinical challenge. Diagnosis of true RH should be established after a careful evaluation. Various pharmacologic and nonpharmacologic measures should be instituted judiciously. Newer drugs appear promising. Machine learning and artificial intelligence are likely to play a role in assisting clinicians in diagnosis and management of true RH in near future, leading to improved outcomes and better health for patients with RH.

ONLINE REFERENCES

Please scan the QR code provided at the end of the table of contents for References of this chapter.

CHAPTER 44

Endovascular Interventions for Secondary Hypertension: Update 2024

Sanjay Tyagi, Vivek Kumar, Amit Mittal

ABSTRACT

Secondary hypertension (HTN) is elevated blood pressure (BP) secondary to an identifiable cause. Though the prevalence of secondary HTN is relatively low, it comprises the subset of HTN that is potentially treatable. Endovascular interventions have emerged as potential therapeutic options for specific secondary HTN subtypes. Clinical workup to identify potentially reversible causes for nonendocrine secondary HTN is essential. These reversible causes include coarctation of aorta, Takayasu disease (aortoarteritis), and renal artery stenosis. In this chapter, we discuss the current status and clinical outcomes of these endovascular interventions and highlight areas for future research.

Keywords: Secondary hypertension, endovascular interventions, renal artery stenosis, Takayasu arteritis, aortic coarctation

INTRODUCTION

Secondary hypertension (HTN) occurs in about 5–10% of patients with HTN.[1] It results from specific, identifiable conditions such as renal parenchymal disease, renal artery stenosis, aortic coarctation, and endocrine disorders.[2] The prevalence of secondary HTN is bimodal and it is most prevalent at the extremes of age. It accounts for 70–85% of HTN cases in children <12 years of age and approximately 17% of cases in adults aged 65 and older.[2,3] Identification of the etiology and pathophysiology of secondary HTN is essential. It does not just guide toward the appropriate therapy but in some subsets, the treatment may result in a complete cure of HTN and elimination of antihypertensive therapy. Management includes pharmacological therapy and lifestyle modifications. However, endovascular interventions have gained traction as potential treatment options, offering minimally invasive alternatives to surgical revascularization in patients with secondary HTN due to vascular stenosis.

RENOVASCULAR HYPERTENSION

Renovascular hypertension (RVH) is one of the most common causes of secondary HTN and can result in resistant HTN. HTN can occur due to stenosis of the unilateral or bilateral renal arteries.[5] Atherosclerosis is the cause of renal artery stenosis (RAS) in elderly. In younger populations, especially females, RAS is usually due to Takayasu's arteritis (TA) or to fibromuscular dysplasia (FMD).[6]

Renal artery stenosis reduces blood flow to the affected kidney, triggering renin–angiotensin–aldosterone system (RAAS) and leading to HTN.[7] Persistent reduced renal blood flow leads to renal ischemia, worsens renal failure, and contributes to disease progression. Percutaneous revascularization is recommended along with medical therapy in selected patients to improve renal perfusion.

The first renal angioplasty in India for TA was performed by Dr Sanjay Tyagi at GB Pant Hospital in 1986 and the first case series of angioplasty in 27 patients with RAS was published in 1989.[6] Most of these patients (21/27) were of TA, four had atherosclerotic RAS while other two had FMD. The angiographic success rate in this early series was 94.4%.

Atherosclerotic Renal Artery Stenosis

Randomized controlled trials comparing medical therapy with percutaneous transluminal renal angioplasty (PTRA) to medical therapy alone have failed to show a benefit of atherosclerotic PTRA; however, the patients with the most severe RAS, who would be more likely to benefit from PTRA, might not have been enrolled in these trials. Severe RAS with HTN is associated with an increased risk of progressive decline in renal function, cardiac destabilization syndromes including "flash" pulmonary edema, and recurrent congestive heart failure. PTRA with stenting has been shown to be helpful in such patients with severe RAS.[1]

Several trials have evaluated the impact of renal artery angioplasty on BP control. The ASTRAL trial, a landmark study, found no significant difference in BP reduction between angioplasty and optimal medical therapy alone.[8,9] Similarly, the CORAL trial showed that angioplasty combined with stenting did not offer substantial long-term benefits over medical management in terms of BP control.[10] In contrast, observational studies have reported positive outcomes, including improvements in BP and renal function following angioplasty.[11] The variability in outcomes highlights the importance of patient selection and procedural technique. JACC appropriate use criteria (AUC) recommends renal artery intervention with hemodynamically significant RAS defined as RAS with 70–99% stenosis or RAS with 50–69% stenosis associated with hemodynamic significance **(Figs. 1A and B)**.[11]

The endovascular technique of PTRA with or without stenting is one of the standard treatments for RAS. According to the AUC, scenarios in which revascularization is appropriate are for patients who present with acute decompensated heart failure with flash pulmonary edema, bilateral RAS alongside worsening kidney function, CKD with unilateral RAS associated with worsening renal function, and patients with hypertension who remain uncontrolled despite optimized medical therapy.[12] Another indication could be RAS in solitary functioning kidney. A meta-analysis study showed that renal artery stent placement could stabilize or even improve renal function with a benefit rate of 77% **(Figs. 2A and B)**.[13]

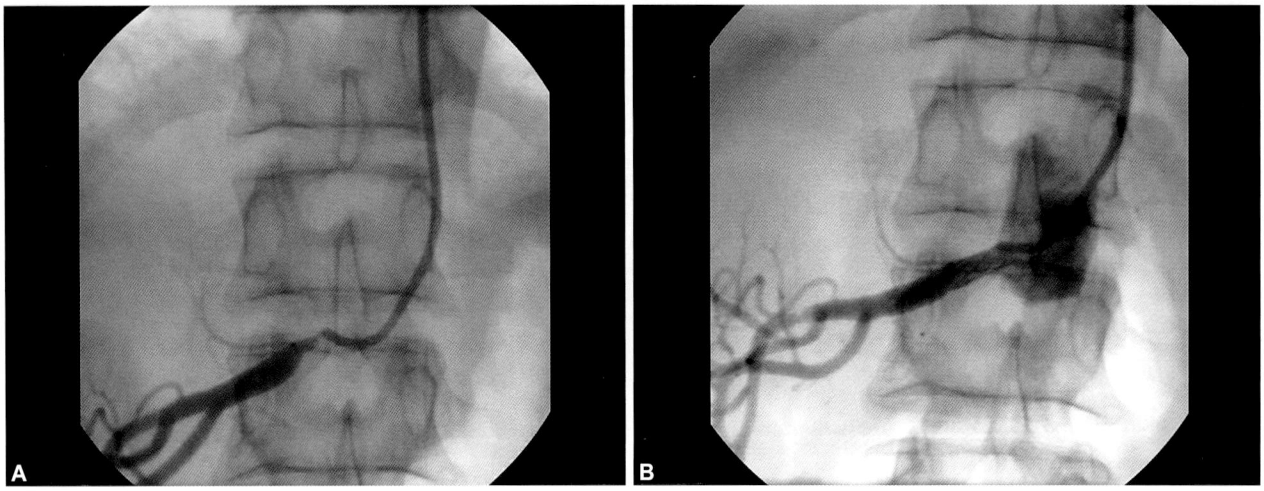

FIGS. 1A AND B: (A) Atherosclerotic right renal artery stenting by brachial approach in an elderly patient with hypertension, renal failure, solitary functioning kidney, and occlusion of infrarenal aorta. (B) Patient had improvement in hypertension and renal failure after angioplasty.

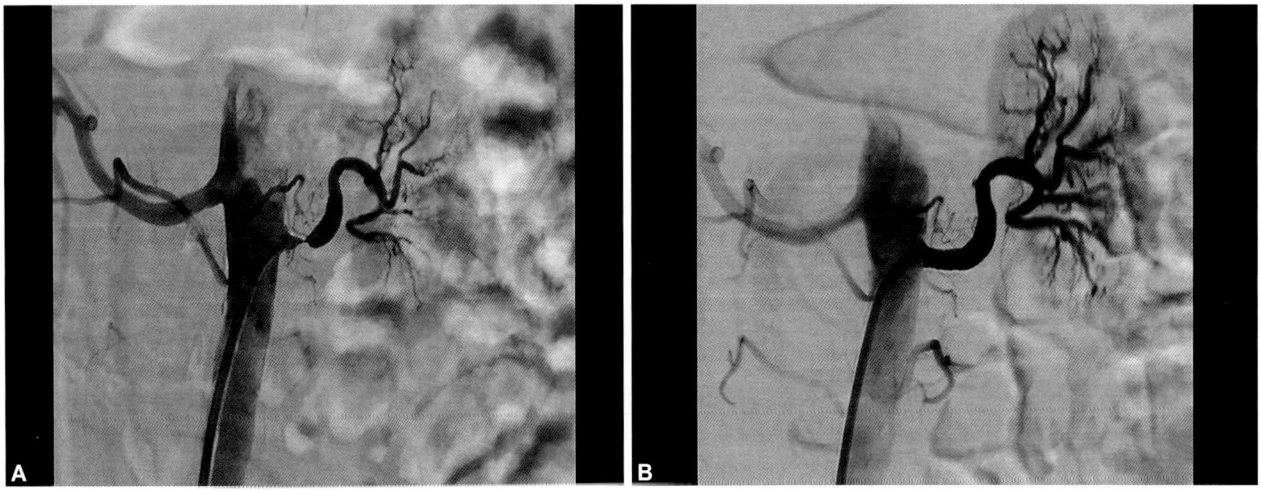

FIGS. 2A AND B: Atherosclerotic left renal artery stenting by femoral approach in a patient with refractory hypertension. Patient had reduction in antihypertensive medications.

Contraindications to Renal Revascularization

Contraindications to renal revascularization include refusal of consent, advanced disease (creatinine level >3–4 mg/dL or kidney length <8 cm), limited life expectancy, generally poor surgical or PTRA candidates (e.g., bleeding diathesis) and pregnancy.[5]

NON-ATHEROSCLEROTIC RAS

Fibromuscular dysplasia: FMD is less common cause of RVH in India than in Western countries. Medial FMD has string-of-bead appearance on angiography. Balloon angioplasty (BA) has been the traditional treatment of choice for renal artery fibromuscular medial dysplastic lesions and stents are rarely required.

In our experience, BA alone is sufficient in most cases **(Figs. 3A and B)** with improvement in HTN. The procedural success rate is 82–100% and restenosis occurs in about 10% of cases. Clinical results show cure of HTN in about 58% of patients, improvement in 35%, and failure in 7%.[13]

TAKAYASU'S DISEASE (NONSPECIFIC AORTOARTERITIS)

The pathogenesis of HTN in TA is complex and multifactorial. Important factors are RAS, followed by stenosis of the thoracic descending aorta, abdominal aorta, noncompliant aorta, and severe aortic regurgitation. Aorta is one of the key vessels responsible for BP regulation because of its elastic component. Dense fibrosis leads to loss of elasticity of aorta in TA. This is an important contributor to HTN in TA. Monitoring and control of BP may be difficult in cases with absent or reduced pulses in upper extremities. BP measurements should be made in the unaffected extremities.

In medical therapy for HTN in patients with Takayasu's disease, drugs are used based on severity of HTN. Combined medical treatments of glucocorticoids and conventional disease-modifying antirheumatic drugs should be used in patients with disease activity for early control of inflammation. Biological disease-modifying antirheumatic drugs should be used in patients with refractory disease activity.[7]

Percutaneous transluminal angioplasty is preferred for patients with renal and aorta stenosis.[14] Results are best in severe, discrete stenosis. It produces marked improvement in HTN. Surgical treatment is limited to total occlusion or long-segment stenosis. It should preferably be done after remission induction if angioplasty is not possible **(Figs. 4A and B)**.[7]

Hypertension secondary to TA in a large cohort was retrospectively analyzed in a single-center study in China in 381 TA patients with HTN.[15] Diagnosis of HTN was according to clinic BP or the central BP measured during angiography. RAS was the most common cause (264, 69.3%), followed by the thoracic descending aorta stenosis (98, 25.7%), abdominal aorta stenosis (78, 20.5%), and severe aortic regurgitation (45, 11.8%). More than two kinds of pathologies were found in 98 (25.7%) patients.[15]

At our center (GB Pant PGI), in three decades, a total of 267 renal angioplasty procedures were performed for 353 stenotic lesions in patients with TA.[16] BA had a procedural success rate of 89.3%. Cutting balloon was used in one-third of cases, which improved the success rate. Renal artery stenting was reserved as a bailout procedure. 89% of patients with procedural success showed good clinical response and improvement in HTN. Periprocedural complications including local-site complications occurred in 5.4% of patients. There was no procedure-related mortality. The

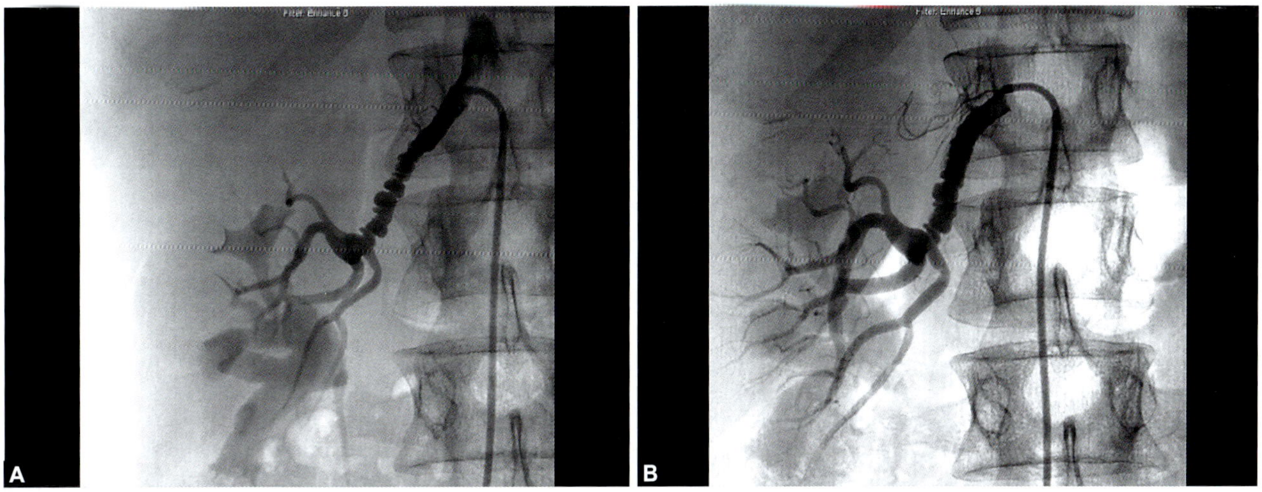

FIGS. 3A AND B: Balloon angioplasty for renal artery medial fibromuscular dysplasia in a young woman with severe hypertension. (A) String-of-bead appearance before and (B) improvement in lumen after balloon angioplasty.

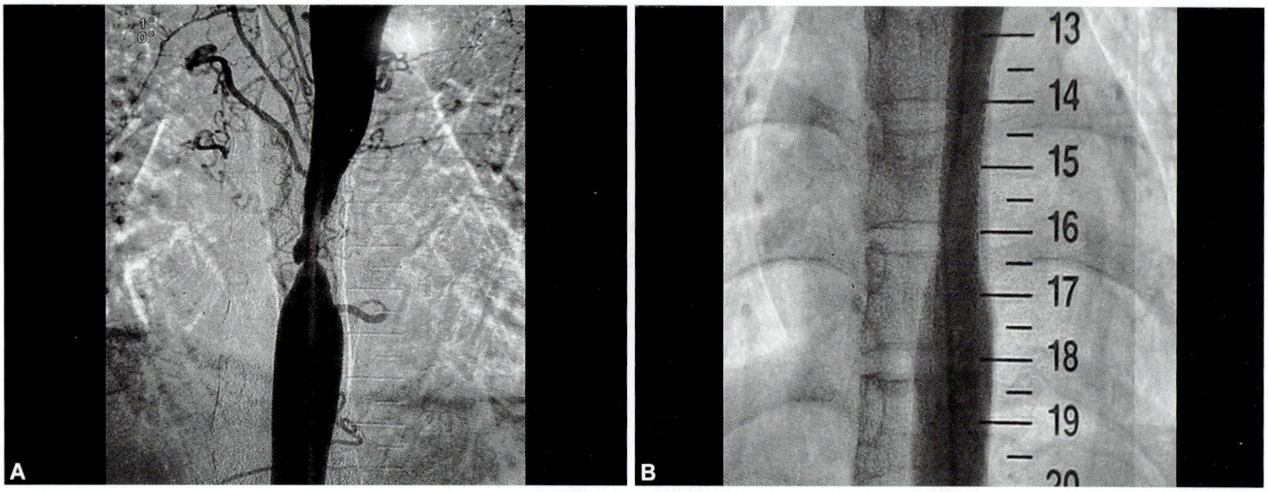

FIGS. 4A AND B: A young girl presented to emergency with severe HTN and CVA due to cerebral hemorrhage. (A) Her angiogram showed severe stenosis of thoracic aorta, (B) which was treated by endovascular balloon angioplasty and stenting with relief of stenosis and no residual gradient in thoracic aorta. Her blood pressure normalized and she does not require any antihypertensive medications even on long-term follow-up.

restenosis rate at a median of 27.7 months was 18.2%, with active disease and length of stenosis being the most important predictor of restenosis. Restenosis was almost associated with recurrence of HTN. Repeat angioplasty, was attempted in all patients with restenosis, mostly with cutting balloon improvement in HTN.[16]

While a lot is said about the high restenosis rates in TA, a word must also be added about the phenomenon of late beneficial remodeling observed in some patients, whereby one is pleasantly surprised to find the follow-up angiogram showing actually better results than what had been achieved immediately postprocedure **(Fig. 5)**.

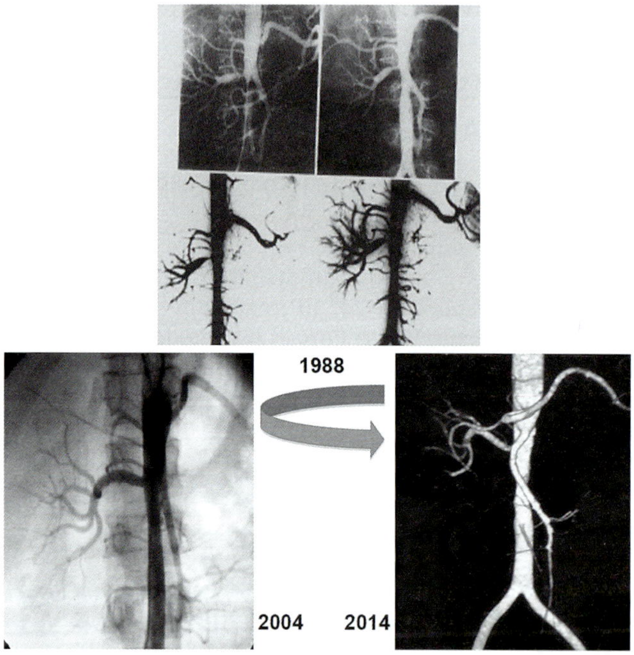

FIG. 5: Long-term follow-up after balloon angioplasty of right renal artery in a patient with Takayasu's arteritis and resistant hypertension: Excellent long-term results 26 years after initial procedure. Of special note is the late beneficial remodeling due to which lumen diameter on follow-up is even better than immediately postprocedure.

RVH in Indian Children

A number of series from India, including ours, show aortoarteritis to be the most common cause of RVH in children in our country. Overall, anywhere between 3 and 10% of children referred for evaluation of severe HTN are subsequently found to have clinically significant renovascular lesions.[2] Vis-à-vis adults, children with RVH have a shorter duration of disease, are more likely to present with malignant HTN, heart failure or hypertensive encephalopathy, have less severe disease angiographically, and respond better to revascularization.

In a series of 35 consecutive children with RVH published by us,[17] 31 (88.6%) were due to aortoarteritis and 4 (11.4%) were attributable to juvenile idiopathic fibromuscular disease. Thus, we concluded that TA is the most common cause of RVH in children in our country as opposed to Western countries where FMD is the most common cause of RVH in children. Overall BA was technically successful in 31 (88.6%) patients. Although restenosis at a mean follow-up of 23 months was to the tune of 25.8%, the restenosed lesions could be easily redilated. 93.1% of patients with technically successful procedure had a beneficial BP response on long-term follow-up, which included complete cure of HTN in about one-third. BP response was better in the FMD group as compared to aortoarteritis group **(Figs. 6A and B)**.[17]

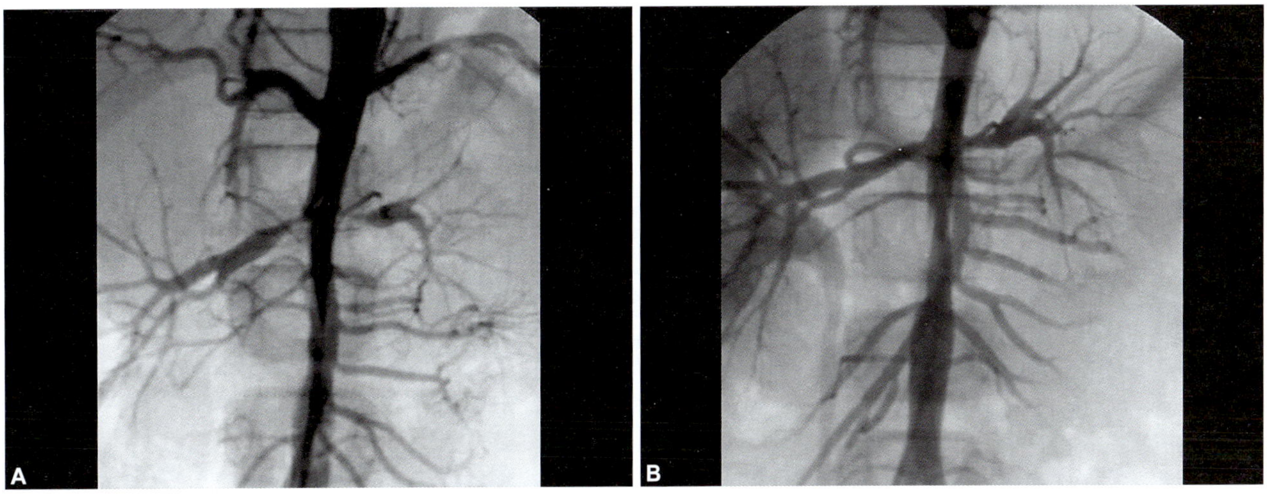

FIGS. 6A AND B: (A) Bilateral ostial renal artery stenosis due to aortoarteritis in a young girl with severe hypertension and (B) marked improvement in luminal diameter after cutting balloon angioplasty with normalization of blood pressure.

As in case of adults, effort should be made to intervene only in the quiescent phase of aortoarteritis, except in severe HTN with heart failure where it needs to be done without waiting for complete cessation of disease activity. Renal stenting in TA should be reserved as bailout for flow-limiting dissection.

In pediatric age group, TA is more often the cause of RAS as compared to FMD in our country. Relief of RAS by BA produces marked improvement in HTN in these subgroups of patients. It is safe and highly effective, and therefore, should be the treatment of choice in pediatric renovascular HTN.

CONGENITAL COARCTATION OF AORTA

Aortic coarctation impedes blood flow and can lead to secondary HTN, particularly affecting the upper body. The treatment of HTN in coarctation of the aorta (CoA) besides drugs is managed by early surgical or transcatheter repair to reduce the risk of irreversible aortopathy and refractory HTN.[4] It improves BP in addition to other associated risks of premature coronary artery disease, stroke, aortic aneurysm, dissection, and rupture.

Transcatheter BA and endovascular stent placement offer less invasive approaches compared to surgery for the treatment of CoA for adolescents and young adults.[18] Endovascular stent implantation is safe and effective in improving suboptimal results after BA for CoA. Self-expandable stents are easier to implant and are adapted better to the wall of the aorta, and most patients had similar efficacy in reducing coarctation as balloon-expandable stents.[19,20] Endovascular stenting of aortic coarctation has shown promising results in terms of reducing BP and improving patient outcomes.[19-21] Surgical treatment is used in infancy due to higher chances of recoarctation after BA **(Figs. 7 and 8)**.

The COAST trial demonstrated that endovascular repair with the NuMED Cheatham Platinum Stent® for treatment of CoA, was effective and was associated with a lower procedural risk.[22] The subsequent COAST II trial [Covered Cheatham-Platinum Stents (CCPS) for Prevention or Treatment of Aortic Wall Injury Associated with Coarctation of the Aorta Trial] established the importance of covered CP stent. The CCPS could effectively treat and potentially prevent AWI associated with CoA.[23] Recently long-term outcomes of stent implantation trials in CoA including both COAST and COAST II trials cohorts were published.[24] It showed that coarctation stenting was effective at maintaining obstruction relief up to 60 months postimplant with reduction in the number of patients requiring antihypertensive medication. An increase in stent fractures and reinterventions was observed between medium and long-term follow-up.

Hypertension in CoA: Persistent HTN is seen after repair of native CoA in adults and is associated with suboptimal LVMI regression and cardiovascular events.[25] Many long-term complications are related to HTN, which is a common finding late after coarctation repair. In a systemic review by Panzer J et al., the prevalence of hypertension after CoA repair was found to be around 47%, ranging from 20 to 70% in various studies.[26] The prevalence of HTN after CoA repair is substantial and progressive, and higher routine 24-hour BP measurement is recommended in the follow-up of patients after CoA repair to identify HTN.[25] LV diastolic dysfunction and LVH are common in patients with repaired CoA, even in the absence of HTN, and correlates with worse long-term outcome. Residual HTN has been linked to several mechanisms, including abnormal geometry of the aortic arch or hypoplasia of the arch, hyperactivation of the renin–angiotensin system, and attenuation of baroreflexes.[26] Optimal BP control with medical therapy after CoA repair may result in improved clinical outcomes.

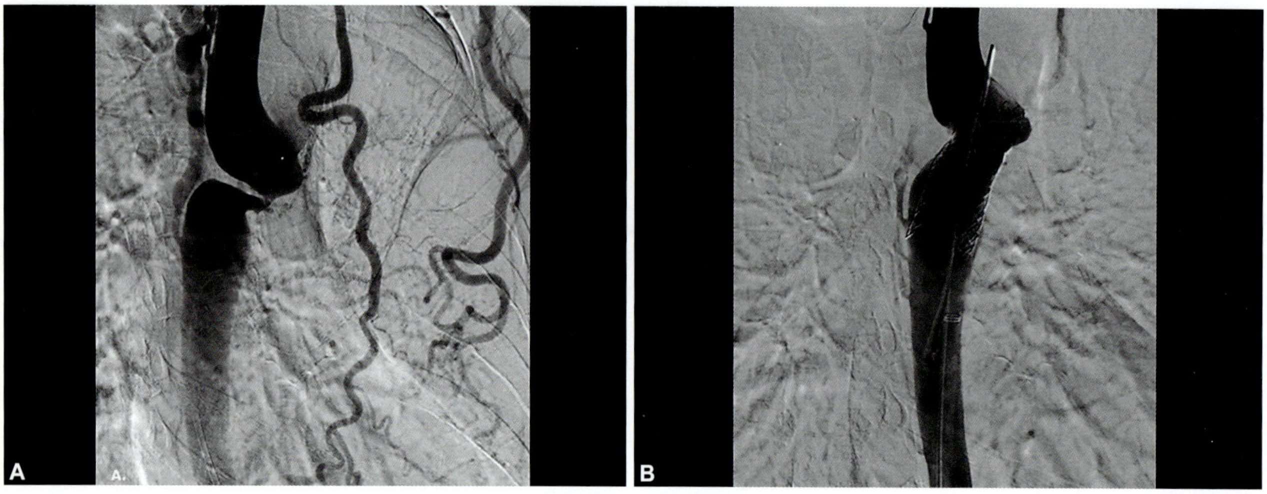

FIGS. 7A AND B: Pre (A) and post (B) stenting digital subtraction angiography (DSA) image. (A) Presenting DSA showing tight postductal coarctation of the aorta with large collaterals and (B) Poststenting DSA showing a reduction in collaterals and well-expanded coarctation segment after aortic stent implantation. Patient had marked improvement in hypertension after stent implantation with reversal of paraparesis.[21]

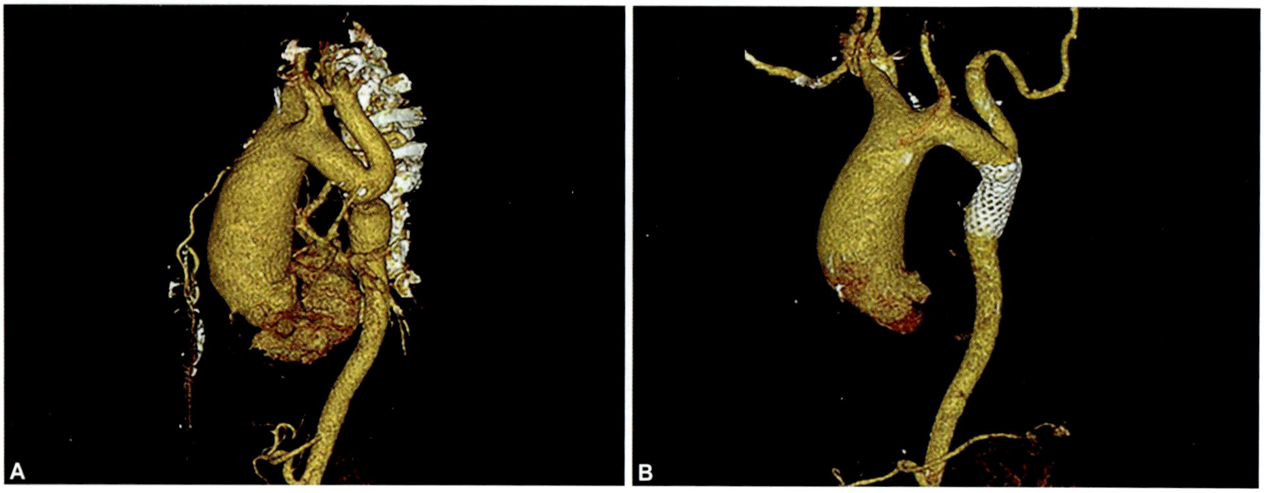

FIGS. 8A AND B: Pre (A) and post (B) stenting multidetector computed tomography angiography images. (A) 3D volume-rendered colored projection showing tight postductal coarctation of the aorta with post stenotic dilation, prominent tortuous anterior abdominal wall, and posterior intraspinal collaterals and (B) Post stenting 3D volume-rendered colored projection showing stent across the coarct with complete resolution of stenosis.[21]

CONCLUSION

Future research should focus on optimizing patient selection criteria, refining techniques, and assessing long-term outcomes of endovascular interventions in management of secondary HTN. Large-scale, multicenter trials will be essential to validate current findings and establish best practices. Endovascular interventions offer promising options for managing secondary HTN due to vascular obstruction, with ongoing advancements enhancing their efficacy and safety.

ONLINE REFERENCES

Please scan the QR code provided at the end of the table of contents for References of this chapter.

CHAPTER

45

Hypertensive Crisis: Clinical Diagnosis and Management

Vishal Batra, Bhushan Shah

ABSTRACT

Hypertensive crises are critical for morbidity and mortality, requiring prompt recognition and early treatment. Management varies depending on presentation, with guidelines aiming for evidence-based recommendations. Treatment focuses on maintaining optimal perfusion and avoiding hypoperfusion in patients with impaired autoregulatory mechanisms. Controlling blood pressure is essential to prevent recurrence.

Keywords: Hypertensive, morbidity and mortality guidelines

INTRODUCTION

Hypertensive crisis comprehensively has two different categories, hypertensive urgency and hypertensive emergency (HE). Both groups present with severely elevated blood pressure (BP), but the differences lie in the presence of end-organ damage (EOD). Distinguishing between the two is important because they require different intensities of therapy.

- *Hypertensive emergency:* The 7th Report of the Joint National Committee on Prevention, Detection, Evaluation, and Treatment of High Blood Pressure (JNC-7) defines it as "characterized by acute elevations in systolic or diastolic blood pressure (SBP/DBP) (>180 mm Hg or >120 mm Hg), associated with impending or progressive target organ damage or dysfunction."
- *Hypertensive urgency:* The JNC-7 defines it as "those situations associated with severe elevations in BP without progressive target EOD or dysfunction."
- The updated JNC-8 did not change these definitions. The important thing to remember is that there is no absolute value of BP that separates the two syndromes. Instead, the most important distinction is whether there is evidence of impending or progressive EOD, which defines an emergency.

RISK FACTORS

Hypertensive crises can present de novo in patients without any known history of hypertension (HTN), and in patients who have untreated and/or uncontrolled HTN, with the uncontrolled group being more common. Secondary causes of HTN can lead to hypertensive crisis more often than spontaneous evolution in patients with essential HTN. Secondary causes include renovascular HTN, acute glomerulonephritis, renal vasculitis, chronic kidney disease, alcohol or recreational drug abuse, concomitant medications, medication withdrawal, and pheochromocytoma.

CLINICAL ASSESSMENT

Detailed medical history including pertinent past medical history and physical examination are the cornerstones for the successful management of a hypertensive crisis. Hypertensive emergencies may occur with a lower value of BP especially if the rise is rapid in a patient with low baseline BP. It is important to rule out transient physiological rise in BP such as white coat HTN and anxiety-related elevations.

HISTORY

- History should include whether the patient was diagnosed with HTN previously; baseline BP; and any previous EOD particularly renal or cerebrovascular damage.
- Documents of past and present antihypertensive drug treatments and review of compliance.
- Intake of recreational drug usage, illicit drug usage (cocaine, methamphetamine, and ephedra) or abrupt stoppage of β-blockers.

- Symptoms suggestive of EOD include chest pain [acute coronary syndrome (ACS)/aortic dissection], shortness of breath (acute pulmonary edema), back pain (aortic dissection), and neurologic symptoms such as headache, blurring of vision, and seizures.
- Also, note any recent head trauma or injuries.

PHYSICAL EXAMINATION

- The BP measurement should be done in both arms.
- Always check the supine and standing BP to assess volume status as patients presenting with HE may be intravascularly volume depleted due to pressure natriuresis.
- *Peripheral pulse examination:* Assess and compare peripheral pulses for irregularities, absence, and delays.
- Key to diagnosing malignant HTN is a good fundus examination.
- A diastolic murmur gives a clue to aortic insufficiency seen in patients with aortic dissection. The systolic murmur of mitral regurgitation too may point toward ischemic rupture/dysfunction of a papillary muscle. Signs of acute heart failure (elevated jugular venous pressure, LV S3 gallop). The presence of rales is suggestive of pulmonary edema.
- Look for abdominal tenderness and masses and auscultate for abdominal bruits.
- Common concerning signs and symptoms of target EOD include neurologic deficits (dizziness, visual changes, severe headache, alterations in mental status, and seizures), cardiopulmonary abnormalities (severe chest pain, palpitations, edema, new murmurs, jugular venous distension, and crackles), and renal damage (decreased urine output).

INVESTIGATIONS

Laboratory studies to assess for target EOD, potential secondary HTN, and other cardiovascular risk factors should be conducted. Hypokalemic metabolic alkalosis may be a result of intravascular volume depletion and secondary hyperaldosteronism. Findings of proteinuria, hematuria, increased serum creatinine, hypokalemic metabolic alkalosis, and hemolytic anemia should alert physicians to the renal involvement of hypertensive crises. Suspicion of heart failure should lead to measurement of brain natriuretic profile (BNP)/N-terminal prohormone of brain natriuretic peptide (NT-proBNP).

Tests evaluating for secondary HTN include plasma and/or urine metanephrines in case of clinical suspicion of pheochromocytoma. Tests for primary hyperaldosteronism (plasma aldosterone and renin levels) may be helpful before initiating medications which may otherwise complicate interpretation—24-hour urinary cortisol for Cushing's if clinically suspected.

OTHER DIAGNOSTIC TESTS

An electrocardiogram (ECG) should be performed to assess for evidence of left ventricular hypertrophy, myocardial ischemia or infarction, and arrhythmias. A chest radiograph should be obtained to evaluate for pulmonary edema as well as widened mediastinum, which suggests aortic dissection.

Imaging

Patients presenting with neurological symptoms should undergo an urgent CT or MRI of the brain to rule out stroke or space-occupying lesions. A CT aortogram can help diagnose aortic dissection. For patients with elevated creatinine, renal imaging, including renal artery Doppler, is useful to assess for renovascular lesions.

Secondary HTN may not always present with clear signs and symptoms, so it is important to screen for secondary causes during subsequent follow-up, even if they are not clinically suspected.

MANAGEMENT

Principles of Management of Hypertensive Crisis

The specific diagnosis and type of EOD direct the choice of treatment, its target, and the rapidity of BP reduction. We need to be careful with BP reduction considering the benefits and risks of rapid BP reduction and worsening of acute EOD. It is crucial to understand the autoregulation of blood flow, which maintains a consistent supply to vital organs across a wide range of arterial pressures. This is particularly important for high-flow, low-resistance organs such as the brain and kidneys. In individuals with normal BP, autoregulation typically operates within a range of about 50–150 mm Hg of mean arterial pressure (MAP).[1] However, in cases of chronic HTN, the autoregulatory range shifts to higher MAP levels.[2] Consequently, if BP drops suddenly below this adjusted range due to intravenous (IV) therapy or short-acting medications like sublingual nifedipine, vital organs may not receive adequate blood flow. This can lead to severe complications such as cortical blindness, stroke, and myocardial infarction.[3,4]

Hypertensive Emergencies

General Principles

Patients experiencing hypertensive emergencies require immediate care and should be admitted to a high-dependency or intensive care unit for continuous BP monitoring and intravenous medication management. Treatment should start simultaneously with the assessment. According to international guidelines, which are based on autoregulatory theory due to a lack of comparative studies on BP reduction rates, the goal in the first 6–24 hours is to achieve a partial reduction in MAP, aiming for a decrease of no >20–25% and a drop in DBP of 10–15% or to a level of 100–110 mm Hg, except in cases of acute aortic syndromes. For patients with aortic dissection, rapidly lowering SBP to at least 120 mm Hg within 20 minutes can be life-saving. Monitoring urine output, acid-base balance, renal function, and neurological status is crucial for assessing end-organ perfusion. If there is excessive BP reduction, it is important to promptly stop intravenous medications, and if necessary, use vasopressors, IV fluids, or both. Long-acting antihypertensive medications should be started or resumed alongside IV therapy to ensure a smooth transition, reduce the duration of IV treatment and intensive care, and minimize the risk of rebound HTN, which is linked to higher mortality. While the optimal timing for initiating or resuming oral medications is uncertain, starting them 6–12 hours after beginning IV therapy is a practical approach, as the risk of hypotension is highest during the first 6 hours.[5] Long-acting oral drugs should follow standard guidelines for managing chronic HTN. For parenteral medications used in hypertensive crises, see **Table 1** for details on dosage, benefits, potential side effects, and contraindications.

Hypertensive Emergency States/ Syndromes (Tables 2 and 3)

Neurologic Emergencies

Hypertensive Encephalopathy

Hypertensive encephalopathy is a serious but fortunately rare condition characterized by transient neurological symptoms that occur with a sudden increase in BP. The most common cause is uncontrolled HTN. The pathophysiology involves a rapid, severe rise in BP leading to autoregulatory failure, which increases intracranial pressure, disrupts the blood–brain barrier, and causes arteriolar vasodilation, cerebral edema, and petechial micro-hemorrhages, followed by vasoconstriction. Symptoms commonly include severe generalized headaches, lethargy, drowsiness, nausea, and vomiting, though these are not specific to HE. More indicative symptoms are confusion, visual disturbances, seizures, and transient focal neurological deficits. Papilledema is often observed on fundus examination. Since HE is a diagnosis of exclusion, it is crucial to rule out intracranial hemorrhage (ICH) and acute ischemic stroke (AIS), which can also present with elevated BP and focal neurological deficits. CT imaging of the brain is useful for excluding ICH. While CT may show cerebral edema, MRI typically reveals symmetrical, subcortical, parieto-occipital hyperintense lesions, consistent with posterior reversible leukoencephalopathy syndrome (PRES). Although PRES is commonly associated with hypertensive encephalopathy and eclampsia, it can also occur without HTN, e.g., in association with cytotoxic or immunosuppressive therapy. Most patients see resolution of symptoms within a few hours with proper BP management.

The first-line treatments are IV labetalol and nicardipine, with nitroprusside as an alternative option.[6]

Intracerebral Hemorrhage

Intracerebral hemorrhage is linked to a 40% mortality rate within 1 month.[7] The risk is further elevated in individuals with intracranial aneurysms and those on anticoagulant therapy. Diagnosis is confirmed with a CT scan. Treatment principles for HTN in intracerebral hemorrhage focus on preventing neurological deterioration due to rebleeding or hematoma expansion while managing the risk of cerebral hypoperfusion from rapid BP reduction. The AHA/ACC (2017) guidelines suggest reducing BP to no <140 mm Hg within 6 hours for patients with a SBP ranging from 150 to 220 mm Hg.[8] The ESC/ESH (2023) guidelines recommend that for patients presenting within 6 hours of symptom onset, SBP should be reduced to below 140/90 mm Hg using IV therapy to prevent hematoma expansion and improve neurological outcomes. For those presenting >6 hours after onset with an SBP <220 mm Hg, a slow and moderate reduction of BP with IV therapy over several hours is preferred over more aggressive measures. In patients presenting >6 hours after onset with an SBP of 220 mm Hg or higher, a cautious reduction to below 180 mm Hg via IV drugs is advised to enhance functional recovery.[9] The NICE guidelines recommend lowering SBP to 140 mm Hg or below within 1 hour of treatment initiation, ensuring the reduction does not exceed 60 mm Hg, and maintaining this target for 7 days, except in cases with suspected underlying structural issues, a Glasgow Coma Scale (GCS) score <6, planned early neurosurgical intervention, or a massive hematoma with a poor prognosis. For patients presenting within 6 hours of intracerebral hemorrhage, maintaining a BP between 150 and 220 mm Hg is advised.[10]

Several large trials and meta-analyses have compared aggressive versus conservative BP reduction strategies. The largest study, the Intensive Blood Pressure Reduction in Acute Cerebral Hemorrhage Trial II (INTERACT II) involving 2,839 participants, compared intensive SBP reduction to below 140 mm Hg within 1 hour with standard reduction to below 180 mm Hg within 1 hour in patients with acute intracerebral hemorrhage . This trial found no difference in the primary outcomes of mortality or severe disability between the two groups. However, 3 months after randomization, the intensive reduction group had better functional outcomes.[11] Similarly, the Antihypertensive Treatment of Acute Cerebral Hemorrhage II (ATACH II) trial, which included 1,000 patients, compared aggressive BP reduction to a target SBP of 110–139 mm Hg within the first 2 hours with a control group targeting SBP of 140–179 mm Hg. This trial also found no difference in outcomes between the two approaches.[12,13] The drug of choice is IV labetalol, administered in a high-dependency unit unless contraindicated, with monitoring of neuro-observations and renal function.

TABLE 1: Drugs used in treatment of hypertensive emergencies.

Drug	Class	Dose	Onset of action	Half-life (T½)	Duration of action	Effect/Advantage	Side effects	Contraindications
Nicardipine	Dihydropyridine calcium channel blocker, vasodilator	5–15 mg/h IV drip; adjust by 2.5 mg/h every 5–15 minutes	Rapid onset (2–5 minutes)	2–4 hours	2–6 hours	• Dilates coronary vessels, can use with known CAD • Used without invasive BP monitoring	• Headache, flushing, dizziness, hypotension, digital dysesthesias • Abrupt withdrawal can cause or worsen angina or hypertension • Metabolized in liver, caution in cirrhotics	Contraindicated in patients with acute coronary ischemia (because of reflex tachycardia)
Clevidipine	Ultra-short-acting dihydropyridine calcium channel blocker, vasodilator	1–16 mg/h IV drip; double dose every 90 seconds, more slowly as BP approaches goal	Rapid onset (2–4 minutes)	1 minute	Effect lasts 5–15 minutes after stopping	• Ultra-short acting with rapid onset, offset of effect • Mild/no reflex tachycardia • Metabolism independent of renal and hepatic function • Arterial line not required • Can give peripherally	Atrial fibrillation, headache, nausea, vomiting, insomnia, and fever	Contraindicated in patients with acute coronary ischemia (because of reflex tachycardia) and in patients with allergy to soy or eggs; may increase triglyceride levels (it is a lipid emulsion)
Labetalol	Combined nonselective β-blocker and α-1 blocker (IV β–α blocking ratio, approximately 7:1)	10–20 mg IV bolus followed by drip; may repeat at same dose or double dose after 10 minutes before starting drip; 0.5–10 mg/min IV drip; adjust drip every 15 minutes; for intermittent boluses, 10–80 mg IV every 10 minutes (maximum cumulative dose, 300 mg)	Rapid onset (5 minutes)	5.5 hours	3–6 hours, sometimes longer at higher doses	• Good for patients with altered mental functions as it does not cause sedation or increased intracranial pressure • Low risk of causing excessive hypotension • Particularly useful in pheochromocytoma and other hyperadrenergic states	Bradycardia, dizziness, drowsiness, nausea	Contraindicated in patients with heart failure, bradycardia or heart block, asthma or severe airway reactivity; caution in cocaine overdose

Continued

Continued

Drug	Class	Dose	Onset of action	Half-life (T½)	Duration of action	Effect/Advantage	Side effects	Contraindications
Esmolol	Selective β-1 blocker	500–1,000 μg/kg bolus, followed by 100–300 μg/kg/min IV drip; adjust drip by 50 μg/kg/min every 5 minutes	Rapid onset (2–10 minutes)	10 minutes	10–30 minutes	• Particularly useful when cardiac contractility and work is to be reduced like in aortic dissection • Often used to manage intraoperative and postoperative hypertension	Bradycardia, nausea, and injection site pain	Contraindicated in patients with heart failure, bradycardia, or heart block, asthma, cocaine overdose
Metoprolol	Selective β-1 blocker	2.5–5 mg IV every 5 minutes (maximum total dose, 15 mg), then every 4–6 hours	Onset, ~5 minutes; peak, 30–60 minutes	4–6 hours	4–6 hours	Preferred in patients with aortic dissection, concurrent tachyarrhythmias	• AV blocks, bronchoconstriction • Fatigue, sexual dysfunction, and mental depression • Worsen glucose tolerance	Contraindicated in patients with heart failure, bradycardia or heart block, asthma, and cocaine overdose
Nitroglycerin	Nitrate donor, mixed venous, and arteriolar dilator with predominant venous effects	10–400 μg/min IV drip; adjust by 10–20 μg/min every 5–15 minutes	Rapid onset 5–10 minutes	1–2 minutes	5–10 minutes; with prolonged use, a higher dose may be needed for same effect	Dilates coronary vessels	• Ineffective arterial vasodilator • HA, hypotension, and tachycardia	Contraindicated in patients with right ventricular infarction
Nitroprusside	Direct vasodilator with predominant arteriolar effects	0.25–10 μg/kg/min IV drip; adjust by 0.5 μg/kg/min every 5 minutes	Rapid onset 1–2 minutes	2 minutes	3–4 minutes after infusion stopped	Large amount of experience with use	• Nausea/vomiting, muscle twitching, and diaphoresis • Cyanide toxicity, especially with renal insufficiency and prolonged infusions (>48 hours) • Inactivated by light • Requires invasive intra-arterial BP monitoring • Use cautiously with ↑ICP as can worsen • Careful with ACS as can cause coronary steal	Contraindicated in pregnancy (risk of fetal cyanide toxicity); use with impaired renal function may lead to thiocyanate toxicity, and use in liver disease may lead to cyanide intoxication, which may occur with higher doses or prolonged infusions; may cause methemoglobinemia (dose-dependent), increased intracranial pressure

Continued

Continued

Drug	Class	Dose	Onset of action	Half-life (T½)	Duration of action	Effect/Advantage	Side effects	Contraindications
Hydralazine	Direct arterial vasodilator	5–20 mg IV every 15–20 minutes, then every 3–4 hours (maximum dose, 20 mg per dose)	Usual onset within 20 minutes and peak within 1 hour; often demands a β-blocker or other negative chronotropic agent to control reflex tachycardia	1.5–3 hours	3–6 hours	Increases uterine blood flow	• Flushing, HA, and nausea • Significant reflex tachycardia • Has precipitated MI • Use cautiously in CKD, CAD, and CVD	Use should be avoided in most cases; may worsen ischemia (owing to reflex tachycardia and possible coronary steal); unpredictable BP responses, often excessive
Fenoldopam	Peripheral, dopamine-1 receptor agonist, causes vasodilation especially in renal, cardiac, and splanchnic beds	0.1 µg/kg/min to maximum 1.6 µg/kg/min. Titrate in 0.05–0.1 µg/kg/min increments	10 minutes Maximum effect in 30 minutes	5–10 minutes	1 hour	• Increases renal blood flow, improving CrCl especially in setting of impaired renal function • Used without invasive BP monitoring	• Reflex tachycardia • HA, dizziness, flushing, and nausea • Worsening angina • Atrial fibrillation • Tachyphylaxis after 48 hours • Contraindicated in glaucoma as causes dose-related increase in IOP	Contraindicated in myocardial ischemia, glaucoma, and intracranial hypertension
Enalaprilat	ACE-I	1.25 mg IV at 4–6 hours intervals, maximum 5 mg in 6 hours	15 minutes to 4 hours	11 hours	12–24 hours	• Good choice in hyperlipidemia patients • Abrupt discontinuation not associated with rapid increase in BP	• BP response variable, unpredictable, and not dose related • May not peak for 4 hours • Contraindicated in pregnancy	Contraindicated in pregnancy, patients with history of angioedema, hypersensitivity to any drug component, bilateral RAS
Phentolamine	α-adrenergic blocker	5–20 mg for hypertensive crisis, 5 mg IV 1–2 hours.	Immediate	19 minutes	15–30 minutes	Pheochromocytoma	Expansion of extracellular fluid; Weight gain; Postural hypotension; Drowsiness	May precipitate postural fall of blood pressure

TABLE 2: Recommended intensity of lowering of blood pressure in hypertensive emergencies and drug of choice.

Category	Intensity of BP reduction	Agent of choice	Alternative agent
Aortic emergencies	Intense reduction SBP<120 mm Hg	Esmolol and nicardipine	Clevidipine and labetalol
Hemorrhagic stroke	Moderate reduction of SBP 140–180 mm Hg	Nicardipine	Clevidipine and labetalol
Subarachnoid hemorrhage	Gradual reduction	Nicardipine	Clevidipine and labetalol
Ischemic stroke	Moderate reduction, reduce MAP by 15% in 1 hour	Nicardipine and labetalol	Clevidipine
Myocardial infarction, acute pulmonary edema	• Moderate reduction • MAP reduction 15–25%	• Nitroglycerine • Labetalol • Furosemide	• Esmolol • Nicardipine • Clevidipine
Hypertensive encephalopathy	MAP reduction by 20–25%	Nicardipine	Labetalol and clevidipine
Acute kidney Injury	MAP reduction by 20–25%	Labetalol and nicardipine	Clevidipine
Pheochromocytoma	MAP reduction by 20–25%	Phentolamine	• Nicardipine • Clevidipine • Labetalol

Acute Ischemic Stroke (AIS)

AIS can sometimes cause a rise in BP in individuals with chronic HTN, though it is uncertain whether this increase is a compensatory mechanism to maintain cerebral perfusion pressure (CPP) or if it is harmful. As with other hypertensive emergencies, a rapid and significant reduction in BP can decrease cerebral blood flow, potentially causing cerebral infarction or ischemia around a hematoma. Conversely, extremely high BP can exacerbate cerebral edema and elevate the risk of hemorrhagic transformation. Randomized controlled trials and subsequent meta-analyses have not demonstrated the benefits of targeting specific BP reductions.[14,15] For acute management, IV labetalol, possibly in combination with IV nicardipine or IV glyceryl trinitrate (GTN), is recommended. BP reduction should be considered in specific situations according to guidelines from the ESO, AHA/ACC and ESC/ESH.[7-9]

- *If BP is 220/120 mm Hg in the acute phase:* Cautious and slow BP reduction (lower MAP by no >15% over 24 hours) to maintain perfusion of the penumbra.
- *AIS patients are eligible for IV thrombolysis or mechanical thrombectomy:* Reduction of BP to 185/105 mm Hg and maintaining a BP <185/105 mm Hg for at least 24 hours.
- AIS patients are not eligible for IV thrombolysis or mechanical thrombectomy and SBP <220/120 mm Hg abstain from BP lowering in the first 72 hours because, under these circumstances, no benefit of a BP reduction has been consistently reported.
- For stable patients, who have BP readings of >140/90 mm Hg >3 days after an AIS, initiation of BP-lowering medications should be considered.

Subarachnoid Hemorrhage (SAH)

SAH is associated with significant morbidity and mortality, with mortality rates reaching 50–60% within the first few months, primarily due to cerebral vasospasm and delayed cerebral ischemia.[16] Agents that preferentially dilate cerebral blood vessels, thereby reducing vasospasm and delaying ischemia, are preferred. Oral nimodipine is recommended for most patients with nontraumatic SAH, as clinical trials and meta-analyses have shown it improves neurological outcomes.[17] The evidence supporting other calcium channel blockers (whether oral or IV) for SAH management is currently limited. Inducing hypotension in SAH is linked to poor outcomes, and there is no evidence that reducing BP is beneficial in this context. Decisions about prescribing or continuing antihypertensive therapy should consider the clinical situation, history of hypotension, and the need to balance the risk of rebleeding against the potential for hypotension.

Cardiac Hypertensive Emergencies

Acute Coronary Syndrome

In patients presenting with HE involving myocardial ischemia or infarction, elevated BP increases myocardial oxygen demand. Rapid or excessive lowering of BP may reduce myocardial oxygen supply. Evidence is mixed regarding the impact of admission BP on patient outcomes, and the benefits of specific BP targets immediately following ACS remain unclear. For patients with high BP and concurrent ACS, guidelines suggest reducing MAP by 15–25% over 1–2 hours, followed by a more gradual decrease while preparing for potential emergency interventions. It is important to avoid lowering DBP below 70 mm Hg. IV GTN and/or IV labetalol or esmolol are preferred treatments. Nitroprusside should be avoided in cases of ACS.

Acute Pulmonary Edema

A hypertensive crisis can present with symptoms of acute heart failure. Conditions such as ischemic heart disease and bilateral renal artery stenosis may increase the risk of heart failure. Treatment should be tailored to the

TABLE 3: Blood pressure targets and recommendation according to various guidelines in hypertensive emergencies.

Hypertensive crisis state	ESC/ESH (2023) guidelines	AHA guidelines	NICE guidelines	ISH (2020) guidelines
Malignant hypertension (MHT)/accelerated hypertension without hypertensive encephalopathy	• Reduce mean arterial pressure (MAP) 20–25% over several hours • *Drug of choice:* labetalol or nicardipine	Not explicitly defined		MAP reduction by 20–25% with labetalol or nicardipine over several hours
Hypertensive encephalopathy	Immediately reduce MAP by 20–25% with labetalol or nicardipine	For all hypertensive emergencies with a few exceptions, reduce BP by maximum 25% over first hour, then to 160/100–110 mm Hg over next 2–6 hours then to normal over 24–48 hours		Immediate • MAP reduction by 20–25% with labetalol or nicardipine
Ischemic stroke	If BP >220/120 mm Hg or if considered for thrombolytic therapy and BP >185/110 mm Hg reduce MAP 15% in 1 hour	Lower SBP to <185 mm Hg and DBP <110 mm Hg before initiation of IV thrombolysis. Maintain BP <180/105 mm Hg for first 24 hours after IV thrombosis. If BP >220/120 mm Hg reduce MAP 15% in 24 hours.	• BP reduction to 185/110 mm Hg considered in people who are candidates for IV thrombolysis • Antihypertensive treatment only if overlap with another hypertensive emergency	• If BP >220/120 mm Hg or if considered for thrombolytic therapy and BP >185/110 mm Hg-1 hour • MAP reduction by 15% with labetalol or nicardipine
Intracerebral hemorrhage	If SBP >180 mm Hg, immediate reduction to 130–180 mm Hg range (especially if initial BP ≥220 mm Hg) with labetalol or nicardipine	AHA 2024—Recommendation of a specific target was not a Class 1 recommendation. In patients with acute spontaneous ICH pharmacological BP lowering is initiated within 1 hour of hospital arrival and with the target BP reached within 2 hours of hospital arrival with the following exceptions: • Patients <18 or ≥90 years of age • Presenting systolic BP <150 or >220 mm Hg • Initial GCS score <5 • Hematoma volume ≥60 mL • Patients transferred from another hospital Avoiding peaks and large variability in SBP, can be beneficial for improving functional outcomes. Lowering systolic BP below 140 mm Hg may be harmful	If presented within 6 hours of ICH and SBP 150–220 mm Hg, reduce BP rapidly. If presented beyond 6 hours after stroke, consider same targets if SBP >220 mm Hg. To consider risk of harm case-by-case	• Acute hemorrhagic stroke with SBP >180 mm Hg • Immediate 130 < SBP < 180 mm Hg with Labetalol • Nicardipine

Continued

Continued

Hypertensive crisis state	ESC/ESH (2023) guidelines	AHA guidelines	NICE guidelines	ISH (2020) guidelines
Acute coronary syndrome (ACS), acute pulmonary edema/hypertensive heart failure	• Reduce SBP to <140 mm Hg immediately on both conditions • ACS treated with GTN, labetalol • Pulmonary edema treated with GTN or nitroprusside (with loop diuretic)	ACS treated with esmolol or labetalol, GTN, and nicardipine. Pulmonary edema treated with clevidipine, GTN, or nitroprusside		Immediate • SBP<140 mm Hg with nitroglycerine or labetalol, Pulmonary edema treated with GTN or nitroprusside (with loop diuretic)
Acute aortic disease	Immediately reduce SBP to <120 mm Hg and heart rate to <60 BPM with esmolol and nitroprusside or GTN or nicardipine	Reduce SBP to <120 mm Hg within 20 minutes with esmolol or labetalol		Immediate • SBP <120 mm Hg and heart rate <60 BPM with esmolol and nitroglycerin or nitroprusside or nicardipine
Severe preeclampsia	Reduce BP to <160/105 mm Hg in the first hour (immediate) with labetalol or nicardipine and magnesium sulfate	Rapid lowering. Reduce SBP to <140 mm Hg in the first hour	Severe hypertension in pregnancy is >160/110 mm Hg. Aim for BP <135/85 mm Hg	Immediate • SBP <160 mm Hg and DBP <105 mm Hg via labetalol or nicardipine and magnesium sulfate

underlying cause and associated pathophysiology. Patients may not always exhibit overt signs of pulmonary edema. Diuretics, particularly loop diuretics such as furosemide and bumetanide, are essential in managing heart failure. Treatment aims for a gradual reduction in BP (a fall in MAP of 15–25%) over several hours, as recommended by most guidelines. The AHA guidelines suggest managing pulmonary edema with medications such as clevidipine, nitroglycerin, nitroprusside, or enalaprilat.[8] According to ESC guidelines, in patients with heart failure, BP should be reduced to a SBP of <140 mm Hg if it is 140/90 mm Hg or higher.[9] Nitroprusside can also be an effective, though it should be avoided in patients with concurrent renal and liver failure. β-blockers are contraindicated in cases of acute pulmonary edema.

Aortic Dissection

Aortic dissection is a severe condition with very high mortality rates if not promptly treated. It is often precipitated by genetic factors, chronic HTN, aging, and atherosclerosis. For acute uncomplicated type B and chronic aortic dissections, medical management is typically preferred. The primary treatment goal is to reduce heart rate to below 60 beats per minute and lower BP using β-blockers. This approach decreases the cyclical stress on the aortic wall and the dissection flap. International guidelines and position statements suggest reducing SBP to <120 mm Hg (*target range:* 90–120 mm Hg) within 1–2 hours, despite the lack of randomized controlled trial data supporting this target.[18] Notably, hypotension, defined as an SBP below 90 mm Hg, is linked to increased mortality in both type A and type B dissections, with odds ratios of 1.95 (1.08–3.52) and 6.43 (2.18–18.98), respectively.[19] Nondihydropyridine calcium channel blockers are a useful alternative for patients who cannot tolerate β-blockers. IV β-blockers (such as labetalol or esmolol) are preferred due to their shorter half-lives and are usually the first choice for lowering BP. Vasodilators that can cause tachycardia, such as nitroprusside and GTN, should only be used after β-blockade.

Hyperadrenergic Crisis and Pheochromocytoma

In patients experiencing HE due to catecholamine excess from pheochromocytoma, cocaine, or amphetamine overdose, or clonidine withdrawal syndrome, the presentation can include symptoms such as elevated BP, episodic palpitations, sweating, pallor, severe headaches, anxiety, tremors, a sense of impending doom, nausea, vomiting, and abdominal pain. Episodes typically develop over several minutes and subside within 15–60 minutes. BP may be normal at baseline or accompanied by existing essential HTN. During adrenergic crises, BP may rise transiently, but it can usually be safely normalized within a few hours.

Management should focus on reversing sympathetic stimulation and correcting volume contraction due to pressure natriuresis. In stable patients, the first-line treatment involves full oral α-blockade, such as with phenoxybenzamine, which is continued as part of presurgical preparation. If phenoxybenzamine is unavailable, doxazosin may be used as an alternative.[20] β-blockade should be avoided until α-blockade is achieved, but selective or nonselective β-blockers may be used to manage tachycardia or as prophylaxis in patients with preexisting ischemic heart disease or arrhythmias. For acute BP control in crises, IV phentolamine, a ganglion blocker, may be useful, and labetalol can be used rarely, though its α-blockade may be incomplete.

Hypertensive Emergency Associated with Renal Failure

Acute kidney injury can be a cause or a consequence of HE. Although IV nitroprusside is widely used, it can cause cyanide or thiocyanate toxicity. Parental fenoldopam mesylate (a dopamine-1 receptor agonist) has shown promising results and enhanced safety.

CONCLUSION

Hypertensive crises lead to significant morbidity and mortality, making prompt recognition and early treatment essential to prevent progressive EOD. Management of acute hypertensive crises varies widely depending on the presentation. High-quality evidence is lacking, and available studies do not definitively support specific rates of BP reduction or particular medications. Guidelines for managing acute hypertensive states aim to provide evidence-based and consistent recommendations to ensure high-quality patient care. While hypertensive emergencies can present in various ways, the primary difference across groups lies in the intensity of BP reduction targets. Treatment focuses on maintaining optimal perfusion and avoiding hypoperfusion in patients with impaired autoregulatory mechanisms. When no target organ damage is present, a conservative approach with outpatient management is generally preferable. Controlling BP is crucial to prevent the recurrence of hypertensive emergencies or urgencies.

ONLINE REFERENCES

Please scan the QR code provided at the end of the table of contents for References of this chapter.

CHAPTER

46

Hypertension in Chronic Kidney Disease: Management Dilemmas

Dharmendra Jain, K Arun Kumar, Umesh K Pandey, Suyash Tripathi, Soumik Ghosh, Rajpal Prajapati

ABSTRACT

Most patients with chronic kidney disease (CKD) have hypertension, which is both a cause and an effect of CKD. Controlling hypertension is crucial because it lowers the risk of cardiovascular disease (CVD) and slows the progression of CKD. There is no agreement on the ideal blood pressure (BP) targets provided by current guidelines. Consequently, when deciding how to care for specific patients, it is essential to comprehend the evidence utilized to develop these guidelines. Nonpharmacological therapies can help but they are rarely enough to achieve optimal BP control. To reach their desired BP, patients with CKD and hypertension may need to take multiple antihypertensive drugs. When starting therapy, it is important to take into account the additional BP-independent renoprotective and/or cardioprotective activity that some pharmaceutical treatments offer. Additional difficulties arise when managing hypertension during hemodialysis and after kidney transplantation. Crucially, meeting BP goals, lowering the risk of CVD, and delaying the course of CKD all depend on an individualized, evidence-based management strategy.

Keywords: Chronic kidney disease (CKD), hypertension, pathophysiology, diagnosis, management

INTRODUCTION

When kidney abnormalities are persistent for at least 3 months and have an impact on health, they are referred to as chronic kidney disease (CKD). Cause, glomerular filtration rate (GFR) category (G1–G5), and albuminuria category (A1–A3)—abbreviated as CGA—are the three criteria used to classify CKD.[1] The idea of a "CGA" categorization of CKD based on etiology (C), kidney function level as assessed by GFR (G), and degree of albuminuria (A) was first introduced in the KDIGO 2012 guideline. The CGA classification established the groundwork for subsequent developments in CKD management, therapy, research, and risk assessment. Since then, studies have shown that higher specific stages or categories of CKD, which are defined by the independent levels of albuminuria and GFR, indicate a higher relative risk (RR) for unfavorable outcomes.[2,3]

CHRONIC KIDNEY DISEASE AND HYPERTENSION

Adverse cardiovascular and cerebrovascular outcomes are increased by the complicated relationship between hypertension and CKD. The primary contributor to the worldwide burden of disease at the moment is hypertension, a global public health issue. It is the most modifiable risk factor for renal failure, heart disease, and stroke.[4] The term hypertension refers to a blood pressure (BP) level where, in younger, middle-aged, and older individuals, the office systolic BP values are ≥140 mm Hg and/or diastolic BP values are ≥90 mm Hg, and the benefits of treatment clearly outweigh the hazards of treatment.[5]

Prevalence

Only 54% of persons with hypertension are diagnosed, 42% receive treatment, and only 21% have their hypertension under control, according to the WHO Global Report on hypertension.[6] In India, the prevalence is between 24 and 30% in urban regions and between 12 and 14% in rural areas. By 2025, 1.56 billion persons worldwide are expected to have high BP.[7]

PATHOPHYSIOLOGY OF HYPERTENSION IN CHRONIC KIDNEY DISEASE

Reduced nephron mass, increased sodium retention and extracellular volume expansion, overactivity of the sympathetic nervous system, activation of hormones such as the renin–angiotensin–aldosterone system (RAAS), endothelial dysfunction, increased intracellular calcium level, and reversal of hypoxia-induced vasodilation are some of the complex factors that contribute to the pathophysiology of hypertension in CKD.[8]

Role of Renin–Angiotensin–Aldosterone System

An essential regulator of blood volume, electrolyte balance, and systemic vascular resistance is the RAAS. The RAAS is known to be more active in CKD patients. Blood flow in peritubular capillaries is diminished in the downstream direction of sclerosed glomeruli. Glomeruli in these areas oversecrete renin in response to the decreased effective blood flow, which raises the levels of angiotensin II in the blood.[9] Angiotensin II directly constricts blood vessels, raising BP and systemic vascular resistance. Additionally, angiotensin II stimulates sodium reabsorption in the collecting duct and the proximal tubule (via aldosterone). Moreover, sodium retention results from impaired sodium excretion brought on by a net reduction of total GFR. Through both volume-dependent and volume-independent processes, sodium retention results in hypertension. The most prevalent one of these is diabetic nephropathy.[10]

Sympathetic Nervous System Overactivity

Renal juxtaglomerular cells in CKD are stimulated to produce renin due to the overactivity of the SNS. Renal ischemia not only causes sodium retention to activate the SNS, but also stimulates renal afferent nerves via adenosine.[11]

Role of the Vasculature in Hypertension in Chronic Kidney Disease

Patients with CKD have their vessels constantly exposed to a variety of hormones, factors, and uremic toxins that cause vascular dysfunction which leads to HTN which is frequently challenging and resistant to medication management.[12] Endothelial dysfunction not only can lead to the development of CVD but also facilitates the advancement of CKD by causing endothelial cell malfunction and disintegration in glomerular capillaries, especially those in the renal medulla.[13]

Other Risk Factors Causing Hypertension

The inability to produce calcitriol, the bioactive form of vitamin D, as well as phosphate excretion impairment works together to cause elevated parathyroid hormone (PTH) levels and parathyroid hyperplasia.[12]

Erythropoietin is linked to improved pressor responsiveness to norepinephrine and Ang II, increased cytosolic calcium in VSMCs, elevated blood serotonin or endothelin levels, increased vasoconstricting (PGF2α and TxA2), and decreased vasorelaxing PGI2 release.[14] Endothelial cell viability and function can be impacted by *uremic toxins* through the induction of endothelial cell death as well as the mitigation of its migration and proliferation.[15]

DIAGNOSIS AND DIAGNOSTIC CHALLENGES

Correct BP measurement is essential for both CKD diagnosis and treatment. For the validation of aberrant BP readings, 24-hour ambulatory BP monitoring (ABPM) is recommended.

Ambulatory Blood Pressure Monitoring

The 24-hour, daytime, and nocturnal readings including BP variables like dipping and a drop in BP of >10% while you sleep are more accurately estimated by ABPM. In individuals with CKD, nocturnal hypertension and nondipping status are common and linked to an increased risk of cardiovascular morbidity and mortality.[16]

Role of Biomarkers and Imaging in Diagnosis

Traditional indicators for estimating GFR and evaluating kidney function include serum creatinine and cystatin C, cystatin C especially when creatinine levels are influenced by muscle mass. Kidney injury molecule-1 (KIM-1) and neutrophil gelatinase-associated lipocalin (NGAL) are two more newly discovered biomarkers. Additionally, proteinuria—a major sign of kidney impairment and a risk factor for cardiovascular events—is disclosed by the urine albumin-to-creatinine ratio.[17]

Imaging techniques: Renal ultrasonography is a popular noninvasive imaging technique that can reveal details about the size, structure, and presence of kidney cysts or blockages. Modern imaging methods, such as computed tomography (CT) and magnetic resonance imaging (MRI), provide precise cross-sectional views of the kidneys, making it possible to diagnose renal artery stenosis—a disease that can lead to secondary hypertension and make appropriate treatment decisions.[18] Contrast-enhanced ultrasonography (CEUS), which offers real-time imaging of renal blood flow and perfusion without the dangers associated with ionizing radiation or nephrotoxic contrast chemicals, is one example of a recent improvement.[19]

Diagnostic Criteria for Hypertension in Chronic Kidney Disease Patients (Conflicting Guidelines)

Regarding BP thresholds and targets for hypertensive medication therapy in CKD, there are three main guidelines: (1) ACC/AHA/AAPA/ABC/ACPM/AGS/APhA/ASH/ASPC/

NMA/PCNA Guideline for the Prevention, Detection, Evaluation, and Management of High Blood Pressure in Adults, (2) European Society of Cardiology (ESC)/ European Society of Hypertension (ESH) Guidelines for the Management of Arterial Hypertension, and (3) Kidney Disease: Improving Global Outcomes (KDIGO) guidelines.[20]

MANAGEMENT: THERAPEUTIC GOALS AND GUIDELINES

Management of hypertension presents several therapeutic problems, especially in those who have comorbidities. This chapter explores four primary challenges in the management of hypertension: Managing comorbid conditions like diabetes, CVD, and obesity; setting target BP goals; addressing difficulties in medication adherence and polypharmacy; and striking a balance between BP control and kidney function preservation.

According to the KDIGO guidelines for 2021, limiting dietary sodium intake to <90 mg/day is an effective non-pharmacological intervention for hypertension management. The next stage in managing hypertension is to start antihypertensive medication if BP is still uncontrolled. The 2021 KDIGO guidelines strongly (Level 1B) propose that the first-choice antihypertensive medication for individuals with high BP, CKD, and extremely high albuminuria be an ACEI or an ARB.[21]

For proper BP control, the majority of patients need to take numerous drugs. As a result, long-acting dihydropyridine calcium channel blockers (CCBs) or diuretics can be used as second-line therapy; patients exhibiting clinical indications or symptoms of volume excess are more suited for the latter. The combination of a dihydropyridine CCB, a diuretic, and a RAS blocker is completed by third-line therapy in the algorithm. It is better to employ single-pill combinations since they ease treatment burden, enhance treatment adherence, and result in higher rates of BP management.[22]

KDIGO 2024 guidelines: A complete treatment strategy should be implemented for individuals with CKD in order to lower their risk of the disease's progression and the consequences that come with it. Encouragement should be given to them to engage in physical exercise that is appropriate for their level of tolerance and cardiovascular health, to reach an ideal body mass index (BMI), and to abstain from tobacco usage. When appropriate and feasible, referrals to healthcare professionals and programs (such as psychologists, registered dietitians, pharmacists, physical and occupational therapists, and smoking cessation programs) should be made.[1]

It is recommended that individuals with CKD engage in moderate-to-intense physical exercise for a minimum of 150 min/week or to an extent that is appropriate for their cardiovascular and physical tolerance (1D). Diets should include less ultraprocessed food and more plant-based meals than animal-based foods. In persons with CKD G3–G5 (2C), 0.8 g/kg body weight/day of protein should be recommended. Systolic BP (SBP) aims <120 mm Hg (where tolerated) to be used in the treatment and high BP utilizing standardized office BP measurement (2B).[22]

Nonpharmacologic Management

Nonpharmacologic management involves altering one's way of life, such as adopting a special diet and cutting back on alcohol, salt, and saturated fat. It has also been shown that weight loss, increasing physical activity, and meal timing restrictions work. Certain conventional techniques, such as transcendental meditation, yoga, and acupuncture, are beneficial.[23] Additional therapies have been added, such as home monitoring, biofeedback, acupuncture, quitting smoking, and dietary supplements (e.g., garlic, cocoa, vitamin C, coenzyme Q10, omega-3 fatty acids, calcium, potassium, and magnesium).[24] It is advised to follow a diet low in fat dairy products, chicken, fish, legumes, nontropical vegetable oils, and nuts and to limit the intake of sweets, sugar-sweetened beverages, and red meat. Instead, a diet high in whole grains, more vegetables, and fruits is advised.[25]

A 10 kg weight loss may result in a 5–20 mm Hg drop in SBP.[26] Smoking immediately raises sympathetic nerve activity, which raises BP, heart rate, and myocardial contractility, all of which increase the need for oxygen in the heart.[27] It is believed that relaxation techniques can assist lessen the stress and physiologic arousal that the autonomic nervous system produces, which will drop BP. Stretching, breathing, meditation, and postural movements are all part of yoga.[28]

Pharmacologic Management

Antihypertensive drugs are typically needed in addition to nonpharmacological therapies. Reaching BP targets often requires combination medication therapy.[29] Patients with CKD benefit greatly from ACE inhibitors and angiotensin II receptor blockers (ARBs), as they have both cardioprotective and renoprotective qualities. RAAS blockage can lower systolic BP by about 20 mm Hg.[30] Diuretics have been demonstrated to improve arterial stiffness and left ventricular mass index and minimize volume expansion.[31] Dihydropyridine and nondihydropyridine CCBs are both helpful in controlling hypertension.[32]

Beta-adrenoceptor antagonists effectively lower BP by affecting the dysregulated sympathetic nervous system. In combination with medication, peripherally acting α-blockers (α-adrenoceptor antagonists) such as doxazosin and prazocin are frequently utilized to manage hypertension in patients with CKD.[33] The theory is that evening dosage could reverse the nondipping nocturnal BP observed in CKD, as the timing of antihypertensive drugs can affect the diurnal fluctuation of BP.[34]

Challenges in Combination Therapy

A simultaneous intervention at multiple pathophysiological levels is required to achieve therapeutic success. The true difficulty in managing hypertension is actually polytherapy, which interferes with the patient's so-called compliance, that is, their cooperation and appropriate obedience to medical advice. They are notably advised for patient populations with diabetes, CKD, or a high risk of CVD.[35]

Emerging Therapies

New Antidiabetic Agents with Cardiovascular and Renal Protection

These drugs include glucagon-like peptide-1 (GLP-1) receptor agonists and sodium-glucose cotransporter-2 inhibitors (SGLT-2i). Thus, SGLT-2i have been demonstrated to decrease glomerular hyperfiltration, lower BP, lower plasma uric acid levels, and lower body weight in addition to decreasing blood glucose and boosting glycosuria.[36]

Endothelin Receptor Antagonists

In fact, endothelin-1 binds to ET-receptors A and B, which are expressed in distinct nephron segments. The former causes vasoconstriction, inflammation, oxidative stress, activation of podocytes, and other consequences, whereas the latter has the opposite effects. An excess of ET-1 is produced in CKD, which causes albuminuria, increased efferent vascular tone, angiotensin II production stimulation, and ultimately glomerular hyperfiltration. Therefore, in addition to RAAS inhibitors, addressing these hemodynamic and nonhemodynamic mechanisms may be useful in treating nondiabetic or diabetic CKD.[37]

Device-based Therapy for Hypertension

Out of a number of interventional strategies, the most important is renal denervation, in light of the critical roles played by the kidney and the sympathetic nervous system in the onset and maintenance of hypertension.[38]

Management Dilemmas and Controversies

A number of debates concerning the best way to treat patients with CKD are being called into question by recent research and clinical studies. These include whether iron and erythropoiesis-stimulating agents (ESAs) are appropriate for treating anemia and whether vitamin D supplementation is beneficial for preventing CKD-bone mineral disorder (CKD BMD).[39]

Risks versus Benefits of Intensive Blood Pressure Control

Although the guidelines advocated for individualized decision-making, they also covered populations like individuals with severe CKD that were either underrepresented or completely excluded from large therapeutic studies. The SPRINT (Systolic Blood Pressure Intervention Trial) yielded mixed results on the benefits and risks of rigorous BP control on CVD and mortality in individuals with CKD.[40]

Treatment of Complications of Chronic Kidney Disease

Particularly in oliguric patients and those with decreased aldosterone secretion, hyperkalemia in CKD might arise. Hyperkalemia may be caused by hypoaldosteronism, tissue deterioration, and potassium intake in the diet. Hyperkalemia may also be brought on by medications like nonselective beta-blockers and ACE inhibitors. A frequent side effect of advanced CKD is metabolic acidosis. Osteopenia, increased protein catabolism, and secondary hyperparathyroidism would be the outcomes of chronic metabolic acidosis. A substantial risk factor for CVD is CKD and the risk rises with CKD severity. Epicardial adipose tissue (EAT) thickness and the incidence of CVD events are significantly correlated, according to a substantial body of research.[41]

Bone and Mineral Disorders

A common CKD consequence brought on by a lower phosphorus filtration load is hyperphosphatemia. As a result, secondary hyperparathyroidism is brought on by an increase in parathyroid hormone (PTH) secretion. Normalization of calcium and phosphorus is the outcome of hyperparathyroidism, although bone is lost in the process. This leads to renal osteodystrophy. Thus, dietary phosphorus restriction and phosphorus binders are utilized to treat secondary hyperparathyroidism.

Typically, normocytic normochromic anemia is seen in CKD. It is mostly caused by decreased red cell survival as well as decreased erythropoietin synthesis from decreased functional renal mass. For patients with CKD III, CKD IV and CKD V, hemoglobin should be checked every 6 months, and for dialysis patients, it should be done every 3 months. When hemoglobin is <10, iron saturation is at least 25%, and ferritin is >200 ng/mL, ESAs should be taken into consideration for individuals with CKD. The target hemoglobin concentration for dialysis patients is between 10 and 11.5 g/dL.

Treatment of Complications of End-stage Renal Disease

Poor protein intake and anorexia are the main causes of malnutrition in ESRD. In an ESRD, the daily calorie intake should be at least 30–35 kcal/kg. One of the complications of low platelet function is uremic hemorrhage. Desmopressin (dDAVP), cryoprecipitate, and estrogen are the therapies that are employed. Dialysis should be started if there is evidence of uremia, which can manifest as uremic pericarditis.[42]

Complications of Renal Transplantation

Complications pertaining to the gastrointestinal, neurological, renal, and cardiovascular systems are hypertension, dyslipidemia, heart failure, arrhythmias, left ventricular hypertrophy, coronary artery disease from recently diagnosed diabetes mellitus, and renal failure. Neurologic problems include neoplastic disease, neuromuscular disease, central nervous system (CNS) infections, stroke, and posterior reversible encephalopathy syndrome. The following are examples of GI complications: Infection, cancer (post-transplant lymphoproliferative condition), mucosal injury, ulceration, perforation, pancreatitis, biliary tract illness, and diverticular disease.[43]

MULTIDISCIPLINARY APPROACH

Research indicates that treating with an interprofessional team that includes a dietitian, pharmacist, nurse staff, primary care practitioner, and community health workers reduces patient morbidity, reduces expenses, and assures better results.[44]

FUTURE DIRECTIONS AND RESEARCH

In low- and middle-income countries (LMICs), a more integrated, multidisciplinary, and sustainable approach to CKD care should be encouraged. In the context of chronic diseases,[45] chronic care models (CCM) seek to advance integrated, patient-centered, culturally sensitive, evidence-based, and economically efficient healthcare delivery. In order to provide patients with standard, repeatable, sustainable, and cost-effective care while improving outcomes like kidney failure or death, the adoption of CCMs in CKD management is particularly relevant in LMICs with localized clinical information systems and political/governmental resources.

CONCLUSION

To effectively target these objectives, it is helpful to understand the pathophysiological mechanisms causing hypertension in patients with CKD. Current guidelines support therapies for either cardioprotection, renoprotection, or both, but they do not provide a consensus on ideal BP levels. Likewise, pharmaceutical treatments intended to accomplish these goals provide varying levels of risk mitigation contingent upon patient attributes. The best options for managing chronic disease management in these settings continue to be early disease detection, preventive measures, and the use of integrative approaches due to the cost of patient care and the unavailability and inaccessibility of various kidney replacement therapy modalities due to economic challenges. For these preventative efforts to be successful, the governments of LMICs must enhance their primary healthcare systems and fortify their noncommunicable disease programs.

ONLINE REFERENCES

Please scan the QR code provided at the end of the table of contents for References of this chapter.

CHAPTER

47

Management of Hypertension in Pregnant and Postpartum Patients

Chhabi Satpathy, Biraja Prasad Beura, Hemant Kumar Satpathy, Trinath Kumar Mishra

ABSTRACT

Hypertensive disorders of pregnancy (HDP) remain one of the major causes of pregnancy-related morbidity and mortality worldwide. Independent of traditional cardiovascular disease risk factors, HDP-affected persons are also at an increased risk for cardiovascular diseases later in life. Evidence obtained from trials has refined the target blood pressure and timing of delivery to manage chronic hypertension and preeclampsia with nonsevere features. In patients with history of HDP, it is important to develop strategic lifestyle and therapeutic interventions to reduce the risk of future cardiovascular disease. This is an opportunity to identify patients with underlying, often unrecognized, cardiovascular risk factors during pregnancy and postpartum. This chapter discusses the current guidelines and research data on the prevention, diagnosis, management, and postnatal follow-up of HDP.

Keywords: Hypertension, pregnancy, preeclampsia

INTRODUCTION

Hypertensive disorders of pregnancy (HDP) complicate up to 10% of pregnancies and represent a significant cause of perinatal morbidity and mortality.[1,2] In India, 18.35% of maternal morbidity and 0.96% of maternal mortality are attributed to HDP.[3] These numbers will likely increase in the coming years due to increasing frequency of obesity and advanced age in pregnant persons. There is regional variation in the prevalence of HDP in India: It is most commonly found in North India and least commonly in East India. This variation may be due to differences in availability and utilization of antenatal care services, lifestyle, dietary factors, or physical activity.

CLASSIFICATION

The term HDP includes chronic hypertension, gestational hypertension, preeclampsia/eclampsia, and preeclampsia superimposed on chronic hypertension **(Table 1)**.

TABLE 1: Diagnostic criteria for various HDP.

HDP	Diagnostic criteria
Gestational hypertension	• New-onset SBP ≥ 140 mm Hg and/or DBP ≥ 90 mm Hg on at least two occasions 4 hours apart after 20 weeks of gestation in a previously normotensive individual And without proteinuria and no clinical features of preeclampsia-related EOD (e.g., thrombocytopenia, AKI, elevated liver transaminases, pulmonary edema, cerebral or visual symptoms)
Preeclampsia	• New-onset SBP ≥ 140 mm Hg and/or DBP ≥ 90 mm Hg on at least two occasions 4 hours apart after 20 weeks of gestation in a previously normotensive individual; patients with SBP ≥ 160 mm Hg and/or DBP ≥ 110 mm Hg should have BP confirmed within a short interval (minutes) to facilitate timely administration of AHT

Continued

Continued

HDP	Diagnostic criteria
	And proteinuria [≥300 mg per 24-hour urine collection (or this amount extrapolated from a timed collection), or protein:creatinine ratio ≥ 0.3 or urine dipstick reading ≥ 2+ (if other quantitative methods are unavailable)] • In a patient with new-onset hypertension without proteinuria, the diagnosis of preeclampsia can still be made if any features of severe disease are present
Preeclampsia with severe features	In a patient with preeclampsia, presence of any of the following findings is a feature of severe disease: • SBP ≥ 160 mm Hg and/or DBP ≥ 110 mm Hg on two occasions at least 4 hours apart (unless AHT is initiated before this time) • Thrombocytopenia (platelet count < 1 lakh/μL) • Impaired LFT as indicated by liver transaminase levels at least twice the normal concentration or severe persistent right upper quadrant or epigastric pain unresponsive to medication and not accounted for by alternative diagnoses, or both • AKI [serum creatinine concentration > 1.1 mg/dL (97 μmol/L) or doubling of the serum creatinine concentration in the absence of other kidney disease] • Pulmonary edema • Persistent cerebral or visual disturbances
Eclampsia	A generalized seizure in a patient with preeclampsia that cannot be attributed to other causes
HELLP syndrome	• Hemolysis, elevated liver enzymes, and low platelets • Hypertension may be present (HELLP in such cases is often considered as a variant)
Chronic (preexisting) hypertension	Hypertension diagnosed or present before pregnancy or on at least two occasions before 20 weeks of gestation; hypertension that is first diagnosed during pregnancy and persists for at least 12 weeks postpartum is also considered chronic hypertension • BP criteria during pregnancy: SBP ≥ 140 mm Hg and/or DBP ≥ 90 mm Hg • Prepregnancy and 12 weeks postpartum BP criteria are: ○ Stage 1: SBP 130–139 mm Hg or DBP 80–89 mm Hg ○ Stage 2: SBP ≥ 140 mm Hg or DBP ≥ 90 mm Hg
Chronic hypertension with superimposed preeclampsia	Any of the following findings in a patient with chronic hypertension: • A sudden increase in BP that was previously well controlled or an escalation of AHT to control BP • New onset of proteinuria or a sudden increase in proteinuria in a patient with known proteinuria before or early in pregnancy • Significant new EOD consistent with preeclampsia after 20 weeks of gestation or postpartum
Chronic hypertension with superimposed preeclampsia with severe features	Any of the following findings in a patient with chronic hypertension and superimposed preeclampsia: • SBP ≥ 160 mm Hg and/or DBP > 110 mm Hg despite escalation of AHT • Thrombocytopenia (platelet count < 1 lakh/μL) • Impaired LFT as indicated by liver transaminase levels at least twice the normal concentration or severe persistent right upper quadrant or epigastric pain unresponsive to medication and not accounted for by alternative diagnoses, or both • New-onset or worsening renal insufficiency • Pulmonary edema • Persistent cerebral or visual disturbances

(AHT: antihypertensive therapy; AKI: acute kidney injury; BP: blood pressure; DBP: diastolic blood pressure; EOD: end-organ dysfunction; HDP: hypertensive disorders of pregnancy; LFT: liver function test; SBP: systolic blood pressure)

SCREENING TESTS

Besides risk factors based on history, several studies have evaluated the role of biophysical markers (uterine artery Doppler studies), biochemical markers (sFlt-1/PIGF), or a combination of the two as potential signs of preeclampsia.[4] Unfortunately, most of these studies have low predictive value and, thus, these tests have limited clinical application. As per the American College of Obstetricians and Gynecologists (ACOG) Clinical Practice Update on biomarker prediction of preeclampsia with severe features, there is insufficient data to recommend management strategies after a positive or negative sFlt-1/PIGF. Based on PRAECIS trial,[5] if this ratio is used, it is applicable only for symptomatic, hospitalized patients between 23 and 35 weeks of gestation. A positive ratio of >40 is not diagnostic of preeclampsia with severe features. On the contrary, a negative ratio of <40 has a high negative predictive value (95%) for developing preeclampsia with severe features in the next 2 weeks. However, it is important to note that the ratio should not replace the current clinical criteria for diagnosing or ruling out preeclampsia with severe features. Rather, it should be considered as a complementary test to the current diagnostic workup.

PREVENTION OF PREECLAMPSIA

Unfortunately, no interventions have been unequivocally proven effective in eliminating the risk of preeclampsia at this time. The Society for Maternal-Fetal Medicine (SMFM) and ACOG support the US Preventive Services Task Force (USPSTF) guideline for prevention of preeclampsia. Low doses of aspirin (81 mg/day) initiated before 28 weeks of gestation, preferably between 12 and 16 weeks, are recommended for prophylaxis in pregnant persons at a high risk of preeclampsia **(Table 2)**. This strategy may also be considered for persons with more than one moderate risk factor **(Table 2)**.

There is no official consensus regarding the optimal dose of aspirin. Some authorities recommend a higher dosage (100–150 mg).[6,7] Furthermore, there is no consensus with regards to the timing of discontinuation of aspirin: 36th week of gestation versus at delivery. Besides aspirin, calcium supplementation (1.5–2 g/day, orally) may be considered for the prevention of preeclampsia particularly in pregnant persons with low baseline calcium intake,[8] to be commenced at the first antenatal clinic. Regarding the role of bed rest, there is currently no data to support its effectiveness[9] and, thus, it should not be routinely recommended.

ANTEPARTUM MANAGEMENT OF HYPERTENSION

Chronic Hypertension

Preconception counseling should be provided to all patients with chronic hypertension to adequately control BP, rule out possible secondary causes of hypertension **(Box 1)**, evaluate for end-organ damage, optimize comorbidities, avoid medications considered unsafe in pregnancy [angiotensin-converting enzyme inhibitors (ACEIs), angiotensin receptor blockers (ARBs), spironolactone, etc.], and inform them about the high risk of developing preeclampsia (20–50%) and other complications **(Box 2)**.[10-12]

Patients with preexisting hypertension and normal renal function who have nonsevere hypertension (140–159/90–109 mm Hg) are at low risk for cardiovascular complications. Besides initiating aspirin for preeclampsia prevention at the end of the first trimester, one should offer at-risk patients baseline preeclampsia blood and urine studies such as complete blood count (CBC), renal/liver function, and urine protein/creatinine ratio along with baseline electrocardiogram (ECG)/echocardiography **(Box 3)**. From a fetal standpoint, the pregnant patient will require early ultrasound (USG) for good pregnancy dating, serial fetal growth by USG, and antepartum fetal testing initiated from 32 weeks of gestation—particularly for patients on BP medication.

Nonpharmacological hypertension management strategies, such as dietary and lifestyle interventions, during pregnancy have minimal effect on pregnancy outcome. In some patients, BP medications are withdrawn in the first half of pregnancy due to the physiological fall in BP. However, close monitoring and resumption of treatment are essential, if necessary. In terms of treatment benefit, tight versus less-

TABLE 2: Preeclampsia risk assessment from medical history.

Risk category	Risk factors	Recommendation
High	• History of preeclampsia, especially when accompanied by an adverse outcome • Multifetal gestation • Chronic hypertension • Type 1 or 2 diabetes • Renal disease • Autoimmune disease (SLE, APLAs)	Low-dose aspirin if the patient has ≥1 of these RFs
Moderate	• Nulliparity • Obesity (BMI > 30 kg/m^2) • Family history of preeclampsia (mother/sister) • Sociodemographic features (low socioeconomic status, African-American race) • Age ≥ 35 years • Personal history factors (e.g., LBW or SGA, previous adverse pregnancy outcome, >10-year pregnancy interval)	Low-dose aspirin considered if the patient has >1 of these moderate RFs
Low	Previous uncomplicated full-term delivery	Low-dose aspirin not recommended

(APLAs: antiphospholipid antibody syndrome; BMI: body mass index; LBW: low birth weight; RFs: risk factors; SGA: small for gestational age; SLE: systemic lupus erythematosus)

BOX 1 Prediction of type of hypertension from history.

Primary hypertension:
- Gradual increase in BP with a slow rate of rise in BP
- Lifestyle factors favoring higher BP (e.g., weight gain, high dietary sodium intake, sedentary lifestyle, excessive consumption of alcohol)
- Family history of hypertension

Secondary hypertension:
- BP lability, episodic pallor, and dizziness—pheochromocytoma
- Snoring or hypersomnolence—OSA
- Weight loss, palpitations, heat intolerance—hyperthyroidism
- Muscle cramps or weakness—aldosteronism (primary or secondary) causing hypokalemia
- Edema, frequent urination, fatigue—kidney disease
- Central obesity, round face, easy bruisability—Cushing's syndrome
- History of coarctation repair, upper limb hypertension associated with coarctation
- Medication or substance use—alcohol, NSAIDs, cocaine, amphetamines
- Absence of family history of hypertension

(BP: blood pressure; NSAIDs: nonsteroidal anti-inflammatory drugs; OSA: obstructive sleep apnea)

BOX 2 Complications of chronic hypertension in pregnancy.

Maternal:
- MI
- Pulmonary edema
- Stroke
- Renal insufficiency
- Preeclampsia
- Placental abruption
- Cesarean delivery
- PPH
- Gestational diabetes
- Death

Fetal and neonatal:
- Growth retardation
- Preterm birth
- Low birth weight
- Congenital anomalies (esophageal atresia, heart defects, etc.)
- IUD
- Stillbirth or perinatal death

(IUD: intrauterine death; MI: myocardial infarction; PPH: postpartum hemorrhage)

tight control of hypertension in pregnancy in the Control of Hypertension in Pregnancy Study (CHIPS) was associated with less severe hypertension. Yet, it showed no difference in the risk of adverse perinatal outcomes and overall serious complications.[13] However, a secondary analysis of the data showed that patients developing severe hypertension had higher rates of adverse perinatal outcomes. Recent systematic review, network meta-analyses, and trial sequential analyses found that all commonly prescribed antihypertensive drugs in pregnancy reduce the risk of severe hypertension, but labetalol may also decrease the development of proteinuria/preeclampsia and fetal/newborn death.[14] In the CHAP trial—a multicenter, randomized controlled trial in pregnant persons with chronic hypertension—a strategy of targeting BP < 140/90 mm Hg was associated with better pregnancy outcomes than reserving treatment for only severe-range BP (>160/90 mm Hg) without an increased risk for fetal growth restriction.[15] Refer to **Tables 3 and 4** for common medications used for maintaining BP control in pregnancy and those used for hypertensive urgency/emergency. For long-term maintenance treatment of pregnant persons, oral labetalol and nifedipine are preferred over all other antihypertensives. Beta-blockers appear to have side effects such as fetal bradycardia, growth retardation, and hypoglycemia compared to calcium antagonists, with atenolol best avoided. The use of ACEIs, ARBs, renin inhibitors, and mineralocorticoid receptor antagonists is also best avoided. Diuretic use, though not contraindicated, is usually not preferred in pregnancy in the absence of pulmonary edema because it results in intravascular volume depletion.

BOX 3 Basic laboratory tests for evaluation of chronic hypertension in pregnancy.

- CBC
- Serum AST and ALT
- Serum creatinine
- BUN
- Serum electrolytes, especially potassium
- Spot urine protein:creatinine ratio or 24-hour urine total protein and creatinine as indicated
- TFT
- ECG and echocardiogram as appropriate

(ALT: alanine aminotransferase; AST: aspartate aminotransferase; BUN: blood urea nitrogen; CBC: complete blood count; ECG: electrocardiogram; TFT: thyroid function test)

Diagnostic uncertainty often arises in differentiating between transient severe-range elevation of BP in a patient with chronic hypertension, superimposed preeclampsia in absence of symptoms, and laboratory findings suggestive of preeclampsia with severe features. In this difficult situation, the clinician should presume preeclampsia first and evaluate the pregnant patient in an inpatient setting with fetal heart rate monitoring, USG for fetal growth, serial preeclampsia blood/urine studies, and serial BP assessment at frequent intervals. In the absence of severe-range BP, these patients are delivered at 37–39 weeks of gestation **(Table 5)**.

TABLE 3: Common oral antihypertensive medications used in pregnancy.

Drug	Initiation dose	Maximum dosage	Remarks
Labetalol	100–200 mg twice daily	200–2,400 mg/day in two to three divided doses	• Potential bronchoconstrictive effects • Avoided in women with asthma, known myocardial disease, bradycardia, heart block
Nifedipine	30–60 mg once daily (extended release)	30–120 mg/day extended-release preparation	• Do not use sublingual form • Immediate-release formulation reserved for control of severe acutely elevated blood pressure in hospitalized patients
Methyldopa	250 mg twice or three times daily	500–3,000 mg/day in two to four divided doses	• Side effects: Depression, sedation, dizziness • Not very effective in control of severe hypertension compared to other drugs
Hydrochlorothiazide		25–50 mg daily	Second- or third-line agent

TABLE 4: Antihypertensive drugs used for acute blood pressure control in pregnancy.

Drug	Route	Dosage	Onset of action	Remarks
Labetalol	IV	10–20 mg and then 20–80 mg every 10–30 minutes to a maximum cumulative dose of 300 mg; or constant infusion 1–2 mg/min	1–2 minutes	• Less adverse effects than with other agents • Avoided in women with asthma, known myocardial disease, bradycardia, heart block
Hydralazine	IV/IM	5 mg IV or IM, and then 5–10 mg IV every 20–40 minutes to a maximum cumulative dose of 20 mg; or constant infusion of 0.5–10 mg/h	10–20 minutes	Higher or frequent dosage causes maternal hypotension, headache, and abnormal FHR tracings
Nifedipine (immediate release)	Oral	10–20 mg, repeat in 20 minutes if required; then 10–20 mg every 2–6 hours; maximum daily dose is 180 mg	5–10 minutes	

(FHR: fetal heart rate; IM: intramuscularly; IV: intravenously)

TABLE 5: Recommendations for timing of delivery.

Hypertensive disorders of pregnancy	General timing	Precise timing
Chronic hypertension: Isolated, uncomplicated, controlled without medications	Early term/full term	38 0/7 to 39 6/7 weeks of gestation
Chronic hypertension: Isolated, uncomplicated, controlled with medications	Early term/full term	37 0/7 to 39 6/7 weeks of gestation
Chronic hypertension: Difficult to control—requiring frequent drug adjustments	Late preterm/early term	36 0/7 to 37 6/7 weeks of gestation
Gestational hypertension, without severe-range BP	Early term	37 0/7 weeks of gestation or at diagnosis if diagnosed later
Gestational hypertension, with severe-range BP	Late preterm	34 0/7 weeks of gestation or at diagnosis if diagnosed later
Preeclampsia without severe features	Early term	37 0/7 weeks of gestation or at diagnosis if diagnosed later
Preeclampsia with severe features, stable maternal and fetal conditions, after fetal viability including superimposed preeclampsia	Late preterm	34 0/7 weeks of gestation or at diagnosis if diagnosed later
Preeclampsia with severe features, unstable or complicated, after fetal viability—including superimposed preeclampsia and HELLP	Soon after maternal stabilization	Soon after maternal stabilization
Preeclampsia with severe features, before viability	Soon after maternal stabilization	Soon after maternal stabilization

(BP: blood pressure; HELLP: hemolysis, elevated liver enzymes, low platelet)

Gestational Hypertension/Preeclampsia without Severe Features/Chronic Hypertension with Superimposed Preeclampsia without Severe Features

These three conditions are considered as mild hypertensive diseases of pregnancy with similar modes of management. Most of these patients are seen on an outpatient basis, with weekly prenatal visits for evaluation. Fetal monitoring includes weekly antepartum testing and USG for amniotic fluid volume along with fetal growth assessment once a month. Evaluation of the pregnant patient consists of blood/urine studies (platelet count, serum creatinine, liver enzymes, and urine protein) and monitoring for signs and symptoms of severe disease, including BP. However, if there is a suspicion of disease progression, the blood work is repeated sooner. If outpatient monitoring remains reassuring, delivery can be planned at 37 0/7 weeks of gestation **(Table 5)**.

Gestational Hypertension with Severe-range BP/Preeclampsia with Severe Features/Chronic Hypertension with Superimposed Preeclampsia with Severe Features

These conditions are considered to be severe diseases associated with grave prognoses if not promptly addressed. They should always be managed as inpatients with frequent monitoring of BP, symptoms of severe disease, and preeclampsia laboratories. Treatment within 30–60 minutes of persistent (>15 minutes) severe-range BP (>160/90 mm Hg) should be prioritized to avoid complications. To treat severe-range BP, intravenous labetalol or hydralazine and oral nifedipine are the most commonly used drugs. Sublingual administration of short-acting nifedipine is contraindicated. Sodium nitroprusside is usually avoided for hypertensive urgency/emergency as its prolonged use is associated with fetal cyanide poisoning. A recent Cochrane systematic review found no significant difference with regards to safety and efficacy between hydralazine and labetalol or between hydralazine and calcium channel blocker.[16] As their clinical status can deteriorate fast, these patients are always delivered by 34 0/7 weeks of gestation. If their condition allows expectant management for 48 hours, steroids are given for fetal lung maturity prior to delivery. As noted in **Table 5**, if there are circumstances such as fetal demise or pulmonary edema, these patients are delivered right away irrespective of steroid prophylaxis. Only when the symptoms of severe disease completely resolve, BP remains controlled with or without medicines, and preeclampsia blood work normalizes, one can offer expectant management till 34 0/7 weeks of gestation.

INTRAPARTUM

Delivery in pregnant patients with mild hypertensive disease is associated with improved outcomes. This includes gestational hypertension without severe-range BP, chronic hypertension with or without mild superimposed preeclampsia when on BP medications, and preeclampsia without severe features beyond 37 weeks of gestation. On the contrary, severe preeclampsia requires prompt delivery, particularly after 34 0/7 weeks of gestation. In patients with eclamptic seizure, immediate delivery is recommended after the patient is stabilized. Vaginal delivery is the preferred route for most of these patients. The decision to perform cesarean delivery should be made individually, based on the anticipated probability of successful vaginal delivery and on the nature and rate of progression of the preeclampsia disease state in the presence of severe features.

In addition to managing labor, two other important goals of intrapartum management are controlling severe-range BP and preventing seizures in patients with severe disease. During labor and delivery, antihypertensive treatment should continue with the aim of keeping systolic BP < 160 mm Hg and diastolic BP < 90 mm Hg. For patients with severe disease, IV magnesium should be given for seizure prophylaxis, which is continued intrapartum and the first 24 hours postpartum. Regarding labor analgesia or anesthesia, regional block is preferred over general anesthesia; however, regional block is contraindicated in the presence of platelet count < 70,000/mL, coagulopathy, or anticoagulant use.[17] General anesthesia is generally avoided in HDP because of increased risk of aspiration, failed intubation from pharyngolaryngeal edema, and stroke from elevation of BP during both intubation and extubation.

POSTPARTUM CARE

Hypertensive disorders of pregnancy may begin antepartum or they can be of new onset during the postpartum period. One must be cognizant of transient elevation in BP in patients who were previously normotensive. This could be due to pain (because of inadequate analgesia), drugs (nonsteroidal anti-inflammatory drugs, ergots, or ephedrine), intravenous fluids, mobilization of extravascular fluid into the intravascular compartment, or restoration of nonpregnant vascular tone. Mild hypertension postpartum usually resolves spontaneously. However, late-presentation preeclampsia is a possibility and should not ignored; inadequate treatment leads to higher readmission rates and increased morbidity and mortality. As in the antepartum period, the preferred medication used for postpartum BP management is nifedipine or labetalol. In comparison to labetalol, the hospital readmission rate is lower with nifedipine.[18] ACEIs and ARBs are usually avoided, particularly during lactation. When needed for specific indications, one may safely use certain ACEIs such as enalapril. Diuretics must be used with caution, as they will decrease milk production. For postpartum pain control, NSAIDs are preferred over opioid analgesics; although there is theoretical concern about the worsening of BP with their use, overall data support their safety for use in the postpartum period in patients with HDP.[19,20]

In addition to adequate BP control, IV magnesium should be initiated or continued for at least 24 hours from the time of delivery, for seizure prophylaxis in patients with severe HDP. Breastfeeding, apart from providing optimal nutrition for newborns, has many important benefits for patients who are at risk of future cardiovascular diseases (CVDs). Longer breastfeeding duration can provide protective effects against preclinical CVDs.[21] Therefore, healthcare professionals should provide relevant education on lactation-associated cardiovascular benefits to promote and support breastfeeding for this high-risk population.

SUBSEQUENT CARDIOVASCULAR DISEASE AND PREVENTION STRATEGIES

Patients with hypertensive disease of pregnancy have a nearly twofold long-term increased risk for CVD.[22-24] This includes risk for chronic hypertension, myocardial infarction, congestive heart failure, stroke, peripheral arterial disease, and cardiovascular mortality. The risk is higher in patients who have had severe preeclampsia, earlier disease onset, and recurring disease. The exact mechanism which accounts for this increased risk for CVD remains unexplained; therefore, these patients require long-term follow-up and lifestyle modifications. The American Heart Association (AHA) has proposed a transition of postpartum care for patients with HDP from their obstetricians to their primary care providers starting 3 months after delivery to assess cardiovascular risk factors.[25] It has additionally been emphasized that thorough documentation of pregnancy complications in medical records and coordination between obstetricians and primary care providers or cardiologists are key for optimal care. For patients with a past record of preterm preeclampsia or recurrent preeclampsia, the ACOG recommends annual assessment of their blood pressure, BMI, glucose, and lipid profile.[26]

CONCLUSION

Globally, HDP are a major cause of morbidity and mortality in the pregnant patient and fetus. The development of more accurate screening tools coupled with targeted aspirin prophylaxis could significantly reduce the number of cases of preterm preeclampsia. Placental growth factor–based testing has been shown to improve the accuracy of preeclampsia diagnosis in patients with HDP and identification of those patients at the highest risk of complications. Future research may offer further refinement of disease phenotypes and progress in the development of much-needed treatments to ameliorate the disease process and prolong gestation in preterm preeclampsia. Although the link between HDP and CVD is well established, the most effective screening strategy and the types of interventions that can help reduce future risk of CVD remain unproven. Further research is required if we are to improve the long-term CVD profile for the millions of patients affected by HDP today.

ONLINE REFERENCES

Please scan the QR code provided at the end of the table of contents for References of this chapter.

CHAPTER 48

Grappling with Hypertension Management in the Old, Very Old, and Frail Patients: A Double-edged Sword

C Venkata S Ram

ABSTRACT

Hypertension management recommendations for older and frail patients are largely derived from trials involving younger or relatively healthy patients, with methodology intended to determine when the benefit for treatment initiation is reached. Many of these "healthy" older patients benefit from intensive blood pressure (BP) management. There is, however, a paucity of prospective data on intensive BP management in "real-world" older patients in whom comorbidities and polypharmacy are the norm. In complex and frail older patients, it is becoming clear that intensive management is often inappropriate and may cause harm as one size does not fit all. Good clinical judgment is therefore critical to individualize management in a way that is appropriate to the patient's circumstances, improves their quality of life (QoL), and is cognizant of their values, goals, and concerns.

Keywords: Hypertension, elderly, frailty, orthostatic hypotension, personalized medicine

INTRODUCTION

Hypertension becomes increasingly common with advancing age. In an American cohort, the prevalence of systolic blood pressure (SBP) ≥ 140 mm Hg or diastolic blood pressure (DBP) ≥ 90 mm Hg was 27.3% in participants aged < 60 years and 71% in those aged ≥ 80 years.[1] As populations age, the proportion of people with elevated blood pressure (BP) levels increases. In India, there were 15 million people aged ≥ 80 years in 2023, with the number projected to increase to 55.9 million in 2050.[2]

Elevated BP levels in aging populations have enormous healthcare repercussions. The relationship between increasing BP levels and the risk of stroke, coronary artery disease, arrhythmias, heart failure (HF), and chronic kidney disease is continuous and applicable to all ages and ethnicities.[3] Throughout middle and older age, elevated BP levels are strongly and directly linked to cardiovascular (CV) and all-cause mortality, without evidence of a threshold until at least 115/75 mm Hg.[4] Elevated SBP was the second leading contributor to global disease burden in 2021.[5] Elevated BP levels are also a modifiable risk factor for dementia and loss of autonomy later in life.[6,7]

Stiffening of the arterial wall **(Table 1)**, resulting in decreased capacitance and limited recoil through the cardiac cycle, is the major cause of elevated SBP in patients aged > 60 years.[7,8] Concurrently, DBP tends to stabilize or decrease beyond age 60 years, leading to an increase in pulse pressure.[7] Older patients often display increased sensitivity to sodium, causing vasoconstriction and increased peripheral vascular resistance.[9] Age-related reductions in the glomerular filtration rate (GFR) can also potentiate the effects of medical treatment, including antihypertensive drugs. Later in life, reduced left ventricular compliance and cardiac fibrosis may result in diminished cardiac output during physical activity and reduced venous return.[9]

Importantly for hypertension management, age-related reductions in baroreflex sensitivity may increase the risk of orthostatic hypotension. In a large cohort,

TABLE 1: Cardiorenal neurohemodynamic factors in the elderly.

↑ Arterial stiffness (pulse pressure)	Cardiac fibrosis
↓ Baroreflex sensitivity	↓ Musculoskeletal mobility
Postprandial hypotension	BP fluctuations
↑ Sensitivity to salt	↓ GFR
↓ Cognition	↓ Postural BP

(BP: blood pressure; GFR: glomerular filtration rate)

orthostatic hypotension was present in 6.9% of people aged ≥ 50 years, and in 18.5% of those aged ≥ 80 years.[10] Likewise, postprandial hypotension may emerge later in life, with both forms of hypotension potentially being asymptomatic at younger ages when cerebral blood flow can be maintained by autoregulatory mechanisms.[9]

While elevated BP levels become more common with advancing age, there is also evidence that BP decreases in the last years of life.[11] In 46,634 participants with an average age of death of 82.4 years, both SBP and DBP peaked 14–18 years before death and then progressively declined, with the steepest decrease occurring in the last 2 years of life. Overall, 64% of participants experienced a decrease in SBP > –10 mm Hg, which was not attributable to antihypertensive treatment. This particular understanding is very important from a management perspective.

EVIDENCE THAT TREATMENT IMPROVES OUTCOMES IN THE ELDERLY

It is now known that the age-related increase in BP levels can be blunted via the early introduction of antihypertensive therapy.[12,13] Furthermore, randomized, placebo-controlled trials provide robust evidence that treating elevated BP decreases CV events in patients aged ≥ 60 years.[14-19] More recently, the Hypertension in the Very Elderly Trial (HYVET) found that in patients aged ≥ 80 years, treating hypertension resulted in a 30% reduction in strokes, a 21% reduction in all-cause mortality, and a 64% reduction in HF, compared to placebo.[20]

The landmark Systolic Blood Pressure Intervention Trial (SPRINT) investigated intensive BP management (SBP < 120 mm Hg) versus standard management (SBP < 140 mm Hg) in ambulatory, nondiabetic patients aged ≥ 75 years.[21] Through a median of 3.14 years, the mean SBP was 123.4 mm Hg in the intensive treatment arm and 134.8 mm Hg in the standard treatment arm. The intensive target was associated with significantly lower rates of nonfatal and fatal major adverse CV events (MACE) and all-cause mortality. Further exploratory analysis suggested that this benefit extended to participants who were frail or had reduced gait speed **(Fig. 1)**. The overall rate of serious adverse effects was 48.4% and 48.3% in the intensive and standard arms, respectively. Specifically, the rates of hypotension (2.4% vs. 1.4%), syncope (3.0% vs. 2.4%), electrolyte abnormalities (4.0% vs. 2.7%), and renal events (5.5% vs. 4.0%) were all higher in the intensive arm but not statistically significantly different between the groups.

Secondary analysis of SPRINT found that patients with higher baseline Montreal Cognitive Assessment (MoCA) scores derived a strong benefit from intensive BP treatment, as measured by a composite of CV disease (CVD) and mortality ($p < 0.001$), whereas there was no appreciable benefit in patients with lower MoCA scores.[22]

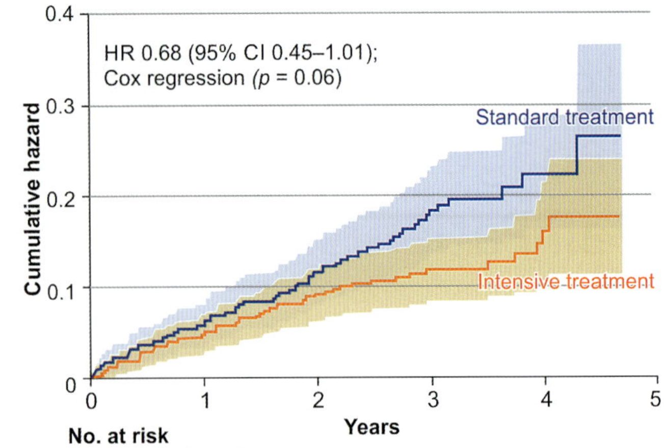

No. at risk
Type of treatment

Standard	375	338	305	177	49
Intensive	440	398	371	223	71

FIG. 1: Cumulative hazard for nonfatal and fatal MACE and all-cause mortality in frail patients in SPRINT receiving standard or intensive blood pressure treatment.

(MACE: major adverse cardiovascular events; SPRINT: Systolic Blood Pressure Intervention Trial)

Source: Adapted from Williamson et al.[21]

A second study, SPRINT MIND, assessed the effect of intensive BP control on the risk of probable dementia.[23] Over a median of 5.1 years, intensive treatment did not significantly reduce the risk of dementia; however, it did reduce the risk of mild cognitive impairment. SPRINT MIND was terminated early due to the reduction in CV events in the intensive treatment arm.

Most recently, the Strategy of Blood Pressure Intervention in Elderly Hypertensive Patients (STEP) trial randomized patients aged 60–80 years to a SBP target of 110 to <130 or 130 to <150 mm Hg.[24] The primary outcome was a composite of stroke, acute coronary syndrome, decompensated HF, coronary revascularization, atrial fibrillation, or CV mortality. Significantly fewer CV events were reported in patients receiving intensive treatment **(Fig. 2)**, with similar rates of adverse effects and renal outcomes, other than hypotension, which was more frequent in the intensive arm.

Post hoc analysis of STEP revealed that the CV risk was significantly lower in the patients in the intensive arm who achieved the SBP target, compared with those in the standard treatment arm who achieved the target ($p < 0.001$).[25] Furthermore, patients in the intensive treatment arm who were unable to meet the target had approximately double the CV risk as those in the same arm who did meet the target.

Confounding Effect of Frailty

Frailty is a multifaceted clinical concept with components that can change over time.[7,26] It is defined as a multisystem, multidimensional condition characterized by decreased functional reserves and increased vulnerability to stress and acute adverse events.[27] It is distinct but may overlap with multimorbidity, disability, and dementia. Frailty is itself an independent risk factor for adverse CV outcomes **(Figs. 3A and B)**, including in older patients without CVD.[27-29]

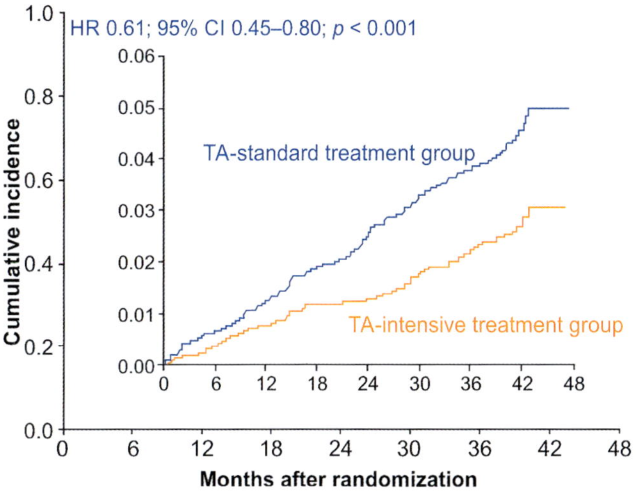

FIG. 2: Cumulative incidence of the primary outcome in target-achieved subgroups.

Source: Adapted from Deng et al. (2023).

The prevalence of frailty is estimated at 7% of the general population.[30]

Despite SPRINT findings of a potential CV mortality and all-cause mortality benefit associated with intensive BP management in frail patients, the extent of this effect remains to be determined as many frail patients were excluded from the trial.[21,31] Longitudinal data from a large cohort aged ≥ 75 years indicate a U-shaped correlation between SBP and DBP with mortality, with higher SBP associated with lower mortality in participants with impaired activities of daily living (ADL).[28] A similar relationship was reported with impaired Mini-Mental State Examination (MMSE).[28] Prospective analysis of the primary healthcare records of a large dataset found that BP < 130/80 mm Hg in patients aged ≥ 75 years was associated with excess mortality, while SBP 150–159 mm Hg was not associated with increased mortality beyond age 85 years or in patients aged 75–84 years with moderate/severe frailty.[32] Another study also reported a tendency toward reduced all-cause mortality in older frail patients with SBP ≥ 130 mm Hg, suggestive of a protective effect.[33] Data from the Atherosclerosis Risk in Communities (ARIC) also show that while SBP ≥ 140 mm Hg was associated with mortality in participants with good function aged < 65 and ≥65 years, hypertension was not associated with mortality in those with impaired function aged < 65 years,

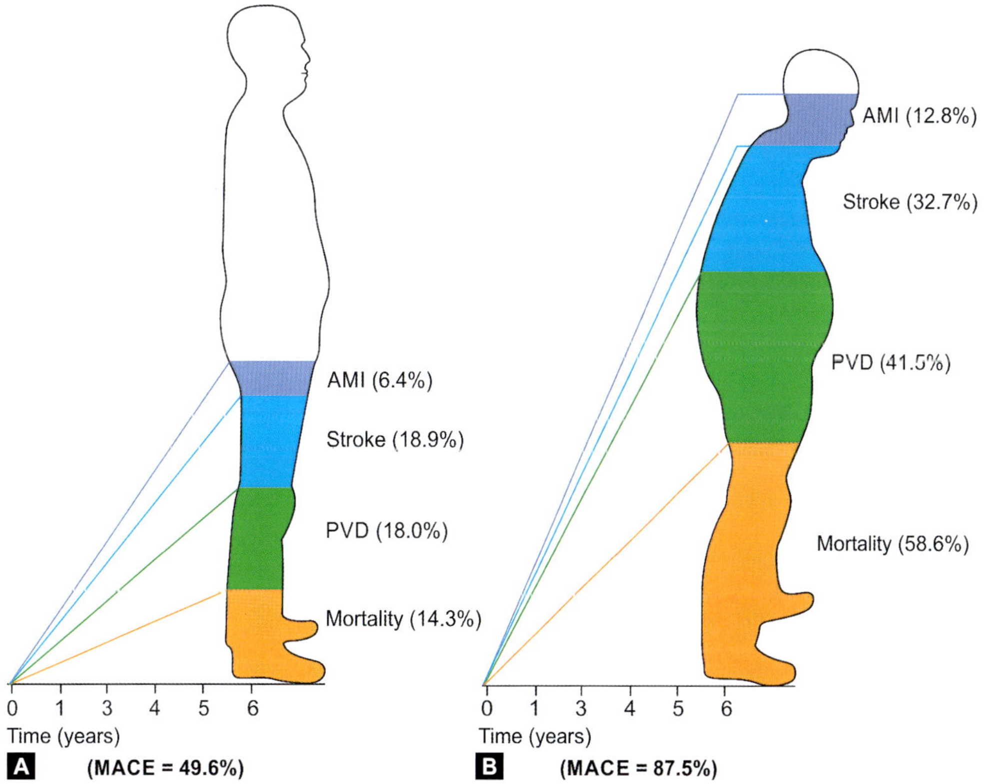

FIGS. 3A AND B: The cumulative incidence of CV outcomes in (A) frail and (B) nonfrail people aged ≥ 65 years over 6 years of follow-up from the National Health and Aging Trends Study (NHATS).

(AMI: acute myocardial infarction; CV: cardiovascular; MACE: major adverse cardiovascular events; PVD: peripheral vascular disease)

Source: Adapted from Damluji et al.[29]

and in participants with impaired function aged ≥ 65 years, hypertension was protective against mortality.[34] Notably, another observational study found that while frailty is a strong risk factor for all-cause and CV mortality, in frail patients there was no association between traditional risk factors and mortality, and frailty could not be used to identify patients who might benefit from CV risk management.[35]

PROBLEM WITH CLINICAL TRIALS

Most clinical trials exclude frail patients or those aged > 80 years or with comorbidities, including orthostatic hypotension and dementia.[6,36] In reality, many older patients have quite different clinical characteristics and medical histories than those enrolled in trials, making it hard for clinicians to balance the risks and benefits of treatment **(Fig. 4)**. For example, SPRINT excluded patients with diabetes, previous stroke, symptomatic HF, dementia, expected survival < 3 years, recent unintentional weight loss, and orthostatic hypotension and those residing in nursing homes.[21] Interestingly, analysis of The Irish Longitudinal Study on Ageing (TILDA) using SPRINT eligibility criteria found that community-dwelling participants aged ≥ 75 years had rates of syncope and injurious falls approximately fivefold higher than those in the standard care group in SPRINT.[37]

Intensive Control and Adverse Outcomes

The potential for harm in older frail patients due to hypertensive management strategies formulated from relatively healthy populations is increasingly clear. Data from the Berlin Initiative Study shows that in patients with a mean age of 81 years, BP levels < 140/90 mm Hg were associated with an increased risk of all-cause mortality, compared to non-normalized levels (60.3 vs. 48.5 per 1,000/year; HR 1.26; 95% CI 1.04–1.54).[39] An increased mortality risk was also reported in patients aged ≥ 80 years and those with previous CV events, but not in patients aged 70–79 years or those without prior CV events.

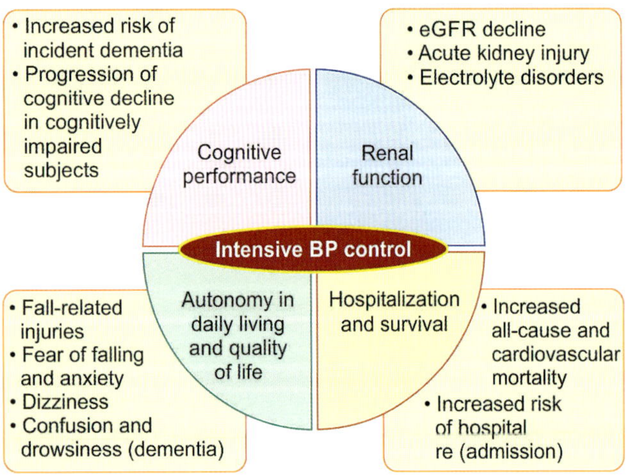

FIG. 4: Potential risks of intensive blood pressure (BP) control in older adults.

Source: Adapted from Rivasi et al.[38]

Intensive BP control often requires aggressive treatment and a high medication burden. A post hoc analysis of the STEP trial found that treatment with three or more different antihypertensive medicines was associated with worse SBP control and an increased risk of adverse CV outcomes, compared to low medication burden.[40] This effect was consistent in both the intensive and the standard treatment arms. Another study of nursing home residents aged > 80 years reported a significant interaction between SBP < 130 mm Hg and treatment with ≥2 antihypertensive medicines and increased mortality, compared to other residents ($p < 0.001$).[41]

Incomplete Reporting of Adverse Effects

There is also evidence that the adverse effects of antihypertensive treatment in older patients may be under-reported in clinical trials due to study methodology. However, a meta-analysis identified four high-quality trials of intensive antihypertensive treatment in patients aged ≥ 65 years.[42] Compared with standard strategies, intensive treatment was associated with a 29% reduction in MACE, a 33% reduction in CV mortality, and a 37% reduction in HF, with no difference in rates of stroke or myocardial infarction (MI). Data on adverse events, however, were limited, not uniform and event definitions varied across trials. Overall, the results suggested an increased risk of renal failure associated with intensive treatment and a possibility of increased hypotension and syncope. A subgroup analysis of SPRINT found that in participants with an estimated GFR ≥ 60 mL/min/1.73 m^2, intensive SBP-lowering therapy increased the risk of renal events, although this was outweighed by the CV and all-cause mortality benefits **(Fig. 5)**.[43]

PRECISION MEDICINE: THIS IS THE WAY FORWARD

Comorbidities are present in >80% of people by age 85 years, with approximately half having ≥4 medical conditions and one in five having ≥6 medical conditions.[44,45] Comorbidities inevitably mean polypharmacy and approximately 20% of adults aged ≥ 65 years in the community can be expected to be taking >10 daily medicines.[46] Polypharmacy is itself a risk factor for hypertension, HF, electrolyte disturbances, falls, hospitalization, and premature mortality.[47]

Due to the functional heterogeneity of older patients as a cohort and the clinical complexity of some individuals **(Box 1)**, a "one-size-fits all" approach to BP management not only is inappropriate but may also cause iatrogenic harm. Best practice therefore requires an individualized approach, with biological age being of greater clinical significance than chronological age.[13,31]

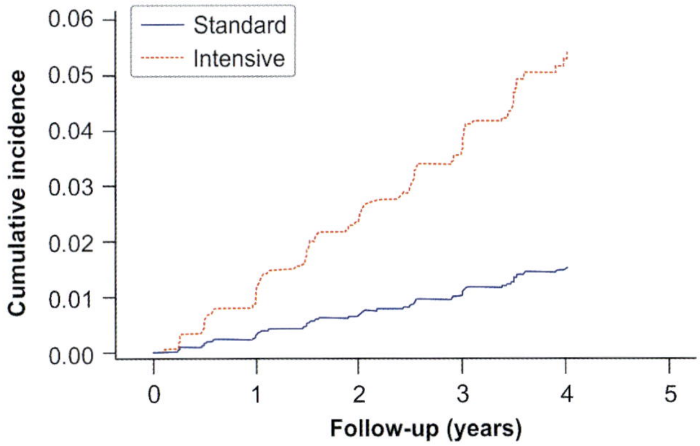

FIG. 5: Cumulative incidence of incident chronic kidney disease in the standard and intensive treatment arms of SPRINT.

(SPRINT: Systolic Blood Pressure Intervention Trial)

Source: Adapted from Beddhu et al.[43]

BOX 1 **Special considerations and unknown factors in elderly patients.**

- Orthostatic hypotension
- Falls
- Mobility
- Cognitive function
- Comorbidities
- Polypharmacy
- Dementia, cognitive input
- Decreased life expectancy (<2 years)
- History of falls
- Mobility disorders
- Frailty

An individualized approach begins with shared decision-making. This requires consideration of the patient's circumstances, including their values, goals, concerns, and quality of life (QoL).[9] Patients should be provided with easily understandable information on which to base decisions about their care. Shared decision-making may improve safety, treatment adherence, and patient satisfaction, and it may also save health resources.[7,9] The precision medicine or personalized medicine vis-à-vis standard individualized medicine may offer significant benefit in future care, as the machine learning or deep learning from big data from multiple inputs like clinical findings, genomics, protein omics, and transcriptomes will guide a clinician in selecting a specific medicine or group medicines in a particular patient.

HOW LOW TO GO?

The European Society of Hypertension (ESH) (2023) recommendations for BP targets in older patients are provided in **Table 2**.[3] There are, however, several safety qualifications:[3]

TABLE 2: BP targets for older groups of patients.

Patients	Recommendation	CoR
Aged 65–79 years	The primary goal of treatment is to lower BP < 140/80 mm Hg	I
	Lowering SBP < 130 mm Hg may be considered if treatment is well tolerated	
Aged 65–79 years with ISH	The primary goal is to lower SBP to 140–150 mm Hg and DBP < 80 mm Hg	I
	Lowering office SBP to 130–139 mm Hg may be considered if well tolerated, but cautiously if DBP is already < 70 mm Hg	II
Aged ≥ 80 years	Lower office SBP to 140–150 mm Hg and DBP < 80 mm Hg	I
	Lowering SBP to 130–139 mm Hg may be considered if treatment is well-tolerated, but cautiously if DBP is already <70 mm Hg	II
Frail	The target for office SBP and DBP should be individualized	I

(BP: blood pressure; CoR: class of recommendation; DBP: diastolic blood pressure; ISH: isolated systolic hypertension; SBP: systolic blood pressure)

Source: Adapted from Mancia et al.[3]

- Do not aim for office SBP < 120 mm Hg or DBP < 70 mm Hg.
- In patients with DBP < 70 mm Hg, SBP should still be lowered, but cautiously, if on-treatment SBP is still well above target.
- Reducing treatment can be considered in patients aged ≥ 80 years with SBP < 120 mm Hg or in the presence of severe orthostatic hypotension or a high level of frailty.

A Pragmatic Approach: Choosing the Middle Course

In older or frail patients with recently diagnosed hypertension, a thorough history and examination should confirm that the elevation is persistent, exclude secondary causes, detect any orthostatic hypotension, and assess the patient's global CV risk and functional status (see the section "Identifying Frailty").[7,8] Older patients who are already receiving antihypertensive treatment should also be regularly assessed for frailty.

Lifestyle modifications, including appropriate mild exercise, ideally in a group setting, should be introduced alongside antihypertensive therapy in older or frail patients.[3] Weight loss in patients aged > 80 years should be avoided, except for those who are obese. Salt restriction is also not

TABLE 3: Factors affecting medication adherence in the elderly.

Forgetfulness	Medical domain
Polypharmacy	Physical domain
Personal "beliefs"	Cognitive domain
Adverse effects	Social domain
Psychological status	

recommended as it may lead to a loss of appetite, although individuals with NaCl consumption > 10 g/day can be advised to restrict their intake.[3]

For each medicine introduced, consideration should be given to the following:[47]

- Do the potential benefits outweigh the potential adverse effects, including drug–drug interactions?
- Is the patient likely to benefit given his/her life expectancy?
- Is the medicine superior to all other medicines or nonpharmacological interventions?

Initiating antihypertensive medicines in older patients is a risk factor for falls.[48] The "start low, go slow" mantra should therefore be adopted, with gradual dose titration and frequent monitoring to detect adverse effects, especially orthostatic hypotension.[8,47]

Nonadherence is reported to increase beyond 80 years, possibly due to declining cognitive function, depression, evolving goals and beliefs, probable familial apathy, and potentially adverse effects **(Table 3)**.[9] In older frail patients, adherence to antihypertensive treatment appears to be protective against CV and all-cause mortality.[49] Strategies to improve treatment adherence include the provision of appropriate educational material, the use of combination medicines, regimen simplification, medication compliance aids, regular follow-up, discussions with caregivers, electronic reminders, and telemedicine.[3,7,8,26]

Step-down Therapy

The decision to step-down medicines should be individualized and requires an understanding of the patient's values and consideration of the benefits and risks associated with each treatment. High-quality communication is necessary to ensure that the patients and their families do not feel abandoned or misunderstand the strategy. Step-down therapy may be appropriate in patients with a history of falls, cognitive impairment, frailty, immobility, significant orthostatic hypotension, and life expectancy < 2 years or in patients aged ≥ 80 years with SBP < 120 mm Hg.[3,7] Where possible, antihypertensive medicine withdrawal should be tapered to prevent rebound hypertension.[47]

Little evidence is available on the effects of stepping-down antihypertensive medicines in older patients. Withdrawing diuretics removes a significant risk factor for electrolyte disorders, including hypokalemia and hyponatremia. Withdrawing low-dose beta-blockers appears to have little effect on BP, at least over a 12-week period.[50] A meta-analysis found no evidence of an effect on all-cause mortality and MI following discontinuation of antihypertensive medicines for the primary prevention of CVD, although the evidence was "low" to "very low" certainty.[51]

Identifying Frailty

Many different screening tools have been created to identify frailty. The Essential Frailty Toolset was developed for patients undergoing coronary bypass surgery by assessing strength, cognitive ability, nutritional status, and a multisystem proxy. Other screening tools include the 5-minute gait speed test, the handgrip strength test, the Physical Activity Questionnaire, the Fried Frailty Index, and the Clinical Frailty Scale.

CONCLUSION

With advancing age, the severity and complexity of medical conditions increases, thereby increasing the complexity of care. Within aging populations, the need for precision medicine continues to grow, as does the need for sound clinical judgment to individualize care for old, very old, and fragile patients. Managing hypertension in these patients is certainly not an "all-or-none phenomenon"; rather, it is deciding how to best treat individuals.

ACKNOWLEDGMENT

The author thanks Mr Mark Caswell for his expert editorial assistance and verification of the source references.

ONLINE REFERENCES

Please scan the QR code provided at the end of the table of contents for References of this chapter.

CHAPTER 49

Chronic Orthostatic Intolerance and POTS Syndrome: Update 2024

Sura Kishore Mishra, Siddhartha Pandey

ABSTRACT

Chronic orthostatic intolerance (COI) and postural orthostatic tachycardia syndrome (POTS) are disorders frequently involving young females with disabling symptoms of orthostatic intolerance, such as lightheadedness, fatigue, headache, exercise intolerance, dyspnea, and tachycardia. The symptom onset is precipitated when the patient assumes an upright posture. Chronic orthostatic intolerance with tachycardia is termed POTS. Various etiological factors have been proposed for COI and POTS and treatment is planned as per the pathophysiological mechanism involved.

Keywords: COI, POTS, exercise intolerance.

INTRODUCTION

Chronic orthostatic intolerance (COI) is defined as "the development of symptoms of orthostatic intolerance like light-headedness, headache, fatigue, neurocognitive/sleep disorders, exercise intolerance, weakness, hyperpnea/dyspnea, tremulousness, nausea/abdominal pain, and sweating without tachycardia during upright posture and relieved by recumbence". The various forms of chronic orthostatic intolerance have been discussed in the subsequent section.[1] COI is usually seen in patients of the younger age group (14–50 years), 75–80% of which are women.[2]

Postural orthostatic tachycardia syndrome (POTS) is a multisystem disorder involving the autonomic nervous system and has symptoms of orthostatic intolerance and tachycardia while standing without hypotension, and the symptoms improve after returning to supine position.[3]

DEFINITION AND DIAGNOSTIC CRITERIA

POTS

- Defined by major international neurologic, autonomic, cardiac, and pediatric societies as:[3] A sustained increase in heart rate (HR) of more than 30 beats/min within 10 minutes of standing or head-up tilt. For the age group of 12–19 years, the required HR increment is at least 40 beats/min.
- An absence of orthostatic hypotension [i.e., no sustained systolic blood pressure (BP) drop of 20 mm Hg or more]
- Frequent symptoms of orthostatic intolerance during standing, with rapid improvement upon return to the supine position. Symptoms may include light-headedness, palpitations, tremulousness, generalized weakness, blurred vision, and fatigue.
- Symptoms for a duration of at least 3 months
- Ruling out other causes of sinus tachycardia such as anxiety disorders, hyperventilation, anorexia nervosa, anemia, fever, pain, dehydration, infection, hyperthyroidism, pheochromocytoma, medications, or severe deconditioning due to prolonged bedrest

POTS Plus

POTS Plus includes all the criteria for POTS; however, in addition, these patients can have noncardiovascular symptoms. These symptoms include:

- Nausea, vomiting, food intolerances, and gastric hyper- or hypomobility (diarrhea or constipation)
- Headache, paresthesia, numbness, neuropathic pain, bladder/incontinence, and urinary retention
- Severe chronic pain
- Joint hypermobility
- Flushing/anaphylaxis symptoms

Postural Symptoms without Tachycardia

Postural symptoms without tachycardia (PSWT) includes patients with orthostatic symptoms without tachycardia, along with additional non-cardiovascular symptoms similar to POTS plus.

Postural Tachycardia of Other Cause

Patients with postural tachycardia of other cause (PTOC) have all the criteria for POTS, but there is a secondary cause for the excessive orthostatic tachycardia that excludes a diagnosis of POTS. Underlying conditions include:

- Anemia and hypovolemia (dehydration or blood loss)
- Endocrine disorders like Addison's disease, hyperthyroidism, pheochromocytoma, and Cushing syndrome
- Anxiety and panic attacks
- Medications
- Recreational drugs
- Prolonged or sustained bed rest

CLINICAL ASSOCIATIONS AND PATHOPHYSIOLOGICAL MECHANISM OF POTS

A number of pathophysiological mechanisms have been proposed in patients with POTS, including autonomic dysfunction,[4] hypovolemia,[5] hyperadrenergic stimulation,[6] and deconditioning.[7] Patients with POTS have associated positive autoantibodies, and about 20% of them have a history of an autoimmune disorder such as Hashimoto's thyroiditis, rheumatoid arthritis, or Sjögren syndrome.[8,9] Recently, some research has shown the presence of autoantibodies against G-protein-coupled receptors in patients with POTS. These antibodies include anti-adrenergic receptor antibodies (anti-ADR) and anti-muscarinic receptor antibodies. The most common pattern of involvement was anti-ADR (ADR-R A1) antibodies, while the elevation of anti-muscarinic receptor antibodies was dependent on anti-ADR antibodies.[10] There has been an association between immune dysfunction and POTS that includes post-infectious [Ebstein–Barr virus, mycoplasma, or severe acute respiratory syndrome coronavirus 2 (SARS-CoV-2)][11,12] or autoimmune disorders (celiac disease, Hashimoto's disease, Sjögren syndrome, and systemic lupus erythematosus).[8,13, 14] The incidence of POTS in survivors of COVID is around 2–14% and around 60% of patients experience POTS-like symptoms, such as tachycardia and palpitations, within 6–8 months after infection. Ehler–Danlos syndrome has also been associated with POTS. Recently after the COVID-19 pandemic, the American Autonomic Society has proposed the term "Long-COVID POTS" that occurs 12 weeks post SARS-CoV-2 infection. The symptoms include palpitations, breathlessness, chest discomfort, fatigue, pain, orthostatic intolerance, sleep disturbance, cognitive impairment, abdominal discomfort, diarrhea, joint pains, anxiety, depression, and headache along with excessive tachycardia.[15,16] The pathophysiological mechanisms involved are similar as discussed but more of immune dysregulation **(Table 1)**.

EVALUATION

The assessment of patients with POTS starts with confirming the diagnosis, identifying the etiology if any, associated comorbidities, the pathophysiological mechanism involved, and excluding other causes of orthostatic intolerance. Clinical history is crucial to identify possible causes, associated conditions, and precipitating factors. It should also focus on dietary intake (salt and fluid), medication history **(Box 1)**, functional capacity, and autonomic symptoms. The presentation of POTS can be acute (<1 month), subacute (1–3 months), and chronic (>3 months).[1] The physical

TABLE 1: Pathophysiological mechanisms of postural orthostatic tachycardia syndrome (POTS).

Type	Mechanism	Clinical findings
Peripheral autonomic denervation	Restricted autonomic neuropathy of small and distal postganglionic autonomic fibers: • Sympathetic tone impairment • Reduce vasoconstriction • Compensatory tachycardia	Autonomic dysfunction
Hypovolemia	• Reduced plasma volume and red blood cell volume • Decreased plasma renin activity and aldosterone levels	24-hour urine sodium < 170 mmol
Deconditioning	Reduced LV mass, stroke volume, and blood volume	• Systolic blood pressure increase <10 mm Hg • Excessive phase IV overshoot on the Valsalva maneuver
Hyperadrenergic	Norepinephrine receptor deficiency	Objective cardiovascular deconditioning on stress test
Antibodies and immunology	• Postinfectious (viral) • Autoimmune (Hashimoto's disease, Sjögren syndrome, SLE, celiac)	

BOX 1 Medications mimicking symptoms of POTS.

- Beta blockers
- Calcium channel blockers
- Alpha blockers
- Serotonin and norepinephrine reuptake inhibitors (SNRI)
- Tricyclic antidepressants (TCAs)
- Phenothiazines
- ACE inhibitors/angiotensin receptor blockers*

*Angiotensin-convertase enzyme.

examination includes measuring vital signs in an orthostatic condition for a period of 10 minutes, especially the heart rate and signs of orthostatic intolerance.

INVESTIGATIONS

The investigations should be used as a tool to identify the etiology and associated conditions. It mainly focuses on hematological, cardiovascular, neurological, and autonomic testing. The hematological investigations include a complete work-up including tests for electrolytes, renal function, thyroid function tests, and cortisol levels to identify underlying causes like autoimmune disorders. Cardiovascular testing includes electrocardiography (ECG), echocardiography, and Holter monitoring and should be done if there is a strong suspicion of any structural heart disease or an arrhythmia. Autonomic testing should be done in patients having autonomic symptoms that include Valsalva maneuver, tilt-table test, quantitative sudomotor axonal test, antibodies against beta receptors, and nicotinic receptors. Neuroimaging and electroencephalography should be considered if there are any neurological deficits or suspected neurological causes, such as multisystem atrophy (MSA-p) **(Table 2)**.[17]

MANAGEMENT

The main aspect of the management of POTS depends on the underlying mechanism and patient education regarding factors responsible for the worsening of symptoms. Management includes non-pharmacological and pharmacological strategies.

Non-pharmacological Management

Non-pharmacological strategies focus on educating patients regarding precipitating factors, such as environmental temperature, dehydration, post-prandial state, and alcohol intake. Attention should be given to avoid medications **(Box 1)** that can worsen the symptoms and sinus tachycardia. Adequate fluid intake (2–3 L/day)[18] is important to maintain blood volume; sodium intake can be increased to 3–10 g daily using salt tablets or electrolyte solutions, and exercise to increase cardiovascular conditioning is important.[19]

TABLE 2: Investigations.

Clinical	Orthostatic measurement of vital signs (heart rate, blood pressure) for 10 minutes
Hematological	• Complete blood count • Renal function • Electrolytes • Thyroid function test • Cortisol (morning levels)
Cardiovascular	• Electrocardiography (ECG) • Echocardiography • Holter • Exercise testing
Neurological and autonomic	• Neuroimaging (MRI) • Electroencephalogram • Valsalva maneuver • Tilt-table test • Quantitative sudomotor axon reflex test (QSART) • 24-hour urine sodium • Blood volume measurements • Antiadrenergic and muscarinic antibodies

TABLE 3: Pharmacological therapy.

Blood volume expanders	• Fludrocortisone: 0.1–0.2 mg daily • IV saline
Heart rate lowering agents	• Propranolol: 10–20 mg orally QID • Ivabradine: 2.5–7.5 mg orally BD • Pyridostigmine: 30–60 mg orally TID
Vasoconstrictors	• Midodrine: 2.5–15 mg orally TID • Octreotide: 10–30 mg long acting intramuscular injection • Methylphenidate: 10 mg 2–3 times orally a day
Sympatholytic drugs	• Clonidine: 0.1–0.2 mg orally BD or TID or patch • Methyldopa: 125–250 mg orally BD

The use of compression garments to provide a pressure of 20–40 mm Hg can also be used for symptomatic improvement.

Pharmacological Management

The pharmacologic therapies are directed to reduce the disabling symptoms experienced by the patients. The agents are selected according to the underlying mechanism of POTS and symptoms. Currently, there are no FDA-approved medications for POTS. However, certain medications have been used for treatment that include blood volume expanders, heart rate lowering agents, vasoconstrictors, and sympatholytic drugs **(Table 3 and Flowchart 1)**.

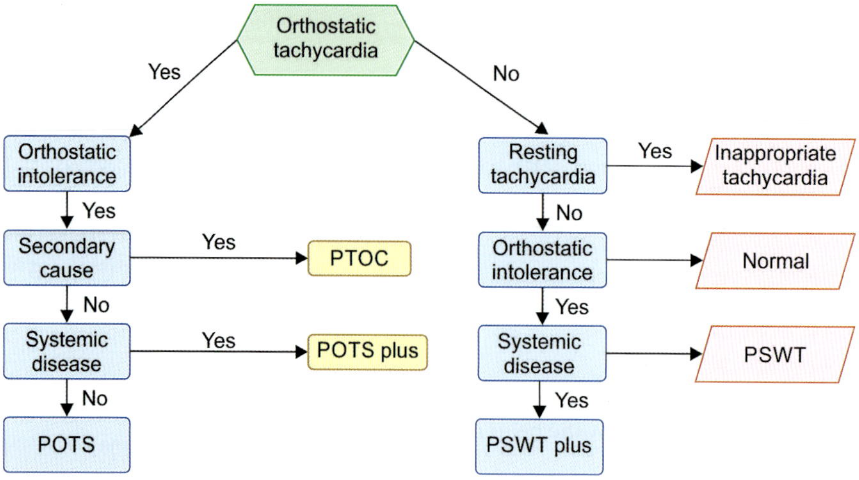

FLOWCHART 1: Diagnostic algorithm.

(POTS: postural orthostatic tachycardia syndrome; PSWT: postural symptoms without tachycardia; PTOC: postural tachycardia of other cause)

CONCLUSION

COI and POTS are conditions with symptoms that are very common in day-to-day life. The symptoms of orthostatic intolerance are non-specific and are usually ignored. Its association with various disorders makes it difficult to diagnose. Therefore, the diagnosis is usually missed and needs proper evaluation including history, clinical, and other examinations. The appropriate diagnosis might help in successfully managing such patients and to find out the secondary causes if any. Especially, after the COVID-19 pandemic such cases have risen and further research is required in this field to find out the etiology and to improve the diagnostic methods.

ONLINE REFERENCES

Please scan the QR code provided at the end of the table of contents for References of this chapter.

CHAPTER

50

Orthostatic Hypotension: Evaluation and Management

Vijay Garg, Shivangi Tiwari, Monika Jain, Ghanshyam Sharma

ABSTRACT

Maintaining blood pressure when assuming an upright posture requires quick cardiovascular adjustments, primarily driven by the autonomic nervous system. When these compensatory mechanisms fail, it can lead to orthostatic hypotension (OH). OH is characterized by a sustained drop in systolic blood pressure of >20 mm Hg or diastolic blood pressure of >10 mm Hg within 3 minutes of standing or during a head-up tilt greater than 60°. It is particularly prevalent among the elderly and is associated with increased risks of cardiovascular and cerebrovascular complications. Consequently, recognizing OH in clinical practice is crucial. Diagnosing OH involves measuring blood pressure in both supine and standing positions. A practical alternative in clinical settings is to measure blood pressure while seated and then standing, although this may yield smaller depressor responses due to reduced gravitational stress. Simultaneous measurement of heart rate responses to standing is essential to evaluate baroreflex function. Patients with OH might experience symptoms of cerebral hypoperfusion upon standing, leading to syncope and falls, although many patients remain asymptomatic. Once OH is diagnosed, it is important to review potentially harmful medications and comorbid conditions and assess for neurogenic autonomic dysfunction to determine underlying causes. Treatment should follow a structured, stepwise approach, beginning with nonpharmacological strategies (such as lifestyle changes and physical countermeasures) and progressing to pharmacological treatments (such as midodrine, droxidopa, or fludrocortisone) for patients with severe OH. The primary treatment goal should be to alleviate symptoms and enhance functional status rather than aiming for specific blood pressure targets.

Keywords: Orthostatic hypotension, syncope, pressure diuresis, baroreceptors, coat-hanger headache, treatment algorithm, management of orthostatic hypotension

INTRODUCTION

Orthostatic hypotension (OH) is a cardiovascular condition characterized by a persistent drop of at least 20 mm Hg in systolic blood pressure (SBP) or 10 mm Hg in diastolic blood pressure (DBP) within 3 minutes of standing or during head-up tilt-table testing.[1] The clinical importance of OH has gained recognition in recent years due to its negative impact on quality of life and overall prognosis.[2] OH can result in severe symptoms, falls, fractures, syncope, cognitive decline, increased hospitalizations among the elderly, and a higher mortality risk.[3,4] Hence, timely assessment and appropriate management of OH are crucial.[5]

It is noteworthy that even healthy individuals might experience a temporary drop in blood pressure (BP) immediately upon standing (within 15 seconds, known as "initial orthostatic hypotension"), which often only requires training the patient to stand up slowly. Conversely, some patients may develop OH after a delay, with symptoms appearing only after standing for 3 minutes ("delayed OH").[4] **Figures 1A and B** depicts the temporal relationship between BP and heart rate (HR) for classic and delayed OH, respectively.

PREVALENCE OF ORTHOSTATIC HYPOTENSION

The prevalence of OH varies depending on the population studied, but it is strongly correlated with age. In the general population, the prevalence of OH is <5% below the age of 50 years and increases to around 20% among individuals above the age of 70 years.[3] Several studies have reported an association between age and the prevalence of OH, with

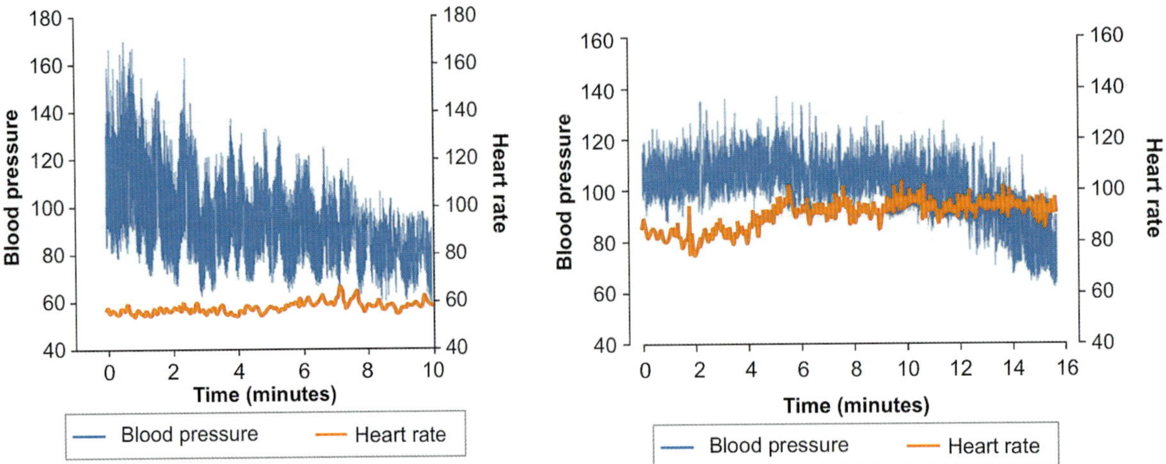

A sustained reduction of at least 20 mm Hg of systolic blood pressure or 10 mm Hg of diastolic blood pressure within 3 minutes of standing or head-up tilt-table testing.

A

A sustained reduction in blood pressure that occurs after 3 minutes of standing or upright tilt.

B

FIGS. 1A AND B: Temporal relationship between blood pressure and heart rate for (A) classic and (B) delayed orthostatic hypotension.

a higher prevalence observed in older individuals.[6] The prevalence increases exponentially with increasing age due to sedentary lifestyles, associated neurodegenerative disorders such as Parkinson's disease, other comorbidities such as diabetes, and aging-related impairment in autonomic function.[4] A community-based study conducted in South India found that the prevalence of OH among elderly individuals was 9.6%.[7] Saedon et al. discovered that one in five older people in a community setting is affected by OH, while almost one in four older individuals in long-term care experiences this condition.[8] Additionally, Tran et al. conducted a systematic review that involved 13 studies with a total of 5,465 participants, and they found that the initial prevalence of OH was high among older adults in general populations (27.8%) and geriatric outpatients (35.2%).[9]

RISK FACTORS OF ORTHOSTATIC HYPOTENSION

Several important risk factors have been identified in patients with OH. These risk factors can help identify individuals who may be more prone to developing OH or experiencing its associated symptoms. Some of the key risk factors include the following:[10]

- *Syncopal episode or unexplained falls:* Syncopal episodes refer to transient loss of consciousness, often caused by a sudden drop in BP. Unexplained falls can also be an indicator of underlying OH.
- *Neurodegenerative disorders associated with autonomic dysfunction:* Certain neurodegenerative disorders, such as dementia with Lewy bodies, multiple system atrophy, Parkinson's disease, and pure autonomic failure, are known to be associated with autonomic dysfunction, which can increase the risk of developing OH.
- *Frail older adults or those taking multiple medications:* Frailty and polypharmacy can contribute to autonomic dysregulation and make individuals more susceptible to OH.
- *Peripheral neuropathies with autonomic dysfunction:* Conditions like amyloidosis, diabetes mellitus, and HIV that are associated with peripheral neuropathies can also lead to autonomic dysfunction and increase the risk of developing OH.
- *Postural (orthostatic) dizziness or nonspecific symptoms on standing:* Individuals who experience postural dizziness or nonspecific symptoms that occur specifically when standing may be at an increased risk of OH. These symptoms can include lightheadedness, dizziness, or feeling faint upon standing, indicating possible OH.

PATHOPHYSIOLOGY OF ORTHOSTATIC HYPOTENSION

Orthostatic hypotension occurs due to a failure of the normal compensatory mechanisms that regulate BP upon assuming an upright posture. The pathophysiology of OH involves multiple levels of dysfunction within the autonomic nervous system, including baroreceptors, autonomic afferents, central processing, autonomic efferents, and peripheral sympathetic receptors.[3]

When a person stands up, approximately 500–1,000 mL of blood shifts from the central intravascular compartment to the peripheral vasculature, specifically the lower extremities and splanchnic bed. This shift of blood reduces venous return to the heart (preload). In response, under normal conditions, compensatory mechanisms activate to maintain BP and perfusion to vital organs (such as the brain).

The compensatory mechanisms in a healthy individual include a slight increase in HR, venoconstriction (constriction of veins), and arteriolar constriction. These mechanisms help preserve SBP, slightly increase DBP, maintain effective venous return, and ensure an adequate cardiac output.[3] **Figures 2A and B** illustrates the anatomy and physiology of BP control in the normal state and autonomic failure.

However, in individuals with OH, there is a failure in these compensatory mechanisms. Dysfunction can occur at various levels of the autonomic reflex pathway. Baroreceptors, which sense changes in BP, may not function properly. Autonomic afferents (sensory nerves) that transmit signals from the baroreceptors to the central processing centers may be impaired. Central processing centers in the brain may not adequately integrate and respond to the signals received. Autonomic efferent (motor nerves) that carry signals from the central processing centers to the peripheral organs, including the heart and blood vessels, may be affected. Peripheral sympathetic receptors (involved in vasoconstriction) may not respond appropriately.

The dysregulation of these autonomic reflexes can lead to a decrease in BP upon standing, resulting in inadequate perfusion to the upper body and brain. This can lead to symptoms of OH, such as lightheadedness, dizziness, syncope (fainting), and potential complications.[3,4] **Figure 3** outlines the pathophysiology involved in OH.

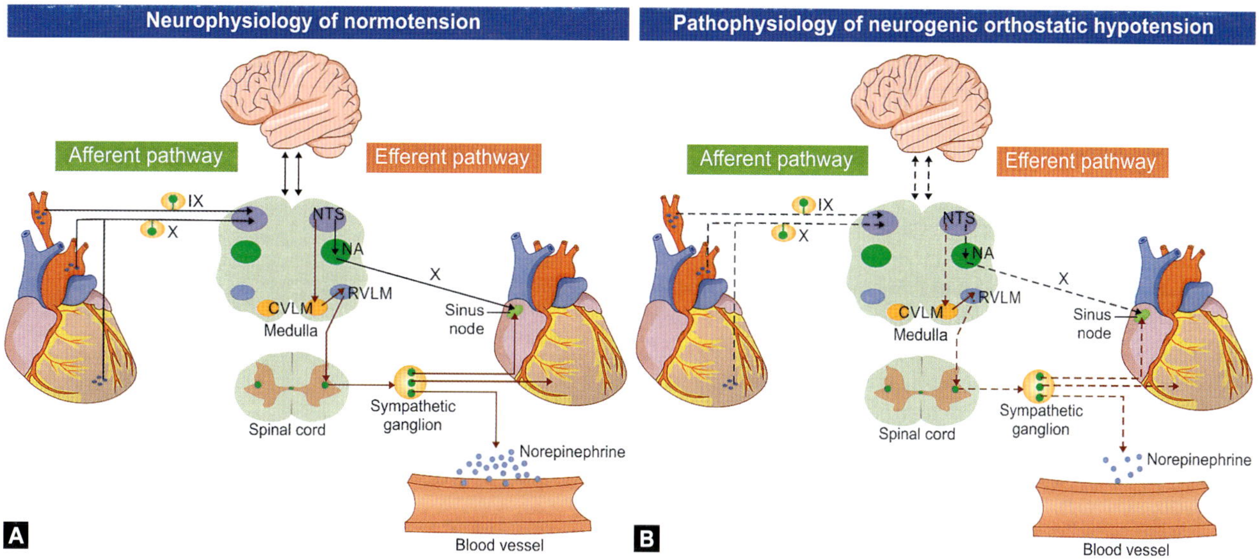

FIGS. 2A AND B: Anatomy and physiology of blood pressure control in the normal state and autonomic failure.

Source: Freeman R, Abuzinadah AR, Gibbons C, et al. Orthostatic hypotension: JACC state-of-the-art review. J Am Coll Cardiol. 2018;72(11):1294-309.[1]

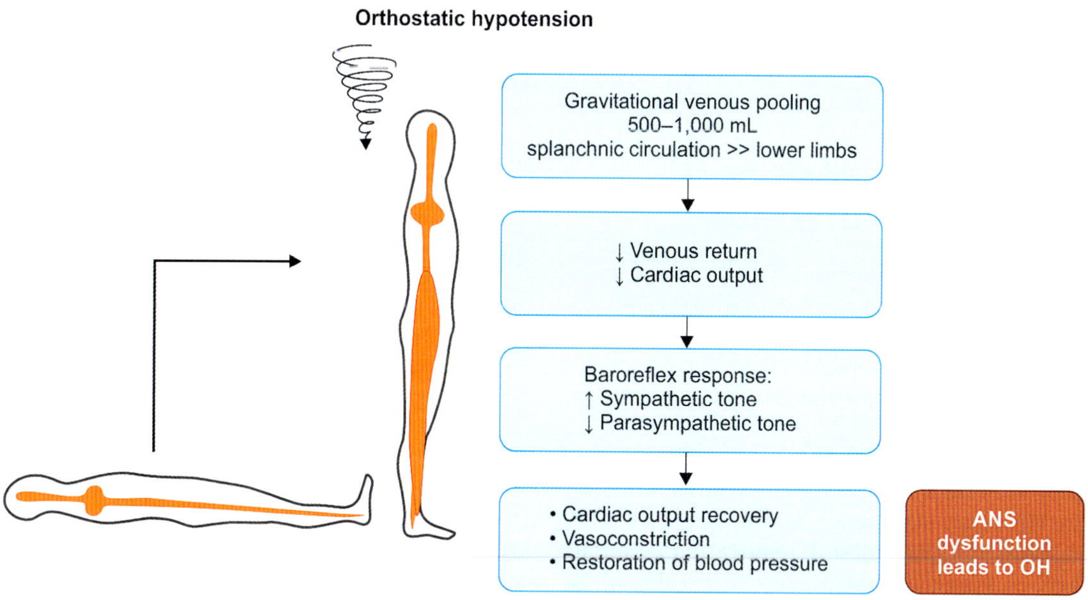

FIG. 3: Mechanisms involved in the pathophysiology of orthostatic hypotension.

(ANS: autonomic nervous system)

CLINICAL PRESENTATION OF ORTHOSTATIC HYPOTENSION

Orthostatic hypotension can present with a range of symptoms, although not all individuals with OH will experience symptoms. The symptoms can be attributed to the drop in SBP or other underlying mechanisms. Common symptoms of OH are included in **Box 1**.

Symptoms of OH never start while supine, occur only on standing, and are relieved by sitting or lying down.

These symptoms may be more pronounced early in the morning after awakening because of nighttime pressure diuresis with volume depletion.[4] It is important to note that symptoms can vary in severity among individuals and may fluctuate throughout the day.[10]

BOX 1 Symptoms of orthostatic hypotension.

- Lightheadedness (dizziness, wooziness, vertigo)
- Syncope or presyncope
- Fatigue
- Visual blurring and visual dimming
- Cognitive impairment
- Neck and shoulder pain ("coat-hanger headache")
- Chest pain
- Dyspnea in upright position

CLASSIFICATION OF ORTHOSTATIC HYPOTENSION

Fedorowski et al.[3] proposed a classification system for OH based on predominant underlying pathophysiological mechanisms. This classification includes the following:[3]

- *Neurogenic OH:* This refers to OH caused by dysfunction or damage to the autonomic nervous system, which regulates BP. Conditions associated with neurogenic OH include neurodegenerative disorders (Parkinson's disease, multiple system atrophy, pure autonomic failure), peripheral neuropathies, and autonomic nervous system disorders.
- *Cardiogenic OH:* This occurs due to impaired cardiac function, such as reduced cardiac output or abnormal heart rhythms. Cardiac conditions that can contribute to cardiogenic OH include heart failure, arrhythmias, and structural heart diseases.
- *Mixed OH:* This refers to a combination of neurogenic and cardiogenic mechanisms contributing to OH. This classification is used when both neurogenic and cardiogenic factors play a role in the development of OH.

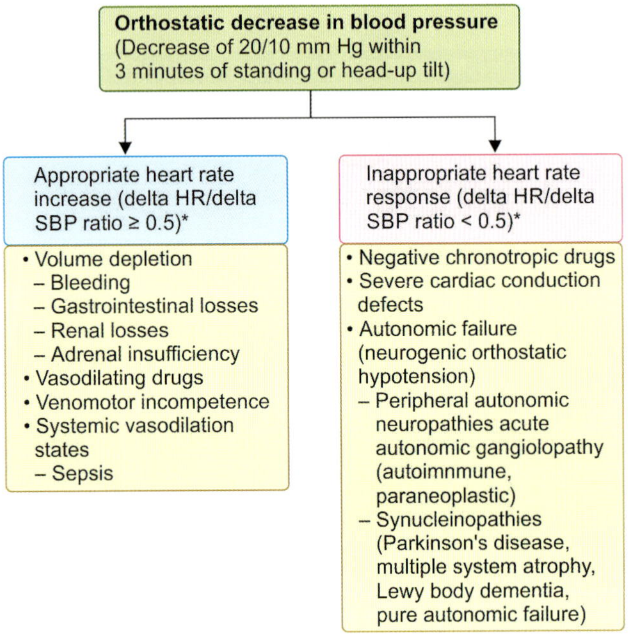

*Delta HR/delta SBP ratio is the ratio of the change in heart rate divided by the change in systolic blood pressure with standing or head-up tilt. Most patients with neurogenic orthostatic hypotension have a ratio < 0.3. Most patients with a normal autonomic response have a ratio > 1.0.

FLOWCHART 1: Approach for evaluation of orthostatic hypotension.

EVALUATION/DIAGNOSIS OF ORTHOSTATIC HYPOTENSION

Accurate evaluation and diagnosis of OH involve specific procedures. BP and HR measurements are taken with the patient in a supine position after at least 5 minutes of rest. The patient is then tilted up or asked to stand, and BP and HR are measured at 1 and 3 minutes after assuming the upright posture.

The evaluation focuses on assessing the HR response of the patient. If there is an appropriate HR response (an increase in HR upon standing), common causes such as volume depletion, vasodilator medications, venous insufficiency, or systemic vasodilatory states should be considered. If the HR response is inadequate (no increase in HR or a decrease), potential causes can include the use of negative chronotropic drugs, cardiac conduction defects, or autonomic failure (neurogenic OH). **Flowchart 1** represents the evaluation approach for OH.[3]

These diagnostic assessments help in identifying the underlying mechanisms and potential causes contributing to OH, guiding appropriate management strategies. The diagnostic algorithm for OH is represented in **Flowchart 2.**[11,12]

SUPINE HYPERTENSION AND PRESSURE DIURESIS

Supine hypertension, which is defined as a SBP of 140 mm Hg or higher and a DBP of 90 mm Hg or higher, is often observed in patients with neurogenic OH. When renal perfusion pressure is elevated, the kidneys respond by reducing the reabsorption of sodium in the proximal tubules. This mechanism is known as pressure natriuresis. Consequently, nighttime supine hypertension leads to nocturnal diuresis and a decrease in overall volume, causing patients to lose around 1,500 mL of urine overnight. This urinary loss contributes to the worsening of daytime OH, which is why patients typically experience more severe symptoms in the morning. On the other hand, adopting a head-up tilt position during sleep can reduce nocturnal diuresis and result in an improvement in symptoms. This phenomenon is highly relevant to the hospitalized patients, who are often confined to bed during the daytime because of their risk of falls.[4]

MANAGEMENT OF ORTHOSTATIC HYPOTENSION

The primary objectives of managing OH are to alleviate symptoms, enhance standing tolerance, and improve overall physical function and activity. These goals should take precedence over solely focusing on optimizing standing BP. Additionally, patient education plays a crucial role in the management process. Key management principles are summarized in **Table 1**.

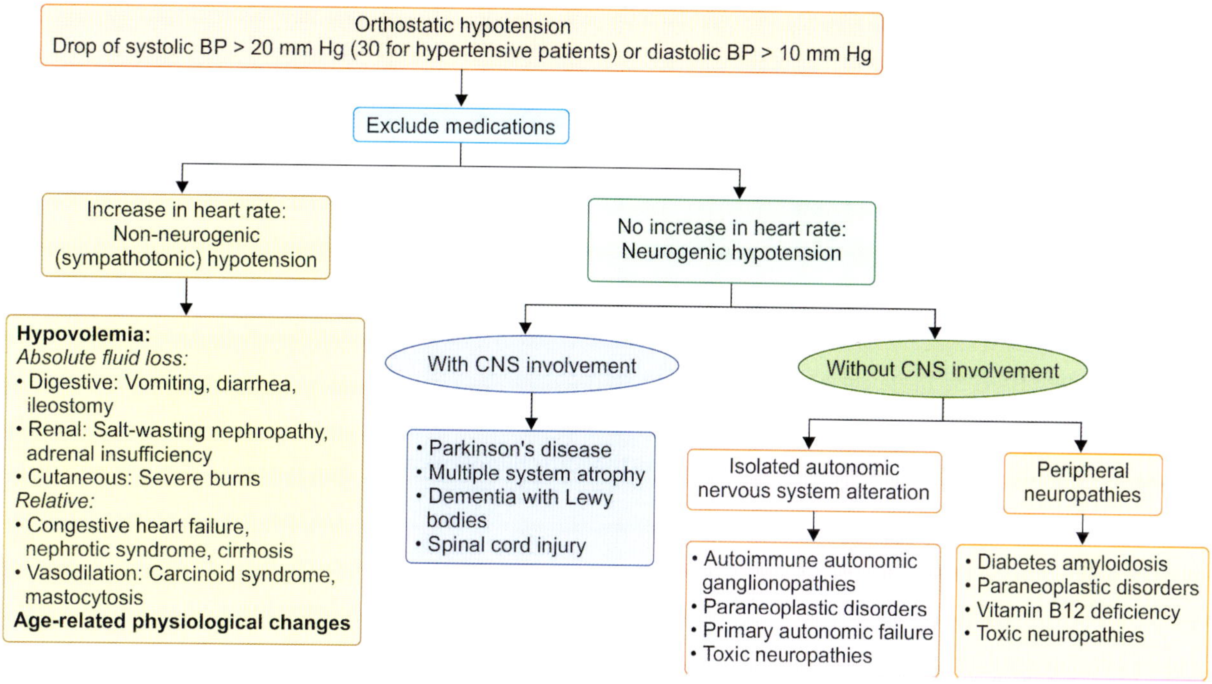

FLOWCHART 2: Diagnostic algorithm for orthostatic hypotension.

TABLE 1: Key principles of managing orthostatic hypotension.

Principle of management	Intervention
General principles of management	• Educate on trigger avoidance and self-management, e.g., patient diaries • Review medications for potential exacerbation of OH • Treat anemia, vitamin B12 deficiency, and optimize underlying causes of autonomic neuropathy (HIV/amyloidosis/diabetes)
Nonpharmacological measures	• Promote fluid repletion (2–2.5 L) with 500 mL bolus if necessary • Encourage salt repletion (4–10 g/day) • Recommend compression garments with abdominal compression • Instruct physical countermaneuvers • Illustrate head-up sleeping (at least 10°)
Pharmacological measures	• Administer volume expanders like fludrocortisone • Use sympathomimetics like midodrine • Explore alternative agents such as droxidopa, atomoxetine, and pyridostigmine

The "American Society for Hypertension" in 2013 proposed a stepwise approach on how to treat OH patients **(Flowchart 3)**.[12]

Treatment of OH relies on nonpharmacological measures as its fundamental basis and advocates for their mandatory incorporation. The nonpharmacological interventions are listed in **Box 2**.

The pharmacological interventions are listed in **Table 2**. **Flowchart 4** summarizes the management of OH.

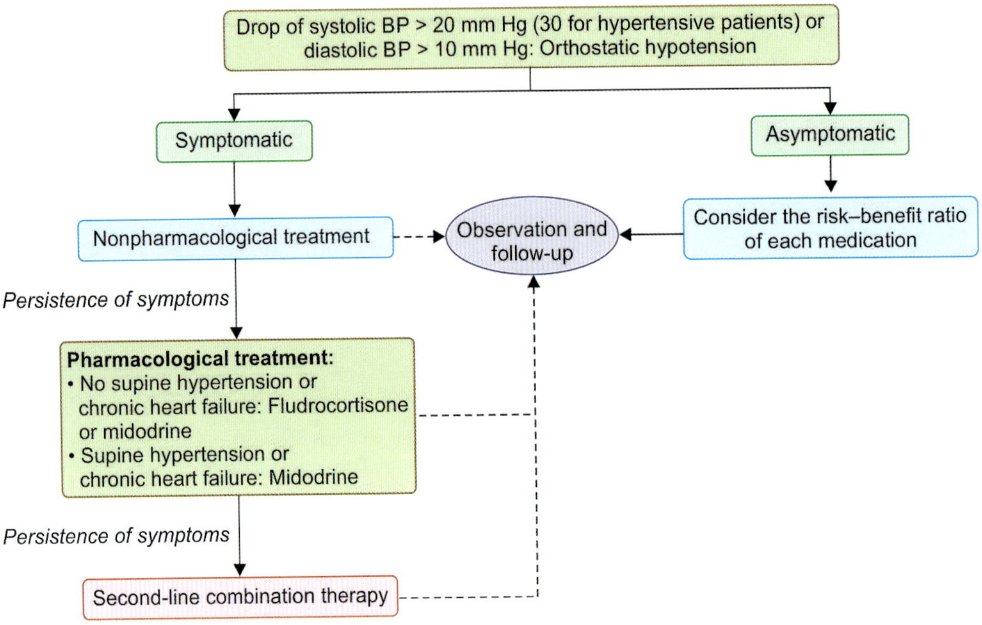

FLOWCHART 3: Treatment algorithm for orthostatic hypotension.

BOX 2 **List of nonpharmacological interventions for orthostatic hypotension.**

Patient and family education for:

- Explanation of symptoms and their causes
- Safety measures to prevent falls related to orthostatic hypotension
- Advice to avoid straining during urination and bowel movements
- Encouragement to keep a diary of physical activity and meals, as well as monitoring blood pressure to identify patterns and potential issues

Methods to prevent symptoms and emergency management:

- Crossing legs upon standing
- Abdominal and leg muscle pumping/contractions
- Bending forward or squatting

Activity and positioning:

- Limit prolonged periods of sitting or standing. If inactive for an extended time, engage in ankle pumps and alternate crossing and uncrossing the legs
- Avoid sudden transitions from lying down to standing or from sitting to standing
- Rise gradually from a seated position to a standing position

Drinking fluids to ensure hydration:

- Extra intake of water may be helpful for reducing symptoms before getting up in the morning, before exercising, or after eating
- However, it is important to note that bolus drinking may not be suitable for patients at risk of fluid overload, such as those with heart failure or end-stage kidney disease

Avoid indiscriminate recommendation for:

- Lower limb compression stockings
- Sleeping with head of bed elevated
- Increasing salt in diet

TABLE 2: Main drugs used for treatment of symptomatic patients with orthostatic hypotension.

Drugs	Mechanism of action	Dosing	Adverse events
Droxidopa	Norepinephrine precursor	100–600 mg TID*	Headache, nausea, supine hypertension
Midodrine	α1-adrenoreceptor agonist	2.5–10 mg BID or TID*	Goose bumps, paresthesia, pruritus, supine hypertension, urinary urgency
Fludrocortisone	Mineralocorticoid	0.05–0.3 mg QD	Supine hypertension and hypokalemia
Pyridostigmine	Acetylcholinesterase inhibitor	30–60 mg BID or TID	Gastrointestinal symptoms, urinary urgency
Atomoxetine	Norepinephrine reuptake inhibitor	18 mg QD	Supine hypertension, urinary urgency
Octreotide	Somatostatin analog	0.2–1.6 mg/kg QD, subcutaneous	Injection site discomfort, erythema, gastrointestinal disturbances, cholelithiasis, hyperglycemia, supine hypertension
Desmopressin	V1a and V2 receptor agonists, vasopressin analog	• *Nasal spray*: 5–40 mg QD • *Oral*: 100–800 mg QD	Limited data about safety
Ephedrine/ pseudoephedrine	Direct and indirect α1-adrenoreceptor agonist	25/30–50/60 mg 3 × per day	Nausea, supine hypertension

*Food and Drug Administration approved.

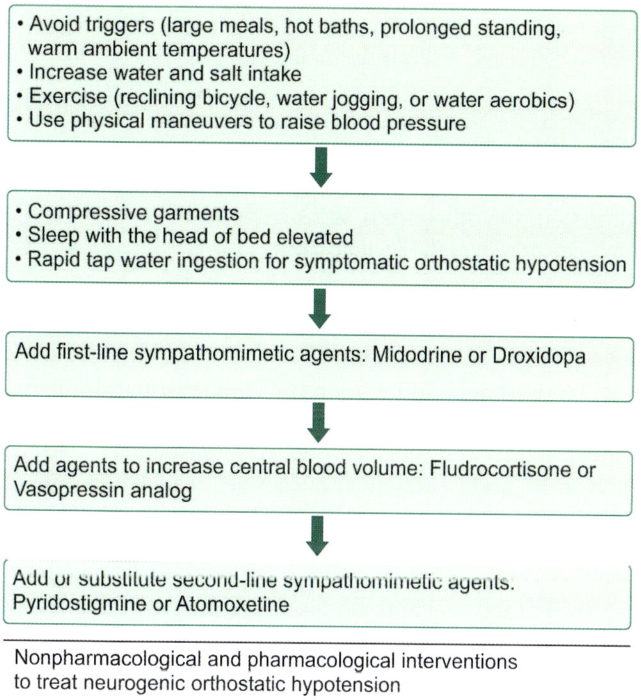

FLOWCHART 4: Treatment algorithm for neurogenic orthostatic hypotension.

MONITORING AND FOLLOW-UP

Evaluation of treatment success involves the assessment of various parameters, including symptoms, falls, quality of life, side effects, and changes in BP. If a medication fails to provide symptomatic relief or causes intolerable side effects, it should be substituted with an alternative medication and undergo further review. It is important to titrate drug doses to the lowest effective dose and regularly reassess their efficacy. Patients should be informed and motivated to adhere to their prescribed medication regimen to ensure optimal outcomes.

CONCLUSION

Orthostatic hypotension is a commonly encountered condition, often overlooked, and can be associated with neurological and cardiac diseases. To approach this potentially complex condition in a practical manner, it is suggested to classify OH into neurogenic, cardiogenic, and mixed forms. OH is particularly prevalent among the elderly population, and its prevalence tends to increase with age. The evaluation of OH requires a comprehensive understanding of the underlying pathophysiology of the disease. Treatment strategies for OH depend on the specific causative mechanisms involved. Nonpharmacological measures form the foundation of OH treatment and should be an integral and mandatory component of OH management. By employing a combination of nonpharmacological and pharmacological interventions, significant improvements can be achieved in the symptoms of OH and the quality of life of affected patients. Currently, only two drugs, namely midodrine and droxidopa, are approved for the treatment of OH. If a medication fails to provide symptomatic benefits or causes intolerable side effects in the management of OH, it should be substituted with an alternative drug and undergo re-evaluation. Adherence to prescribed medications is of utmost importance in the effective management of OH.

ONLINE REFERENCES

Please scan the QR code provided at the end of the table of contents for References of this chapter.

CHAPTER

51

Newer Antihypertensive Drugs

Vijay Kumar Chopra

ABSTRACT

Despite the availability of several classes of drugs, uncontrolled hypertension continues to be a challenge and is a significant contributor to cardiovascular morbidity and mortality. In most of the instances, it is due to inadequate doses, side effects, noncompliance with the drugs, or failure to observe lifestyle changes. However, there are many patients where, despite all measures, the blood pressure continues to be high. Newer techniques such as renal denervation have been advocated but different trials have given conflicting results. Several new classes of drugs have become available or are in different stages of clinical trials. sacubitril/valsartan, which is a well-established drug for heart failure, has been shown to be a powerful antihypertensive agent and is approved for this use in some countries. Of the other drugs, aldosterone synthase inhibitors appear to be promising but more data is needed before they can be recommended for clinical use.

Keywords: Side effects, cardiovascular morbidity, sacubitril/valsartan, newer techniques

INTRODUCTION

Hypertension is the most common cardiovascular disease and contributes significantly to the morbidity and mortality. Estimates of its prevalence vary in different countries, but it is recognized that its incidence is higher in the middle- or low-economy countries. In the fifth National Family Health Survey among 1,691,036 respondents from 28 states, eight union territories, and 707 districts of India, carried out in 2020–2021, 52.6% were women and the mean age was 41.6 years. The results showed that 28.1% had hypertension, of whom 36.9% were diagnosed. Of these, 44.7% were on treatment and among them only 52.5% had a BP of <140/90. Several factors are responsible for the poor control of hypertension. Some of these are use of a large number of drugs, poor adherence to therapy, and side effects of these drugs. Utilization of double- or triple-drug combination can help in improving compliance in many of these patients. The recent guidelines recommend starting treatment with a RAAS inhibitor along with a calcium channel blocker and the addition of a thiazide diuretic, if blood pressure (BP) remains high. If hypertension is still not under control, then an MRA can be added. Alternately, drugs such as beta-blockers, alpha-blockers, loop diuretics or clonidine can be used depending upon the clinical situation. Renal denervation is another strategy which has had a chequered career, but can be considered in truly resistant HT. Various preventive and treatment strategies are available, but there is a significant lack of awareness of the serious implications of uncontrolled hypertension in the population and the medical community.

Even if the available strategies are diligently employed, there are always patients whose BP remains uncontrolled, and there is a need for developing newer therapies, which can help these patients Therefore, as in all other branches of medicines, the quest for newer, more effective and safer treatments goes on.

Several newer drugs are now available or under investigation with the object to treat true resistant hypertension. In this review, we will focus on the following different strategies, which act through different pathways. The main pathophysiological mechanism of these newer agents is shown in **Figure 1**.

- *New use for HF drug*: ARNI
- *Aldosterone synthase inhibitors*: Baxdrostat
- *mRNA interference drug*: Zilebesiran
- *Inhibitor of aminopeptidase A*: Firibastat
- *Endothelin antagonist*: Aprocitentan

EFFECTS OF ARNI

This is a well-established drug now for treatment for heart failure, but this was originally developed as a treatment for hypertension. This is not surprising, considering its powerful vasodilator action and other mechanisms by which it lowers BP **(Fig. 1)**. In fact, the first trial for its efficacy in the management of hypertension was published well before the landmark PARADIGM trial for HFrEF. In 2010, 1,215 patients were enrolled and over an 8-week treatment period, there was a greater reduction of BP with sacubitril/valsartan (S/V) as compared to valsartan **(Fig. 2)**. However, it was not pursued as an antihypertensive agent at that time.[1]

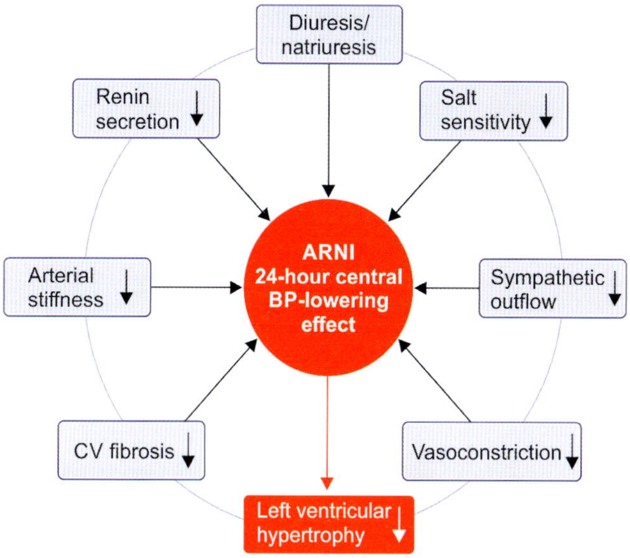

FIG. 1: Mechanisms of actions of ARNI.

Source: Kario K, Williams B. Angiotensin receptor-neprilysin inhibitors for hypertension-hemodynamic effects and relevance to hypertensive heart disease. Hypertens Res. 2022;45(7):1097-110.

Parameter[2] was the first randomized trial comparing sacubitril/valsartan versus an ARB, Olmesartan, on the central aortic pressures and hemodynamics in elderly patients. It showed that S/V was significantly more effective than conventional ARB in lowering brachial and central aortic systolic pulse pressures.

In the post hoc analysis of Paragon-HF[3] trial the effect of S/V in patients of apparent resistant hypertension was compared with Valsartan. Apparent resistant hypertension was (defined as systolic BP > 140, over 135 if diabetic) despite treatment with valsartan, diuretic, MRA, and a calcium channel blocker. In 731 patients, thus, analyzed the reduction of BP was greater with S/V when compared to valsartan at week 4 and 16. Up to 47% patients reached normal BP with ARNI as compared to 34% with Valsartan. The difference was more prominent in MRA-resistant HT. S/V has been shown to reduce arterial stiffness more than ARBs, which may be important in RHT.

A lack of dip in the nocturnal BP is an important risk factor in patients of hypertension. In a study of 632 in Japan patients by Kazuomi Kario,[4] ambulatory BP monitoring was carried at baseline and on follow-up to compare the effect of S/V versus olmesartan. It demonstrated that changes in 24-hour daytime and nighttime ambulatory SBP and DBP were

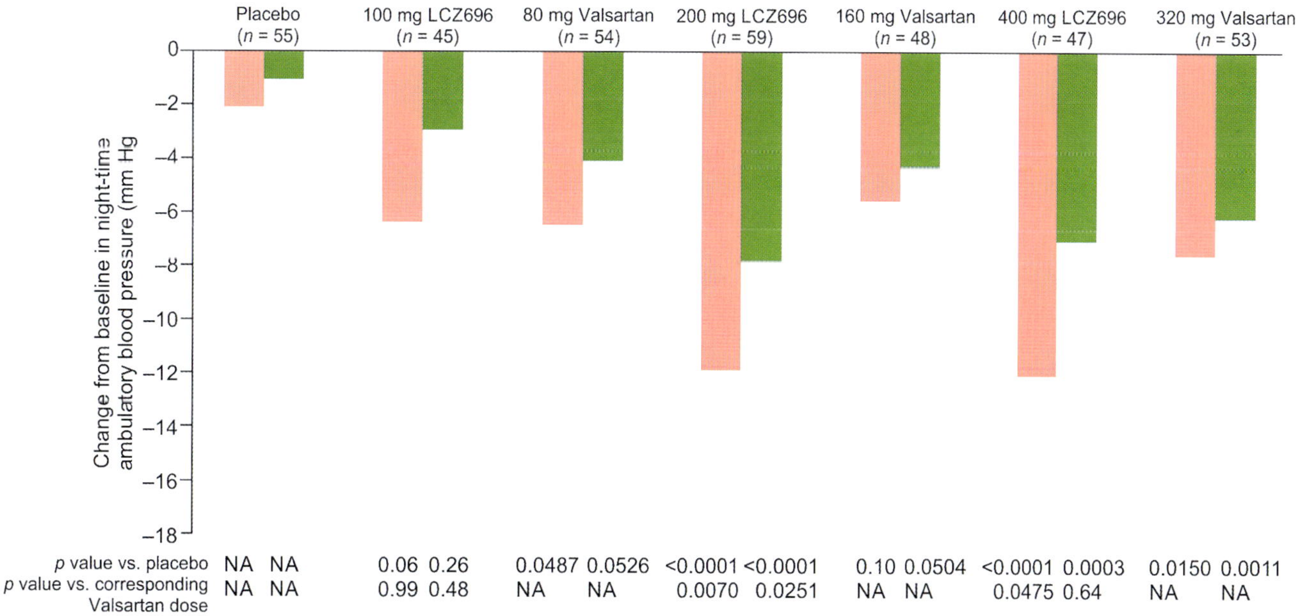

FIG. 2: Comparison of antihypertensive effects of ARNI versus valsartan.

Source: Ruilope LM, Dukat A, Lacourciere Y, et al. Blood-pressure reduction with LCZ696, a novel dual-acting inhibitor of the angiotensin II receptor and neprilysin: a randomised, double-blind, placebo-controlled, active comparator study. Lancet. 2010;375(9722):1255-66.

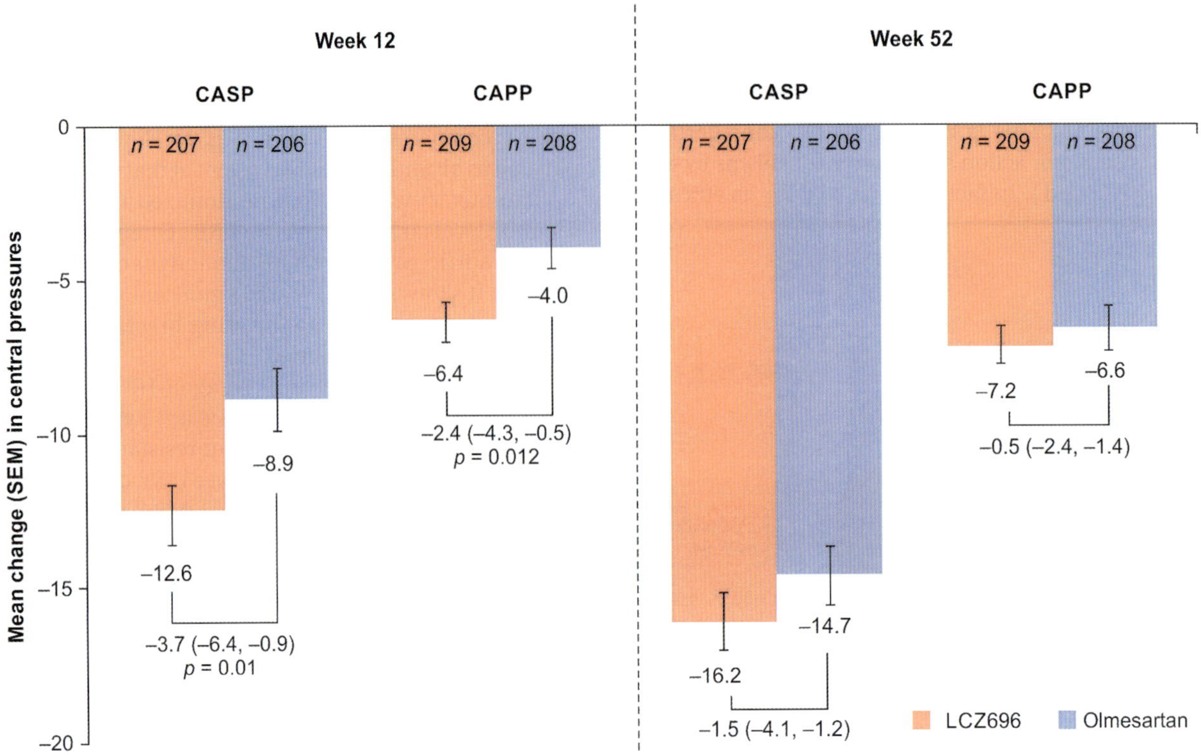

FIG. 3: Comparison of antihypertensive effects of ARNI versus olmesartan.

Source: Williams B, Cockcroft JR, Kario K, et al. Effects of sacubitril/valsartan versus olmesartan on central hemodynamics in the elderly with systolic hypertension. Hypertension. 2017;69(3):411-20.

more significant with S/V compared to olmesartan. The effect was even pronounced in nondippers as compared to dippers. This effect is likely to be useful in preventing future CV events. The drug is already approved in treatment of hypertension in Japan and China and is likely to be approved in other countries as well **(Fig. 3)**.

ALDOSTERONE SYNTHASE INHIBITORS

Aldosterone is a key component of RAAS. It is produced in zona glomerulosa of adrenal cortex. High levels of angiotensin-II and ACTH result in increased production of aldosterone. It is involved in fluid and electrolyte balance and increases sodium and water retention at distal convoluted tubules in kidneys. It also causes vasoconstriction and increased fibrosis, all of which contribute to hypertension. The rate-limiting enzyme responsible in the synthetic pathway from 18-OH corticosterone to aldosterone is aldosterone synthase. Recently, inhibition of ASI has been proposed as a strategy to control aldosterone-dependent hypertension. Several trials have been carried out targeting this pathway.

The first agent to be tried in this class was osilodrostat. In this proof-of-concept study,[5] dose-dependent reduction of BP and correction of hypokalemia in patients with primary aldosteronism were observed. However, eplerenone resulted in larger reduction of BP. Subsequent trials too did not yield, particularly encouraging results for this drug.

Selective inhibition of aldosterone synthase is difficult because it shares 93% sequence similarity with another enzyme that catalyzes cortisol synthesis. The current attention in this class of drugs is focused on baxdrostat, which shows high selectivity for inhibiting aldosterone synthesis without affecting cortisol levels as compared to the previous ASI agents.[6,7] Baxdrostat binds to the active site of the enzyme, preventing the enzyme to catalyze the conversion of corticosterone to aldosterone, thus reducing aldosterone levels and decreasing activity of the RAAS system, which is a key regulator of BP. In phase 1 studies, baxdrostat demonstrated high selectivity for aldosterone synthase inhibition (100:1) compared with cortisol synthesis and reduced plasma aldosterone levels without affecting cortisol levels, a property lacking in other unselective mineralocorticoid receptor antagonists such as spironolactone.

After the initial small studies, Brig HTN, a multicenter, randomized placebo-controlled dose finding trial was conducted. It randomized 275 patients with uncontrolled hypertension taking three or more antihypertensive drugs on maximally tolerated doses including a diuretic. Three doses—0.5 mg, 1 mg and 2 mg—were tested.[8] After 12 weeks, the trial was stopped by DSMB for overwhelming superiority. Doses of 2 and 1 mg produced a significant reduction in BP. This was accompanied by reduction in aldosterone levels and compensatory rise in Renin activity. Importantly, serum cortisol levels did not change, indicating its selective inhibition of aldosterone production. Currently, a new large trial Bax-HT[9] is under way, which is enrolling patients on uncontrolled hypertension on 2 drugs or resistant hypertension on three or more drugs of which one has to be a diuretic in both the arms.

ENDOTHELIN A/ENDOTHELIN B RECEPTOR ANTAGONISTS: ETA, ETB

Endothelin-1 is a vasoconstrictor peptide which is produced in several tissues, particularly in the endothelium of blood vessels. Its action on receptors in smooth muscles causes vasoconstriction and on endothelial receptors leads to vasodilatation.[9] ET-1 production is increased in hypertension and endothelial dysfunction. Blocking this pathway has been another approach to treatment of hypertension. The studies with bosentan and darusentan showed conflicting results. ERAs appear to be more effective in low-renin conditions.[10] Aprocicentan is a dual Endothelial A and B receptor blocker. After the initial studies showed encouraging results, a large randomized double-blind placebo-controlled trial, PRECISION, was started and reported in 2022. About 730 patients with resistant hypertension were randomized to receive 12.5 mg or 25 mg aprocitentan or placebo.[11] At 4 weeks, both doses resulted in a modest systolic and diastolic BP reduction by –3.8/–3.9 with 12.5 mg and –3.7/4.5 with 25 mg aprocitentan, however, results in fluid retention in some patients which could be of concern in patients with heart failure or renal diseases. Further investigations in the role of this class of drugs are continuing.

NONSTEROIDAL MRAs

Both spironolactone and eplerenone are effective in reducing BP by blocking the binding of aldosterone to its receptors which are present in several tissues including the kidneys. However, their use gets limited in the presence of hyperkalemia and CKD. Spironolactone also has side effects such as gynecomastia and sexual disorders. Finerenone, a nonsteroidal MRA has been shown to be effective in providing renal protection in patients with marked albuminuria and advanced CKD as seen in the FIDELIO-CKD trial in patients with diabetic kidney disease.[12] These results were complemented by the FIGARO-DKD trial, which enrolled patients with type-2 diabetes with severe CKD and moderate albuminuria or mild CKD with severely elevated albuminuria.[13] In a pooled post hoc analysis of both these trials, patients with RHT and GFR of 25–45 mL/min/1.73 m^2 and baseline K between 4.3 and 5.1, experienced systolic BP reduction by –7.1 with finerenone and –1.3 by placebo ($p < 0.0001$).[14] An additional advantage of the drug is the absence of adverse effects of steroids. Coupled with safety in these high-risk patients, it is a promising drug for RHT. In recent studies, finerenone has demonstrated favorable outcomes in this patient population. Compared to other mineralocorticoid receptor antagonists such as spironolactone, it has been linked to a decreased incidence of hyperkalemia and treatment discontinuation. FINE-ARTS, a trial, which demonstrated the efficacy of finerenone reducing the composite end points of reduction in mortality and heart failure-related hospitalizations in patients with heart failure with mildly reduced and preserved ejection fraction[15] was recently published. This further strengthens the role of this agent in controlling BP while simultaneously reducing hospitalizations due to heart failure.[15]

Preclinical investigations have revealed that finerenone possesses anti-inflammatory and antifibrotic properties. Also by reducing proinflammatory mediators and fibrosis in the kidney and heart, finerenone may contribute to the management of resistant hypertension. Recently a large trial, Fine-ARTS, was published which explored the role of finerenone in patients with HFpEF.[15] The trial met its combined primary end-point of reducing HHF and death with a significant p value ($p < 0.006$). The benefit was driven by reduction in HHF with a modest mortality reduction. Considering that hypertension is an important contributor to HFpEF, the use of Finerenone in hypertension becomes promising.

It is important to note that finerenone appears does not affect systolic BP in those with diabetic renal impairment. This suggests that its beneficial effects extend beyond BP control alone. Additionally, mineralocorticoid receptor antagonists, including finerenone, have shown potential in slowing the progression of CKD, treating refractory hypertension, and providing cardiorenal protection. As compared to the currently available aldosterone receptor blockers such as eplerenone and spironolactone, it has a lower relative affinity to other steroid hormone receptors, and therefore it has fewer side effects including gynecomastia, impotence and poor libido.

ZILBESIRAN

Among new approaches to target the RAS are agents that inhibit angiotensinogen (AGT) RNA translation, or small-interfering RNA (siRNA) that function via the RNA interference pathway. AGT is primarily synthesized by the liver and is the sole precursor of all angiotensin peptides. RAAS inhibition with this approach may limit compensatory angiotensin activation associated with angiotensin-converting enzyme inhibition or angiotensin-receptor blockade. Among the novel drugs being developed for hypertension is Zilebesiran.

It is an investigational RNA interference therapeutic agent (siRNA) that binds with high affinity to the hepatic asialoglycoprotein receptor, resulting in specific reduction in hepatic angiotensinogen messenger RNA (mRNA) levels, thereby reducing the production of angiotensinogen.[16] Moreover, with hepatocyte-targeted delivery, extrahepatic angiotensinogen effects may be preserved, limiting off-target effects in the kidney and other tissues.[17] By its unique mechanism of action, it suppresses angiotensin up to 6 months. This consistent and prolonged pharmacodynamic effects offer the potential for sustained reduction of BP over a 24-hour period and for months, with twice yearly or quarterly subcutaneous administration. In a phase 1 study KARDIA-1 involving patients with hypertension, dose-related decreases in both serum angiotensinogen levels and BP after single subcutaneous doses of Zilebesiran were observed, that were sustained for up to 24 weeks.[18] KARDIA-2 study was presented in April 2024 in which Zilebesiran was tested on top of the standard medical care in inadequately controlled hypertension. It enrolled 672 patients (average age, 59 years; 43% women; 28% Black individuals) who had elevated BP, despite already taking antihypertensive medications. The average baseline BP was 143 mm Hg. The study's primary endpoint was the change in average 24-hour ambulatory systolic BP at 3 months. Zilebesiran resulted in statistically significant additional reductions in their 24-hour ambulatory systolic BP compared with placebo. The incremental reduction in BP as compared to indapamide: 12 mm Hg, amlodipine: 9.7 mm Hg and olmesartan: 4 mm Hg. Differences were sustained up to month 6 in the indapamide and amlodipine cohorts. Addition of zilebesiran to any of these drugs did not result in any new serious safety concerns with regard to K, BP, or AKI. KARDIA-3 is a new ongoing study which will test the efficacy and safety of zilebesiran in patients with hypertension uncontrolled on two to four antihypertensive drugs with high cardiovascular risk or advanced chronic kidney disease.

FIRIBASTAT

Unlike the other drugs targeting the systemic RAAS, this drug is an aminopeptidase inhibitor which acts centrally by lowering the conversion of angiotensin II to angiotensin III in the brain.[19] Reduction in angiotensin III levels in the brain results in lowering of BP. A phase III trial of firibastat, a first-in-class inhibitor of APA in the brain (FRESH), was carried out.[20] The trial randomized 514 patients in 11 countries who had SBP 140–180 mm Hg, despite treatment with at least two classes of antihypertensive agents (difficult to treat) or at least three classes (resistant) including a diuretic. After 12 weeks of treatment, there was no difference in the active and placebo arms in office BP and ambulatory monitoring of BP. Because of these results, another larger trial testing the same drug, (REFRESH) trial, was prematurely interrupted and dropped.

CONCLUSION

Hypertension is the most common cardiovascular disorder and is a significant contributor to cardiovascular morbidity and mortality. Despite the availability of several classes of drug, the BP is uncontrolled in a vast majority of patients. While adoption of healthy lifestyle and appropriate use of the available antihypertensive drugs results in good control of BP, in practical terms this is not achieved. The quest for newer antihypertensive agents goes on and several novel drugs are under investigation. S/V is a powerful vasodilator and is often effective where the other drugs have not been successful. Aldosterone synthase inhibitors, mRNA interference drugs such as zilebesiran, inhibitor of aminopeptidase-a, fibribistat and endothelin antagonist aprocitentan are some of the promising drugs which are under clinical trials, but not yet available for clinical use. There is also added interest in the available drugs such as S/V and finerenone due to their demonstrable benefits in hypertension.

ONLINE REFERENCES

Please scan the QR code provided at the end of the table of contents for References of this chapter.

SECTION 6

Heart Failure

Section Outline

CHAPTER

52

Heart Failure: Definition, Terminology, and New Concepts in Recent Guidelines

Gaurav Tripathi, Dipankar Das, Sulabh Chandrakar

ABSTRACT

Heart failure is increasing in prevalence in many countries with aging populations. Fortunately, remarkable scientific advances have been made in the past few years that have led to new treatments and improved prognosis for patients with heart failure. This review examines these changes with a focus on the definition, newer classification, and some recent updates in the concept of heart failure management. Introduction of a universal definition of heart failure, to improve communication among clinicians, researchers, and general population, similar to a universal definition of MI, has been a key milestone in the recent past. Proper classification and staging of heart failure have been emphasized by various guidelines recently in view of vast difference in management of different types of heart failure in different stages. This chapter emphasizes evidence published since the recent heart failure guidelines of the European Society of Cardiology and American College of Cardiology/American Heart Association/Heart Failure Society of America in 2021 and 2024.

Keywords: Heart failure, stages of heart failure, heart failure with reduced ejection fraction, heart failure with preserved ejection fraction, heart failure with midrange ejection fraction, definition of heart failure, improved ejection fraction

INTRODUCTION

What defines a heart failure (HF) is difficult to standardize. There is significant heterogeneity regarding the specific criteria to diagnose HF. Criteria used to define HF in clinical trials have also been highly variable. Definitions of HF had already been provided by the American College of Cardiology/American Heart Association (ACC/AHA) in the year 2013,[1] the Heart Failure Association of the European Society of Cardiology (HFA/ESC) in 2016,[2] and the Japanese Heart Failure Society (JHFS) in 2017.[3] All these definitions shared a common platform in that they identified HF as a clinical syndrome, comprising a cluster of signs and symptoms. The definitions included three basic elements: Evidence of structural problem in the heart, history of symptoms commonly reported in HF, and objective signs commonly seen in HF. However, a number of gaps remained in diagnosing HF based on these definitions. This type of definition is hard to apply in public health or epidemiological settings because of the subjective nature of the symptoms and also because these symptoms are often not specific to a single disease (e.g., fatigue and dyspnea). There is also the unfeasibility (invasive) or unreliability of measurements of cardiac output or filling pressures. For a definition to be useful by a nonspecialist, it should be easily assessable and have low interobserver variability.

Growing evidence suggests lagging behind by clinicians to implement the guideline-directed medical therapy (GDMT); the need of the hour was for a universal definition of HF.[4] So in 2020, a writing committee comprising members of the Heart Failure Society of America (HFSA), the HFA/ESC, and the JHFS assembled a consensus document resulting in the new universal definition and classification of HF.[5]

UNIVERSAL DEFINITION OF HEART FAILURE (FLOWCHART 1)

Heart failure is a clinical syndrome with current or prior:

- Symptoms and/or signs caused by a structural and/or functional cardiac abnormality [as determined by a left ventricular ejection fraction (LVEF) < 50%, abnormal cardiac chamber enlargement, *E/e'* of >15, moderate/severe ventricular hypertrophy or moderate/severe valvular obstructive or regurgitant lesion]

- And corroborated by at least one of the following:
  - Elevated natriuretic peptide levels
  - Objective evidence of cardiogenic pulmonary or systemic congestion by diagnostic modalities, such as imaging (e.g., by chest radiograph or elevated filling pressures by echocardiography) or hemodynamic measurement (e.g., right heart catheterization, pulmonary artery catheter) at rest or with provocation (e.g., exercise).

This definition seems comprehensive and forms a base for further subclassifications.

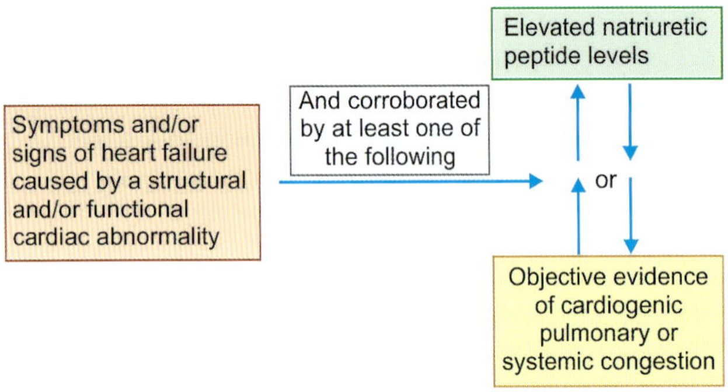

FLOWCHART 1: Universal definition of heart failure.

STAGES OF HEART FAILURE CONTINUUM (FLOWCHART 2)

Classifying HF by stage allows a clinician to communicate with patients in a more practical manner:

- *Stage A (at risk for HF)*: Patients at risk for HF but without current or prior symptoms or signs of HF and without structural cardiac changes or elevated biomarkers of heart disease. Examples of patients in this category are those with hypertension, diabetes, obesity, atherosclerotic cardiovascular (CV) disease, positive family history of cardiomyopathy, exposure to cardiotoxins, etc.
- *Stage B (pre-HF)*: Patients without current or prior symptoms or signs of HF with evidence of one of the following:
  - *Structural heart disease*: For example, left ventricular hypertrophy, cardiac chamber enlargement, ventricular wall motion abnormality, valvular heart disease, myocardial tissue abnormality (e.g., late gadolinium enhancement)
  - *Abnormal cardiac function*: For example, reduced right or left ventricular systolic function, abnormal diastolic dysfunction, evidence of increased filling pressures (by invasive or noninvasive measures)
  - Elevated natriuretic peptide levels
- *Stage C (HF)*: Patients with current or prior symptoms and/or signs of HF caused by a structural and/or functional cardiac abnormality

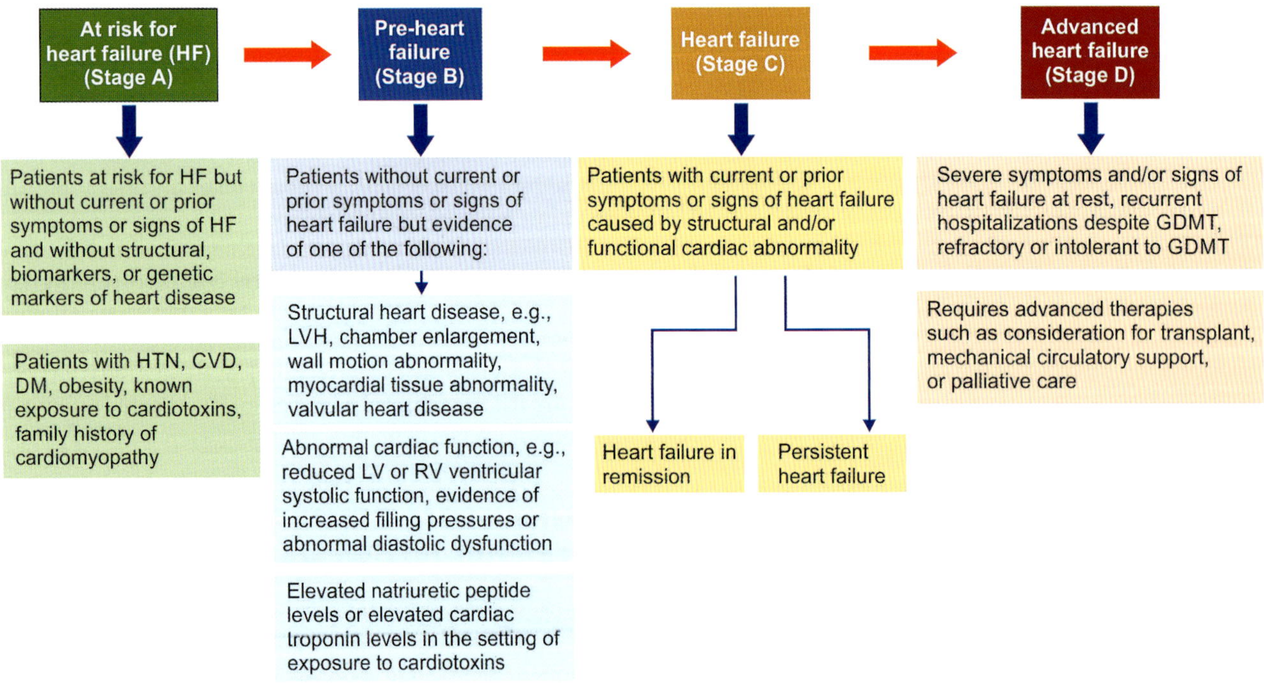

FLOWCHART 2: Stages in progression of heart failure.

- *Stage D (advanced HF)*: Severe symptoms and/or signs of HF at rest, recurrent hospitalizations despite GDMT, refractory or intolerant to GDMT, requiring advanced therapies such as consideration for transplantation, mechanical circulatory support, or palliative care

CLASSIFICATION BY LEFT VENTRICULAR EJECTION FRACTION

Argument to classify HF based on LVEF is to differentiate patients who belong to a particular subgroup of HF who are known to respond to life-prolonging therapies/GDMT based on randomized controlled trials. The following is the revised classification of HF based on LVEF:

- *HF with reduced ejection fraction (HFrEF):* Symptomatic HF with LVEF ≤ 40%
- *HF with mildly reduced ejection fraction (HFmrEF):* Symptomatic HF with LVEF 41–49% (previously labeled as HF with midrange ejection fraction)
- *HF with preserved ejection fraction (HFpEF):* Symptomatic HF with LVEF ≥ 50%
- *HF with improved ejection fraction (HFimpEF):* Symptomatic HF with a baseline LVEF of ≤40%, a ≥10-point increase from baseline LVEF, and a second measurement of LVEF of >40%

The terminology of "*stable HF*" should no longer be used, as patients are expected to improve with GDMT. These patients should have further optimization of therapies despite stability, because there is evidence for much more improvement in outcomes with additional therapies. Such patients should be termed "*persistent HF.*" "*HF in remission*" or NYHA functional class I should be reserved for patients who have resolution of symptoms and signs of HF along with resolution of previously present structural and functional heart disease after a phase of symptomatic HF. The term "*recovered HF*" should be used for patients who have persistent resolution of HF symptoms and signs, and normalization of cardiac structure, function, and biomarker profile after resolution and treatment of a fully reversible cause (e.g., tachycardiomyopathy, peripartum cardiomyopathy, Takotsubo syndrome, viral myocarditis).

ACUTE HEART FAILURE

Acute heart failure (AHF) refers to rapid or gradual onset of symptoms and/or signs of HF, severe enough for the patient to seek urgent medical attention, leading to an unplanned hospital admission or an emergency department visit.[6] It may be the first manifestation of HF (new onset) or, more commonly, due to an acute decompensation of chronic HF. Clinical presentation of AHF can be classified into four different presentations with possible overlaps between them:

1. Acute decompensated HF—this is the most common presentation.
2. Acute pulmonary edema
3. Isolated right ventricular failure
4. Cardiogenic shock

NEW CONCEPTS IN GUIDELINES

Management of Heart Failure with Reduced Ejection Fraction

The concept of HFrEF and its associated treatment poses a huge challenge to the clinician and can often feel daunting. Many opportunities are often missed to improve the patient outcomes. Based on new data that are emerging on the go, many new concepts have arisen and found their way into the guidelines. The new 2024 ACC Expert Consensus Decision Pathway of HFrEF tries to streamline patient care for optimal outcomes.[7] Some of the pivotal issues are discussed below.

Sequence to Initiate/Switch GDMT

The four established pillars of therapy for HFrEF (class I recommendations) include angiotensin-converting enzyme inhibitors (ACEI)/angiotensin receptor blocker (ARB)/ angiotensin II receptor/neprilysin inhibitors (ARNI), mineralocorticoid receptor antagonists (MRAs), sodium-glucose cotransporter (SGLT) inhibitors, and beta blockers.[8] Vericiguat is considered the fifth harmony of HF therapy and is currently given a class IIB recommendation for use in select high-risk patients with recent worsening of HF already on GDMT.[8,9] An ideal time to initiate these drugs is during the index hospitalization. But a question arises of which medication to start first. There is no order that needs to be followed and the clinician should add or titrate agents based on each patient's need.

Uptitration of doses of these medicines should be done as rapidly as possible with the aim of reaching the target dose or maximally tolerated dose ideally no longer than within 3 months. Initiation of ARNI is often best tolerated when the patient is still "wet," whereas beta blockers are better tolerated by a "dry" patient. All patients on ACEI or ARB, even if stable, should be shifted to ARNI, if there are no contraindications like prior angioedema. A 36-hour washout period is necessary to convert from ACEI, but not ARB, to ARNI. For SGLT inhibitor initiation, recent updates have lowered the cutoff of eGFR to <25 mL/min/1.73 m^2 for only dapagliflozin and sotagliflozin, with no lower cutoff for empagliflozin.[10] Based on the VICTORIA trial, vericiguat is a class IIb indication for worsening HF symptoms on maximally tolerated GDMT.[11]

Achieving Optimal Therapy with Multiple Drugs

Maximum benefits are obtained if GDMT is rapidly initiated and titrated to tolerated doses.[12] More than one drug may be started at a time or, in certain cases, all four classes may be started at once. Beta blockers should be adjusted every 1–2 weeks, if there is no evidence of HF decompensation.

ARNI doses can be increased every week, sometimes necessitating decreasing the loop diuretic doses simultaneously. MRA should be added to patients who are already taking ARNI (or ACEI/ARB) and beta blockers. Achieving maximally tolerated doses of other medicines is not a prerequisite to start MRA or SGLT inhibitor. SGLT inhibitors are used in a fixed dose; dose titration is not required. Loop diuretic dosage needs to be adjusted with initiation of SGLT inhibitors. For select patients, when used, vericiguat should be uptitrated every 2 weeks.

Common hindrances to initiate and titrate GDMT include abnormal kidney function and/or hyperkalemia. Low-potassium diet and use of SGLT inhibitors should be prioritized in such settings. Newer potassium binders, patiromer and sodium zirconium cyclosilicate, are now US FDA approved and may be used.[13] Starting dose of ARNI should be 50 mg twice daily if the eGFR is <30 mL/min/1.73 m^2. MRA is contraindicated if eGFR is <30 mL/min/1.73 m^2, potassium is >5.0 mEq/L, or creatinine is >2.5 mg/dL in men or >2.0 mg/dL in women. Kidney function test and potassium should be assessed within 1–2 weeks after initiation or increase in the dose of ARNI. The patient should be assessed clinically every 3–6 months and more frequently if unstable. For stable patients on optimal doses of GDMT, an echocardiogram should be repeated after 3–6 months.

When to Stop GDMT

For patients whose LVEF reaches normal, a question arises as to whether to stop the GDMT. The TRED-HF studied this question. It found that almost half of the patients withdrawn from GDMT had a relapse of their cardiomyopathy within 6 months.[14] So GDMT should be continued once initiated, irrespective of the LVEF, until and unless a reversible cause of LV dysfunction could be named, for example, sepsis-mediated or tachycardia-mediated cardiomyopathy.

Referral to a HF Specialist

Remembering the acronym "*I-NEED-HELP*" can assist in decision-making for referral to a heat failure specialist:

- *I:* Intravenous inotropes
- *N:* NYHA IIIB/IV or persistently elevated natriuretic peptides
- *E:* End-organ dysfunction
- *E:* Ejection fraction < 35%
- *D:* Defibrillator shocks
- *H:* Hospitalization > 1
- *E:* Edema despite escalating diuretic agents
- *L:* Low blood pressure, high heart rate
- *P:* Prognostic medication—progressive intolerance or downtitration of GDMT

Improve Adherence to Drugs

Fundamental to the therapeutic effectiveness of GDMT is that the patients are taking medicines regularly. Nonadherence is reported to be around 20–50%.[15] Reasons are many for nonadherence, like perceived lack of effect, poor health literacy, cognitive impairment, cost-related issues, and frequency of dosing. Such nonadherence is associated with worse outcomes in HF. Recent guidelines promote regular assessment of drug compliance. Blaming patients for nonadherence is counterproductive and inappropriate. To improve compliance, six categories of interventions have been identified: (i) Patient education, (ii) medication regimen management, (iii) clinical pharmacist consultation for chronic disease management, (iv) cognitive behavioral therapies, (v) medication-taking reminders, and (vi) incentives to promote adherence.

Manage Common Comorbidities

Heart failure patients, particularly the elderly, have many CV and non-CV comorbidities that effect their prognosis. Examples are many and not limited to conditions like hypertension, diabetes, chronic kidney disease, atrial fibrillation, coronary artery disease, anemia/iron deficiency/sleep disorders, and chronic lung disease. The presence of multiple other comorbidities increases the symptom burden, contributes to the progression of an underlying disease, and also becomes the reason for recurrent hospitalizations. Vaccination for influenza and pneumonia has shown marked improvements in mortality and hospitalization outcomes for HF patients.[16]

Integrate Palliative Care and Transition to Hospice Care

Advances in HF care have slowed the progression of the disease but have failed to completely cure it. Patients with HF remain at a risk of poor prognosis, with a 1-year mortality of 15–30% and a 3-year mortality of 30–50%.[17] Clinicians should shoulder the responsibility for an end-of-life plan based on the values and goals of the patient and family. Worsening disease as indicated by recurrent hospitalization or progressive intolerance of medications due to hypotension or kidney dysfunction should trigger preparation toward palliative care. Withholding some therapies like reducing ARNI in the setting of symptomatic hypotension and deactivation of defibrillator therapy, while adding some therapies that are usually not recommended, like opioids for refractory dyspnea, may sometimes be needed for symptom relief and quality of life. These steps should be individualized and made in consent with the patients and their caregivers.

Heart failure with reduced ejection fraction remains a leading cause of morbidity and mortality globally. Management requires a multidisciplinary approach. With the advent of available diagnostics and therapeutics, many questions have emerged regarding optimal utilization of these newer approaches to patient care. The 2024 ACC/AHA guidelines for HF management help to streamline care to realize best possible patient outcomes.

Management of Heart Failure with Preserved Ejection Fraction

The overall incidence of HF appears to be stable in the United States or even declining. However, the incidence of HFpEF continues to rise. It now accounts for >50% of cases of HF. HFpEF is often under-recognized, so a correct diagnosis is mandatory. To bridge the existing communication gap between CV and primary care clinicians who jointly manage patients with HFpEF, the ACC has published the 2023 ACC Expert Consensus Decision Pathway on management of heart failure with preserved ejection fraction.[18]

Diagnosis of HFpEF

Heart failure with preserved ejection fraction diagnosis requires symptoms and/or signs of HF caused by structural/functional abnormalities and at least one of the following:

- Elevated natriuretic peptides
- Objective evidence of cardiogenic pulmonary or systemic congestion

However, diagnosing HFpEF is more difficult as an echocardiogram may not show obvious abnormalities and the natriuretic peptides may be falsely low in situations such as obesity. Given the lack of a definite test to diagnose HFpEF, use of a clinical scoring system may be helpful. One such scoring system is the *H_2FPEF score*.[19] The six components of the *H_2FPEF score* are:

1. *H:* Heavy (BMI > 30 kg/m^2)—2
2. *H:* On >2 antihypertensives—1
3. *F:* Fibrillation (atrial)—3
4. *P:* Pulmonary hypertension—1 (PASP > 35 mm Hg on echocardiography)
5. *E:* Elderly (age > 60 years)—1
6. *F:* Filling pressure (*E/e'* > 9 on echo)—1

A score of 6 or more is highly suggestive of HFpEF.

Management of HFpEF

Management focuses on:

- Risk stratification and management of comorbidities, including diabetes, hypertension, AF, CAD, CKD, etc.
- Nonpharmacological management like exercise and weight loss
- Symptom management and disease-modifying therapy with loop diuretics, MRAs, SGLT inhibitors, ARNIs, and ARBs

Although historically discouraging, recent clinical trials have demonstrated the benefit of GDMT in HFpEF.[8]

- SGLT-2i significantly reduces the risk of hospitalization for HF and CV deaths across all EF groups. This group of drugs appears to be safe and effective when started in index hospitalization for acutely decompensated HF, once stable clinically. It has a class IIa recommendation in the 2022 AHA/ACC/HFSA HF guidelines.
- MRA significantly improves diastolic function and also reduces the risk of hospitalization in HFpEF. Monitoring of potassium and kidney function is necessary. It has a class IIb recommendation.
- ARNI has a class IIB recommendation for patients with HFpEF.
- ARB may be used, where ARNI is contraindicated, for example, in angioedema.
- Loop diuretics should be used judiciously to reduce congestion and improve symptoms.

Referral to Advanced HF Specialists

The acronym to assist in decision-making for HF specialist referral is *INHALE*:

- *I:* In need of diagnosis (lack of conventional risk factors)
- *N:* Nonresponsive to diuretics or medical therapy; high natriuretic peptides
- *H:* Hospitalized frequently for HF (>2 hospitalizations in the past year)
- *A:* Acute or chronic end-organ dysfunction
- *L:* Low blood pressure (systolic BP < 100 mm Hg)
- *E:* Evidence of HFpEF mimics

Heart failure with preserved ejection fraction is a complex condition with multiple overlapping comorbidities. Timely diagnosis and implementation of therapies are the prerequisite for optimal outcomes.

CONCLUSION

The universal definition of HF is comprehensive and practical enough to form the base that allows further subclassifications and that can encompass formal disease stages, with universal applicability, prognostic and therapeutic validity, and an acceptable sensitivity and specificity. Identifying various classes of HF is important to individualize treatment and follow GDMT in respective class of HF. Staging of HF helps identifying at-risk patients (Stage A) to apply preventive measures, from asymptomatic (Stage B) to symptomatic (Stages C and D) patients, where clinicians need to initiate GDMT and HF devices as and when required. Recent updates also shed important information about ensuring optimal initiation, escalation, adherence, and referral of HFrEF patients. Scoring in patients suspected of HFpEF will help taking a more objective approach for diagnosing HFpEF.

ONLINE REFERENCES

Please scan the QR code provided at the end of the table of contents for References of this chapter.

CHAPTER 53

Transformation of Guidelines of Heart Failure from Dropsy to Remodeling

Mrinal Kanti Das

ABSTRACT

The present history of the journey of heart failure (HF) with the transformation of the guidelines has been derived from the various records obtained from the literature of yesteryears, dwelling with the healing practices several millennia ago. The fascinating journey through various changing models of pathophysiology, disease, and health reflects the human minds which are ever truth-seeking. This quest for the truth led to the modern canvas of pillars of therapy for HF based on hemodynamic, neurohormonal modulation, remodeling of the heart and panvascular system, and advances in technology with device therapy, assist devices, and artificial heart. They could be incorporated, because the drugs and devices demonstrated robust evidences of bettering and modifying the disease and the natural history of HF, which influenced the guidelines from time to time. Many more are yet to come with advancement of artificial intelligence (AI) and quantum computations, which will be guided by yet-unimagined mechanistic and statistical models. This chapter attempts to explore the human histories of success and failure, which transformed the formulations of guidelines over the years.

Keywords: Heart failure (HF), guidelines, guideline-directed therapy (GDT)

INTRODUCTION

Heart failure (HF) is a major public health problem, affecting 26 million people worldwide. It is the end stage of all the diseases of the heart and is a major cause of morbidity and mortality.

A huge number of guidelines have happened over many years and have been formulated from time to time by the physicians to guide the principles of treatment of a particular disease, based on the conception about the pathophysiology, availability of the drugs at the particular point of time, and the personal real-life experience and the so-called intuition of a physician, without necessarily being supported by any concrete evidence. This personal experience or intuitions many a time amounted to whims and show of power in the past, which could not be questioned because of the authority imposed by a particular physician. During the remotest era, physicians, pharaohs, and commoners believed that *"magic is effective together with medicine; medicine is effective together with magic."*[1] Along the line of the cultures, the medicine in those days was also combined with magical incantations and the drug formulations often contained unproved ingredients for certain diseases. The ingredients of the prescriptions of the ancient Egyptians contained extracts from plants, trees, fruits, and several mineral substances. Those days, eggs, liver, hair, milk, animal horns and fat, honey, and wax were also used in drug preparation. They were administered as gels, infusions, pills, gargles, snuffs, poultices, or suppositories.

However, with changing time, the evidence-based medicine started flourishing. The stakeholders of health found the opportunity to impose the formulation of guideline or standard operating procedure (SOP) with the help of evidences and thus routinize the clinical practice often lowering the quality of treatment. The stakeholders comprising the administrators, governments, physicians' bodies, insurance company, etc., could reduce the cost of therapy because of the generalization of the treatment. Often, these guidelines could modify the treatment by the physicians only modestly. But the fallacy also cropped up because of the nonadherence of guidelines by most of the physicians, though many of them were aware of them. Fowkes and Roberts in 1984 and many others conceptualized the implication of moral character in management practice and initiated medical and financial auditing, which could reduce the cost by €6 billion in those days. For over the last two decades, almost all organizations of cardiologists across the globe formulated different guidelines for the physicians and those responsible for care of the patients with HF. These bodies have, from time to time, updated those guidelines or published consensus documents on certain management principles which have changed the paradigm of therapy for HF. The following descriptions are intended to dwell upon the interesting and intriguing history and science of development of the guidelines for HF management.[2,3]

HISTORICAL JOURNEY OF HEART FAILURE

From the Valley of Queens to Valsartan

The documentation of HF was first reported by Italian Egyptologist Ernesto Schiaparelli way back in 1479 BCE. In 2015, archaeologists after exploration of a plundered tomb in the Valley of the Queens found a 3,500-year-old ancient mummy in Egypt and revealed the evidence of accumulation of water by pathological tests, in the lungs, likely to be the effect of the HF. It was the oldest recorded case of HF. The mummy consisted only of a head and internal organs in the glass container. Nebiri, "Chief of Stables," was a middle-aged man (approximately 40–60 years old), when he expired. Computed tomography scan and three-dimensional skull reconstruction revealed in him severe periodontal disease with massive abscesses. The histology of Nebiri's lungs revealed: (1) "HF" cells and (2) fluid in the air sacs presently called pulmonary edema. Histochemical tests ruled out acid-fast bacilli or other granulomatous diseases including tuberculosis. From these findings, the researchers opined that Nebiri could have died from acute decompensation of chronic left-sided HF due to chronic hypertension.[4]

On the other side of the world, in China, "*The Yellow Emperor's Classic of Internal Medicine*" discussed dropsical swellings as early as 2600 BC.[5]

Hippocrates in 425–360 BCE also recognized some of the features of congestive heart failure (CHF) by hearing the sounds akin to "boiling vinegar" by putting his ears on the chest of a person. He also proposed and executed treatment by draining the fluid from the lungs by making a hole in the ribcage.[6]

Greek physician Galen and early Egyptian physicians recognized that the heart contracts and found the channels known as arteries, believed to distribute heat and air to the body. They however could not find any relationship between edema, dyspnea, and anasarca. Ibn al-Nafis in the thirteenth century first discovered the pulmonary circulation. He described the blood movement from the right to the left side of the heart via the lungs.

William Harvey in the seventeenth century made his revolutionary conclusion that blood circulates in channels in series from right to left through the lungs and then from left to right by the pumping or contracting function of the heart muscle, thus making the heart as the pivot of the circulatory system. He conclusively showed that arteries and veins form a complete circuit, which starts at the heart and leads back to the heart, a revelation which was epoch-making and responsible for all the future understanding about the heart and circulatory system. He also observed that a dilated heart was associated with HF.[7]

Sir William Withering in 1785 first published his observations on use of *foxglove* in patients suffering from anasarca or generalized swelling of body and used the term *"dropsy."* The extracts from the leaves increased the power of contraction of the heart and thus increased the urine formation known as diuresis, thereby reducing swelling of the body and breathlessness associated with the swelling. Later on, the glycoside digitalis was isolated from the extracts, which was attributed to the increased contractility of the heart muscles. Further later on, it was found by research works that the inhibition of sodium-potassium-ATPase pump on the heart muscle membrane receptors resulted in the influx of calcium via calmodulin, causing the coupling of the actin-myosin complex, responsible for the contraction of the heart muscles. For the last 220 years, digitalis remained as a mainstay of HF therapy.[8]

Ernest Henry Starling brought physics in the mechanism of heart function in 1910 and opined that as the muscles get elongated or dilated up to a certain extent, the contractile function increases. This was referred to as Starling's law of the heart. This gave way to the principle that as the end-diastolic volume increases, cardiac performance increases to a point. This explained the HF with dilated heart with abnormal contractile function, but could not explain the HF in patients without dilation of the ventricle.[9] In 1940–1960, the journey of cardiac catheterization and surgery revealed many aspects of HF in rheumatic and congenital heart diseases, in terms of hemodynamic abnormalities, but failed to explain HF with obstructive coronary arteries or hypertension or without any evidence of obvious cause.[10,11] From these inputs, the concept of remodeling came into the picture. It was conceived that remodeling can happen in different ways like concentric or eccentric hypertrophy of the heart without external dilatation and dilated heart with increase in length of the muscles at the cost of strength and width. Remodeling and reverse remodeling are considered very important in the progression or deterioration, treatment responses, and further consequences in HF and related conditions.[12] The concept of remodeling later on enthused workers to propose different names of the HF. This concept of remodeling and prior and postremodeling events at heart and cellular levels is depicted in **Flowchart 1** and **Figure 1**.

Historically, Röntgen's discovery of X-rays **(Figs. 2A to C)** and Einthoven's development of electrocardiography in the 1890s led to quantum improvements in the investigation and treatment of HF.

The subsequent advent of echocardiography, cardiac catheterization, and nuclear medicine has since improved the diagnosis and study of patients with HF and immensely contributed to the development of the diagnostic and therapeutic guidelines in later period of time.

The Framingham Heart Study, carried out since 1948, has been the most reliable and important longitudinal source of data on the epidemiology of HF. One of the seminal papers describing the epidemiology of CHF arose out of Framingham. McKee et al. authored a paper in 1971, where they described the criteria for diagnosing HF. The criteria have continued to be used till date in clinical and epidemiologic studies. The paper also stated that hypertension is an important precursor for HF and those patients with hypertension developing CHF have a poor prognosis. This is possibly the first attempt to structuralize the disease called heart failure.[13]

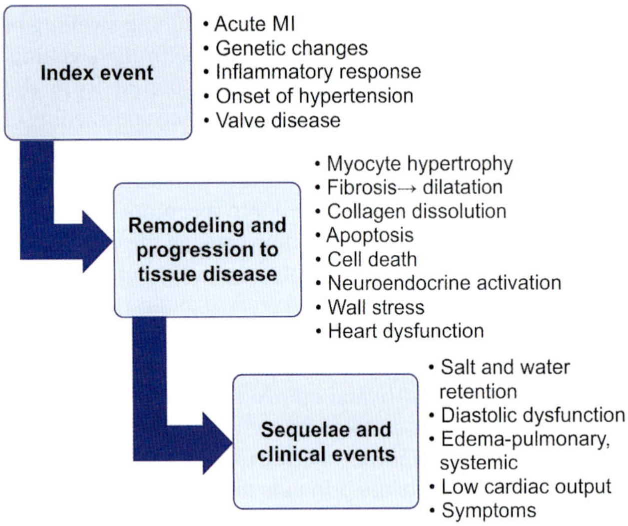

FLOWCHART 1: Preremodeling events, remodeling, and the aftermath.

Between the 1970s and the 1980s, researchers termed the HF as a syndrome which meant simultaneous dysfunctions of multiple organs including the heart, lungs, liver, kidneys, gut, endocrine and exocrine organs, and peripheral muscles resulting in features of congestive disorders and constellation of symptoms due to dysfunction of several organ systems, rather than due specifically to the heart. The terminologies like forward failure, backward failure, left HF, right HF, high-output failure, and low-output failure with specific clinical signs and symptoms were thus coined explaining the various clinical pictures of HF.[1]

During the same period, the concept of activation of the neuroendocrine system with increased sympathomimetic activity became accepted as the pathophysiological mechanism of HF. That prompted the use of beta blocker (BB) as a therapeutic option, which could take care of the exaggerated sympathomimetic activities including high heart rate and downregulation of the beta receptors. However, its use deteriorated the patient's profile and thus BB was labeled as a contraindicated drug for HF till the mid-1980s. Interestingly, later on, it was found that in certain subsets of HF like high-output failure or hypertensive HF, there was increased cardiac output with amelioration of symptoms. Presently, certain BBs with vasodilating properties are put in the guidelines as mandatory. Simultaneously, drugs that lowered aldosterone were found to have favorable response on HF, operating through the mechanisms of weak diuretic

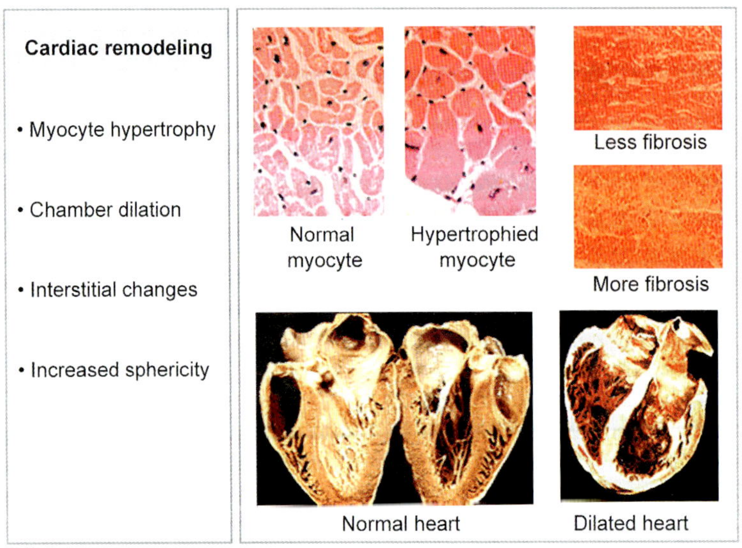

FIG. 1: Cellular and mechanical remodeling.

effect, and inhibition of the renin–angiotensin system. Then came the angiotensin-converting enzyme (ACE) inhibitors which also had a beneficial effect on HF. The CONSENSUS-1 study (1987) unequivocally showed a survival benefit of ACE inhibition in HF.[14] The angiotensin II receptor blockers were the natural extension of the RAS inhibiting group of drugs.

*A summary of the historical perspectives of concepts and therapeutics of HF is given in **Box 1**.*

HEART FAILURE MILIEU

Based on all this information, an attempt has been made to come to a consensus idea about the various facets of HF to explain the definition of HF, which is basically a failure in the part of the heart to perform its normal activities. This has been shown in **Figures 3A and B** depicting various facets and summary of HF syndrome.[15]

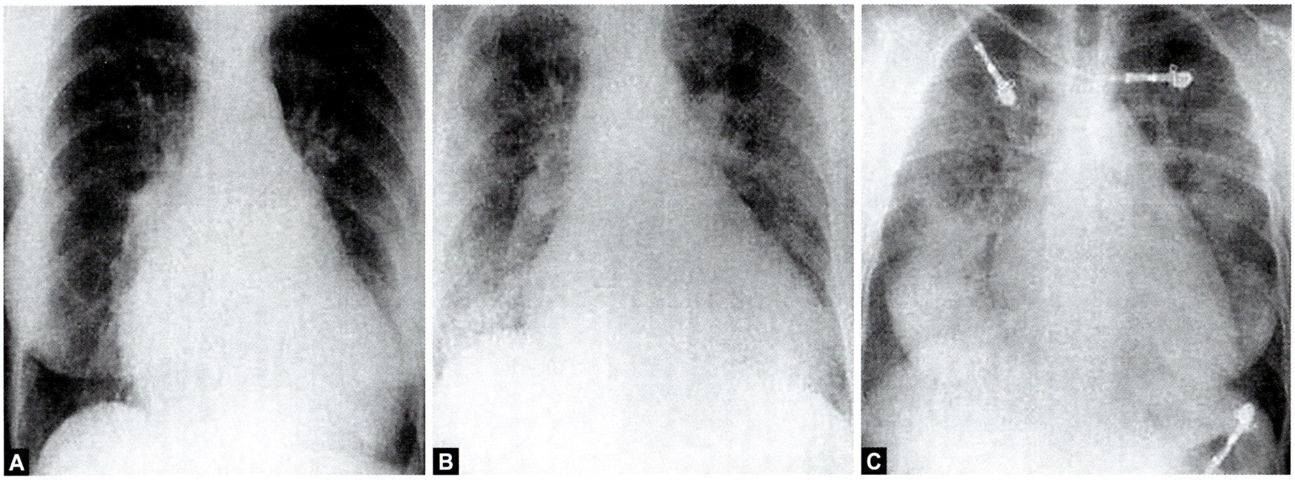

FIGS. 2A TO C: (A) Pulmonary blood flow redistribution. Engorgement of the upper lobe vessels with elevated pulmonary venous pressure. (B) Pulmonary interstitial edema. The vessels are indistinct and enlarged with peribronchial cuffing. (C) Pulmonary alveolar edema. The central perihilar opacities called "bat wing" edema caused by cardiovascular or fluid overload.

BOX 1 Nocturnal hypertension are detailed.

I. *HF is a dropsical state with generalized fluid accumulation in the body*
   a. Loop diuretic therapy
   b. Lymphatic drainage tube insertion
   c. Thoracic or abdominal cavity drainage
   d. Foxglove tea and era
II. *HF is due to failure of central heart pump function*
   a. Cardiac glycoside pharmacotherapy
   b. Inotropic and inodilator therapy
   c. Heart transplant
   d. Mechanical ventricular-assist devices or artificial heart
III. *HF is precipitated by decompensation of ventricular hypertrophy*
   a. Antihypertensive therapy
   b. Surgical repair of the valves
IV. *HF is due to circulatory dysfunction*
   a. Vasodilators to augment peripheral blood flow and organ perfusion
V. *HF is the result of endocrine abnormalities*
   a. Sympathetic overstimulation blocking by beta blockers (BB)

Continued

Continued

   b. Angiotensin-converting enzyme inhibitor (ACEi) therapy
   c. Angiotensin-converting enzyme receptor blocker (ARB) therapy
   d. Mineralocorticoid receptor antagonist (MRA) therapy
   e. Angiotensin receptor–neprilysin inhibitor (ARNI)
VI. *HF is an inflammatory disorder*
   a. Cytokine modulating agents
VII. *HF is a complex milieu of pump failure, remodeling, hormonal, cytokine, and neurohormonal perturbation with circulatory insufficiency*
   a. Five pillars of HF therapy: Diuretics, beta blocker, ARNI/ACEi/ARB, MRA, SGLT-2 inhibitor
   b. Vericiguat
   c. Ivabradine
   d. Digoxin
   e. Isosorbide dinitrate + hydralazine combo
   f. CRTP/CRTD/AICD
   g. Coronary revascularization, valve repairs like MitraClip, or valve replacement
   h. LV assist devices, cardiac transplant, or artificial heart

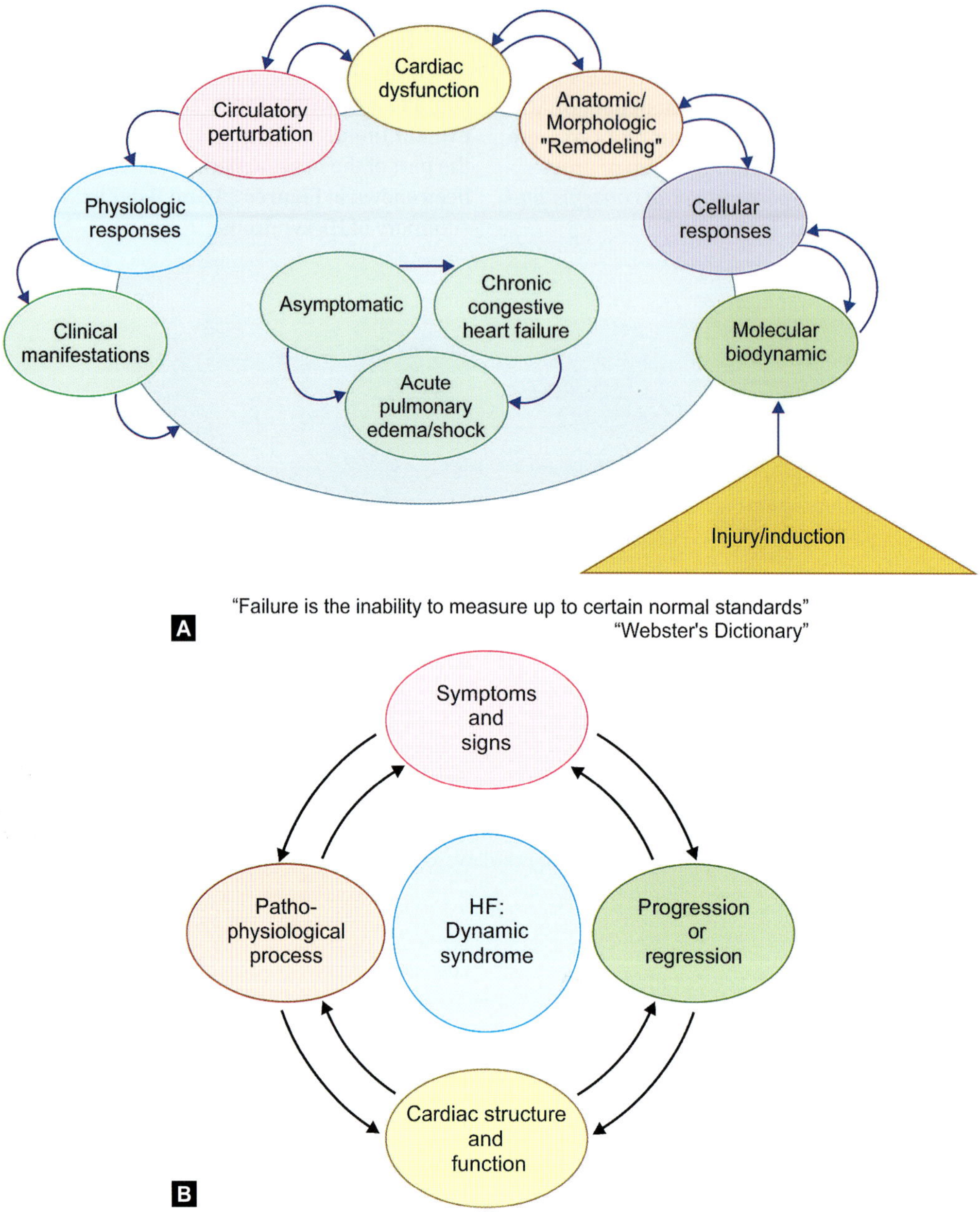

FIGS. 3A AND B: Heart failure (HF) milieu[16] (modified).

CONCEPT OF HEART FAILURE IN THE LIGHT OF EJECTION FRACTION[16]

The concept of ejection fraction (EF) developed over a long period of time starting with the concept of dilatation of the left ventricle by Sir William Harvey and later on by various workers with the help of cardiac catheterization and other tests including echocardiography which formed the stellar procedure in the diagnostic armamentarium of HF. **Figures 4 and 5** are suggestive of the pathways to the concept of EF.

But the EF could not explain many things related to HF. There were heterogenous responses to medications. Some were responders; some were nonresponders. This led to the concept of "clusters" based on phenotyping and phenomapping. The guideline-directed treatments were proposed toward the specific cluster, which offered personalized care of HF patients. The HFpEF was clustered into three types based on environmental factors, comorbidities, and genetic susceptibility: Type 1, exercise-induced increase in LA pressure; type 2, volume overload; and type 3, pulmonary hypertension and RV failure. The

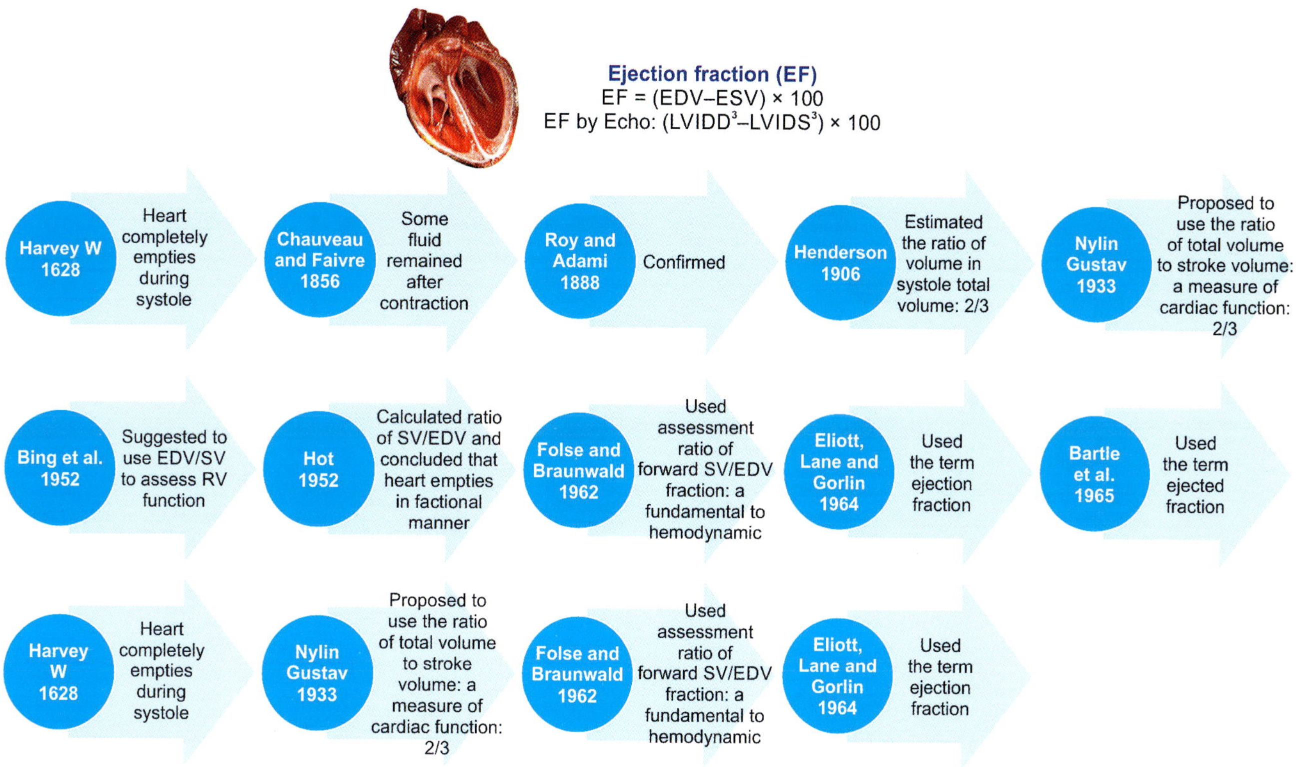

FIG. 4: Pathways of the development of the concept of ejection fraction (EF).

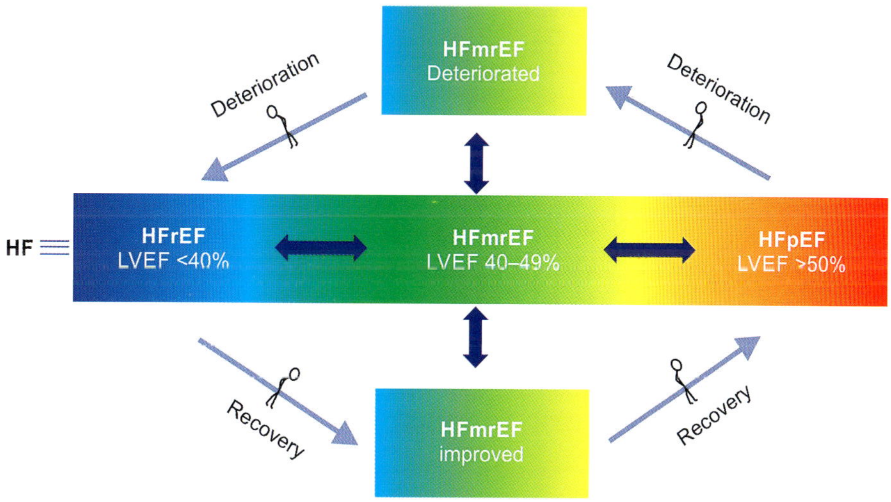

FIG. 5: Continuum of concept of EF leading to different classes of HF.
(HF: heart failure; EF: ejection fraction)

concept of clusters is still evolving and is shown in **Figure 6** and **Table 1**. It highlights Kaplan–Meier curve for the composite of clinical events of different clusters on the right side of **Figure 6** along with various clinical clusters in the middle. **Table 1** highlights different clusters based on echocardiographic and clinical domains in addition to the clinical and echo accumulative scores.[17]

STAGES OF HEART FAILURE

Figure 7 shows the different stages of HF. This forms the foundation stone for the management of HF at different phases and all the guidelines have been mostly focused on this classification hovering around for more than a decade. It depicts both clinical stagings and the therapeutic options.[18]

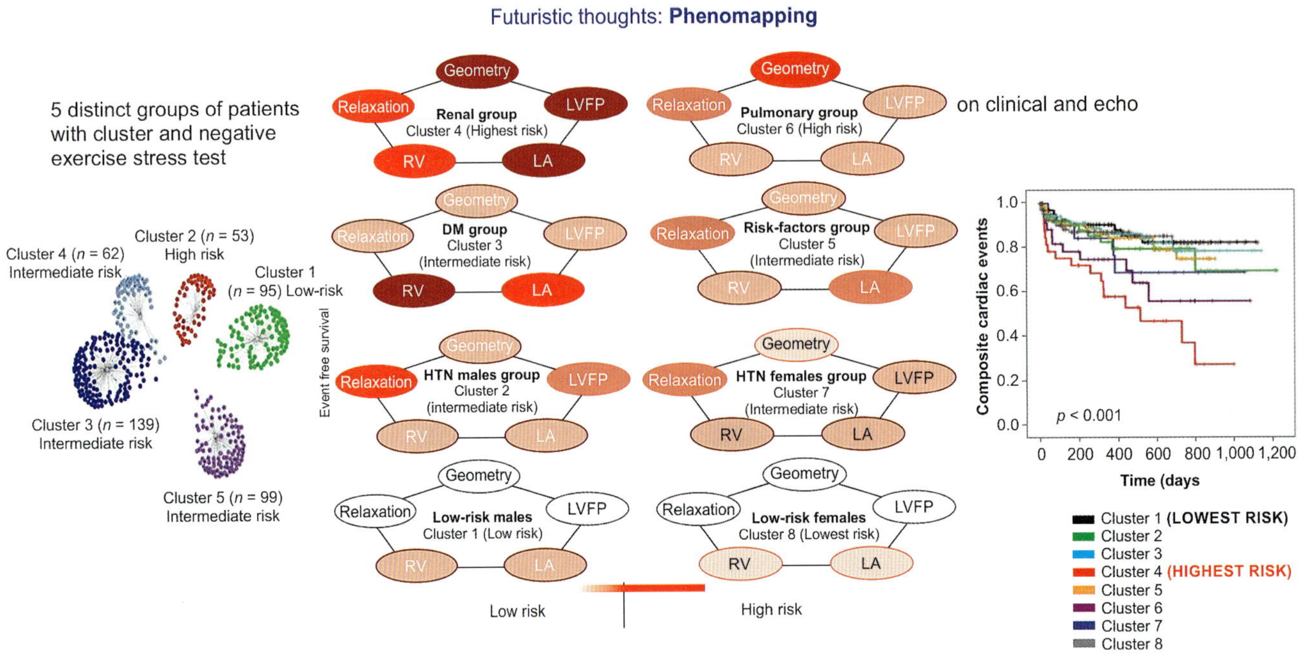

FIG. 6: Clusters of HF and risk status.
Source: Adapted from Omar et al.[17]

TABLE 1: Different clusters based on echocardiographic and clinical domains in addition to the clinical and echo accumulative scores.

Domain	Cluster 1 (*n* = 82)	Cluster 2 (*n* = 68)	Cluster 3 (*n* = 23)	Cluster 4 (*n* = 35)	Cluster 5 (*n* = 90)	Cluster 6 (*n* = 37)	Cluster 7 (*n* = 107)	Cluster 8 (*n* = 114)
Systolic domain	+	+	++	++	+	++	+++	++
Geometry	*n*	+	+	++	+	++	+	*n*
Relaxation	*n*	+	+	++	+	+	+	*n*
LVFP	*n*	*n*	*n*	+++	++	*n*	++	*n*
RVSP	+	+	++	+++	+	++	+	+
LA	+	++	+++	++++	++	+	+	*n*
Clinical score	3.7 ± 1.9	6.3 ± 1.9	4.2 ± 2.4	8.3 ± 2.6	6.21 ± 2.3	6.6 ± 2.4	4.1 ± 1.9	1.8 ± 1.6
Echo	3.5 ± 1.7	4.5 ± 1.9	4.9 ± 2.7	7.3 ± 2.3	5 ± 1.9	4 ± 1.8	4.6 ± 1.8	3.6 ± 1.7
Cardiac death	1 (1)	4 (6)	2 (9)	9 (26)	4 (4)	2 (5)	1 (1)	2 (2)
Rehospitalization	9 (11)	11 (16)	4 (17)	12 (34)	14 (16)	11 (30)	16 (15)	14 (12)
Composite	9 (11)	11 (16)	5 (22)	17 (49)	15 (17)	11 (30)	16 (15)	15 (13)

EVOLUTION OF THE CONCEPT OF GUIDELINES[19]

Though there were no guidelines per se during the 1980s, standard teaching on management of HF was focused on restriction of fluid intake, bed rest, oxygen therapy, diuretics, digitalis, and morphine in an acute HF state. Apart from these, the goals of treatment of HF also included heart-healthy lifestyle changes; treating the underlying diseases such as coronary artery disease, high blood pressure, atrial fibrillation, diabetes, or valvular heart disease; and using devices and surgical procedures, along with ongoing care. Although our comprehension of HF has remarkably improved and we traversed a long way so far with new thoughts and treatment schedules that improved survival, hospitalizations for HF are still high, readmissions are frequent, and sudden deaths are common. Essentially, cure for HF is still eluding. The author himself learnt the same approach during the early 1980s. But in course of time, guideline-directed therapy (GDT) came in and is in full force.

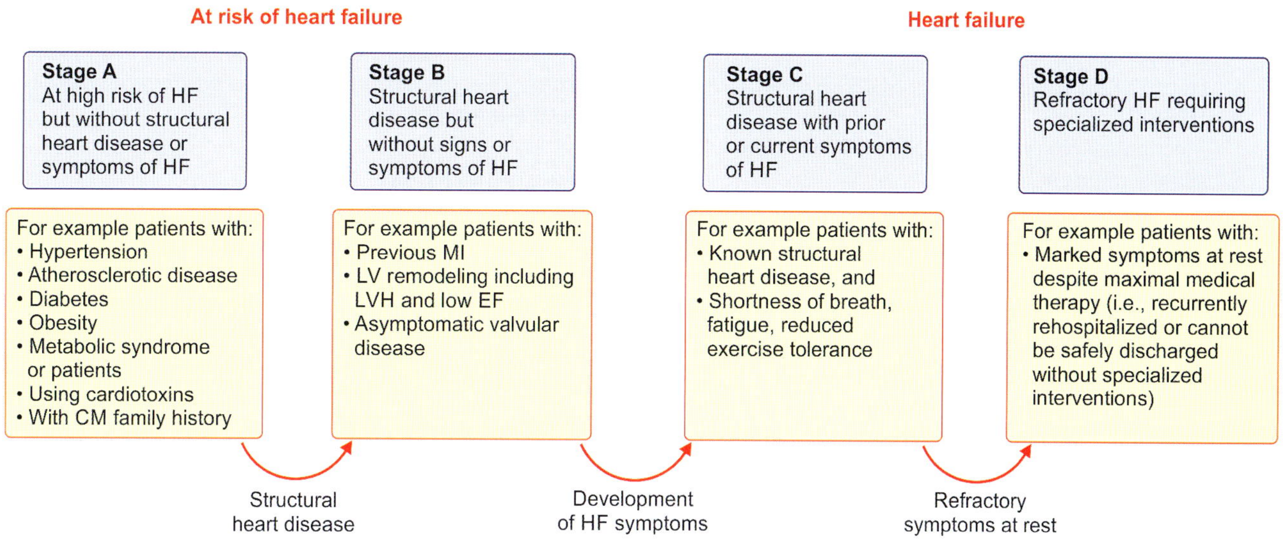

FIG. 7: Different stages of heart failure (HF).
Source: Adapted from Jessup et al. (2009).[18]

The term "clinical practice guidelines," very commonly used nowadays, started as a concept only recently since 1990 with the better understanding of the pathology and pathophysiology of HF along with natural history of the disease with the help of the various noninvasive and invasive diagnostic procedures and therapeutic measures. The National Academy of Medicine (NAM), earlier known as the Institute of Medicine, used the term "clinical practice guideline" along with eight attributes of good practice guidelines. In 1992, a category for practice guidelines was added to the National Library of Medicine's PubMed and in 2003, the GRADE approach (Grading of Recommendations, Assessment, Development, and Evaluation) for rating guideline recommendations was developed, hastening the movement for evidence-based medicine that had begun in 1981. In 2011, the NAM defined clinical practice guidelines and set criteria for establishing them. They unequivocally expressed that the recommendation statements intended to optimize patient care are based on a thorough systematic review of the available evidences and an assessment of the benefits and harms of alternative care options.

The whole exercise of the guidelines was:
- Based on systematic literature reviews
- Developed by a multidisciplinary, expert panel
- To include patient representation and values
- Explicit, transparent, minimizing bias and conflict of interest
- To provide clear explanation of alternative options
- To provide ratings of the quality of evidence and the strength of recommendations
- To be reconsidered and revised whenever there was important new evidence

These approaches and criteria have subsequently been widely disseminated and adhered to in most fields of medicine, including HF. Recommendations and evidences combined together have led to the universally accepted nomenclatures. For example, guideline recommendations are typically graded as Class I, Class II, and Class III and evidences as A or B. Very recently, a new addition "E" has been made implying the "expert opinion" to accommodate consensus view by many experts in the same field.

ARE THERE SIMILARITIES OR DISSIMILARITIES IN DIFFERENT GUIDELINES?[20]

There are very few of these. Most of them follow the same level of evidences. Since the two guidelines by the ESC and ACC/AHA/HFSA are widely followed across the globe, the similarities or dissimilarities are cited below:
- *Similarities*:
  - Same diagnostic tools
  - Optimal management of risk factors and similar management for asymptomatic HF
  - Four pillars for HFrEF and HFmrEF: renin-angiotensin-aldosterone system inhibitors (RAASi) + BB + mineralocorticoid receptor antagonist (MRA) + sodium-glucose cotransporter-2 inhibitors (SGLT 2i)
  - HFpEF: Comorbidity management by both
  - Acute and advanced HF: Same approach
- *Dissimilarities*:
  - Prediction of disease trajectory: Mentioned only in ACC/AHA/HFSA GL
  - For diagnosis: Different levels of evidence for BNP/NT-proBNP
  - Stage A versus stage B
  - ACC/AHA/HFSA: Different QRS intervals for cardiac resynchronization therapy (CRT) and different levels

of evidence for implantable cardioverter-defibrillator (ICD)

- HFpEF: RAASi + BB + MRA + SGLT-2i by ACC/AHA/HFSA GL
- Mechanical circulatory supports (MCS) in two GL are slightly different.

IMPACTS OF THE GUIDELINES ON HEART FAILURE OUTCOMES[21,22]

Despite many shortcomings including nonadherence and differing statements by different organizations, a meta-analysis of 57 trials from 1987 to 2015 of guideline-directed medical therapy (GDMT) HF demonstrated benefits: 56% reduction in all-cause mortality with ACE inhibitor + BB + MRA compared with placebo and 63% reduction with ARNI + BB + MRA.

OTHER BENEFITS

Data on more than 40,000 HFrEF patients in 12 clinical trials showed a sharp decline in the rate of sudden death over the years as new agents were incorporated into GDMT. The cumulative incidence of sudden death within 90 days after randomization plunged from 2.4% in the earliest trial to 1.0% in the most recent one. *International clinical practice guidelines therefore strongly recommend the prescription of HF GDMT at target doses.*

CONCLUSION

Heart failure is a complex syndrome and the understanding of the disease has evolved over centuries of researches and studies. There is complex interaction between epigenetics (environmental factors), comorbidities, genomics, cytokines inducing inflammation, and remodeling of the heart which loses its normal function of supplying oxygen and nutrition to tissues and organs and thus generates a precarious situation with multiple symptoms and clinical, mechanical, and biochemical changes in the body. The history of the changing concepts is fascinating, but there is a lot to achieve even after the formulations of the guidelines by different cardiovascular societies in both diagnostic and therapeutic milieu. Being complex in nature, "one size does not fit all" may be the reality of life and artificial intelligence (AI)-based evaluation and therapy may augment the clinician's effort in not-so-far future in mitigating the menacing disease in terms of both morbidity and mortality.

ONLINE REFERENCES

Please scan the QR code provided at the end of the table of contents for References of this chapter.

CHAPTER

54

Heart Failure and Left Ventricular Remodeling: Current Understanding

Abraham Oomman, Narra Lavanya

ABSTRACT

Heart failure (HF) is a clinical syndrome characterized by structural and functional abnormalities culminating in ventricular filling or ejection of blood being impaired as compared to the requirement of an individual.[1] HF burden related to traditional risk factors is increasing. HF is a primary contributor to cardiovascular mortality and morbidity. Left ventricular (LV) remodeling is one of the pathologies encountered in the progression of HF. It is driven by adaptation of cardiac myocytes via structural, functional, cellular, and molecular changes to their surroundings. This chapter highlights the mechanism of LV remodeling, reverse remodeling, latest diagnostic tools, and effective treatment options for patients with HF and LV remodeling.

Keywords: Heart failure, left ventricular remodeling, left ventricular reverse remodeling

INTRODUCTION

Heart failure (HF) is a condition in which there are physiological and structural abnormalities of ventricular filling or ejection of blood. The most common causes of HF include hypertension, diabetes mellitus, valvular heart disease, myocardial ischemia, cardiomyopathy, pulmonary hypertension, sleep apnea, excessive drug or alcohol use, obesity, and congenital heart disease.[2] We propose a universal definition of heart failure (HF with aging population), HF will affect a large number of individuals globally.

Heart failure is divided into three categories based on left ventricular ejection fraction (LVEF). Nearly one-half of patients with HF have HF with preserved ejection fraction (HFpEF) with an LVEF ≥ 50%, while the remaining account for HF with reduced ejection fraction (HFrEF) with an LVEF ≤ 40%.[3] HF with midrange ejection fraction (HFmrEF) with an ejection fraction (EF) range from 41 to 49% accounts for 10–25% of the population.[4] HF with recovered EF (HFrecEF) refers to patients with improvement in LVEF spontaneously or that which occurs after the use of guideline-directed medical therapy (GDMT) and device therapy.[5]

Cardiac remodeling was initially described by Jean-Nicolas Corvisart in 1806. He described two types of left ventricular (LV) dilatation: (1) Active with thick walls and increased force; and (2) Passive with thinning and decreased force.[6] LV remodeling is influenced by three crucial factors: Changes in myocyte biology, alterations in myocardial structure, and modifications in LV chamber shape. While initially observed following a myocardial infarction (MI), it can also occur in reaction to different types of myocardial injury.[7,8]

PATHOPHYSIOLOGY OF LEFT VENTRICULAR REMODELING

Remodeling refers to a process in which mechanical, neurohormonal, and genetic factors drive molecular and structural alterations that contribute to changes in size, shape, and function of the ventricle. The pathological hallmarks include hypertrophy, interstitial fibrosis, and myocyte loss. Molecular alterations involve elevated levels of inflammatory cytokines, heightened oxidative stress, and enhanced matrix metalloproteinase (MMP) activity.

Initially adaptive, these changes when sustained may contribute to irreversible damage and HF progression[9,10] **(Box 1)**.[1]

BOX 1 Mechanisms involved in the appearance and progression of cardiac remodeling in IHD.[11]

- *Inflammation*:
  - Increased in inflammatory cytokines—TNF-α, IL-6, 2, and 1β
- *Oxidative stress*:
  - Increased activity of MMPs
- *Neurohormonal activation*:
  - Activation of SNS, RAAS, and ADH
- *Fibrosis and cell death*:
  - Myocyte hypertrophy
  - Myocyte necrosis or apoptosis

(ADH: antidiuretic hormone; IL: interleukin; MMPs: matrix metalloproteinases; RAAS: renin–angiotensin–aldosterone system; SNS: sympathetic nervous system; TNF-α: tumor necrosis factor-alpha)

Remodeling may manifest as either physiological or pathological, entailing an increase in myocardial mass. Physiological remodeling denotes alterations in heart dimensions due to physiological stimuli such as exercise (athlete's heart) and pregnancy. Conversely, pathological remodeling arises as a result of an underlying cardiac stressor. This may involve a condition of volume overload like valvular regurgitation or a situation of pressure overload such as hypertension or aortic stenosis. Pathological remodeling can also occur following myocardial injury, as observed in MI.[12]

Chamber remodeling entails various pathological changes including infarct thinning and stretching, local metabolic changes, and remote myocyte growth and fibrosis. Initially compensatory, these changes progress to irreversible stages over time, leading to deteriorating LV stress and dysfunction.

LEFT VENTRICULAR REVERSE REMODELING

The term left ventricular reverse remodeling (LVRR) was first used in medical literature by Barry and Arlene Levine in 1997.[13]

Left ventricular reverse remodeling is thought to occur as a result of removal of the triggering injury/insult that contributes to remodeling and/or institution of interventions that mitigate exacerbating factors, hemodynamic load, maladaptive neurohormonal activation, etc., that drive remodeling. The changes in genome expression result in molecular and cellular alterations that modify tissue and organs. Patients with HF go on from a trajectory of normal heart to that of HF and then either have myocardial remission and recovery due to LVRR or spiral down to a vicious cycle of recurrent HF and end-stage heart disease.

ASSESSMENT OF FACETS OF LEFT VENTRICULAR REVERSE REMODELING

Cardiac Biomarkers

Biomarkers are valuable tools in clinical practice for assessing the severity of HF, predicting prognosis, and monitoring response to treatment. Their use in combination with imaging techniques and clinical assessment provides a comprehensive approach to managing patients with heart disease. Some key biomarkers commonly used are as follows:

- *Brain natriuretic peptide (BNP) and N-terminal proBNP (NT-proBNP)*: BNP is released from the ventricles (particularly from the LV) in response to increased wall stress, whereas NT-proBNP is a stable fragment of BNP and is more commonly used. Elevated levels of both these biomarkers correlate with increased LV filling pressures and indicate myocardial stress and volume overload. Greater improvement in the LVEF and reduced LV volumes were seen in patients with greater reduction in NT-proBNP levels ≤ 1,000 pg/mL.[14]
- *Cardiac troponins (cTnT and cTnI)*: Troponins are released into the bloodstream following myocardial injury or damage. Persistent elevation suggests ongoing myocardial injury or stress. hs-Troponin T values < 11 pg/mL and hs-troponin I < 11 pg/mL were associated with lower CV event rate and higher-frequency reverse remodeling.[15]
- *Galectin-3*: It is involved in the inflammatory processes within the myocardium. Elevated levels (values > 20 ng/mL) indicate adverse cardiac remodeling, including fibrosis and ventricular dysfunction. It serves as a prognostic marker in HF patients.
- *Soluble ST2 (ST2)*: ST2 is a member of the interleukin-1 receptor family and is involved in inflammatory and fibrotic responses. Elevated levels (>35 ng/mL) are associated with adverse outcomes in HF.[16]

The other potential biomarkers include bone morphogenetic protein (BMP)-1, carboxy-terminal propeptide of type I procollagen (PICP), tissue inhibitor of metalloproteinases (TIMP)-1, MMP-9, osteoglycin (mimecan), and insulin-like growth factor–binding protein 7.

Echocardiography

- *Two-dimensional (2D) echocardiography (echo)*: It is a widely available and easy-to-use bedside tool. 2D echo has been proven superior to M-mode in normal subjects and those with abnormal LV geometry.[17] The drawbacks are that it is subject to geometric assumptions and is operator-dependent.
- *Three-dimensional (3D) echo*: 3D echo overcomes geometric assumptions and operator dependence of 2D echo. Its measurements of LV mass, volume, and LVEF

correlate well with cardiac magnetic resonance imaging (CMR).[18]

- *Contrast-enhanced and speckle tracking echo*: Contrast-enhanced echo improves visualization of cardiac structures and function, while speckle tracking echo offers quantitative assessment of myocardial mechanics, both playing significant roles in enhancing the diagnostic capabilities of echo in clinical practice. They allow rapid quantification of global LV dyssynchrony, aiding in the assessment of cardiac function.[19]
- *LV global longitudinal strain (LVGLS)*: It is a sensitive marker of LV systolic function. It is useful in reclassifying baseline function across different EF ranges and may predict mortality better, especially when EF is >35%. Improvement in LVGLS indicates response to treatment and reverse remodeling.[20]
- *Left atrial reservoir strain (LARS)*: It indicates LV diastolic function and its improvement indicates reverse remodeling.[21]

In clinical practice, these echocardiographic techniques play a crucial role in assessing treatment response and guiding therapeutic decisions aimed at promoting LVRR and improving patient outcomes.

Cardiac Magnetic Resonance Imaging

Cardiac magnetic resonance imaging is the gold standard modality when evaluating functional and volumetric metrics. The degree of late gadolinium enhancement (LGE) indicates whether or not myocardial fibrosis is present. Reverse remodeling and LGE have an inverse relationship.[22] The prognosis is worse for patients with LGE and EF > 35% than for those without LGE and EF between 21 and 35%.

Although guidelines suggest that LGE-negative patients with LVEF between 21 and 35% should receive a primary prevention implantable cardioverter-defibrillator (ICD), these patients had a lower risk for arrhythmic events and sudden cardiac death. Conversely, among patients with LVEF > 35%, the presence of LGE with high-risk distribution was associated with intermediate to high risk, suggesting that these patients might benefit from ICD.[23]

Molecular Imaging

Myocardial fibrosis in response to myocardial injury plays an important role in LV remodeling. ^{68}Ga-labeled fibroblast activation protein (FAP) inhibitor (FAPi) is a positron emission tomography (PET) tracer, and it has gained interest in recent years for its potential in detecting myocardial fibrosis. It can differentiate between active and chronic diseases and assess disease progression. The degree of FAPi uptake decreases with the increase in myocardial fibrosis, thus suggesting that ^{68}Ga-FAPi PET selectively identifies active myocardial fibrosis. Thus, detection of early FAP expression may aid in treatment decision making in HF patients.[24]

BOX 2 Surgical techniques and devices for ventricular restoration and reconstruction.[25]

- *Surgical exclusion*:
  - Batista procedure
  - Aneurysmectomy
  - Revivent TC
- *Constraint*:
  - Acorn
  - Paracor
- *Reshaping*:
  - Myocor
  - AccuCinch
  - Cardiac success
  - MIRTH
- *Partitioning*:
  - Parachute
  - Eucardia

(MIRTH: myocardial intramural remodeling by transvenous tether)

PROMOTING REVERSE REMODELING

Revascularization

Timely revascularization after an MI—through thrombolysis, percutaneous coronary intervention (PCI), or coronary artery bypass grafting (CABG)—is crucial to mitigate adverse ventricular remodeling. Early revascularization has been associated with better outcomes, smaller infarct size, and improved LV function. Various surgical techniques and devices have been explored for ventricular restoration and reconstruction following an MI **(Box 2)**.[25]

EFFECT OF DRUGS ON LEFT VENTRICULAR REVERSE REMODELING

Left ventricular reverse remodeling can occur either by withdrawing the noxious stimulus causing cardiac injury or by introducing therapies that can halt or slow LV remodeling. Neurohormonal activation is the main culprit in LV remodeling and its inhibition is associated with improved LV function and LVRR.

RAAS Inhibitors

Angiotensin II (Ang II) promotes sodium retention and induces both renal and systemic vasoconstriction. Inhibiting the RAAS through angiotensin-converting enzyme inhibitors (ACEIs), angiotensin receptor blockers (ARBs), or angiotensin receptor-neprilysin inhibitors (ARNIs) has been shown to significantly enhance survival in HF patients by counteracting Ang II effects.

The SOLVD trial compared the ACEI enalapril to a placebo in HF patients receiving standard treatment. Results indicated that enalapril led to a significant reduction in both mortality and hospitalization for HF. In the CHARM-Alternative trial, candesartan was well tolerated and demonstrated a reduction in CV mortality and morbidity in symptomatic HF patients who could not tolerate ACE inhibitors.[26,27]

Angiotensin Receptor–Neprilysin Inhibitor

A study by Moon et al.[28] found that adding ARNI to GDMT in patients with HFrEF resulted in lower rates of CV death and HF hospitalization, along with improvements in LVGLS and LV area remodeling score over 6 months.

The PARADIGM-HF trial established that ARNI was superior to enalapril in reducing HF hospitalizations, CV mortality, and all-cause mortality in HFrEF patients. The sacubitril/valsartan combination also led to reduced NT-proBNP levels, though its impact on LV remodeling remains unclear.[29]

The PROVE-HF trial showed that even low doses of sacubitril/valsartan decreased NT-proBNP levels, increased LVEF, and reduced left atrial volume index (LAVI) and *E/e′* ratio (filling pressures). Despite patients mostly receiving contemporary GDMT, ARNI initiation was linked to reverse cardiac remodeling, suggesting that a reduction in NT-proBNP following ARNI treatment may indicate potential for reverse cardiac remodeling.[30]

Beta-blockers

Beta-blockers (β-blockers) mitigate systemic catecholamine stimulation, lower heart rate, decrease myocardial energy demand, and reduce LV remodeling by decreasing LV mass. The reduction in LV remodeling (LVRR) from β-blockers improves LV shape and function, and reduces functional mitral regurgitation (MR).[31] Large-scale trials, including studies on carvedilol, metoprolol, and bisoprolol, demonstrated that adding cardioselective β-blockers to standard GDMT reduces mortality in both ischemic and nonischemic HF patients.[32-34]

Mineralocorticoid Receptor Antagonists

Mineralocorticoid receptor antagonists (MRAs) help alleviate endothelial dysfunction, salt and water retention, and electrolyte imbalances. Adding selective or nonselective MRAs to GDMT decreases rates of HF hospitalizations, mortality, and sudden cardiac death.[35] The RALES trial showed that adding 25 mg of spironolactone to GDMT in HFrEF patients resulted in reduced CV mortality, fewer HF hospitalizations, and improved HF symptoms.[36]

Sodium-glucose Cotransporter-2 Inhibitors

Sodium-glucose cotransporter-2 inhibitors (SGLT-2i) reduce LV remodeling in HF by decreasing extracellular matrix (ECM) synthesis and myocardial fibrosis. Both dapagliflozin and empagliflozin have been shown to reduce ECM remodeling and promote antifibrotic markers, thereby limiting LV remodeling and HF progression.[37]

The EMPA-TROPISM study found that empagliflozin significantly reversed LV remodeling by decreasing LV volumes and hypertrophy, increasing LVEF, and causing less structural remodeling compared to placebo in nondiabetic HFrEF patients.[38] Conversely, the EMPA-HEART trial reported LV mass regression in diabetic patients without HF.[39] However, the REFORM trial showed no improvement in LV remodeling with dapagliflozin in diabetic HF patients, likely due to including those with relatively preserved LVEF and less dilated LV.[40] However, the DAPA-MODA trial showed beneficial effects on remodeling with dapagliflozin.

Vericiguat

Heart failure often leads to reduced soluble guanylate cyclase (sGC) activity, lowering intracellular cyclic guanosine monophosphate (cGMP) levels, and disrupting cGMP-dependent signaling, which negatively impacts cardiac function. Vericiguat, a novel drug, stimulates sGC activity, restoring cGMP levels. The VICTORIA Echocardiographic Substudy demonstrated significant improvements in LV structure and function over 8 months in high-risk HFrEF patients with recent worsening HF.[41] Further studies are needed to confirm the benefits of vericiguat on LVRR.

DEVICE THERAPY IN LEFT VENTRICULAR REVERSE REMODELING

Cardiac Resynchronization Therapy

Left bundle branch block (LBBB) leads to intraventricular dyssynchrony and abnormal septal motion, which contributes to pathological LV remodeling. This remodeling is characterized by increased LV volumes, diminished diastolic filling, and prolonged duration of MR.[42]

Cardiac resynchronization therapy (CRT) has become a well-established treatment for patients with symptomatic HFrEF, with LBBB and LVEF of <35% with a QRS duration exceeding 150 ms despite optimal GDMT. It is known to improve symptoms and lower morbidity and mortality (Class I, Level A recommendation). Similarly, for those with LBBB and a QRS duration between 139 and 149 ms despite GDMT, CRT improves symptoms and reduces morbidity and mortality (Class IIa, Level B recommendation). One of CRT's primary mechanisms of action is its ability to reverse LV remodeling (LVRR).[43]

Mitral Valve Repair/Replacement

Significant MR is a key predictor of progressive LV remodeling. Persistent moderate-to-severe MR, despite GDMT or CRT, is linked to a poor prognosis. Such patients should be considered for therapeutic options like surgical or percutaneous mitral valve repair or replacement.

Percutaneous Valve-based Therapies

MitraClip: Percutaneous Edge-to-Edge Mitral Valve

The COAPT trial using MitraClip demonstrated that LVRR at 6 months was associated with improved clinical outcomes in patients with HF and severe MR. However, the transcatheter edge-to-edge repair did not significantly affect the extent of residual MR or the LVRR after 2 years.[44]

Carillon and Transcatheter Annular Reduction Therapy (ARTO)

The Carillon device reproduces surgical annuloplasty with a coronary sinus (CS)-based device with shaping ribbon, whereas the ARTO is a CS device that tethers the anteroposterior dimension of the mitral annulus. Both these devices reduce the degree of MR and improve the functional status of HF patients.[45]

Transcatheter Aortic Valve Replacement

Multiple CMR studies demonstrated a reduction in LV end-diastolic volume index (LVEDVi) and indexed left ventricular end-systolic volume index (LVESVi) post-transcatheter aortic valve replacement (TAVR). TAVR has been found to regress diffuse myocardial fibrosis and reduce myocyte hypertrophy. Moreover, 5 years post-TAVR, the degree of LV mass reduction was associated with less all-cause mortality and HF hospitalization.[45]

Left Ventricular Assist Device

The left ventricular assist device (LVAD) is a mechanical circulatory support system that can lead to significant LVRR, particularly in younger HF patients, women, and those with nonischemic HF of short duration. Although LVRR can be substantial enough to allow for the withdrawal of LVAD therapy, relapses can occur due to persistent molecular and cellular changes. Nevertheless, LVAD therapy has been shown to improve biventricular function, decrease hospitalizations for HF, and enhance exercise tolerance.[46]

PREDICTORS OF LEFT VENTRICULAR REVERSE REMODELING

The indicators of LVRR include female sex, nonischemic etiology, idiopathic cardiomyopathy, shorter disease duration, higher baseline systolic blood pressure, shorter disease duration, absence of LBBB, NT-proBNP < 1,000 pg/mL, sST-2 < 48 ng/mL, and absence of LGE on CMR.

Various reverse remodeling criteria on echo and CMR are in use including a relative percent change of LVESVi of 15% or more, absolute LVEF increase of at least 10% or 15%, relative percent change of LVEDVi of 10% or more, relative LV end-diastolic volume (LVEDV) reduction or at least 10%, relative LVESVi reduction of 20% or more, or again relative LV end-systolic volume (LVESV) reduction of at least 40%. This shows the lack of a standard definition to assess LVRR and a need for more specific criteria to define the response to modern guideline-directed therapy.

The therapeutic interventions described above show improvements in LVEF and LV size as evidenced by various landmark clinical trials. Most of these changes reflect sequential benefits of each intervention on top of prior therapy **(Table 1)**.[47]

TABLE 1: LVEF improvements and LV size reduction expected with therapeutic interventions targeting LVRR.[47]

Modality (drug/device)	LVEF improvement with LVRR	LV size reduction with LVRR
ACE/ARB	1–4%	LVEDV: 12–13 mL/m^2; LVESV: 13 mL/m^2
BB	4–12%	LVESV: 4.8 mL/m^2
MRA	4%	LVEDV: 17.3 mL/m^2; LVESV: 18.5 mL/m^2
ARNI	9–15%	LVEDV: 12.25 mL/m^2; LVESV: 15.29 mL/m^2
SGLT-2i	1–6%	LV mass index: 2.6–13.7 g/m^2
CRT	2–24%	LVEDVi: 21 mL/m^2; LVESVi: 18.4 mL/m^2
MitraClip	3%	LVEDVi: 26 mL/m^2; LVESVi: 16 mL/m^2

(LVEDV: left ventricular end-diastolic volume; LVEDVi: left ventricular end-diastolic volume index; LVESV: left ventricular end-systolic volume; LVESVi: left ventricular end-systolic volume index)

POSSIBLE FUTURE TREATMENTS FOR LEFT VENTRICULAR HEALING AND REMODELING FOLLOWING MYOCARDIAL INFARCTION

- Cardiac microRNA-132-3p (miR-132) is a noncoding RNA which plays a major role in LV remodeling. It is involved in multiple signaling pathways and appears to be a promising molecular target in HF management. The levels of miR-132 are increased in patients with HF. CDR132L is an antisense oligonucleotide-based ncRNA inhibitor that targets microRNA-132. In a study by Täubel et al., CDR132L was found to reduce the miR-132 levels, improve the LVEF, and reduce NT-proBNP levels and QRS duration ultimately causing LVRR. Further studies are needed in this regard.[48]

- Myeloid-derived growth factor (MYDGF) and endoplasmic reticulum membrane protein complex subunit 10 (EMC10) are proteins produced by marrow-derived monocytes and macrophages that promote cardiac myocyte survival and angiogenesis. They were found to reduce infarct size and improve the heart function and survival in mice with acute MI. Further research is needed to establish the role of these proteins in ischemic tissue repair.[49,50]
- Gene-based therapy with a gene delivery system (a plasmid or viral origin) in combination with adequate proangiogenic genes can serve as a promising tool for successful cardiac tissue by stimulating blood vessel growth, increasing tissue perfusion and recovery, and reducing apoptosis. Adeno-associated virus is the most commonly used vector. Gene therapy is a promising therapy but may take several years for beneficial effects to manifest.[51]

CONCLUSION

Cardiac remodeling is a key driver for HF progression. Predictors of adverse remodeling include male sex, ischemic etiology, longer HF duration, higher LVEF, presence of LGE, and high or rising biomarker levels. Predictors of LV remodeling and LVRR should be assessed using a multimodality approach.

Reverse remodeling can be enhanced by appropriate application of GDMT. Device-based therapy may further enhance reverse remodeling. Both the extent and the pace of reverse remodeling are correlated with reductions in mortality and HF events. Reverse remodeling may lead to two distinct clinical outcomes, namely myocardial remission and, less often, complete recovery. Further research is needed for identifying potential mechanistic pathways and optimize patient selection for available therapies promoting LVRR and myocardial recovery.

ONLINE REFERENCES

Please scan the QR code provided at the end of the table of contents for References of this chapter.

CHAPTER

55

Diuretic Therapy for Patients with Heart Failure: Update 2024

Subhasis Roy Chowdhury, Arijit Ghosh, Mainak Mukhopadhyay

ABSTRACT

Increased extracellular fluid is the final common pathway leading to the signs and symptoms of heart failure (HF). Diuretics continue to be the cornerstone of therapy for congestion despite recent advances in drugs for neurohormonal modulation. Despite being in use for more than half a century there is a lack of robust clinical trial evidence. Hence, we need to base our clinical decisions on consensus, guidelines, and an understanding of renal physiology and pharmacology of the available drugs. Recent trials such as DOSE, ADVOR (Acetazolamide in Acute Decompensated Heart Failure with Volume Overload), CLOROTIC, and TRANSFORM have tried to address some of these issues. This write-up attempts to summarize the latest and most relevant data regarding diuretic use in HF.

Keywords: Loop diuretics, natriuresis, decongestion, heart failure, acetazolamide

INTRODUCTION

Heart failure (HF) management has been inundated with growing evidence of the benefits of newer modalities of neurohormonal inhibition over the past few years. It is widely agreed that worsening quality of life indicators in chronic HF patients and hospitalizations for acute decompensation adversely affect survival.[1,2] Both of these occur due to congestion and diuretics continue to be the cornerstone and perhaps the only option for decongestive therapy in current practice. Despite this, trials to fill the knowledge gaps regarding the use, dosage, benefits, and treatment goals of diuretics in HF are scanty. The chapter tries to unearth this evidence base.

LOOP DIURETICS

Loop diuretics (LDs) have the advantage of being the most potent and short-acting agents and hence continue to be the drugs of first choice in acute or chronic conditions.

Which loop diuretic is preferred?

TRANSFORM-HF (Effect of Torsemide vs. Furosemide After Discharge on All-Cause Mortality in Patients Hospitalized with Heart Failure) trial: 2,859 patients were randomized to receive either one of the LD and followed up for a median period of 17 months for mortality and repeat hospitalizations. No difference was noted in the primary or secondary outcomes. Most patients took 80 mg equivalent of oral frusemide per day. Though the trial unraveled the dire prognosis after hospitalization for HF (26% mortality in both arms), it could not shed light on the possibility of inadequate decongestation being the etiology as it did not document symptoms or diuresis.[3]

What is the correct dose of loop diuretics?

Oral doses required for chronic heart failure with reduced ejection fraction (HFrEF) range from 20–600 mg frusemide and 10–200 mg torsemide **(Table 1)**. Reasons for such wide variations include (1) change of LV function with time and comorbidities, (2) coprescription of ARNI, sodium-glucose cotransporter-2 inhibitor (SGLT-2i), and MRA which have a diuretic effect, and (3) development of diuretic resistance. Contrary to some observational studies documenting worse clinical outcomes with higher doses of LD used,[4] insights from the TIME-CHF study highlighted that if treatment intensification translated into clinical decongestion, then outcomes were better.[5] In fact, high LD at baseline or at 6 months was not identified as an independent predictor of survival or repeat hospitalization.

TABLE 1: Doses of oral diuretics used in chronic heart failure.

Drugs	Initial daily dose	Maximum daily dose
Loop diuretics		
Furosemide	24–40 mg once/twice	600 mg
Torsemide	10–20 mg once	200 mg
Thiazide diuretics		
Hydrochlorothiazide	25 mg once/twice	200 mg
Chlorthalidone	12.5–25 mg once	100 mg
Chlorothiazide	250–500 mg once/twice	1,000 mg
Metolazone	2.5 mg	20 mg
Indapamide	2.5 mg	5 mg

The dosing and strategy of frusemide in acute decompensated heart failure (ADHF) was studied in the *DOSE (Diuretic Optimization Strategies Evaluation)* trial.[6] It enrolled 308 patients in a double-blinded, multicentric, 2 × 2 design and randomized them 1:1:1 to receive high dose (2.5 × preadmission) or low dose (1 × preadmission) and twice daily bolus or continuous infusion. Changes in symptoms and serum creatinine at 72 hours were observed. Though high doses led to greater diuresis and weight loss, there was no significant difference in the primary endpoint of the patient's symptom global assessment or change in creatinine. In fact, worsening renal function (defined as an increase in plasma creatinine > 0.3 mg/dL within 72 hours) was more frequent in the high-dose arm, although subsequent analyses showed that an initial rise in plasma creatinine was associated with better, rather than worse, long-term clinical outcome.[11] Continuous infusion was associated with a lesser likelihood of the need for dose intensification but without any difference in the primary outcomes compared to bolus.

Diuretic dose follows a law of diminishing returns, that is, doses above a certain threshold do not induce greater diuresis.[7] In fact, poor natriuretic response is associated with worse renal parameters, inadequate decongestion, and poor prognosis.

The PUSH-AHF (Pragmatic Urinary Sodium-based Algorithm in Acute Heart Failure) trial compared natriuresis-guided versus nonguided therapy in ADHF. Though the first primary endpoint of increased natriuresis was met (409 ± 178 mmol vs. 345 ± 202 mmol, $p = 0.0061$); however, there were no significant differences between the two arms for the combined endpoint of time to all-cause mortality or first HF rehospitalization.[8]

Hence, a practical approach, proposed by the ESC, based on consensus rather than robust evidence, advocates initial low doses of LD and frequent natriuretic-response-monitored escalation, till a significant negative fluid balance is obtained **(Flowchart 1)**.[9]

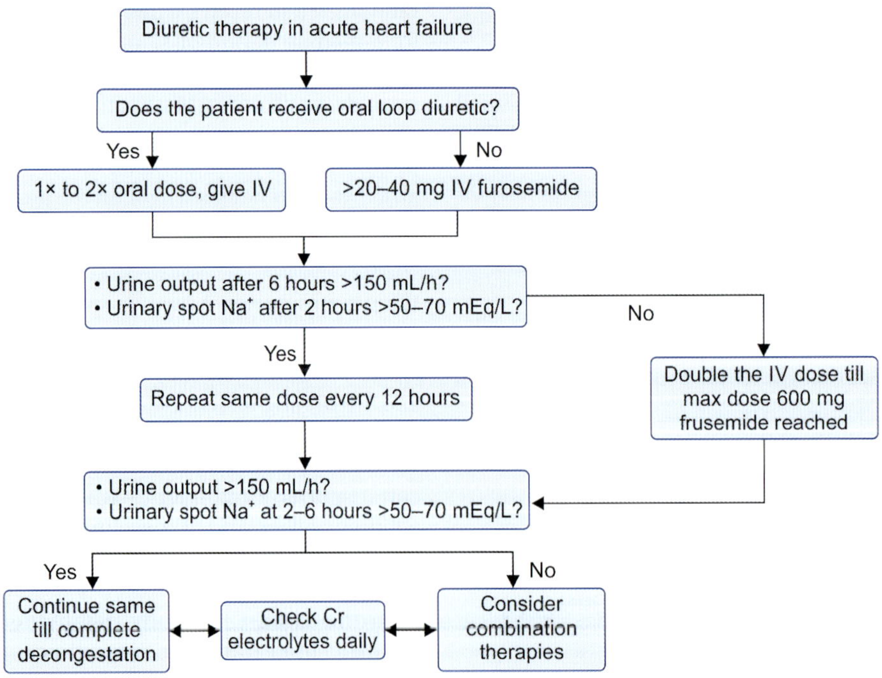

FLOWCHART 1: Dosing strategy of diuretics in acute heart failure.

Source: Adapted from McDonagh TA, et al. (2016).[9]

What is the role of outpatient-department (OPD)-based parenteral LD therapy?

The concept of "Frusemide Lounges" where patients are canulated and given IV frusemide and discharged home is unheard of in India. However, this forms one of the definitions of "Worsening HF," an evolving concept and a potential target for newer drugs, such as vericiguat. Such utilities lessen the burden on the healthcare system and should be explored.[10]

Diuretic Resistance

A quantitative definition for diuretic resistance is absent. The pathophysiology of the prerenal and renal factors contributing to resistance is also poorly understood. Though braking mechanisms, hypoperfusion, and high sodium intake are proposed as the contributing factors, an interventional evidence base is lacking. It is widely believed that renal mechanisms, especially at the post-loop of Henle level are a dominant driver of diuretic resistance in HF.[11] Strategies to improve diuretic resistance include natriuretic response-based optimization of LD followed by sequential nephron blocking tactics. Though metolazone is a common empiric choice, other types of thiazides or thiazide-like diuretics appear to have equal efficacy without evidence of superiority for one agent, even in patients with low estimated glomerular filtration rate (eGFR).

Can diuretics be withdrawn in stable chronic HF patients?

Rohde et al. evaluated the safety and tolerability of withdrawal of low-dose LD in stable HF patients in a multicentric randomized trial in Brazil. It demonstrated that in patients with low-risk features (oral frusemide dose <80 mg daily, no recent HF hospitalizations, and optimized HF therapy) withdrawal of LD was not associated with worsening symptoms or the need to reinstitute diuretic therapy compared with continuation of diuretic agents.[12]

THIAZIDE AND THIAZIDE-LIKE DIURETICS

Though guidelines widely agree upon thiazides/thiazide-like diuretics (TLDs) as potent adjuncts to LD, differences of opinion persist regarding early versus late initiation. Hypotension, renal dysfunction, and dyselectrolytemia are cited as disadvantages of more aggressive diuresis using combination therapy.

The CLOROTIC[13] trial compared the addition of varying doses of oral HCTZ versus placebo to IV frusemide in decompensated patients (n = 230). Coprimary endpoints were body weight and patient-reported symptoms at 3 days. Patients in the HCTZ arm showed more diuresis (1,775 mL vs. 1,400 mL; $p = 0.05$), greater weight loss (–2.5 kg vs. –1.5 kg, $p < 0.001$), more frequent hypokalemia (44.7% vs. 19.0% $p < 0.001$) and more frequent renal impairment (46.5% vs. 17.2%; $p < 0.001$). There was no significant difference in patient-reported dyspnea, length of hospital stays, or mortality. No difference was noted according to baseline LV function. Premature termination of the trial due to slow recruitment precluded assessment of safety issues and hence failed to influence guidelines.

ACETAZOLAMIDE

Interest in this carbonic anhydrase inhibitor acting at the proximal convoluted tubule (PCT) has been rekindled after the ADVOR trial.[14] ADHF Patients (n = 519) with NT-proBNP > 1,000 were randomized to receive 500 mg IV acetazolamide or placebo in addition to iv frusemide, stratified according to their LV function (<40% or >40%). The primary endpoint was successful decongestion within 3 days after randomization and without an indication for escalation of decongestive therapy. Secondary endpoints included a composite of death from any cause or rehospitalization for HF during 3 months of follow-up. The use of acetazolamide led to a higher incidence of decongestion (42.2% vs. 30.5%; $p < 0.001$), higher cumulative urine output and natriuresis, and shorter hospital stays but without any difference in death or rehospitalization rates.

A particularly interesting point to note was that the primary endpoint was achieved in the acetazolamide arm in the subgroup receiving < 120 mg IV frusemide per day (n = 263; HR 1.78) and not in the subgroup receiving > 120 mg IV furosemide per day (n = 252; HR: 1.08), highlighting how acetazolamide, and not LD, was the dominant driving force of diuresis in these patients.[15] However, pending more robust data regarding clinical outcomes and safety, acetazolamide is not included in the guidelines for acute HF currently.

SODIUM-GLUCOSE COTRANSPORTER-2 INHIBITORS

The diuretic effects of SGLT-2i and the potency of this class to influence clinical outcomes along the entire spectrum of LV function of HF are well established. (EMPEROR–PRESERVED and DELIVER trial).

All trials of empagliflozin in hospitalized HF patients (EMPAG-HF, EMPA-RESPONSE-AHF, and EMPULSE) have documented a small but significant increase in diuresis compared to placebo.

EMPULSE trial compared empagliflozin versus placebo in hospitalized patients after stabilization (mean 3 days) and assessed them by a stratified win ratio, defined as a composite of death, number of HF events, time to first HF event, and change in KCCQ total symptom score (KCCQ-TSS) from baseline to 90 days. Significant clinical benefit was documented with empagliflozin (53.9% vs. 39.7%). It was also associated with improved weight loss, fewer deaths, improvement in quality of life, and greater reduction in body weight. There were no safety concerns with empagliflozin.[16]

A small but intriguing trial comparing metolazone to dapagliflozin to overcome diuretic resistance (DAPA-RESIST) has documented equal efficacy of both agents with decreased incidence of hyponatremia and rising creatinine with SGLT-2i.[17]

TOLVAPTAN

It acts on the AVP V2 receptors in cells in the collecting duct. Comparison of tolvaptan with placebo or other adjunctive diuretics in the EVEREST, TACTICS, SECRETs of CHF, and the 3T trial have shown no added diuretic benefits of the drug and at best a suggestion for use in resistant hyponatremia.[15]

OTHER DRUGS

Angiotensin receptor-neprilysin inhibitor (ARNI) and MRA have diuretic properties; however, their role as pillars of HF therapy is more well-defined and hence are an essential part of therapy in HF anyway.

Digoxin, oral steroids, and oral salt supplementation remain theoretical and interesting propositions as adjunct diuretics and may stimulate trials in the future.

CONCLUSION

There is a lack of consensus regarding the starting dose and method of administration (bolus/infusion) of LD in hospitalized patients. Similarly, the diuretic dose at discharge and duration of therapy are also empirical. Though guidelines stress on euvolemia at discharge, there is no agreement on whether ultrasound should be used to confirm decongestion.

The evolution of outpatient intravenous LDs and alternative routes of administration require validation in future trials. Novel diuretic combination strategies need to be evaluated for efficacy and safety.

In conclusion, diuretics need to be revisited at a physiological and fundamental research level to direct future clinical trials. That may lead to safer and sustained clinical outcomes for acute and chronic HF patients.

ONLINE REFERENCES

Please scan the QR code provided at the end of the table of contents for References of this chapter.

CHAPTER

56

Emerging Drugs in Heart Failure beyond SGLT-2 Inhibitors

PS Banerjee, Tanmay Mukhopadhyay, Gourav Bhattacharya

ABSTRACT

Heart failure (HF) is a complex clinical syndrome characterized by symptoms such as breathlessness, ankle swelling, and fatigue, often accompanied by elevated JVP, pulmonary crackles, and peripheral edema. It affects 1–2% of the population, particularly the elderly. HF pathophysiology is demonstrated through various models, including cardiorenal, hemodynamic, and neurohormonal models. HF is classified based on left ventricular ejection fraction (LVEF) and is often treated with foundational therapies such as renin angiotensin-aldosterone system inhibitors, beta-blockers, mineralocorticoid receptor antagonists, and sodium-glucose cotransporter-2 inhibitors. However, CV mortality remains high in HF patients.

Keywords: Heart failure, LVEF, mortality, sodium-glucose cotransporter-2 inhibitors

INTRODUCTION

Heart failure (HF) is a complex clinical syndrome resulting from structural and functional impairment of ventricular filling or ejection of blood or both as outlined in the ACC/AHA definition.

The ESC guidelines define HF as "a clinical syndrome characterized by typical symptoms (breathlessness, ankle swelling, and fatigue) that may be accompanied by signs (elevated JVP, pulmonary crackles, and peripheral edema) caused by a structural and/or functional cardiac abnormality, resulting in a reduced cardiac output and/or elevated intracardiac pressures at rest or during stress."

Heart failure involves 1–2% of the population more in the elderly.[1] HF pathophysiology can be demonstrated by various models. Initially, focus was on the cardiorenal model, and later on hemodynamic model.[2] In the last 30 years, the neurohormonal model, i.e., disruption of neurohormonal activation and peripheral feedbacks having catalytic function in HF patients has taken a pivotal role.

Clinically, HF is usually classified based on left ventricular ejection fraction (LVEF) into HF with reduced ejection fraction (HFrEF, LVEF < 40%), HF with preserved ejection fraction (HFpEF, LVEF ≥ 50%), and HF with mid-range ejection fraction (HFmrEF, LVEF 40–49%).[3] The most recent HF guidelines recommend the use of a foundational therapy including renin-angiotensin-aldosterone system inhibitors (RAASi), beta-blockers (BBs), mineralocorticoid receptor antagonists (MRAs) and sodium-glucose cotransporter-2 inhibitors (SGLT-2i) to improve outcomes and reduce HF-related events in HFrEF patients. Recently, SGLT-2i have also been shown to influence prognosis in HF patients with HFmrEF and HFpEF. Still, CV mortality remains high[4] in these patients, as these drugs are targeted toward the traditional receptors or enzymes, deviating away from the pathophysiologic "phenotypes." The synthesis of newer drugs for HF should happen from novel targets of myocardial energetics (as cardiomyocyte, interstitium, cardiac metabolism, GCs-cGMP pathway, mitochondrial function and intracellular calcium handling),[5] thus shifting the focus back from the periphery to the failing heart muscle **(Fig. 1)**.

CURRENT THERAPEUTIC TARGETS

Sympathetic Nervous System

Heart failure is characterized by an overactivation of the sympathetic nervous system (SNS), originally focused at restoring the circulatory homeostasis. Habitual stimulation of SNS causes a systemic slipover of catecholamines. Norepinephrine stimulates beta-1 adrenergic receptor, thus, improving myocardial contraction and relaxation through a cascade of events. The role of alpha1 receptors

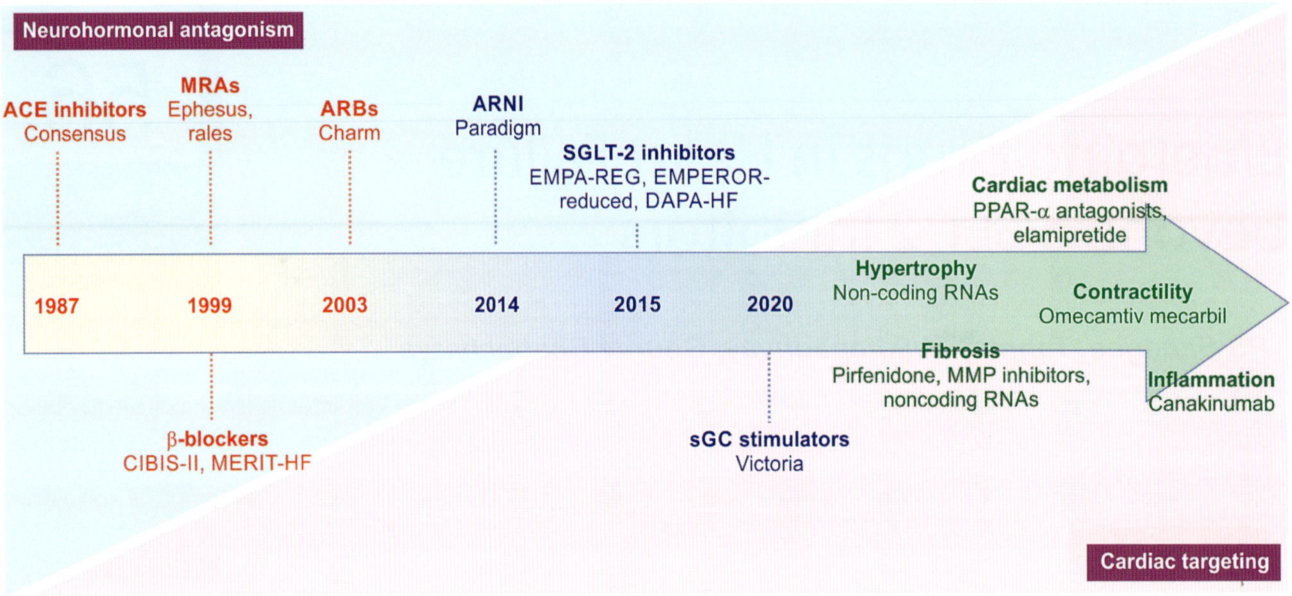

FIG. 1: Gradual development of drugs in HF, showing the shift from neurohormonal antagonism to specific cardiac targeting. BOLD RED: Current guideline recommended drugs; BOLD BLUE: drugs with evidence-based outcome benefit in HF; GREEN: novel possible targets.

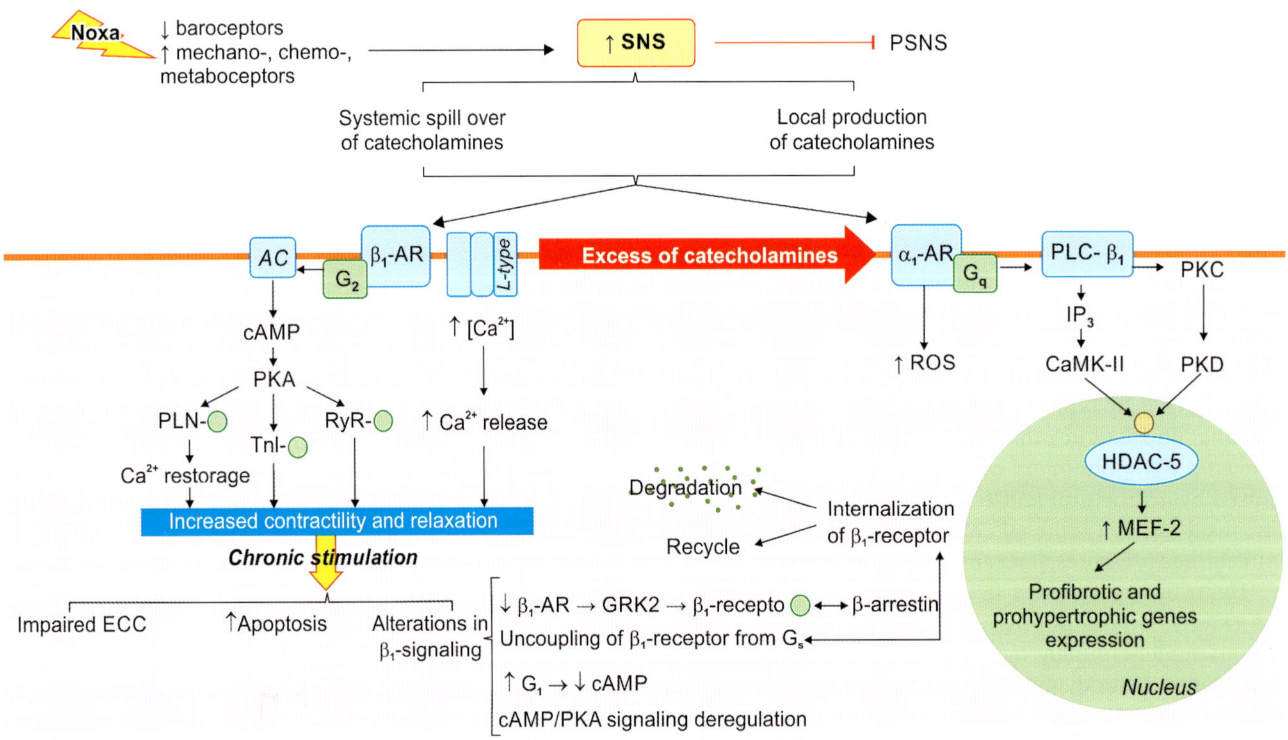

FIG. 2: Molecular signaling of SNS pathway in failing heart.

is less understood, and there is proof that they may hold vital adaptive functions, promoting cardiomyocyte survival and protecting against adverse remodeling.[6] Conversely, persistent stimulation of beta-1-adrenergic receptor antagonizes excitation-contraction coupling (ECC) and enhances apoptosis. Inhibition of adrenergic receptors is effectively achieved by beta-blockers. Specifically, beta-blockers cause a reduction in myocardial oxygen consumption and prevent the dangerous effects of a long-standing adrenergic stimulation **(Fig. 2)**.

Renin–Angiotensin–Aldosterone System

Renin and Angiotensins

Renin–angiotensin–aldosterone system (RAAS) is one of the main drivers in HF pathophysiology through various mechanisms as shown in **Figure 3**. Angiotensin receptor 1 (AT-1) as well as numerous angiotensins (II, III, and IV) are responsible for vasoconstriction, inflammation, proliferation and atherosclerosis. AT-2 counteracts these detrimental actions substantially via vasodilation. RAAS antagonism plays a crucial part in the neurohormonal blockade in HF. Compared to ACE inhibitors, ARBs have a downstream activity as they prevent Ang-II from binding to AT-1, thus, resulting in additional antifibrotic effects versus ACE inhibitors. But, the evidence is weak in favor of ARBs compared to ACE inhibitors in HF patients. The direct renin inhibitor aliskiren did not reduce the hard endpoints. Finally, combined angiotensin receptor and neprilysin inhibition has become the first option among drugs acting on RAAS.

Aldosterone

It is a steroid hormone produced by adrenal cortex. Its signaling includes genomic and nongenomic actions mediated by intracellular and membrane-bound mineralocorticoid receptors (MRs), respectively. MRAs, due to their antifibrotic and antihypertrophic actions, were proven useful in cardiovascular diseases and in HF. Currently available molecules have either a steroidal (i.e., spironolactone and eplerenone) or non-steroidal structure (i.e., finerenone).

Endothelin

Endothelin binds to receptors, ET-A and ET-B, both expressed in heart and vessels. The major role of ET-A on cardiomyocytes is mediating hypertrophy, fibrosis, and favoring the onset of arrhythmias.[7] In the vasculature, ET-B induces fibrosis, acting along with ET-A as well as causes vasoconstriction in vSMCs via protein kinase C. Despite the involvement of endothelin in the causation of target organ damage, numerous medicines blocking ET-A and/or ET-B (i.e., Bosentan, Sitaxentan) displayed no benefits compared to placebo, while some others were shown to be dangerous, both in acute and chronic HF.

Antidiuretic Hormone

The antidiuretic hormone (ADH) pathway has been considered one of the main pathophysiological determinants of HF, especially in advanced stages, when hyponatremia is more common.[8] Despite this assumption, the important clinical studies targeting ADH system have shown dubious results, with nonsignificant progress in hard endpoints. Conivaptan is a nonselective, intravenous V1a and V2 antagonist, whereas Tolvaptan is a selective V2 antagonist, which has been shown to regulate serum sodium levels in acute and chronic HF.

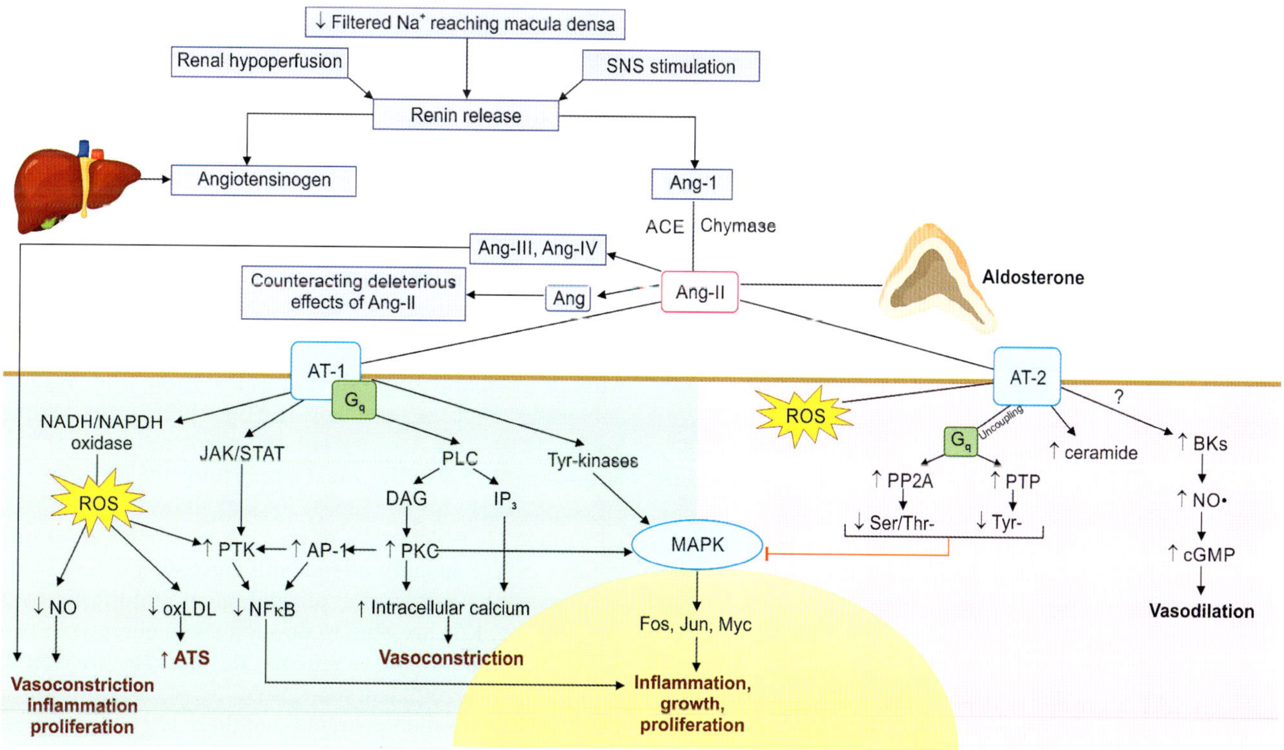

FIG. 3: Molecular cascade of the RAAS in HF.

Natriuretic Peptides

The natriuretic peptide system represents the leading counter regulatory axis, with diuretic, natriuretic, vasodilative, and antifibrotic actions.[9] The main driver of its release is increased atrial or ventricular wall tension. They induce renal vasodilation, natriuresis, and diuresis via dilation of the afferent and constriction of the efferent arteriole, reduce sodium-water reabsorption and inhibit RAAS and ADH signaling pathways. Initially, exogenous natriuretic peptides were administered. Despite few optimistic results in the beginning, the largest trial on *nesiritide* (a recombinant form of BNP) failed to demonstrate benefit versus placebo, and showed poor tolerance (e.g., hypotension and worsening renal function), leading to approval withdrawal. Neprilysin inhibitors did not prove to be effective when used alone in HF. Therefore, neprilysin inhibitors were first tested in combination with ACE inhibitors as omapatrilat which proved to be harmful due to increased risk of angioedema. Conversely, the association of neprilysin inhibitor and ARB proved effective and safe, and represents the only available neurohormonal modulator to date providing both antagonism of RAAS pathway and potentiation of the natriuretic peptide axis as shown in the landmark trial PARADIGM-HF.

Sodium Glucose Cotransporter-2 Inhibitors

Sodium glucose cotransporter-2 (SGLT-2) inhibitors were specifically designed for the treatment of type 2 DM as they promote renal glucose excretion by inhibiting reabsorption. Actually, they have been shown to be effective in the context of HFrEF, even in the absence of diabetes as demonstrated in the EMPEROR-Reduced and the DAPA-HF trials. They showed a lower risk of cardiovascular death and HF hospitalization and a slower decline in renal function with empagliflozin and dapagliflozin as compared to placebo, irrespective of the presence of diabetes mellitus.

Sodium glucose cotransporter-2 inhibitors mitigate oxidative stress, inflammation, and fibrosis in the whole cardiovascular system, and ameliorate glomerular hypertension, thus preventing shear stress-related renal damage. Moreover, they reduced cardiac cytosolic Na^+ and Ca^{2+} concentrations through inhibition of Na^+/H^+ exchanger, promote weight loss by inducing a fasting-like state with increased production of ketones, an advantageous substrate for the failing heart. Finally, SGLT-2 inhibitors may antagonize sympathetic activation, as they decrease renal and cardiac levels of tyrosine hydroxylase and norepinephrine, and their hypotensive effect is maintained, irrespective of renal function.

NOVEL THERAPEUTIC TARGETS

The development of new drugs for HF must arise from novel targets (cardiomyocyte, myocardial interstitium, cardiac metabolism, GCs-cGMP pathway, mitochondrial function and intracellular calcium regulation),[5] identified through gradual and better understanding of the complicated pathophysiological changes occurring in the failing cardiomyocyte **(Fig. 4)**.[10]

Nitric Oxide Synthase and Guanylate Cyclase

In HF, nitric oxide (NO) production is greatly decreased due to several mechanisms, which include inhibition of endothelial NO synthase and deactivation by ROS, particularly superoxide dismutase. All this leads to vasoconstriction and increased cardiac preload and afterload, higher muscular and vascular stiffness and adverse remodeling. In the myocardium, NO mitigates the action of the calcium channel, (SERCA) pump, and sarcoplasmic reticulum and ryanodine receptor, with an impact on mitochondrial metabolism.[11] Therefore, restoring NO-sGC-cGMP (cyclic guanosine monophosphate) pathway plays an important role to decrease the HF burden. There are three classes of drugs with different mechanisms of action: Drugs directly acting on the soluble form of GC and are named as activators (cinaciguat) and stimulators (vericiguat and riociguat), others reduce cGMP degradation, the phosphodiesterase 5 inhibitors (such as sildenafil).

Vericiguat was tested in phase II SOCRATES PRESERVED[12] and REDUCED studies[13] and recently also in the phase III VICTORIA study, with reduction of the composite endpoint of all-cause mortality or HF hospitalization versus placebo in subjects with worsening HFrEF. Therefore, this medicine is also recommended in the existing HF guidelines (COR II, LOE B). In the VITALITY-HFpEF trial, vericiguat has failed to improve the quality of life in HFpEF patients. Patients with a recent worsening HF event and a baseline NT proBNP value ≥ 8,000 pg/mL are the ones who benefit the most from this drug.

Cardiac Metabolism

The heart produces and consumes approximately 6 kg of ATP every day and has high oxygen demand to maintain its work. It is capable of producing ATP starting from various substrates, such as fatty acid (FA), carbohydrate, ketone bodies (KB), and, less frequently, pyruvate, lactate, and amino acids. FA is the most important but less energy-efficient source for the heart. Beta-oxidation of FA (FAO) consumes 11–12% further oxygen for producing the same volume of ATP in comparison with glucose. A recent study showed that heart under physiological conditions uses less glucose. KBs are able to develop more energy per two carbons in comparison to glucose; despite they are overall energetically less efficient than latter.

Clinical trials demonstrated that there is a 30% decrease in ATP levels in the failing myocardium, with respect to healthy myocardium with a shift toward increased glucose

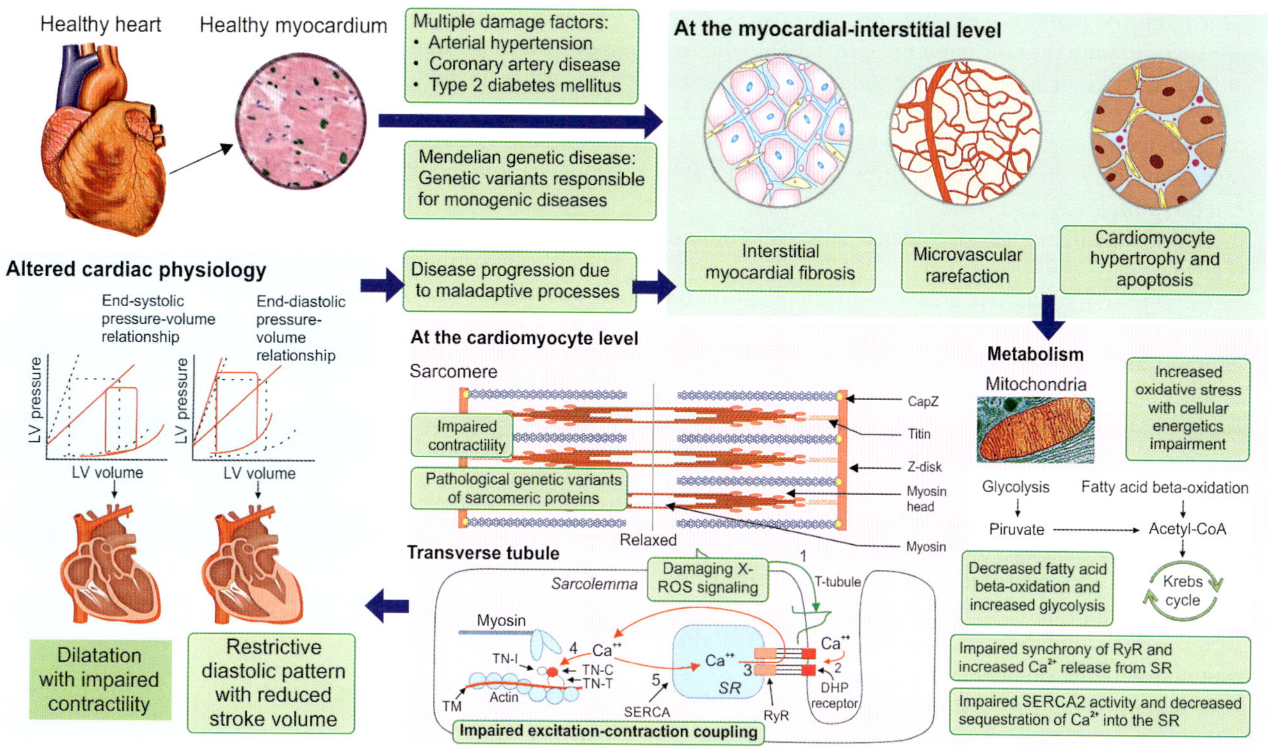

FIG. 4: Cardiac energetics and potential cardiac targets in the failing heart.

consumption. This metabolic switch indirectly induces glycolysis and at the same time causes a decrease in glucose oxidation. As HF progresses, glucose oxidation is also reduced, paving the pathway for KB to be the main energy resource for cardiac metabolism. The final goal is to ensure the best possible energy efficiency, both allowing better inotropy and lusitropy and avoiding further energy loss. There are five main paths that can be pursued in therapy targeting cardiac metabolism in HF:

1. *Inhibition of FA uptake by cardiomyocytes*: Carnitine palmitoyl-transferase (CPT1) is the limiting enzyme for FA oxidation regulating FA entrance into mitochondria. *Etomoxir and perhexiline,* two CPT1 inhibitors, result in decreased FA oxidation and increased glucose oxidation. In a small pilot study, it has been suggested that etomoxir can improve cardiac performance in HF patients. Perhexiline was previously used to treat angina pectoris. It also improved VO2max, LVEF, and myocardial energetics in HF. The ongoing RESOLVE-HCM trial will clarify if perhexiline is able to revert LVH in symptomatic HCM patients.[14] On the other hand, the HYPER trial assessed the role of perhexiline as a metabolic modulator in patients with LVH secondary to AS undergoing surgical aortic valve replacement (SAVR). Use of CPT1 inhibitors is limited due to their potential neurotoxic and hepatotoxic side effects.
2. *Reduction of FA oxidation*: *Trimetazidine (TMZ)* plays a competitive inhibition of 3-ketoacyl coenzyme A thiolase, the final enzyme of FA oxidation and has been used for stable angina. TMZ has been shown to reduce free FA oxidation, antagonize oxidative phosphorylation, and improve glucose utilization and ATP production and has been associated with improvements in functional class and LVEF[15] in HF patients. Furthermore, TMZ showed more beneficial effects in patients with metabolic disorders associated with increased FFA oxidation, such as in obesity and diabetes mellitus.
3. *Reduction of circulating FA levels:* β-blockers (metoprolol and carvedilol) showed to improve cardiac performance and survival in patients with HF by reducing myocardial FA use[16] and increasing carbohydrate oxidation. *Niacin* could antagonize myocardial FA oxidation by decreasing circulating FA levels. However, studies about the nicotinic acid derivative *Acipimox* in ischemic and nonischemic HF[17] showed both a significantly reduced cardiac function and efficiency and a significant decline in circulating FA. Reduction of FA delivery to the cardiac muscle through peroxisome proliferator-activated receptor (PPAR) α and PPARγ agonists *(fibrates and thiazolidinediones)* has been connected to the risk of new or aggravated HF.
4. *Increase of glucose oxidation:* Pyruvate dehydrogenase kinase (PDK) inhibitor, *dichloroacetate (DCA),* an analog of pyruvate, leads to an increase in PDK function and thus, promotes glucose oxidation, but it demonstrated no benefit on LV performance or exercise capacity in HF patients.[18] Moreover, DCA's chronic neurotoxicity limits its trial in human studies.

Glucagon-like peptide-1 receptor agonists (GLP-1RAs) are recommended in all patients with T2DM who are at high CV risk or have an atherosclerotic CV disease (ASCVD), as they may prevent the development of HF through increasing glucose uptake and its utilization by myocardial cells. The CV effects attributable to GLP1-RAs can be summarized as:

- Antagonizing inflammation, oxidative stress and atherosclerosis
- Counteracting oxidative stress-induced endothelial dysfunction and counteracting thrombosis
- Diuretic and natriuretic effect
- Renin–angiotensin–aldosterone effect

Human studies do not provide sufficient proof to support the hypothesis that this mechanism induced by GLP-1RAs therapy mediates cardioprotection. The STEP HFpEF trial showed in obese patients with HFpEF, treatment with *semaglutide* (2.4 mg) resulted in greater reductions in symptoms and physical limitations, more improvement in exercise capacity, and increased weight loss than placebo. Another trial CARDIO SEMA is ongoing studying similar effects.

5. *Increase of ketone oxidation*: The recent evidences suggest a beneficial effect of therapeutic ketosis, in particular in HFrEF. Increased ketone levels are reached with fasting, ketogenic diet, medium-chain triglyceride (MCT), 1,3-butanediol, ketone salts (KSs), or ketone ester (KE) supplementation. Remarkably, it has also been reported that SGLT-2i can augment circulating ketone levels and cardiac energetics. It may modulate the NLRP3 inflammasome through increasing circulating ketones, thereby reducing inflammation in the failing heart.

Mitochondrial Function

Mitochondria play a pivotal role in the cardiac pathophysiology by affecting cardiac function and metabolism. In HF models, increase of ROS, the prolonged opening of the mitochondrial permeability transition pore (mPTP) and aberrant mitochondrial dysfunction[19] are detrimental to mitochondrial metabolism and adversely affect cardiac structure and function. There is new data justifying the use of molecules targeting mitochondrial fission and fusion in different CV diseases.[20] The latest challenge is to convert these new molecules into medications, viz., *peroxisome proliferator-activated receptor γ coactivator 1* alpha *(PGC-1α), nuclear erythroid 2-related factor 2 (Nrf2),* adenosine A1 receptor (A1AR) agonists such as *capadenoson, neladenoson and N6-cyclopentyladenosine (CPA), and elamipretide.*

In pathophysiology of HF, mitochondria-induced cell apoptosis seems to play a pivotal role. Thus, identifying mitochondria-related genes (*mito-RGs*) based on transcriptome sequencing data may be used as potential novel markers and pharmacological targets for HF. *NADH: ubiquinone oxidoreductase core subunit S1 (Ndufs1)* expression is decreased in the HF. Cardiac-specific Ndufs1 overexpression betters cardiac function and ameliorates myocardial fibrosis. *Empagliflozin* improve mitochondrial biogenesis, enhancing mitochondrial oxidative phosphorylation (OXPHOS), reducing ROS production, attenuating apoptosis, and increasing autophagy.

Mitochondrial Ca^{2+} regulation may play a pivotal role for cardiomyocyte contractions as well as cell death induction. Possible pharmacological targets are at the level of the *MICU1-dependent calcium uptake by the mtCU ($Ca2^{+}$ uniporter)* and mitochondria localized circular RNAs (*circRNAs*) such as circSamd4.

Endoplasmic reticulum-mitochondria contacts (*ERMCs*) may contribute to preserve the normal cellular function and may be a new target for antiremodeling drugs in HF.

Coenzyme Q10/ Mito Q promotes the synthesis of ATP in the mitochondria by taking part in redox reactions within the electron transport chain. Administering coenzyme Q10, studied in Q-SYMBIO study, resulted in a reduced rate of both cardiovascular- and all-cause mortality and with less hospitalization.

Myocardial Contractility

Myosin modulators are a novel set of molecules that directly increases contractility and cardiac output, to relieve HF symptoms without altering calcium signaling and without the adverse effects of traditional inotropes. *Omecamtiv mecarbil (OM)* is a selective cardiac myosin activator that enhances myocardial contractility by stimulating the ATPase activity of myosin, thus favoring the formation and stabilization of actin myosin cross-bridges.

In the GALACTIC HF trial, among patients with HFrEF, those who received OM had a lesser incidence of a composite of a heart failure event or CV death than those who received placebo. Unlike other drugs specific for HFrEF, OM did not affect blood pressure, renal function or potassium levels. Prolonged (20 weeks) treatment with OM was also associated with serum troponin increase in the phase II study COSMIC-HF[21] while in the GALACTIC-HF patients with severe HF experienced a greater rate of cardiac infarction, especially if their HF had an ischemic origin. *Danicamtiv*, another myosin activator, plays similar effects on cardiac myosin and is undergoing trial.

Cardiac myosin activators could be an attractive therapeutic option, especially for subjects with lower blood pressure values, reduced kidney function, lower LVEF values, and at high risk of recurrent hospitalization. However, patients in atrial fibrillation and flutter at baseline were less likely to get benefitted.

Drugs Acting on Intracellular Calcium Dysregulation

The sarcoplasmic reticulum of cardiomyocytes has poor calcium content, partly as a result of a reduced SERCA Isoform 2a pump activity.

Istaroxime, a new HF drug, acts through a dual pathway: Na^+/K^+ ATPase blockage and potentiation of Ca^{2+} uptake into sarcoplasmic reticulum (SR) mediated by the SERCA2a. This is at the basis of its inotropic and lusitropic effects, due to the ability of dissociating SERCA from its inhibitory protein phospholamban with a lower risk of Ca^{2+} triggered arrhythmias.

In the HORIZON-HF trial 120 patients with acute HF have been treated with intravenous istaroxime or placebo in a 3:1 ratio. All three dosages of istaroxime were associated with a decrease in pulmonary capillary wedge pressure, but cardiac index improved only at the highest dose, that also was associated with a lusitropic effect. Unlike traditional inotropes, these effects resulted in an increase systolic blood pressure but not in heart rate. The CUPID 2 study showed that patients receiving the high dose of SERCA2a complementary DNA by intracoronary infusion had favorable outcomes as regards symptoms and NT-proBNP levels. After 1 year, researchers registered a significant increase in time to clinical events, and faster CV hospitalizations with the high-dose treatment versus placebo and, after 36 months, a reduction in the risk of recurrent CV events by 82%. The MUSIC-HFrEF1 is an ongoing trial.

JTV519 (K201) is a drug consolidating the closed state of ryanodine receptor by improving its affinity to calstabin, thus preventing spontaneous diastolic calcium leakage.[22] In animal myocardial infarction model and pacing-induced HF, K201 has been shown to attenuate significantly the development of cardiac dysfunction and ventricular remodeling.

In vitro studies have showed the inotropic and lusitropic effects of *nitroxyl (HNO) donors* that act increasing calcium sensitivity and calcium handling efficiency. HNO-induced increase of myocardial Ca^{2+} cycling and function is due to the posttranslational adaptation of thiol residues belonging to proteins such as SERCA2a, ryanodine receptors, phospholamban and myofilaments. HNO also induces a peripheral vasodilation through the endothelial soluble guanylate cyclase but does not cause tachyphylaxis. The STAND-UP AHF trial evaluated the effects of *Cimlanod* (a HNO donor) in patients hospitalized for AHF. Its intravenous infusion may reduce systemic pressure and intracardiac filling pressures, and may increase cardiac index (CI);[23] however, these did not last beyond the end of treatment. Moreover Lang et al. hypothesized that the CI improvement could come from a vasodilatory effect rather than to an inotropic property of cimlanod.

Myocytes in HF show an upregulated activity of this exchanger and an increased intracellular concentration of Na^+, with a consequent increment of intracellular Ca^+. Increasing evidence suggests that *NHE-1 inhibitors* such as cariporide, eniporide, and zoniporide may protect against cardiac hypertrophy, ischemia/reperfusion injury, and myocardial infarction.

Treatments Targeting Hypertrophy and Fibrosis

Historically, RAAS inhibitors and beta-blockers antagonize cellular hypertrophy.[24] The current research is studying the antihypertrophic effects of molecules acting directly on the cardiomyocyte, targeting vital signaling pathways that alter gene expression, protein function, and redox imbalance **(Fig. 5)**. These agents include histone deacetylase inhibitors, a wide spectrum of prohypertrophic microRNAs and several other small molecules such as rapamycin, inhibitors of Rho kinase.

Contrary to the traditional view in which fibrosis is considered a secondary phenomenon; recent evidences indicate a primary role of cardiac fibroblasts in myocardial disease. Cardiac fibrosis is linked to cardiac dysfunction, increased risk of arrhythmia, and poor outcomes. Despite the use of ACE inhibitors and MRAs, a residual fibrotic activity is still observed in HF. Novel antifibrotic agents are currently under investigation, specifically targeting connective tissue growth factors (e.g., TGF-β1 by *pirfenidone*), galectin-3 (e.g., by *antisense RNA*), matrix metalloproteinases, and cell reprogramming via *non-coding RNAs.*

HFpEF: A THERAPEUTIC CHALLENGE

Unlike in HFrEF, neurohormonal blockade did not decrease mortality in patients with HFpEF. However, barring cohorts from Georgia and Russia in the TOPCAT trial, the use of *spironolactone* significantly reduced mortality in this setting. Till date, treatment of risk factors and underlying disease is the most beneficial therapeutic modality for HFpEF patients. Notably, *tafamidis,* a pharmacological transthyretin stabilizer, improved outcome of patients affected by transthyretin-related cardiac amyloidosis, a progressively more recognized clinical phenotype of HFpEF

SUMMARY

Figures 6 and 7 summarizes the list of potential novel drugs and their mechanism.

FUTURE PERSPECTIVES

Novel therapeutic options address well-known pathophysiological mechanisms such as neurohormonal deregulation and the NO-GC-cGMP system. Specific transient receptor potential cation channel subfamily V (TRPV)-4 blocker, GSK2798745, has shown promising results in a model of chronic HF, possibly by interfering with TGF β1-induced activation of myofibroblasts. In the future of HF therapy, stem cells, micro-RNA, and epigenetics are likely to become novel cornerstone and to allow a tailored approach. As an example, micro-RNAs-34 family encloses many subtypes of

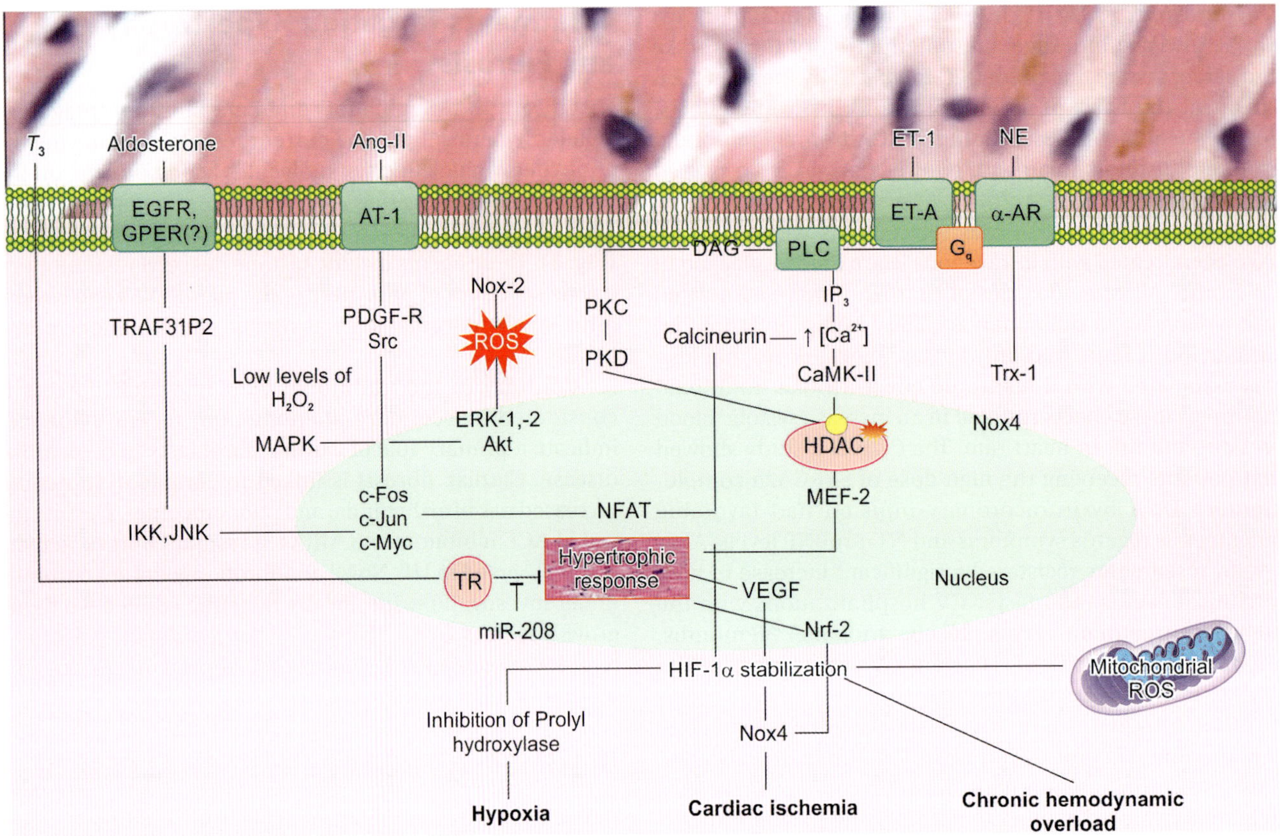

FIG. 5: Important molecular cascades for cardiac hypertrophy resulting from both hemodynamic and nonhemodynamic factors.

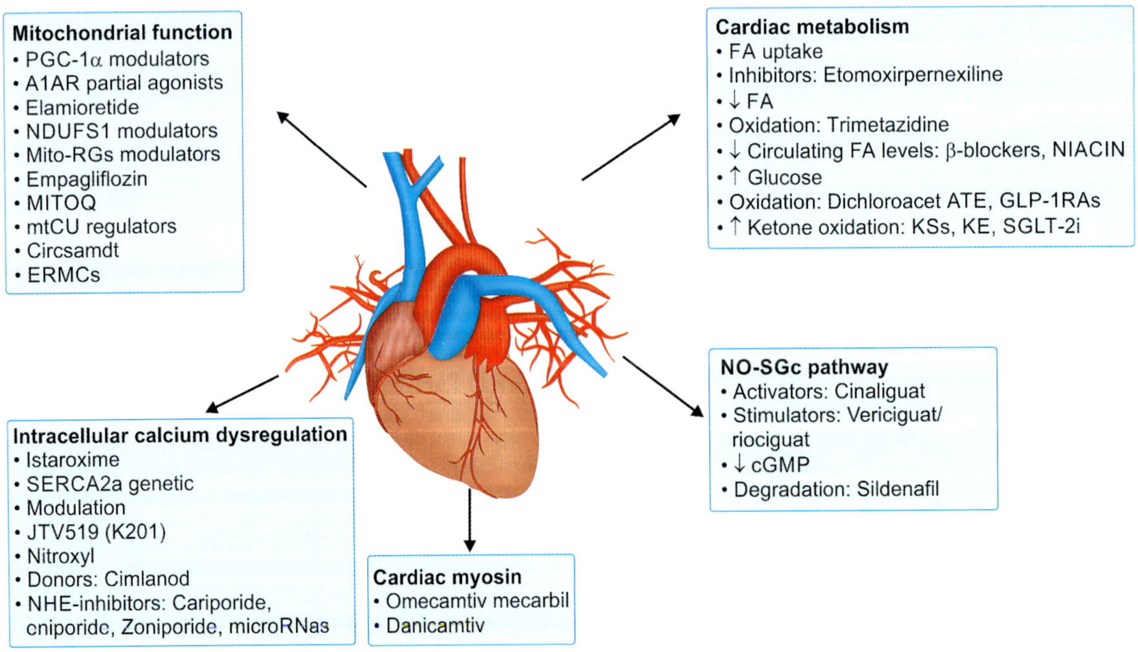

FIG. 6: Summary figure (list of potential new drugs).

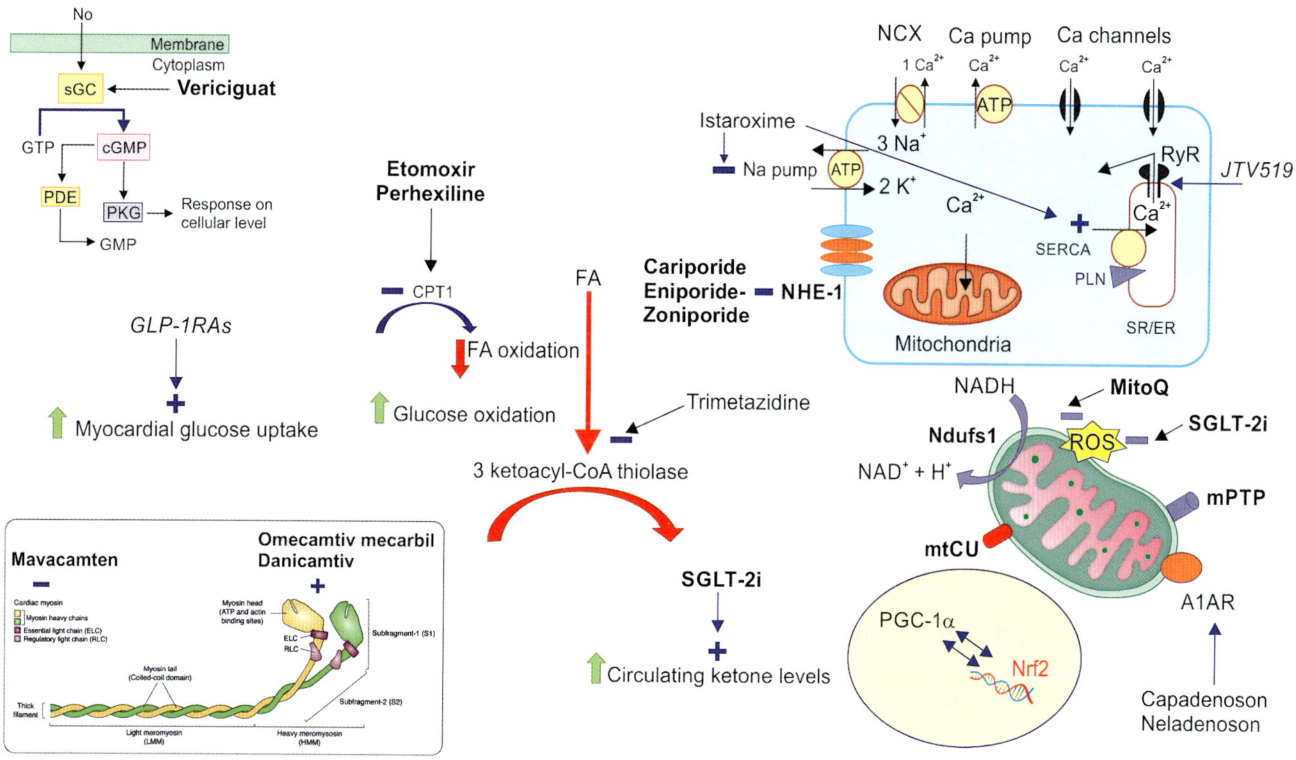

FIG. 7: Figure summarizing the mechanism of actions of different drugs.

micro-RNAs whom are involved in fibroblast survival and growth factors secretion (i.e., micro-RNA-21)[25] and in the activity of calmodulin kinase (i.e., micro-RNA-1).[26] As shown in the RIMECARD trial, the use of umbilical cord stem cells was safe in patients with stable HFrEF under optimal medical treatment, and improvements in LVEF, functional status and quality of life were observed.

CONCLUSION

Heart failure is a complex, multisystemic syndrome with a dramatic social and economic impact. Since decades, HF therapeutics has been following the interpretative pathophysiological models. After initial strategies targeting inotropism and congestion, and neurohormonal antagonism addressing dysregulation of peripheral feedbacks, novel therapeutic approaches have been recently developed, directed to the heart muscle. Drugs acting at a second-messenger levels, such as vericiguat, as well as other drugs acting on myocardial energetic and mitochondrial function, including elamipretide or omecamtiv mecarbil may then represent in the next future some additive, synergistic tools to improve patient outcome. Effective, evidence-based drugs from the fields of stem cells, micro-RNAs, and epigenetic remodulation are awaited in the next decades. In the next future, individual profiling and dissection of the activation of specific pathophysiological pathways of organ damage may represent the base for a tailored treatment of HF.

ONLINE REFERENCES

Please scan the QR code provided at the end of the table of contents for References of this chapter.

CHAPTER

57

Personalized Therapeutic Approach in Heart Failure with Reduced Ejection Fraction

Navjyot Kaur, KK Talwar

ABSTRACT

As per the latest guidelines on heart failure with reduced ejection fraction (HFrEF), the four drug classes, namely renin–angiotensin–aldosterone inhibitors [angiotensin receptor neprilysin inhibitor (ARNI)/angiotensin-converting enzyme inhibitor (ACEi) and angiotensin receptor blocker (ARB)], sodium-glucose cotransporter-2 inhibitors (SGLT-2i), mineralocorticoid receptor antagonists (MRAs), and beta blockers, form the foundation of therapy for HFrEF and have been associated with improvement in morbidity and mortality. However, beyond the trials, the implementation of this drug therapy has been challenging due to complex clinical and biochemical profile of patients with HFrEF leading to a large gap. To overcome this, a personalized approach to HFrEF therapy has been recently advocated by the European Society of Cardiology in a consensus statement, which appears promising and would allow for initiation and titration of drug therapy without the fear of intolerance and potential complications.

Keywords: Guideline-directed medical therapy, heart failure with reduced ejection fraction (HFrEF), patient profile, personalized, rapid sequencing

INTRODUCTION

Heart failure (HF) continues to remain an important health issue with an estimated global prevalence of 37.7 million.[1] The universal definition of HF (2021) defines it as a "clinical syndrome with symptoms and/or signs caused by a structural and/or functional cardiac abnormality and corroborated by either elevated natriuretic peptide levels and/or objective evidence of pulmonary or systemic congestion."[2] Left ventricular ejection fraction (LVEF) is used to further classify it as HF with reduced ejection fraction (HFrEF) when LVEF is ≤40%, HF with mildly reduced ejection fraction (HFmEF) when LVEF is between 41% and 49%, HF with preserved ejection fraction (HFpEF) when LVEF is ≥50%, and HF with improved ejection fraction (HFimpEF) when baseline LVEF is ≤40% and there is a ≥10-point increase from baseline LVEF along with a second measurement of LVEF > 40%.[2]

Management of HFrEF has undergone a paradigm shift in the last two decades. With introduction of new drugs like angiotensin receptor neprilysin inhibitor (ARNI)[3] and sodium-glucose cotransporter-2 inhibitors (SGLT-2i),[4] the whole armamentarium to treat HFrEF has changed and now they are the part of four pillars of HFrEF therapy along with beta blockers and mineralocorticoid receptor antagonist (MRA).[5] In fact, ARNI are preferred and have virtually replaced other renin–angiotensin–aldosterone inhibitors (RAASi), i.e., angiotensin-converting enzyme inhibitor (ACEi) and angiotensin receptor blocker (ARB). We have new drugs like ivabradine, vericiguat, omecamtiv mecarbil, sotagliflozin, and finerenone to further optimize the treatment in special situations.[6-10] Though the loop diuretics (furosemide or torsemide) have failed to show any mortality benefit, they remain the cornerstone of decongestion therapy in worsening HF.[5] The patients refractory to loop diuretics might require thiazide-like diuretics, e.g., metolazone, and in refractory hyponatremia, vasopressor 2 antagonists like tolvaptan may help.[5]

WHAT LED TO THE CONCEPT OF PATIENT PROFILING IN HFREF?

While the current guidelines give class I recommendation for all four drug classes in HFrEF, it remains challenging to introduce all four drugs in target dosages in daily clinical practice,[5,11] which has been highlighted in various registries.[12-18] Several studies support rapid sequencing of drugs for HFrEF as opposed to the conventional approach of uptitrating a drug class before adding a new one.[19,20] To implement rapid sequencing of drugs, multiple strategies have been advocated and published,[21-23] and one of these strategies is to define the phenotypic profile of the patient based on various clinical and biochemical parameters.[21,24,25] The factors which commonly interfere with initiation and uptitration of HF drugs are heart rate (HR), low blood pressure (BP), impaired renal function, and serum potassium.[21,25] In 2021, Rosano et al. published a position paper in which they advocated a personalized drug treatment based on patient profile rather than a "one-size-fits-all" approach.[21] Their aim is that all patients with HFrEF get a regimen as close to guideline-directed medical therapy (GDMT) as possible. They recommended 11 patient profiles based on HR, BP, renal function, potassium levels, and presence of atrial fibrillation (AF), which can guide the clinicians in initiation, uptitration, and correct sequencing of drug therapy in individual patients.[21,25] Various studies have shown that initiation and rapid sequencing of all four drug classes at lower doses are more effective than fully uptitrating a single drug class before adding a new one.[25,26]

WORSENING HEART FAILURE

Heart failure with reduced ejection fraction patients admitted with fluid overload often require parenteral loop diuretics, which may be switched to oral dosages after achieving sufficient diuresis. If the patient has concomitant cardiogenic shock, parenteral vasopressor support may be required. Noradrenaline is used as a first-line drug followed by adrenaline. If mean arterial pressure (MAP) is ≥65 mm Hg, dobutamine may be added to augment cardiac output. Dopamine should be used only if there is associated bradycardia and vasopressin is best avoided. In patients on long-term beta blockers and those with significant pulmonary hypertension, levosimendan or milrinone is preferred. During any admission for worsening HF, every reversible cause should be looked for and corrected, which includes reinforcement of compliance with medication and diet, ruling out infection/thyroid disorders, and also ruling out anemia. The current guidelines recommend the correction of iron deficiency in HFrEF with parenteral iron, irrespective of hemoglobin levels, to improve the functional status.[1] After stabilization, each patient should be profiled as per the clinical and biochemical parameters, should be started on GDMT, and should be observed for at least 48 hours before discharge.[5] Vericiguat may be initiated before discharge in selected patients to reduce HF-associated hospitalizations.

RECOMMENDATIONS AS PER PATIENT PROFILE (TABLE 1)

Profile 1: Patients with Low BP and High HR (Sinus Rhythm)

Symptomatic hypotension and low BP (<90/60 mm Hg) comprise this group and represent 10% in clinical trials but constitute higher percentage in clinical practice.[25] Target HR in HFrEF is 60–70/min (sinus rhythm). All vasodilators like nitrates should be stopped; hypovolemia and infection should be ruled out. If the patient is dry, the dose of diuretics may be reduced. Inotropes may be required to stabilize BP before initiating the main pillars of drugs. Out of all drug classes for HFrEF, ARNI has the most potent antihypertensive effect and is contraindicated in patients with SBP < 100 mm Hg; ACEi or ARBs can be used instead. MRA and SGLT-2i have minimal effect on BP and should be started/optimized.[27-29] Among MRAs, eplerenone may be preferred over spironolactone as it has a lower antihypertensive effect.[30,31] After ruling out congestion, beta blockers should be added to target HR of 60–70/min. The beta blockers with less vasodilatory action like bisoprolol or metoprolol CR/XL may be preferred.[32] If the HR still remains high or the patient does not tolerate beta blockers, ivabradine may be added. In patients with erectile dysfunction and those with obstructive airway disease, nebivolol is preferred.[21]

Profile 2: Patients with Low BP and Low HR

Intervention is required only if the patient has symptomatic hypotension. After stabilizing BP with inotropes (if necessary), MRA (eplerenone preferred) and SGLT-2i should be initiated and their dosages should be optimized. The dose of diuretics should be reduced in the absence of congestion. If ARNI is not tolerated, ACEi/ARB should be tried. Rule out hypothyroidism and hyperkalemia as a cause of bradycardia. The dose of beta blockers (metoprolol XL/CR or bisoprolol preferred) should be reduced only if HR < 50/min or the patient has symptomatic bradycardia.

Profile 3: Patients with Normal BP and Low HR

Stop drugs with a negative chronotropic and inotropic effect like nondihydropyridine calcium channel blockers (verapamil and diltiazem) and antiarrhythmic drugs. One must rule out hyperkalemia and hypothyroidism. The dose of beta blockers might require reduction if HR rate remains <50 bpm or the patient has symptomatic bradycardia. ARNI, SGLT-2i, and MRA should be continued and optimized to targeted dose.

TABLE 1: Heart failure with reduced ejection fraction (normal renal function): Personalized therapy.[21,25,32]

Profile 1: Low BP and high HR (NSR)	Profile 2: Low BP and low HR (NSR)	Profile 3: Normal BP and high HR (NSR)	Profile 4: Normal BP and low HR (NSR)	Profile 5: AF, target HR >70/min
• Stabilize • Rule out congestion • Inotropes/diuretics may be required	• Stabilize • Rule out hypothyroidism and hyperkalemia • Avoid drugs with negative inotropic/chronotropic action • Inotropes may be required	• Rule out infection/congestion/hyperthyroidism • Avoid drugs with beta-agonist action	• Rule out hyperkalemia/hypothyroidism • Avoid drugs with negative chronotropic action	• Stabilize • Inotropes may be required if BP is low • *New-onset AF*: Chemical cardioversion in hemodynamically stable and synchronized cardioversion in hemodynamically unstable or failed chemical cardioversion
• Beta blockers (metoprolol XL and bisoprolol preferred) • Ivabradine may be added if beta blockers are not tolerated or HR not controlled	• Ivabradine may be stopped (if the patient is taking the drug) • Dose of beta blockers may require reduction or stoppage	• Optimize dosages of beta blockers • May add ivabradine	• Ivabradine may be stopped (if the patient is taking the drug) • Dose of beta blockers may require reduction or stoppage	• Beta blockers • Digoxin (if BP is low) • Amiodarone may be required
SGLT-2i	SGLT-2i	• RAASi • ARNI preferred	• RAASi • ARNI preferred	• RAASi • If systolic BP < 90 mm Hg: ACEi/ARB • If systolic BP > 100 mm Hg: ARNI
MRA (eplerenone preferred)	MRA (eplerenone preferred)	SGLT-2i	SGLT-2i	SGLT-2i
• RAASi • If systolic BP < 90 mm Hg: ACEi/ARB • If systolic BP >100 mm Hg: ARNI	• RAASi • If systolic BP < 90 mm Hg: ACEi/ARB • If systolic BP > 100 mm Hg: ARNI	MRA (Aldactone/eplerenone)	MRA (Aldactone/eplerenone)	• MRA (Aldactone/eplerenone) • Eplerenone preferred in low BP
Vericiguat may be added				• *Consider*: ○ Catheter ablation ○ AV nodal ablation with CRT

(ACEi: angiotensin-converting enzyme inhibitor; AF: atrial fibrillation; ARB: angiotensin receptor blocker; ARNI: angiotensin receptor neprilysin inhibitor; AV: atrioventricular; BP: blood pressure; CRT: cardiac resynchronization therapy; HR: heart rate; MRA: mineralocorticoid receptor antagonist; NSR: normal sinus rhythm; RAASi: renin–angiotensin–aldosterone inhibitor; SGLT-2i: sodium-glucose cotransporter-2 inhibitor)

Profile 4: Patients with Normal BP and High HR

The aim should be to use target dosages of beta blockers and if the HR still remains >70/min (sinus), ivabradine may be added. An attempt should be made to uptitrate the ARNI to target dosages.[5] MRA and SGLT-2i should be continued.

Profile 5: Patients with AF

This group is different as HR is not a predictor of mortality in this group, unlike the patients in sinus rhythm and the target resting HR is >70/min. Also, there is not much evidence on the benefit of beta blockers in this group;[33,34] hence, an attempt to uptitrate the beta blockers to target dosages may have a detrimental effect, as ventricular rates of <70/min have been associated with a poorer outcome.[35] In patients with normal BP, the dosages of ARNI/ACEi/ARB, MRA, and SGLT-2i should be optimized. In patients with low BP, beta blockers may be discontinued or reduced and digoxin may be used for HR control. This strategy would allow the introduction or uptitration of drugs such as ARNI/ACEi/ARB which have a definite impact on mortality and morbidity. Oral anticoagulation is almost always indicated unless there are certain contraindications.

Rate versus Rhythm Control in Patients with AF

The answer is far from having been answered in various trials. AF can cause HFrEF and it can be secondary to left ventricular dysfunction. AF in HFrEF is associated with a worse prognosis and warrants GDMT for both HFrEF and AF.

In acute-onset AF, an attempt should be made to restore the rhythm. In hemodynamically stable patients, chemical cardioversion with amiodarone is preferred; the upfront electrical cardioversion is reserved for hemodynamically unstable patients and in patients refractory to chemical cardioversion. An attempt must be made to rule out left atrial/left atrial appendage clot before cardioversion to prevent cardioembolic stroke, and all these patients should be adequately anticoagulated.

In patients with chronic AF, catheter ablation (CA) remains the most effective strategy, though the success rate ranges from 46 to 59% in persistent AF.[36,37] The patients who are likely to benefit from CA are the ones in whom AF-mediated cardiomyopathy is suspected, patients in NYHA class I/II, with no significant left ventricular scar or atrial fibrosis on cardiac MRI, and younger patients with few/no comorbidities and with paroxysmal or new persistent AF.[37] In patients who are less likely to benefit from CA, the options available are rate control or atrioventricular node ablation with cardiac resynchronization therapy (CRT). The HFrEF with AF patients undergoing cardiac surgery should be considered for concomitant surgical AF ablation. An interdisciplinary approach involving electrophysiologists is recommended in patients with HFrEF and AF.[37]

Profile 6: Patients with CKD

All four drug classes for HFrEF can be administered for patients with CKD with eGFR of 30 mL/min/1.73 m^2 or more, with a clear benefit in mortality. The indication for stopping ACEi/ARBs is if creatinine increases by >100% or to >3.5 mg/dL, or eGFR <20 mL/min/1.73 m^2. Sacubitril/valsartan and MRAs can be administered down to eGFR of 30 mL/min/1.73 m^2, provided potassium is ≤5.0 mEq/L for MRAs and ≤5.5 mEq/L for ARNI.[19] The selective nonsteroidal MRA, finerenone, has shown promise in reducing cardiovascular events in HFrEF patients with CKD and diabetes mellitus.[10] It has been given class I recommendation for preventing HF hospitalization in this subgroup.[5] The potassium level should be checked at weeks 1 and 4 after initiation/uptitrating the MRAs and periodically thereafter. In patients in whom RAASi are contraindicated, Isolazine (combination of hydralazine and nitrate) should be used.[5] SGLT-2i (empagliflozin and dapagliflozin) have shown to be safe and effective in improving cardiovascular and renal outcomes up to eGFR >20–25 mL/min/1.73 m^2. In addition, they also decrease the potassium, so they are a good combination to be given with MRAs and other RAASi like ARNI/ACEi/ARB. The initial minor fall in eGFR after starting a SGLT-2i should not lead to discontinuation of this therapy, as this reversible reduction in eGFR is actually associated with long-term beneficial effect on kidney function.[38] Beta blockers can be safely used in patients with CKD and are found to have mortality benefit. Newer agents omecamtiv mecarbil and vericiguat can be initiated in patients with an eGFR > 20 and >15 mL/min/1.73 m^2, respectively.[7,8] Potassium binders (patiromer and sodium zirconium cyclosilicate) reduce serum potassium in HFrEF and CKD patients treated with RAASi; however, there is no evidence of their positive impact on prognosis.[39] **Tables 2 and 3** summarize the drug therapy for HFrEF in CKD patients and worsening kidney function, respectively.

Profile 7: Predischarge Patient

After hospitalization for worsening HF, if the patients were beta-blocker naïve, then these should not be first-line drugs and these drugs may be added on subsequent hospital visits rather than on discharge.[40] SGLT-2i and MRAs can be introduced safely. In addition, ACEi or ARNI may be added in patients with a systolic BP of >90 or >100 mm Hg, respectively. Sotagliflozin, a combined SGLT-1 and SGLT-2 inhibitor, when initiated before or just after discharge, reduced the combined end point of cardiovascular mortality and hospitalization for HF in diabetic patients hospitalized for worsening HF.[9] The newer drugs like vericiguat when added to selected patients before discharge can contribute to decongestion and can eventually allow safer initiation of beta blockers.[7] They have shown to reduce HF-related hospitalizations. The patients with LBBB and wide QRS should be made aware of device therapy like CRT and conduction system pacing and should be offered the same

TABLE 2: Heart failure with reduced ejection fraction and abnormal kidney function.[21,25,32]

Drug	eGFR >30 mL/min/1.73 m^2	eGFR 20–30 mL/min/1.73 m^2	eGFR <20 mL/min/1.73 m^2
ARNI	Recommended	Not recommended	Not recommended
ACEi	Recommended	Recommended (in low dose)	Not recommended*
MRA	Recommended	Not recommended	Not recommended
Beta blocker	Recommended	Recommended	Recommended
SGLT-2i	Recommended	Recommended	Not recommended
Isolazine	Recommended	Recommended	Recommended

*ACEi may be used in end-stage kidney disease, especially on dialysis.

(ACEi: angiotensin-converting enzyme inhibitor; ARNI: angiotensin receptor neprilysin inhibitor; MRA: mineralocorticoid receptor antagonist; SGLT2i: sodium-glucose cotransporter-2 inhibitor)

TABLE 3: Heart failure with reduced ejection fraction and worsening kidney function.[21,25,32]

Increase in serum creatinine from baseline (%)	Creatinine (mg/dL)	eGFR (mL/min/1.73 m^2)	Potassium (mEq/L)	GDMT modification
<50	<3.0	>25 (<10% decline from baseline)	<5.5	No change
50–100	3.0–3.5	20–25	5.5–6.0	Temporarily reduce the dose of ACEi/ARNI/MRA by half
>100	>3.5	<20	>6.0	• Stop ACEi/ARNI/MRA • SGLT-2i may be required to be stopped for worsening kidney function (with eGFR <20 mL/min/1.73 m^2)

Note: General measures: Stop nephrotoxic drugs, maintain euvolemic status, and withdraw potassium supplements/potassium-retaining drugs like amiloride (in case of hyperkalemia).

(ACEi: angiotensin-converting enzyme inhibitor; ARNI: angiotensin receptor neprilysin inhibitor; GDMT: guideline-directed medical therapy; MRA: mineralocorticoid receptor antagonist; SGLT-2i: sodium-glucose cotransporter-2 inhibitor)

after an optimal trial of GDMT. Those in more advanced stage HF (stage D) may be considered for left ventricular assist device or cardiac transplantation.

CONCLUSION

Various studies have established that GDMT has a major impact on morbidity and mortality of HFrEF patients and have also established that the combination therapy is better than a single drug in maximal dosages. Rather than following a single sequencing strategy for all HFrEF patients, a personalized approach based on the patient's clinical and biochemical profile offers a more practical approach to initiate and titrate the drugs in HFrEF patients without the fear of significant adverse events. However, more studies would be required to evaluate this strategy.

ONLINE REFERENCES

Please scan the QR code provided at the end of the table of contents for References of this chapter.

CHAPTER

58

Efficacy of Ferric Carboxymaltose Treatment of Heart Failure in Iron Deficiency

Pintu Nahata, Nadeem Akhtar

ABSTRACT

Iron deficiency is prevalent in heart failure and is associated with adverse clinical outcomes, regardless of anemia status. This chapter discusses the mechanisms of iron deficiency in heart failure, including reduced intake, impaired uptake, and increased loss, along with neurohormonal activation. The role of inflammation, hepcidin regulation, and genetic factors are examined to understand the systemic and cellular impacts of iron deficiency in heart failure.

Recent clinical trials have demonstrated the benefits of intravenous iron, particularly ferric carboxymaltose (FCM), in improving exercise capacity, quality of life, and reducing hospitalizations in heart failure patients with iron deficiency. These studies, including FAIR-HF, CONFIRM-HF, EFFECT-HF, and AFFIRM-AHF, provide evidence supporting the use of intravenous (IV) iron in this population.

The chapter also explores the challenges of oral iron supplementation, including its limited efficacy due to inflammation and hepcidin-mediated iron sequestration. Safety concerns associated with IV iron therapy, such as infection risk and hypophosphatemia, are discussed.

Emerging evidence suggests that IV iron therapy can play a crucial role in managing iron deficiency in heart failure, improving patient outcomes, and reducing healthcare burden. As ongoing and future randomized controlled trials (RCTs) continue to shed light on this therapeutic approach, the current guidelines are likely to evolve, emphasizing the need for routine iron status assessments and targeted interventions in heart failure management.

Keywords: Ventricular tachycardia, ripple mapping, catheter ablation, pulse field ablation, stereotaxic radiotherapy

INTRODUCTION

Iron exists in two primary oxidative states, ferrous (Fe^{2+}) and ferric (Fe^{3+}), and is indispensable for numerous cellular functions due to its ability to undergo redox cycling among these states. Additionally, it serves as a vital cofactor in numerous enzymatic reactions that occur during oxygen intake, storage, transport, and oxidative metabolism, including oxygen transport by hemoglobin (Hb). Iron deficiency (ID) can significantly impact physiological processes across all mammalian cells, highlighting its critical role in health and disease, particularly in patients with heart failure (HF).[1,2]

Iron deficiency and anemia are among the most common comorbidities with HF, impacting the clinical outcomes and potential management strategies.[3,4] The severity of these comorbidities has also been associated with a poor prognosis, with increasing severity being linked to increased death rates. Anemia in HF, often linked with ID, but not always present in tandem with ID, contributes significantly to poor prognosis and increased mortality rates. Interestingly in HF, there is a limited correlation between ID and traditional red cell indices. This discrepancy underscores the necessity of assessing iron status comprehensively, regardless of erythropoietic parameters to effectively manage ID in HF patients.[5]

Heart failure can be categorized into two main types based on ejection fraction: HF with reduced ejection fraction (HFrEF) and HF with preserved ejection fraction (HFpEF). Both types commonly present with ID, affecting up to 59% of cases in ambulatory settings even among nonanemic HF patients. This underscores the need for routine assessment and targeted interventions to address ID and improve overall patient prognosis, irrespective of HF subtype.

The interplay between iron metabolism and HF is complex and multifaceted. Research continues to explore the mechanisms by which ID exacerbates HF symptoms and affects patient prognosis. Emerging evidence suggests that iron supplementation, particularly IV formulations such as ferric carboxymaltose (FCM), can significantly improve exercise capacity, quality of life (QoL), and reduce hospitalizations in HF patients due to its efficacy in replenishing iron stores and improving symptoms in HF patients with ID.[6-8] Evaluating the efficacy and safety of FCM in this context is crucial for optimizing therapeutic strategies and enhancing patient outcomes.

PREVALENCE

Anemia prevalence in HF varies with disease severity and patient demographics. Regardless of whether a patient has HFrEF or HFpEF, approximately 30% of stable patients and 50% of hospitalized patients experience anemia. In contrast, the general population has a prevalence of <10%, though it increases with age, reaching 20% in individuals aged 85 years and older.[3]

Even among ambulatory HF patients who are not anemic, ID is notably more prevalent than anemia with a frequency as high as 59%. The prevalence of ID in nonanemic individuals with acute HF is even higher, reported at 57% in males and 79% in females.[5]

Understanding the prevalence and clinical implications of ID in HF is essential for guiding evidence-based management approaches. This chapter explores recent advancements in the treatment of ID with FCM in HF, focusing on its role in improving symptoms, reducing hospitalizations, and enhancing QoL across HF subtypes.

DIAGNOSIS OF IRON-DEFICIENCY ANEMIA IN HEART FAILURE

Iron deficiency in HF can manifest as either functional ID, caused by hepcidin-induced sequestration of iron reserves in hepatocytes or macrophages, or absolute ID, resulting from dietary deficits or blood loss.[4,9] The European Society of Cardiology has adopted a widely used definition of ID, defining it as either ferritin < 100 μg/L (indicating absolute ID) or ferritin levels between 100 and 300 μg/L with transferrin saturation (TSAT) < 20% (reflecting functional ID). However, this conceptualization has been debated due to its lack of validation against a universally accepted standard, particularly in acute HF patients.[10]

Both subtypes of ID impair iron availability to tissues, impacting critical biological processes such as erythropoiesis, assessable through reduced iron staining on bone marrow biopsy, considered the gold standard for diagnosis. However, due to its invasive nature, clinical practice typically relies on serum iron indicators: Ferritin, iron levels, and TSAT.[4,9] Recently, serum-soluble transferrin receptor (sTfR) levels have been proposed as a more sensitive but less specific alternative to serum ferritin, offering a better correlation with iron status and being less influenced by inflammation. Despite its promising results, sTfR testing remains less accessible and its clinical advantage over conventional measures of iron status such as serum ferritin and TSAT is still debatable and under evaluation.[1] In practice, therefore, serum ferritin and TSAT remain the cornerstone for diagnosing IDA in HF, providing crucial insights into iron status and guiding appropriate management strategies.

Transferrin Saturation[11,12]

Transferrin saturation is a crucial biochemical indicator of body iron status, accounting for both plasma iron and its primary transport protein, transferrin. The formula for calculating TSAT is as follows **(Box 1)**.

A TSAT value of 25–35% is considered normal. Deviations from this range can indicate ID or overload, making TSAT a valuable marker for assessing iron status in various clinical contexts, including HF.

Serum Ferritin[9,13]

Serum ferritin, an acute phase reactant, is a widely used marker for assessing body iron stores. However, its levels can fluctuate significantly due to hepcidin levels and inflammatory states, complicating its reliability in inflammatory conditions. This variability is particularly challenging in diagnosing functional ID.

It has long been believed that HF is a chronic inflammatory condition, with elevated levels of inflammatory cytokines such as tumor necrosis factor-alpha (TNF-α), interleukin-1 (IL-1), and interleukin-6 (IL-6). These inflammatory markers can influence serum ferritin levels, making it difficult to distinguish between inflammation-related increases and actual iron stores.

In the context of HF, the criteria for ID used in clinical trials are based on findings from IV iron studies in chronic kidney disease. The generally accepted criteria for ID in HF, which were first utilized in the FAIR-HF trial in 2008, include:

- Ferritin < 100 ng/mL, indicating absolute ID
- Ferritin 100–299 ng/mL with TSAT < 20%, indicating functional ID

BOX 1 Calculation of transferrin saturation percentage.

Transferrin saturation (TSAT%) = [Serum Fe (μg/dL)/Transferrin (mg/dL)] × 70.9

– [Serum Fe (μmol/L)/Transferrin (mg/dL)] × 398

PATHOGENESIS OF IRON DEFICIENCY IN HEART FAILURE

Heart failure is significantly influenced by ID due to the high metabolic activity of cardiac myocytes, making them particularly sensitive to low iron levels. Reduced myocardial iron reserves can be partly attributed to the downregulation of the transferrin receptor in HF, likely resulting from elevated catecholamine and aldosterone levels frequently observed in HF.[14]

Hepcidin plays a pivotal role in the complex pathophysiology of ID in HF. During periods of absolute ID, hepcidin is typically downregulated to enhance ferroportin (FPN)-mediated mechanisms of iron release by reticuloendothelial system macrophages and absorption by enterocytes. However, the chronic release of inflammatory mediators in conditions such as HF suppresses bone marrow function and stimulates increased hepcidin production by hepatocytes. This overexpression of hepcidin, despite apparently adequate total body iron stores, leads to functional, rather than absolute, ID anemia (IDA). This also explains the ineffectiveness of oral iron supplementation in individuals with ID and HF **(Fig. 1)**.[1,14-18]

Hepcidin levels can be used to categorize anemia into two groups—high- and low-hepcidin anemia. Chronic elevation of hepcidin inhibits iron absorption and recycling, reducing iron availability for erythropoiesis and causing IDA. Conversely, low hepcidin levels cause iron overload, characterized by inadequate erythropoiesis. These two categories of anemia arise from distinct pathophysiological mechanisms **(Fig. 2)**.

Since luminal pH affects iron reduction, substances that alter pH, such as proton pump inhibitors, can hinder nonheme iron absorption. Hepcidin regulates the iron exporter FPN, which releases iron into the bloodstream or stores it in ferritin within the enterocyte. Elevated hepcidin levels cause FPN internalization, leading to iron sequestration inside enterocytes and hindering iron absorption into the circulation. Hypoxia-inducible factor 2 (HIF-2) regulates the transcription of iron transport mechanisms such as DCytB, DMT1, and FPN. Dysregulation of HIF-2 in HF can impair iron regulation. Gut microbial metabolites may also impact systemic iron homeostasis by reducing HIF-2 expression. Gastrointestinal (GI) pathology, such as colon cancer, can lead to systemic ID through increased iron loss. Myocardial ID in the heart results from neurohormonal stimulation, downregulating iron-regulatory proteins (IRP1/2). Hepcidin and IRP1/2 regulate cardiac iron circulation and their faulty regulation results in decreased iron absorption and increased iron release **(Fig. 3 and Flowchart 1)**.[7]

RECENT RECOMMENDATIONS FOR THE MANAGEMENT OF ANEMIA (FLOWCHART 2)

The primary objectives of IDA treatment should be diagnosing and treating the underlying condition causing anemia. If the underlying issue is chronic, addressing the ID alone may result in recurrence. However, iron replacement can help patients quickly offset their IDA symptoms during diagnostic evaluation or while treating the underlying cause.

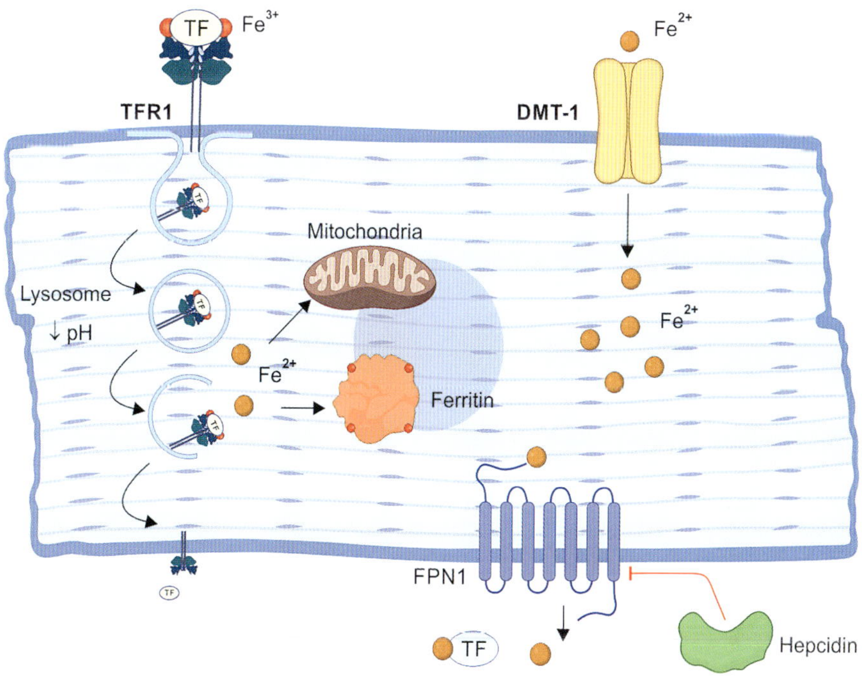

FIG. 1: Regulation of cellular iron.[9]

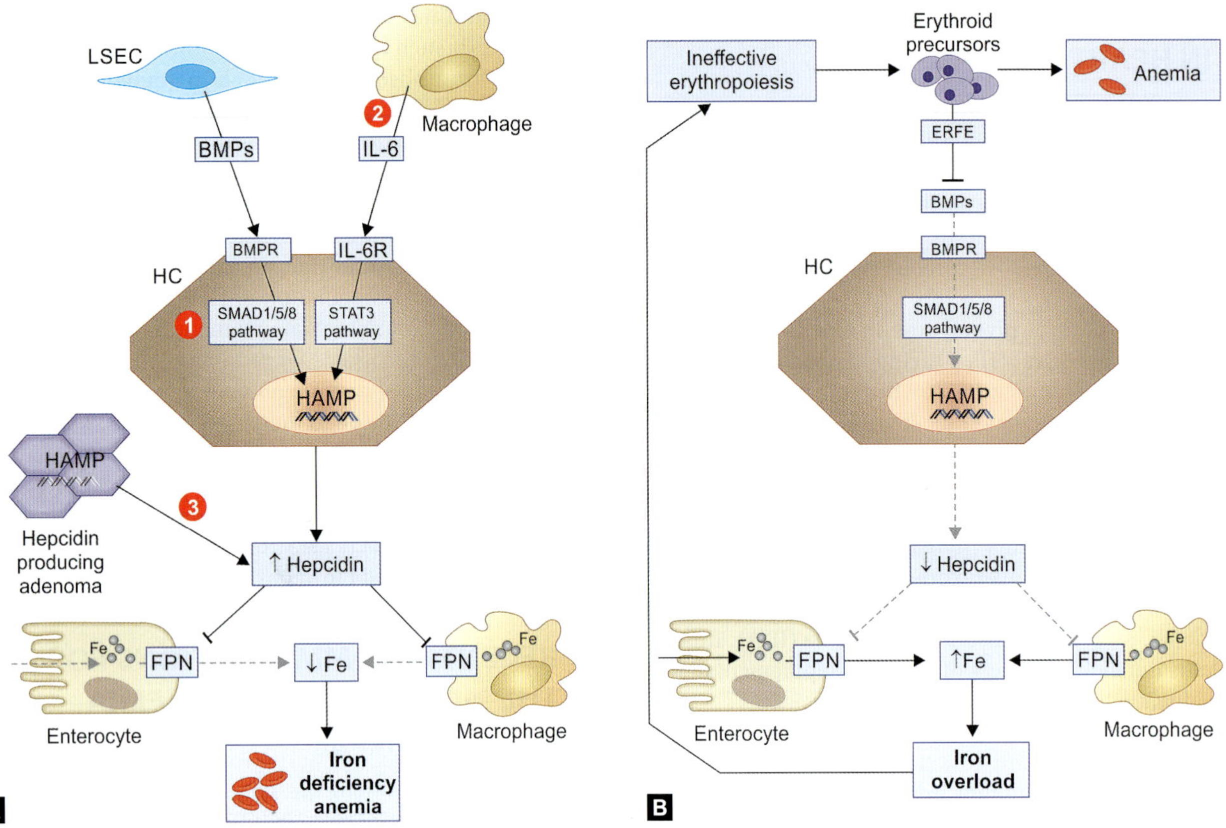

FIGS. 2A AND B: Mechanism of action of anemias (high and low hepcidin).[17]

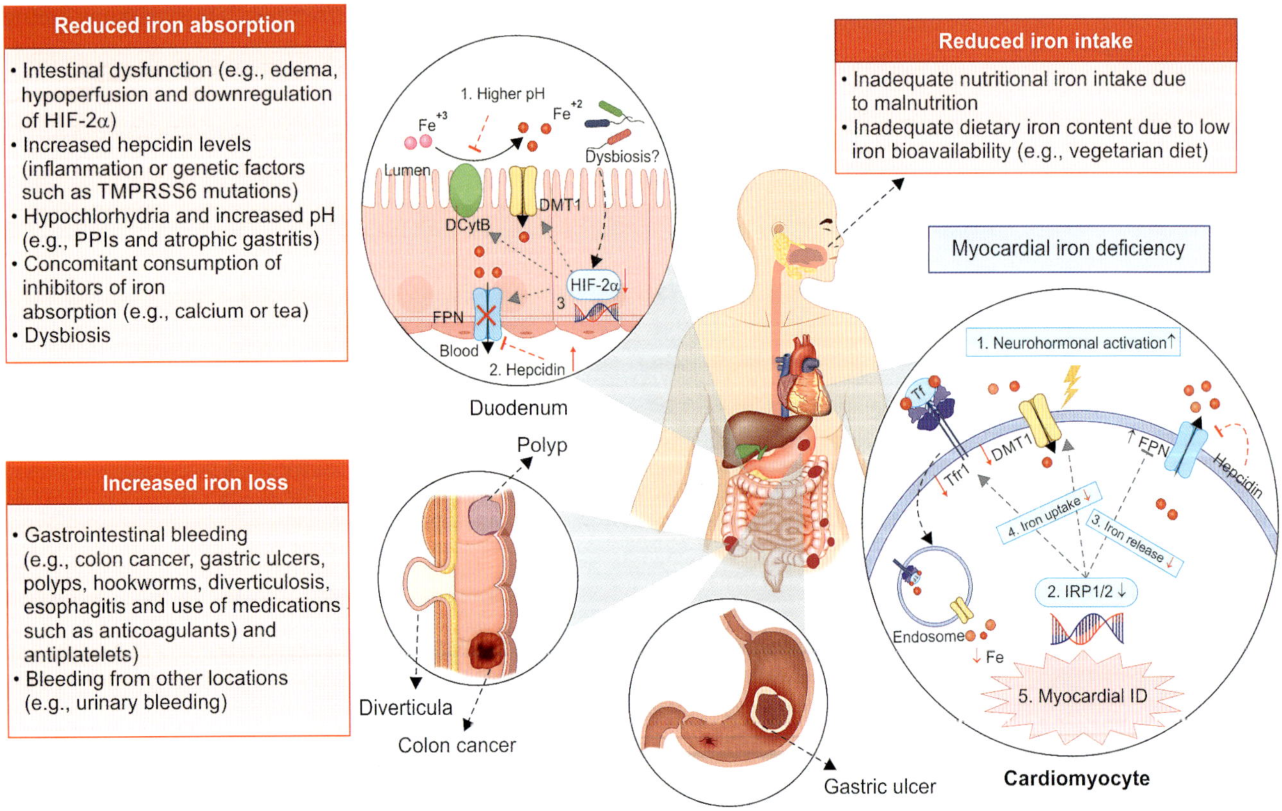

FIG. 3: Current overview of the factors behind iron deficiency in heart failure.[7]

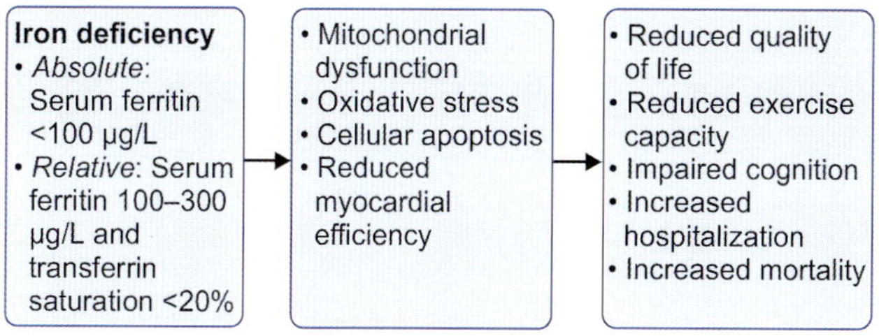

FLOWCHART 1: Effects of iron deficiency.[1]

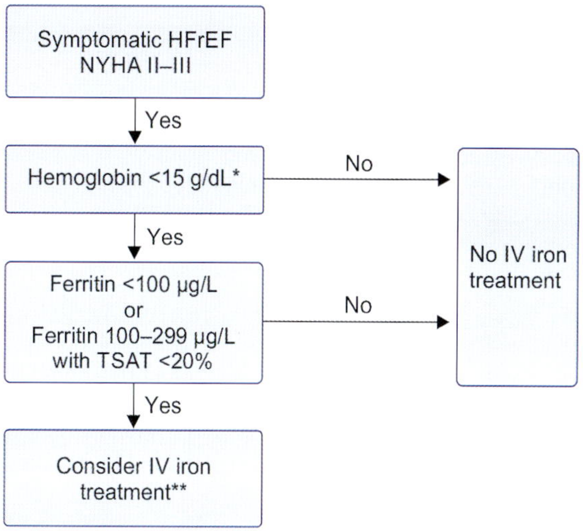

*If significant anemia, initiate evaluation.
**Reevaluate iron status after 3–6 months.

FLOWCHART 2: Treatment strategy for treatment of IDA in individuals with heart failure (HF) as based on expert consensus recommendations and the ESC guidelines.[15]

Both enteral and parenteral iron replacement methods have their advantages and disadvantages. Sufficient iron must be provided to replenish the body's deficiency. The Ganzoni formula can be used to determine the required iron dose to raise Hb levels:

$$\text{Iron deficit (mg)} = \text{Bodyweight (kg)} \times (\text{target Hb} - \text{actual Hb}) \text{ (g/dL)} \times 2.4 + \text{iron storage depot (mg)}$$

FERRIC CARBOXYMALTOSE

Ferric carboxymaltose is a new form of iron that is free of dextran and is composed of a ferrous hydroxide core stabilized by a carbohydrate shell. Administered intravenously, it enables the reticuloendothelial system's cells to receive iron under controlled conditions, facilitating the distribution of iron-binding proteins. FCM is useful in treating IDA because it delivers a high dosage of iron in a short amount of time.[19]

It is indicated for the treatment of IDA in adults unable to tolerate oral iron, those not responding favorably to oral iron, or those with nondialysis-dependent chronic kidney disease. A maximum dose of 750 mg is permissible in adults. It can be repeated after a week for a maximal total dose of 1,500 mg per course. Repeat courses can be administered in case of recurrence of IDA. It is diluted in normal saline and administered slowly intravenously at a rate of 100 mg/min over at least 15 minutes.[3]

Subsequent small-scale randomized controlled trials (RCTs) were prompted by early research, and these included FAIR-HF (Ferinject Assessment in Patients with Iron Deficiency and Chronic Heart Failure), CONFIRM-HF (Ferric Carboxymaltose Evaluation on Performance in Patients With Iron Deficiency in Combination With Chronic Heart Failure), and EFFECT-HF (Effect of Ferric Carboxymaltose on Exercise Capacity in Patients With Heart Failure and Iron Deficiency). Taken as a whole, these RCTs demonstrated improved functional capacity, patient-reported symptoms, and QoL metrics with IV iron in patients with IDA and HFrEF.[9,20,21]

ACUTE DECOMPENSATED HEART FAILURE AND INTRAVENOUS IRON SUPPLEMENTATION

The AFFIRM-AHF was a double-blind study that lacked a matching placebo for IV FCM. 1,108 patients with ID who were hospitalized for HF and had an LVEF < 50% were randomly assigned 1:1 to receive IV FCM or a placebo, with further doses administered as needed for a maximum of 24 weeks. The primary outcome, which was the composite of total hospitalization for HF and cardiovascular mortality, was monitored for 52 weeks. With 293 primary events (57.2 per 100 patient-years) in the treatment arm and 372 (72.5 per 100 patient-years) in the control arm [rate ratio (RR) 0.79, 95% CI 0.62–1.01, $p = 0{\cdot}059$], this trial just missed its main goal. Furthermore, no significant difference was observed in the rate of CV death between the groups. The authors summarized that IV FCM was safe to use in cases of acute HF and decreased the likelihood of HF hospitalization but had no discernible impact on the risk of CV death.[21]

Fifty Southeast Asian patients, irrespective of LVEF, were included in the PRACTICE-ASIA-HF study and, prior to their discharge, were randomly assigned 1:1 to receive either a single 1,000 mg dose of IV FCM or a single dose of IV saline. A single IV FCM dose increased the functional capacity when compared to a placebo. Furthermore, the QoL scores of both groups were comparable **(Tables 1 and 2)**.[22]

SAFETY CONCERNS WITH INTRAVENOUS IRON

Intravenous iron infusions bypass the usual hepcidin-mediated regulatory mechanism of iron absorption in the intestine, delivering iron directly into the bloodstream. This causes nontransferrin-bound iron to grow quickly in healthy individuals, and since elemental iron is reactive and releases free radicals, endothelial cells and tissues may be harmed. When IV iron was administered to humans,

TABLE 1: Intravenous iron therapy and trials.[21,23-28]

	FAIR-HF	CONFIRM-HF	EFFECT-HF	AFFIRM-AHF	IRON CRT	HEART FID
Year of publication	2009	2015	2017	2020	2021	2023
Number of subjects	459	301	172	1,108	34	1,532
HF diagnosis	HFrEF	HFrEF	HFrEF	Acute decompensated HF	Stable HF	Ambulatory, optimally treated CHF
Treatment versus control	2:1 FCM:placebo	1:1 FCM:placebo	1:1 FCM:placebo	1:1 FCM:placebo	1:1 FCM:placebo	1:1 FCM:placebo
Duration of follow-up	24 weeks	52 weeks	24 weeks	52 weeks	24 weeks	1.9 years
Dosage	IV FCM 200 mg weekly till iron repletion was achieved, thereafter, every 4 weeks	IV FCM 500–2,000 mg based on Hb and weight	IV FCM 500–1,000 mg based on Hb and weight	500–1,500 mg FCM based on Hb and weight	Patients needing a dose > 1,000 mg received remaining dose after 1–2 weeks of the initial dose	750 mg on days 0 and 7
Inclusion criteria	LVEF ≤ 45% NYHA II–III Hb between 9.5 and 13.5 g/dL	LVEF ≤ 45% NYHA II–III elevated natriuretic peptides Hb < 15 g/dL	LVEF ≤ 45% NYHA II–III Elevated natriuretic peptides peak VO_2 of 10–20 mL/kg/min	LVEF < 50% Hospitalized for HF	LVEF < 45%, NYHA class ≥ H, those who received cardiac resynchronization therapy	NYHA II–IV. LVEF ≤ 40% within 24 months or ≤30% within 36 months of screening. Hb > 9 g/dL and <13.5 (females) or <15 (males)
Primary outcome	Changes in self-reported Patient Global Assessment and NYHA class from baseline to week 24	Change in 6 MWT distance from baseline to week 24	Change in peak VO_2 (mL/min/kg) from baseline to week 24	Composite of total HF hospitalizations and CV death up to 52 weeks after randomization	Change in LVEF from baseline to 3-month follow-up	Composite of death and hospitalization for HF (12 months) and change in 6MWT distance (6 months)

TABLE 2: Current guidelines regarding use of intravenous iron in heart failure.[10,29]

Guidelines group	Year of publication	Recommendations	Class/Level of evidence
European Society of Cardiology	2021; updated	Symptomatic patients with HFrEF and HFmrEF and ID → consider IV iron supplementation to reduce HF symptoms and improve QoL	I/A
	2023	Consider IV iron supplementation with FCM or ferric derisomaltose to reduce risk of HF hospitalization	IIa/A
American Heart Association/ American College of Cardiology	2022	IV iron may improve functional status and QoL in HF patients (NYHA class II and III and IDA: ferritin < 100 µg/mL, or 100–299 µg/mL if TSAT < 20%	IIb/B-R
Scottish Intercollegiate Guidelines Network	2017	IV iron should be considered in HFrEF patients with either NYHA class III and LVEF ≤ 45% or NYHA class II and LVEF ≤ 40% along with Hb 9.5–13.5 g/dL	1+++

it caused a decrease in flow-mediated vasodilation, a direct indicator of endothelial cell damage compared to a placebo.[9] Furthermore, there is evidence that IV iron therapy increases the risk of infection compared to oral iron therapy or no therapy at all (RR 1.16; 95% CI 1.03–1.29; $i^2 = 36\%$).[30]

Hypophosphatemia and increased levels of fibroblast growth factor (FGF) 23 have been associated with IV iron. Increased FGF-23 blunts the renal absorption of phosphate, which can lead to low serum phosphate levels, resulting in bone resorption and ultimately osteomalacia.[31] Concerns have also been raised about the possibility that IV iron loading, which has been confirmed in several animal models, may accelerate the onset and spread of cancer as cancer cells are heavily dependent on iron for growth.[32] Additionally, ferroptosis—a nonapoptotic form of cell death directly related to iron—could be exacerbated by administration of exogenous IV iron. Ferroptosis has been linked to various types of cardiovascular disease, such as doxorubicin-mediated cardiomyopathy and ischemic/reperfusion injury.[33,34]

ORAL IRON SUPPLEMENTATION (TABLE 3)

Oral iron therapy (ferrous fumarate or sulfate) is an inexpensive and practical substitute for IV iron. Currently, there is no evidence to support its usage in HFrEF. Lewis et al. conducted a large trial named IRONOUT-HF to examine the effects of high-dose oral iron on exercise capacity over a 16-week period in a randomized study with 225 participants. The 6MWT distance, NT-proBNP levels, and the Kansas City Cardiomyopathy Questionnaire did not significantly change across treatment groups, and high-dose oral iron did not affect exercise capacity at 16 weeks as compared to placebo. It was determined that the data did not support giving HFrEF patients oral iron supplements.[14]

A meta-analysis evaluated the effectiveness and safety of oral iron in individuals with HF and IDA. Patients with HF were observed to be more vulnerable to injury, and iron could negatively impact GI organs. However, following oral iron administration, there was no rise in side effects in the experimental group as compared to the control arm. Therefore, the findings recommend that oral iron supplementation is safe to use in individuals with HF.[36] In the examined studies, oral iron supplementation was given at a dose of 200–600 mg daily, which, when taking into consideration restricted GI tract intake, is 10–20 times the oral iron's absorption capacity. Unexpectedly, the total oral iron dosage in the IRON-HF trial was about 38 times that of IV iron.[14,35] However, IV iron is significantly more efficacious than oral iron supplementation in terms of iron storage status. The IRONOUT experiment revealed extremely high baseline hepcidin levels, which may limit the iron absorption in the skeletal muscle and cardiomyocytes by suppressing the TSAT and ferritin increase following oral iron supplementation, thus rendering it ineffective in enhancing exercise function and iron storage status.[37,38]

Iron deficiency in HF has significant consequences that extend beyond anemia. One of the key issues in HF is an energy deficit, largely due to mitochondrial dysfunction. Evidence increasingly shows that ID exacerbates mitochondrial impairment, further depleting the already scarce energy reserves in HF patients. Traditional pharmacological treatments for HF primarily aim to reduce the heart's workload rather than enhancing its energy production capacity. Addressing ID directly targets this energy deficiency by improving mitochondrial function, thereby offering a unique therapeutic avenue. ID is relatively straightforward to diagnose and treat, making it an attractive target for therapeutic intervention in HF, with potential benefits in preventing cardiac remodeling and improving overall patient outcomes.[39]

TABLE 3: Clinical trials involving oral iron.[14,35,36]

	IRON HF	IRONOUT HF	IRON 5
Year of publication	2013	2017	2022
Number of participants	23	255	24
Inclusion criteria	LVEF < 40%, NYHA II–IV, Hb between 9 and 12 g/dL, ID (ferritin < 500 µg/mL, TSAT < 20%)	LVEF ≤ 40% NYHA II–IV, ID (ferritin 15–100 ng/mL or ferritin 100–299 ng/mL with TSAT < 20%)	LVEF < 45%, NYHA II–III, Hb between <13 g/dL for men and <12 g/dL for women, ED (ferritin < 100 ng/mL or ferritin 100–300 ng/mL with TSAT < 20%)
Intervention	Iron sucrose 200 mg weekly for 5 weeks versus oral ferrous sulfate 200 mg three times daily for 8 weeks	Oral iron polysaccharide 150 mg twice daily for 16 weeks	Ferrous sulfate 200 mg three times daily for 12 weeks
Comparator	Placebo	Placebo	Placebo
Follow-up	12 weeks	16 weeks	12 weeks
Primary outcomes	No change in pVO_2 in either study group. Early termination of study due to funding challenges and competing studies	No change in pVO_2	Significant improvement in 6MWTD in treatment arm

UPCOMING RANDOMIZED CONTROLLED TRIAL OF IRON DEFICIENCY IN HEART FAILURE AND NOVEL FINDINGS

In comparison to other oral iron forms, oral sucrosomial iron was found to have a better GI side effect profile and to improve serum iron indices and Hb levels comparable to IV iron in a recent nonrandomized, open-label study.[36] Two clinical trials comparing FCM to sucrosomial iron are further studying patients with ID with either HFpEF [PREFER-HF (Effects of Iron Therapy in HFpEF and ID); NCT03833336] or HFrEF (IVOFER-HF; EudraCT 2017-005053-37). Furthermore, new research indicates that reducing the dosage or extending the schedule of dosing to every alternate day may enhance oral iron absorption while also perhaps enhancing GI tolerance.[40]

- *PREFER-HF (Effects of Iron Therapy in HFpEF and Iron Deficiency)*
  - *Objective*: To evaluate the effects of iron therapy on HFpEF and ID
  - *Clinical trial identifier*: NCT03833336
- *IVOFER-HF*
  - *Objective*: To compare the efficacy of IV FCM versus oral sucrosomial iron in patients with ID and HFrEF
  - *Clinical trial identifier*: EudraCT 2017-005053-37
- *IRONMAN*
  - *Objective*: To investigate the long-term effects of IV iron treatment on morbidity and mortality in patients with HF
  - *Clinical trial identifier*: ISRCTN23024455
- *FAIR-HF2 (Ferric Carboxymaltose Assessment in Patients with ID and Chronic Heart Failure)*
  - *Objective*: To assess the long-term impact of FCM on hospitalization and mortality in patients with HF and ID
  - *Clinical trial identifier*: NCT03036462
- *HEART-FID (Ferric Carboxymaltose in Heart Failure Patients with ID)*
  - *Objective*: To determine the effects of FCM on clinical outcomes in HF patients with ID
  - *Clinical trial identifier*: NCT03037931
- *IRON-HF (Oral Iron in Heart Failure)*
  - *Objective*: To evaluate the efficacy and safety of oral iron therapy in patients with HF and ID
  - *Clinical trial identifier*: NCT03875943
- *IRONMAN-JAPAN*
  - *Objective*: To explore the impact of IV iron therapy on Japanese patients with HF and ID
  - *Clinical trial identifier*: Not specified (local registry)
- *AFFIRM-AHF (Ferric Carboxymaltose in Acute Heart Failure)*
  - *Objective*: To evaluate the effect of IV FCM on reducing the risk of recurrent hospitalizations and cardiovascular death in iron-deficient patients admitted for acute HF
  - *Clinical trial identifier*: NCT02937454
  - *Status*: Completed (recently published)

KEY POINTS

- *Study designs*: These RCTs vary in design, including comparisons between IV and oral iron therapies, long-term outcome studies, and evaluations in different HF subtypes (HFpEF and HFrEF).
- *Primary outcomes*: Common outcomes being assessed include hospitalization rates, mortality, exercise capacity, QoL, and iron repletion effectiveness.
- *Therapeutic interventions*: The trials focus on FCM and oral sucrosomial iron as primary interventions.

These trials aim to provide further evidence on the efficacy and safety of iron supplementation in HF patients, potentially influencing future guidelines and treatment strategies **(Fig. 4)**.

CONCLUSION

Iron deficiency is a common and significant concern in HF patients, strongly associated with a worse prognosis. Patients with HFrEF and concurrent ID benefit substantially from IV iron therapy; multiple trials have demonstrated improvements in hospitalizations, NYHA functional class, QoL scores, and exercise capacity. As ongoing research continues to highlight the crucial role of IV iron in managing patients with both ID and HF, current guidelines are likely to evolve. FCM offers a therapeutic option with the highest concentration of iron in a single IV dose, a favorable side effect profile, and the ability to rapidly and effectively replenish iron stores.

Testing for IDA in all symptomatic HFrEF patients is reasonable. A complete blood count should also be carried out. IV FCM can be infused over a 15-minute period or given as a bolus injection upon diagnosis of IDA. It may be used up to a Hb content of 15 g/dL. The weekly dose should not exceed 1,000 mg; 0.9% sodium chloride can be used to dilute the medication. After the injection, the patient's ferritin level usually rises sharply, often surpassing 500 mg/L, then declines very slowly over weeks to months. After 3–6 months, it is helpful to reevaluate the iron status. However, it is unknown if this window of time is ideal, and it is unclear if doses of 1,000 mg or more are best for every patient.[16]

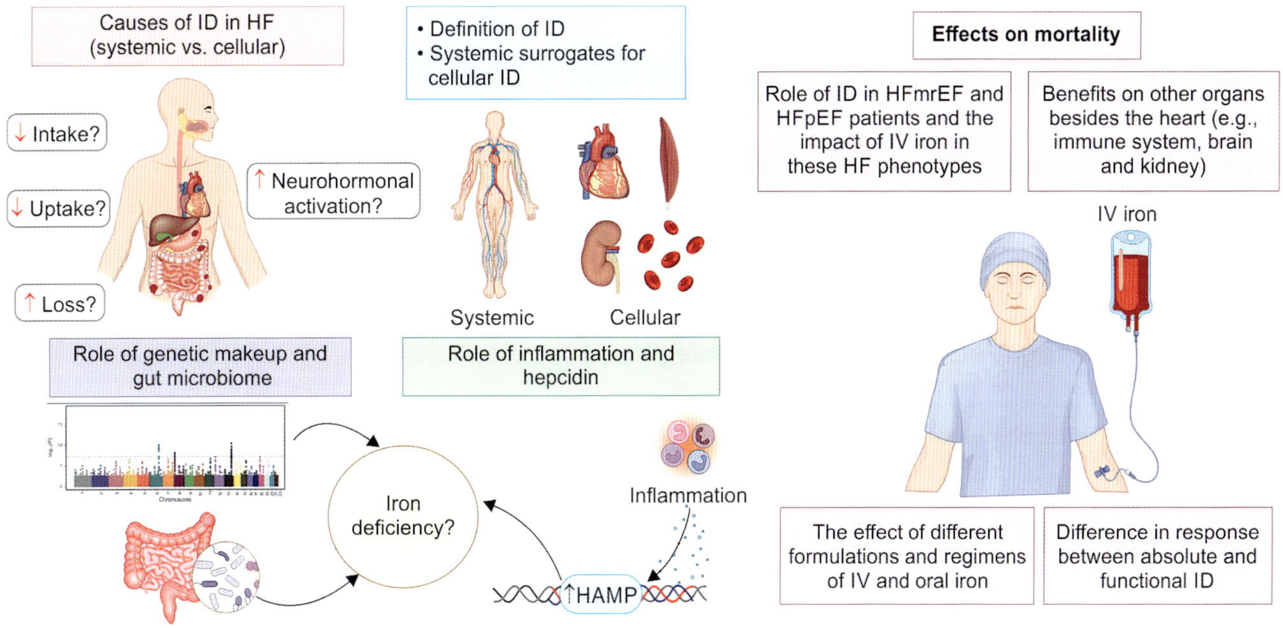

FIG. 4: Future directions and gaps in current knowledge regarding ID in HF.[10]

ONLINE REFERENCES

Please scan the QR code provided at the end of the table of contents for References of this chapter.

CHAPTER

59

Heart Failure with Preserved Ejection Fraction Diagnosis and Management: Where do We Stand in 2024

Sarumathi Thangavel, Ravikumar Rathnagiri

ABSTRACT

The HFpEF has been gaining more recognition in the last decade. Despite that, it still remains a challenge to diagnose HFpEF as it is a diagnosis of exclusion. Until recently, there were no proven therapies for HFpEF. After years of negative or equivocal trials, there has been a breakthrough in terms of HFpEF treatment with sodium-glucose cotransporter-2 inhibitors (SGLT-2i) which has clearly shown to be beneficial. Hence, there is increasing urgency to accurately diagnose HFpEF and initiate guideline-directed medical therapy (GDMT) in a timely fashion. In this chapter, we will discuss the pathophysiology, diagnosis, and treatment of HFpEF.

Keywords: HFpEF, SGLT-2i, heart failure

INTRODUCTION

An estimated 5–6 million adults in the United States are living with heart failure (HF). Around the world it is estimated that 64 million adults are living with HF and roughly half of that number is believed to be secondary to HFpEF which is defined by those with left ventricular ejection fraction (LVEF) >50%.[1] HFpEF like heart failure with reduced ejection fraction (HFrEF) is associated with significant morbidity and mortality. Despite an overall decline in the incidence of HF, the incidence of HFpEF continues to be on the rise.[2,3]

UNIVERSAL DEFINITION OF HEART FAILURE

Since 2021, HF has been universally defined as the signs and symptoms of HF caused by structural or functional cardiac abnormalities along with one of two criteria. (1) Elevated natriuretic peptides, (2) Signs of cardiogenic pulmonary congestion or systemic congestion.[4]

CLASSIFICATION OF HEART FAILURE BASED ON LEFT VENTRICULAR EJECTION FRACTION (FIG. 1)

The classification is based on consensus from the US Heart Failure Collaboratory and Academic Research Consortium, as supported by the universal definition of HF.[4-6]

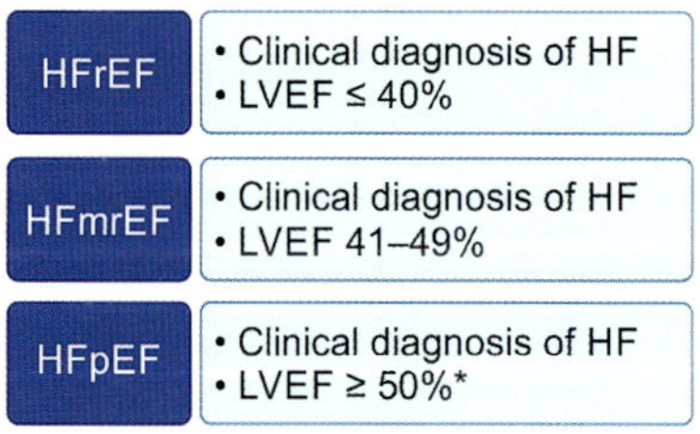

*Heart failure should not be attributable to an underlying cause such as an infiltrative cardiomyopathy, hypertrophic cardiomyopathy, valvular disease, pericardial disease, or high-output HF.

FIG. 1: Classification of heart failure based on left ventricular ejection fraction.

The presence of diastolic dysfunction on echocardiogram is not adequate proof to diagnose a person with HFpEF. Clinical signs of HF must be present to make the diagnosis.

HFpEF mimics: Clinical diagnosis of HF and LVEF ≥50% with a primary noncardiac cause (kidney or liver disease) or an underlying cardiac cause (infiltrative cardiomyopathy, hypertrophic cardiomyopathy, valvular disease, pericardial disease, or high-output HF).

Those who fall under heart failure with mildly reduced ejection fraction (HFmrEF) comprises of those with worsening HFpEF or improving HFrEF titled heart failure with improving ejection fraction (HFimpEF).

PATHOPHYSIOLOGY

Pathophysiology of HFpEF is less well-understood. Initially, HFpEF was believed to be secondary to hypertension as the majority of patients diagnosed with HFpEF had underlying hypertension. But this does not explain all of the HFpEF patients. After this came the inflammation theory, as most of the HFpEF patients have inflammatory comorbidities such as diabetes, chronic kidney disease (CKD), obesity, lung disease, etc. This can cause microvascular inflammation and an increase in interleukin-6, tumor necrosis factor-α, and/or soluble suppression of tumorigenesis-2, better known as sST2. This in turn leads to impaired myocardial perfusion leading to fibrosis and stiffness of the underlying myocardium. The inflammation also leads to oxidative stress which can impair nitric oxide production and its downstream signaling → soluble guanylate cyclase and cyclic GMP production which in turn causes diastolic dysfunction. Another theory is that the inflammation can impair the unfolded protein response which can impair the heart ability to clear dysfunctional proteins leading to diastolic dysfunction.

DIAGNOSIS

Challenges with Diagnosis

Despite the universal definition of HF, diagnosis of HFpEF continues to be a challenge.

When a patient presents with dyspnea and/or edema, noncardiac sources have to be ruled out namely cirrhosis, renal disease (nephrotic syndrome), pulmonary causes, venous insufficiency, medication side effect, obesity, etc. And after this, if the patient meets the universal definition of HF, then rule out HFpEF mimics (cardiac and noncardiac causes) as detailed earlier. Then apply the H2FPEF score[7] to assess the probability and/or confirm the diagnosis of H2FPEF score. See **Flowchart 1** for suggested algorithm for diagnostic approach to HFpEF (adapted from the 2023 ACC Expert consensus in the management of HF).[8]

H2FPEF Score

It is a validated tool using the gold standard invasive exercise hemodynamics and it has six components including body mass index, hypertension, atrial fibrillation, pulmonary hypertension (pulmonary artery systolic pressure—PASP >35 mm Hg on Doppler echocardiography), age >60 years and filling pressures on echocardiography. Each component is given a score and a total score of 6 or more is highly suggestive of HFpEF (see **Tables 1 and 2**). It is practical and easy to use since clinical history and echocardiographic parameter are all that are needed to use this score.

HFA-PEFF Algorithm

Another score based on expert consensus from European Society of Cardiology (ESC) with no validation is the HFA-PEFF.[9] This has four steps as detailed in **Figure 2**. This score necessitates natriuretic peptide levels to establish diagnosis

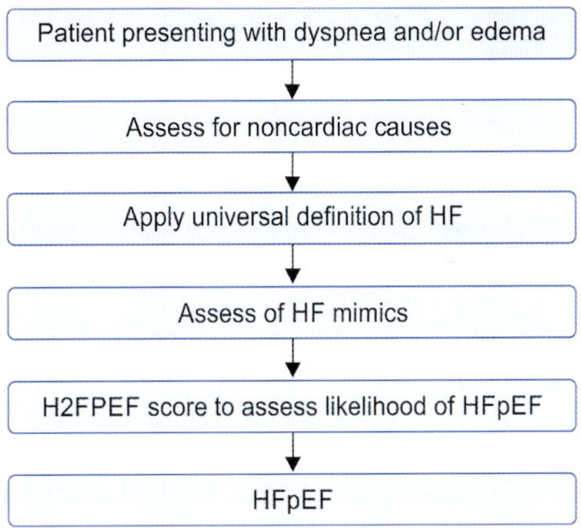

FLOWCHART 1: Diagnostic approach to heart failure with preserved ejection fraction.

TABLE 1: H2FPEF score.

Comorbidity/clinical variable	Points
Heavy (BMI ≥30 kg/m²)	2
Hypertension (>2 medications)	1
Atrial ***F***ibrillation	3
Pulmonary Hypertension (PASP >35 mm Hg on TTE)	1
Elder (Age >60 years)	1
Filling pressure (E/e′ >9 on Doppler echocardiography)	1
H2FPEF score = Sum of total points (0–9)	

TABLE 2: H2FPEF total score and probability of HFpEF.

Total score	HFpEF probability in percentage (%)
3	>50%
4	>70%
5	>80%
≥6	>90%

P Pretest assessment	• Signs and symptoms of HF • Comorbidities/risk factors • ECG • Standard echocardiography • Natriuretic peptides • Ergometry/6 minute walk testing/ Cardiopulmonary testing
E Echo and biomarkers	• Comprehensive echocardiography • Natriuretic peptides
F1 Functional testing in case of uncertainty	• Diastolic stress test (exercise stress echocardiography) • Invasive hemodynamic measurements
F2 Final etiology	• Cardiovascular magnetic resonance • Cardiac and noncardiac biopsies • Scintigraphy/CT/PET • Genetic testing • Specific laboratory testing

Functional	**Morphological**	**Biomarker (Sinus rhythm**	**Biomarker (Atrial fibrillation)**
1. Septal e' <7 cm/s or lateral e' <10 cm/s or 2. Average E/e' ≥ 15 3. TR velocity > 2.8 m/s (PASP >35 mm Hg)	***1. LAVI >34 mL/m² 2. LVMI ≥149/122 g/m² (m/w) and RWT >0.42***	***NT-proBNP >220 pg/mL or BNP >80 pg/mL***	***NT-proBNP > 660 pg/mL or BNP >240 pg/mL***
1. Average E/e' 9–14 2. GLS <16%	1. LAVI 29–34 mL/m² 2. LVMI >115/95 g/m² (m/w) 3. RWT >0.42 4. LV wall thickness ≥12 mm	NT-proBNP 125–220 pg/mL or BNP 35–80 pg/mL	NT-proBNP 365–660 pg/mL or BNP 105–240 pg/mL
Major criteria (italics)—2 points Minor criteria (nonitalics)—1 point			
Total score: ≥5 points: HFpEF **2–4 points: Diastolic stress test or invasive hemodynamics**			

FIG. 2: HFA-PEFF score.

and a score of ≥5 established the diagnosis of HFpEF. However, if there is uncertainty in the diagnosis then one can consider diastolic stress testing or invasive hemodynamics to confirm the diagnosis of HFpEF. Prior to any invasive testing, a trial of GDMT is reasonable and response can be assessed. Cardiac MRI, PET scan, PYP scan, endomyocardial biopsies, and genetic testing can be considered in a selective few to rule out cardiac cause of HFpEF mimics.

The challenges with the HFA-PEFF algorithm is that HFpEF has been shown to have lower natriuretic peptide levels compared to HFrEF and obese individuals have low natriuretic peptide levels which makes using the HFA-PEFF score challenging. Nevertheless, both these scoring systems can be utilized in the clinical decision making for diagnosis of HFpEF. Clinical judgment must be used when scoring systems show low or intermediate probability but patient has overt signs of HF on clinical exam.

MANAGEMENT

Back in the 2001 ESC guidelines, there was still ongoing debate about whether or not HF can occur secondary to diastolic dysfunction (note the terminology, diastolic dysfunction, and not HFpEF) and there was little or no evidence as to how to treat it.[10] All this changed after the landmark paper was published by Zyle et al. in 2004,[11] who showed that compared to the control group, left ventricular end diastolic pressure was significantly increased in patients with diastolic HF at the same left ventricular diastolic volume. In 2012, ESC had used the term HFpEF to describe patients with LVEF ≥40%.[12] In 2016 ESC guidelines, that was further subdivided into HFmrEF (LVEF 40–49%) and HFpEF for LVEF ≥50%.[13]

Finally in the 2021 guidelines, both ESC and ACC/AHA guidelines included MRA, ARB, ACEi, ARNI, and evidence based β-blockers as class IIb indications for HFmrEF.[14,16] ACC/AHA 2021 guidelines however included MRA, ARB, and ARNI as class IIb indications for HFpEF as well, and also included SGLT-2i as class IIa as the results of EMPEROR-preserved and DELIVER trials were published just prior to release of the 2021 ACC/AHA guidelines. In the 2023 focused update, ESC included SGLT-2i as class I recommendation for HFpEF along with diuretics and treatment of cardiovascular comorbidities contributing to HFpEF.[15] The ACC/AHA 2022 updated guidelines and 2023 expert consensus document[8] continue to have the same recommendations as the 2021 ACC/AHA guidelines.[16,6] We will take a brief look into the evidence behind approval of these classes of drugs.

HISTORY OF HEART FAILURE WITH PRESERVED EJECTION FRACTION TRIALS

Before approval of SGLT-2i for HFpEF, historically, none of the prior randomized controlled trials for the treatment of HFpEF have achieved their primary endpoints. These include PEP-CHF (perindopril), CHARM-Preserved (candesartan), I-PRESERVE (irbesartan), TOPCAT (spironolactone), DIG-Preserved (digoxin), and PARAGON-HF (sacubitril/valsartan).[17-22]

Although nebivolol significantly reduced the combined primary endpoint of all-cause mortality or CV hospital admission in the SENIORS trial,[23] this trial included only 15% with an LVEF >50%. What we learnt from all these negative or equivocal trials was that the pathophysiology for HFpEF was very different from the pathophysiology for HFrEF, and neurohormonal blockade was not the key as in HFrEF.

Trials targeting the nitric oxide-cyclic guanosine monophosphate pathway have also failed to improve exercise capacity or quality of life in HFpEF, e.g., NEAT-HFpEF, RELAX, INDIE-HFpEF, VITALITY-HFpEF, and CAPACITY-HFpEF which studied the drugs isosorbide mononitrate, sildenafil, inorganic nitrite, vericiguat, and praliciguat, respectively.[24-28] So perhaps these HFpEF patients need to undergo further phenotyping and need tailor therapies based on the underlying cause.

WHAT DO THE CURRENT GUIDELINES SAY?

Pharmacological Management

Diuretics

Diuretics continue to have a class I recommendation for treatment of HFpEF both in the 2022 ACC/AHA HF guidelines and 2023 ESC guidelines for treatment of chronic HF. **Flowchart 2** adapted from the 2023 ACC Expert consensus in the management of HF.[8]

Sodium-glucose Cotransporter-2 Inhibitors

As we all are aware, SGLT-2 inhibitors were originally studied as an antidiabetic drug but given the cardiovascular benefits, it has currently been approved to be used across entire spectrum of LVEF. What is remarkable is the that the DELIVER[29] and the EMPEROR-Preserved[30] trials have made history being first of a kind in terms of showing tremendous benefit in reducing HF hospitalizations and CV death in patients with LVEF >40% regardless of the presence or absence of diabetes. The PRESERVED-HF evaluated HFpEF patients with LVEF >50% and showed the same benefits.[31] This was again proven in the SOLOIST-WHF (sotagliflozin) and EMPULSE (empagliflozin) trials which studied safety and efficacy of SGLT-2i in patients with acute HF and was shown to reduce HF hospitalizations, urgent care visits, and ultimately reduced cardiovascular death.[32,33] Currently, the ESC guidelines have given a class I recommendation and ACC/AHA has given a class IIa recommendation for SGLT-2i.[6,8,15,16] The currently approved drugs are dapagliflozin 10 mg once a day and empagliflozin 10 mg once a day. The drugs are contraindicated in patients with diabetes mellitus type 1 and in patients with severe CKD.

Mineralocorticoid Antagonists

The MRA, specifically spironolactone was approved for use in HFpEF patients based on the results of the TOPCAT trial.[20] The trial was conducted across North America and Russia/Georgia and included 3,445 patients. The trial did not meet the primary endpoint but a subgroup analysis of the patients that were enrolled in North America showed reduction in HF hospitalizations. The benefit was also more profound in men with LVEF <60%, lower range of BNP/proBNP and across all LVEF spectrum in women. Based on this, MRA currently has a class IIb recommendation in the ACC/AHA guidelines whereas they are not part of HFpEF treatment in the ESC guidelines.[6,8,15,16] The starting dose of spironolactone is 25 mg once a day with a goal dose of 50 mg once a day. Caution should be exercised in patients with CKD and hyperkalemia.

Angiotensin Receptor–Neprilysin Inhibitors

Sacubitril inhibits neprilysin, an enzyme that inactivates several important vasoactive peptides that contribute to the pathogenesis and progression of HF, including natriuretic peptides, bradykinin, and substance P. Combination with

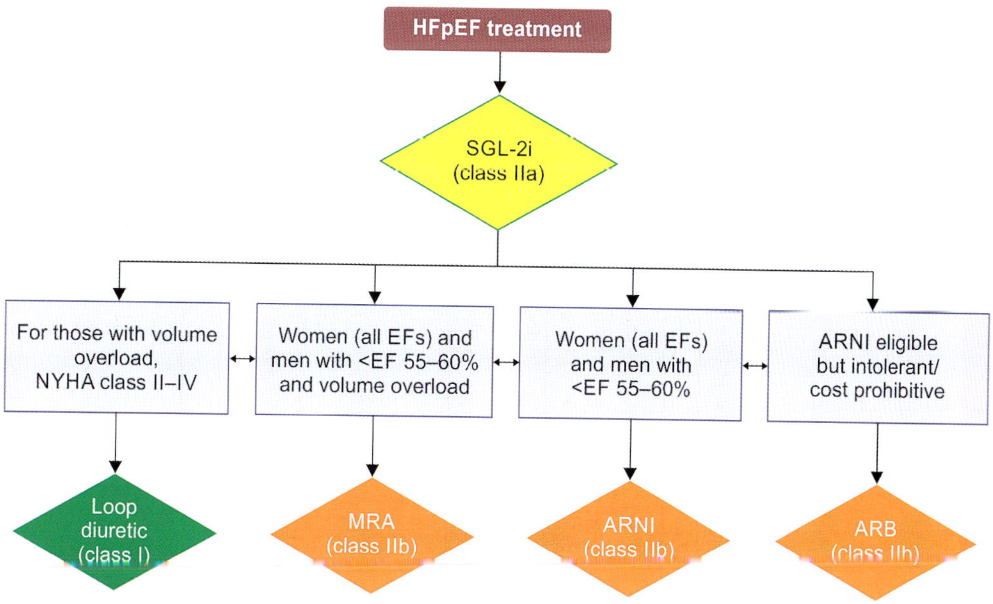

FLOWCHART 2: ACC/AHA guidelines for the treatment of HFpEF.

valsartan is necessary because neprilysin inhibition increases angiotensin levels, which could offset the vasodilatory effect of sacubitril unless also inhibited. Sacubitril/valsartan provides modest additional benefit compared with valsartan in individuals with HFpEF. ARNI was studied against valsartan in patients with LVEF ≥45% in the PARAGON-HF trial.[22] The trial showed reduction in HF hospitalization and CV death but the results were not statistically significant. But subgroup analysis showed that there was indeed a benefit in women across all LVEF spectrum and in men with LVEF 45–57%. Based on this the FDA made an expanded indication that ARNI can be used to adults patients with chronic HF who has LVEF below normal range. Based on this data, ARNI currently has a class IIb recommendation in the ACC/AHA guidelines whereas they are not part of HFpEF treatment in the ESC guidelines.[6,8,15,16] The recommended starting dose of ARNI is 24–26 mg twice a day with a target dose of 96–101 mg twice a day.

Angiotensin Receptor Blockers

In patients who do not tolerate ARNI or where the cost is prohibitory, ARB can be used because of the results of the CHARM trial.[18] ACE inhibitors are however contraindicated as PEP-CHF trial was a negative trial in HFpEF patients.[17] The recommended ARB is candesartan with a starting dose of 4–8 mg once a day to be increased to a target dose of 32 mg once a day.

Nonpharmacological Management

Device Therapies

Pulmonary Artery Pressure Monitoring

The pulmonary artery (PA) sensor monitoring is a IIb recommendation in the 2022 ACC/AHA guidelines in the management of HF and this is based on the results of CHAMPION-HF and GUIDE-HF trial.[34,35] It is currently recommended for patients with (1) Persistent NYHA class III symptoms, (2) Cardiorenal syndrome, (3) Those with obesity, lung disease which make it difficult to assess dyspneic symptoms, and (4) Those with significant liability in their volume status. This device is currently not available in India.

Other Devices

Other device interventions for HFpEF such as blood volume analysis, interatrial shunting devices, splanchnic nerve ablation, or cardiac contractility modulation are under evaluation; their benefits remain ambiguous.[36-38]

Management of Comorbidities

Management of comorbidities play a large role in the management of HFpEF as it is a heterogeneous disease with various phenotypes and it is as important as pharmacological therapy in the management of HFpEF.

Management of hypertension with a goal BP of <130/80. ARB, ARNI, and MRA should be the first choice of agents given their proven benefit in HFpEF patients. For patients with atrial fibrillation, β-blockers, and nondihydropyridine calcium channel blockers can be used for rate control. Rate versus rhythm control to be decided based on symptoms. Digoxin can also be used for rate control. Aggressive rate control is not recommended as it impacts stroke volume.

For patients with type 2 diabetes, SGLT-2i should be the first line of therapy. Alternatively, glucagon like peptide-1 receptor agonists can be used if patients have underlying obesity too. Weight loss and aerobic exercise are recommended for those patients with obesity as it helps with improvement in functional capacity. Those with sleep apnea should be referred to a sleep specialist. Patients with CKD should be initiated on ARNI, SGLT-2i based on their eGFR. Renin angiotensin inhibitors and SGLT-2i will slow the progression of renal disease. CKD should be managed with the help of a nephrologist.

CONCLUSION

The HFpEF is a complex heterogeneous disease with various phenotypes and it differs between geographical locations. A prospective cohort study using Asian HF registry showed that the Asian patients with HF are much younger and have lower BMI compared to the US counterparts. The study further categorized the patients into five phenotypes and they were very different from the usual phenotypes of the western world.[39]

Currently approved therapies are diuretics, SGLT-2i, and management of comorbidities. There are many drugs being investigated down the pipeline like a soluble guanylate cyclase stimulator, agents that loosen the bonds between proteins and glycosylation end products, and gene therapy to increase the level of SERCA2 protein in the myocardium.[40] As we continue to unravel the mysteries surrounding the management of HFpEF, clinicians should make every effort to diagnose HFpEF and exclude cardiac and noncardiac mimics of HFpEF as the treatment is different in each case. Referral should be made to advanced HF providers when necessary, especially when there is a strong suspicion for cardiac mimics of HFpEF which needs specialized care.

ONLINE REFERENCES

Please scan the QR code provided at the end of the table of contents for References of this chapter.

Heart Failure with Preserved Ejection Fraction and Left Atrial Atriopathy: Diagnostic, Prognostic, and Therapeutic Implications

CHAPTER 60

HK Chopra, Manish Bansal, Ravi R Kasliwal

ABSTRACT

Heart failure with preserved ejection fraction (HFpEF) is a clinical syndrome characterized by intermittent or sustained elevation in left ventricular filling pressure (LVFP), despite preserved left ventricular ejection fraction. Although elevated LVFP is the core abnormality seen in HFpEF, it is often associated with several other cardiac and noncardiac pathophysiological abnormalities that collectively produce the phenotype of HFpEF. Left atrial (LA) remodeling is an integral abnormality in HFpEF and is the direct consequence of intermittent or sustained elevation of LVFP. Echocardiography is an excellent modality for assessing LA remodeling. LA volume is the traditional parameter used for this purpose, whereas LA strain has recently emerged as a valuable tool with many advantages over LA volume. Both these parameters are highly useful for diagnosing left ventricular diastolic dysfunction and HFpEF. They also have excellent prognostic utility and predict the risk of atrial fibrillation, heart failure, stroke, and cardiovascular as well as all-cause mortality in a wide variety of clinical settings, including the patients with HFpEF.

Keywords: Diastolic dysfunction, left atrial volume, left ventricular

INTRODUCTION

Heart failure with preserved ejection fraction (HFpEF) is a clinical syndrome characterized by intermittent or sustained elevation in left ventricular filling pressure (LVFP), despite preserved left ventricular ejection fraction (LVEF). Although elevated LVFP is the core abnormality seen in HFpEF, it is often associated with several other cardiac and noncardiac pathophysiological abnormalities that collectively produce the phenotype of HFpEF. Multitude of the underlying mechanisms make it quite a heterogenous condition and difficult to diagnose.[1-3]

Since the left atrium and left ventricle are in direct continuity with each other during diastole, the elevated LVFP exposes the left atrium to increased afterload which results in progressive left atrial (LA) remodeling. The extent of such LA remodeling correlates with the severity and chronicity of the increased LVFP.[4-6] Hence, LA remodeling serves as an excellent measure of the cumulative extent of the underlying left ventricular (LV) damage and is a useful parameter to aid the diagnosis of HFpEF. It is also an excellent prognostic marker and predicts various adverse cardiac consequences seen in HFpEF. For these reasons, there has been a considerable interest in evaluating the presence and severity of the LA remodeling in HFpEF.

Echocardiography is the most useful modality for assessing LA remodeling. Echocardiographically, LA remodeling can be recognized in the form of LA dilation and/or LA dysfunction. This chapter describes the role of echocardiography in assessing left atriopathy in HFpEF.

LEFT ATRIAL ENLARGEMENT

Chronic exposure to increased LVFP leads to progressive enlargement of the LA size and hence, LA enlargement has been one of the most important echocardiographic features of LV diastolic dysfunction and HFpEF.[4-6] Due to its ability to reflect chronically elevated LVFP, LA size is also considered to be the glycosylated hemoglobin of LV diastolic function.

Earlier, the anteroposterior diameter of the left atrium derived from the parasternal long-axis view was the main measurement used for diagnosing LA enlargement. However, the LA enlargement in the anteroposterior dimension is usually constrained because of the presence of the sternum anteriorly and the spine posteriorly. Hence, the LA anteroposterior diameter often underestimates the extent of the LA dilatation, and no guideline currently recommends its use. Instead, the LA volume (LAV) is considered the current gold standard for quantifying the LA size.[7]

Echocardiographic Estimation of Left Atrial Volume

Previous guidelines had recommended the biplane area-length method for calculating LAV.[8] However, this method was relatively cumbersome, precluding its widespread adoption. To overcome this challenge, the current guidelines now recommend the biplane Simpson's method for estimating LAV.[7] A recent study including 467 patients showed that LAV was significantly associated with all-cause and cardiovascular mortality, regardless of the method used for its estimation.[9]

Left atrial volume estimation using the biplane Simpson's method is a simple technique **(Fig. 1)**. First, the LA-focused apical four- and two-chamber views need to be acquired. The images need to be optimized to avoid the LA foreshortening. This can be confirmed by ensuring that the LA base appears wider than the mitral annular plane. Once the two LA views have been obtained, LAV can be estimated by tracing the endocardial border in end-systole (ventricular systole) in both these views. When tracing the LA endocardial border, care should be taken to avoid entering the pulmonary veins or the LA appendage. The border is traced from one end of the mitral annulus to the other, and the echocardiography machine automatically joins the two ends with a straight line. The LAV thus obtained is indexed to the body surface area to yield the LA volume index (LAVI), which is the standard measure used for all the diagnostic and prognostic purposes. The upper limit of normal for LAVI is 34 mL/m^2 for both genders, and any value exceeding this indicates LA enlargement.[7]

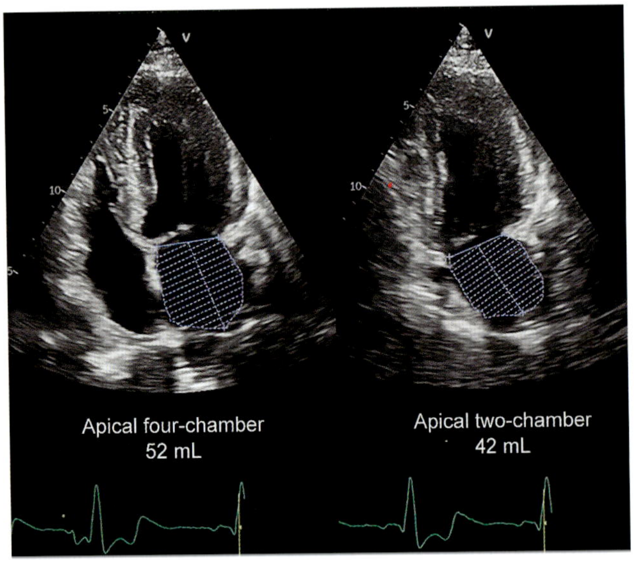

FIG. 1: Measurement of left atrial volume using the biplane Simpson's method. The average left atrial volume in this patient was 47 mL.

Diagnostic Utility of Left Atrial Volume Index

Left atrial enlargement is quite common in heart failure (HF), occurring in most patients with HF with reduced ejection fraction (HFrEF) and nearly 50–66% patients with HFpEF.[10,11] Persistent elevation of LVFP is the main driving force for LA enlargement, though atrial fibrillation (AF) and mitral regurgitation may also contribute to this. In the absence of an alternate cause (such as AF or mitral regurgitation), LA enlargement is virtually diagnostic of advanced LV diastolic dysfunction and is an important clue to the presence of HFpEF. In one study, LAVI had the highest area under the curve for diagnosing HFpEF as compared to LV global longitudinal strain and the ratio of mitral inflow early diastolic velocity (E) to mitral annular early diastolic velocity (e') (E/e').[12]

For diagnosing HFpEF, it is essential to demonstrate some cardiac structural abnormality (typically LV hypertrophy or increased LAVI) that could explain the congestive physiology. The HFA-PEFF algorithm proposed by the Heart Failure Association of the European Society of Cardiology includes increased LAVI as one of the diagnostic criteria. A value > 34 mL/m^2 is considered a major criterion and assigned two points, whereas LAVI in the range of 29–34 mL/m^2 is considered a minor criterion and is assigned one point.[13] The other guidelines have also included increased LAVI as one of the diagnostic criteria for HFpEF.[14] Besides this, increased LAVI has also been one of the eligibility criteria for inclusion in the major randomized trials evaluating various therapeutic agents in HFpEF.[15,16]

It is however noteworthy that unlike HFrEF, in HFpEF, LAVI is correlated with less number of clinical, echocardiographic, and biochemical parameters, reflecting pathophysiological complexity of HFpEF.[17] In another study involving patients with HFpEF, the relationship between LAVI and natriuretic peptides was not consistent and varied according to the mitral E/e'.[18]

Prognostic Value of Left Atrial Volume Index

Left atrial size (LA diameter in older studies and LAV or LAVI in the recent studies) is a strong predictor of adverse cardiovascular outcomes. It is associated with increased risk of AF, HF hospitalizations, stroke, and cardiovascular as well as all-cause mortality.[4,10,11,19-33] The prognostic value of LAVI has been demonstrated in a wide variety of patient subgroups and even in the general population.[27]

In a study including 1,554 elderly subjects with no prior AF, LAV was independently predictive of first ischemic stroke and even death.[27] In another study, LAVI measured in patients undergoing cardiac magnetic resonance (CMR) imaging for various indications was associated with all-cause mortality.[34] In a large study of 36,561 patients with preserved LVEF but with or without raised LVFP, LAVI was associated with all-cause mortality regardless of the LV geometry.[35] Other studies have also demonstrated LAVI to be a predictor of all-cause mortality and major adverse cardiovascular events in patients without LV systolic dysfunction or AF.[36] A meta-analysis of several studies including patients with HF showed that each 10 mL/m^2 increase in baseline LAVI was associated with a 22% increased adjusted hazard of all-cause mortality.[37]

Left atrial volume index can also be used to monitor disease progression in HFpEF. In a study of 409 patients with HFpEF, improvement in LAVI was associated with a lower rate of HF hospitalization over a follow-up of 22 months, as compared to the patients with stable or increased LAVI.[38]

Increased LAVI is a strong predictor of new-onset AF or AF recurrence after interventions. A meta-analysis showed that LAVI was a good predictor of AF recurrence after electrical cardioversion.[39] Another meta-analysis showed that among patients undergoing radiofrequency ablation for AF, those who had recurrence had higher LAVI. Larger LAVI increased the odds of having AF recurrence after ablation.[40] LAVI also predicts AF recurrence after other modes of ablation.[41-43]

Left atrial volume index has useful diagnostic and prognostic value in patients with stroke. Raised LAVI is associated with cardioembolic stroke and AF in patients presenting with cryptogenic stroke.[44,45] It is also associated with the LA appendage thrombus.[46,47]

Apart from the above, the prognostic utility of LAVI has been demonstrated in many other clinical settings. LAVI predicts adverse events (aortic valve replacement of death) in asymptomatic patients with moderate or severe aortic stenosis.[48] It also predicts improvement in natriuretic peptides following transcatheter aortic valve replacement in severe aortic stenosis.[49] In a meta-analysis involving 2,191 patients, LAVI predicted response to CRT.[50]

Limitations

Although LAVI has been the most valuable measure of LA remodeling, it has several limitations. The use of improper views and incorrect endocardial border tracing can lead to measurement variability. In addition, the time and effort required to perform LAVI estimation (albeit small) discourage its routine measurement. Several different techniques such as the use of three-dimensional echocardiography and automated image recognition and analysis are being developed to overcome these challenges.[51-55] Some investigators have also tried to validate methods to derive LAVI from LA diameter.[51-55]

Another limitation of LAVI is that it is not sensitive to detect milder forms of LV diastolic dysfunction. It is also not responsive to dynamic changes in the LVFP. In addition, it has already been mentioned that due to the complex nature of HFpEF, the relationship between LAVI and LVFP is not perfect. A significant scatter has been demonstrated between LAVI and LVFP in patients with HFpEF.[56] This problem is also reflected in a relatively inconsistent correlation between LAVI and other echocardiographic and biochemical parameters in HFpEF.[17,18]

LEFT ATRIAL STRAIN

The advent of speckle tracking echocardiography (STE) has allowed a simple option for quantifying myocardial deformation during echocardiography. Originally developed for the assessment of LV function assessment, the technique has subsequently been expanded to other cardiac chambers, such as the right ventricle and left atrium. LA strain has emerged as a very useful tool for the assessment of LV diastolic function and has several advantages over LAVI, as discussed below.

Measurement and Interpretation of Left Atrial Strain

Since STE is a grayscale-based technique, conventional grayscale echocardiography images are used for LA strain measurement. The LA-focused apical four- or two-chamber view acquired at a frame rate of 50–80 frames/s is needed. A good-quality electrocardiogram (ECG) with well-visible P waves is essential. The image sector should be narrowed to improve the lateral resolution. Artifacts should be minimized.

Once a satisfactory image has been acquired, it is analyzed using the LA strain quantification tool available on the echocardiography machine. If a dedicated option for the left atrium is not available, then the LV strain tool may also be used, but it would require transferring the image to a workstation.

The first step in the image analysis is to generate a region of intertest (ROI). It is generated by tracing the LA endocardial border from one end of the mitral annulus to the other, in the same manner as done for LAV quantification. The software then automatically creates an ROI that covers the LA wall. Typically, a 3-mm-wide ROI is created, but it may be modified as needed. The ROI should follow the LA contour and cover the LA myocardium without extending into the pericardium. The system will then process the data and display the cine image showing the LA wall tracking. If the tracking appears proper, it can be accepted to generate the LA strain curve.

The above method utilizes the beginning of the QRS as the reference point, which is the default method. A P-wave-based method is also available but is not used for a variety of reasons. Using the QRS as the reference point, a positive LA strain curve is generated as depicted in **Figures 2 and 3**. The strain curve starts at the zero baseline and the value increases as the left atrium enlarges during the ventricular systole to reach the peak value just before the mitral valve opening

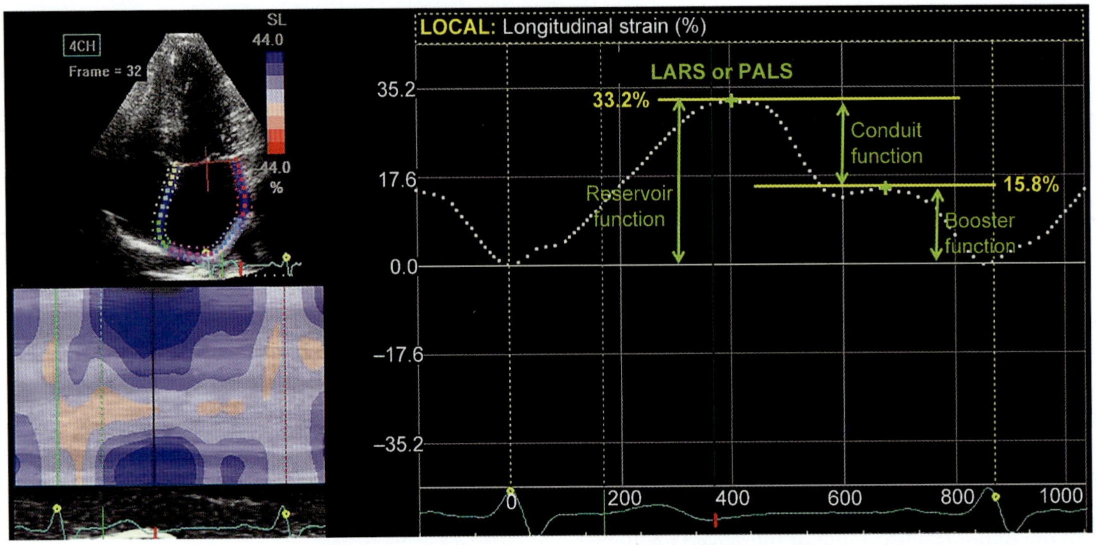

FIG. 2: Left atrial strain measurement using QRS as the reference point. There is an initial positive wave during ventricular systole which is followed by reduction in strain during early rapid filling phase and subsequently during active atrial contraction. The reservoir strain was calculated as 33.2%, conduit strain as 15.8–33.2 = −17.4%, and contraction strain as 0–15.8 = −15.8%.

(LARS: left atrial reservoir strain; PALS: peak atrial longitudinal strain)

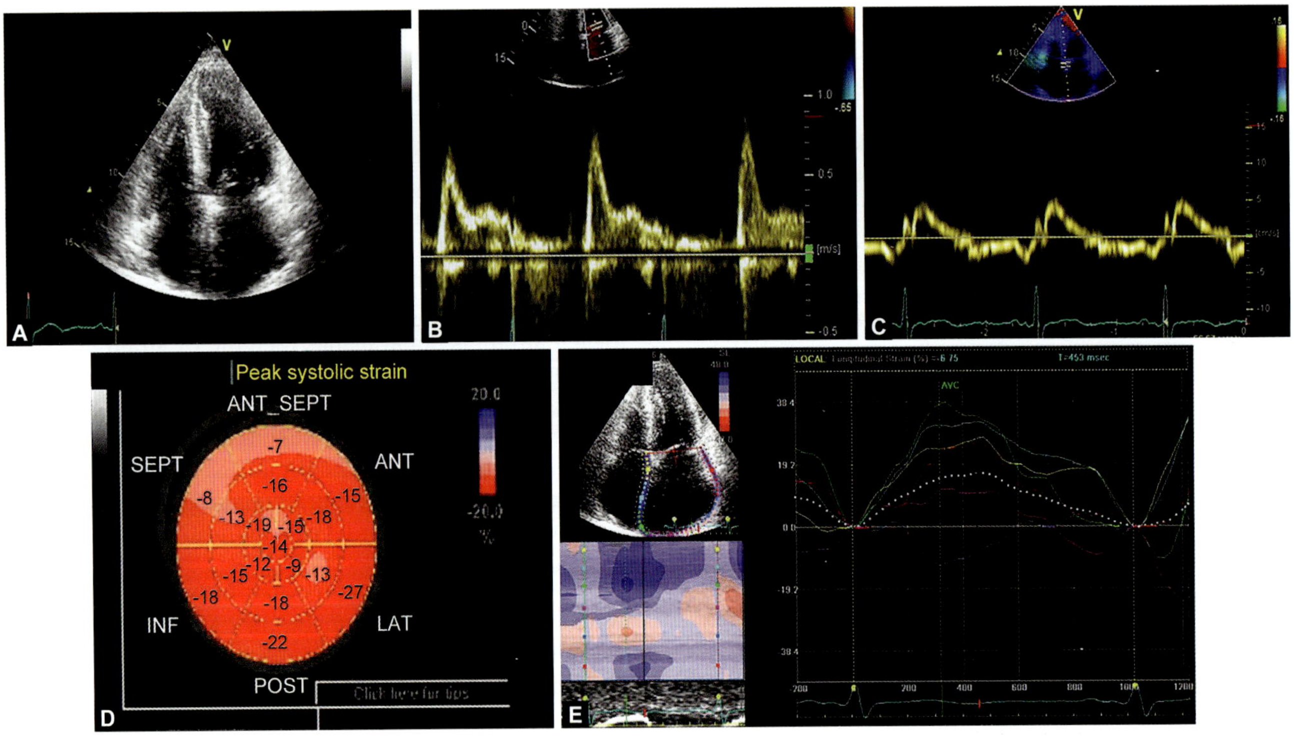

FIGS. 3A TO E: A typical patient with heart failure with preserved ejection fraction. (A) The left ventricle is hypertrophied, normal size, whereas the left atrium is markedly dilated. (B) Mitral inflow early diastolic wave is tall and steep, late diastolic wave is small, and an "L" wave is also present. (C) Mitral annular early diastolic velocity is markedly reduced. (D) Mild reduced (−15.5%) left ventricular global longitudinal strain. (E) Markedly reduced (17%) left atrial reservoir strain.

(coinciding with the T wave on the ECG). This peak value is referred to as the peak atrial longitudinal strain (PALS) or simply the LA reservoir strain (LARS). Reservoir strain is clinically the most important LA strain parameter.

Once the mitral valve opens, the LA strain rapidly decreases and reaches a plateau during the diastasis. Subsequently, as the left atrium contracts with the onset of the P wave, the LA strain decreases further and reaches the baseline by the end of the ventricular diastole. The difference between the reservoir strain and the strain value during diastasis is known as "conduit strain" and the difference between the diastasis and the baseline value (i.e., zero) is known as "contraction strain."

A meta-analysis of 40 studies showed that the normal value of LARS is 39% (95% confidence interval 38–41%).[57] However, the lower limit of the normal has been reported to be approximately 22–23%, which varies according to the age and gender.[58]

Diagnostic Utility

Left atrial strain serves as a measure of the cumulative LA overload and is a sensitive measure of LA dysfunction and remodeling. Hemodynamic studies have shown that LARS correlates well with invasively measured LVFP and may have better accuracy than mitral *E*/*e*′.[59] Studies using CMR have demonstrated that LA strain correlates with the myocardial fibrosis.[60]

Numerous studies have demonstrated that abnormalities of LA strain occur earlier than the increase in the LA size, because the latter requires a sustained elevation of LA afterload for a long time. For the same reason, LA strain is also more responsive to the changes in LVFP. It is more of an instantaneous measure of LVFP, unlike LAVI which predominantly reflects only the chronic abnormalities.[61]

Left atrial strain is particularly useful in the evaluation of LV diastolic dysfunction and HFpEF. The American Society of Echocardiography in 2016 published guidelines for the assessment of LV diastolic dysfunction.[62] Algorithms for stepwise assessment of LVFP and grading of LV diastolic dysfunction were proposed. Although the 2016 guidelines provided better accuracy and clarity than the previous guidelines published in 2009,[63] several challenges were recognized. Most importantly, using these guidelines, a sizeable proportion of individuals are diagnosed as having indeterminate LV diastolic dysfunction. The incorporation of LARS, either in addition to or in place of LAVI, significantly reduces this uncertainty.[64]

Morris et al. studied 517 patients who were in sinus rhythm and were at risk for developing LV diastolic dysfunction due to various reasons.[64] Among those with normal LAVI, LV diastolic dysfunction and reduced LARS were present in 80% and 29.4%, respectively. The addition of LARS increased the sensitivity to detect LV diastolic dysfunction, compared to the conventional parameters. More important, reduced LARS (i.e., <23%) was significantly associated with worse functional class, even when LAVI was normal. These findings were further corroborated by another retrospective analysis which showed that reduced LA strain was significantly associated with the risk of HF hospitalization at 2 years, even after adjusting for LAVI.[64] Another study showed that LARS had superior ability compared to LAVI for distinguishing between the different grades of LV diastolic dysfunction.[65] Similar findings have been reported in other studies as well.[66]

In a study of 669 consecutive patients with LVEF ≥ 50% undergoing exercise echocardiography, LARS correlated well with the LVFP at rest and during exercise.[67] It was lowest in patients with raised LVFP at rest, intermediate in those with increased LVFP only during exercise, and highest among those who had normal LVFP even on exercise. Furthermore, the addition of LARS significantly improved the accuracy of the HFA-PEFF algorithm for diagnosing HFpEF. Another study showed that LARS was a more sensitive marker of HF than LAVI and was abnormal in many patients with both HFpEF and HFrEF, despite normal LAVI.[66] A large study from South Korea showed good correlation between H_2FPEF score and LARS.[68] Other studies have also shown good agreement, or even incremental value, of LARS over various HFpEF diagnostic algorithms.[69-71] LA strain also correlates with symptomatic status and exercise capacity in HF, regardless of the LVEF.[72-75] It can also distinguish between noncardiac and cardiac causes of dyspnea.

Prognostic Utility and Therapeutic Implications

Several studies have demonstrated that LA strain is a good predictor of the risk of HF hospitalization and AF.[64,76-78] Park et al. analyzed data on 2,461 patients in sinus rhythm out of 4,312 consecutive patients admitted with acute HF. Reduced LARS (<18%) was a significant predictor of AF risk over a follow-up of 5 years. The authors also developed a score (HAS-BAP) which had good accuracy for predicting the AF risk.[76] Reduced LA strain has also been shown to predict AF in many other settings.[77-82] LA strain also predicts recurrence of AF after cardioversion or catheter ablation and may thus help in patient selection for these procedures.[83-88]

Left atrial strain has also been shown to predict the risk of stroke in patients with paroxysmal or persistent AF and has incremental value over CHA_2DS_2-VASc score for this purpose.[89,90] Although LA strain is currently not included in the algorithms used for guiding anticoagulation in AF, it can potentially be helpful for this purpose.

Apart from AF, LA strain also predicts other adverse cardiovascular events.[75,91] In a study of 100 patients with HFpEF, LA strain predicted a composite of all-cause death, myocardial infarction, and hospitalization due to decompensated HF over a mean follow-up of 4.4 ± 1.9 years.[91] LA strain has also been incorporated into machine-learning algorithms to improve the prediction of adverse clinical outcomes.[92] It has also been used for assessing the impact of various HF therapies on LA remodeling.[93,94]

Limitations

Despite the many advantages of LA strain, it has some important limitations as well. First, there are many technical issues that compromise its accuracy. The left atrium is situated in the far field of the image sector resulting in lower resolution, the LA wall is thin and difficult to track, the interatrial septum is often mobile, and there are several echocardiographic dropouts due to fossa ovalis, pulmonary veins, and LA appendage. All these issues contribute to the intraobserver and interobserver variability in the measurement of LA strain. Second, the relationship between LARS and LVFP is weaker in patients with HFpEF as compared to those with reduced LVEF. And last, unlike the LAVI, LA strain currently has much less data to support its regular use.

CONCLUSION

Left atrial remodeling is an integral abnormality in HFpEF and is the direct consequence of intermittent or sustained elevation of LVFP. Echocardiography is an excellent modality for assessing LA remodeling. LAVI is the traditional parameter used for this purpose, whereas LARS has recently emerged as a valuable tool with many advantages over LAVI. Both these parameters are highly useful for diagnosing LV diastolic dysfunction and HFpEF. They also have excellent prognostic utility and predict the risk of AF, HF, stroke, and cardiovascular as well as all-cause mortality in a wide variety of clinical settings, including patients with HFpEF.

ONLINE REFERENCES

Please scan the QR code provided at the end of the table of contents for References of this chapter.

CHAPTER

61

Cardiovascular–kidney–metabolic Syndrome: Pathophysiology

Prakas Chandra Mondal

ABSTRACT

Cardiometabolic risk is a complex array of interconnected and sometimes mutually inclusive traditional risk factors such as dyslipidemia, hypertension, obesity, insulin resistance, hyperglycemia, and behavioral factors such as smoking, physical inactivity, and unhealthy dietary habits. Nonmodifiable risk factors such as family history, age, sex, and ethnicity are also play significant role in risk clustering. Substantial overlap between metabolic, cardiovascular, and kidney diseases leads to a new disease condition known as cardiovascular–kidney–metabolic (CKM) syndrome, which also includes the time before the onset of symptoms and social determinants of health during its screening. People with adverse social determinants of health have higher prevalence of poor cardiovascular–kidney–metabolic health. A holistic approach for an integrated management of this CKM syndrome will have synergistic effects on patient's health and significant outcome improvements.

Keywords: Cardiorenal, social determinants of health, chronic kidney disease, glycation end products

INTRODUCTION

Cardiovascular–kidney–metabolic (CKM) syndrome is a progressive condition, usually begins early in life with accumulation of excess and dysfunctional adipose tissue with resultant adverse changes in internal milieu in the form of inflammation, oxidative stress, and insulin resistance.

Unlike metabolic or cardiorenal syndromes, CKM syndrome includes the time before the onset of symptoms, stressing the importance of screening for metabolic factors at an early age, which not only include biological factors but also the social determinants of health (SDOH) that effects clinical outcomes. These include environmental, social, psychological factors, and also financial hardships that can put an individual at increased health risk.[1]

STAGES OF CKM SYNDROME[2]

- *Stage-0*: No risk factors
  Individuals are typically young, asymptomatic with normal body weight, no metabolic risk factors or diagnoses of CKD or CVD.
- *Stage-1*: Excess or dysfunctional adipose tissue
  Individuals have increased body fat, abdominal obesity, may have prediabetes. No other metabolic risk factors or any diagnoses of CKD or CVD
- *Stage-2*: Metabolic risk factors and CKD.
  Individuals have developed additional metabolic risk factors such as hypertension, type 2 diabetes mellitus, metabolic syndrome, dyslipidemia, or CKD
- *Stage-3*: Subclinical CVD in CKM syndrome
  Individuals have metabolic risk factors from the earlier stages, may have symptoms and will test positive for subclinical diagnoses of heart disease, heart failure (HF), or peripheral artery disease (PAD).
- *Stage-4*: Clinical CVD in CKM syndrome
  Individuals have cardiovascular disease, ischemic stroke, clinical HF, PAD, and atrial fibrillation.

RISK-ENHANCING FACTORS FOR CKM SYNDROME[3]

- High-risk demographic groups such as South Asian ethnicity and lower socioeconomic status

- High burden of SDOH
- Chronic inflammatory conditions, e.g., psoriasis, rheumatoid arthritis, lupus, and HIV/AIDS
- Mental health disorders such as depression and anxiety
- Sleep disorders like obstructive sleep apnea.
- *Sex-specific risk enhancers (beyond gestational diabetes in stage-1):*
  - History of premature menopause (age < 40 years).
  - History of adverse pregnancy outcomes (e.g., hypertensive disorders of pregnancy, preterm birth, small for gestational age)
  - Polycystic ovarian syndrome
  - Erectile dysfunction
  - Elevated high-sensitivity C-reactive protein
  - Family history of diabetes and kidney failure

PATHOBIOLOGICAL PATHWAYS

Adipose Tissue Dysfunction

Adipose tissue dysfunction is a long-term positive energy balance, leading to weight gain and increased adipocyte size. Adipocyte hypertrophy is accompanied by disturbances in lipid metabolism and altered adipokine secretion, i.e., a shift toward a proinflammatory phenotype. Adipose tissue is a complex organ with marked effect on whole body metabolic physiology and expansion of adipose tissue does not necessarily translate into increased metabolic and cardiovascular disease risk.[4] A proportion of obese subjects are relative protected against worsening of metabolic health signifying that adipose tissue dysfunction rather than body fat mass is the key factor in the pathogenesis of obesity-related metabolic and CVDs.[5] Impairment in adipose tissue lipid metabolism, a decreased adipose tissue blood flow (ATBF), and an increased production of proinflammatory cytokines by hypertrophic adipocytes and infiltrating adaptive and innate immune cells are major functional characteristics of dysfunctional adipose tissue. Adipose tissue dysfunction is accompanied by lipid spillover in the circulation and ectopic fat storage in nonadipose tissues. These impairments induce local as well as systemic insulin resistance, thereby affecting metabolic health.

Adipose Tissue Hypoxia

Adipose tissue angiogenesis is insufficient to maintain normoxia in the entire fat depot during progressive development of obesity leading to tissue hypoxia. A lower expression of angiogenic genes such as *VEGF* and lower capillary density is observed in abdominal subcutaneous adipose tissue of obese as compared to lean subjects.[6] Fasting and postprandial ATBF is decreased in obese insulin-resistant subjects as compared to lean insulin-sensitive subjects.[7] Rarely, the diameter of hypertrophic adipocytes in obesity exceeds the normal diffusion distance of oxygen in tissues (100–200 μm).[8] Adipose tissue hypoxia has a positive correlation with gene expression for proinflammatory markers.

Parameters Associated with Adipose Tissue Dysfunction

- *Visceral adiposity index:*[9] A sex-dependent mathematical model, which estimates visceral functionality based on BMI, waist circumference, triglycerides, and HDL level. It is a marker of adipose tissue dysfunction and able to identify metabolic risk before metabolic syndrome or cardiovascular complication develop. But it needs validation in non-Caucasian people and also not useful with triglyceride level > 300 mg% or very high BMI > 40 kg/m^2.
- *Hypertriglyceridemic waist*: This indicates simultaneous presence of an increased waist circumference and elevated fasting triglyceride level. It is indicative of higher risk of cardiovascular disease and type 2 diabetes.[10]
- *Metabolic flexibility*: It is defined as the ability of an organism to adapt substrate oxidation to substrate availability and can be measured through the changes in respiratory quotient under metabolic changes such as overnight fasting. Metabolic inflexibility has been proposed as a pathophysiological mechanism for ectopic lipid accumulation and insulin resistance.[11]
- *Biomarkers*: Adiponectin and leptin are well-studied adipokines. Adiponectin is considered as a favorable adipokine because its actions are related with decreased inflammation, improving insulin sensitivity, and reducing hepatic gluconeogenesis. In obesity and diabetes, adiponectin levels are decreased. Leptin is proinflammatory adipokine that induces monocyte proliferation and stimulate proinflammatory cytokine secretion. Adiponectin/Leptin (A/L) ratio has emerged as a marker of adipocyte health. A decreased A/L ratio is associated with a deleterious secretory profile of adipose tissue.[12]

Endoplasmic Reticulum Stress

Physiologic stresses such as increased secretory load or pathological stresses such as the presence of mutated proteins that cannot get folded properly in the endoplasmic reticulum can lead to imbalance between the demand for protein folding and capacity for protein folding which lead to endoplasmic reticulum stress. Stress leads to activation of signal transduction pathways called unfolded protein response (UPR). These are implicated as the pathogenetic pathway for cardiomyocyte apoptosis, atherosclerosis in individuals with diabetes and progression of diabetic kidney disease.[13]

Oxidative Stress

Reactive oxygen species (ROS) and reactive nitrogen species (NOS) are generated physiologically to regulate cell growth and differentiation, smooth muscle relaxation, and inhibition of platelet adhesion. Imbalance in redox homeostasis leads to a proinflammatory and profibrotic environment, which leads to disruptions in insulin metabolic signaling, diminished endothelial-mediated vasorelaxation, and a wide variety of structural and functional abnormalities in cardiovascular and renal systems.[14]

mTOR/S6 Kinase-1 Signaling Pathway

Overnutrition characterized by excessive consumption of high-fat and high-carbohydrate foods and the presence of aldosterone and angiotensin-II can promote insulin resistance through activation of mammalian target of the rapamycin m*TOR*/S6 kinase-1 signaling pathway in cardiovascular tissue and the kidney thereby contributing to the intricate connection of CKM syndrome.[15]

Pathogenetic Pathways Linking Type 2 Diabetes Mellitus to Cardiorenal Damage

- *Unifying hypothesis*:[16] Excessive intracellular glucose flux (glucotoxicity) leads to mitochondrial superoxide production and exacerbation of oxidative stress. Increased ROS production causes tissue damage through activation of the polyol and hexosamine pathways. "ROS" also lead to the formation of advanced glycation end products from nonenzymatic glycation of proteins.
- Advanced glycation end products can damage the heart, the blood vessels and the kidney both directly, causing cross-linking of matrix proteins and higher tissue stiffness, indirectly via receptors leading to activation of signaling pathways. Thus advanced glycation end products are involved in the pathogenesis of diabetic cardiomyopathy, atherosclerosis, and diabetic kidney disease.[17]
- Activation of local renin angiotensin in the myocardium and in the kidney promotes vasoconstriction, fibrosis, and exacerbation of organ dysfunction.
- "*Nutrient abundance*": Diabetes is a state of nutrient abundance, characterized by aberrant activation of nutrient sensing pathways such as sirtuins and mTOR-downregulating cytoprotective responses and promoting organ damage.[18]
- *Metabolic shift*: Insulin resistance is associated with a metabolic shift toward free fatty acid oxidation which is more oxygen consuming, leading to impaired metabolic flexibility and reduced energetic efficiency. Increased uptake of free fatty acids leads to accumulation of intracellular triglycerols, promoting lipotoxicity and apoptosis.[19]
- *Epicardial adipose tissue* has got paracrine effect in myocardial metabolism, protecting it from free fatty acid overload. Diabetes has been associated with pathological changes in its volume and cytokine secretory profile which are potential drivers of diabetes associated cardio-vascular diseases.[20]
- *Diabetic cardiomyopathy is one of two forms*: (1) restrictive, i.e., HFpEF-like phenotype, which is more common in women and obesity, linked to coronary endothelial inflammation. (2) dilated, i.e., HFrEF phenotype associated with myocyte loss.

IMPACT OF DIABETES MELLITUS ON KIDNEY FUNCTION

Diabetic nephropathy is redefined as "diabetic kidney disease" and includes all forms of renal abnormalities occurring in diabetes.

- Glomerular hyperfiltration
- *Podocyte damage*: Pathological changes in podocytes such as dedifferentiation, detachment, and foot process effacement. Dysfunctional podocytes lead to glomerular basement thickening with alteration in its filtration function leading to albuminuria.[21]
- *Mesangial cell damage*: Mesangial cells become hypertrophied, proliferate, and increase the synthesis of matrix proteins leading to diabetic glomerulopathy.[22]
  Nonalbuminuric diabetic kidney disease: Secondary to macrovascular damage and tubulointerstitial damage[23]

BIDIRECTIONAL CARDIORENAL INTERPLAY

Acute or chronic dysfunction of one leads to acute or chronic dysfunction of the other. Deceased cardiac output, effective hypovolemia, and excess vasoconstrictive mediators lead to chronic renal hypoperfusion and decreased e-GFR leading to initiation and progression of kidney dysfunction. Conversely, sodium and water retention, RAAS activation increases cardiac pre- and afterloads. Uremic toxins and chronic inflammation lead to cardiac remodeling and dysfunction.[24]

CARDIOVASCULAR DYSFUNCTION AND ONSET OF TYPE 2 DIABETES MELLITUS

Cardiovascular dysfunction can promote metabolic alterations and new-onset diabetes mellitus. Proposed mechanisms include endothelial dysfunction, insulin-resistant state of heart failure, pancreatic beta-cell loss with high natriuretic peptides and proinflammatory cytokines. Reduced skeletal muscle mass and muscle hypoperfusion lead to reduced peripheral glucose utilization.

KIDNEY DYSFUNCTION AND TYPE 2 DIABETES ONSET

Kidney disease can promote metabolic dysregulation and new-onset diabetes mellitus. Proposed mechanisms include:

- Defective insulin signaling pathway[25]
- Postreceptor defect involving signal transduction protein

- Uremic toxins such as urea, p-cresyl sulfate, and asymmetric dimethylarginine
- Vitamin D deficiency[26] modulates calcium in beta cell and increases expression of insulin receptors

NEW RISK PREDICTION EQUATION BASED ON CKM SYNDROME

Khan et al. developed and validated new, sex-specific and race-specific risk equations known as *prevent equations*. Five key factors were included, viz., systolic blood pressure, total cholesterol, high-density lipoprotein cholesterol, BMI, and eGFR. The *prevent* equations provide CVD risk estimates over timeperiods of 10 and 30 years. They include e-GFR as a risk predictor and adjust for competing risk of non-CVD death. If clinically indicated, additional models include other CKM factors such as u-ACR, hemoglobin A1c, and social determinants of health.[27]

CONCLUSION

Cardiovascular, kidney and metabolic diseases interact at the pathophysiological level leading to a clinical overlap manifested in the broader CKM syndrome. Activation of shared underlying mechanism initiates a detrimental cycle, perpetuating disease process and escalating morbidity and mortality. A holistic approach with integrated multidisciplinary collaboration in CKM care is needed rather than isolated treatment of individual diseases. Further research is crucial for better understanding of CKM pathophysiology, especially interethnic variations in risk and exploring social determinants and their interconnections.

ONLINE REFERENCES

Please scan the QR code provided at the end of the table of contents for References of this chapter.

CHAPTER

62

Advanced Heart Failure: Diagnosis and Management

Lekha Adik Pathak, Ronak V Ruparelia

ABSTRACT

Advanced heart failure incidence is increasing with recent advances in cardiac care and mortality remains high in developing as well as developed countries. It is of utmost importance for all clinicians to have a clear idea about the diagnosis and treatment of advanced heart failure. The four pillars of heart failure management play a central role in the management of advanced heart failure. Beyond this, certain newer medications have also shown encouraging reports in management. Nonetheless, invasive and surgical approach for the management of advanced heart failure also needs to be kept in mind while treating such cases.

Keywords: Advanced heart failure, SGLT-2 inhibitors, vericiguat in heart failure

INTRODUCTION

"Advanced" heart failure (HF) means clinical syndrome characterized by persistent or progressive symptoms of ventricular dysfunction despite guideline-directed medical therapy (GDMT). The prevalence of advanced HF is increasing due to increasing number of patients with risk factor for cardiovascular (CV) disease and the aging of population. 1 year mortality has been reported from 25% to as high as 75% among various literature. In this chapter, we will focus on the diagnosis and management of advanced HF.

CLASSIFYING ADVANCED HEART FAILURE

Multiple classification system has been described. NYHA class is the most commonly used classification. NYHA class IV defines those with symptoms at rest and with any physical activity. Another commonly used classification system is by the ACC/AHA, which describes stage D HF as those who require specialized treatment due to refractory symptoms despite optimal medical management. Another one is the INTERMACS classification system which was developed to risk stratify patients with advanced HF to better define prognosis and urgency of intervention. These classification systems should be used in parallel to precisely define where a HF patient lies on the spectrum of progressive disease and how frequently he may need advanced line of care.

According to the HF Association of European Society of Cardiology, all the following criteria must be met to define advanced or end-stage HF despite optimal medical therapy.

- Severe and persistent symptoms of HF (NYHA class III or IV)
- Severe cardiac dysfunction characterized by at least one of the following criteria:
    - Reduced left ventricular ejection fraction (LVEF) ≤ 30%
    - Isolated right ventricular failure
    - Inoperable severe valvular disease
    - Inoperable severe congenital defects
    - Persistently high (or increasing) levels of brain natriuretic peptide (BNP) or N-terminal pro-BNP (NT-proBNP) and presence of severe diastolic dysfunction or structural abnormalities of the left ventricle
- Episodes of pulmonary or systemic congestion requiring high-dose intravenous diuretics or episodes of reduced cardiac output that require inotropic support or the use of vasoactive drugs or malignant arrhythmias causing >1 unplanned visit to the doctor or hospitalization in the last 12 months.
- Significant exercise intolerance with the inability to perform physical activity or the 6-minute walk test

(6MWT) or the peak oxygen consumption (peak VO_2) on the exercise test < 12–14 mL/kg/min, which are assumed to be of cardiac etiology.

Dunley et al.[1] studied 6,836 patients, out of which 936 (13.7%) had end-stage HF. Among these, only 42.3% had reduced ejection fraction,14.3% had mildly reduced ejection fraction, and 43.4% had preserved ejection fraction. Prevalence of advanced HF increased with age and was higher in men. Median survival was 12.2 months from the day of diagnosis.

APPROACH TO PATIENTS WITH ADVANCED HEART FAILURE

Heart failure is characterized by the retention of fluid and sodium, which in turn leads to congestion of lungs or peripheries in case of left and right HF, respectively. Left ventricular failure presents with dyspnea, orthopnea, and paroxysmal nocturnal dyspnea that progresses to dyspnea at rest and at minimal activity. Advanced HF patients usually have tachycardia and tachypnea and at times they are cyanotic. The most common symptoms of right HF are fatigue, heaviness in legs, and abdominal fullness. Signs of right HF are pitting edema, ascites, hepatomegaly, and increased jugular venous pressure. Patients with advanced HF characteristically have raised left ventricular filling pressure and reduced cardiac output, resulting in systemic hypoperfusion. Bendopnea (dyspnea on bending over) is considered a specific symptom of end-advanced HF. On the other hand, crepitation remains absent in >80% of patients with advanced HF.[2] Other clinical manifestations of advanced HF include exercise intolerance, unintentional weight loss, recurrent ventricular arrhythmias, refractory volume overload, hypotension, and hampered perfusion despite optimal therapy.[3]

TREATMENT OF ADVANCED HEART FAILURE

As per guidelines, all four pillars of HF therapy [ARNI, beta-blockers, MRA, and sodium-glucose cotransporter-2 inhibitors (SGLT-2i)] should be uptitrated to maximum possible dose, but often advanced HF patients cannot tolerate this due to hypotension and associated renal dysfunction.

- *Beta-blockers*: 2,298 patients with severe LV dysfunction (LVEF 25%) and significant symptoms (NYHA class III and IV) were evaluated in the COPERNICUS study which concluded that patients on carvedilol have significant reduction in mortality. In routine practice, beta-blockers with high CV selectivity such as bisoprolol and metoprolol are used frequently.
- *Angiotensin receptor and neprilysin inhibitor (ARNI)*: Sacubitril/valsartan showed significant reduction in hospitalization (21%) and mortality (20%) as compared to enalapril in PARADIGM-HF trial. Dose of ARNI needs to be carefully monitored in patients with advanced HF as they are prone to have hypotension and frequent renal dysfunctions.
- *Mineralocorticoid receptor antagonists*: In the RALES study, the use of spironolactone resulted in reduced mortality and hospitalization in patients with end-stage HF. The effectiveness of the use of spironolactone has also been recorded in patients with impaired renal function or moderate hyperkalemia. It is necessary to regularly control serum potassium levels. Eplerenone, a more selective MRA than spironolactone, is a better choice due to a lower side effect rate.
- *SGLT-2i:* They are new drugs in the treatment of chronic HF. Their positive effect on major CV outcomes in HF, regardless of the presence of diabetes, was proven by two studies, the EMPEROR-Reduced for empagliflozin and DAPA-HF for dapagliflozin. SGLT-2i are the only group of drugs that affects HF prognosis across the ejection fraction spectrum with a good safety profile, multiple beneficial effects, and simple dosing. Various mechanisms by which SGLT-2i acts are natriuresis, reduction of endothelial dysfunction, reduction of proinflammatory cytokine production, reduction of oxidative stress, and reduction of albuminuria.
- *Decongestion*: They are primarily given for decongestion and improvement of the symptoms of advanced HF. In order to achieve the desired effect, it is necessary to progressively increase the dose due to resistance, and one of the main mechanisms of resistance is remodeling of the nephron due to prolonged treatment with diuretics. In the case of resistance, the first therapeutic option is to increase the oral dose of loop diuretics, and patients with an inadequate response should receive intravenous diuretics with an initial dose higher than the oral one. Resistance to diuretics and deterioration of renal function are indicators of end-stage HF and the need for advanced treatment.[4] Ultrafiltration or hemodialysis is the next therapy for the treatment of fluid overload which can be helpful for patients who do not respond adequately to diuretic therapy.
- *Ivabradine*: An If channel blocker in the sinoatrial node can be given to HF patients who are in sinus rhythm with heart rate > 70 beats/min and who cannot tolerate beta-blockers.
- *Vericiguat*: It is a soluble guanylate cyclase (sGC) stimulator which increases nitric oxide production. It achieves its effect by directly stimulating sGC independently of nitric oxide and sensitizes sGC to endogenous nitric oxide. This stabilizes the binding of nitric oxide to the binding site. The VICTORIA study included patients with worsening symptoms and HFrEF who had recently been hospitalized or who had received intravenous diuretic therapy. Vericiguat reduced HF hospitalization as compared with placebo (27.4% vs. 29.6%), while it reduced

composite endpoint (CV death or first HF hospitalization) as compared to placebo (35.5% vs. 38.5%). It has been shown that the use of vericiguat will reduce the primary composite endpoint and its components in patients with NT-proBNP level < 8,000 pg/mL and that vericiguat has the most significant therapeutic effect at NT-proBNP level < 4,000 pg/mL.

- *Others*:
  - Digoxin can be used particularly in HFrEF patients with atrial fibrillation.
  - Iron hydroxy maltose intravenously is recommended in the presence of anemia. A routine evaluation of iron profile is recommended in patients with advanced HF.
- *Inotropic support*: It is used to increase cardiac contractility and cardiac output as a result. They also have a vasodilating or vasoconstricting effect depending on the specific drug and dose. They are used in severe HF manifestations, sometimes with the parallel need to give vasoconstrictors. However, routine use of inotropic support is not recommended as it does not have any effect on prognosis. Beta-adrenergic agonists, phosphodiesterase III inhibitors, and calcium sensitizers are the few inotropic agents which are being used for advanced HF. The most commonly used inotropes are dobutamine, milrinone, and levosimendan. According to a meta-analysis, long-term use of inotrope infusion resulted in an improvement of the NYHA class in patients with end-stage HF and reduced ejection fraction; however, no significant statistical difference in mortality compared to controls was recorded. There is limited evidence of the risks and benefits of inotrope infusion in nonhospitalized patients with end-stage HF. When deciding on the continuous use of inotrope infusion, it is necessary to consider the need for symptom relief as well as the patient's wishes.
  - *Dobutamine*: It increases cardiac output and decreases pulmonary capillary pressure. It is recommended in patients with reduced cardiac output and reduced organ perfusion. In the FIRST study, it was reported that continuous intravenous dobutamine was associated with a higher 6-month mortality rate in patients with end-stage HF.
  - *Milrinone*: Milrinone is a phosphodiesterase 3 inhibitor that increases intracellular calcium concentration and has an inotropic and vasodilating effect. The vasodilating effect may result in hypotension and additional hypoperfusion in patients who are already hypotensive. Nevertheless, milrinone is the therapy of choice for patients with systemic and pulmonary hypertension and reduced cardiac output and for those who need inotropic support due to the aggravation of disease and beta receptors that have been blocked by the earlier use of beta-blockers. The OPTIME-CHF study evaluated 951 patients and showed that there was no significant difference in mortality and rehospitalization, but the use of milrinone was significantly associated with higher incidence of hypotension and arrhythmias.
  - *Levosimendan*: It enhances the sensitivity of myocytes to calcium but has no effect on intracellular calcium concentration. It activates ATP-sensitive potassium channels of smooth muscles and mitochondria and consequently causes systemic and pulmonary vasodilation. It is also cardioprotective. Conventional inotropes such as beta-adrenergic agonists and phosphodiesterase 3 inhibitors increase the concentration of serum calcium and consequently, their use entails a higher risk of ventricular arrhythmias. Given the prolonged effect, even up to 14 days, it can be used as a periodic maintenance infusion for patients with end-stage HF. The PERSIST study showed improvement in quality of life and a decrease in NT-proBNP level in patients receiving levosimendan. While the LevoRep study showed no significant improvement in functional capacity or quality of life, the LION-HEART study showed that levosimendan reduces NT-proBNP level and reduces hospitalization as compared to placebo. It is considered that levosimendan infusion is well tolerated and can be considered as maintenance therapy in patients with advanced HF who are not eligible for heart transplant and LVAD implantation.

ADVANCED TREATMENT OF HEART FAILURE/ROLE OF HEART FAILURE CLINICS

It comprises primarily heart transplantation and mechanical circulatory support (MCS) implantation. Clinical indicators suggestive of progression include the use of inotropic support, NYHA class III or IV, persistently elevated natriuretic peptides, end-organ dysfunction, LVEF <20%, frequent defibrillation shocks, more than one hospitalization in the last 12 months, persistent edema, persistently low arterial pressure, and GDMT intolerance. It is important to point out that more than two hospitalizations in the last 12 months indicate a very high risk of a bad outcome with 1 year mortality as high as 40%. Timely referral to specialized HF centers is of utmost importance to improve outcomes. The most commonly used risk assessment models for nonhospitalized patients with end-stage HF are the Heart Failure Survival Score (HFSS) and the Seattle Heart Failure Model (SHFM), which are used to evaluate patients for heart transplantation. SHFM has been shown to reduce 1 year mortality and the need for urgent transplantation and LVAD implantation, so it is used in combination with cardiopulmonary exercise tests while deciding on listing for transplantation. Several risk stratification models have been proposed for selecting patients for MCS implantation; however, most models are focused on specific devices and do not take into account other important conditions such as patient frailty and psychosocial support. If patients do not tolerate GDMT and are still significantly symptomatic, it is necessary to consider heart transplantation and MCS implantation as the next therapeutic option. Extracorporeal membrane oxygenation (ECMO) can also be considered in patients with sudden deterioration of end organs as a short-term therapy along with inotropic and vasodilators.

- *Heart transplant*: It is the gold standard treatment of advanced HF which significantly improves patients' quality of life. Post transplantation, 1 year survival is reported to be about 90% with a median survival of 12.5% years. The main limiting factor for heart transplant is limited availability of donors. Another challenge is primary graft dysfunction and antibody-mediated rejection in post-transplantation period along with cardiac allograft vasculopathy and late graft dysfunction. Detailed discussion of heart transplant is out of the scope of this chapter.
- *MCS*: It can be implanted percutaneously or surgically and there are devices for short-term and long-term use. Short-term devices are used over several days or weeks in order to achieve cardiogenic shock stabilization, most often as a bridge to decision (BTD) or a bridge to recovery (BTR). Care for patients with implanted short-term devices is very complex and requires a decision to remove the device if there is no recovery of function and no exit strategy. Long-term devices are used in carefully selected patients as a bridge therapy until heart transplantation [bridge to transplantation (BTT)] or a bridge to candidacy (BTC), and the number of implanted devices as destination therapy (DT) in patients who are not candidates for transplantation is increasing. Candidates for this type of treatment of advanced HF are patients with persistent severe symptoms despite optimal therapy, without severe right ventricular dysfunction and/or severe tricuspid regurgitation, with a stable psychosocial status and without contraindications, and who also meet at least one of the following criteria:
  1. LVEF < 25% and unable to tolerate exercise or if the patient is able to perform a cardiopulmonary exercise test with a peak $VO_2 < 12$ mL/kg/min and/or <50% of the predicted maximum VO_2
  2. ≥3 hospitalizations in the previous 12 months without a clear precipitating cause
  3. Dependence on intravenous inotropic support or a short-term MCS
  4. Progressive end-organ dysfunction (deterioration of renal and/or liver function, type 2 pulmonary hypertension, and cardiac cachexia) due to reduced perfusion and not to inadequately low ventricular filling pressure (PCWP ≥ 20 mm Hg, systolic blood pressure ≤ 90 mm Hg, and cardiac index ≤ 2 L/min/m^2).

Absolute contraindications for implanting a device are irreversible neurological injuries, systemic diseases that affect survival, disseminated malignant disease with a low chance of survival, severe coagulopathies, existing contraindications for the use of anticoagulant therapy, significant aortic or peripheral arterial disease, and significant cognitive and/or psychosocial problems.

PALLIATIVE CARE

It aims at improving the quality of life of patients by providing physical, emotional, psychosocial, and spiritual support to patients as well as caregivers. It targets mainly patients who are not eligible for active treatment. The main objectives of palliative care are to control symptoms, reduce distress, not hasten or delay death, and provide support and help for patients to live as actively and as well as possible until death. The PAL-HF study enrolled 150 patients with advanced HF and showed that interdisciplinary palliative care results in better quality of life and reduction of anxiety and depression.

CONCLUSION

Advanced HF is associated with poor prognosis despite having advanced treatment possibilities. Timely referral to HF specialized centers is the key to success by improving selection chances for advanced therapeutic options before the end-organ damage sets in. Palliative care with multi-disciplinary approach is also as important as pharmacological management. Despite all these, many patients continue to suffer from this clinical syndrome with a malignant course.

ONLINE REFERENCES

Please scan the QR code provided at the end of the table of contents for References of this chapter.

CHAPTER

63

Challenges in Management of Heart Failure in End-stage Renal Disease Patients

DP Sinha, Kaushik Manna, Navanil Biswas

ABSTRACT

Heart failure and chronic kidney disease are two very debilitating chronic disorders, which, when occur together, present a serious health problem to both the patient and his/her treating physician. The presence of one complicates the management of the other in various aspects including diagnosis, assessment of volume status, and therapy to be administered. This becomes more significant in patients with end-stage renal disease. The main handicap is the lack of trials involving this particular subgroup of patients, with most information derived from observational data or post hoc analyses. There is no "one-size-fits-all" approach that can be applied, and it takes maximum collaboration between the cardiologist and the nephrologist to optimally manage these very sick patients. This chapter aims to provide a brief summary of the main challenges faced while treating them, along with the ways how we can overcome these challenges to some extent.

Keywords: Heart failure, chronic kidney disease, end-stage renal disease, challenges

INTRODUCTION

Patients unfortunate enough to suffer from the dual burden of heart failure (HF) and chronic kidney disease (CKD) have been observed to experience unacceptably high rates of symptoms, frequent hospitalizations, as well as cardiovascular events including death. *It has been estimated that almost 50% of HF patients have coexisting CKD. Conversely, up to 70% of CKD patients and almost 36% of dialysis patients have HF.* This can be explained by the fact that both these morbid diseases share the same traditional (diabetes, hypertension, obesity) as well as nontraditional risk factors (inflammation, anemia, metabolic disturbances).[1] *The challenges faced in treating such patients are further compounded in patients with end-stage renal disease (ESRD), defined by the Kidney Disease: Improving Global Outcomes (KDIGO) Work Group as those having their eGFR <15 mL/min/1.73 m^2, i.e., Stage 5 CKD.*

The prognosis of such HF patients is heavily dependent on renal function, with the mortality and prevalence of HF directly proportional to the stage of CKD. Worsening renal function is an independent predictor of inpatient mortality in acute HF patients and also influences the duration of hospital stay and rates of readmission. HF is responsible for precipitating CKD by reducing renal blood flow, altering renal hemodynamics, and causing ischemic injury. CKD influences HF by causing LV remodeling, fibrosis, and cardiac dysfunction through the multifaceted effects of fluid retention and overload, anemia, uremia, and overactivation of the sympathetic nervous system and renin–angiotensin–aldosterone system (RAAS),[2] as depicted in **Figure 1**. Thus, treating such patients comes with its own unique set of problems and challenges, which are described in detail next.

CHALLENGE: USE OF BIOMARKERS IN THE DIAGNOSIS AND PROGNOSTICATION OF DISEASE

Natriuretic peptides (NPs) are the principal biomarker used in HF, both for diagnosis and for prognostication. Unfortunately, CKD is one of the common reasons of high NP levels, leading to their weakened utility as a diagnostic tool. Hence, the cutoff may need to be raised in patients with eGFR < 60 mL/min/1.73 m^2 for detecting HF. As there is strong correlation between the degree of renal dysfunction

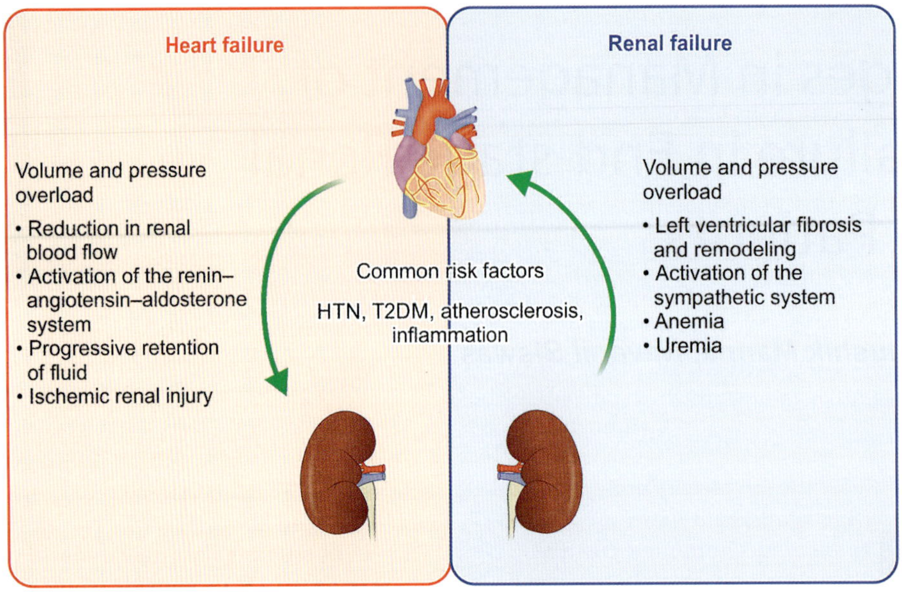

FIG. 1: A schematic representation of the various interdependent and intricate pathways showing how heart failure and kidney failure affect each other.

Source: Modified from Ryan DK, Banerjee D, Jouhra F. Management of heart failure in patients with chronic kidney disease. Eur Cardiol. 2022;17:e17.[2]

and age, *NT-proBNP levels based on age-adjusted cutoffs have been seen to be sufficient. For BNP, increasing the cutoff to 200 from 100 pg/mL in these patients is necessary*, as the effect of renal dysfunction on BNP is much lesser. *Lastly, in patients on dialysis, NP testing should be discouraged.*[3]

Often, it becomes necessary to determine the etiology of HF. Biomarkers are used for excluding acute ischemic injury as a probable cause of HF. However, it must be kept in mind that *troponins, just like NPs, are usually elevated in such patients, leading commonly to false-positive results.* Using more cardiac-specific biomarkers like *creatine kinase (CK) and CK-MB* might be more specific in unearthing an ischemic injury.[4]

CHALLENGE: USE OF VARIOUS IMAGING MODALITIES FOR DETERMINING THE SEVERITY AND ETIOLOGY OF HF

There is a host of different imaging modalities used in HF patients, but not all of them are safe in patients with CKD and need to be used with caution and in moderation. *Ischemic heart disease is the most common cause of HF in CKD patients. Transthoracic echocardiography* is most commonly used and is safe, but *stress echocardiography* (with both exercise and dobutamine) often gives equivocal results, is less helpful, and needs to be interpreted carefully.[5]

Both *invasive* and *CT-coronary angiography* use iodinated contrast which is excreted by the kidneys and is nephrotoxic. Contrast-induced kidney dysfunction results in increased all-cause mortality. Though not a problem in patients already on dialysis, strategies to minimize the amount of contrast used during diagnostic angiography and during percutaneous intervention *by IVUS guidance and preprocedure and postprocedure hydration based on left ventricular end-diastolic pressure (LVEDP)* are some of the techniques which can be applied on patients not on dialysis. Similarly, *cardiac magnetic resonance (CMR)* uses gadolinium contrast, which is highly nephrotoxic, and carries the risk of developing nephrogenic systemic fibrosis in CKD patients. However, the risk is low with Group II agents like gadobutrol and gadoteridol, but they are less widely available. Nuclear scans like *positron emission tomography (PET) and single photon emission computed tomography (SPECT)* appear to be safe but are very expensive and not commonly available.[6]

CHALLENGE: DIAGNOSIS AND CLASSIFICATION OF HF-RELATED CONGESTION IN ESRD PATIENTS WHO ARE ALREADY VOLUME OVERLOADED

Chronic kidney disease patients have impaired sodium and water excretion, leading to volume overload which causes edema and dyspnea. HF patients also have pulmonary and systemic congestion due to impaired cardiac function. It is clinically important to distinguish this volume overload into cardiac and noncardiac components, as it carries prognostic significance and also influences treatment. *The two most upcoming methodologies in assessing them are bioimpedance*

TABLE 1: The proposed classification by the Acute Dialysis Quality Initiative (ADQI) XI Workgroup with respect to chronic heart failure in chronic kidney disease (CKD) patients.[8]

Class	Echocardiographic heart disease	Presence of dyspnea	Relief of dyspnea with RRT or UT
1	Yes	Not	
2R	Yes	On exercise	Yes
2NR	Yes	On exercise	Not
3R	Yes	With daily life activities	Yes
3NR	Yes	With daily life activities	Not
4R	Yes	At rest	Yes
4NR	Yes	At rest	Not

analysis for the assessment of overhydration and the use of lung ultrasound for detecting pulmonary congestion.[7]

Another point to remember is that in ESRD patients, the symptoms of volume overload are not static and change very quickly depending on methods of volume removal like dialysis. This causes severe limitation to the definition and staging of HF by the European Society of Cardiology (ESC) guidelines. *To overcome this challenge, the Acute Dialysis Quality Initiative (ADQI) XI Working Group has proposed a new classification for this subgroup of patients (HF with ESRD), putting emphasis on the timing of assessment and the frequency of dialysis*[8] **(Table 1)**. The advantage of this system is that it allows physicians to identify high-risk patients who require more intensive monitoring and the probability of them requiring advanced therapies.

CHALLENGE: MANAGEMENT OF VOLUME OVERLOAD IN THESE PATIENTS AND ITS EFFECT ON THE FAILING HEART

Management of volume overload in patients with HF and ESRD is quite challenging and requires a multidisciplinary effort and a combination of diet and fluid restriction, diuretics, and frequent dialysis. A comprehensive clinical assessment to determine the predialysis volume status and the dry weight is required. *The symptoms of dyspnea, orthopnea, bendopnea, early satiety, abdominal distension, poor appetite, and interdialytic weight gain can guide the fluid removal goals.* [Hazard ratio (HR) for all-cause death is 0.67 for <1 kg weight gain compared to 1.25 for >4 kg weight gain].[9]

It should be remembered that though diuretics are class I indications in HF patients for decongestion and improvement of symptoms, those with CKD, particularly ESRD, usually have a *diuretic-resistant state*. This may lead to using a higher diuretic dose, which causes intravascular volume depletion and damages the remaining functioning nephrons and consequently worsens renal damage. Indeed, a number of trials including *UNLOAD*[10] (Ultrafiltration Versus Intravenous Diuretics in Decompensated Heart Failure), *CUORE*[11] (Continuous Ultrafiltration for Congestive Heart Failure), and *AVOID-HF*[12] (Aquapheresis Versus Intravenous Diuretics and Hospitalization for Heart Failure) demonstrated *greater benefits with ultrafiltration rather than with diuretics in patients with CKD with HF.*

Though dialysis is very effective in removing excess fluid, it *is often curtailed by intradialytic hypotension and peripheral cramping caused by overaggressive ultrafiltration.* This fluctuation in blood pressure causes myocardial stunning, cardiac arrhythmias, and further deterioration of cardiac function.[13] *Strategies that can be used to mitigate this are*:

- Longer dialysis runs
- Increasing the frequency of hemodialysis to almost-daily dialysis
- Lowering the temperature of the dialysate
- Discontinuation of antihypertensive drugs with no proven mortality benefit
- Holding antihypertensive drugs on the day of dialysis
- Use of midodrine or fludrocortisone
- Peritoneal dialysis rather than hemodialysis

Using more frequent dialysis with shorter interdialytic intervals is less harmful. A meta-analysis comparing 32,056 patients receiving alternate-day dialysis to daily dialysis showed significant ($p < 0.001$) increase in all-cause mortality (22.1% vs. 18.0%), cardiac mortality (10.2% vs. 7.5%), HF hospitalizations (29.9% vs. 16.9%), and arrhythmic hospitalizations (20.9% vs. 11.0%) in patients receiving alternate-day dialysis.[14] *Peritoneal dialysis* allows gradual fluid shifts and hence lesser hypotensive episodes and is *the preferred method in patients with HF having unstable hemodynamics.*[15] However, there are no randomized controlled trials (RCTs) to back up this claim, although it has been noticed in many observational studies. *Home dialysis has been observed to have a significant reduction in HF hospitalization and CV mortality.*[16]

Arteriovenous fistula (AVF), a mainstay in dialytic treatment of CKD patients, is also potentially harmful in HF patients. This is because these fistulas effectively *function as left-to-right extracardiac shunts, causing a high output state that significantly increases cardiac workload and increases the progression of HF.* Besides causing left ventricular hypertrophy (LVH), LV dilatation, and reduction of LV ejection fraction, it also causes increase in pulmonary hypertension and deterioration of RV function, which is associated with a fourfold increase in mortality risk [HR 3.9 (1.7–9.2)].[17] Excessive deterioration of cardiac function might lead to ligating these fistulas, especially those that are not being used, like in stable renal transplant recipients. *Other measures like partial banding, placement of hemoclips over the venous outflow, or the Miller procedure* can also be considered in cases where HF deterioration can be proven to be due to volume overload. In such patients, in worst-case scenarios, the risk of infection, morbidity, and mortality associated with an indwelling central venous catheter should be weighed against and compared to the risk of HF progression in the "fistula first" approach.[18]

CHALLENGE: EXCLUSION OF THIS SUBGROUP OF PATIENTS FROM MOST LARGE RCTS LEADING TO PAUCITY OF EVIDENCE

The major and most important stumbling block in the treatment of these extremely high-risk patients is the exclusion of this subgroup from major trials of HF patients. Though a number of drugs and other modalities of treatment have shown proven benefits in HF patients, very few studies have actually included patients having CKD stages 4 and 5 or those receiving dialysis, hence providing very limited data on their safety and efficacy. Ours being mainly an evidence-based management discipline, this lack of evidence and guidelines has led to potential suboptimal management and undertreatment. Indeed, Pandey et al. in the *Get-With-The-Guidelines-Heart Failure (GWTG-HF) registry* showed that patients with heart failure with reduced ejection fraction (HFrEF) on dialysis are less likely to receive guideline-directed medical therapy (GDMT) than patients with normal renal function.

It is therefore imperative for major cardiology and nephrology professional societies to develop best clinical practice models and international guidelines to address this critical need and bridge this information gap. This entails including HF with ESRD patients in dedicated large RCTs, increasing research funding in both these specialties for establishing the benefits of current therapies, and developing new therapies, as well as starting dedicated cardiorenal interdisciplinary teams for the management of such patients, in both the inpatient and outpatient settings.

CHALLENGE: DIFFICULTY IN IMPLEMENTING STANDARD HF DRUGS IN PATIENTS WITH ESKD AND ITS POTENTIAL PITFALLS

Thanks to groundbreaking research and meticulously planned clinical trials, we now have in our armamentarium a host of drugs that have showed unprecedented benefit in HF patients. Unfortunately, the same cannot be said in patients with HF who have CKD. All the trials involving the main HF drugs like ACEi, ARBs, ARNIs, beta blockers, MRAs, and SGLT-2i seem to have excluded those with lower eGFRs <30 mL/min/1.73 m^2. The few studies that have been conducted show conflicting results and did not achieve statistical significance. None of them show any benefit with respect to all-cause mortality, while data only exists for ACEi, SGLT-2i, vericiguat, and digoxin showing some reduction in CV mortality and HF hospitalizations in patients with Stage 4 CKD[19] **(Fig. 2)**. No established data exist for patients with ESKD (Stage 5 CKD).

The main concern preventing widespread use of HF drugs in CKD patients is the concern regarding hyperkalemia and other renal side effects like transient worsening of renal function. However, it must be borne in mind that adequate data exists establishing the efficacy of all these drugs in CKD Stages 1–3 (eGFR > 30 mL/min/1.73 m^2), and these side effects should not be a barrier in depriving patients of these drugs. There are clear prognostic benefits of using these drugs, and judicious monitoring of renal function and potassium levels is warranted in such patients, especially with drugs affecting the RAAS pathway. *Most studies show that an increase in creatinine of up to 50% above baseline or >3 mg/dL or eGFR < 25 mL/min/1.73 m^2 is acceptable and expected. The established cutoff for withdrawing these drugs is a rise in serum potassium > 5.5 mEq/L or a rise in creatinine by 100% above baseline or a drop in eGFR to < 20 mL/min/1.73 m^2.*[20]

The drugs or therapies that can be used in ESRD patients are narrowed down to *beta blockers (mainly carvedilol), hydralazine and isosorbide dinitrate* [*A-HeFT trial* (African-American Heart Failure Trial)], *ivabradine and digoxin* to some extent, and *IV iron therapy* (in patients with anemia and transferrin saturation < 30% and ferritin < 500 µg/L) as seen in *PIVOTAL* (The Proactive IV Iron Therapy in Haemodialysis Patients) trial.[21]

CHALLENGE: USE OF VARIOUS CARDIAC DEVICES IN THESE MORIBUND PATIENTS WITH POOR PROGNOSIS AND POOR QUALITY OF LIFE

The use of many cardiac devices like *implantable cardioverter defibrillator (ICD) and cardiac resynchronization therapy (CRT)* which have become the norm in patients with HFrEF (EF < 35%) have to be rethought when being applied to patients with ESRD. *Additional problems faced by this populace include high chance of infections, high bleeding risk, poor quality of life (QoL), and limited life expectancy, as well as possibility of device dysfunction due to hyperkalemia and other metabolic disturbances.* Here also, due to exclusion of such patients from key pivotal trials, the evidence remains unclear and conflicting.

With respect to *ICDs*, a cohort study including 303 patients on dialysis by Pun et al.[22] showed no benefit at 1- and 3-year follow-up, while a study by Hiremath et al.[23] on 100 dialysis patients showed significant reduction in all-cause mortality. *Thus, the implantation of ICD for primary*

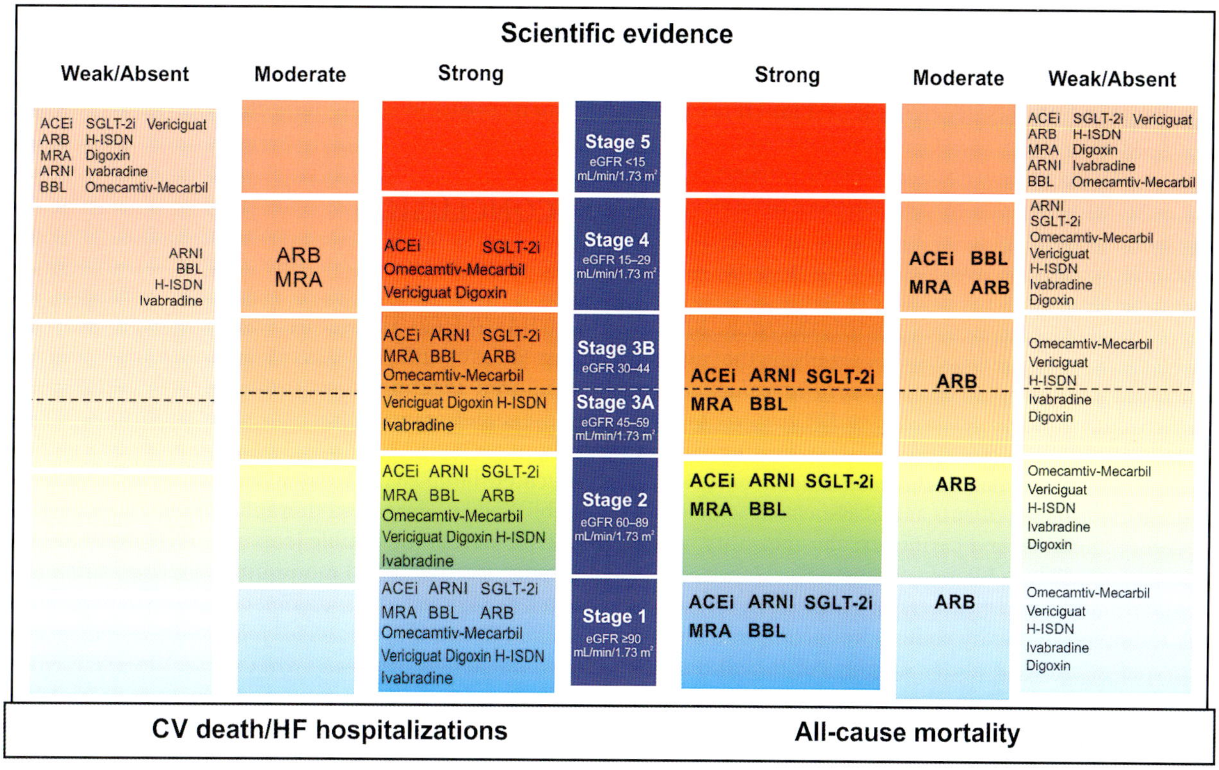

FIG. 2: An overview of the evidence base of the various drugs used in HFrEF with respect to different stages of CKD.

Source: Modified from Beldhuis IE, Lam CSP, Testani JM, et al. Evidence-based medical therapy in patients with heart failure with reduced ejection fraction and chronic kidney disease. Circulation. 2022;145(9):693-712.[19]

prevention in these moribund patients should generally be avoided in light of insufficient data till clear guidelines become available. Similarly for *CRTs*, the meager data available from case-control studies and retrospective analysis showed conflicting results, resulting in questionable benefit of CRTs in such patients. Of note, a large retrospective study of 11,000 subjects with advanced CKD conducted by Friedman et al. comparing CRT-D and ICDs showed clear benefits ranging across all stages of CKD.[24]

More advanced devices like *left ventricular assist devices (LVAD)* are *generally not recommended* in these patients in light of increasing mortality rates, poor prognosis, and other LVAD-related complications.[25] Hence, peritoneal dialysis and more frequent hemodialysis seem more safer options. Similarly, a nationwide retrospective study of 11,000 patients involving *transcatheter mitral valve repair (TMVR) using MitraClip* showed futility when used in advanced CKD patients and associated with higher in-hospital mortality, higher bleeding rates, increased readmission rates, and increased requirement of blood transfusion.[26] A smaller study of 2,000 patients however, showed significant reduction of in-hospital mortality rates.

Dialysis-dependent acute renal failure post heart transplantation is an important clinical issue. Post-transplant dialysis is associated with a higher risk of complications, increased cost of care, and fivefold higher risk of mortality. Hence, in patients with HF and CKD, a *simultaneous heart and kidney transplantation (SHKT)* is generally recommended and results in greater survival benefits, clinical benefits, and lower risk of rejection compared to only heart transplant recipients.[27]

CHALLENGE: CONTROL OF HYPERKALEMIA AND HYPERTENSION IN SUCH PATIENTS WITH HIGH PROPENSITY TO DEVELOP THE SAME

Hyperkalemia in CKD patients is very common, *occurring usually due to poor dietary adherence, higher catabolism rates, and as a side effect of various drugs like the RAAS inhibitors* which are the mainstay of therapy in these patients. Often, it leads to discontinuation of these drugs leading to poor prognosis and undertreatment. *The various strategies that can reduce the incidence of hyperkalemia include:*

- Limiting intake of potassium-rich foods
- Correction of metabolic acidosis
- Reduction of dialysate potassium concentrations
- Using novel potassium binders like patiromer or sodium zirconium silicate

Indeed, various trials involving these potassium binders like the *PEARL-HF* (Evaluation of Patiromer in Heart Failure

Patients), *OPAL-HK* (Patiromer in Patients with Kidney Disease and Hyperkalemia Receiving RAAS inhibitors), and the famous *DIAMOND* (Patiromer for the Management of Hyperkalemia in Subjects Receiving RAASi for HFrEF) trial showed that the use of these drugs in conjunction with RAAS inhibitors is associated with *lesser incidences of hyperkalemia, lower discontinuation rates, better adherence to GDMT, and improved prognosis.*[28]

Hypertension and its control remains a major challenge in CKD patients with and without HF. Recent studies have shown a U-shaped curve between predialysis systolic BP and mortality in those undergoing dialysis, signifying that neither too-high nor too-low BP is desirable. *Due to large fluctuations in BP, the evidence points to taking the BP measured in the morning after dialysis as the standard and titrating therapy according to it. Ambulatory BP measurement remains the gold standard for these patients* and is associated with better prediction of all-cause and cardiovascular mortality, when compared to peridialysis BP measurement.[29]

Nonpharmacological measures for control of hypertension include reduction in dietary sodium, reduction in dialysate sodium, and attainment of dry weight. Peritoneal dialysis seems to be better than hemodialysis in this regard too and achieves more stable BP control. Pharmacological therapy with antihypertensive drugs remains the cornerstone therapy, with limited use of RAAS inhibitors and more frequent use of prazosin and other central sympatholytics like clonidine.

CONCLUSION

Information regarding the treatment and prognosis of HF patients with CKD is disheartening with various trials like the *CHAMP-HF* (CHAnge the Management of Patients with Heart Failure) and *BIOSTAT-CHF* (A Systems Biology Study to Tailored Treatment in Chronic Heart Failure) pointing out the undertreatment and suboptimal utilization of GDMT in these patients.[30] There is an urgent critical need to have dedicated large RCTs to assess the efficacy and safety of established HF drugs and therapies in ESKD patients. These patients, having the double jeopardy of HF and ESKD, need intensive treatment and monitoring. *The acquisition of more knowledge, correct interpretation of changes in renal function, and modification of treatment following the evidence-based HF management strategies are essential to overcome these challenges.*

ONLINE REFERENCES

Please scan the QR code provided at the end of the table of contents for References of this chapter.

CHAPTER

64

Revascularization in Heart Failure: Current Concept

Vidyut Jain, Avani Jain

ABSTRACT

Heart failure (HF) is a prevalent condition primarily resulting from ischemic heart disease. Efforts are consistently made to enhance cardiac output in affected patients to mitigate morbidity and mortality rates. While revascularization through various procedures can be beneficial for a failing heart, the outcomes can be inconsistent. Both percutaneous intervention and coronary artery bypass grafting (CABG) are recognized therapeutic options following a thorough evaluation of patients. It is important to note that comparable data are scarce from prior randomized controlled trials (RCTs) regarding reperfusion through percutaneous coronary intervention (PCI) versus CABG in this subset of patients. PCI offers a minimally invasive method for coronary revascularization; however, it is essential to examine the findings from the REVIVED and BSCI2 studies for high-risk PCI in ischemic left ventricular (LV) failure patients. Currently, the growing expertise in surgical techniques has demonstrated favorable long-term outcomes for CABG in patients with LV dysfunction but immediate postoperative complications pose challenges. Conversely, recent advancements in PCI technology for complex lesions for reperfusion have enabled comparable results in high-risk heart failure cases. The advantages and limitations of both treatment modalities must be assessed on an individual basis by the heart team.

Keywords: Heart failure, coronary artery bypass surgery

INTRODUCTION

Ischemic heart disease stands as the leading cause of heart failure (HF) with reduced ejection fraction (EF), and is associated with a poor prognosis and higher mortality rate, despite advancements in all pathways of medical treatment. Real-world data involving 156,013 patients in US hospitals corroborate that 59% of HF patients have coronary artery disease (CAD) as the underlying cause.[1,2] Despite the availability of optimal medical therapy (OMT), mortality rates from ischemic systolic HF remain significantly high, reaching up to 41% within 5 years of follow-up, often complicated by recurrent hospitalizations.[3] In majority of patients undergoing revascularization via PCI, the decision-making process is influenced by the operator's experience and an understanding of observational data from previous studies, similar to surgical interventions. Surgical interventions are designed to achieve complete revascularization, alongside the correction of ventricular geometry, and if necessary, the management of mitral valve insufficiency, to optimize patient outcomes. This varied clinical approach, which seeks to attain similar results, is essential for integrating new therapies within this patient population.[4]

In addressing HF resulting from ischemic heart disease, the strategy involves pinpointing the chronically ischemic regions, and if viable, restoring myocardial perfusion to meet metabolic demands and enhance the function of hibernating myocardium.[5] Myocytes possess an adaptive ability to sustain viability even under conditions of limited nutrient availability. Once perfusion is restored, there is a reversal of mitochondrial dysfunction and the dysregulation of the sarcoplasmic reticulum, ultimately leading to increased ATP production in the hibernating myocardium and the prevention of cell apoptosis.[6] Achieving revascularization in ischemic segments initiates a process of reverse left ventricular (LV) remodeling, resulting in a decrease in residual LV volume and an enhancement of contractile function. Furthermore, revascularization can reverse LV remodeling, contributing to improvements in both LV volume and contractile performance.[7] Viability assessments are conducted to evaluate hibernating myocardium, utilizing various anatomical, physiological, or functional criteria. Several functional characteristics of hibernation have been identified to determine myocardial viability and assist in recognizing patients likely to benefit from enhanced LV function.[8] Viability tests are routinely advised for all ischemic HF patients who are candidates for myocardial revascularization; however, their clinical utility has not been substantiated in randomized controlled trials (RCTs). In the STICH trial, a study focused on viability testing did not reveal any differential treatment advantages from revascularization through surgical methods.[9]

Exceptions are known to affect the interpretation such as clinical condition and decision, types of viability tests such as single photon emission[3] computed tomography or dobutamine or cardiac magnetic resonance assessment of viability. All these newer modalities of viability will be evaluated to some extent in the AIMI-HF study. This study is likely to enroll the eligible patients for randomization to either single photon emission computed tomography (SPECT) or cardiac magnetic resonance or positron emission tomography (PET) for viability assessment.[10] The single imaging technique of viability for subsequent revascularization is not accepted and it is usually at the discretion of the heart team to decide which patient will benefit from the procedure. Viable testing in clinical practice is not only to refuse an eligible patient but also to avoid revascularization of potential nonviable segments of the myocardium. It may be considered a pathway for targeted revascularization.[11] In a substudy of the ISCHEMIA (International Study of Comparative Health Effectiveness with Medical and Invasive Approaches) trial involving symptomatic HF patients with an EF of 45% also suggested better outcomes with invasive over conservative therapy but not applicable in patients with severe LV dysfunction which excluded patients of severe LV dysfunction.[12]

SURGICAL REVASCULARIZATION: CORONARY ARTERY BYPASS GRAFTING

The most commonly used modality of revascularization for HF due to ischemic heart disease in the last 4 decades is coronary artery bypass grafting (CABG). The initial observational study conducted by the Duke Databank revealed that patients who underwent surgical intervention exhibited superior outcomes compared to those receiving medical treatment for ischemic HF, demonstrating notable survival advantages. It is crucial to highlight that these patients did not receive medical therapies such as β-blockers, ACE inhibitors, ARNI, MRAs, and SGLT2 inhibitors, all of which have been associated with mortality benefits.[13] In the surgical cohort, data from the STICH trial analyzed 1,212 patients who underwent CABG due to LV dysfunction [left ventricular ejection fraction (LVEF) <35%] and CAD. The mean age of the patient was about 60 years. The primary endpoint assessed was all-cause mortality and long-term survival free from cardiac hospitalization. Although the CABG group exhibited a threefold increase in 30-day mortality, but over 5-year period, all-cause mortality rates were comparable between the medical and surgical groups, with the CABG group experiencing fewer cardiovascular deaths, myocardial infarctions (MIs), and hospitalizations. In patients who were followed for 10 years, a significant reduction in all-cause mortality was found within whom CABG was done. Further analysis of the STICH data revealed that the most substantial mortality benefits were observed in younger patients.[14] Additionally, there was a marked improvement in quality of life, as measured by the KQCCC score, among those treated with CABG.[15] In the STICH trial, myocardial viability was evaluated using dobutamine stress echocardiography (DSE) and SPECT to determine clinical outcomes. Myocardial viability assessed by SPECT was classified as extensive if >11 segments were identified as viable, while fewer segments indicated "no viable myocardium." DSE defined viability as the presence of >5 dysfunctional segments exhibiting contractile reserve. Based on these criteria, patients with extensive viability appeared to derive significant benefits from CABG at the 10-year follow-up; however, the statistical power to confirm this finding was limited.[16]

The survival advantage associated with CABG stems from its ability to safeguard the remaining viable myocardium against future MIs, rather than solely facilitating functional recovery.[17] Consequently, identifying viable myocardial segments remains crucial in the stage wise planning of surgical revascularization. The PARR-2 study was conducted to evaluate the influence of myocardial viability assessed through PET imaging and to predict improvements in LVEF following surgical intervention.[18,19] Notably, this study included a higher proportion of patients undergoing surgical revascularization, with 48% compared to 35% in the control group; however, no significant differences in cardiac events were observed. While a reduction in the rate of cardiac rehospitalization was noted—39% in the PET group versus 46% in the standard care group—there was no discernible effect on overall or cardiac mortality.[14] Nevertheless, patients exhibiting more extensive myocardial viability (>7% of hibernating myocardium) appeared to derive the greatest benefit from myocardial revascularization, with a 1-year event rate of 13% compared to 56% in those who did not undergo revascularization ($p = 0.015$).[19]

PERCUTANEOUS APPROACH OF REVASCULARIZATION

The REVIVED-BCIS2 trial involved 700 patients suffering from severe CAD and included a follow-up period of 3 years. Participants were randomly assigned to receive either PCI combined with OMT or OMT alone. The primary outcome, which encompassed all-cause mortality or hospitalization due to HF, was observed in 37.2% of the PCI plus OMT group, compared to 38.0% in the group receiving only OMT (p = 0.96). These results were consistent across all subgroups. In terms of secondary outcomes, all-cause mortality was recorded at 31.7% for the PCI plus OMT group, while it was 32.6% for the OMT alone group (p = not significant). The occurrence of acute MI was 10.7% in the PCI plus OMT group, in contrast to 10.8% in the OMT alone group (p = NS). No significant enhancement in LVEF was noted at the 12-month mark, with a mean difference of merely 0.9 percentage points (p = NS). The rates of all-cause death or aborted sudden death were also comparable, with 41.6% in the PCI plus OMT group versus 40.2% in the OMT alone group (p = NS). Among patients exhibiting LV systolic dysfunction and extensive CAD, multivessel PCI did not yield improvements in all-cause mortality or LV systolic function; however, this approach did not indicate any harm.[20] Neither complete anatomical revascularization nor viability-guided revascularization demonstrated better outcomes compared to OMT. Furthermore, PCI did not significantly reduce the risk of potentially fatal ventricular arrhythmias. The ongoing PROTECT IV trial (NCT04763200) aims to investigate the effects of intra-aortic balloon pump (IABP) or Impella-supported PCI in 1,252 high-risk CAD patients. Participants include those with chronic coronary syndromes or non-ST-segment elevation acute coronary syndromes with an LVEF of 40% or less, as well as those with ST-segment elevation MI and an LVEF below 30%. The primary endpoint of this trial is a composite measure that includes all-cause mortality, stroke, durable left ventricular assist device (LVAD) or heart transplant, and myocardial infarct.[21]

CHIP-BCIS3 (Controlled Trial of High-risk Coronary Intervention with Percutaneous Left Ventricular Unloading) is a prospective, multicenter, open-label RCT that aims to determine whether a strategy of elective percutaneous LV unloading is superior to standard care (no planned mechanical circulatory support) in patients undergoing nonemergent high-risk PCI which is ongoing and will analyze the outcome.[22]

HOW TO OPTIMIZE PERCUTANEOUS CORONARY INTERVENTION?

To get optimal result of PCI, physiology-guided PCI procedure is appealing, as evidenced by the FAME-2 trial, which highlighted the advantages of fractional flow reserve (FFR)-guided PCI over medical management for patients with hemodynamically significant lesions. This is particularly relevant for the primary composite outcome of death, MI, or urgent revascularization. Initial findings from this trial, with a mean follow-up of 7 months, indicated a decrease in unplanned revascularization rates. Furthermore, long-term follow-up at 5 years suggested a reduction in MI (hazard ratio 0.66, 95% confidence interval 0.43–1.00).[23] Conversely, the recent FAME 3 trial indicated that FFR-guided PCI did not demonstrate noninferiority to CABG for patients with three-vessel CAD concerning the 1-year endpoint of death, MI, or stroke. It is crucial to recognize that only 18% of participants in the FAME trial had low LVEF, thus limiting the applicability of these results to patients with low LVEF undergoing PCI. The introduction of nonhyperemic indices for assessing coronary stenosis severity is anticipated to facilitate the adoption of intracoronary physiology by eliminating barriers to implementation, particularly the necessity for pharmacological vasodilators. The instantaneous wave free ratio (iFR) has demonstrated comparable outcomes to FFR in two large-scale RCTs involving a total of 4,529 patients.[24,25] These studies did not exclude individuals with HF; however, only 6% had a history of congestive HF, and 19% presented with reduced LVEF. Resting indices may offer a theoretical advantage over hyperemic indices for patients with HF, as they are less influenced by elevated filling pressures. Nonetheless, the impact of these theoretical advantages on clinical outcomes in HF patients remains uncertain. Lastly, noninvasive physiological lesion assessment methods, such as FFR computed tomography (FFR-CT) and quantitative flow ratio (QFR), may eliminate the need for invasive physiological assessments for better outcome of PCI.[26]

Recent advancements in stent technology, particularly with second-generation drug-eluting stent (DES) platforms, have demonstrated remarkable clinical outcomes, showcasing enhanced safety and efficiency compared to their first-generation counterparts. These improvements stem from technological innovations such as bioresorbable scaffolds, polymer-free DES, and bioresorbable polymer-based DES. Research indicates that ultrathin-strut DES is linked to a 15% decrease in target lesion failure and a 25% decrease in target vessel failure, primarily due to reductions in both target lesion and target vessel revascularization procedures. Additionally, there were fewer reported cases of MI and stent thrombosis. The implementation of thinner strut stents, along with the utilization of intracoronary imaging to refine PCI outcomes, may also facilitate a reduction in the duration of dual antiplatelet therapy. This is particularly significant for patients with HF, who are frequently at an elevated risk of bleeding.[27]

COMPLEX LESION SUCH AS CHRONIC TOTAL OCCLUSION AND LEFT VENTRICULAR DYSFUNCTION

In chronic CAD, CTO lesions in the presence of LV dysfunction are difficult to handle for performer, as these cases are more complex, takes longer procedural time, and successful outcome is not always favorable. At present there are no data to support over CABG by RCT. In the EURO-CTO,

PCI led to greater symptomatic improvement and quality of life than medical therapy and such cases are accepted as per feasibility.[28]

BRIDGING THE GAPS

The current evidence regarding revascularization in ischemic cardiomyopathy raises important questions. As the first, patient enrolled in the STICH trial almost over 20 years ago surgical arm fared better but in the present scenario with better medical options and interventional procedural success in complex cases of extensive CAD with LV dysfunction, one must consider every case on individual basis. The MASS-VI (HF) study (ISRCTN77449548) has completed its recruitment phase, targeting 600 patients suffering from angina, multivessel disease, and an LVEF of 35% or lower, who will be randomized to receive either CABG or OMT.[29] The primary endpoint of this study is a composite measure that includes all-cause mortality, nonfatal MI, stroke, and episodes of unstable angina necessitating further intervention over 5 years.

This inquiry will also be addressed by the STICH 3.0 consortium, which proposes a series of seven independently funded trials at the country level (NCT05427370 and NCT05329285) aimed at directly comparing PCI with CABG in patients experiencing ischemic LV dysfunction. Results from these trials are anticipated after 4 years.[30]

CONCLUSION

Patients with advanced CAD and LV dysfunction frequently encounter significant challenges. It is widely recognized that CABG provides a more comprehensive solution for this patient population, enhancing long-term outcomes when patients are carefully selected based on their comorbidities, to achieve complete revascularization, and if necessary, addressing mitral valve abnormalities and LV geometry. While PCI is acknowledged for delivering immediate and safe outcomes in complex cases, it is crucial to consider the interplay between myocardial viability, ischemia, and the anatomical severity of the disease. The adjunctive use of devices such as Impella and IABPs often facilitates the management of intricate angioplasty procedures, with findings to be reported in the PROTECT IV trial. Additionally, the results from the MASS-VI (HF) study, which compares OMT and CABG in patients with angina and LV dysfunction over a 5-year follow-up, will contribute to this ongoing discussion. The forthcoming STICH 3.0 trial, which will evaluate and compare PCI and CABG in the context of ischemic LV dysfunction, is expected to yield results by 2029.

ONLINE REFERENCES

Please scan the QR code provided at the end of the table of contents for References of this chapter.

CHAPTER

65

Revascularization for Heart Failure

Vivekanand S Gajapati

ABSTRACT

Ischemic heart disease is estimated to account for over two-thirds of heart failure (HF) patients and is associated with poor prognosis despite optimal medical treatment. Coronary revascularization has been shown to improve myocardial function and prognosis in ischemic cardiomyopathy (ICM). In patients with ischemic HF, blood flow restoration of viable but ischemic myocardium might reverse the hibernation of the myocardium and prevent future spontaneous myocardial infarction (MI). Patients with ICM have been largely excluded from randomized trials of revascularization in stable coronary artery disease (CAD). Coronary artery bypass graft surgery (CABG) has been the main mode of revascularization in patients with extensive CAD and reduced ejection fraction (EF) based on STICH trial. Recent development in the interventional cardiology has led to overall increase of percutaneous coronary intervention (PCI) procedures in treatment of ischemic heart failure with reduced ejection fraction (HFrEF). The beneficial effect of PCI in ICM has been challenged by recently published REVIVED-BCIS2 trial which demonstrated no added benefit of PCI over optimal medical therapy. A multidisciplinary approach is needed to tailor treatment strategy in these patients, based on ability to achieve complete revascularization.

Keywords: Coronary artery bypass surgery, ischemic cardiomyopathy, myocardial revascularization, myocardial viability, percutaneous coronary intervention

INTRODUCTION

Coronary artery disease (CAD) remains the most common cause of HFrEF. Ischemic etiology is estimated to account for over two-thirds of all heart failure (HF) cases and is associated with impaired quality of life and poor prognosis.[1,2] Pharmacological and device therapy are the main modalities of treatment of HF with reduced ejection fraction. Revascularization should be offered to patients with impaired left ventricular function who present with angina or acute coronary syndrome.

There is limited evidence to support revascularization in patients with stable ischemic HF and minimal symptoms. Separating true ischemic HF from bystander CAD in nonischemic HF is frequently challenging. The preferred choice of revascularization (PCI or CABG) depend on age, sex, comorbidities, and coronary anatomy. Severe LV dysfunction is associated with increased procedural mortality and morbidity following surgical or percutaneous revascularization. CABG surgery has been the important mode of revascularization in patients with multivessel CAD and HFrEF. However, recent advances in the interventional cardiology led to an overall increase of PCI in treatment of ischemic HFrEF. It is essential to understand the better modality for coronary revascularization in this unique and growing patient population to improve outcomes.

ROLE OF REVASCULARIZATION

Ischemic cardiomyopathy is left ventricular dysfunction due to atherosclerotic CAD. It incorporates many clinical, imaging, and angiographic features. Revascularization, particularly CABG, is recommended for patients with ischemic HFrEF based on the assumption that blood flow restoration of viable but ischemic myocardium might reverse the left ventricular dysfunction.[3] The potential mechanism of improving pumping function is the reversal of myocardial hibernation, an adaptive process triggered by repeated episodes of ischemia. Myocardial viability testing is the prospective identification of myocardium which is likely to be hibernating and it is one of the important considerations when adopting revascularization strategy.

A large meta-analysis demonstrated a strong association between myocardial viability and improved survival after revascularization in patients with chronic CAD and left ventricular dysfunction.[4]

TYPES OF REVASCULARIZATION

Coronary Artery Bypass Graft

Patients with ischemic cardiomyopathy frequently presents with complex and extensive CAD, which often makes surgical revascularization the preferred mode of invasive treatment. The contemporary evidence on the role of CABG comes from the results of the STICH (Surgical Treatment of Ischemic Heart Failure) trial which randomized 1,212 patients with ischemic cardiomyopathy <35% LVEF to either CABG or medical therapy.[5,6] At the first prespecified analysis at 5-years, there was no significant difference in primary outcomes of all-cause mortality between groups. There was only borderline significance in the secondary endpoint of cardiovascular mortality. When followed up for 10 years, there was significant reduction of all-cause mortality in CABG arm (7% absolute reduction), which translated into 17 months median increase in survival.

The STICH remains a landmark trial but there were several limitations which limits us to generalize its conclusions in routine clinical practice. Increasing age is known to be an important predictor of worse outcomes in patients with HF. Patients in STICH were younger than most contemporary registries of HF (the mean age was 60 years). Younger cohorts derived more beneficial outcomes than those over the age of 65 years. The use of medical and device therapy did not reflect contemporary practice with very low rates of ICD implantations and poor adherence to medical therapy. Presence of three vessel disease, LVEF <27% and LV end systolic volume >79 mL/m^2 were associated with greater benefit from CABG. Surprisingly, the presence of angina, ischemia, viability, and diabetes did not appear to benefit more from CABG. Myocardial viability testing was not mandatory in STICH trial. Moreover, the evidence of viability was not associated with improved outcomes in HF patients undergoing CABG.[7,8] In conclusion, CABG is an effective mode of revascularization in selected cases and its modest benefit can be distinguished from the increased mortality due to the surgical procedure beyond 5 years.

Percutaneous Coronary Intervention

The PCI is now emerging as an important mode of revascularization in patients with ischemic cardiomyopathy due to technological development and advancing experience. The role of PCI have expanded to more complex cases such as left main disease, multivessel disease, and chronic total occlusions. The number of patients with ischemic HFs undergoing PCI has increased compared to those referred for CABG[9,10] even though most randomized clinical trials comparing CABG and PCI in stable patients have excluded patients with reduced LVEF.[11,12] The long-term outcomes are unknown in patients undergoing PCI for ischemic HF.[13] The theoretical advantage of PCI compared to CABG cannot be extrapolated as the mechanism of revascularization are substantially different. PCI may not achieve complete revascularization compared to CABG. Although PCI is considered to be associated with lesser mortality and morbidity than CABG, no robust comparisons have been made in patients with HF.

The US and European Society of Cardiology (ESC) guidelines recommend CABG as the preferred revascularization option in patients with ischemic HF.[14,15] CABG is superior to PCI according to ESC guidelines, while the US guidelines do not comment on PCI but recommend CABG. Still PCI is extensively performed in daily practice due to preference of patients, refusal by surgeons, and feasibility of PCI.

More recently published large, randomized revascularization for ischemic ventricular dysfunction (REVIVED) trial provided critical evidence on the possible role of PCI in patients with ischemic cardiomyopathy. It showed no significant prognostic impact of PCI over OMT.[16] A total of seven hundred patients with LVEF ≤35% with extensive CAD suitable for PCI, and confirmed myocardial viability, were enrolled in the study. The primary outcome (composite of all-cause mortality and HF hospitalization) over a median of 41 months was comparable between the groups (PCI 37.2% vs. OMT 38.0%). Furthermore, there was no difference in LVEF between the groups at 6 and 12 months. Longer term follow-up is planned, but late benefit is unlikely to emerge as 3.4 year follow-up did not show any discernible effect. However, the results need to be interpreted carefully as there are some major concerns. The trial included only patients with confirmed myocardial viability but previous studies did not demonstrate the benefit of revascularization guided by viability testing. Scar burden, but not viability predicts likelihood of LV function recovery. Therefore, based on myocardial viability alone, it is difficult to identify patients with HFrEF who might benefit from PCI.[17,18] Patients enrolled in REVIVED-BCIS2 were 10 year older than those enrolled in STICH trial. Further analyses of REVIVED data are awaited, which will answer some of the questions, for example, the extent of ischemia versus myocardial jeopardy (67% of patients had no angina). BCIS jeopardy score which was used by investigators to define angiographic eligibility was not validated in HFrEF patients. It was hypothesized that PCI on top of optimal medical treatment would offer the benefits of revascularization without early mortality associated with CABG.

In REVIVED trial, despite inclusion of patients with left main disease PCI was not associated with increased early mortality. Periprocedural MI constituted approximately 40% of all MIs in PCI arm. There was two-fold increase of spontaneous MI which was observed in the optimal medical treatment group when compared to PCI (5.2% vs. 9.3%). Therefore, overall MI rates at the end were similar in both the groups (OMT 10.8% vs. PCI 10.7%).

The concept of recovery of myocardial hibernation with revascularization will be disproven considering the above trial is yet to be answered. The medical management of heart failure is evolving rapidly with the introduction of new therapies such as sodium-glucose cotransporter-2 (SGLT-2) inhibitors. The important role of OMT in HFrEF patients has been emerged as one of the significant findings of the REVIVED trial but role of SGLT-2 inhibitors has not been addressed by this trial.

CONCLUSION

Ischemic cardiomyopathy is associated with high morbidity and mortality and the identification of an ischemic substrate can help decision-making process and improve patient's outcomes. To date, the evidence base for coronary revascularization in ischemic LV dysfunction is largely informed by observational data. There is an absence of direct randomized controlled trial evidence comparing revascularization strategies in these patient population. This may illustrate why, despite the guidelines and the large body of observational evidence supporting CABG in favor of PCI, high PCI rates have been observed in this patient population in the real world. Better understanding this discrepancy between theory and practice will require direct randomized evidence of PCI versus CABG in this specific patient population.

Revascularization decisions in patients with reduced LVEF have so far been largely based on STICH trial that showed a benefit of CABG over OMT alone. The beneficial effect of CABG is observed after extended observation (10 years) and therefore it should be performed in carefully selected patients with acceptable perioperative risk. REVIVED trial confirmed the importance of contemporary pharmacological treatment in the HFrEF setting. But it demonstrated that in stable asymptomatic patients with confirmed myocardial viability PCI added no benefit in reduction of all-cause mortality or HF hospitalization rates. that is why, extended follow-up and more detailed analyses of this study are crucial to confirm these results in the long-term observation and identify potential subgroups of patients in whom PCI might be beneficial.

Both REVIVED-BCIS2 and STITCH trials challenge the hypothesis of hibernating myocardium amenable to functional improvement following successful revascularization that would ultimately improve prognosis. Assessment of myocardial viability does not aid the selection of patients who will benefit or not from the PCI for ischemic cardiomyopathy. So, REVIVED-BCIS2 also challenged long-held beliefs on myocardial viability prior to PCI.

The decision on revascularization in ischemic cardiomyopathy often cannot be made based on the guidelines. Therefore, tailored treatment approach is essential with multidisciplinary approach **(Flowchart 1)**. These decisions should be based on ability to achieve complete revascularization which may not be accomplished in certain patients.

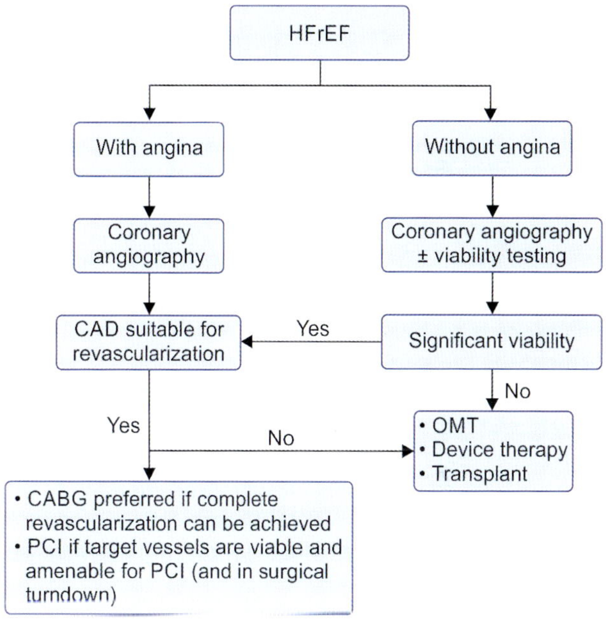

FLOWCHART 1: Tailored management algorithm for patients with ischemic heart failure with reduced ejection fraction (HFrEF).
(CABG: coronary artery bypass grafting; CAD: coronary artery disease; OMT: optimal medical therapy; PCI: percutaneous coronary intervention)

ONLINE REFERENCES

Please scan the QR code provided at the end of the table of contents for References of this chapter.

CHAPTER

66

Acute Heart Failure: Management

SN Routray, NK Mohanty

ABSTRACT

Acute heart failure (AHF) is a life-threatening condition characterized by the rapid onset or worsening of heart failure symptoms, necessitating immediate medical intervention. This chapter explores the comprehensive management of AHF, emphasizing initial stabilization, pharmacological treatment, nonpharmacological interventions, and long-term care strategies. Initial stabilization focuses on airway, breathing, and circulation (ABC), often requiring oxygen therapy and ventilatory support. Pharmacological treatment includes the administration of diuretics, vasodilators, inotropes, and other agents such as beta-blockers, ACE inhibitors, ARBs, and MRAs, each tailored to the patient's hemodynamic status and underlying etiology. Nonpharmacological interventions, such as ultrafiltration, dialysis, and mechanical circulatory support (MCS), are crucial for patients unresponsive to standard therapies. Hospitalization criteria for AHF are based on severe symptoms, hemodynamic instability, and the need for intensive monitoring and treatment. Inhospital management involves continuous monitoring of vital signs, fluid balance, renal function, and hemodynamic status. Discharge criteria emphasize the resolution of acute symptoms, stabilization of hemodynamics, and the establishment of a follow-up care plan. Prognostic factors influencing outcomes include left ventricular ejection fraction (LVEF), renal function, serum sodium levels, and response to treatment. Strategies to reduce readmission rates involve optimizing discharge planning, patient education, and multidisciplinary follow-up care. Special populations, such as the elderly and patients with comorbidities, require tailored management approaches to address their unique needs. Considerations for specific etiologies, such as ischemic heart disease and cardiomyopathies, guide targeted therapeutic interventions. This chapter underscores the importance of a multidisciplinary approach in the management of AHF to improve patient outcomes and reduce healthcare burden.

Keywords: Acute heart failure, management, initial stabilization, pharmacological treatment, ischemic heart disease, cardiomyopathies

INTRODUCTION

Acute heart failure (AHF) is a serious illness that requires immediate medical attention due to the abrupt onset or development of heart failure symptoms and signs. AHF can manifest as a chronic heart failure exacerbation or a de novo presentation, with profound implications for patient prognosis. In order to improve prognosis and lessen the burden of this condition on global healthcare systems, effective management measures are essential.

Acute heart failure is defined as the abrupt onset or acute decompensation of chronic heart failure. It shows up as symptoms like extreme dyspnea, fluid retention, and exhaustion, which are brought on by the heart's incapacity to pump blood effectively enough to fulfil the body's demands.[1] Based on the underlying cause, hemodynamic state, and clinical presentation, AHF can be further subdivided.

Acute heart failure is a prevalent condition with significant implications for public health. Epidemiological studies indicate that AHF is responsible for a substantial number of emergency hospital admissions, particularly among older adults. The incidence of AHF varies globally, influenced by factors such as age distribution, prevalence of risk factors, and healthcare access. In developed countries,

AHF remains one of the leading causes of hospitalization among individuals over the age of 65 years.[2]

The impact of AHF on morbidity and mortality is profound. Patients with AHF often experience a high burden of symptoms and a marked decline in quality of life. Despite advances in treatment, the prognosis for AHF remains poor, with high rates of inhospital mortality and readmissions. Long-term outcomes are also concerning, with many patients facing chronic heart failure progression and increased risk of death. Therefore, timely diagnosis and effective management of AHF are critical to improving patient outcomes and reducing healthcare costs.

PATHOPHYSIOLOGY

Pathophysiology of AHF is given in **Fig. 1**.

Acute heart failure is caused by a complicated interaction among a number of systemic and cardiac variables. Important mechanisms consist of:

- *Myocardial dysfunction*: Reduced cardiac contractility due to myocardial ischemia, infarction, or cardiomyopathies leads to decreased cardiac output.
- *Volume overload*: Excessive fluid accumulation, often due to renal dysfunction or increased preload, exacerbates heart failure symptoms.
- *Increased afterload*: Elevated systemic vascular resistance, commonly seen in hypertensive emergencies, impedes left ventricular ejection.
- *Neurohormonal activation*: Activation of the renin-angiotensin-aldosterone system (RAAS) and sympathetic nervous system (SNS) contributes to fluid retention, vasoconstriction, and adverse cardiac remodeling.

COMMON ETIOLOGIES AND RISK FACTORS

Several etiologies and risk factors are associated with the development of AHF, including:

- *Ischemic heart disease*: The two main causes of AHF are chronic coronary artery disease and acute myocardial infarction.
- *Hypertension*: Uncontrolled hypertension increases the risk of left ventricular hypertrophy and subsequent heart failure.
- *Valvular heart disease*: Conditions such as aortic stenosis or mitral regurgitation can precipitate AHF.
- *Cardiomyopathies*: Dilated, hypertrophic, and restrictive cardiomyopathies contribute to impaired cardiac function.
- *Arrhythmias*: Atrial fibrillation, ventricular tachycardia, and other arrhythmias can lead to acute decompensation.
- *Infections*: Myocarditis and sepsis are notable infectious causes of AHF.
- *Noncardiac factors*: Pulmonary embolism, anemia, and thyrotoxicosis can precipitate or exacerbate heart failure.

CLINICAL PRESENTATION

The clinical presentation of AHF **(Table 1)** is often dramatic, with patients presenting with a constellation of symptoms and signs, including:

- *Dyspnea*: Severe dyspnea, particularly during physical activity or when lying flat
- *Edema*: Swelling of the lower extremities and, in severe cases, generalized body swelling (anasarca)

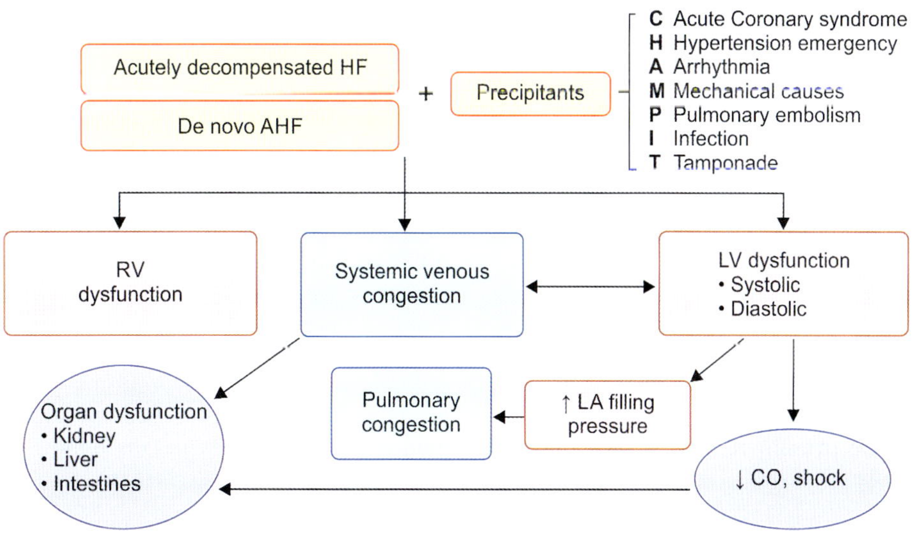

FIG. 1: Pathophysiology of acute heart failure (AHF).

TABLE 1: Signs and biology of AHF.

Symptoms	Signs
• Dyspnea • Orthopnea • Paroxysmal nocturnal dyspnea • Reduced exercise tolerance • Fatigue	• Elevated jugular venous pressure • Hepatojugular reflux • Third heart sound (gallop rhythm) • Laterally displaced apical impulse • Peripheral edema • Pulmonary rales
Parameters	
Chest X-ray	• Diffuse ground-glass opacity • Cardiomegaly • Kerley B-lines • Pleural effusion
LUS	B-lines (3 or more in 2 or more bilateral lung zones)
ECG	• LV hypertrophy • Q waves • Widened QRS complex • Arrhythmias • Signs of AMI
Echocardiography	• LVEF (≤40%: HFrEF, ≥ 50%: HFpEF) • LV and LA size • E/e' ratio > 9 • RV function • Regional wall motion abnormalities (e.g., underlying CAD, Takotsubo, and myocarditis) • Mechanical causes (e.g., myocardial rupture, valve regurgitation, and tamponade)
Natriuretic peptides	• BNP ≥ 100 pg/mL • NT-proBNP ≥ 300 pg/mL • MR-proANP ≥ 120 pg/mL

(AHF: acute heart failure; AMI: acute myocardial infarction; BNP: B-type natriuretic peptide; CAD: coronary artery disease; E/e': early filling velocity on transmitral Doppler/early relaxation velocity on tissue Doppler; ECG: electrocardiogram; LA: left atrium; LUS: lung ultrasound; LV: left ventricle; MR-proANP: mid-regional pro-atrial natriuretic peptide; NT-proBNP: N-terminal pro-B-type natriuretic peptide; RV: right ventricle)

- *Fatigue*: Extreme tiredness and reduced exercise tolerance
- *Cough*: Often productive of frothy, pink-tinged sputum in pulmonary edema
- *Chest pain*: May be present if AHF is secondary to myocardial ischemia

CLASSIFICATION BASED ON CLINICAL PRESENTATION

Acute heart failure can be classified based on clinical presentation into different categories to guide management:

- *Wet versus dry*: This classification is based on the presence (wet) or absence (dry) of volume overload symptoms such as edema and pulmonary congestion.
- *Warm versus cold*: This classification assesses perfusion status. "Warm" indicates adequate perfusion with normal or high cardiac output, while "cold" suggests hypoperfusion with low cardiac output.

DIAGNOSIS

Accurate and prompt diagnosis of AHF is critical for effective management and improving patient outcomes. To determine the degree and underlying causes of heart failure, the diagnostic approach combines imaging techniques, laboratory testing, clinical evaluation, and hemodynamic monitoring.

CLINICAL EVALUATION

A detailed medical history and physical examination are necessary for the first diagnosis of AHF. A thorough medical history should be obtained by clinicians, with special attention to prior heart disease, hypertension, diabetes, and other cardiovascular risk factors. A history of recent weight gain, reduced exercise tolerance, and orthopnea (difficulty breathing when lying flat) are key indicators of AHF. During the physical examination, healthcare providers assess for signs of fluid overload, such as jugular venous distention, peripheral edema, and pulmonary crackles. The presence of a third heart sound (S3) on auscultation is also suggestive of AHF. Identifying these clinical signs helps differentiate AHF from other conditions presenting with similar symptoms, such as chronic obstructive pulmonary disease (COPD) or pneumonia.

Patients with AHF typically present with a range of symptoms that reflect both systemic and pulmonary congestion. Dyspnea, or shortness of breath, is the most common symptom and may be accompanied by paroxysmal nocturnal dyspnea, where patients wake up suddenly at night gasping for air. Fatigue and weakness are also prevalent due to reduced cardiac output and impaired perfusion of vital organs. Other symptoms include cough, often producing frothy, pink-tinged sputum in cases of severe pulmonary edema, and chest discomfort, which may indicate underlying ischemic heart disease.

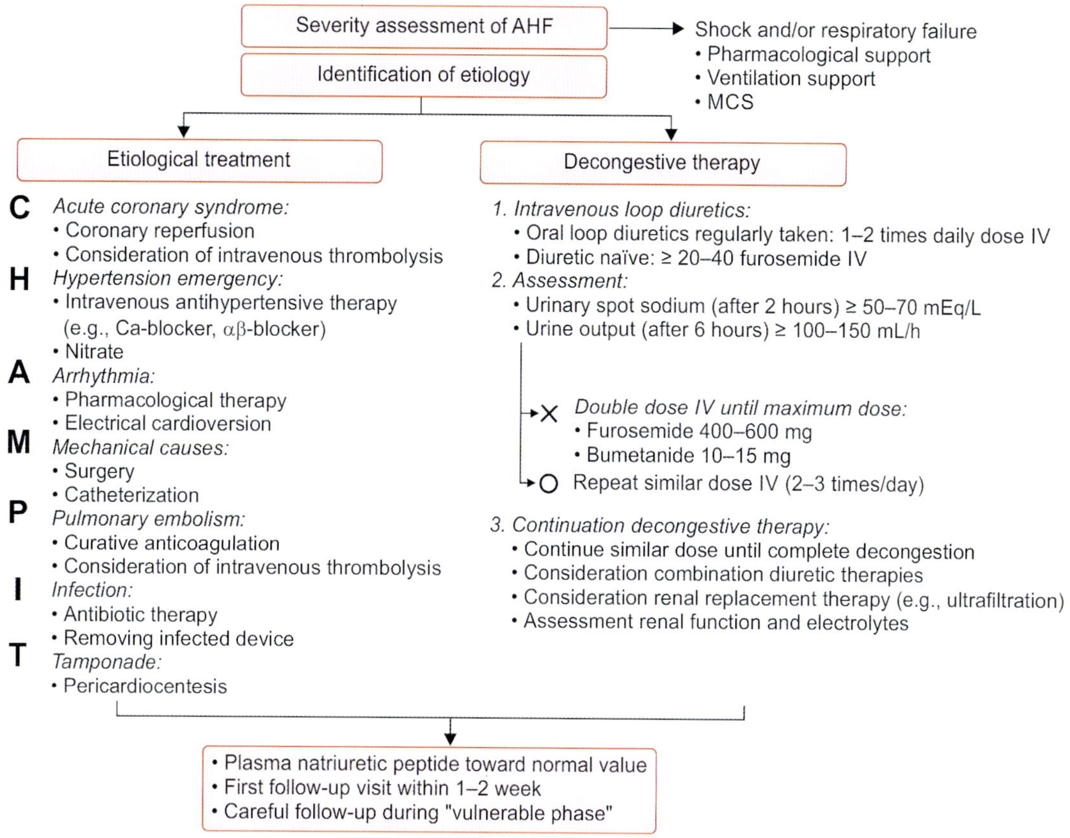

FLOWCHART 1: Severity evaluation of acute heart failure (AHF).

ASSESSMENT OF SEVERITY

The severity evaluation of AHF is given in **Flowchart 1**.

DIAGNOSTIC TOOLS

Lab testing is essential for both the diagnosis and treatment of AHF. It is especially helpful to measure levels of N-terminal pro BNP (NT-proBNP) or BNP (B-type natriuretic peptide). Increased ventricular wall stress is indicated by elevated levels of these biomarkers, which are also highly correlated with heart failure.[3] These tests are useful not just for diagnosis but also for determining the degree of AHF and tracking the effectiveness of treatment. Routine blood tests can help detect any problems or comorbid illnesses by revealing vital information about the patient's overall health status, including electrolytes, liver function, and renal function.

Imaging studies are essential for confirming the diagnosis of AHF and evaluating the underlying cardiac structure and function. A chest X-ray is often the first imaging modality used, revealing signs of pulmonary congestion, cardiomegaly (enlarged heart), and pleural effusions. Echocardiography is the gold standard for assessing cardiac function and structure. It provides detailed information about left and right ventricular function, valvular abnormalities, and the presence of pericardial effusion. Doppler imaging can further evaluate blood flow patterns, which is crucial for diagnosing diastolic dysfunction and estimating pulmonary artery pressures.

In more complex or severe cases of AHF, invasive hemodynamic monitoring may be required. Direct assessment of cardiac output, systemic vascular resistance, and pulmonary artery pressures is possible with pulmonary artery catheterization, commonly referred to as a Swan-Ganz catheter. This data is essential for directing fluid management in critically sick patients and for customizing advanced therapeutic strategies, such as the use of inotropes or vasodilators. While not routinely used in all cases, hemodynamic monitoring is particularly valuable in patients who are not responding to initial treatments or those with ambiguous clinical presentations.

MANAGEMENT

The management of AHF is multifaceted, aiming to stabilize the patient, relieve symptoms, improve hemodynamics, and address the underlying causes. Effective management requires a combination of initial stabilization, pharmacological treatment, and nonpharmacological interventions to optimize patient outcomes.

Initial Stabilization

The initial management of AHF focuses on the ABCs: Airway, breathing, and circulation. Ensuring a patent airway is paramount, and patients may require assistance with breathing. Supplemental oxygen is often administered to maintain adequate oxygenation, particularly in those with hypoxemia. To relieve respiratory distress and lessen the effort of breathing, noninvasive or invasive ventilatory support—such as mechanical ventilation or continuous positive airway pressure (CPAP)—may be required in extreme circumstances. In order to sustain blood pressure and perfusion, circulatory support includes keeping an eye on vital signs, setting up an intravenous access, and giving out fluids or medicine.

The foundation of first AHF care is oxygen therapy. Improving tissue oxygenation and treating hypoxemia are the objectives. Reducing the need for intubation and mechanical breathing might be especially beneficial when using a high-flow nasal cannula or noninvasive ventilation (NIV) techniques like bilevel positive airway pressure (BiPAP) or CPAP. NIV reduces lung congestion and eases dyspnea by enhancing gas exchange and lessening the effort required to breathe.

Pharmacological Treatment

The first-line treatment for volume overload in AHF is diuretics **(Flowchart 2)**. Furosemide is one example of a loop diuretic that is frequently used to increase diuresis and lower preload. Based on renal function and congestion severity, diuretic dosage should be customized.[4] To prevent problems such electrolyte imbalances and declining renal function, close observation of urine output, electrolytes, and renal function is necessary.

Vasodilators, such as nitroprusside and nitrates (such as nitroglycerine), are used to lower preload and afterload, enhance cardiac output, and lessen congestion symptoms. Patients with severe mitral regurgitation or hypertensive crisis benefit most from these medications. To avoid hypotension, the dosage and type of vasodilator should be carefully chosen, and blood pressure should be continuously monitored.

Patients with reduced cardiac output and hypoperfusion symptoms despite normal filling pressures should be treated with inotropic drugs such milrinone and dobutamine. Arrhythmias and an increase in the oxygen demand of the heart are just two of the serious hazards associated with inotropes, even if they can enhance cardiac output and organ perfusion. As such, their use ought to be restricted to the smallest amount of time required and saved for particular symptoms.

Angiotensin-converting enzyme inhibitors, beta-blockers, angiotensin receptor blockers (ARBs), and mineralocorticoid receptor antagonists (MRAs) are key players in the treatment of chronic heart failure. Their function in AHF is more complex. In most circumstances, beta-blockers should be continued unless there is severe decompensation; nevertheless, the patient's hemodynamic stability and renal function will determine when to start or continue using ACE inhibitors, ARBs, and MRAs. By reducing the course of the disease and altering neurohormonal activation, these medications contribute to better long-term results.

Nonpharmacological Interventions

In patients with severe volume overload unresponsive to pharmacological therapy, ultrafiltration, and dialysis can be effective alternatives. Ultrafiltration helps in removing excess fluid, reducing congestion, and improving symptoms. This intervention is particularly useful in patients with concomitant renal dysfunction where diuretics are less effective.

Mechanical circulatory support including intra-aortic balloon pumps (IABP) and ventricular assist devices (VADs), may be indicated in patients with refractory cardiogenic shock or severe decompensation not responsive to medical therapy.[5] These devices provide temporary support to maintain adequate perfusion and cardiac output while definitive treatment strategies, such as cardiac transplantation or recovery of myocardial function, are pursued.

Long-term management of AHF involves educating patients about lifestyle modifications to prevent recurrent episodes. This includes dietary sodium restriction, fluid management, regular physical activity, and adherence to prescribed medications. Patient education should also emphasize recognizing early symptoms of decompensation and seeking prompt medical attention. Regular follow-up and monitoring are essential to ensure adherence to lifestyle changes and optimize treatment regimens.

HOSPITALIZATION AND MONITORING

Patients with AHF frequently need to be hospitalized because of the severity of their symptoms and the requirement for close observation and medical attention. A patient's overall stability and some clinical criteria are taken into consideration while deciding whether to accept them.

When a patient with AHF shows symptoms of severe volume overload, marked hypoxemia, or hemodynamic instability, they are usually admitted to the hospital. Additional signs and symptoms include evidence of end-organ malfunction (e.g., renal failure and altered mental status), severe dyspnea, particularly if accompanied by hypoxia or hypercapnia, and the requirement for intravenous medicine or extensive monitoring that cannot be supplied in an outpatient setting.[6] Hospitalization is also recommended

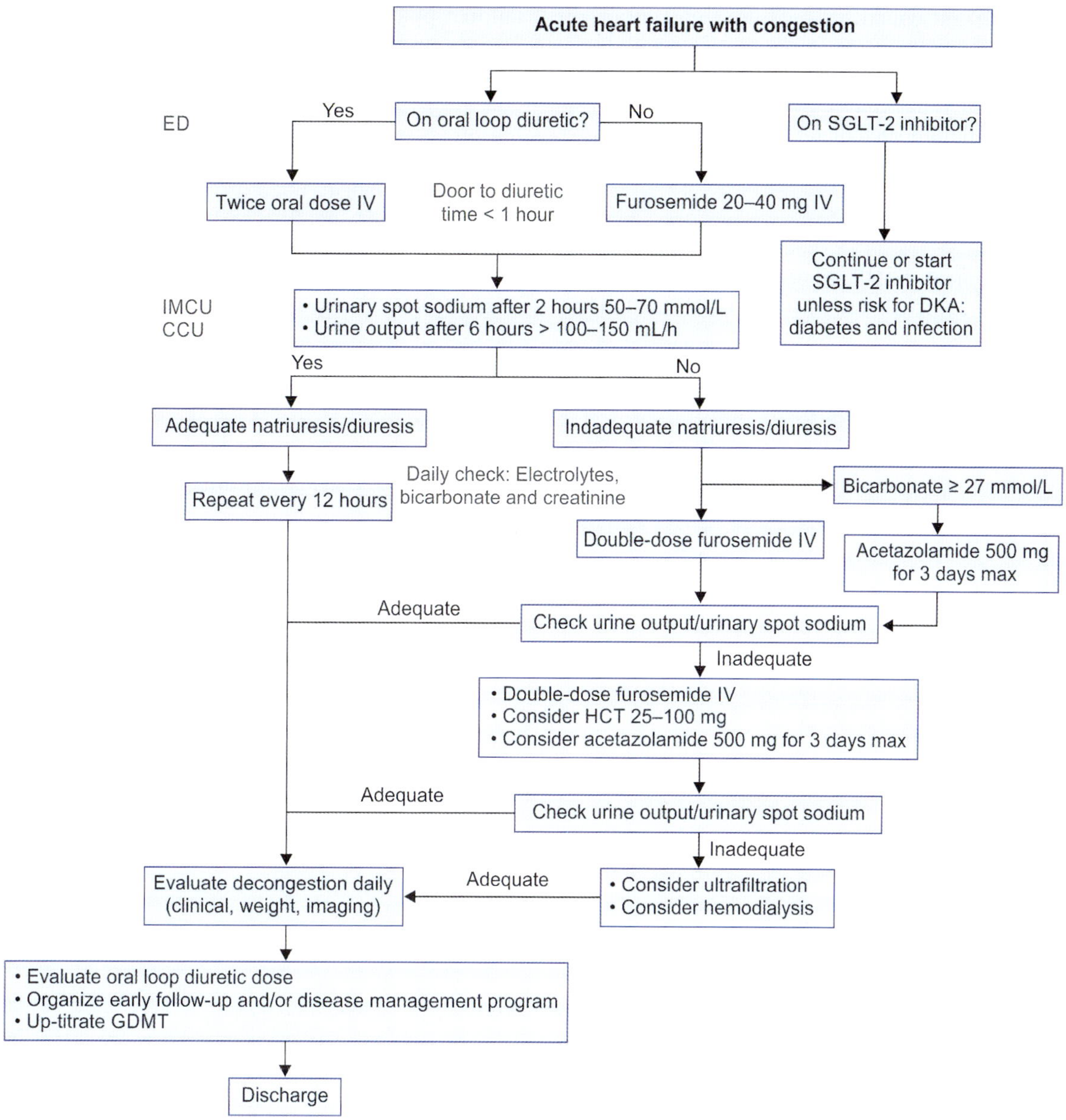

FLOWCHART 2: A depiction of the new treatment algorithm for the optimal decongestion strategy.[5]

(CCU: coronary care unit; DKA: diabetic ketoacidosis; ED: emergency department; GDMT: guideline-directed medical therapy; HCT: hydrochlorothiazide; IMCU: intermediate care unit; SGLT-2: sodium-glucose cotransporter-2)

Source: With permission from Collins et al. (2015).[5]

for patients who have a high risk of adverse outcomes, such as those who have recently experienced a myocardial infarction or uncontrolled hypertension.

Discharging a patient from the hospital requires careful consideration to ensure they are stable and can be safely managed as an outpatient. Criteria for discharge include the resolution of acute symptoms, stabilization of hemodynamics, and a significant reduction in congestion, as evidenced by decreased edema and improved respiratory status. Patients should be on an optimized oral medication regimen, with any intravenous medications successfully transitioned to oral therapy. Additionally, they should have a follow-up plan in place, including scheduled visits with a heart failure specialist, and being educated about managing their condition at home, recognizing early signs of decompensation, and adhering to lifestyle modifications.

PROGNOSIS AND FOLLOW-UP

The severity of the initial presentation, the underlying cause of heart failure, and the existence of concomitant disorders are some of the variables that affect a patient's prognosis when they have AHF. Serum sodium levels, renal function, left ventricular ejection fraction (LVEF), and the patient's reaction to the first course of treatment are important prognostic variables. The prognosis for patients with intact LVEF is often better than that of those with diminished LVEF. Furthermore, outcomes may be negatively impacted by concomitant conditions such diabetes, chronic renal illness, and chronic obstructive lung disease.

CONCLUSION

Effective management of AHF requires a comprehensive and multidisciplinary approach that includes initial stabilization, tailored pharmacological and nonpharmacological treatments, and careful long-term follow-up. Early identification and prompt intervention are crucial to improving patient outcomes, reducing morbidity and mortality, and minimizing hospital readmissions. Special consideration must be given to elderly patients and those with comorbidities, as well as to the specific etiologies underlying heart failure. By integrating these strategies, healthcare providers can enhance the quality of care for patients with AHF, ultimately leading to better health outcomes and a reduced burden on healthcare systems.

ONLINE REFERENCES

Please scan the QR code provided at the end of the table of contents for References of this chapter.

CHAPTER

67

Worsening Heart Failure: Advances in Management

Punitha Lakxmi Ramesh, Harikrishnan S

ABSTRACT

Worsening heart failure (WHF) represents a significant deterioration in patients with established HF, marked by increased hospitalizations and adverse outcomes. Although first defined in recent guidelines, its management lacks specificity, despite its high morbidity and mortality. WHF precipitated by both cardiovascular and non-cardiovascular factors, necessitates a comprehensive approach including decongestion, guideline-directed medical therapy (GDMT), and patient-centered strategies like telemonitoring, PAP devices, and nurse-led HF clinics. Recent advancements in wearable technology, inotropes, diuretic strategies, and cardiac contractility modulation provide promising avenues for preventing HF exacerbations and improving long-term outcomes.

Keywords: WHF, American College of Cardiology, guidelines, treatment

INTRODUCTION

Worsening heart failure (WHF) is deterioration of signs and symptoms in a patient with preexisting heart failure (HF), despite previous stable guideline-directed medical therapy (GDMT). The presentation may be as an urgent hospitalization or emergency department (ED), or outpatient (OP) visit, mostly requiring intensification of therapy, with intravenous (IV) or oral diuretics.[1]

It was first recognized in scientific literature in the 2021 update of the European Society of Cardiology (ESC) practice guidelines and later in the 2022 American College of Cardiology (ACC)/American Heart Association (AHA) guidelines considered as a potential trajectory among patients with stage C HF going to stage D HF. However, no specific management recommendations were included.

Nearly 25% of patients hospitalized for WHF succumb or are readmitted within 30 days of discharge.[2] WHF patients receiving treatment in the OP/ED also have the same risk as those hospitalized as evident from the secondary analysis of MADIT-CRT and PARADIGM-HF. WHF is linked to a significantly higher risk of adverse outcomes compared to new-onset HF. Specifically, WHF is associated with an increased combined risk of all-cause mortality or HF readmission (37%), all-cause mortality (22%), and HF readmission (81%).[3] Thus, their prevention is a major target in the current treatment of HF.

PRINCIPLES OF MANAGEMENT OF WORSENING HEART FAILURE

- Identification and management of precipitants
- Decongestion with diuretics
- Initiation and optimization of GDMT to maximum tolerated doses by close monitoring

PRECIPITANTS OF WORSENING HEART FAILURE

Worsening heart failure can be triggered by both cardiovascular (CV) and non-CV factors. The most common triggers as per REPORT-HF registry[4] are summarized in **Table 1**. These conditions are frequently overlooked during initial hospital evaluations, where the primary focus is often on treating decongestion. It is important to emphasize on lifestyle modification with a DASH diet, weight loss to achieve a BMI < 35 kg/m^2, moderate salt restriction < 5,750 mg/day, smoking cessation, and avoidance of alcohol. Fluid restriction (1.5–2 L) can be advised in patients with severe HF/hyponatremia to relieve symptoms and congestion. Intake must be appropriately adjusted during periods of high heat/humidity and nausea/vomiting. Engaging in a supervised exercise-based, cardiac rehabilitation program improves functional status and quality of life (QoL).[5]

TABLE 1: Precipitants of worsening heart failure (WHF).

Precipitant	%
Unknown	48
Acute coronary syndrome	13
Pneumonia/Infection	10
Arrhythmia	10
Nonadherence to medication/diet	9
Uncontrolled hypertension	6
Worsening renal function	2
Medication-related WHF	1
Pulmonary embolism	1

IDENTIFICATION OF PATIENTS WITH WORSENING HEART FAILURE

Despite advancements in HF therapy, patients discharged after decompensation remain at high risk for readmission (30%) and mortality (10%) within the next 3 months. Failure to achieve and document euvolemia prior to discharge was associated with more short-term readmissions. 24% of patients hospitalized for HF have signs of congestion at discharge. Persistent congestion at 4–6 weeks is predictive of poor prognosis **(Table 2)**.[6]

Recent interventions have thus concentrated on the transition between inpatient and OP care. These include intensive nursing support, telemonitoring, expedited follow-up, and enhanced patient education.[7]

STRATEGIES TO PREVENT WORSENING HEART FAILURE

Heart Failure Clinics and Heart Failure Nurse-based Follow-up

An HF clinic is an organized setup attached to hospitals that provides protocol-based evaluation and follow-up for HF patients. Typically nurse-led, these clinics emphasize early detection of HF symptoms by nurses and allied professionals **(Box 1)**. Regular telephonic follow-ups help identify early signs of worsening, such as rapid weight gain, worsening of NYHA class, or decreased urine output. If deterioration is suspected, patients are advised to visit the hospital for further assessment and management. This approach has proven effective in reducing all-cause mortality, hospital readmissions, and shortening hospital stays while offering emotional support and reassurance to patients.[8]

Digital Health—Telehealth

Digital health has the potential to shift healthcare systems toward a patient-centric, preventive approach, prioritizing health maintenance over crisis management. Remote consultations via video or phone reduce travel, facilitate medication adjustments, and provide direct education and support. While cloud-based technologies have limitations for patients with decompensated symptoms, AI-driven technologies enable objective home examinations. HF nurses can use these platforms to review stable patients and identify those needing urgent in-person consultations. The study by Knoll et al.[9] demonstrated that participants in telehealth programs had significantly reduced all-cause mortality (5.8% vs. 11.0%; $p < 0.001$), fewer HF hospitalizations [17.9 vs. 21.8/100 patient-years (PY); $p < 0.001$], all-cause hospitalizations (129.0 vs. 133.2/100 PY; $p = 0.015$), and shorter hospital stays.

Pulmonary Artery Pressure Monitoring Devices

Remote monitoring of congestion markers, such as pulmonary artery pressure (PAP) or left atrial pressure, offers a proactive approach to early detection of WHF, enabling timely pharmacological intervention to prevent hospitalization. Elevated PAP, associated with congestion, precedes clinical symptoms, making it a promising early marker for impending HF-related hospitalizations. FDA-approved devices such as CardioMEMS HF system and Cordella PAP sensor

TABLE 2: Risk factors of residual congestion at discharge and/or for HF readmission.

Clinical factors	Therapy related	Laboratory	ECG/Imaging	Comorbidities
• NYHA class > 2 • ≥1 HF hospitalization within 6 months • SBP < 90 mm Hg • Tachycardia • Inadequate weight loss	• GDMT discontinuation during hospitalization • Intolerance to GDMT • High diuretic dose	• Renal dysfunction • Electrolyte disturbance • BNP > 250 pg/mL • NT-proBNP >1,500 pg/mL • Anemia	• QRS duration > 130 ms without CRT • Ventricular arrhythmias • LVEF < 20% • High pulmonary pressure/LV filling pressures • Moderate/severe TR • IVC > 21 mm • B-lines > 15	• Diabetes mellitus • Valvular heart disease • Coronary artery disease • Atrial fibrillation • Pulmonary disease • Frailty

(BNP: B-type natriuretic peptide; CRT: cardiac resynchronization therapy; EF: ejection fraction; GDMT: guideline-directed medical therapy; IVC: inferior vena cava; LV: left ventricle; NT-proBNP: N-terminal pro-B-type natriuretic peptide; NYHA: New York Heart Association; SBP: systolic blood pressure; TR: tricuspid regurgitation)

BOX 1 Warning signs of worsening heart failure (WHF).

- Sudden weight gain (2–3 pounds in 1 day or ≥5 pounds in 1 week)
- Extra swelling in the feet or ankles
- Swelling or pain in the abdomen
- Loss of appetite
- Reduced urine output
- Shortness of breath not related to exercise
- Discomfort or trouble breathing when lying flat
- Waking up short of breath
- Chest discomfort
- Coughing or wheezing
- Increased fatigue
- Mental confusion

transmit real-time data to healthcare providers, enabling medication adjustments to prevent exacerbations. These are recommended in HFpEF or HFrEF with NYHA class III symptoms, at least 1 HF-related hospitalization in the preceding year, despite receiving at least 3 months of optimal GDMT, ESC class IIb, level B **(Table 3)**.[11,12] It involves three key phases:[13]

1. *Immediate postimplant period (0–7 days)*: Establish baseline pulmonary artery diastolic pressure (PADP) ranges
2. *Optimization phase*: Intensive medication management, close monitoring (two to three times per week) to achieve PADP goals
3. *Maintenance period*: Adjust neurohormonal drugs, vasodilators, and diuretics as needed to maintain or improve PADP, and reassess PADP goals

TABLE 3: Remote monitoring devices for heart failure.

Study	Number	Follow-up	Outcomes	Adverse events (AE)
CardioMEMS				
CHAMPION (2017), randomized	550 HFrEF	18 months	• 28% reduction in HFH • 32% lower mortality	99% free from device-related complications
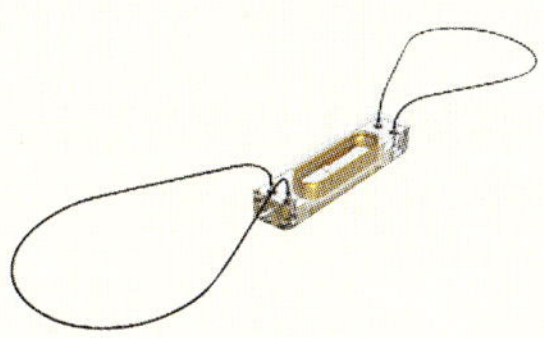 GUIDE HF (2022), randomized	1,000–various groups of HF	12 months	• 19% reduction of a composite of all-cause mortality and HF events • 28% reduction in HFH • Similar benefits in HFrEF and HFpEF	No device-related AE
Cordella				
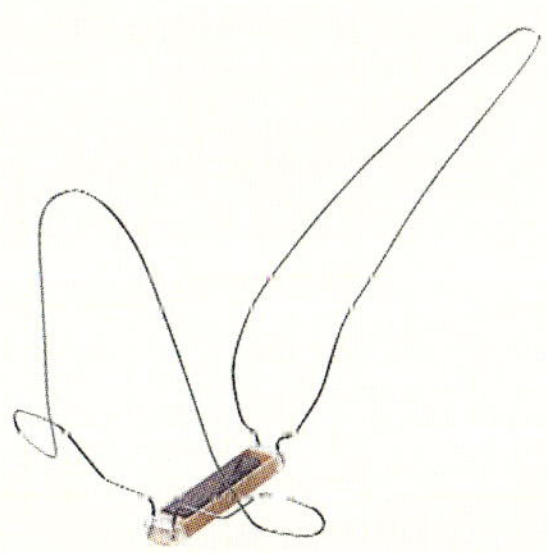 SIRONA 2 (2024), open label	70	12 months	• Mean PAP difference between Cordella and Cath being 2.9 ± 7.3 mm Hg • Hospitalizations and mortality were low (0.33 event/patient/year)	98.4% freedom from device/system-related complications
V-LAP				
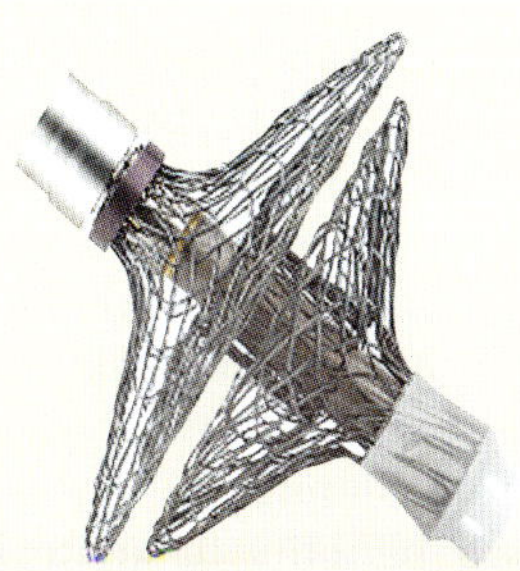 VECTOR-HF (2023), open label[10]	30	12 months	• Mean LAP difference between V-LAP and Cath is −0.22 ± 4.92 mm Hg • 32% reached NYHA class II at 6 months and 60% by 12 months • 6MWD improved by 67 and 99 m at 6 and 12 months, respectively, freedom from short-term MACNE was 97%	3% device-related CVA

(CVA: cerebrovascular accident; MACNE: major adverse cardiac and neurological event)

Cardiovascular Implantable Electronic Device Based Monitoring

Algorithms in cardiovascular implantable electronic devices (CIEDs) can monitor congestion by measuring thoracic impedance, eliminating the need for extra hardware. However, no randomized trials have definitively shown a reduction in hospitalization and mortality rates. The HeartLogic™ algorithm (Boston Scientific) monitors multiple parameters such as heart sounds, respiration rate, intrathoracic impedance, nighttime heart rate, and physical activity, to detect impending HF decompensation. Pulmonary congestion, which alters impedance, can also be detected by algorithms such as Optivol™ (Medtronic), CorVue™ (Abbott), and BIO-Link™ (Biotronik), aiding in early intervention. The sensitivity and specificity of CIED-based remote monitoring to identify WHF are 98.6% (92.5–100.0%) and 63.4% (55.2–71.0%), respectively.[14]

Wearable Devices

These externally applied sensors capture functional or physiological data continuously and can be integrated into accessories such as watches, clothing, or skin patches. They work alongside devices such as smartphones to collect, analyze, or transmit the data.

Ambulatory ECG monitoring to detect arrhythmias can now be performed via a wearable patch, e.g., Carnation™ patch and VivaLNK™. Electrodes can also be woven into a "smart textile" vest for prolonged multilead ECG monitoring, e.g., Cardioskin™.[15]

Remote dielectric sensing (ReDS) system is a novel electromagnetic technology that noninvasively quantifies changes in lung fluid concentration. ReDS SAFE HF trial demonstrated improved prognosis 1-month post discharge, primarily due to reduced HF readmissions.[16]

The swelling of soft tissues in the vocal tract and folds results in altered speech which can be detected by digital speech technology (e.g., HearO). It can predict HF events with 82% accuracy 18 days prior to clinical event, while daily weight monitoring had an accuracy of 10–20%.

Improving Treatment Compliance

An effective treatment plan requires both physicians to devise appropriate strategies and patients to adhere to their prescribed regimen. Poor medication adherence (<80%) is associated with higher all-cause mortality and major CV hospitalizations (HR 2.19; 95% CI 1.72-2.79; $p < 0.0001$).

Patients with depressive symptoms or limited knowledge of their condition often struggle with adherence. Regular health education during hospitalization, utilizing printed materials, enhances understanding and supports GDMT implementation. Postdischarge education via mobile phones, websites, and social media further improves adherence. Addressing psychological issues, such as anxiety or depression, through therapy is essential.

Financial constraints also hinder GDMT adoption, particularly in developing countries with inadequate insurance coverage, making access to costly medications challenging, forcing patients to forgo essential medications or use less expensive alternatives, such as substituting angiotensin receptor/neprilysin inhibitors (ARNI) with renin-angiotensin-aldosterone system inhibitors (RAASi). Integrating ARNI and sodium-glucose cotransporter-2 inhibitors (SGLT-2i) into GDMT poses economic challenges due to high costs. But the benefit obtained by the addition of these two drugs is substantial and should be considered while prescribing GDMT. The Medical Expenditure Panel Survey indicates that 33% of patients experience financial distress from medical expenses, with 13.2% unable to afford such costs.

MANAGEMENT OF WORSENING HEART FAILURE

The cornerstone of management of WHF is uptitrating the diuretics followed by titration of GDMT. The typical strategy involves administering an IV dose of loop diuretics at 2.5 times the patient's current oral dosage.

INNOVATIVE COMBINATIONS WITH DIURETICS FOR DECONGESTION

Door-to-furosemide time ≤1 hour, lowered short-term risk of HF hospitalizations or CV death.[17] According to the DOSE trial, administering a higher dose of diuretics (2.5 times the oral dose) significantly improved dyspnea, increased weight loss, and substantial reduction in serum natriuretic peptides.

Emergence of diuretic resistance is of great concern and predicts increased risk of mortality, readmission, and renal complications resulting from HF. Pathophysiological mechanisms resulting in diuretic resistance are:[18]

- Elevated daily sodium intake exceeding the salt loss caused by diuretics
- Hyponatremia or hypokalemic metabolic alkalosis
- Reflex activation of renal nerves
- Acidosis and hypoalbuminemia affecting drug delivery
- Decreased dietary salt intake
- Repeated administration of furosemide reducing renal tubular response or affecting its pharmacodynamics

Sodium-glucose cotransporter-2 inhibitors promote osmotic diuresis by acting on the proximal tubule, complementing the action of loop diuretics on interstitial fluid reduction. This improves diuretic efficacy and facilitates decongestion as demonstrated by various studies **(Table 4)**.[19-21] Additionally, acetazolamide, a carbonic anhydrase inhibitor, has shown benefits in acute HF cases, as demonstrated by the ADVOR[22] trial **(Table 4)**. A triple diuretic strategy, combining loop diuretics with

TABLE 4: Drugs for worsening heart failure.

Study	Drug	Follow-up	Outcomes	Adverse effects
Acetazolamide				
ADVOR (2022), randomized	259—acetazolamide 260—placebo	3 months	• 46% successful decongestion • 42% successful decongestion without escalation therapy • Hospitalization duration: 8.8 days (acetazolamide) vs. 9.9 days (placebo) • Death or rehospitalization for heart failure reduced by 7%	Similar incidences of renal safety endpoint, hypokalemia, and hypotension between groups
Empagliflozin				
EMPA-RESPONSE-AHF (2020), randomized	• 41—empagliflozin 10 mg/day for 30 days • 39—placebo	• Primary outcomes – day 4 • Secondary outcomes – 60 days	• Urinary output until day 4 was significantly greater with empagliflozin vs. placebo [difference 3,449 (95% confidence interval 578–6321) mL; $p < 0.01$] • Empagliflozin reduced a combined endpoint of in-hospital worsening HF, rehospitalization for HF, or death at 60 days compared with placebo [4 (10%) vs. 13 (33%); $p = 0.014$]	• Lower number of cardiovascular AEs in empagliflozin group ($p = 0.046$) • No excess UTI or other adverse effects with empagliflozin • No difference in renal events or WRF between groups
EMPAG-HF (2022), randomized	30—empagliflozin 25 mg OD for 5 days 30—placebo	30 days	• 25% increased cumulative urine output over 5 days • Greater reduction in NT-proBNP	No statistically significant differences in the occurrence of safety events between the two groups
EMPLUSE (2023), randomized	• 265 in each treatment arm • Empagliflozin 10 mg/day for 90 days	90 days	Empagliflozin significantly reduced congestion at all time points, days 15, 30, and 90 were: for WL −1.97 (−2.86, −1.08), −1.74 (−2.73, −0.74); −1.53 (−2.75, −0.31) kg, respectively (all $p < 0.05$)	Not assessed
Thiazide diuretics				
CLOROTIC (2023), randomized	• IV furosemide+ HCTZ (114) • IV furosemide+ placebo (116)	90 days	• Higher weight loss at 72 hours – 2.3 versus 1.5 kg • No significant differences in patient-reported dyspnea • HCTZ showed greater 24 hours diuresis (1,775 vs. 1,400 mL) and weight loss for each 40 mg of furosemide • No differences in mortality or rehospitalizations	Frequent renal impairment with HCTZ

Continued

Continued

Study	Drug	Follow-up	Outcomes	Adverse effects
Vericiguat				
VICTORIA (2020), randomized	2,526—vericiguat 2,524—placebo	10.8 months	10% reduced in death from CV causes or first HF hospitalization	• *SAE*: 32.8% vericiguat vs. 34.8% placebo • *Anemia*: 7.6% vericiguat vs. 5.7% placebo
Levosimendan				
LeoDor (2023), randomized	38—6-hour levosimendan infusion q2 weeks 57—24-hour levosimendan infusion q3 weeks 53—placebo	• 14 weeks (primary outcome) • 26 weeks (secondary outcome)	• No significant difference in global rank score between groups (mean rank: 72.55 for levosimendan vs. 73.81 for placebo; $p = 0.863$) • Higher proportion of patients with ≥10-point increase in KCCQ-OSS in levosimendan group (63.5% vs. 41.7%, $p = 0.037$) • No significant differences in KCCQ-CSS, NYHA class, EQ-5D VAS	• Hypotension in 9.7% levosimendan infusions, 11.1% placebo ($p = 0.564$) • Tachycardia, new-onset AF, and NSVT were higher in levosimendan group • Adverse events were higher in the 24-hour infusion group
LION HEART (2018), randomized	48—levosimendan 6-hour infusion q2 weeks 21—placebo	12 weeks	• Significant reduction in NT-proBNP levels with levosimendan ($p < 0.001$) • Significant reduction in HF (HR 0.25, $p = 0.001$), CV, and all-cause hospitalizations in the levosimendan group • QoL (EQ-5D VAS): Less decline in HRQoL in the levosimendan group ($p = 0.022$)	• Deaths: 31% (levosimendan) vs. 38% (placebo), $p = 0.781$ • Hypotension requiring infusion reduction/discontinuation is more frequent with levosimendan, but not statistically significant

(UTI: urinary tract infection; WL: weight loss)

IV acetazolamide from admission to day 3 and adding an SGLT-2i from day 3 onward, can be an effective approach.

Finerenone, a nonsteroidal mineralocorticoid receptor antagonist (MRA) inhibits RAASi, thus reducing the risk of myocardial and renal fibrosis. It is highly selective for its receptors, offering a better safety profile and a reduced incidence of hyperkalemia and gynecomastia. It can be used as a substitute for eplerenone in HF patients with diabetes mellitus and/or chronic kidney disease (CKD) as evidenced by the ARTS-HF trial.[23]

INOTROPES—LEVOSIMENDAN

Levosimendan is an inodilator that enhances cardiac troponin C sensitivity to calcium, improving systolic function without impairing diastolic relaxation. Metabolized in the liver into an active form with a 75–80-hour half-life, its CV effects persist for 7–9 days postdiscontinuation. It induces vasodilation in pulmonary, coronary, and peripheral arteries by activating potassium channels in smooth muscle cells. The repetitive administration of levosimendan and hemodynamic stabilization in patients with worsening HF remains controversial, and further studies are needed **(Table 4)**.[24,25]

SHORT STAY UNITS

Short stay units (SSUs) have emerged as an appealing alternative to direct discharge from ED because they enable clinicians to monitor initial response to therapy and make informed decisions regarding disposition. 41.9% of patients in the SSU group subsequently require further management with hospitalization after initial treatment.[26]

FOUR PILLARS OF HEART FAILURE

Achieving optimal doses of beta-blockers (BB), RAASi/ARNI, MRA, and SGLT-2i is essential for effective, sustainable decongestion and improved QoL. Quadruple therapy has been shown to reduce mortality by 73% over 2 years, even with maximally tolerated doses. For patients with WHF and no contraindications, initiating and escalating quadruple therapy to target or maximum tolerated doses (50–99% of the target) within 4–6 weeks is crucial.[27]

The STRONG HF trial showed that patients on an intensive treatment strategy, involving rapid uptitration of GDMT to 100% within 2 weeks postdischarge and close follow-up with four OP visits over 2 months, had a 34% relative and 8.1% absolute risk reduction in all-cause death or HF readmission. CV death, HF readmission, and all-cause death decreased by 26%, 44%, and 16%, respectively, with improved symptoms and QoL.[28]

Not all patients will reach the target dose for every medication, as seen in clinical trials. Therefore, it is essential to carefully adjust medications to the maximum dose each patient can tolerate. The potential obstacles to the optimization of GDMT are clinical inertia, physiological limitations (hypotension, bradyarrhythmia, renal dysfunction, and electrolyte imbalance), comorbidities, nonadherence, cost, socioeconomic status, psychological condition, and frailty.[29,30]

Guideline-directed medical therapy prescription rates drop to 62.7% in patients with systolic blood pressure (SBP) below 100 mm Hg. Orthostatic hypotension, especially drug-induced, is a major concern during GDMT titration, particularly in the elderly. ARNIs should be used with caution in patients with SBP under 100 mm Hg to maintain adequate organ perfusion. The COPERNICUS trial found that BB did not further lower BP in patients with SBP between 85 and 95 mm Hg compared to placebo. MRAs and SGLT-2i generally have mild antihypertensive effects and rarely require discontinuation due to hypotension.

Only 15% of patients with an eGFR of 45–60 mL/min/1.73 m^2 and 5% with an eGFR of 30–45 mL/min/1.73 m^2 receive BB, ACEI/ARB/ARNI, or MRA after HF admission. An initial drop in eGFR, termed pseudo-WRF, is not indicative of structural damage or adverse outcomes. The ESC guidelines recommend continuing GDMT if creatinine rise is <50%, remains <3 mg/dL, with eGFR > 25 mL/min/1.73 m^2. Treatment should be stopped if creatinine rises over 50% or exceeds 3.5 mg/dL. For eGFR above 15 mL/min/1.73 m^2, hydralazine with isosorbide dinitrate combination is an alternate option.[30]

Hyperkalemia often leads to discontinuation of RAASi, in 0.4–10% patients. Dose reduction is recommended for potassium levels between 5.5 and 6 mEq/L, temporary cessation if levels exceed 6 mEq/L, and resuming therapy once levels fall below 5.5 mEq/L. New treatments such as patiromer and sodium zirconium cyclosilicate can help manage hyperkalemia while maintaining therapy. Routine laboratory tests for creatinine, urea, eGFR, and electrolytes should be performed 14 days after drug titration and every 4 months thereafter.[30]

Simultaneous/rapid-sequence initiation of medications has additive effects and maximizes tolerance to each other. Swapping an RAASi to ARNI decreases the risk of hyperkalemia. SGLT-2i therapy prevents hyperkalemia and slows the progression of renal disease. These strategies reduce the risk of discontinuation of MRA.

SOLUBLE GUANYLATE CYCLASE STIMULATORS

The ongoing inflammation, oxidative stress, and endothelial dysfunction reduce nitric oxide (NO) and NO-dependent intracellular cGMP production. Direct soluble guanylate cyclase (sGC) stimulators (vericiguat) bind to sGC receptors (located on myocardial cells) and enhance the cGMP pathway which in turn activates protein kinase G (PKG) and results in vasodilation, anti-inflammatory, antifibrotic, and antiremodeling (inhibits hypertrophy) effect. The meta-analysis by Abuelazm et al.,[31] which included 8 RCTs and 7,307 patients, showed that vericiguat 10 mg effectively reduced the composite CV mortality and HF hospitalization [RR 0.88, 95% CI (0.79; 0.98)] with no significant AE compared to placebo. Though it was effective in HFrEF [RR 0.87, 95% CI (0.78; 0.97)], it was not promising in HFpEF [RR 0.69, 95% CI (0.15; 3.05)]. It has been recommended for use in patients with WHF despite optimized GDMT in 2021 ESC HF guidelines (class IIb).

Various renal cells, including glomerular arterioles, granular cells, descending vasa recta, fibroblasts, and podocytes, express sGC. Its activation can modulate renal blood flow, regulate the function of glomerular and tubular compartments, and reduce inflammation and renal fibrosis.

Its efficacy was demonstrated by the VICTORIA trial **(Table 4)**.[32] It should be used with caution in patients with clinically unstable advanced HF, with multiple comorbidities and NT-proBNP values > 5,314 pg/mL. It can be initiated upfront with quadruple therapy as quintuple therapy or can be reserved for a subsequent WHF event despite optimal GDMT.

HYDRALAZINE-ISOSORBIDE DINITRATE

Hydralazine, known for its antioxidant properties, induces vasodilation of arteries and arterioles without affecting venous smooth muscle. ISDN metabolized to NO relaxes vascular smooth muscle in arteries and veins, including coronary arteries. This combination reduces afterload and preload, enhances cardiac output, and decreases myocardial workload. Hydralazine mitigates nitrate tolerance, a common issue with long-term nitrate use, making this combination therapy potentially beneficial for CKD patients with HF. It reduced mortality by 52% and CV death and sudden cardiac death by 38% each. In contrast, HF admission and MI were more frequent in patients treated with hydralazine-isosorbide dinitrate (H-ISDN) (195.5 and 18.0 events/100-PY) compared with nonusers (73.4 and 10.2 events/100-PY).[33]

OMECAMTIV MECARBIL

Omecamtiv mecarbil is a cardiac myosin activator, which enhances cardiac contractility without modifying intracellular Ca^{2+} concentration or myocardial oxygen consumption. It recruits myosin heads ready to bind to actin in the systolic phase, extends systolic ejection time, and improves cardiac output. It does not impair renal function or potassium homeostasis, thus facilitating its administration in these patients. In the GALACTIC HF trial, the time to first HF event or CV death was reduced by 20% in HF patients with NYHA II–IV and EF < 35%, with 25 mg twice daily of omecamtiv.[34]

IRON SUPPLEMENTATION

The 2023 ESC guidelines recommend IV iron supplementation for symptomatic HFrEF or HFmrEF patients with iron deficiency to improve symptoms and QoL (class I) and reduce the risk of HF hospitalization (class IIa). Secondary analyses of the AFFIRM AHF trial showed that IV ferric carboxymaltose provided benefits similar to placebo, regardless of baseline hemoglobin levels, and was slightly more effective in patients with ischemic compared to nonischemic etiology. A prespecified analysis of the IRONMAN trial, which censored follow-up due to the COVID-19 pandemic, found that IV ferric derisomaltose significantly reduced the primary outcome of recurrent HFH and CV death.[35]

Sodium-glucose cotransporter-2 inhibitors have anti-inflammatory effects which reduce oxidative stress, lower hepcidin levels, and promote iron mobilization from intracellular stores. It also increases erythropoietin. This is linked with increased hemoglobin and hematocrit levels. A retrospective, single-center analysis of 160 patients with HFrEF showed that combined treatment with IV iron and SGLT-2i resulted in a greater increase in hemoglobin and hematocrit compared to IV iron alone.[36]

VACCINATION

Influenza infection is a potential risk factor for recurrent major CV event affecting >20% patients with confirmed CV disease, and >50% of these repeated events represent HF. Influenza vaccination reduced all-cause deaths, CV deaths, and pneumonia by 21%, 23%, and 49%, respectively, during periods of peak influenza circulation.[37]

CARDIAC CONTRACTILITY MODULATION

Patients who are not candidates for cardiac resynchronization therapy (CRT) or do not respond to CRT may benefit from cardiac contractility modulation (CCM) therapy. Excessive sympathetic nervous system activation impairs calcium channels in the heart, reducing contractility. CCM delivers biphasic electrical signals to the right ventricular septum during the refractory period, enhancing calcium influx in myocytes and improving contractile function. The OPTIMIZER device (Impulse Dynamics) delivers high-voltage signals and is FDA-approved for patients with LVEF of 20–45%, NYHA class III symptoms, who are on appropriate GDMT and without CRT.

CONCLUSION

Managing WHF requires a comprehensive approach that includes identifying and addressing precipitants, improving patient compliance, effective decongestion strategies, and optimizing GDMT. Advances in remote monitoring and telehealth, along with novel therapeutic agents and strategies, hold promise for improving outcomes in this high-risk patient population. Continued research and guideline updates are necessary to refine these approaches and ensure that patients with WHF receive the best possible care.

ONLINE REFERENCES

Please scan the QR code provided at the end of the table of contents for References of this chapter.

CHAPTER

68

Inflammation in Heart Failure: Pathophysiology and Therapeutic Strategies

Jayagopal PB

ABSTRACT

Heart failure (HF) is emerging as a significant entity that needs to be tackled by physicians. Though many pathophysiological entities such as ischemic heart disease, hypertension, diabetes, and chronic kidney disease all contribute to the development of heart failure; the focus has mostly been on the effects of renin-angiotensin and sympathetic pathways. The present-day therapy is centered around addressing this axis. However, a lot of development has occurred in the field of systemic inflammation. The advancements in the studies contributing to inflammation in heart failure are increasing. The present chapter describes the current understanding of the pathogenesis of inflammation in heart failure and various strategies that could be utilized to address this.

Keywords: Inflammation, heart failure, inflammatory biomarkers

INTRODUCTION

Heart failure (HF) has been known to be associated with systemic inflammation.[1] It is not only thought to be responsible for the development of HF but also found to be associated with progression. Many studies have looked into this and tried therapies with little success. Traditionally, the symptom status and ejection fraction by imaging were thought to be predictors of poor outcomes.[2] Present-day studies on HFpEF and inflammation as a cause and target for therapy are gaining acceptance.

Inflammation in HF has been observed both in acute and chronic states. One measure routinely employed in clinical trials is the C-reactive protein (CRP) and high-sensitive CRP (hsCRP). The TIME-CHF trial had elevated mean hsCRP levels of 6.6 and 8.5 mg/mL in both reduced and preserved HF groups.[3] The RELAX trial also had a high percentage of elevated CRP.[4] Acute HF patients were also noticed to have higher hsCRP levels.[5] HFpEF has been found to have higher hsCRP levels and inflammation compared to HFrEF.[6] Thus, the newer studies target this subgroup of HF patients.

PATHOPHYSIOLOGICAL MECHANISMS

Many newer and novel markers are being studied in HF **(Box 1)**. These act by stimulating key pathways and activating inflammatory cytokines **(Flowchart 1)**.

Tumor Necrosis Factor

Experimental studies have shown that infusions of TNF-α produce left ventricular (LV) dysfunction through its negative inotropic effects.[7] This is known to impair both systolic and

BOX 1 Biomarkers and heart failure.

Inflammatory biomarkers:
- ESR/CRP
- Neutrophils
- Cytokines—IL-1, IL-6, IL-8, IL-18, IL-1β, IL-1RA, and IL-33
- Uric acid
- Galectin-3
- RAAS biomarkers—angiotensin II and aldosterone
- Natriuretic peptides—BNP and NT-proBNP

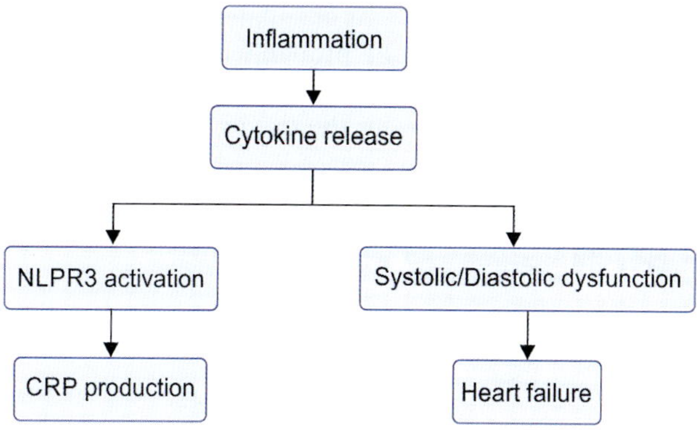

FLOWCHART 1: Pathophysiological mechanism of inflammation.

TABLE: 1: Role of other organs in inflammation.

Organs	Pro-inflammatory cytokines
Kidney	IL-6, RAS activation
Brain	TNF-α
Lungs	C-reactive protein, interleukins (IL-1-β, IL-6, IL-8, and IL-12), chemokines, and TNF-α
Skeletal muscle	TNF-α, IL-1β, IL-6, IL-2, and sphingosine, and angiotensin II
Intestine	IL-6 and TNF-α
Liver	IL-6
Adipose tissue	TNF-α, IL-6, IL-1β, and MCP-1

diastolic function and is reversible. Many mechanisms, such as the uncoupling of beta-adrenergic receptors and depletion of intracellular calcium, are responsible. Myocardial hypertrophy and fibrosis are also implicated through activation of metalloproteinases.[8] However, some beneficial effects in preventing cell death have also been noticed through the effect on nuclear factor kappa B, which is a key effector of TNF.[9]

Interleukin-1

This is an established signaling pathway for reducing systolic and diastolic function through the effects on calcium channels. Beta-adrenergic receptors are desensitized; thus, the ill effects lead to systolic dysfunction. The contractile reserve is also affected due to the impairment of calcium reuptake.[10,11]

Interleukin-6

Interleukin-6 (IL-6) as a target has recently been identified based on the mechanism in the liver through inflammasome activation NLRP3, thus leading to the production of CRP.[12]

Endothelium

Endothelial inflammation leads to a reduction in NO release and a decrease in protein kinase G activity, which, in turn, affects the function of the titin-binding protein. The wall tension then increases, leading to diastolic dysfunction. Adhesion molecules are also implicated, leading to collagen deposition and stiffness. All these are conceptually good targets for HFpEF therapy.[13]

Immune System

Both humoral and innate immunity are affected in HF. Damaged host cells and pathogens release damage-associated molecular patterns (DAMP) and pathogen-associated molecular patterns (PAMP). These are recognized by specific ligands on the cardiac myocytes-pattern recognition receptors (TLR4), and the interaction and signaling lead to cytokine and inflammasome activation (NLRP3). The clinical picture is high hsCRP.[14]

Anticardiac antibodies against beta-adrenergic receptors, troponin, and myosin have all been observed. It has been seen in 60% of nonischemic cardiomyopathy and end-stage HF patients; in LV assist device patients, this is as high as 90%.[15] Once removed by immunoadsorption, the cardiac index improves. Combined free light chains kappa and lambda are high in HF. This is responsible for cardiac apoptosis.[16]

Role of Other Organs in Heart Failure

It is now recognized that there is interaction between various organs and crosstalk responsible for HF, particularly in HFpEF groups with many comorbidities. It is interesting to note that proinflammatory cytokines, immune response, and adipose tissue all contribute **(Table 1)**.[17,18]

High PET FDG uptake in postmyocardial infarction (MI) has opened research in HF. Proinflammatory cytokines may be showered from the spleen and migrate to the heart. Splenectomy in such cases has been shown to increase EF.[19]

Obesity has long been documented as a source of various cytokines, including IL-1, IL-6, and TNF. Visceral fat is recognized as a source of inflammatory pathways, and this clinical expression is a novel target of HFpEF.[20]

PULMONARY VASCULATURE AND HYPERTENSION

Pulmonary arterial hypertension is often associated with HF in both reduced and preserved groups (75% and 83%, respectively), as shown by Lam et al., many factors such as high left-sided pressures, passive increase, and pulsatile distension are contributory.[21,22] Many inflammatory markers such as IL-1, IL-6, CRP, and TNF-α are elevated in PH.[23] Macrophage migration inhibitory factor (MIF) is known to be elevated and associated with a bad prognosis.[24]

SKELETAL MUSCLE

Cachexia seen in HF is due to skeletal muscle wasting. Apoptosis and muscle atrophy, like in inflammatory conditions, are also seen. All these have been associated with increased IL-6, TNF, and angiotensin II.[25,26]

KIDNEYS

Present-day therapy revolves around sodium absorption and SGLT-2I treatment. The epithelial sodium channel (ENaC) is responsible, and elevated IL-6 levels have been associated with diuretic resistance.[27] As seen in some studies, AKI and cardiorenal syndrome may all be related to high IL-6 levels.[28] The various hemodynamic effects in HF are known to be a source of inflammation and thus lead to high levels of IL-6, TNF, and angiotensin II release. Mitochondrial dysfunction and NRLP3 activation are key steps.[29]

Gastrointestinal System

Heart failure leads to gut mucosal ischemia through low cardiac output or venous congestion.[30] This alters gut permeability and leads to endotoxin release. This stimulates the release of various inflammatory markers such as IL-6 and TNF through the activation of TLR4. All these trigger systemic inflammation. Gut microbiomes are affected, and studies have shown the depletion of butyrate-producing bacteria. This has anti-inflammatory effects and regulates T cells. Modifying this gut microbiome is a potential target in HF therapy.[31]

INFLAMMATION AND TREATMENT OF HEART FAILURE

Guideline-directed Medical Therapy

This is the cornerstone of HFrEF treatment, which is done through the RAS and sympathetic pathway.[32] It has been clearly shown that these lead to a reduction in inflammatory markers. Angiotensin II is implicated in inflammation. It has been observed that enalapril reduces IL-6 levels post-MI, thus preventing LV remodeling. Olmesartan in hypertension treatment reduces CRP levels. The use of ACE leads to a 2.6-fold decrease in CRP levels.[33] Recently, angiotensin receptor neprilysin inhibitor therapy has been shown to reduce IL-6 and metalloproteinase levels. Treatment with ARNI is also known to decrease sST2 in the PIONEER-HF trial.[34] However, no direct effects on inflammation have been proven. Similarly, mineralocorticoid receptor stimulation has been associated with releasing inflammatory markers. MRA has no effect on CRP and uric acid. Data on anti-inflammatory agents is not precise. However, studies showing positive effects are lacking.[35] β-blocker therapy in dilated cardiomyopathy patients has shown a reduction in TNF. It is known to reduce IL-1 and IL-6. However, the best evidence is a reduction in CRP levels.[36] As elucidated earlier, the newer SGLT-2 inhibition in HFpEF probably has some effects by reducing inflammatory markers. About 10 of 12 studies showed decreased CRP with the use of SGLT-2. However, the mechanism is not very clear.[37]

STATINS

This reduces inflammatory markers like CRP, as shown in the JUPITER trial.[38] The NO release and improvement in endothelial function are contributory. The release of inflammatory markers is evident. Though initial observational studies in post-MI had shown a 26% reduction in hospitalization with atorvastatin, studies with rosuvastatin have provided only neutral results.[39] The UNIVERSE and CORONA studies showed no improvement in LV function, mortality benefits or reduction in HF hospitalizations.[40,41] The same results came from the GISSI-HF study.[42]

Xanthine Oxidase Inhibitors

Uric acid is supposed to activate the inflammasomes and lead to an increase in IL-6.[43] However, studies with allopurinol or oxypurinol have not been encouraging. There was not only a mortality benefit, but the quality of life and exercise capacity did not improve.[44]

Methotrexate

The first evidence that methotrexate is an anti-inflammatory agent came from studies in rheumatoid arthritis, where there was a reduction in CV events. However, there was no reduction in HFH. Moreover, smaller trials with methotrexate in ischemic cardiomyopathy did not reduce CRP or IL-6 levels.[45]

Colchicine

The efficacy of colchicine as an anti-inflammatory agent is unquestionable. The latest trials in MI provide ample proof of that (COLCOT and LODOCOT).[46,47] However, in the context of HF studies, no significant decrease in CRP levels has been shown in HF.[48] Moreover, this cannot be used in the cardiorenal subset, which is frequent in HF. This indicates that despite colchicine therapy, there is a residual inflammatory risk.[49]

ANTI-TUMOR NECROSIS FACTOR THERAPY

Though the role of TNF is well established in HF, the usage of anti-TNF agents has been dismal. The RENEWAL and ATTACH trials showed no benefit and, on the contrary, increased mortality and hospitalization. There are many theories concerning this, perhaps related to the usage of dosage medications.[50,51]

Anti-interleukin-1 Therapy

The first study was in a small number of patients with rheumatoid arthritis. Anakinra therapy was found to be associated with greater recovery of LV function.[52] Similar effects of anakinra in acute decompensated HF treated with daily injections were seen.[53] These are encouraging studies, but more extensive randomized trials are needed. Similar results with IL-2/IL-23 inhibition are observed in small studies. Ustekinumab was found to improve the global longitudinal strain.[54]

Interleukin-1β signaling has been implicated in the pathogenesis of HF, and elevated concentrations of IL-1β through its effect on NLRP3 inflammasome is known to reduce LV systolic function. Thus, inhibition of this pathway helps improve LV function. A subanalysis of the CANTOS trial has shown a 38% reduction in HF hospitalization and a 32% reduction in death and HFH. This is really encouraging.[55]

Interleukin-6 Inhibition

One of the significant developments in research has been the IL-6 pathway activating the NLRP3 inflammasome and thus leading to elevated CRP. The results from the RESCUE study showed that ziltivekimab, a human monoclonal antibody against IL-6, reduces high-sensitivity CRP in patients with high atherosclerotic risk.[56] The ongoing HERMES trial using the monoclonal antibody ziltivekimab in HFpEF would also shed light on this.

GLUCAGON-LIKE PEPTIDE-1 AGONISTS

The SELECT trial has opened up a lot of interest in HF therapy. Semaglutide, an antidiabetic drug, was used in obesity and now has shown promising data in HFpEF through its anti-inflammatory efficacy. This has opened up avenues in HF research, particularly in inflammatory pathways.[57]

CONCLUSION

Inflammation is present in both acute and chronic HF. The interaction between various organs and systems contributes to the severity of HF. Many newer and novel biomarkers are being investigated in HF to improve diagnosis, enhance prognosis, and optimize treatment monitoring. Inflammation plays a crucial role in the pathophysiology of HF. Targeting inflammation has emerged as a promising therapeutic strategy for HF treatment.

ONLINE REFERENCES

Please scan the QR code provided at the end of the table of contents for References of this chapter.

CHAPTER

69

Aging-associated Cardiovascular Changes and Their Relationship to Heart Failure

Vijaya Kumar Varada, Bhanu Duggal, Rupendra Nath Saha

ABSTRACT

The aging population is increasing across the world, especially in developed countries, and the management of their illness significantly differs compared to their counterpart and requires special attention in terms of diagnosis, treatment, and prognosis. Most of the trials include the age group of 18–75 years for the management of hypertension, heart failure (HF), and coronary artery disease. Very few trials are performed in the aging population and their management options are highly individualized and beyond the scope of this chapter. However, most common aging-related cardiovascular system disorders are covered along with their anatomical factors, physiology, pathology, aging markers, diagnostic modalities, and management.

Keywords: Aging population, cardiovascular disorders, pathophysiology in aging, biomarkers, comorbidities management, polypharmacy, medication adherence

INTRODUCTION

As per the National Commission on Population of India, the proportion of elderly individuals in the population was 8–9% in 2011 and could potentially rise to 18% by 2036. Due to the world's growing aging population, 34 countries are predicted to have >20% of their population over 65 years by 2030. An important resource for any society is the elderly people.

There is no accurate definition for age limit and aging process. It depends on chronological, social, and functional factors. Defining the elderly as age >65 years was based on socioeconomic and political decisions. Since aging is a progressive biological process, it was often thought to start when a person could no longer actively contribute to society. In developing nations such as India, old age is mostly defined by societal roles.

PATHOPHYSIOLOGY

Cardiomyocyte Death and Regeneration

Research has shown that the rate of renewal of adult cardiomyocytes ranges from 0.5 to 2% annually. It was discovered that this regeneration decreased with age, suggesting a reduced capacity to offset the loss of cardiomyocytes.[1]

Mitochondrial Dysfunction

In addition to providing the heart muscle ATP, mitochondria also play a critical role in controlling cardiomyocyte survival. One of the main characteristics of cardiac aging is mitochondrial dysfunction, which is the intersection of several important senescence-related processes. HF may be mostly caused by the general decrease in mitochondrial activity that comes with aging of the heart, which raises the formation of reactive oxygen species (ROS).[2]

Cellular Senescence and Inflammation

Cells experiencing cellular senescence endure irreversible cell cycle arrest, functional decline, and the acquisition of a proinflammatory phenotype. This state is brought on by telomere attrition as a result of repetitive replication or by other types of cellular stress. Senescent cells gradually build up in tissues over the course of life and have negative paracrine effects on nearby cells as well as systemic impacts on adjacent tissues and organs. The senescence-associated secretory phenotype (SASP), which is responsible for the release of insoluble extracellular matrix components, proteases, and proinflammatory cytokines, mediates these effects. In addition to promoting inflammation, SASP signaling also causes cell death and senescence in other cells.[3,4]

MOLECULAR MECHANISMS OF HEART FAILURE DURING AGING

Telomere Shortening and Damage

Telomeres are repeats of deoxyribonucleic acid (DNA) that act as protective ends for chromosomes. The enzyme telomerase, which is made up of a catalytic subunit (TERT) and an RNA component (TERC), is responsible for creating telomeres. Around 104 telomeres shorten in response to oxidative stress, inflammation, and aging, as well as other stresses. Extremely short telomeres cause DNA damage, cellular senescence, and cell death by destabilizing the shelterin complex and upsetting the telomeric DNA structure.[2,5]

Secreted Factors

In the chronic systemic inflammation leading to HF, the role of proinflammatory SASP factors like IL-1α, IL-1β, IL-6, and CXCL1 has been thoroughly studied.[1,6]

Epigenetic Mutations

The term "epigenetics" describes somatically acquired changes in gene function that arise from modifications in DNA methylation, histone modifications, or chromatin remodeling rather than from variations in DNA sequence. As a defining feature of aging, epigenetic modifications probably have a role in cardiac aging and cardiovascular illness in general.[1,6]

Noncoding Ribonucleic Acid

Functional RNA molecules that are transcribed from DNA but not translated into proteins are known as noncoding RNAs (ncRNAs). Endogenous tiny ncRNAs known as microRNAs (miRNAs) are around 22 nucleotides long and function as post-transcriptional regulators by attaching to messenger RNA (mRNA) to either promote or hinder mRNA translation. It has been discovered that many miRNAs play pathophysiological roles in HF.[1]

Somatic Deoxyribonucleic Acid Mutations

Over time, somatic DNA mutations accumulate in various tissues, serving as both a marker of aging and a possible cause of heart illnesses and aging. Mitochondrial DNA has a limited capacity for repair and a high rate of mutation can lead to cardiac cellular aging. Perhaps the most well-researched somatic DNA mutations in cardiac aging and disease, around 170 mitochondrial genetic mutations affect mitochondrial biogenesis and raise free radical production.[1,2]

TABLE 1: Structural changes in cardiac myocardium in young versus aged people.

Tissue	Young myocardium	Aged myocardium
Vascularity	Normal	Reduced
Myofibril number	More	Relatively less
Size of myofibril	Less	Relatively large
Collagen	Less	Abundant
Fibrous tissue	Scarce	Plenty
Inflammation	Less	More

AGING-RELATED CARDIOVASCULAR SYSTEM CHANGES

- *Structural changes*: Vascular stiffening, increased left ventricular (LV) wall thickness and fibrosis, leading to diastolic dysfunction and increased afterload **(Table 1)**
- *Functional changes*: Variations in the maximum heart rate, sympathetic signaling, contractility, extended diastolic relaxation, prolonged systolic contraction, and end-systolic volume (ESV and EDV)
- Decreased baroreceptor sensitivity leading to increased risk of orthostatic hypotension with vasodilators
- Increased LV stiffness and peripheral vascular resistance decrease cardiac output with beta blockers.
- Decreased cardiac reserve with exacerbation of HF due to CCBs
- SA and AV node dysfunction
- Decreased body mass, water, albumin, glycoproteins, and increased body fat.[7-9]

FUNCTIONAL CHANGES IN CARDIOVASCULAR SYSTEM

Changes in aerobic capacity and cardiac regulation between the age group of 20 and 80 years in healthy men and women include oxygen consumption ↓(50%), (A-V)O_2 ↓(25%), cardiac index ↓(25%), heart rate ↓(25%), no change in stroke volume, preload EDV ↓(30%), vascular (PVR) ↑(30%), cardiac (ESV) ↑(275%), LV contractility ↓(60%), ejection fraction ↓(15%), plasma catecholamines ↑, cardiac and vascular responses to β-adrenergic stimulation decreases.[3]

Age-related ECG changes—no change in RR interval, P-wave duration minor increase, PR interval increase, no change in QRS duration, QRS axis leftward shift, QRS voltage decrease, QT interval minor increase, T wave voltage decrease.[2]

BIOMARKERS IN AGING

In HF BNP, NT-proBNP, troponin, and CKMB are usual biomarkers that are evaluated for diagnosis, prognosis, and follow-up. However, there are so many other biomarkers that increase in the aging population.[10,11]

Adipokines

Obesity is understood to represent a low-level chronic inflammatory state. Adipokines are proinflammatory cytokines, such as apelin, adiponectin, chemerin, resistin, RBP4, vaspin, visfatin, leptin, omentin-1, LCN-2, and FSTL1 which have been linked to the onset and course of HF in obese patients.[12,13]

Resistin

Serum resistin is primarily released by macrophages, monocytes, and bone marrow. It has a role in multiple processes, such as atherothrombosis, vascular smooth muscle cell proliferation, and endothelial dysfunction, which can lead to the development of hypertension and coronary artery disease.[14]

Erythropoietin

Multifactorial factors like suppression of erythropoiesis in the bone marrow resulting from the chronic inflammatory state associated with HF and bone marrow resistance to endogenous erythropoietin may be the cause of high erythropoietin levels. Increased mortality was correlated with both chronically elevated erythropoietin levels and elevated baseline erythropoietin levels.[15]

Renin–Angiotensin–Aldosterone System

By promoting inflammation, cell growth, and ROS generation at cellular and mitochondrial levels, angiotensin II regulates energy metabolism and affects the onset and progression of cell senescence. Chronic activation of renin–angiotensin–aldosterone system (RAAS) promotes end-stage organ injury, justifying the use of angiotensin-converting enzyme (ACE) inhibitor and angiotensin II receptor blockers (ARBs), which reduce age-associated cardiovascular, renal, and brain damage and preserve mitochondria function.[10,16]

Senescence Marker Protein 30 and Molecular Pathways

Senescence marker protein 30 (SMP30), which is ubiquitously expressed in human organs and preserved across species, has recently been identified as another player in cardioprotection in the setting of aging-associated myocardial changes. They also demonstrated that SMP30 deficiency leads to increased myocardial oxidative stress concomitant with increased NADPH oxidase activity. SMP30, therefore, may tip the redox balance in the aging heart **(Flowchart 1)**.[17]

MANAGEMENT

Hypertension in Aging

An increased systolic blood pressure, widening pulse pressure, and lowered diastolic blood pressure are frequently indicative of the increased wall stiffness and tortuosity of the aorta and major arteries with aging. Increased left atrial dimension, decreased cardiovascular response to catecholamines, decreased LV diastolic volume and filling rate, increased peripheral resistance, decreased baroreceptor sensitivity, and increased characteristic aortic impedance at rest are all more common in older adults with hypertension.[8,9]

A diet with low sodium (<2 g/day) is recommended for the treatment of hypertension in the elderly. A diet high in fruits, vegetables, and low-fat dairy products with less saturated and total fat is recommended, along with quitting

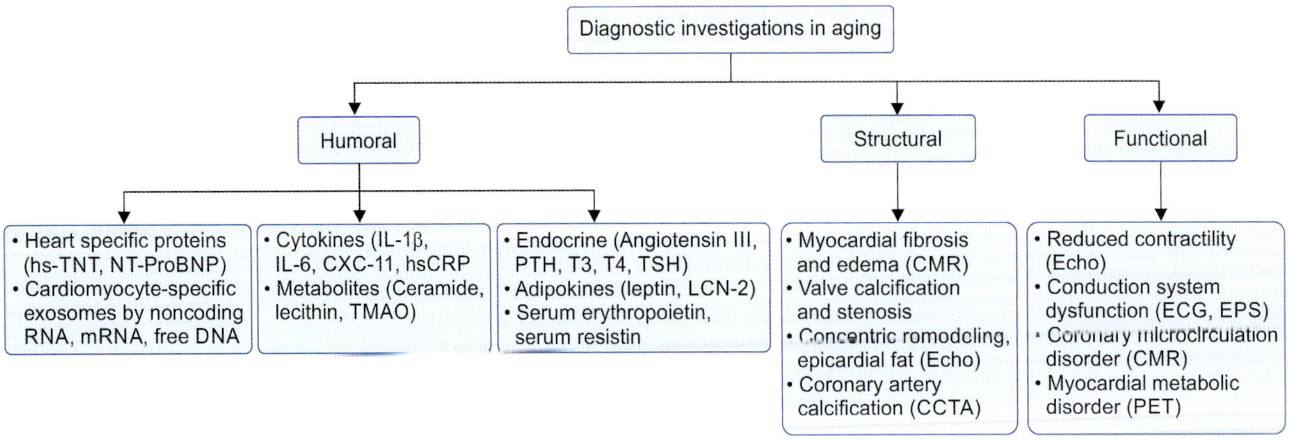

FLOWCHART 1: Humoral, functional, and structural changes of cardiovascular system in the aged population with necessary investigations.

smoking, engaging in regular aerobic exercise, avoiding excessive caffeine, nonsteroidal anti-inflammatory drugs, and glucocorticoids.[7,8]

Patients with diastolic dysfunction who have angina pectoris, myocardial ischemia, complicated ventricular arrhythmias, supraventricular tachyarrhythmias, hypertension, or a history of myocardial infarction may benefit from beta-blocker medication. Patients with diabetes mellitus, atherosclerotic vascular disease, hypertension, and LV hypertrophy are treated with ACE inhibitors, ARNI, or ARBs. Twenty-four-hour ambulatory BP-guided hypertension management and preference to short-acting drugs may decrease the common side effects like syncope and frequent falls observed in this age group.[7,11]

Systolic Heart Failure in Aging Management

Angiotensin-converting Enzyme Inhibitors

According to the recent AHA/ESC guidelines, every patient with LV systolic dysfunction with EF < 40% and HF symptoms should be on ACE inhibitors. Since most patients with LV ejection fractions between 10 and 15% are prone to orthostatic hypotension, it appears that this is the limiting factor when it comes to titrating ACE inhibitors as some degree of autonomic dysfunction also present as a result of other comorbidities with severe LV failure. Since ACE inhibitors are better tolerable when patients are supine, taking them prior to bedtime is preferred. The dose of ACE inhibitors should be decreased when a higher dose of diuretics is used in patients with refractory fluid retention rather than completely stopping them.[10,16]

Angiotensin II Receptor Blockers

Angiotensin II receptor blockers are not evaluated in as many trials as ACE inhibitors; however, recent trials advise using them in patients who are not tolerating ACE inhibitors. Patients who were unable to tolerate the prescribed ACE inhibitors are moved to ARBs (reduction in mortality in the CHARM-Alternative trial). The Val-HeFT (Valsartan Heart Failure Trial) observed a similar benefit, indicating a possible medication class impact.[11,16]

Aldosterone Antagonists

Guidelines state that in patients with reduced LV systolic function, an aldosterone antagonist (spironolactone or eplerenone) should be administered when the patient is stable on beta blockers and ACE inhibitors. It is important to remember that older patients may experience more adverse effects because their baseline renal perfusion is typically lower, and they are more likely to develop hyperkalemia if they are already taking high dosages of ACE inhibitors or ARB. According to the ACC/AHA/ESC, electrolytes and creatinine should be measured 1 week after starting treatment and then every 3 months after that. The routine should thereafter be restarted anytime a patient's medical condition changes.[16]

Beta Blockers

It is recommended that bisoprolol, carvedilol, and sustained-release metoprolol are efficacious in treating HF in the elderly. Rather than stopping beta blockers completely in hospitalized ADHF patients, it should be continued at the same dose or with the amount reduced by half. It has been demonstrated that ivabradine reduces the risk of HF hospitalization in patients with sinus rhythm, LV ejection fraction < 35%, heart rate > 70 beats/min, and NYHA classes II–IV symptoms.

Diuretics

It is advised that the patients take low-dose diuretics and follow a salt-restricted diet (<2 g/day) rather than using high doses of diuretics. In ADHF patients, thiazide diuretics and loop diuretics work synergistically and can be a useful combination. Diuretics do not appear to reduce mortality in long-term trials.

ATRIAL FIBRILLATION IN AGING POPULATION

Elderly AF is also linked to an increased risk of consequences like HF and stroke. The risk of an ischemic stroke is raised by AF on its own by a factor of 4–5. All cardiovascular risk factors have a decreasing risk of stroke with age, with the exception of AF, which has an increasing risk of stroke from 1.5% for people in their sixth decade to 23.5% for those in their ninth decade. Compared to other causes of stroke, AF-related strokes are more deadly, more severe, and more likely to recur.[8,9]

Decision-making between rate and rhythm management is one of the most important therapy decisions. In order to determine the best course of action for AF patients, six significant trials have been conducted. The AFFIRM and HOT CAFÉ trials suggested that rate control was superior to the rhythm control technique; however, the STAF trial displayed a contrary pattern, whereas the PIAF and RACE trials did not demonstrate any variation. The incidence of ischemic strokes and all-cause mortality did not differ between the rate and rhythm control strategies, according to a meta analysis of the first five trials.

Procainamide, dofetilide, and sotalol are mainly eliminated by the kidneys. Either these drugs should be avoided altogether or their dosages should be changed in accordance with the severity of renal impairment, given the increased incidence of renal dysfunction in the aged population. Adipose tissue is the distribution site for the lipophilic medication amiodarone. Amiodarone has a greater volume of distribution, lesser clearance, and a longer elimination half-life in the elderly due to the age-related increase in body fat. Amiodarone with warfarin, digoxin, or quinidine has significant medication interactions that can increase their plasma levels and risk for toxicity, particularly when AF is present in older adults.

Amiodarone increases warfarin's anticoagulant action, necessitating a decrease in the medication's dosage. The elderly have higher serum digoxin concentrations because they have higher total body fat, less muscular mass, and less total body water. Digoxin is also less effectively eliminated by the kidneys as a result of an age-related decrease in the glomerular filtration rate, which lengthens the drug's half-life. Concomitant use of other frequently recommended medications in the elderly, including quinidine, verapamil, warfarin, and diuretics, also raises the levels of digoxin.

The $CHADS_2$ stroke risk index formula includes congestive HF, hypertension, age over 75 years, diabetes, and past cerebral ischemia, all of which were previously found to be independent risk factors for stroke. Previously patients with AF are categorized into low-, intermediate-, and high-risk groups for stroke according to their $CHADS_2$ score. These groups correspond to adjusted yearly stroke rates of 1.9%, 2.8%, and >4%, respectively. In recent years, $CHADS_2$-VASc scores of 0, 1, and ≥2, respectively, are used to classify people into low-, intermediate-, and high-risk categories. These scores translate into adjusted yearly stroke risks of 0%, 0.7%, and >1.9%, respectively. This new scoring method means that elderly individuals with AF who are above 75 years of age will be at high risk for stroke and will need to take oral anticoagulant (OAC) therapy even in the absence of additional risk factors.

Oral anticoagulants are superior to aspirin or combined therapy with clopidogrel (75 mg/day) and aspirin (75–100 mg/day), as shown by several trials. Antiplatelet medicine, in contrast to OACs, appears to be ineffective in preventing strokes after the age of 80 years, and its relative effectiveness for reducing cardiovascular events and stroke declines noticeably with age. This is probably because antiplatelet medications mostly protect against noncardioembolic causes of stroke, which account for 24% of stroke cases in patients with AF, while OACs largely prevent cardioembolic strokes. Antiplatelet medications' ability to prevent strokes is significantly reduced in older adults with AF as the percentage of noncardioembolic strokes declines.

Newer oral anticoagulants, including dabigatran, rivaroxaban, apixaban, and edoxaban, have been recommended for the prevention of thromboembolism in AF. Over the past decade, catheter ablation for AF has emerged as an important treatment option for patients with AF.

POLYPHARMACY IN ELDERLY PEOPLE

A universal definition is presently not available, although polypharmacy is defined as greater than five medications in studies. From 2015 onward, there have been many new groups of drugs recommended for HF management, which improve mortality and morbidity benefits for the patients. This resulted in prescribing a cascade of medication to improve HF outcomes and symptoms, increasing polypharmacy. Especially for HF, four groups of drugs are recommended including beta blockers, SGLT-2 inhibitors, ARNIs, and aldosterone antagonists. Elderly patients had a high risk of AKI, postural hypotension, syncope, and falls leading to fractures. Gradual uptitration of drugs starting at the lowest dose and adding each group of drug weekly may improve medication adherence and prevent side effects.[18]

CONCLUSION

Aging-related cardiovascular disorders and their management are beyond the scope of this chapter. Trials are to be conducted targeting the aged group and separate guidelines need to be published. Common comorbidities like hypertension management significantly differ in terms of recommended diet, target lowering of BP, 24-hour ambulatory BP-guided medical management and judicious use of vasodilators, RAAS inhibitors, beta blockers, and diuretics. Guideline-directed medical therapy for heart failure management guidelines may not be applicable to the aged population, especially those with >75 years of age, and their treatment is highly individualized. Polypharmacy and medication defaulter groups are a major drawback in view of multiorgan involvement and are to be addressed by basic specialties like geriatric medicine and internal medicine. Family support (economically and physically), diet, symptom-directed therapy, palliative management, geriatric physiotherapy, yoga, AYUSH, and naturopathy play a key role in the management of various disorders in the aged population along with medications.

ONLINE REFERENCES

Please scan the QR code provided at the end of the table of contents for References of this chapter.

CHAPTER 70

Statins and Heart Failure: What is the Evidence

Ankit Kumar Sahu, Aditya Kapoor

ABSTRACT

The "cholesterol paradox" in heart failure patients may not be due to advanced heart failure and may not have a significant role in adverse outcomes. Studies such as CORONA and GISSI-HF show that predicting drug efficacy from observational studies doesn't always lead to predictable clinical results. Statins may not show a survival benefit once heart failure is established, as cardiac tissue is too advanced to be modified. Therefore, it is recommended to initiate statins in patients with ischemic heart failure with NYHA Class II–III symptoms.

Keywords: Heart failure, CORONA, GISSI-HF

INTRODUCTION

Statins are a standard part of the therapeutic toolbox for management of coronary artery disease. Apart from their lipid-lowering abilities, statins also have multiple pleiotropic effects that impact neurohormonal activation and cardiac remodeling. In keeping with this, previous large observational studies, registries, and post hoc analyses of primary and secondary prevention trials indicated that statins may be beneficial for the prevention and treatment of heart failure (HF). Although subsequently, two prospective, randomized controlled trials (RCTs) demonstrated that rosuvastatin did not confer any survival advantage in patients with chronic systolic HF, these results should not be interpreted as a universal justification to avoid statins in patients with HF. Low total cholesterol (TC) is reported to be an independent predictor of impaired survival in patients with HF. Similar association of low cholesterol with adverse outcomes has also been noted in patients with sepsis, trauma, postsurgery, multiple organ failure, chronic kidney disease, and the elderly.[1,2] While evidence does suggest that low TC is associated with higher mortality and morbidity in patients with HF, this seems to be *secondary to the underlying patient milieu rather than an independent risk factor of poor outcomes. The Korean registry*[3] *and the recent Lipid Association of India (LAI) guidelines*[1] summarize that low cholesterol may merely be a consequence of advanced HF and have no pathophysiological role in genesis of adverse outcomes related to HF.

The chapter shall focus on the following:
- Data of statins in HF from observational nonrandomized studies and previous primary and secondary prevention trials
- CORONA and GISSI-HF trials and possible reasons for lack of benefit
- Which subset of HF patients would benefit?
- Meta-analysis of statins in HF
- Statins and HF with preserved ejection fraction (HFpEF)
- Guidelines and messages

DATA OF STATINS IN HF FROM OBSERVATIONAL NONRANDOMIZED STUDIES AND PRIMARY AND SECONDARY PREVENTION TRIALS

The rationale of considering statins in HF stems from the fact that a large percentage of patients with LV dysfunction and CHF have underlying CAD and many of these patients have had a myocardial infarction (MI) in the past. Statins are known to reduce the risk of (MI) in primary- and secondary-prevention populations and due to reduction in both first and recurrent ischemic events they also reduce the development of HF.[5-9] Benefits are due to cholesterol lowering and pleiotropic effects of stains, including anti-inflammatory actions, reduction of inflammatory cytokines, reduction of oxidative stress, and improved endothelial function.

Observational Nonrandomized Studies

- Amongst 551 patients with ischemic and nonischemic systolic HF, Horwich et al. reported that statins significantly improved survival (91% vs. 72%, $p < 0.001$) and need for urgent cardiac transplantation (81% vs. 63%, $p < 0.001$ at 1-year).[10]
- The population-based, retrospective Ontario cohort study of approximately 30,000 patients reported that statins when administered to those with newly diagnosed HF (as compared to those with established, long-standing HF), resulted in significant reduction in all-cause mortality (HR 0.67; 95% CI 0.57–0.78).[11]
- Post hoc analysis of the ELITE II database demonstrated that of the 5,200 patients with ischemic and nonischemic HF, significant improvement in survival was noted with statin therapy in both groups.[12]
- Examination of 61,939 US Medicare beneficiaries (≥65 years of age and hospitalized with a primary diagnosis of HF between 1998 and 2001) found that statin prescribed at discharge was associated with significant improvement in mortality at 1-year (HR 0.80; 95% CI 0.76–0.84) and 3-year mortality (HR 0.82; 95% CI 0.79–0.85).[13]
- In a retrospective analysis of the VAL-HeFt trial, Krum et al. reported that all-cause mortality was significantly reduced in patients on statins compared with those who were not (17.9% vs. 20.3%, $p = 0.029$).[14] A similar analysis of the CIBIS-II study, also revealed that statin use was an independent predictor of benefit in HF (HR 0.60; 95% CI 0.39–0.94; $p < 0.05$). Survival was greatest in patients on statin plus bisoprolol as compared to those only on bisoprolol (98.3% vs. 87.2%).[15]

Data from Previous Primary and Secondary Prevention Randomized Controlled Trials

In a meta-analysis of 17 trials with 132,538 patients from various primary and secondary prevention RCTs, *statins were found to modestly reduce the risks of nonfatal HF hospitalizations* (RR 0.90; 95%, CI 0.84–0.97), *and the composite HF outcomes* (RR 0.92; 95% CI 0.85–0.99) *but not HF death* (RR 0.97; 95% CI 0.80–1.17).[16] The benefit on first nonfatal hospitalization for HF was similar whether this was preceded by MI or not. The overall extent of risk reduction was, however, modest (10%), and far lower than the robust benefits on other CHD outcomes.

Message

Collectively, these data from older RCTs and various observational studies provide *"reasonable evidence" that statin use can prevent or delay the onset of HF*, especially when used early in patients at risk of HF (stages A and B, including stable CAD or those with previous/history of ACS). However the following *need to be considered*:

- Many of these primary and secondary prevention trials did not include patients with severe HF and the HF endpoints varied amongst different trials, with some reporting HF death and others reporting nonfatal HF hospitalization, and/or a composite of fatal and nonfatal HF events.
- It is also possible that the benefit attributed to statins was merely a marker of appropriate drug prescription, rather than a direct drug effect. This is supported by the observation that in primary care settings, statin treated subjects are 1.5 times more likely to receive a β-blocker or an ACEI and five times more likely to receive a combination of both than those not on statins.

CORONA AND GISSI-HF TRIALS AND POSSIBLE REASONS FOR LACK OF BENEFIT

- The CORONA (Controlled Rosuvastatin Multinational trial in Heart Failure) included 5,011 patients (≥60 years of age), with ischemic systolic HF, LVEF < 40% (mean 31%), NYHA class II–III (~63% in class III) and randomly assigned them to either 10 mg rosuvastatin ($n = 2,514$) or placebo ($n = 2,497$).[17] At a median follow-up of 32.8 months, there was no significant reduction in the primary endpoint (a composite of CV death, nonfatal MI and nonfatal stroke, HR 0.92; CI 0.83–1.02; $p = 0.12$) or total deaths with rosuvastatin (HR 0.95; 95% CI 0.86–1.05; $p = 0.31$). However in a prespecified secondary analysis, there were fewer hospitalizations for cardiovascular causes in the rosuvastatin group (2,193) than in the placebo group (2,564) (25 vs. 22.9 events/100 patient-years $p < 0.001$). *The study concluded that despite having favorable biological effects (i.e., reduction in LDL-C, TG, and hsCRP and an increase in HDLc) and an acceptable safety profile in moderate-to-severe HF, the long-term clinical outcomes were unaffected.*
- The GISSI-HF (Gruppo italiano per lo studio della sopravvivenza nell'infarto miocardico-Heart Failure) included 4,564 patients (mean age 68 years, 44% >70 years), mean LVEF 33%, NYHA class II–IV (36% class III) with chronic systolic HF.[18] In contrast to the CORONA study, patients were younger, with mixed etiologies of HF (40% ischemic, 35% DCM, 18% HT), had less advanced HF (37% in NYHA class III–IV) and 10% had LVEF > 40%. At a median of 3.9 years, although

there was reduction in LDL-C and hsCRP, there was no reduction in the primary endpoints of time to death, and time to death or admission to hospital for CV reasons. Overall, 29% patients died from any cause in the rosuvastatin group versus 28% in the placebo group (adjusted HR 1.00, $p = 0.943$). In the rosuvastatin group, 57% patients died or were admitted to hospital for cardiovascular reasons compared to 56% in the placebo group (adjusted HR 1.01, $p = 0.903$). *Similar to what was reported by the CORONA study, the GISSI-HF study also established the safety of statins in patients with chronic systolic HF, but did not show any incremental benefits in reducing adverse clinical outcomes.*

Possible Reasons for Lack of Benefit in CORONA and GISSI-HF

- Patients were older and sicker; CORONA—mean age 73 years, 41% > 75 years, GISSSI-HF—mean age 68 years, 43% > 70 years and it was probable that many had established CAD. More than 60% in CORONA and 35% in GISSI-HF had NYHA class II–IV HF. Hence, the patients had moderate-to-severe symptomatic HF rather than symptomatic CAD.
- The annualized mortality was ~10% and ~7.4% in the CORONA and GISSI-HF, respectively.
- The majority of CV deaths was driven by worsening HF and sudden deaths, while the rate of nonfatal MI and stroke was relatively lower in this population.

Message

The plaque stabilization and pleiotropic effects of rosuvastatin are more likely to modify atherothrombotic vascular events such as MI and stroke rather than CV deaths/sudden death, possibly explaining its lack of benefit in the two studies. It is possible that these patients may have had atherosclerotic or myocardial disease that was too advanced to modify, and rosuvastatin might have had more favorable effect in patients with milder HF.

Pooled Data Analysis of Both Trials

Since most patients in CORONA and GISSI-HF experienced death from arrhythmic causes, worsening HF or non-cardiovascular causes, and the number of MI/strokes was low, the ability to detect a statistically significant benefit for statins may have been limited. Feinstein et al. pooled the data from the CORONA and GISSI-HF, to improve the power to detect any statistically significant differences in atherothrombotic events by competing risks analyses.[19] In this pooled analysis of CORONA study (all of whom had ischemic HF) and GISSI-HF study participants with ischemic etiology of HF, a 19% risk reduction in first incident MI's was observed (HR 0.81; 95% CI 0.66–0.99; $p < 0.05$) with rosuvastatin, with a number needed to treat to prevent one MI as 94. *This significant reduction in risk for MI amongst those with ischemic etiology of HF is consistent with previous findings of pooled data of non-HF patients.* However, the absolute risk reduction for MI was comparatively small since only a few patients actually had an MI due to their elevated risks from other causes of death.

WHICH SUBSET OF HF PATIENTS WOULD BENEFIT?

Two subanalysis of the CORONA study focused on the possibility of assessing a threshold point for cardiac biomarkers, below which, patients with HF would demonstrate a favorable outcome and greater benefit with rosuvastatin.

- Of the 5,011 patients enrolled in the CORONA study, 73% had an available NT-proBNP level, was measured in 3,664 (73%). Cleland et al. divided the patient population into tertiles of NT-proBNP (<868, 868–2,347, and > 2,347 pg/mL). Log NT-proBNP was the strongest predictor of clinical every outcome with the HR for death from worsening HF as 1.99; 95% CI 1.71–2.30.[20] *The maximum benefit with rosuvastatin was observed in patients in the lowest tertile of NT-proBNP (<868 pg/mL) with a 35% risk reduction in the primary endpoint* (HR 0.65; 95% CI 0.47–0.88). The effect was entirely driven by fewer MIs, strokes, and CV deaths in the lowest tertile, reflecting fewer atherothrombotic events with rosuvastatin. This benefit was seen independent of the effect of rosuvastatin on lipid profile and hsCRP in each tertile of NT-proBNP.
- Plasma galectin-3 which is part of the family of β-galactoside-binding lectins and plays a regulatory role in fibrogenesis, inflammation, and cell proliferation, is thought to be a marker for irreversible myocardial fibrosis and poor prognosis in HF. It was measured in 29% of the CORONA participants and Gullestad et al. reported that *patients with median galectin-3 (≤19.0 ng/mL), when assigned to rosuvastatin had lower primary event rate* (HR 0.65; 95% CI 0.46–0.92; $p = 0.014$), lower total mortality (HR 0.70; 95% CI 0.50–0.98; $p = 0.038$), and lower event rate of all-cause mortality and HF hospitalizations (HR 0.72; 95% CI 0.54–0.98; $p = 0.017$) compared with placebo.[21] No benefit was observed in patients with higher levels of galectin-3. *A combination of both low galectin-3 and NT-proBNP identified patients with the largest benefit with rosuvastatin* (HR 0.33; 95% CI 0.16–0.67; $p = 0.002$) reflecting the fact that a combination of biomarkers was perhaps a better prognostic marker.

Message

Although statins may not be harmful in patients with advanced HF and can be used in these patients on a case-to-case basis, maximum benefit of rosuvastatin was evident in those with less advanced HF. *Biomarkers such as*

NT-proBNP and galectin-3 can potentially help identify a subset of ischemic HF patients who might benefit from treatment with statins. Initiating statins early in the course of ischemic HF (when the biomarkers are not very high—tertile 1 of CORONA, NT-proBNP < 868 pg/mL, and galectin-3 ≤ 19.0 ng/mL), may be associated with maximum clinical benefit.

META-ANALYSIS OF STATINS IN HF

- In one of the earliest pooled estimate analysis of 13 studies of statins in HF (11 retrospective and 2 prospective), Ramasubbu et al. reported that *statins conferred a significant 26% relative risk reduction of mortality* (HR 0.74; 95% CI 0.68–0.8). Stratified analysis according to etiology of HF demonstrated a*n equal degree of protective efficacy irrespective of etiology* (HR for ischemic HF 0.73; 95% CI 0.65–0.82 vs. HR for non-ischemic HF 0.73; 95% CI 0.61–0.87).[22] The degree of reduction in mortality with statins was similar to that reported in previous trials with angiotensin-converting enzyme inhibitors (ACEIs) (18–44%) and beta-blockers (23–35%)
- Data from 10 prospective RCTs of statins in HF ($n = 10,192$ patients) was analyzed by Lipinski et al. to assess the effect on hospitalization for worsening HF, LVEF, major adverse cardiovascular events, and safety outcomes.[23] Rosuvastatin was used in three trials, atorvastatin in six and simvastatin in one. *No impact on all-cause or cardiovascular mortality was observed; statins significantly reduced hospitalizations for worsening HF* (OR 0.67; $p = 0.008$) and *improved LVEF* (+ 4.2% increase in LVEF, 95% CI 1.3–7.1; $p = 0.004$). *Lipophilic statin (atorvastatin) significantly reduced all-cause mortality* (OR 0.39; $p = 0.004$) and *decreased hospitalization for worsening HF* (OR 0.30; $p < 0.00001$), *while no benefit was seen in those receiving hydrophilic statin (rosuvastatin).*
- Meta-analysis of 17 studies ($n = 88,100$; 2 RCTs and 15 cohort studies) by Bielecka-Dabrowa et al. revealed that *statin use in HF was associated with lower all-cause mortality* (HR 0.77; 95% CI 0.72–0.83; $p < 0.0001$), *CV mortality* (HR 0.82; 95% CI 0.76–0.88; $p < 0.0001$), and *CV hospitalization* (HR 0.78; 95% CI 0.69–0.89; $p = 0.0003$).[24] Benefit was seen both in patients with EF < 40% and EF > 40% (reduction in all-cause mortality 23% and 25%, reduction in CV mortality 14% and 17%, and reduction in CV hospitalizations 20% and 24%, respectively). *The favorable effects on clinical outcomes were larger in magnitude for lipophilic than hydrophilic statins.*

Message

Cumulative evidence from these meta-analysis suggested that statins may have a beneficial effect on CV outcomes irrespective of HF etiology. Although lipophilic statins seem to be more favorable for patients with HF, one needs to remember that rosuvastatin (a hydrophilic statin) was associated with a significant decrease in CV hospitalization in the CORONA trial.

Differences in pleiotropic effects of statins have been attributed to differences in lipophilicity between the types of statins. Lipophilic statins passively diffuse into cells and are distributed throughout the body whereas hydrophilic statins are mainly liver-specific and require active protein transport Low cardiac uptake of hydrophilic rosuvastatin (<1% of liver) versus lipophilic statins (simvastatin, atorvastatin, 80% of liver) has been postulated to explain the observed lack of benefit with rosuvastatin in the two RCT's of chronic systolic HF. Furthermore, lipophilic statins have also been shown to significantly reduce the excess SNS activation in HF and improve electrical stability by modifying ventricular repolarization.

Although previous *meta-analysis showed that lipophilic statins were more effective in HF* in terms of improvement in LVEF, reduction in BNP, all-cause mortality, cardiovascular mortality, and hospitalization for worsening HF, *no randomized trial has been performed with lipophilic statins like atorvastatin in HF, and more studies are needed to clarify this issue.* In contrast to these studies, Imran et al. reported a modestly *reduced risk of incident HF in a large US national database of HF patients, initiated on high-intensity hydrophilic statins* (mainly rosuvastatin) when compared to lipophilic statins.[25] Factors governing this difference include the prostimulatory effects of lipophilic statins on the mineralocorticoid pathway (leading to hypertension and aggravation of HF) and favorable effects of hydrophilic statins on cytokine action and glucose homeostasis. Whether the effects of statins in the setting of HF are a class effect (hydrophilic vs. lipophilic agents), needs clarification by more randomized studies.

HF PRESERVED EF

Limited data are available on the role of statins in patients with HF and preserved systolic function (HFpEF). In one of the first prospective observational studies of HFpEF, Fukuta et al. demonstrated improvement in survival with statins in contrast to no benefit with ACEI, angiotensin-receptor blocker, beta-blocker, or calcium channel blockers.[26] Liu et al. reviewed 11 previously published observational studies of statins in HFpEF ($n = 17,985$ patients) and found that statins were associated with a 40% lower risk of mortality (RR 0.60; 95% CI 0.49–0.74; $p < 0.001$).[27]

Message

In light of paucity of data from RCTs in patients with HFpEF, the decision to start statins should be based upon other indications, like presence of absence of ASCVD and LDL-C above guideline cutoffs.

GUIDELINES

The European Society of Cardiology (ESC) guidelines recommend that based on current evidence, routine administration of statins in patients with HF without other indications for their use (e.g., CAD) is not recommended.[28,29] Since there is no evidence of harm in patients on statin treatment *after the occurrence of HF*, there is no need for discontinuation of therapy if the patients is already on statins. Treatment with statins is recommended in patients at high risk of CV disease or with CV disease in order to prevent or delay the onset of HF, and to prevent HF hospitalizations as Class Ia indication.

The LAI guidelines offer the following comprehensive and detailed recommendations for patients with HF:[4]

- Patients with ischemic HF (NYHA class II–III) should be started on statins.
- If a patients with CAD develops symptomatic HF, statins can be continued, with a goal to achieve 50% reduction in LDL-C.
- Patients of ischemic HF awaiting cardiac transplantation should be given statins.
- Statin therapy is not recommended in advanced HF patients who have a short life expectancy (e.g., because of comorbidities like malignancy).
- Statins are not recommended for advanced severe HF (NYHA class IV), if there are no other indications for starting statins.
- Patients with advanced symptomatic HF need individualized therapy. Although rosuvastatin 10 mg/day was found to be safe in advanced HF patients in CORONA and GISSS-HF, no benefit was observed. In view of the fact that significantly fewer hospitalizations were noted with rosuvastatin in the CORONA study, a statin with potency equivalent to rosuvastatin 10 mg is recommended if statin therapy is deemed necessary for advanced HF patients.
- Statins are not recommended in patients with dilated cardiomyopathy or nonischemic HF solely for the management of HF.

CONCLUSION

A counterintuitive relationship exists between cholesterol and HF wherein low TC is associated with adverse outcomes in these patients. There is reasonable evidence to suggest that this "cholesterol paradox" is merely a consequence of advanced HF and may have no actual role in genesis of adverse outcomes related to HF. The CORONA and GISSI-HF studies show that drawing conclusions of efficacy of drugs from observational studies and post hoc analyses of data does not always translate into predictable clinical results. Whether the results of the CORONA and GISSI-HF studies were due to the hydrophilic properties of rosuvastatin, a true lack of benefit of statins in HF or inclusion of an older and sicker patient population who had severe HF needs to be kept in perspective.

Once HF is established, statins may be less likely to demonstrate a survival benefit, since the disease is simply too advanced to be modified and the cardiac tissue behaves like a *"burnt out organ"*. Such patients have a high mortality burden from nonatherothrombotic causes such as sudden death and progressive HF. Statins administered at a late stage in HF may not have the opportunity to prevent atherothrombotic vascular events such as MI and strokes. Hence, it is prudent to initiate statins in patients of ischemic HF with NYHA class II–III symptoms, especially those with NT-proBNP of a level similar to that found in the first tertile of NT-proBNP in the CORONA study. Initiating statins may not be associated with a significant survival advantage in patients with HF and markedly elevated NT-proBNP that reflects a state of severe advanced HF, which is the beginning of the end, and the end of the beginning.

ONLINE REFERENCES

Please scan the QR code provided at the end of the table of contents for References of this chapter.

SECTION 7

Cardiomyopathy/Myocarditis

Section Outline

CHAPTER

71

Genetics of Cardiomyopathy

Biswajit Majumder, Ratul Ghosh, Somnath Maji

ABSTRACT

Genetic studies have significantly advanced our understanding of cardiomyopathies, and the field of heart failure genetics is rapidly evolving. Research has focused on identifying various genetic markers to predict risk in cardiomyopathy patients. Although this work is ongoing, new genomic technologies and analytical approaches offer exciting opportunities to explore the genetic basis of cardiomyopathies, uncover early signs of the disease, and understand the molecular mechanisms driving cardiac remodeling. With advancements in machine learning and artificial intelligence, the future perspective is extremely promising. Cardiovascular physicians must be aware of the benefits and limitations of integrating genetic test results into preventive treatment strategies for patients with cardiomyopathies presenting with early-stage heart failure. Future research should investigate the biological mechanisms of rare and common gene variants, environmental factors influencing gene expression, and the genotype–phenotype relationship. Significant advancements have been achieved in the field of genetics related to cardiomyopathy, particularly in the areas of hypertrophic cardiomyopathy and dilated cardiomyopathy. However, additional research is necessary to translate these findings into practical applications for everyday clinical practice. The ultimate goal is to improve diagnosis, treatment, and risk stratification for young patients with cardiomyopathies, enabling early intervention and prevention of severe disease consequences such as sudden cardiac death and early onset fatal heart failure.

Keywords: Genetic testing, cardiomyopathy, genetic counseling

INTRODUCTION

Cardiomyopathy has been defined by ESC as "a myocardial disorder in which the heart muscle is structurally and functionally abnormal, in the absence of coronary artery disease, hypertension, valvular disease, and congenital heart disease sufficient to cause the observed myocardial abnormality." In the past decades, significant strides have been made in understanding the genetic factors contributing to cardiomyopathy. Genetic testing has enabled more accurate classification and identification of individuals at risk, even those without symptoms. This progress offers insights into the early stages of cardiomyopathy and its molecular basis. Advancements in genetic tools and techniques open up newer avenues to explore the genetic basis of cardiomyopathies. While ongoing research aims to elucidate variant-specific pathophysiology, it may lead to novel therapeutic targets and personalized medicine approaches. Cardiomyopathies often progress silently, leading to late diagnosis with severe consequences such as heart failure (HF), arrhythmias, and sudden cardiac death (SCD). Identifying genetic risk factors is crucial, enabling early screening and detection of initial signs, potentially preventing or delaying disease progression. Early detection through genetic screening enables timely interventions, such as lifestyle changes, medication, and preventive measures. Genetic counseling and informed reproductive decisions become possible for individuals at risk. By leveraging these advances, physicians can improve outcomes and revolutionize cardiomyopathy management. Genetic testing is advised for individuals with various cardiomyopathies, including hypertrophic cardiomyopathy (HCM), dilated cardiomyopathy (DCM), restrictive cardiomyopathy (RCM), arrhythmogenic right ventricular cardiomyopathy (ARVC), and left ventricular noncompaction cardiomyopathy (LVNC), as well as those patients with extracardiac manifestations.

Research has revealed significant genetic similarities and overlap between these conditions, highlighting the complex relationships between genetic and phenotypic expressions.

HYPERTROPHIC CARDIOMYOPATHY

Hypertrophic cardiomyopathy is one of the most common causes of sudden death in young individuals and significant progress has been made in genetics of HCM. HCM is primarily caused by disease-causing variants [pathogenic variants (PVs)] in genes that encode proteins essential for sarcomere function. These variants exhibit a spectrum of effects, ranging from mild to severe, which influences their ability to manifest as HCM and the variability of symptoms displayed. The genes *MYH7* and *MYBPC3*, which code for β-myosin heavy chain and myosin binding protein C, are the most common genetic culprits behind HCM, accounting for around 40–70% of all cases, with an even higher proportion in large families. Additionally, PVs in genes encoding thin filament proteins contribute to approximately 5% of HCM cases. While the harmful effects of these variants are well established in large families, determining their causality in smaller families and individual cases can be difficult.[1] However, diagnostic certainty increases with identification of a pathogenic or likely pathogenic mutation in genes implicated for HCM **(Table 1)**.

TABLE 1: Genes implicated in HCM.

Group	Gene	Comment
Genes encoding thick filament proteins of the sarcomere	*MYH7*	The gene codes for the β-myosin heavy chain, which comprises about one-third of the sarcomere proteins. The protein has 1,935 amino acids and is ≈220 kDa in molecular weight. Several hundred PVs and LPVs in the *MYH7* gene, primarily missense variants and a few nonsense and indels variants, have been identified in patients with HCM. Overall, PVs in the *MYH7* gene are found in ≈20% of patients with HCM cases but a higher number of large families with HCM (50–70%)[2]
	MYBPC3	The gene codes for myosin-binding protein C, which is associated with both the thick and thin filaments of the sarcomere. The protein has 1,274 amino acids and a molecular weight of ≈140 kDa. Heterozygous mutations in the *MYBPC3* gene are found in about 20% of the HCM cases and in a higher number of large HCM families (50–70%).[2] A notable feature of mutations in the *MYBPC3* gene is the overrepresentation of the truncating mutations, such as indels, splicing, and nonsense mutations, as opposed to other well-established causal genes, whereby the missense mutations prevail[3]
	MYL2, MYL3	Genes encoding myosin light chain were among the first set of genes identified as causes of HCM, but they are uncommon causes for HCM (<1%).[4] These genes are largely tolerant to missense and LoF variants
	TTN	This gene encodes for titin. The gene is intolerant to LoF but tolerant to missense variants. Truncating variants in this gene are major causes of familial and sporadic dilated cardiomyopathy but are rare in HCM[5]
	MYH6	Myosin heavy chain 6 protein, encoded by the *MYH6* gene, comprises <10% of the total myosin heavy chain protein. This gene is mostly tolerant to missense and LoF variants
Genes encoding thin filament proteins	*TNNT2*	This gene encodes for troponin T. Mutation in this gene usually causes less hypertrophy but is associated with increased chances for sudden cardiac death. Mutations are mostly of missense variants[6]
	TNNI3, TNNC1, TPM1	These genes encode for troponin I, troponin C, and tropomyosin 1, respectively. The three genes are partially intolerant to missense and LoF variants and responsible for <1% of cases[6]
	ACTC1	This gene encodes cardiac α-actin 1, which is the least tolerant gene to missense and LoF variants
Genes encoding the protein constituents of the Z lines	*MYOZ2*	This encodes protein myozenin 2, which is tolerant to LoF and missense variants. PV and LPVs in the *MYOZ2* have been implicated in sporadic and familial HCM[7]
	ACTN2	This encodes protein α-actinin 2. The gene is intolerant to LoF variants and is associated with skeletal myopathies
	CSRP3	This encodes protein cysteine and glycine-rich protein 3, which was previously known as muscle LIM protein. Mutation in this gene alone is not causative of HCM but it acts in association with other genes[8]
	TCAP, FHL1	They encode for TTN capping protein and four and a half LIM domain 1 respectively. They are rare causes for HCM and are expected to exert modest effect sizes on the expression of HCM and are unlikely to cause HCM in the absence of skeletal myopathy[9]

Continued

Continued

Group	Gene	Comment
Genes coding for proteins located at the M line	*OBSCN, MYOM2, TRIM63*	They encode for obscurin, myomesin 2, and tripartite motif containing 63, respectively. They are expressed in skeletal and cardiac muscles and are tolerant to LoF and missense variants. They represent very rare causes of HCM (<0.5%)[10]
Gene regulating calcium homeostasis in cardiac muscle	*JPH2, PLN*	They encode for junctophilin 2 and phospholamban, respectively. They are best known to cause DCM (particularly PLN), but a rare truncating variant is often found in cases of HCM[11]
Genes encoding sarcomere-associated proteins	*FLNC, ALPK3, CAV3, CRYAB*	They encode for filamin C, α-kinase 3, caveolin 3, and crystalline αB, respectively. *FLNC* is best known for causing autosomal dominant restrictive cardiomyopathy but rarely causes sporadic cases of HCM. *CAV3* gene is associated with skeletal myopathy and long QT syndrome 9 and various forms of cardiomyopathies, including HCM. *CRYAB* gene has been reported mostly in patients with dilated cardiomyopathy and in a few patients with sporadic HCM[12-14]

CLINICAL IMPORTANCE

Familial cases of HCM have autosomal-dominant inheritance with variable penetrance and expressivity. Cascade genetic testing in family members of individuals with HCM who have a pathogenic/likely pathogenic (P/LP) mutation can significantly clarify their risk of developing the condition. This information guides the frequency of screening, which varies by age, including annual testing during adolescence and early adulthood and testing every 3–5 years in later adulthood. Additionally, identifying a P/LP variant enables the option of preimplantation genetic testing in conjunction with in vitro fertilization, providing further family planning insights. Research has shown that relatives of individuals with HCM who test positive for the genetic mutation are more likely to develop the condition, especially if they are male or display abnormal ECG. Notably, the *TNNI3* gene has a lower likelihood of expressing the disease compared to the *MYBPC3* gene. Furthermore, SCD has not been observed in individuals who carry the genetic mutation but do not exhibit symptoms or signs of HCM. About 60% of individuals with HCM lack a detectable mutation in the sarcomere genes. Research suggests that environmental influences and the interplay of multiple genetic variants may contribute to the development of HCM in these cases. Family members of individuals with "nonfamilial" HCM, where no genetic mutation is identified, may require less frequent screening compared to those with a known genetic mutation. Even in the absence of left ventricular hypertrophy (LVH), individuals who carry genetic variants associated with HCM may exhibit subtle cardiac abnormalities, including diastolic dysfunction, fibrosis, small left ventricle (LV) cavity, increased EF, myocardial crypts, elongated mitral leaflets, myocardial perfusion defects, electrophysiological abnormalities, etc. If these findings are present, it is recommended to intensify clinical monitoring for the potential development of LVH, with follow-up evaluations every 6–12 months to ensure early detection and appropriate management. Individuals with HCM who test positive for sarcomere gene mutations tend to experience an earlier onset of symptoms compared to those without these mutations. They often exhibit more pronounced hypertrophy, fewer instances of left ventricular outflow tract obstruction, and a higher likelihood of cardiac scarring. Additionally, they face an increased risk of developing arrhythmias and HF. However, integrating genetic information into risk assessment tools has proven challenging due to the complex interplay between genetic and clinical factors, such as age and maximum wall thickness, which can influence disease severity and are partially correlated with genotype.

Targeted treatments for HCM have emerged, including cardiac myosin inhibitors such as mavacamten and aficamten. Clinical trials have demonstrated that these medications can significantly enhance exercise capacity and alleviate symptoms in patients with obstructive HCM, surpassing the benefits of a placebo. Recently, it was shown that mavacamten can decrease the need for septal reduction therapy in a notable proportion of patients (VALOR HCM). Gene therapy for HCM is still in its infancy, with ongoing trials exploring the use of adeno-associated viral vectors to deliver DNA or lipid nanoparticles to introduce RNA. However, this innovative approach comes with potential risks, including unintended off-target effects that could lead to somatic cell mutations and increased cancer risk. Other concerns include immune responses to viral vectors, inadequate targeting of cardiomyocytes, and the possibility of neutralization due to preexisting antibodies from prior adenovirus exposures.

DILATED CARDIOMYOPATHY

Dilated cardiomyopathy has a complex and multifaceted genetic landscape. Research suggests that up to 40% of DCM cases may be attributed to genetic factors, with more than 50 different genes identified as contributors. These genes often impact the function of various protein complexes, highlighting the diverse molecular mechanisms underlying this condition.[15-17] Although the implicated genes participate in diverse genetic pathways, they ultimately converge to produce a consistent DCM phenotype. Notably, DCM exhibits a remarkable degree of genetic complexity, with a larger number of associated genes and a wider variety of

TABLE 2: Important genes implicated in DCM.

Gene	Protein	Estimated prevalence	Comments
TTN	Titin	12–25%	Isolated DCM, more common in women than in men. The clinical phenotypes of *TTN* truncating variants include low penetrance, low association with abnormalities in the conduction system, relatively good prognosis, sex differences in prognosis (males have a worse prognosis than females), and a tendency for LV reverse remodeling[18]
LMNA	Lamin A/C	5–10% (up to 30% if conduction disease is also present)	Part of Emery–Dreifuss muscular dystrophy is a relatively high incidence of sudden cardiac death or major ventricular arrhythmias, even before the development of systolic left ventricular dysfunction. ICD may be needed
MYH7	β-myosin heavy chain	4–10%	Primarily HCM; also familial DCM, LVNC, and RCM
MYH6	α-myosin heavy chain	4–6%	Primarily HCM, prognosis variable
MYPN	Myopalladin	3–4%	Usually, isolated DCM, early onset heart failure, and early death
DSP	Desmoplakin	3–4%	Primarily ARVC. However, when it causes DCM, the arrhythmic burden is lower than ARVC
RBM20	RNA-binding protein 20	1–5%	Rapid progression: SCD and end-stage heart failure are common, with a high incidence of ventricular arrhythmias. More severe in males
TNNT2	Troponin T	2–3%	Primarily HCM; also familial DCM, LVNC, and RCM
SCN5A	Sodium channel protein type 5, α subunit	2–3%	Commonly found with Brugada syndrome and LQTS. When found in DCM—early onset, commonly with atrial fibrillation; not associated with the risk of ventricular arrhythmias
TPM1	α-tropomyosin	0.5–1.0%	Primarily HCM; also familial DCM, LVNC, and RCM
FLNC	Filamin C	1–2%	Associated skeletal myopathy, high risk for ventricular arrhythmia, and SCD

genetic variants (including allelic and locus heterogeneity) compared to other cardiomyopathies, making it a uniquely challenging condition to understand and manage. The significant genetic diversity observed in individuals with DCM has crucial implications for clinical practice, given that DCM is a leading cause of HF and associated morbidity and mortality. Most genetic cases of DCM follow an autosomal-dominant inheritance pattern, characterized by variable expression and penetrance. However, less common forms of inheritance, including autosomal-recessive, X-linked-recessive, and mitochondrial patterns, can also occur, adding to the complexity of this condition **(Table 2)**.

GENETIC TESTING

Genetic testing in DCM serves to uncover underlying causes rather than establish a diagnosis. In many cases, identifying a PV does not significantly impact clinical management. However, genetic testing enables the identification of at-risk individuals and informs close surveillance of DCM cases associated with a high risk of SCD. This is particularly valuable in young individuals exhibiting early symptoms of DCM, as aggressive forms of the condition can be challenging to detect at an early stage. It is essential to interpret genetic test results in the context of comprehensive cardiac and systemic evaluations to ensure accurate assessment and management.

ARRHYTHMOGENIC RIGHT VENTRICULAR CARDIOMYOPATHY GENETICS

Arrhythmogenic right ventricular cardiomyopathy is a progressive cardiac condition characterized by the substitution of heart muscle cells with fatty and fibrotic tissue, leading to abnormalities in the structure and function of the right ventricle. While the classical form of ARVC is primarily an autosomal-dominant genetic disorder, accounting for 30–50% of cases with varying expressivity, other rare forms include Naxos disease and Carvajal syndrome. These two conditions are autosomal-recessive inherited diseases. ARVC is a relatively rare condition, affecting approximately 1 in 5,000 individuals in the general population.[19] Despite its prevalence, ARVC often goes unrecognized due to the challenges associated with its diagnosis, leading to a lack of awareness and understanding of this condition.

Patients with ARVC usually have genetic abnormalities in the genes that encode desmosomal proteins. The majority of PVs associated with ARVC occur in the *PKP2* gene (encoding plakophilin-2), accounting for 10–45% of cases, followed by variants in the *DSP* gene (encoding desmoplakin) in 10–15% of cases, *DSG2* (encoding desmoglein-2) in 7–10% of cases, and *DSC2* (encoding desmocollin-2) in approximately 2% of cases.[20-22] In a limited subset of cases, ARVC has been linked to mutations in nondesmosomal genes, including *TMEM43* (encoding transmembrane protein 43) and *PLN* (encoding phospholamban), which play critical roles in cardiac function and structure.[23,24]

Studies have shown that individuals with multiple PVs in key desmosomal genes, a phenomenon known as compound or digenic heterozygosity, experience a more severe disease course. Affecting 6–20% of patients, this genetic profile is linked to earlier disease onset, increased arrhythmic events, and a higher likelihood of left ventricular dysfunction and HF compared to those with a single mutation.[25,26]

HRS/EHRA recommends comprehensive or targeted (*DSC2, DSG2, DSP, JUP, PKP2*, and *TMEM43*) arrhythmogenic cardiomyopathy (ACM)/ARVC genetic testing can be useful for patients satisfying task force diagnostic criteria for ACM/ARVC along with variant-specific cascade screening and phenotypic screening among relatives.[27]

RESTRICTIVE CARDIOMYOPATHY GENETICS

Genes implicated in RCM are similar to those of other cardiomyopathies. RCM is predominantly diagnosed with echocardiography. Familial RCM often follows an autosomal-dominant inheritance pattern, but alternative modes of inheritance, such as autosomal-recessive and compound heterozygous forms, have also been observed. Notably, hereditary RCM may not always present as a distinct genetic cardiomyopathy, but rather as part of a broader phenotypic spectrum, highlighting the complexity and overlap of genetic cardiac disorders.

Pathogenic variants have been described in various sarcomeric genes such as *TTNT2, MYBPC3, MYL2, MYL3*, and *ACTC1*.[28] Recent discoveries have revealed that nonsarcomeric gene variants also contribute to RCM. Specifically, PVs in the *MYPN* and *TTN* genes can lead to myofibrillar disarray and restrictive cardiac physiology.[29] It is suggested that disrupted myofibrillogenesis is a key mechanism driving the development of RCM. Furthermore, PVs in the *FLNC* gene have been identified in multiple families, exhibiting an autosomal-dominant inheritance pattern.[30]

There are various genetic systemic diseases that have restrictive physiology like hereditary amyloidosis (mainly caused by PVs in *TTR* gene, but also in *CST3, FGA, LYZ, GSN, APOA2*, and *APOA1*), metabolic disorders such as glycogen storage diseases, Fabry disease (*GLA*), hemochromatosis (*HFE*), cystinosis, sarcoidosis, lymphoma, Danon's disease (*LAMP2*), and *PRKAG2*-mediated heart disease.[31]

LEFT VENTRICULAR NONCOMPACTION CARDIOMYOPATHY GENETICS

Left ventricular noncompaction cardiomyopathy is a distinct cardiac condition marked by excessive trabeculations within the LV, accompanied by deep recesses between these trabeculations and a thinning of compact epicardium. The majority of cases of LVNC are inherited in an autosomal-dominant pattern, while a smaller proportion follow X-linked or mitochondrial (maternal) inheritance, highlighting the genetic complexity of this condition. A significant proportion of cases, estimated to be around 60–70%, occur sporadically, without a clear family history. Furthermore, while multiple genetic variants have been linked to LVNC, no single gene stands out as the primary contributor, suggesting a complex interplay of genetic factors.[32]

Genetic variants in over 15 genes, including those encoding critical cardiac proteins such as sarcomeric components (*MYH7, MYBPC3, ACTC1, TNNT2*, and *TPM1*), ion channel proteins (*HCN4, SCN5A*), and other key proteins, have been implicated in the development of LVNC, highlighting the diverse genetic landscape of this condition.[33,34] *LMNA* and *RBM20* PVs were associated with worse outcomes **(Table 3)**.[35]

TABLE 3: Important inherited syndromes associated with cardiac disease.

Gene	Protein	Disease	Comment
DMD	Large sarcolemmal protein dystrophin	Duchenne muscular dystrophy	X-linked recessive, early-onset DCM with a history of muscular dystrophy
Mitochondrial	Energy metabolism	MELAS, MERRF	Maternal transmission or autosomal dominant, various systemic manifestations, DCM, heart block
FRDA/FXN	Frataxin	Friedreich ataxia	Cerebellar ataxia, dysarthria, and HCM are among the important manifestations
PRKAG2	5'-AMP-activated protein kinase subunit gamma-2	*PRKAG2*-related cardiomyopathy	Symmetrical nonobstructive hypertrophy, diastolic dysfunction, skeletal myopathy
TTR	Transthyretin	Amyloidosis	HCM phenotype along with systemic manifestations
LAMP2	Lysosome-associated membrane glycoprotein 2	Danon disease	LVH, preexcitation, skeletal myopathy, intellectual disability
PTPN11 *RAF1*	Protein tyrosine phosphatase nonreceptor type 11, serine/threonine kinase	Noonan syndrome	Typical facies, HCM phenotype, dysplastic PS among others
GLA	Galactosidase alpha	Fabry disease	LVH, preexcitation, sinus node dysfunction, and angiokeratoma among other manifestations

CONCLUSION

Despite the ease of obtaining human genome sequence data, challenges persist in harnessing this information for precision medicine. However, advances in validating rare genetic variants and identifying common genetic markers for cardiomyopathy risk have paved the way for integrating genomic data into routine healthcare. Ongoing research aims to address critical questions surrounding the treatment of patients and relatives with detrimental genetic variants, as well as the investigation of therapeutic efficacy. While genotype-phenotype correlations may appear inconsistent due to the late manifestation of traditional phenotypes such as LVH, HF, and SCD, studying earlier disease manifestations can reveal stronger correlations, uncover mechanistic pathways, and potentially lead to disease-modifying treatments. Our hope is that future research will enable genetic testing to identify variants and improve treatment outcomes, ultimately informing a new clinical framework for personalized HF care in cardiomyopathy.

ONLINE REFERENCES

Please scan the QR code provided at the end of the table of contents for References of this chapter.

CHAPTER

72

Dilated Cardiomyopathy: A Review

Tharun David Varghese M, Louie Fischer

ABSTRACT

The short overview of dilated cardiomyopathy in this chapter with a look into pathophysiology, genetics, diagnosis, management, and newer avenues.

Keywords: Dilated cardiomyopathy, heart failure

INTRODUCTION

The definition of dilated cardiomyopathy (DCM) is characterized by left or biventricular dilatation and impaired contraction, which is not explained solely by abnormal loading conditions.[1]

DCM is classified as genetic, mixed, or acquired by the American Heart Association. Familial (40%) and nonfamilial are the forms prescribed by the European Society of Cardiology (ESC).[2,3]

EPIDEMIOLOGY AND RISK FACTORS

Dilated cardiomyopathy is responsible for about 40% of patients in trials for heart failure, those with hospitalization for heart failure, and in patients who are recipients of heart transplant. DCM is responsible for 60% of childhood cardiomyopathies, which are detected during infancy.[4] The prevalence, phenotype, and natural history of DCM can be modulated by the sex of the individual.[5] There are differences in the epidemiological data seen in adult and pediatric DCM. The incidence of DCM in adults is 10 times higher than in children. The causes of the same include less exposure of children to detrimental adult health habits and the long time period with age seen in adults.[6]

The mortality associated with cardiomyopathy in 2010 was 5.9 per 100,000 global population, corresponding to ~403,000 deaths. This was an increase of over 5.4 per 100,000 in 1990.[7] Most of the causes of DCM hospitalizations are related to pump failure. The cardiac deaths are usually related to the development of arrhythmias.[8]

The risk factors as shown by studies for the development of DCM, congestive heart failure, mortality, and poor outcomes in adults include black ethnicity and male gender.[9-11] In the pediatric age group, the incidence is seen to be higher in infants, boys, and African Americans.[12]

Familial Dilated Cardiomyopathy

The term familial DCM is used when two first- or second-degree relatives meet the diagnostic criteria for DCM.[13] The most common inheritance pattern is autosomal dominant. It has been seen that there are cases that may be X-linked or mitochondrial.[4] The cause may be diverse and can be monogenic, polygenic, and multifactorial.

The mutations seen in DCM may affect the intercellular junctions, sarcolemma, cytoskeleton, ion channels, and sarcomere.[14] Recent studies have shown that around 12 genes have definite causation and around 7 genes have moderate level of causation.[15-17] The genetics include a spectrum from Mendelian to polygenic forms. The expression may also be variable, and there may be incomplete and age-related penetrance **(Table 1)**.[18,19]

Nonfamilial Dilated Cardiomyopathy

Myocarditis

Myocarditis is one of the most common causes of acquired DCM. In biopsy, it may be differentiated into lymphocytic, eosinophilic, granulomatous, and giant cell myocarditis. The most common etiological agents for the same include viruses of the enterovirus, parvovirus, and the herpes virus family.

TABLE 1: Genes with definitive dilated cardiomyopathy (DCM) association.

Titin (TTN)	Definitive
Lamin A/C (LMNA)	Definitive
Myosin heavy chain *(MYH7)*	Definitive
Filamin C *(FLNC)*	Definitive
RNA-binding motif-20 *(RBM20)*	Definitive
Troponin-T *(TNNT2)*	Definitive
Troponin-Cl *(TNNC1)*	Definitive
Phospholamban *(PLN)*	Definitive
Desmoplakin (DSP)	Definitive
BLC2-associated athanogene 3 (BAG3)	Definitive

SARS-CoV-2 can also have direct cytotoxicity mediated by cytokines or an autoimmune response.[20,21]

Toxins

The different toxins that cause cardiomyopathy act through different mechanisms of action.

The use of doxorubicin is associated with reactive oxygen-mediated damage, the components of which include DNA strand breaks, lipid peroxidation, and impaired mitochondrial function.[22,23]

Immune checkpoint inhibitors are monoclonal antibodies that bind to immune checkpoints. When there is a transreactive inhibition of vascular and cardiac components, these lead to T-cell-mediated atherosclerosis, myocarditis, and cardiomyopathy.[24]

The use of alcohol is associated with innate immune system activation, oxidative stress, and apoptosis.[25] When it is prolonged, it can result in iron overload and cardiac fibrosis.[26] The cessation of alcohol intake can cause reversal of systolic dysfunction.

The use of agents like cocaine and amphetamines is related to autonomic overactivation, reactive oxygen species, and endothelial dysfunction.[27] The damage done is usually irreversible.[28]

Peripartum Cardiomyopathy

By definition, it is a cardiomyopathy diagnosed in the last month of pregnancy or within 5 months of delivery in the absence of another cause. The risk factors for the development of the same include multiparity, increased maternal age, and hypertensive disorders of pregnancy.

The outcomes are in a spectrum ranging from full recovery to sometimes needing mechanical support or transplantation.[29] There has been found to be genetic similarities between DCM and peripartum cardiomyopathy with the most common being overrepresentation of truncating variants.[30] The development of peripartum cardiomyopathy is a result of both genetic and environmental influence—the so-called multiple hit hypothesis. In this scenario, pregnancy acts as a disease modifier.[31]

SECOND HIT PARADIGM IN DILATED CARDIOMYOPATHY

The finding that most people with so-called pathogenic variants of genes do not develop the disease brought forward the concept of the second hit. The outcomes and severity have been shown to be dependent on the presence of a second genetic or acquired hit. These can either be modifiers, comorbidities, or direct causal acquired factors **(Flowchart 1)**.[32]

PATHOPHYSIOLOGY

Dilated cardiomyopathy is characterized by the development of a spherical LV. This is due to remodeling, scar formation, and fibrosis. The physiology that develops includes increased end-diastolic pressures, reduced ventricular filling, and decrease both in cardiac output and stroke volume. In response to the changing hemodynamics, there is an increase in venous pressures, vascular resistance, and blood volume. The arterial compliance on the other hand is reduced. The preload and the afterload are increased with the elevated afterload leading to increase in wall stress. There is also an associated diastolic dysfunction that accompanies the systolic dysfunction.

HISTORY AND PRESENTATION

The usual presentation is between the ages of 20 and 60 years; though it can be seen in extremes of age. Most patients

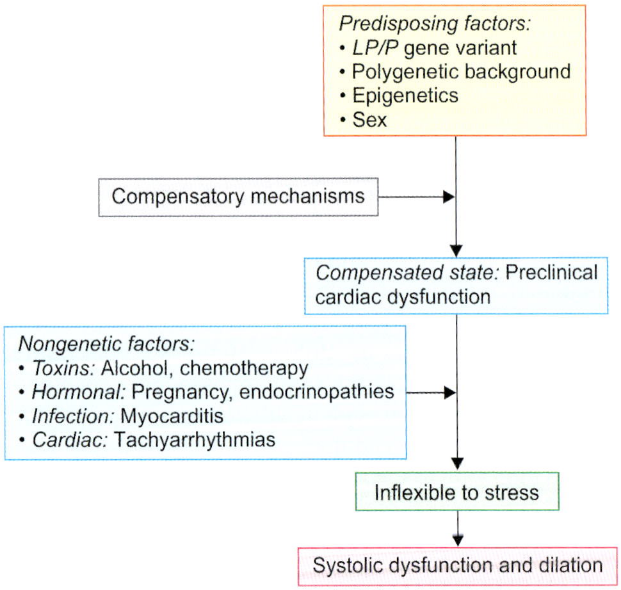

FLOWCHART 1: Second hit paradigm.

have a long latent period. The symptoms with which they present include paroxysmal nocturnal dyspnea, orthopnea, pedal edema, fatigue, and malaise. The other symptoms that are seen in the spectrum include thromboembolic complications, conduction disturbances, arrhythmias, and sudden cardiac death.

The Morphology, Organ involvement, Genetic, Etiology, and Stage (MOGES) classification by the World Heart Federation[33] gives a more complete picture of DCM.

EVALUATION

ECG

The importance of ECG is that in some types the initial presentation may be in the form of conduction abnormalities. There can be generalized ECG abnormalities, which may show left atrial/biatrial enlargement, atrial fibrillation (AF), left ventricular or biventricular enlargement, left axis deviation, left bundle branch block (LBBB), poor R wave progression, ventricular ectopics, and VT/VF **(Table 2)**.

In certain high-risk mutations such as laminin, titin (TTN), filamin, and desmoplakin, it is also essential to take an ambulatory ECG.

ECG findings that are more specific for certain cardiomyopathies include:

- Sinus bradycardia, AF, AV block—laminin mutation
- Lateral T wave inversions, low QRS voltages, and frequent VPC—desmoplakin, filaminin, and phospholamban mutation

Echocardiogram

Echocardiogram is an initial modality of investigation in view of the noninvasive nature. It has importance in both the initial diagnosis and long-term follow-up. The use of both 2D and 3D echocardiogram helps to quantify the LV dilatation and EF. This modality is useful in both RV and LV anatomy, both global and regional. LV enlargement that develops prior to the reduction in EF is considered a prequel to DCM. More subtle changes in LV function can be identified with the use of myocardial deformation imaging. It is especially useful in first-degree relatives. In the pediatric age group, an LVEDD z-score >2 and left ventricular end-systolic diameter (LVESD) z-score >2 are diagnostic. The parameters other than EF and LV dimensions include cardiac fibrosis and left ventricular global longitudinal strain with more prognostic value over LVEF.[34] The use of echocardiogram can also help in identifying subtle changes based on the mutation present. It is seen that sarcomeric variants have reduced global longitudinal strain. This is seen before the reduction in EF happens.[35]

TABLE 2: ECG changes in specific cardiomyopathies.

AV block	• Laminopathy • Emery–Dreifuss 1 • Myocarditis (especially, Chagas disease, Lyme disease, and diphtheria) • Sarcoidosis • Desminopathy • Myotonic dystrophy
Low P wave amplitude	Emery–Dreifuss 1 and 2
Atrial standstill	Emery–Dreifuss 1 and 2
Posterolateral infarction pattern	• Dystrophinopathy • Limb–girdle muscular dystrophy • Sarcoidosis
Extremely low QRS amplitude	*PLN* variant

Cardiac Magnetic Resonance

The use of cardiac magnetic resonance (CMR) is the gold standard for assessment of volumes, systolic function, and tissue characterization. It is noninvasive and in addition to that it is acoustic window-independent. CMR as an addition to echocardiogram helps to characterize the DCM phenotype. Contrast enhancement helps to identify myocardial edema and fibrosis. In diseases like Beckers and Duchene muscular dystrophy, it shows late gadolinium enhancement. This is visible prior to echocardiographic changes.

Depending on the underlying DCM phenotype, different late gadolinium enhancement (LGE) patterns can be seen.

- *TTN related DCM:* No specific pattern of LGE
- *Laminin-related DCM:* Mid-myocardial late gadolinium enhancement of the basal septum
- *Desmoplakin and filamin:* Midmyocardial/subepicardial extensive ring-shaped LGE
- *Chagas disease:* Apical transmural LGE
- *Dystrophinopathies:* Lateral wall epicardial LGE
- *Sarcoidosis:* Subepicardial and midwall LGE at basal septum with extention to inferolateral wall
- *Postmyocarditis:* Subepicardial LGE

T1- and T2-weighed imaging in patients in whom myocarditis is suspected helps in quantifying edema and fibrosis.

T2 mapping is useful in quantifying myocardial iron accumulation in diseases like hemochromatosis, sickle cell disease, and thalassemia major.

When considering CMR as a whole, studies done have shown that the LGE in its presence and extent is a predictor of outcomes independent to and incremental in nature over EF.[36] As was mentioned in regards to echocardiogram, the use of global longitudinal strain is a predictor of outcomes in addition to LGE and EF.[37]

Left atrial conduit strain is a new emerging modality that has shown promise in being an independent prognostic factor, which is better than LVEF and left atrial volume. It is also an incremental measurement to LGE in predicting all-cause mortality and future hospitalizations.[38]

PET-CT

The use of F18 FDG PET CT is useful in assessing viability and active inflammation. It is also a valuable tool for diagnosing cardiac sarcoidosis. A full-body PET-CT may help in identifying autoimmune, inflammatory, or systemic diseases.

Biomarkers

The biomakers that are routinely used for heart failure include natriuretic peptides. These include BNP and NT-pro BNP. The use of the same helps in both the diagnosis as well as to prognosticate heart failure. The other biomarkers which can help include:

- *Creatine kinase:* It is used as a marker of skeletal muscle involvement that is seen in muscular dystrophinopathies. The diseases in the constellation include limb-girdle muscular dystrophy, Beckers and Duchenne. It may also be seen to be elevated in sarcomere-related and mitochondrial cardiomyopathies as well as glycogen-storage disorders.[39]
- *High sensitivity troponin:* It marks the presence of myocardial injury, which can be seen in DCM with added myocardial stress or in acute myocarditis.
- *Others:* Other makers are soluble suppression of tumorigenicity 2 (sST-2, marker of stress), galectin-3 (inflammation and fibrosis), carboxy-terminal propeptide of procollagen type I (PICP and fibrosis), growth differentiation factor-15 (GDF15), inflammation, and fibrosis. The use of these newer markers is still unclear and more research is needed for the same.

Endomyocardial Biopsy

According to the expert consensus of ESC, endomyocardial biopsy (EMB) is recommended in all patients in whom an inflammatory pathology is suspected. It should include the use of immunohistochemistry, viral genome identification, and electron microscopy when there is suspicion of mitochondrial cardiomyopathies. Newer modalities include molecular examination such as microRNA, next-generation sequencing, and gene expression profiling. The main drawback of EMB is the fact that at times, the infiltration is patchy resulting in negative biopsies. A 1–3% complication rate and a 0.5 % rate of serious complications are seen.

Arrythmia Monitoring

Dilated cardiomyopathy as a heterogeneous disease is seen to be associated with sudden cardiac death and arrythmias. It is more prevalent in certain genetic subsets. Symptomatic bradycardia and tachycardia can be seen. For 24- or 48-hour recordings, the use of Holter monitoring is helpful. For prolonged recordings, the use of external and internal loop recorders is helpful. These help identify the patients who would benefit from the use of devices like implantable cardioverter-defibrillator (ICD) and pacemakers.

Genetic Testing

Genetic testing may broadly be divided into **(Flowchart 2)**:

- *Confirmatory/diagnostic testing:* This is done in patients affected with cardiomyopathy. It is done for the following purposes: Diagnosis, prognosis, treatment selection, and reproductive management.
- *Cascade testing:* It is done in clinically unaffected relatives irrespective of age, provided a diagnosis has been made with confidence in the affected individual.
- *Opportunistic screening:* At the moment, it is more used for research context.
- *Polygenic risk scores:* It is used in non-Mendelian cardiomyopathies. In this, many variants that are present across the genome are evaluated, and the score that is obtained is an aggregation of the same.

MANAGEMENT

The aims of management include the reduction of heart failure symptoms, improving cardiac function, and arrhythmia management. Guideline-directed management of heart failure is recommended for patients with DCM **(Flowchart 3)**.

There has been shown to be differences in the response of different genetically medicated DCM to GDMT.

It has been shown that TTN-related DCM shows better early reverse remodeling while laminin-related

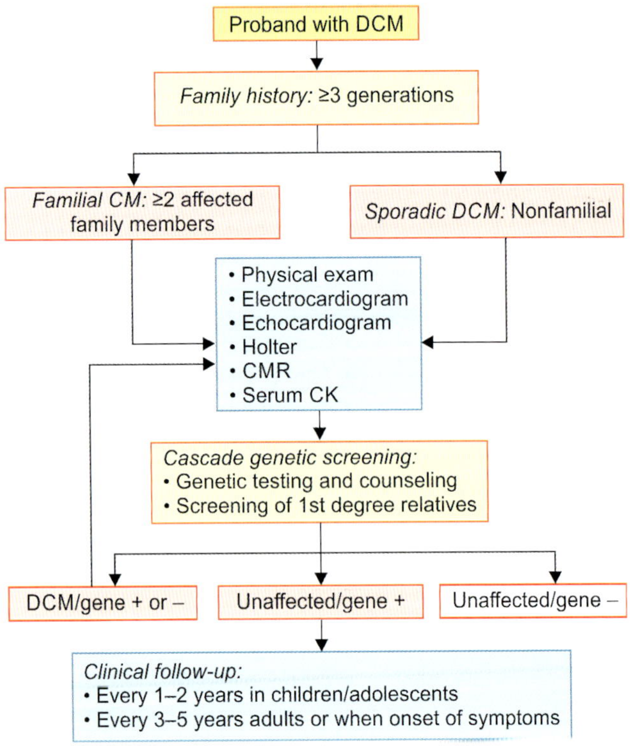

FLOWCHART 2: Genetic testing in dilated cardiomyopathy (DCM). (CK: creatine kinase; CM: cardiomyopathy; CMR: cardiac magnetic resonance)

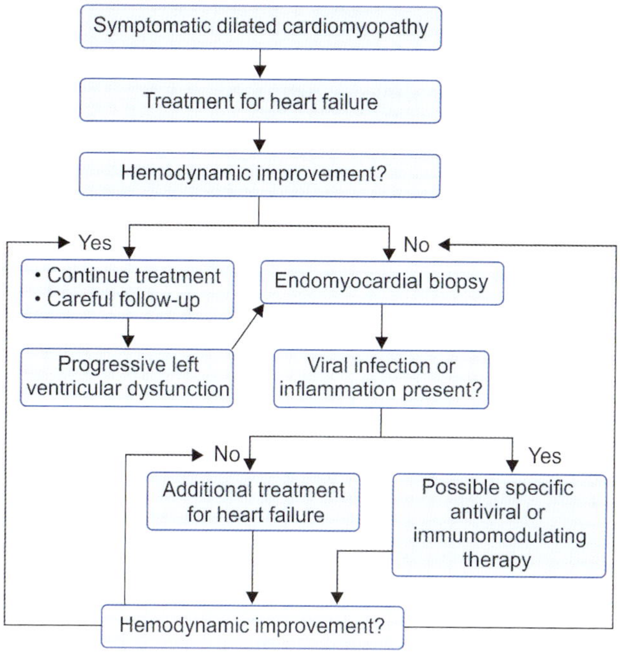

FLOWCHART 3: Management of dilated cardiomyopathy (DCM).

cardiomyopathies are shown to be less amenable to conventional treatment modalities.[40]

The drugs used include diuretics, ACEI, ARB, beta-blockers, mineralocorticoid receptor antagonists, ARNIs, nitrate and hydralazine, ivabradine, digoxin, and SGLT-2 inhibitors. They are administered based on existing heart failure guidelines.

Exercise and Physical Activity

The addition of low-intensity activity is considered a part of cardiac rehabilitation. The selection of patients and the exercise regimen should be judicious. There are certain findings that are not conductive to an exercise regimen. They include:

- LVEF < 45%
- Unexplained syncope
- High-risk genotype—laminin and filamin C
- Frequent ventricular tachyarrhythmias
- Extensive cardiac fibrosis

Device Therapy

Implantable Cardioverter-defibrillator

The DANISH trial did not show improved all-cause survival with the use of prophylactic ICD. There was an age-related difference with patients >the age of 70 years having lower cardiovascular mortality, sudden cardiac death, and all-cause mortality.[41] Hence, the use of an ICD for primary prevention should be decided based on multiple points that include:

- High-risk mutations such as laminin, filamin C, desmoplakin, RBM 20, and phospholamban

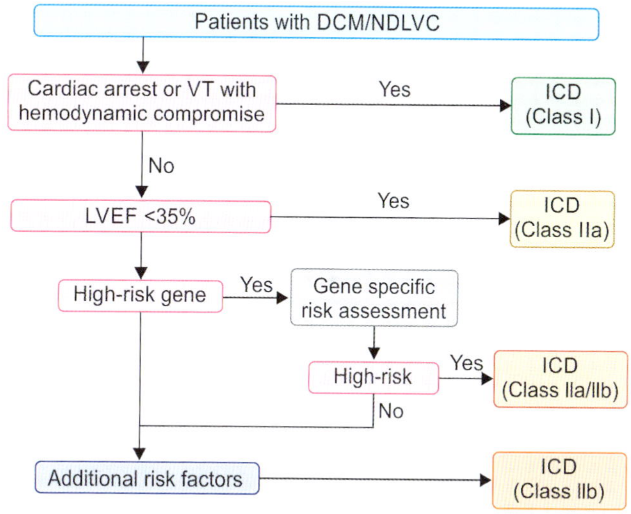

FLOWCHART 4: Implantable cardioverter-defibrillator (ICD) recommendation in dilated cardiomyopathy (DCM).

- Family history of sudden cardiac death
- Myocardial fibrosis and or LGE in CMR
- The severity of systolic dysfunction
- Presence of low grade ventricular ectopy
- History of syncope

The use of risk scores can help to guide the decision. The present ESC recommendations for the use of ICD in DCM are depicted in **Flowchart 4**.

Cardiac Resynchronization Therapy

Cardiac resynchronization therapy (CRT) is a modality of treatment that is indicated in patients with LV systolic dysfunction and ventricular dyssynchrony. It is, at present, indicated in patients who have ≤35% EF in the background of LBBB ECG morphology with a QRS duration of ≥130 milliseconds.

There have been multiple trials evaluating the role of CRT. They have shown that the benefits of therapy are better seen in nonischemic cardiomyopathies, in women, and in LBBB morphology.

Post hoc analysis of trials like COMPANION and MADIT-CRT have shown that patients with heart failure who do not have LBBB but have isolated PR prolongation may also benefit from the procedure.[42,43] Even though the recommendation for CRT is in QRS duration of 130 milliseconds or more, the MADIT-CRT, REVERSE, and RAFT have shown that irrespective of QRS duration there will be a benefit in LBBB.

Arrhythmia Management

The most common is the presence of AF. The addition of AF is associated with more severe symptomatology, increased risk of CVA, and death. In patients with DCM and AF, the use of anticoagulation may be decided based on the CHA2DS2-VASc score. The use of NOACs is preferred over

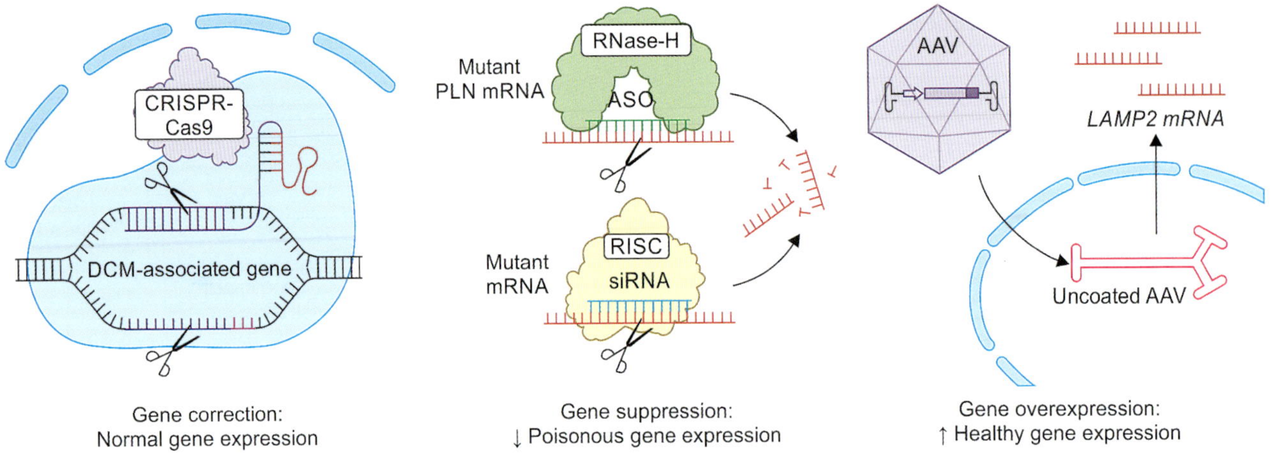

FIG. 1: Gene modification for dilated cardiomyopathy (DCM).

VKAs. In addition to anticoagulation, rate control is also to be considered. This is based on data that show that higher heart rates are associated with worse outcomes. The agents preferred for rate control include beta blockers or digoxin. For the purpose of rhythm control, the use of agents like amiodarone and sotalol can help. Radiofrequency ablation can also be considered.

Mechanical Support and Transplantation

The support devices include left ventricular assist devices (LVAD) and biventricular assist devices. These are being used more because of the increasing prevalence of end-stage heart failure and the less pool of donor hearts. These can be used either as a bridge to transplant or may also be considered as a destination therapy for patients who are not eligible for heart transplants.

The use of orthotopic cardiac transplant may be considered for patients who have advanced heart failure or ventricular arrhythmias, which are refractory to medical/invasive/device therapy, who have no absolute contraindication to the same.

Since the demography of DCM patients is more favorable, they have been shown to have better outcomes compared to ischemic subtypes. This is usually due to the patients being younger and free of usual underlying diseases.[44]

CONCLUSION

The future plan of care would include improving the diagnostic precision with the combination of phenoclustering, omics, and risk stratification. The use of precision diagnosis is useful because of the development of gene-specific therapies, which are in the pipeline. The broad approach is shown in **Figure 1**.

Other areas of research include trials in cardiac regeneration with various strategies being used for the same. They include the use of miRNA and growth factors. The starting cells have included pluripotent stem cells, cardiac progenitor cells, and bone marrow-derived stem cells. They have been found to be safe but with no functional improvement.

ONLINE REFERENCES

Please scan the QR code provided at the end of the table of contents for References of this chapter.

CHAPTER

73

Pacing-induced Cardiomyopathy: Current Treatment Options

Soormpally Vijay, Gautam Sharma

ABSTRACT

Pacing-induced cardiomyopathy (PICM) is a known complication of chronic right ventricular (RV) pacing, occurring in 10–20% of patients, resulting from nonphysiological ventricular activation bypassing the natural conduction system. The incidence is significantly higher in patients with preexisting left ventricular (LV) dysfunction, baseline left bundle branch block (LBBB), high burden of RV pacing, and a wider QRS-paced morphology. The precise definition of PICM varies across studies, creating uncertainty about the optimal management approach. The best management strategy for these patients is to upgrade the device to cardiac resynchronization therapy (CRT) with biventricular pacing or more recently with conduction system pacing, such as His bundle pacing (HBP) or left bundle branch area pacing (LBBAP), along with guideline-directed medical therapy for heart failure.

Keywords: Pacing-induced cardiomyopathy, cardiac resynchronization therapy, His bundle pacing, left bundle branch area pacing

INTRODUCTION

The right ventricle is the preferred site for cardiac pacing in patients who require a pacemaker due to its ease of implantation, improved lead stability, stable capture thresholds, and extensive expertise. Right ventricular (RV) pacing is well tolerated by most patients; however, in a few, chronic RV pacing leads to pacing-induced cardiomyopathy (PICM) due to ventricular dyssynchrony. PICM is associated with an increased risk of developing atrial fibrillation, hospitalization for heart failure (HF), and cardiac death. Therefore, identifying risk factors is crucial for the prevention and early treatment of PICM. In patients with PICM, upgrading to biventricular pacing cardiac resynchronization therapy (BiV-CRT) or conduction system pacing (CSP) promoted reverse remodeling of the left ventricle, resulting in significant improvements in left ventricular ejection fraction (LVEF) and relief HF-related symptoms **(Table 1)**.

DEFINITION

Although there is no universally accepted definition of PICM, the current recommendations define it as a drop in LVEF of at least 10%, beginning with a baseline LVEF above 50% before RV pacing, with a pacing burden of >20%, with no apparent causes for LVEF reduction following RV pacing.[1]

Pacing-induced cardiomyopathy has historically been regarded as a form of heart failure with reduced ejection fraction (HFrEF). Consequently, most studies that report the incidence of PICM incorporate impaired LVEF as part of the diagnostic criteria. Few patients, however, experience negative consequences from RV pacing and develop symptoms due to ventricular dyssynchrony and elevated cardiac filling pressures before a significant reduction in LVEF. So, the development of HF symptoms or the occurrence of HF hospitalizations is important in diagnosing PICM, and few studies support broadening the definition of PICM to include the beginning of HF symptoms following PPM implantation regardless of specific LVEF criteria. This explains the wide variation in the incidence of PICM from different studies and definitions of PICM that emphasize reduced LVEF may represent only the "tip of a larger PICM iceberg."[2,3]

INCIDENCE

Pacing-induced cardiomyopathy occurs in approximately 10–20% of people within 3–4 years of pacemaker implantation. The diversity in incidence across studies is related to

TABLE 1: Central illustration: Pacing-induced cardiomyopathy—definition, incidence, risk factors, and treatment.

Definition	A drop in LVEF of at least 10%, beginning with a baseline LVEF above 50% before RV pacing, with a pacing burden of >20%, with no apparent causes for LVEF reduction following RV pacing
Incidence	• Approximately 10–20% • Variable incidence is related to diversity in defining PICM, percentage of RV pacing, characteristics of the study population, and the follow-up duration • Practically we see only the "tip of the iceberg" 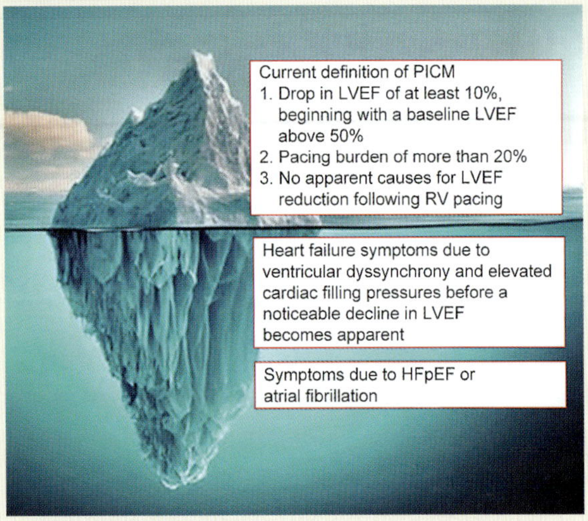
Risk factors	High burden of RV pacing (>20%), preimplant LV dysfunction, older age, coronary artery disease, and wide spontaneous or paced QRS durations
Treatment	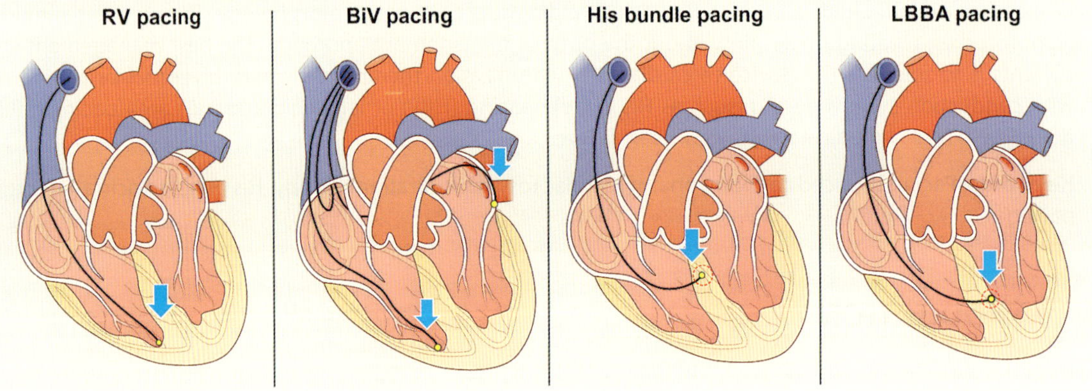

variations in defining PICM, the percentage of RV pacing, the characteristics of the study population, and the follow-up duration.[4-7]

Pacing-induced cardiomyopathy is associated with an increased risk of developing atrial fibrillation and hospitalization due to HF, so using the current guideline definition for PICM, we see only the "tip of the iceberg," necessitating a redefining of PICM.[8]

RISK FACTORS

There is significant variability in individual susceptibility to the harmful effects of RV pacing, emphasizing the need for further research to identify those at the highest risk of developing PICM and to tailor preventive measures accordingly. Strong risk factors include a high percentage of RV pacing (>40%), preexisting left ventricular (LV) dysfunction, wide-paced QRS morphology, old age, and preexisting left bundle branch block (LBBB).

TREATMENT

Initially, it was thought that PICM is the result of RV apical pacing due to very wide QRS, which can be managed with RV septal pacing that resulted in narrowed QRS but none of the studies comparing the RV apex with RV septal pacing showed the clinical benefit of RV septal pacing over apical pacing.[9,10]

The primary strategy for managing patients with PICM is to upgrade their single or dual-lead pacemaker to a cardiac resynchronization therapy [CRT; biventricular pacing or CSP that includes His bundle pacing (HBP), left bundle branch pacing, and left ventricle septal pacing] in addition to the guideline-adjusted medical therapy for HFrEF.

RATIONALE

In RV pacing, the electrical activation bypasses the natural His-Purkinje system, resulting in sluggish transmission of the electrical impulse from myocardium to myocardium through solitary point of conduction. Consequently, areas of the myocardium near the pacing site in the right ventricle receive the electrical activation early and contract earlier. In contrast, segments of the LV farther from the pacing site experience delayed electrical activation and delayed contraction, with the inferior basal region of the left ventricle typically being the latest activating segment. This disparity in electrical activation timing between the right ventricle and the left ventricle results in irregular mechanical contraction resulting in ventricular dyssynchrony that leads to a redistribution of myocardial strain and workload, ultimately causing less efficient overall contraction and potentially inducing PICM.[11]

Cardiac resynchronization therapy with BiV pacing synchronizes the contractions of both the right ventricle and the left ventricle, restoring a more natural and coordinated pattern of electrical activation and mechanical contraction by placing lead in right ventricle and left ventricle at the latest activation point via the coronary sinus (CS). This restores a more natural and coordinated pattern of electrical activation and mechanical contraction. Synchronized contraction decreases stress on the ventricular walls, improves stroke volume, reduces mitral regurgitation, and facilitates reverse remodeling of the LV, reducing its size and improving its shape and function.

In recent advancements, CSP targets either the His-Purkinje system or the left bundle branch area (LBBA) to replicate a more physiological pattern of electrical activation and contraction. This approach engages natural conduction pathways, effectively minimizing and potentially reversing dyssynchrony. The advantages and disadvantages of BiV pacing, CSP versus RV pacing are noted in **Table 2**.

BiV Pacing

Randomized controlled trials (RCTs) and numerous observational studies have demonstrated that upgrading to BiV pacing in patients with PICM reduces HF hospital admissions, significantly improves LVEF, and promotes reverse remodeling. As a result, current ESC guidelines recommend upgrading to BiV pacing for patients with permanent pacemakers or ICDs who develop refractory HF and have LVEF ≤ 35%, as well as those with a substantial burden of RV pacing.[12]

However, BiV pacing poses challenges such as anatomical variations in CS anatomy (including poor target vessels, presence of valves, and tortuosity), potential for diaphragmatic pacing, high pacing thresholds, and the risk of LV lead dislodgement. In cases where BiV pacing is not feasible, CSP serves as an alternative. However, comparative data with RCTs on BiV pacing versus CSP in patients with PICM are still lacking.

His Bundle Pacing

Observational studies have showed that upgrading to HBP in patients with PICM resulted in improvement in HF symptoms, narrowed QRS duration, improvement in LVEF, and reverse remodeling.[13-17]

In one study, HBP resulted in better clinical outcomes, LVEF, and mitral regurgitation than BiV pacing. Even though this is an observational study, theoretically, HBP is the most physiological pacing that resulted in greater improvement than BiV pacing.[14]

But concerns about lead implantation success rate, lead stability, high thresholds, early battery depletion, and a relatively high reimplantation rate have limited its clinical application.

TABLE 2: Pros and cons of BiV pacing and CSP compared to RV pacing.

			Conduction system pacing	
	Conventional RV pacing	**BiV pacing**	**His bundle pacing**	**LBB area pacing**
Advantages	• Ease of implantation • Stability provided by passive fixation leads within the trabeculae of RV	• Overcomes the electromechanical delay between the ventricles • Allows multipoint left ventricular pacing	Most physiological pacing	• Can correct infra-Hisian block • Stable capture thresholds • Enhanced "R"-wave amplitude
Disadvantages	• Nonphysiological pacing • Electromechanical dyssynchrony between the ventricles leading to PICM	• Nonphysiological pacing • Difficulty in obtaining the optimal site of left ventricular pacing because of feasible venous anatomy • High LV lead capture thresholds • LV lead dislodgement • Diaphragmatic pacing	• Unstable lead position • High capture threshold resulting in early battery depletion • Low success rates in infra-Hisian block • Septal scar can affect the success rate • Poor R-wave sensing	• Septal scar can affect the success rate • Lead perforation

Left Bundle Branch Area Pacing

Haung et al. first introduced novel physiological left bundle branch area pacing (LBBAP) in 2017 and raised its importance as it overcomes the pitfalls of HBP. Recent studies have shown that upgradation to LBBAP in PICM patients resulted in reduced incidence of HF admissions, LVEF, LVESV, and death compared to RV pacing.[18-22]

EVIDENCE

Few observational studies showed that, in patients requiring CRT, left bundle branch pacing has been shown to provide better electromechanical resynchronization, better symptomatic improvement, a narrower QRS duration, and echocardiographic response than conventional BiV pacing. Upgrading to LBBAP in PICM patients led to improved cardiac function (lower LVEDD, cardiothoracic ratio, and increased LVEF) and quality of life.[23-26]

CONCERNS WITH LEFT BUNDLE BRANCH AREA PACING

During the procedure, lead perforation into the left ventricle is detected by a sudden rise in capture threshold and a drop in unipolar impedance to <500 Ω. This can be managed by repositioning the lead at a different site. Late lead dislodgements or perforation can occur, necessitating careful follow-up.

The risk of injuring the septal branch of the LAD while screwing the lead is reduced by implanting the lead 1 cm distal to the His bundle region, as is the theoretical risk of systemic thromboembolism from exposing the lead helix to the LV cavity.[27]

HOW TO PREVENT PACING-INDUCED CARDIOMYOPATHY

Reduce Pacing Burden by Device Programming

One of the important risk factors for the development of PICM is the high pacing burden, so we need to utilize all the possible device algorithms to prevent unnecessary RV pacing, especially in sick sinus syndrome and intermittent AV block patients. These include AAI pacing, programming the lowest feasible backup ventricular pacing rate, AV hysteresis, avoiding rate response pacing in individuals with a competent sinus node, and programming rate response that does not lead to nonphysiological heart rates at rest or during activity.[28]

Cardiac Resynchronization Therapy

Is upfront CRT or CSP necessary for all patients requiring a pacemaker? The answer is no. The BIOPACE study showed that the routine use of CRT with BiV pacing in patients with atrioventricular block and a mean LVEF of 55% resulted in no significant difference in hospitalization due to HF and death compared to RV pacing. However, the positive outcomes of the BLOCK-HF study, which compared BiV pacing with RV pacing, were attributed to the high prevalence of LBBB and AFib patients with LVEF <50% in the study population, unlike in the BIOPACE study. This suggests that CRT is most beneficial for these patients.[29,30]

His bundle pacing despite being the most physiological pacing that can prevent PICM, its routine use as a first-line therapy is limited due to its related drawbacks. Although LBBAP has addressed many limitations of HBP, there is still a lack of extensive randomized data on its use as an upfront therapy in patients with AV block and normal LVEF. Long-term data are needed on the stability of capture thresholds, lead integrity, and extractability.[8]

Even though around 10–20% of patients postpacemaker develop PICM, it may not be justifiable to consider these complex, costly procedures upfront in all cases. Moreover, many people can endure the high burden of RV pacing for many years without any noticeable negative consequences. As individual susceptibility to developing PICM varies, much research is needed to identify these individuals at risk of PICM and target them with preventive therapy. So currently, the CRT with BiV pacing or CSP as an upfront device therapy is suited only in individuals with the highest risk of PICM, especially with preexisting LV dysfunction. Current recommendations suggest BiV pacing for patients with an EF of 36–50% who develop AV block and require >40% RV pacing.[31]

CONCLUSION

A decline in LVEF and the development of HF are primary signs of PICM, common complications of permanent RV pacing due to nonphysiological ventricular activation. Although upgrading to BVP is the preferred pacing technique, recent advancements in HBP and LBBP techniques have shown improved outcomes in terms of LVEF, 6MWT, and quality of life in patients with PICM. Compared to HBP, LBBP has a higher success rate and lower reintervention rates. Further studies and research are necessary to establish LBBP as the first-choice technique for patients with AV block and sinus node dysfunction requiring CRT.

ONLINE REFERENCES

Please scan the QR code provided at the end of the table of contents for References of this chapter.

CHAPTER

74

Tachycardiomyopathy: A Not-to-Miss Diagnosis

Jaishankar Krishnamoorthy, Sivashanmuganathan Velu

ABSTRACT

Arrhythmias usually accompany heart failure and LV dysfunction. Arrhythmia and cardiomyopathy (CM) have a cause–effect relationship, in the sense that arrhythmia leads to CM and vice versa. Primary challenge is to identify the extent of arrhythmia contribution to LV dysfunction. Confirmation of arrhythmia-induced cardiomyopathy (AICM) is when CM reverses after cessation of arrhythmia.

Keywords: Heart failure, LV dysfunction, arrhythmia contribution, AICM

INTRODUCTION

Tachycardiomyopathy (T-CM) is defined as a reversible impairment of ventricular function induced by persistent arrhythmia. However, since LV dysfunction can also occur due to dyssynchrony caused by atrial/ventricular ectopics, arrhythmia-induced cardiomyopathy (AICM) is an emerging broad-spectrum terminology.[1,2] AICM is defined as *atrial or ventricular dysfunction—secondary to rapid or asynchronous or irregular myocardial contraction, partially or completely reversed after treatment of the causative arrhythmia* (**Flowchart 1**).[3]

Arrhythmia-induced cardiomyopathy includes T-CM (heart rate >100 beats/min), premature ventricular complex cardiomyopathy (PVC-CM), and atrial fibrillation cardiomyopathy (AF-CM). It occurs due to nonphysiological conduction abnormalities. The term AICM, however, does not include cardiomyopathy (CM) due to right ventricular pacing, left bundle branch block, and pre-excitation.[4,5] Overview of causes/triggers, possible predictors, cellular mediators, and effects of AICM is summarized in **Table 1**.

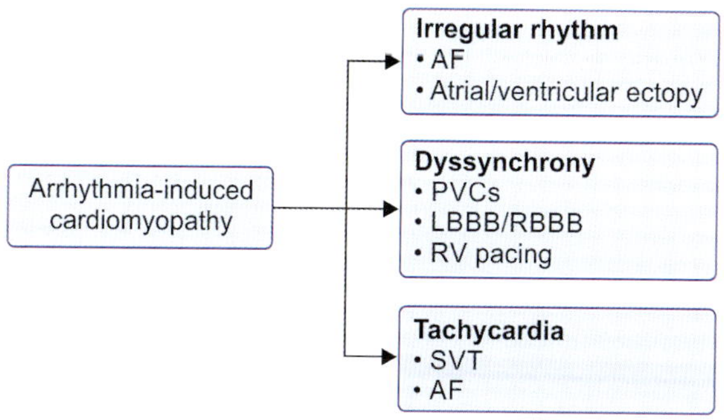

FLOWCHART 1: Arrhythmias leading to cardiomyopathy and the three main mechanisms.[6]

TABLE 1: Overview of causes/triggers, possible predictors, cellular mediators, and effects of AICM.[6]

	T-CM	PVC-CM	AF-CM
Cause/ Triggers	Increased HR	• PESP • LV dyssynchrony • AV dyssynchrony • Irregular HR • Autonomic dysfunction	Loss of atrial boost
Possible predictors	• Type • HR • Duration	• Axis • Burden • CI • VT	Persistent
Cellular mediators	Calcium mishandling, calcium overload		
Effects	Dilated LV, fibrosis, neurohumoral activation, myocyte and electrical remodeling, systolic dysfunction		

(AF-CM: atrial fibrillation cardiomyopathy; AV: atrioventricular; CI: coupling interval; HR: heart rate; LV: left ventricle; PESP: post-extrasystolic potentiation; PVC-CM: premature ventricular complex cardiomyopathy; T-CM: tachycardiomyopathy; VT: ventricular tachycardia)

TACHYCARDIOMYOPATHY

Tachycardiomyopathy is a reversible LV dysfunction due to increased ventricular rate. Factors or possible predictors determining T-CM are type, duration, and rate of arrhythmia.

Incidence and Etiology

Tachycardiomyopathy can occur with incessant or paroxysmal tachycardias. It occurs in 20–50% of patients with PJRT,[7] 37% with incessant atrial tachycardia, 10% with AT,[8] and only 4% with atrial fibrillation (AF). Incidence in AF though is underestimated by selection bias.[9]

The most common cause is supraventricular tachyarrhythmias—AF and atrial flutter with rapid ventricular rate.[6] Less common causes are frequent atrial tachycardia, AVRT, AVNRT, VT, PMT, and sustained sinus tachycardia. In general, faster heart rate and ventricular arrhythmias cause more T-CM.

Pathophysiology

Tachycardiomyopathy is characterized by biventricular dilatation without hypertrophy. Structural and functional myocardial changes **(Fig. 1)** are noted.[10,11] Animal models have demonstrated electrical remodeling and abnormal calcium hemostasis, which causes impaired excitation-contraction coupling. There is reduced calcium transient (calcium uptake and release) which leads to fall in LV function.[12]

Clinical Features

Clinical presentation varies among patients, with dyspnea due to heart failure being the most common presentation.[7,13]

- Heart failure class III/IV: 47%
- Palpitation: 29%
- Syncope: 12%
- No symptoms: 11%
- SCD: 8–12%

After tachycardia initiation **(Fig. 2)**, there is fall of BP and rise of LV end-diastolic pressure/pulmonary artery pressure, which plateaus after 1 week. There is fall of ejection fraction and cardiac output up to 4 weeks when symptomatic heart failure develops.[10]

After tachycardia termination, NT-proBNP starts falling after 1 week.[13] EF and CO start to increase 48 hours after tachycardia termination and improve within 1–3 months when NYHA functional class also improves.

Diagnosis

Factors that point to diagnosis of T-CM include:

- Previously normal EF and LV dysfunction disproportionate to other comorbidities
- No other cause of nonischemic cardiomyopathy found
- Absent LV hypertrophy
- Normal LV dimensions
- Recovery of LV function after tachycardia cessation
- Rapid decline in EF following recurrence of tachycardia

Ambulatory ECG for at least a period of 2 weeks is required for the diagnosis of T-CM. Echo and cardiac magnetic resonance (CMR) help in excluding other etiologies.

Treatment

Guideline-directed medical therapy for heart failure is given. Recovery of systolic function takes 3–6 months after tachycardia elimination. Age, heart rate, baseline EF, and LVEDD are the predictors of recovery.[7]

Arrhythmias and treatment options for AICM are listed in **Table 2**.

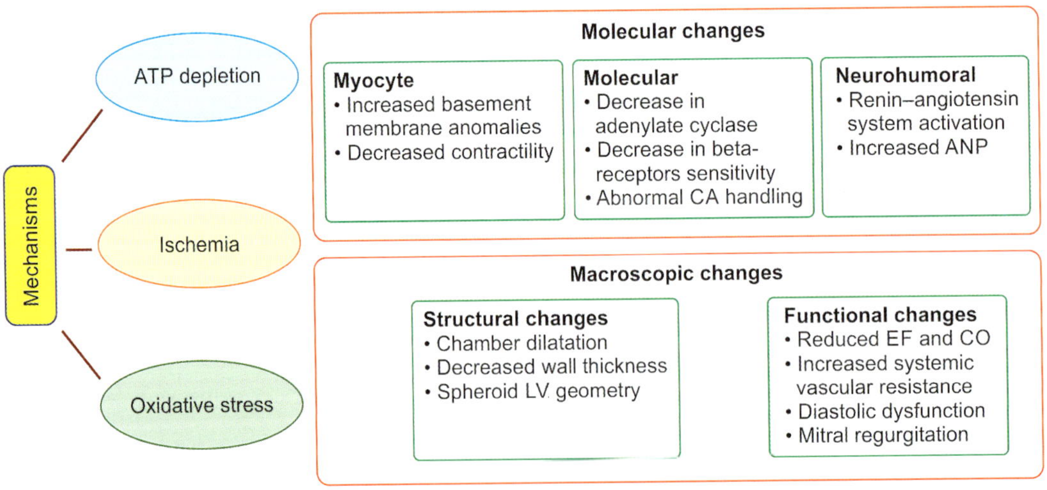

FIG. 1: Mechanisms of tachycardiomyopathy. Molecular, structural, and functional changes in T-CM.[10,11]
(CO: cardiac output; EF: ejection fraction)

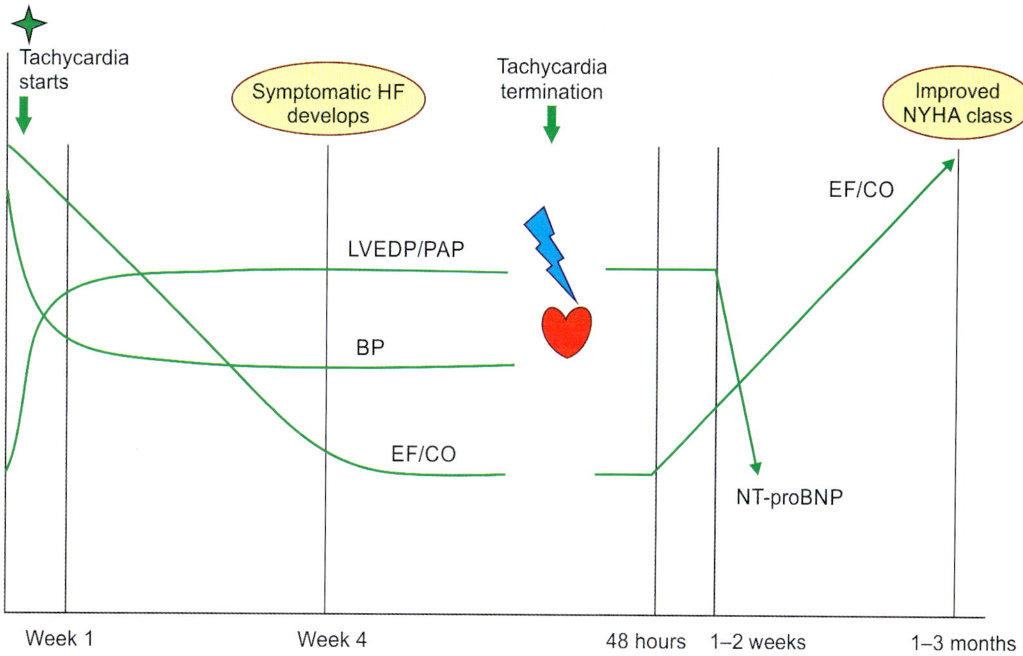

FIG. 2: Timeline of events after initiation and termination of tachyarrhythmia.[10]

TABLE 2: Arrhythmias and treatment options.

Arrhythmia	Treatment
Sinus tachycardia	Beta blocker; treat underlying cause
Atrial fibrillation RVR	Rhythm control (pulmonary vein isolation, AAD) vs. rate control vs. AV nodal ablation
Atrial flutter with RVR	RFA
Atrial tachycardia	RFA vs. AAD
AVRT/AVNRT	RFA
PMT	Reprogram pacemaker
Sustained VT	RFA vs. AAD

(AAD: antiarrhythmic drug; PMT: pacemaker-mediated tachycardia; RFA: radiofrequency ablation; RVR: rapid ventricular response)

ATRIAL FIBRILLATION CARDIOMYOPATHY

Atrial fibrillation cardiomyopathy is defined as LV dysfunction due to paroxysmal or persistent AF despite appropriate rate control.[6] AF can alone lead to CM despite rate control. AF per se can cause heart failure and vice versa. AF duration and irregularity predicts LV dysfunction rather than ventricular rate.

Etiopathogenesis

Two factors play a role in pathogenesis:[6]

1. Heart rate irregularity leads to abnormal Ca^{2+} dynamics.
2. Loss of atrial boost leads to sympathetic activation which in turn causes increased LV filling pressure, secondary MR, and diastolic dysfunction.

There is atrial mitochondrial dysfunction that leads to ATP depletion. This energy deficit and metabolic dysregulation leads to heart failure.

Clinical Presentation and Diagnosis

Atrial fibrillation cardiomyopathy is diagnosed after exclusion of other causes of CM and suspected in patients with nonischemic CM and persistent AF when there is no improvement despite adequate rate control.[6] Diagnosis is confirmed only when LVEF normalizes after AF elimination.

Holter monitoring helps to rule out poor rate control. CMR is used to prognosticate and look for ventricular scar burden. In the CAMERA-MRI trial, scar burden <10% predicted reversibility of LV dysfunction after rhythm control with catheter ablation.

Treatment

Rate versus Rhythm Control

Rhythm control is better (8–18% increase in LVEF). The RACE 3 trial demonstrated that 75% of the intervention group maintained sinus rhythm after 1 year compared to only 63% in conventional group.[14] The AATAC-AF and CASTLE-AF[15] trials suggest ablation is better than medications **(Flowchart 2)**.

Rhythm control by catheter ablation is best when there is no myocardial abnormalities or LA dilatation and ECG shows no conduction or repolarization changes. If any of these are

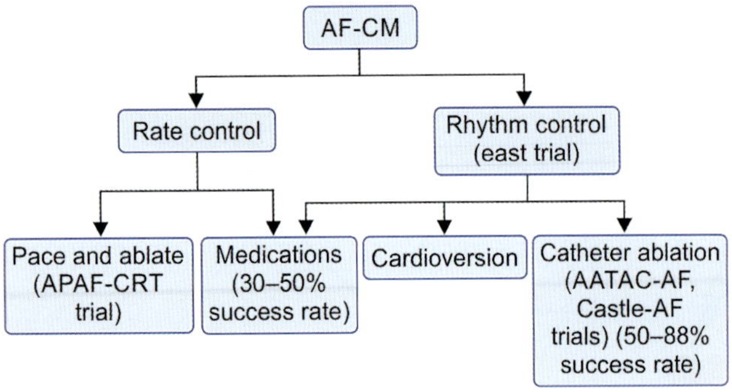

FLOWCHART 2: Atrial fibrillation cardiomyopathy (AF-CM) management options and respective trials for treatment strategies.[16]

present, "*pace and ablate*" is a better option.[17] However, the problem of dyssynchrony with RV pacing will be present that can be overcome by biventricular pacing. In the APAF-CRT trial, patients with AV nodal ablation + CRT pacemaker did well compared to rate control strategy.

PREMATURE VENTRICULAR COMPLEX CARDIOMYOPATHY

Premature ventricular complex cardiomyopathy is defined as LV dysfunction due to frequent VPDs (>10% burden). In superimposed PVC-CM, LVEF falls by at least 10% in a known cardiomyopathy patient. High PVC burden leads to increased incidence of systolic heart failure (six-fold increased risk), mortality, and stroke.

Epidemiology

The incidence of PVC was <1% in patients aged <11 years and >70% in patients aged >70 years.[18] PVC is more prevalent in post-MI, CAD, dilated cardiomyopathy, and heart failure patients. The prevalence of PVC-CM is 7% in patients with >10% burden, although this is an underestimate likely.[18] PVC-CM was found in 9–30% of patients referred for PVC ablation.

Etiopathogenesis

The primary cause of LV dysfunction is disorder of Ca-induced Ca release mechanism itself with alterations of dyad (extracellular Ca^{2+} enters the cell through L-type Ca channel, leading to a rapidly increased calcium concentration in the dyadic space, triggering ryanodine receptors on the sarcoplasmic reticulum to release more calcium and trigger myocyte contraction). The Ca^{2+}-related protein changes were distinct from T-CM. Oxidative phosphorylation in mitochondria is not affected unlike in T-CM where it is reduced. In histopathology, no inflammation, fibrosis, and apoptosis are found as well as no scar in MRI.[19] Hence, it is primarily a *functional abnormality* that is reversible.

The potential triggers for PVC-CM are both intraventricular and extraventricular as described further. The following are the important features of this entity:

- *Post-extrasystolic potentiation:* Post-PVC, there is increased intracellular Ca^{2+} which leads to increased contractility, thereby increasing O_2 consumption. Post-extrasystolic potentiation is inversely proportional to coupling interval. In short coupled PVCs, there is greater intracellular Ca^{2+}, which leads to more potentiation. In animal models, less prominent potentiation leads to more severe PVC-CM.
- *LV dyssynchrony:* Dyssynchrony is directly proportional to coupling interval. So, late coupled PVCs have greater dyssynchrony.[20]
- *Irregular heart rate:* Heart rate is usually normal due to compensatory pause.
- *AV dyssynchrony:* Short coupled PVCs have greater PVC-PCWP augmentation—defined as prominent "a" wave due to atrial contraction against closed AV valve.
- *Autonomic nervous system:* PVCs alone lead to increased sympathetic activity. Variable coupled PVCs cause more adrenergic output than fixed coupled PVCs. The chronic imbalanced sympathetic output and reduced vagal activity leads to an ischemia-like picture.

Post-extrasystolic potentiation and irregular heart rate also occur in frequent PACs but do not manifest with LV dysfunction. So, LV dyssynchrony[20] which occurs in PVCs but not in PACs plays an important role in pathogenesis.

Predictors of Premature Ventricular Complex Cardiomyopathy

- PVC burden[21] >10% in 24 hours
- Epicardial origin
- Variable coupling interval PVCs (due to high cardiac neuronal disturbance)
- QRS > 150 ms
- In RVOT PVCs, higher peak deflection index (time from QRS onset to peak of R in inferior leads divided by QRS duration)[22]
- Male gender
- Lack of symptoms
- >30-month history of palpitations
- Genetic (R222a missense mutation)

The ABC-VT score[23] (maximum 12 points) is used in frequent PVCs >5% burden. It is a risk stratification tool to predict development of LV remodeling and MACE: Low risk: 0–4 points; intermediate risk: 5–8 points; or high risk: 9–12 points.

- Axis (superior): 1 point
- Burden:
    - 10–20%: 2 points
    - >20%: 3 points

- Coupling interval (>500 ms): 4 points
- Ventricular tachycardia: 4 points

Clinical Features

Most of the patients are asymptomatic. Symptoms develop within 4 weeks of onset of ectopics. Some of the patients present with heart failure and rarely syncope. Symptoms are increased if PVC CI ratio[24] (PVC coupling interval/sinus coupling interval) >0.5.

The "*chicken-egg*" story: Most of the time, it is difficult to differentiate whether PVCs induced cardiomyopathy or cardiomyopathy induced PVCs. However, it is always better to treat PVCs if burden is increased because even if cardiomyopathy leads to PVCs, PVCs per se can worsen LV function termed "superimposed PVC-CM."[25]

The following are the features that favor cardiomyopathy leading to PVCs: (1) Old age with known heart disease (CAD, myocarditis), (2) Segmental hypokinesia in echo, (3) Significant scar in MRI, (4) PVC frequency <5,000/day or <5%, (5) Multifocal PVC, (6) Nonspecific QRS pattern, and (7) Post-PVC suppression LV function fails to improve.

Premature ventricular complex cardiomyopathy has LV systolic and diastolic dysfunction, LV dilatation, LA enlargement, and mitral regurgitation that reverses within 2–12 weeks of PVC termination. It has PVC origin from locations as follows, according to one large study: LVOT 28%; RVOT 21%; coronary sinus (epicardial) 24%; mitral 7%; septum 5%; and apex 4%.

Diagnosis

Holter monitoring is used to estimate PVC burden. In general, longer the duration of monitoring, more is the diagnostic yield. PVC prevalence is 1–4% in 10-second ECG, compared to 40–75% in 24- to 48-hour Holter. When compared to 24-hour Holter,[26] 7-day Holter had twice the diagnostic yield of detecting PVC burden of >10%. 24-hour Holter identified only 53% of >10% burden. 47% of patients were missed. Hence, prolonged monitoring is needed to detect PVC burden in suspected cases.

Echo strain imaging can help in early detection.

Cardiac magnetic resonance is used to look for scar burden and can predict response to treatment and prognosticate. No or minimal scar burden will have good response to ablation.[27]

Bhushan/Asirvatham criteria[10] for PVC-CM include the following:

- Young healthy individual without abnormal CV substrate
- >20,000 PVCs/day
- Fascicular or outflow tract VT
- No more than two PVC morphologies
- Preserved wall thickness

Treatment

Premature ventricular complex suppression strategy includes RFA or AADs for high PVC burden (>10,000 beats/day or >10% burden in 24 hours). Asymptomatic high PVC burden is usually followed up closely for LV dysfunction every 6 months. Spontaneous resolution might occur in 12% of patients over 6-month duration.[28]

Radiofrequency ablation is more effective than antiarrhythmics. It has its limitations when PVCs originate from critical structures like papillary muscle, epicardium, coronaries, and conduction system. Successful ablation is when burden is decreased by >80%. Even a <5,000/day target reduction shows dramatic LV function.[29] Current success rate is between 70 and 80%; complication rates are between 5 and 8% for ablation. Improvement in EF postablation is between 10 and 15%. Also, there is reduction in NT-proBNP levels and improvement in renal function.

Antiarrhythmic drugs have higher discontinuation rates due to side effects.[30] While the CAST trial showed increased mortality with class IC used to treat PVCs after MI, the GESICA, CAMIAT, and CHF-STAT trials showed decrease in mortality after MI and NICM with amiodarone.

In case of CRT implant, >0.1% ectopic beats makes them nonresponders; hence, ablation is needed for them. Recurrence after ablation leads to faster and more severe onset of T-CM than the first presentation. So, monitor carefully and continue GDMT for heart failure.

*Management options for AICM are summarized in **Flowchart 3**.*

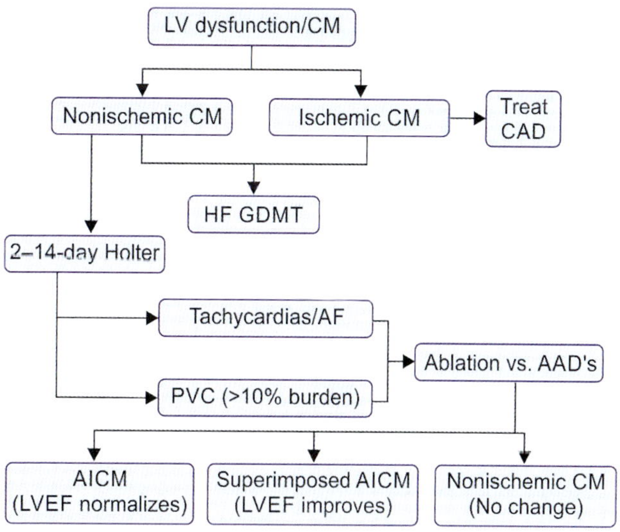

FLOWCHART 3: Management algorithm for suspected AICM and follow-up.[6]

(AAD: antiarrhythmic drugs; CAD: coronary artery disease; GDMT: guideline-directed medical therapy)

CASE VIGNETTE 1

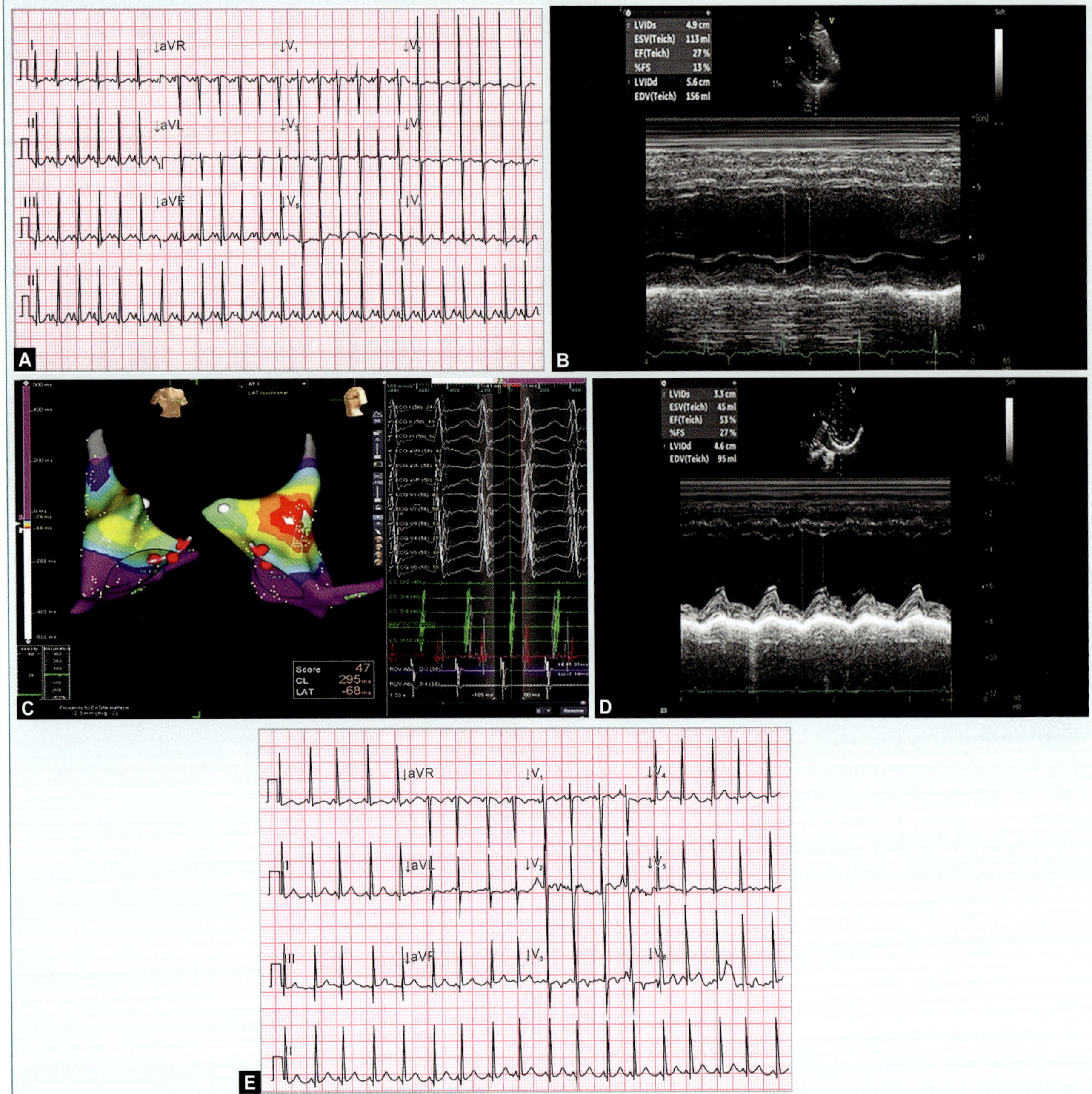

A 10-year-old female child presented with a history of frequent hospitalization for recurrent palpitations and breathlessness. (A) ECG revealed atrial tachycardia. (B) Echo showed severe LV dysfunction. (C) Cardiac MRI showed dilated LV with LV dysfunction and no scarring. She was taken up for EP study using 3D EnSite which revealed earliest activation in the upper septal area of the right atrium. Radiofrequency ablation was done for ectopic atrial tachycardia and sinus rhythm was achieved (E). On follow-up, there was gradual improvement of LV function (D) over a period of 6 months which normalized subsequently.

CASE VIGNETTE 2

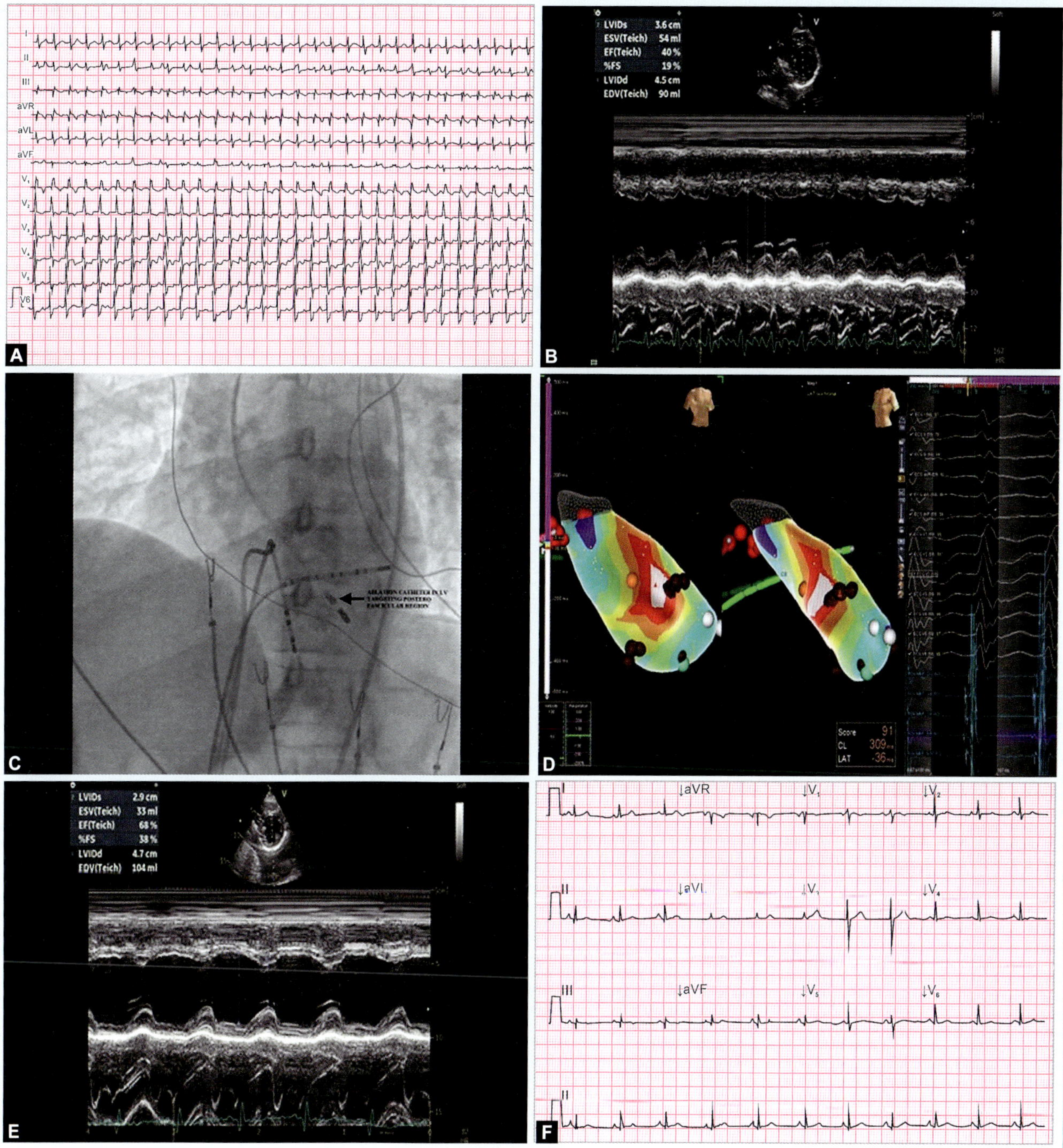

A 26-year-old male presented with complaints of palpitations with tiredness on and off past 2 months. The patient had a similar episode while waiting in OPD; ECG showed relatively narrow QRS tachycardia with RBBB and left-axis deviation (A) which was reverted to sinus rhythm by synchronized cardioversion. (B) Echo revealed global hypokinesia with moderate LV dysfunction. He subsequently underwent (D) EP study using 3D EnSite, which revealed posterofascicular VT. (C) Radiofrequency ablation was done by catheter placed in LV retrograde from the aorta. (F) ECG reverted to sinus rhythm post-RFA. (E) LV function showed dramatic improvement within 2 weeks of follow-up postablation. These cases show that abolition of tachyarrhythmias in the presence of LV dysfunction brings about dramatic reversal of deteriorating LV function, and can even get patients out from transplant list with unrecognized arrhythmic cause for severe LV dysfunction and congestive heart failure.

CONCLUSION

Arrhythmia-induced cardiomyopathy is one of the preventable causes of LV dysfunction with early diagnosis and treatment. AF-CM occurs in spite of adequate rate control, emphasizing the paradigm shift in treatment strategy that rhythm control should be aimed for whenever possible. PVC-CM is diagnosed by extended Holter monitoring and ablation is the treatment of choice. Being a reversible cause of cardiomyopathy, it is imperative to make a prompt and early diagnosis of AICM. High index of suspicion is required for diagnosis which will go a long way in reducing mortality, morbidity, and healthcare spending.

ONLINE REFERENCES

Please scan the QR code provided at the end of the table of contents for References of this chapter.

CHAPTER

75

Reversible Cardiomyopathy

Girish MP, Subrat Kumar Muduli, Mohit D Gupta

ABSTRACT

Up to 50% of cases of heart failure hospitalizations in the elderly are potentially reversible. Reversible cardiomyopathy represents a heterogeneous group of cardiac conditions which differ in many ways. Takotsubo syndrome occurs in postmenopausal females, whereas peripartum cardiomyopathies involve postpartum females. Myocarditis can be seen in any age group. Despite females being more sensitive to alcohol toxicity, males represent most of alcohol cardiomyopathy cases. Stress cardiomyopathy and acute myocarditis can mimic acute ST-elevation myocardial infarction. Alcohol and peripartum cardiomyopathy (PPCM) more commonly present as acute or chronic heart failure. Patients may also present with thromboembolism, refractory shock, and sudden death. Thiamine deficiency can cause high-output heart failure. Treatment of all these conditions should start with guideline-directed medical therapy (GDMT). Specific treatment modalities might include bromocriptine therapy for PPCM, catheter ablation to cure tachyarrhythmias, thiamine supplementation in beriberi heart, etc. Acute refractory heart failure cases may go on to require ventricular-assist devices, wearable ICDs, or even cardiac transplantation. Complete recovery is the rule in conditions like beriberi heart, whereas left ventricular (LV) dysfunction may persist years after tachycardia cessation in arrhythmia-induced cardiomyopathy. In recovered cases, the disease might recur within months to years.

Keywords: Heart failure, cardiomyopathy, reversible, tachycardia, beriberi heart

INTRODUCTION

Cardiomyopathy (CMP) refers to a primary myocardial illness that ultimately leads to cardiac contractile dysfunction. Reversible cardiomyopathies are characterized by partial or complete recovery of cardiac dysfunction with the treatment of underlying triggers. Chamber enlargement and heart failure (HF) are the dominant presenting feature while some patients may present with thromboembolic events, sudden cardiac death, or even mimic an acute coronary syndrome (ACS). In up to 50% of cases of HF hospitalizations in the elderly could be due to a potentially reversible form of CMP.[1] The prognosis of a patient with reversible CMP is much better compared to that of ischemic or nonischemic irreversible causes. Identification and treatment of the underlying cause is the key to the management of such patients.

ETIOLOGY AND PATHOGENESIS

A wide variety of inciting agents have been identified which can cause CMP that is transient and potentially reversible. They differ in their epidemiological associations, clinical presentation, and management strategies. **Table 1** describes the pathogenetic mechanisms and classical diagnostic features of various types of cardiomyopathies which are potentially reversible.

Takotsubo Cardiomyopathy

Also known as stress CMP, Takotsubo cardiomyopathy derives its name from the Japanese word for octopus pot due to its characteristic LV apical ballooning. It is primarily seen in postmenopausal women after an emotional trauma within 1–5 days of the onset of symptoms. Its incidence is on the rise with 15–30 cases diagnosed per 100,000 person-years.[2]

TABLE 1: Pathogenetic mechanisms and diagnostic features of specific forms of cardiomyopathies.

Cardiomyopathy type	Pathogenetic mechanisms	Clinical/Diagnostic clues
Takotsubo CMP	Stress-induced intense sympathetic activation causes direct contraction band form of cellular necrosis and microvascular dysfunction	*History*: Postmenopausal women, preceded by emotional stress *ECG*: Ischemic ST-T changes *ECHO*: Apical ballooning with basal hyperkinesia *CMR*: Absence of any LGE InterTAK criteria can be used
PPCM	16 kD prolactin fragment causing vascular damage and apoptosis	*History*: Last month of pregnancy to 5 months postpartum *ECHO*: Global HK, apical thrombus
TCMP	Tachycardia-induced calcium overload and calcium mishandling	*ECG*: Atrial fibrillation, EAT
ACMP	Direct toxic effects of alcohol on the myocardium, oxidative stress, mitochondrial dysfunction, and acetaldehyde-induced direct toxicity	*History*: Chronic (>5 years) heavy alcohol intake (>80 g/day) *ECHO*: Initially preserved EF with diastolic dysfunction followed by a DCM pattern later
Myocarditis	Maladaptive postviral immune-mediated response, toxin-mediated cardiac damage	*History*: Viral prodrome and illness *CMR*: Intramural rim-like or patchy epicardial LGE *EMB*: Lymphocytic or eosinophilic myocardial infiltrate with myocyte injury/necrosis Dallas criteria can be used to make a diagnosis of active or borderline myocarditis
Beriberi	Thiamine deficiency causes decreased ATP production leading to impaired vasomotor function and decreased SVR which causes a high-output HF	Measurement of erythrocyte thiamine transketolase activity
Keshan disease	Selenium deficiency causes reduced glutathione peroxidase which makes the heart susceptible to oxidative damage and prone to coxsackie virus-mediated damage	Serum selenium levels in endemic areas

Note: A potentially reversible cardiomyopathy can be due to various causes with various pathogenetic mechanisms. LVEF improves after removal or treatment of the underlying cause. From clinical history taking to advanced diagnostic modalities can be used to reach a specific underlying cause. Occasionally multiple causative mechanisms may be responsible in a single patient, e.g., alcohol cardiomyopathy.

(ACMP: alcohol cardiomyopathy; CMP: cardiomyopathy; CMR: cardiac magnetic resonance; EAT: ectopic atrial tachycardia; EMB: endomyocardial biopsy; InterTAK: international takotsubo diagnostic criteria; kD: kilo Dalton; LGE: late gadolinium enhancement; PPCM: peripartum cardiomyopathy; SVR: systemic vascular resistance; TCMP: tachycardia induced cardiomyopathy)

In up to 35% of cases, there may not be an identifiable trigger. Male patients are more likely to be young, without any emotional trigger, and present with atypical variants. Happy heart syndrome refers to its occurrence after a happy pleasant event. Half of stress-induced CMP patients are cases of an acute or a chronic neuropsychiatric disorder. Stress CMP is a form of acute neurogenic stunning of the myocardium. In response to stress, spillover of norepinephrine and neuropeptide Y occurs at the presynaptic ends of neurons from the brainstem ending at the myocardium, and this causes direct injury to cardiomyocytes in the form of contraction band necrosis.[3] Ischemic stunning at the microvascular level due to these neuromodulators might also be responsible.[4] Usually, postmenopausal women have an increased sympathetic drive and endothelial dysfunction, predisposing them to microvascular dysfunction and hence an increased risk for stress CMP. The abundance of beta-adrenergic receptors in the LV apex makes it more susceptible to injury. In many cases of subarachnoid hemorrhage, epilepsy, electroconvulsive therapy, and head injury a similar pattern of cardiac damage is seen. These are known as Takotsubo phenocopies rather than classical neurogenic stunned Takotsubo CMP.[4]

Peripartum Cardiomyopathy

Peripartum cardiomyopathy is another form of reversible CMP described to occur in the last month of pregnancy to 5 months postpartum. The worldwide incidence on average is 1 in every 2,000 live births.[5] In endemic areas such as Nigeria, the incidence is as high as 1 in 100 deliveries compared to Japan where it is as low as 1 in 20,000 deliveries. African ancestry, preeclampsia, multifetal gestation, advanced maternal age, and anemia are risk factors for

PPCM. Most patients develop HF within 1 month of delivery. Maternal prolactin during the last trimester of pregnancy has been proposed to cause cardiac damage in a genetically susceptible individual. In certain oxidative conditions prolactin gets modified into a 16 kD form that in experimental models has been shown to be cardiotoxic. This is the basis of the recently proposed hormonal vascular model to explain the occurrence of PPCM.[6]

Tachycardia Cardiomyopathy

In animal models, rapid ventricular pacing has been proven to cause LV dysfunction as early as 24 hours to 3 weeks of pacing.[7] It occurs primarily in patients with structurally normal heart. Patients with higher heartrates develop tachycardia cardiomyopathy (TCMP) at an early stage. It is rare in patients with inappropriate sinus tachycardia or POTS syndromes due to the unsustained nature of tachycardia. In children, EAT (59%) and PJRT (23%) appear to be common causes of TCMP.[8] Atrial fibrillation (AF) is the most common arrhythmia in adults presenting with HF (up to 50%).[9] Though SVTs are more likely to cause TCMP, ventricular arrhythmia can also cause this. For VPCs, the usual burden for CMP development appears to be >10,000/day. Male sex, VPCs arising from outflow tract, interpolated VPCs, presence of retrograde P waves, patients with homozygous deletion in ACE polymorphism are prone to develop TCMP.[10] Abnormal calcium loading handling is the primary reason for contractility impairment and a decrease in cardiac output. Later it leads to mitral regurgitation, a rise in LVEDP, and cardiac dilation eventually leading to neurohormonal activation.

Alcohol Cardiomyopathy

Alcohol use accounts for around 10% of all cases of nonischemic dilated CMP.[11] Though prevalence in males and females is similar, females appear to be more sensitive to alcohol cardiomyopathy (ACMP) as it can occur at lower levels of alcohol intake. It is classically known to occur at a daily intake of >80 g/day (equivalent to 8 × 300 mL of beer) of alcohol for at least 5 years. In Asian patients due to alcohol dehydrogenase (ALDH) deficiency, toxicity can occur at lower levels. The postulated mechanisms include mitochondrial injury, oxidative damage, and actin-myosin modification in the contractile apparatus of cardiomyocytes. Acetaldehyde is a major metabolite of alcohol, which can cause direct cardiomyocyte injury. Nutritional deficiencies such as thiamine, folate, and magnesium deficiency might also be contributing factors in chronic alcoholics. The cause of Quebec beer drinkers' CMP is an excess of cobalt ingestion added during the brewing process rather than alcohol itself. ACMP in the initial stage is more of a heart failure with preserved ejection fraction (HFpEF) that progresses to heart failure with reduced ejection fraction (HFrEF) on further drinking.

Myocarditis

According to the current WHO classification, myocarditis is clinically and pathologically defined as an inflammatory disease of the myocardium diagnosed by established histological, immunological, and immunohistochemical criteria. Most commonly viral pathogens such as coxsackie, adenovirus, human herpes virus 6 (HHV6), and parvovirus B19 are the responsible agents. A common transmembrane receptor (CTR) exists in these viruses which helps them in their cardiotropism. HIV-infected patients are also known to develop CMP by direct infection of cardiac cells. Multiple cases of COVID-19 and influenza-associated myocarditis have been recently reported.[12] Viral myocarditis is mostly seen in young patients who are otherwise healthy. Bacteria such as borrelia, treponema, mycoplasma, and protozoal infections can also cause damage to the myocardium. Chagas disease, caused by *Trypanosoma cruzi*, is endemic in Latin American countries. Giant cell myocarditis causes a fulminant form of myocarditis with high mortality. Drugs such as anthracycline and cocaine can lead to cardiac dysfunction. Inflammatory cell-mediated damage, direct cellular toxicity, and cytokine-mediated damage are the usual mechanisms responsible for myocyte injury in myocarditis.

Nutritional

Thiamine deficiency can cause a high-output form of HF.[13] Deficiency can be a result of poor intake, poor absorption (chronic alcoholism, gastric bypass surgery), increased loss (excessive vomiting, diarrhea, diuretic agents, renal replacement therapy), or increased consumption (pregnancy, breastfeeding, hyperthyroidism) of thiamine. Chronic alcoholism and a poor dietary intake from polished rice use appear to be dominant forms worldwide.[1] Hypocalcemia from nutritional vitamin D deficiency can also cause cardiac dysfunction by impairing cardiac contractility.[14] Micronutrient deficiency, particularly selenium deficiency, has also been linked to coxsackie-induced viral myocarditis and cardiac dysfunction. Keshan disease is endemic in northeast China where the selenium levels in soil are low.

Miscellaneous

Sepsis, uremia, obesity, and cirrhosis have also been seen to cause depression in cardiac function.

CLINICAL FEATURES AND DIAGNOSIS

Most of the cases present with acute or chronic forms of HF with reduced cardiac output. Takotsubo CMP and viral myocarditis can mimic ACSs due to anginal chest pain and ECG changes similar to ischemia.

A typical patient with stress CMP is a postmenopausal woman who presents with acute or subacute onset of anginal-type chest pain (>75% of cases) and/or shortness of breath (approximately 50%), often with dizziness (>25%) and occasional syncope (5–10%). Apical ballooning **(Figs. 1A to F)** with basal hyperkinesia is classical on echo but focal, midventricular, and biventricular involvement can be seen. Mid ventricular pattern is seen in 10–20% and basal or inverted pattern is seen in <5%. The mid-ventricular pattern is more likely to present with shock. Apical ballooning in the acute stage can cause LVOT obstruction **(Figs. 1A to F)**.[15] LV cine angiography can be done in the absence of contraindications. Coronary angiography is often needed to rule out coronary artery disease. InterTAK diagnostic criteria, HF-ESC criteria, or a modified Mayo Clinic criteria are helpful in making a diagnosis in atypical cases.[16] ECG is abnormal in >95% of cases. 40% have ST elevation in precordial leads. ST elevation in aVR with ST elevation in anteroseptal leads (V1, V2, V3) has a positive predictive value of 100% but a low sensitivity and negative predictive value.[17] Reciprocal changes and abnormal Q waves are usually absent. A minimal rise in peak troponin levels (<10 ng/mL) with severe elevation in natriuretic peptide levels is typical of stress CMP. Around 1–2% of suspected ACS cases are finally diagnosed as stress CMP. InterTAK diagnostic score of >50 is highly specific for Takotsubo CMP.[16] On cardiac MRI absence of LGE is classical of stress CMP compared to ACS/MI.[18]

Clinical presentation of myocarditis is highly variable starting from a subclinical disease to presenting as acute chest pain, severe HF, refractory cardiogenic shock, or sudden death. A viral syndrome involving the respiratory or gastrointestinal tract with associated systemic symptoms might precede the onset of cardiac symptoms. Troponin I and troponin T are more frequently elevated than creatine kinase-MB, with increased levels of troponin I at presentation portending a worse prognosis. ECG changes are mostly nonspecific but may mimic ST elevation MI. Regional wall motion abnormalities can be seen in echocardiography. Cardiac magnetic resonance (CMR) imaging is useful to make a diagnosis. According to the revised LAKE LOUISE criteria, CMR provides strong evidence of acute myocardial inflammation in patients with high clinical pretest probability if at least one criterion in each of the following two categories is positive: A T2-based marker of myocardial edema and a T1-based marker of myocardial damage.[19] LGE imaging in myocarditis has indicated two common patterns of myocardial injury: Either an intramural, rim-like pattern involving the septum or a patchy epicardial distribution involving the lateral free wall of the left ventricle. Endomyocardial biopsy (EMB), using standardized histopathological (Dallas criteria) and immunohistochemical diagnostic criteria, is the current gold standard by which a diagnosis of myocarditis is made. The Dallas criteria yield diagnostic information in only 10–20% of patients. Therefore, immunohistochemistry with the use of a large panel of monoclonal and polyclonal antibodies is now obligatory.[20] LGE-guided biopsy might improve the sensitivity of EMB. PCR techniques can be used to detect viral DNA/RNA in biopsy specimens.

Peripartum CMP and ACMP present with acute or chronic HF features such as dyspnea, orthopnea, and raised JVP. Thromboembolic manifestations can be seen in 7% of cases of PPCM. Sudden death has also been reported. Echocardiographic evidence of LV dysfunction and their temporal association in a pregnant or postpartum lady is adequate to make a diagnosis of PPCM. LV apical thrombus can be seen in 5–20% of cases. ECG-documented episodes of persistent tachyarrhythmias are helpful in making a diagnosis of TCMP. Similarly, a history of excessive alcohol intake for a prolonged duration with echocardiographic evidence of LV dysfunction suggests ACMP.

PROGNOSIS AND RECURRENCE

Stress CMP has an in-hospital mortality of up to 5%. Mid-cavity variants are more likely to present with cardiogenic shock. Recovery of LV function occurs in 2–3 weeks.[15] In apical variants, the recovery rate is >90%. The average recurrence rate is reported as 2–4% per year. It may recur as a different anatomical variant in the same patient. PPCM case recovery takes 3–6 months postpartum but has been described until 48 months after delivery. At 1-year follow-up, the reported mortality rate ranges from 4 to 11%. LV function at diagnosis is the most important parameter for prognosis and LV recovery. In the American IPAC study, 72% of patients recovered to left ventricular ejection fraction (LVEF) > 50% at 12 months.[21] LV dilation, presence of thrombus, RV dysfunction, and African ancestry are additional factors associated with worse outcomes. Preeclampsia lowers 1-year survival but is associated with better LV recovery. ESC EORP PPCM recovery score is used to predict LV function recovery in such patients.[22] In patients with recovered LV function, PPCM recurs in 20% of cases, but in patients with partial or minimal recovery the recurrence rate is >50% with an increase in mortality.

Ventricular function recovery in TCMP patients, following restoration of sinus rhythm, is variable. It depends on the rate and duration of the responsible arrhythmia. The greatest LVEF recovery occurs by 1 month after arrhythmia cessation and then follows a more gradual recovery reaching a complete normalization up to 1 year.[23] Complete recovery may not occur in many patients even years after tachycardia cessation. The impact of recurrent or new tachyarrhythmias on LV function has been poorly assessed with some authors suggesting severe deteriorations in clinical status after recurrence.

Myocarditis has been linked as the cause of sudden cardiac death in young adults in up to 12% of cases. Acute myocarditis in patients who present with HF and mild LV systolic dysfunction typically recover in weeks to months. Among patients who present with significant LV dysfunction, 50% of patients will have complete resolution, 25%

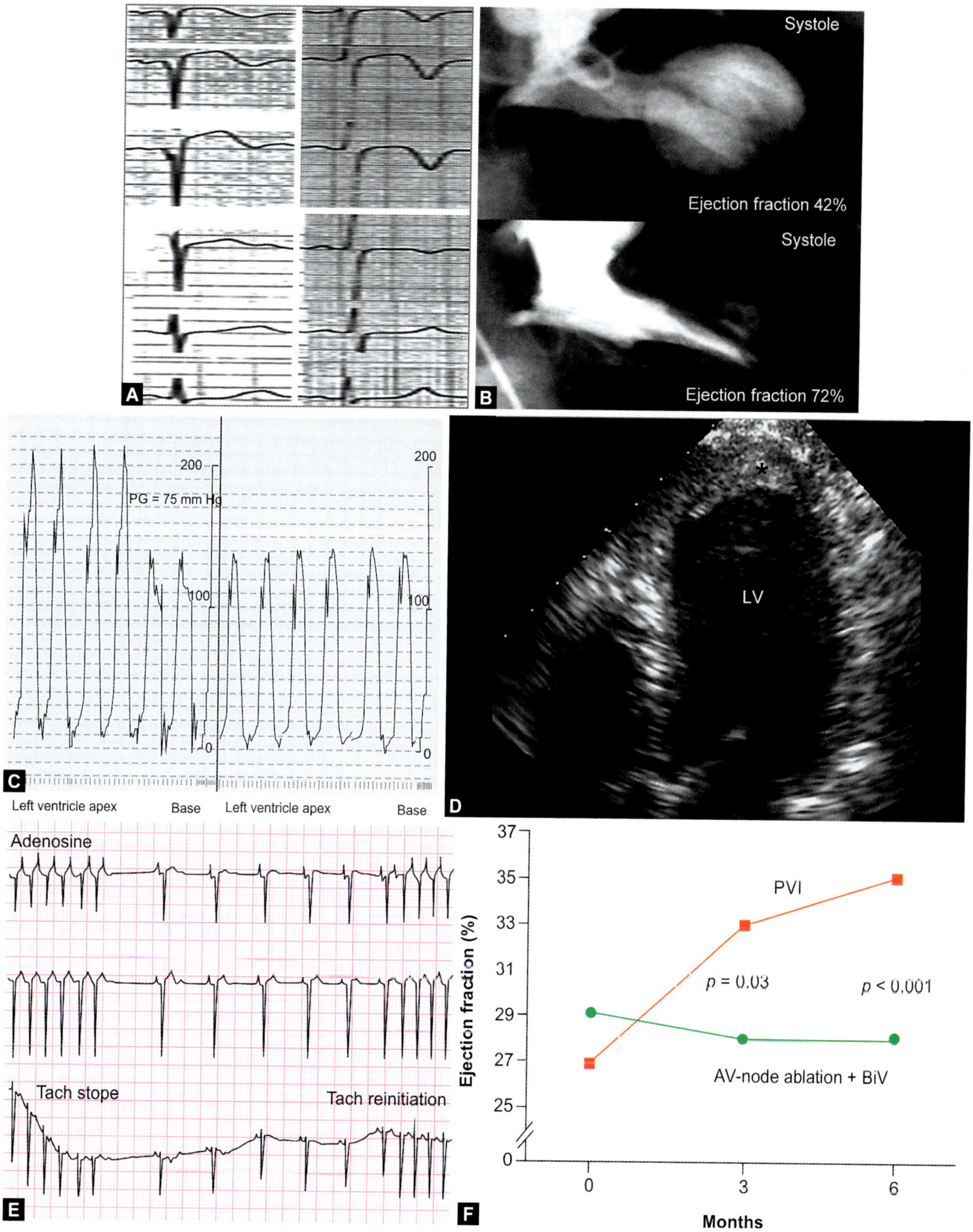

FIGS. 1A TO F: Characteristic clinical findings of individual cardiomyopathies and their spontaneous or post-treatment reversibility. Classical case examples of potentially reversible cardiomyopathies. ST-elevation in V_1–V_6 in acute phase of Takotsubo cardiomyopathy (A) and their normalization in subacute phase (A′).[15] LV apical ballooning (B) and its normalization after 2 weeks (B′) in the same patient. Similar observation of LVOT obstruction in LV pressure trace (C). Apical thrombus in a patient with PPCM (D). Tachycardia termination after IV adenosine in a patient with TCMP and immediate reinitiation of tachycardia (E). Results of PVI in a patient with atrial fibrillation in improving ejection fraction after 6 months (F).[23]

(PPCM: peripartum cardiomyopathy; PVI: pulmonary vein isolation; TCMP: tachycardia cardiomyopathy) will go on to have chronic systolic dysfunction, and 25% will progress toward an end-stage CMP resulting in transplantation or death.[24] Patients with giant-cell myocarditis have a substantially worse prognosis, with <20% of patients surviving 5 years. ACMP has a mortality of 15% at 5 years, much better than idiopathic DCMP. After 10 weeks to 1.5 years of complete abstinence, LVEF starts normalizing.[25] Along with continued alcohol intake, the presence of AF, QRS duration of >140 ms, and absence of beta-blocker therapy are risk factors for poor prognosis.

MANAGEMENT STRATEGIES

General Treatment

The management approach is like that of any other form of HFrEF. Beta-blockers, mineralocorticoid antagonists, and ACE inhibitors/ARBs have proven beneficial in all such cardiomyopathies. Diuretics are essential to reduce congestion. Vasodilators like isolazine are helpful, particularly in the black population or when ACE inhibitors/ARB cannot be used. Though data on ARNI and SGLT inhibitors are lacking, there is little to doubt their effectiveness. In PPCM cases, ACE inhibitors/ARBs and MRAs are contraindicated in pregnancy. Digoxin can be used in refractory cases. Anticoagulation has been advocated for patients with severe LV dysfunction or in patients with AF or LV thrombus. Inotropes are useful during the acute decompensated phase as temporary stabilizing measures. Mechanical assist devices might be required in a few fulminant cases. Subcutaneously placed ICDs are to be avoided keeping in view the reversible nature of CMP. However, wearable ICDs can be used. How long to use GDMT after normalization of ejection fraction is not definitely known but therapy continuation for at least 3 months is the standard approach and can be continued up to 1 year.[26]

Disease-specific Treatment

Takotsubo CMP does not have a specific treatment. Many experts advocate for the use of beta-blockers in patients with increased sympathetic tone, ongoing cardiac symptoms, persistent anxiety, or recurrent episodes in Takotsubo syndrome. Complete abstinence or at least moderation of alcohol consumption improves LVEF in ACMP.[27]

As prolactin plays a pathological role in PPCM, bromocriptine therapy at 2.5 mg once daily for 1 week reduces mortality by improving LVEF. It is a dopamine agonist which reduces serum prolactin levels. In refractory cardiogenic shock cases, therapy can be extended up to 8 weeks. Recently, a new BOARD therapeutic algorithm has been advocated for acute PPCM.[28] A definitive cure to TCMP can be obtained with catheter ablation, and it should be pursued whenever possible. Pulmonary vein isolation by catheter ablation in paroxysmal or persistent AF has been tested in the CASTLE-AF trial and was found to be quite effective in achieving sinus rhythm for a sustained period. It reduced death and HF hospitalization by 40% at 5 years.[29]

In severe fulminant forms of myocarditis causing acute HF, immunosuppression with steroids, azathioprine, and cyclosporine can be helpful. Viral clearance is a must before resorting to immunosuppression. Giant cell myocarditis, eosinophilic forms, and autoimmune forms respond very well to immunosuppression. IVIg therapy improves LV systolic dysfunction in pediatric forms of acute myocarditis and also increases the chances of survival.[30] Beriberi-associated HF can be treated with high doses of thiamine (200 mg thiamine administered intravenously or orally three times a day) till resolution of symptoms which can then be converted to 10 mg/day oral therapy. Similarly, 95% of cases of hypocalcemia-associated CMP improve by achieving normocalcemia.[31] Treatment for each of the reversible causes of cardiomyopathies is described in **Flowchart 1**.

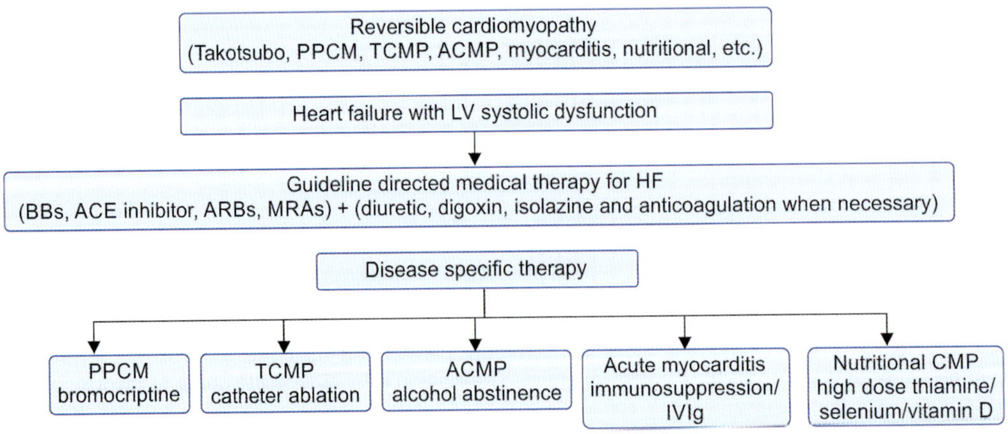

FLOWCHART 1: Management of heart failure in a patient with potentially reversible cardiomyopathy.

Note: Guideline-directed medical therapy (BBs, ACE inhibitors/ARB, MRA) forms an essential part of the management of cardiomyopathies. However, identifying the cause of a potentially reversible CMP can help us guide a specific form of treatment. Bromocriptine therapy for PPCM, catheter ablation for TCMP, and IVIg in pediatric myocarditis has been proven to normalize EF and improve mortality.

(ACMP: alcohol cardiomyopathy; ARB: angiotensin receptor blocker; BB: beta blockers; MRA: mineralocorticoid antagonist; PPCM: peripartum cardiomyopathy; TCMP: tachycardia cardiomyopathy)

CONCLUSION

Up to half of the cases of HF hospitalization are potentially reversible. Causes such as Takotsubo CMP, PPCM, TCMP, and ACMP can be diagnosed using patients' clinical history, ECG changes, and classical echocardiographic features. CMR is quite helpful in diagnosing acute viral myocarditis. EMB is the gold standard for diagnosing myocarditis but should be used with caution. GDMT should be used for each of these forms presenting with HF. Specific forms of treatment such as bromocriptine therapy in PPCM, catheter ablation for TCMP, and thiamine supplementation in beriberi have proven to improve LVEF and improve mortality outcomes. High-dose thiamine supplementation in beriberi heart can cause complete reversal of cardiac dysfunction in most of the patients. This undermines the importance of diagnosing a specific etiology of HF.

ONLINE REFERENCES

Please scan the QR code provided at the end of the table of contents for References of this chapter.

CHAPTER

76

Sudden Death Risk Assessment in Hypertrophic Cardiomyopathy Across Lifespan

Shitij Chaudhary, Aseem Basha, Rakesh Yadav

ABSTRACT

Hypertrophic cardiomyopathy (HCM) is one of the most common causes of sudden cardiac death in young adults. There has been a significant decline in HCM-related all-cause mortality and sudden death overtime due to better screening and management strategies. However, sudden death risk assessment is crucial to identify patients who may derive the maximum benefit from implantable cardioverter defibrillator (ICD) therapy and avoid overtreatment at the same time. In this chapter, we discuss in detail the various clinical variables associated with sudden death and the strategies for risk assessment in HCM.

Keywords: Hypertrophic cardiomyopathy, sudden cardiac death, implantable cardiac defibrillator

INTRODUCTION

Hypertrophic cardiomyopathy (HCM) is the most common genetic cardiac disorder, with a population prevalence ranging from 1:200 to 1:500.[1] Often due to mutations in one of the sarcomeric genes, it is inherited in an autosomal-dominant pattern, with variable expressivity and incomplete penetrance. It has been regarded as one of the most common causes of sudden cardiac death (SCD) in young adults.

MORTALITY IN HYPERTROPHIC CARDIOMYOPATHY

Mortality in HCM is largely due to SCD, heart failure, atrial fibrillation, and thromboembolism besides noncardiac causes. Earlier natural history studies (published between 1960 and 2003) provided all-cause mortality estimates in HCM as high as 3–6% per year and sudden death rates as high as 1.5–3.5% per year.[2] These estimates confer quite a grim outlook on the prognosis associated with this disease. However, recent studies provide estimates of HCM-related all-cause mortality at 1.16% per year (0.53% from cardiac causes) and sudden death rates at 0.23% per year.[3] In a systematic review and meta-analysis, sudden death rates declined by more than twofold between studies from 2015 to 2020 compared to studies from 1985 to 2000 (0.32% per year vs. 0.73% per year).[4]

Such stark differences in mortality rates **(Table 1)**[5-10] may be attributed to tertiary referral bias in older cohorts, the inclusion of patients with milder disease in contemporary studies (diagnosed as a part of better screening strategies including family screening), the evolution of medical and interventional therapies (including surgical myectomy,

TABLE 1: Trends in HCM-related mortality over time.

Cohort	All-cause mortality rates	Sudden death rates
Early HCM referral cohorts:		
• Hardarson et al. (1973) (*n* = 119)[5]	5.5%	3.5%
• Shah et al. (1974) (*n* = 190)[6]	5.0%	2.6%
• McKenna et al. (1981) (*n* = 254)[7]	4.0%	2.2%
• Loogen et al. (1983) (*n* = 339)[8]	2.8%	
• Elliott et al. (2000) (*n* = 368)[9]	2.9%	1.7%
• SGH (1988–2002) (*n* = 956)[2]	2.3%	1.0%
Contemporary HCM cohorts:		
• O'Mahony et al. (2014) (*n* = 3,675)[10]		0.81%
• Maron et al. (2015) (*n* = 1,000)[3]	1.16%	0.23%
• Abdelfattah et al. (2022) (n = 6,393)*[4]		0.32%*

*Systematic review and meta-analysis (mortality rates from studies between 2015 and 2020 included).

alcohol ablation, and heart transplantation), and most importantly, appropriate recognition and management of patients at high risk of sudden death (primary and secondary prevention implantable cardiac defibrillators).

NEED FOR SUDDEN DEATH RISK ASSESSMENT

While the importance of implantable cardioverter defibrillator (ICD) therapy in HCM cannot be undermined, it is imperative to understand that it comes at the expense of high-cost burden, risk of inappropriate shocks, along with device-related and lead-related complications in low-risk patients. Therefore, sudden death risk assessment becomes crucial to identify patients who might derive maximum benefit from ICD therapy and avoid overtreatment at the same time.

CLINICAL VARIABLES ASSOCIATED WITH SUDDEN DEATH

The following clinical variables need to be considered for the assessment of sudden death risk in patients with HCM:

Age of the Patient

The patient's age is an important factor in determining the natural history and clinical course of HCM. Sudden death rates are low in HCM patients >60 years of age, with deaths mainly from noncardiac causes.[11] Childhood-onset HCM, albeit far less common than adult-onset HCM, with an estimated prevalence of 0.24–0.47 per 1,00,000, is associated with a much greater risk of sudden death, in the range of 1–1.5% per year.[12-16] There are data to suggest that the risk of sudden death in HCM is negligible below the age of 6 years and appears to rise beyond 8 years with a peak between 9 and 15 years of age.[17] Based on these data and the narrative set by the media showing HCM-related sudden deaths in young athletes, it appears that sudden death events occur only in the younger age group. However, ICD studies over the years have shown that shocks in HCM can be delayed with only 35% of patients with an ICD receiving appropriate shocks within 5 years of implant and the average age of first ICD therapy at 40 years.[18]

Family History of Sudden Death

Family history is considered significant if one or more first-degree or second-degree relatives have died suddenly, definitively, or likely due to HCM. While the AHA/ACC guidelines specify an age cutoff of <50 years, the ESC guidelines mention an age cutoff of <40 years for the same.[19,20] Multiple sudden deaths in tertiary relatives are also considered significant. While this is one of the factors to consider in adult-onset HCM, studies have shown no association with sudden death in pediatric HCM.[15,16]

Massive Left Ventricular Hypertrophy

Hypertrophic cardiomyopathy in adults is suspected based on an echocardiographic wall thickness of 15 mm or more (or 13 mm in cases of a positive family history and gene mutation carriers), which corresponds to a *z*-score of 6 above the mean. Diagnosis of HCM in children considers a *z*-score cutoff of >2.5 (or >2 in cases of a positive family history and gene mutation carriers).[19]

Massive LVH is defined as a wall thickness of 30 mm or more in any segment in adults or a *z*-score of 20 or more in children (>10 in the presence of another risk factor) and is associated with an increased risk of sudden death in various studies.[15,16,19-22] The risk of sudden death increases progressively with increasing wall thickness.[21,22]

There are data to suggest the discrepancy between measurements of wall thickness by cardiac MRI and transthoracic echocardiography with better correlation between measurements by contrast echocardiography and cardiac MRI.[23,24]

Unexplained Syncope

Syncope of unknown origin adjudged to be not of neurocardiogenic etiology and not due to left ventricular outflow tract obstruction (LVOTO), especially occurring within 6 months of evaluation is considered significant and is associated with increased sudden death risk.[15,16,19,20]

Nonsustained Ventricular Tachycardia

Nonsustained ventricular tachycardia (NSVT) is defined as three or more ventricular beats with a rate of 120 beats/min or more lasting for <30 seconds. The AHA/ACC guidelines specify that more weightages should be given to NSVT runs that are faster (200 beats/min or more), longer (10 beats or more), and frequent (3 runs or more). A VT rate that exceeds the sinus rate by 20% or more should be considered significant for pediatric patients.[19,20]

Left Ventricular Apical Aneurysms

Apical aneurysms are defined as discrete, thinned out, akinetic, or dyskinetic segments in the distal-most portions of the left ventricular cavity. A prevalence of as high as 3% is described in patients with HCM and they are generally associated with midcavitary obstruction.[25] The presence of LV apical aneurysms is associated with an increased risk of sudden death and thromboembolic events.[26]

Left Ventricular Systolic Dysfunction (Hypokinetic Hypertrophic Cardiomyopathy)

The prevalence of left ventricular systolic dysfunction (ejection fraction < 50%) in HCM ranges from 2.4 to 8.7% in various studies, with an annual incidence of 0.39–1.12% and is associated with an increased rate of sudden death events.[27-33]

Late Gadolinium Enhancement on Cardiac Magnetic Resonance Imaging

Late gadolinium enhancement (LGE) on cardiac magnetic resonance imaging (CMRI) represents replacement fibrosis in patients with HCM. The presence of LGE is common with a reported prevalence of 50–60%, but extensive LGE (15% or more) is seen in around 2% of patients with HCM only.[25] While there is heterogeneity among studies, one large study has shown that LGE of 15% or more is associated with an increased risk of sudden deaths even in low-intermediate risk HCM patients.[34] In a meta-analysis that studied the prognostic role of LGE in risk stratification in HCM, the presence of LGE on CMRI was associated with an increased risk of sudden death (odds ratio = 2.93). The extent of LGE was also associated with an increased risk of sudden death with an increase in hazard ratio by 1.56 for every 10% increase in LGE mass. This association remained significant even after adjusting for baseline variables.[35]

Genotype Status

There is significant heterogeneity among studies ascertaining a relationship between genotype status and phenotypic expression because of variable expressivity and incomplete penetrance in HCM. There is some data to suggest that in pediatric HCM, a positive pathogenic variant, especially MYH7 is associated with an increased risk of adverse cardiac outcomes including sudden death.[36] Based on this, the ACC/AHA has given a Class IIa recommendation to include genotype status as one of the variables to calculate sudden death risk in pediatric patients (<16 years of age) with HCM.[19]

Left Atrial Diameter

There are some data to suggest the association of an increased left atrial diameter with an increased sudden death risk and many risk prediction models have incorporated it as one of the variables.[10,15,16]

Left Ventricular Outflow Tract Obstruction

In various studies, the maximal LVOT gradient obtained by transthoracic echocardiography has shown a correlation with sudden death risk and has been incorporated in risk prediction models and calculators.[10,16,37]

Table 2 summarizes the hazard ratios for the various clinical variables associated with sudden death.[35,38]

STRATEGIES FOR SUDDEN DEATH RISK ASSESSMENT

The best strategy for sudden death risk assessment is still a matter of debate. For now, it may be best to apply the "see-saw model" for risk assessment **(Fig. 1)**.[39] The "see-saw" provides a weighted balance between the sensitivity and the specificity of a strategy in identifying high-risk patients eligible for an ICD. While one strategy may identify nearly all high-risk patients eligible for an ICD (high sensitivity), it would entail some low-risk patients receiving an ICD with its possible complications of inappropriate shocks and device-related complications (low specificity). In contrast, another approach with higher specificity would decrease the number of ICDs implanted at the expense of missing some high-risk patients (lower sensitivity).

TABLE 2: Hazard ratios for clinical variables associated with sudden death.

Clinical variable	Hazard ratio (95% CI)	Population attributable risk
Age	0.53 (0.18–1.53)	
Family history of sudden death	2.34 (1.46–3.75)	11.89%
Syncope	2.31 (1.22–4.38)	8.16%
NSVT	2.92 (1.97–4.33)	14.47%
Maximum LV wall thickness	3.17 (1.64–6.13)	
LV outflow obstruction	2.41 (1.55–3.73)	16.44%
LGE on CMRI	3.41 (1.97–5.94)	

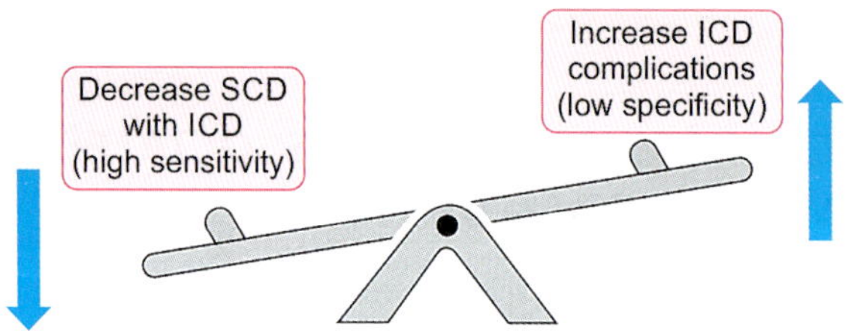

FIG. 1: The "see-saw" model.[39]

Following the "see-saw" model, currently, two different approaches are advocated by the AHA/ACC and the ESC, respectively.

The "major risk marker strategy" advocated by the AHA/ACC utilizes a list of major risk markers to identify high-risk patients (with one or more major risk markers adjudging the patient to be at high risk). After the physician's judgment of patient risk, emphasis is laid on shared decision-making, considering the psychological aspect and the patient's perspective on sudden death risk. An important factor to note is that LGE and CMR-related markers are included in this strategy, which might account for at least 20% of the appropriate ICD shocks and hence a greater sensitivity. This strategy provides a sensitivity of 95% with a specificity of 78%, with greater flexibility to both the physician and the patient.[19,39] **Figure 2** summarizes the AHA/ACC strategy.

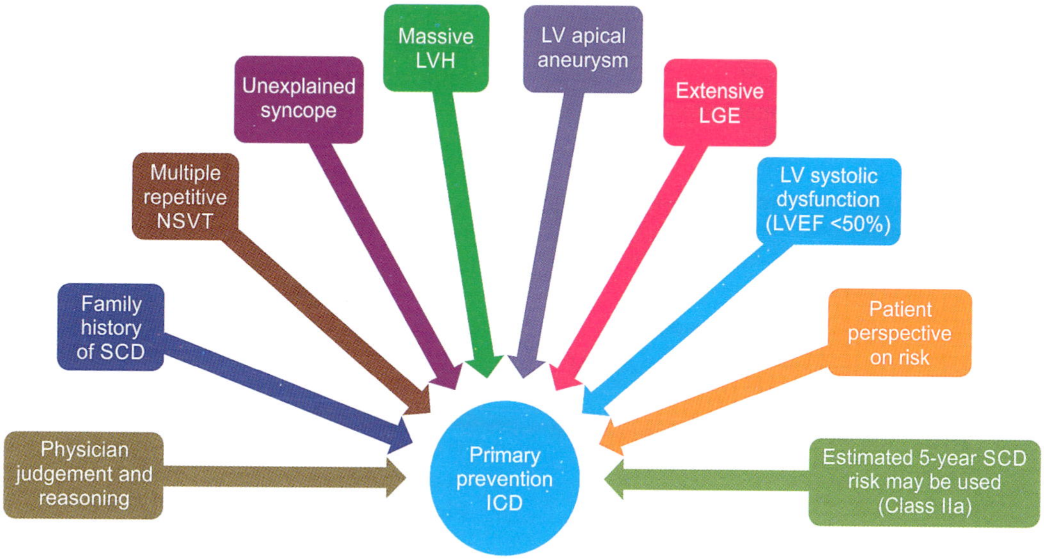

FIG. 2: The ACC/AHA "major risk marker strategy"[19]—presence of one or more major risk markers along with shared decision-making.

On the other hand, the ESC advocates the "risk score" approach, wherein a set of predefined variables is used to calculate the 5-year sudden death risk, and management recommendations are based on whether a patient falls into one of three risk categories: Low (<4%—ICD not indicated), intermediate (4–6%—ICD could be considered), or high (≥6%—ICD should be considered). This approach, albeit more objective, provides less flexibility regarding the patient's perspective on risk and shared decision-making. Also, CMR-related parameters are not directly incorporated into the risk score, which accounts for a lower sensitivity of 34% with a higher specificity of 92% of this strategy. However, the most recent ESC guidelines (2023) provide an opportunity to consider CMR-related parameters (extensive LGE 15% or more) in patients adjudged to be in the low-intermediate risk category based on the risk score **(Flowchart 1)**.

Although the two approaches advocated by the AHA/ACC and the ESC are quite different, both highlight that sudden death risk assessment in HCM is a trade-off between preventing sudden death with appropriate device therapies and device-related complications. Shared decision-making with the patient is also an important part of risk assessment. **Table 3** highlights the important differences between the two approaches.

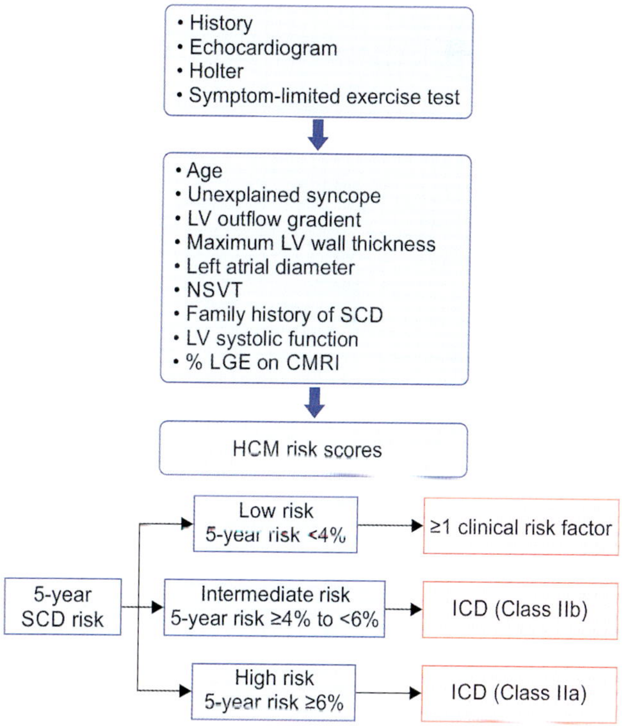

FLOWCHART 1: ESC "risk score" approach.[20]

ASSESSMENT OF SUDDEN DEATH RISK

The first and foremost step in evaluating sudden death risk in HCM is to screen for any compelling indication of an ICD for secondary prevention. Implantation of an ICD is recommended in patients who have survived a cardiac arrest due to VT or VF or who have spontaneously sustained VT with hemodynamic compromise.[20]

Once it has been established that there is no compelling indication for secondary prevention, it is prudent to search for various risk factors and clinical variables (as summarized previously) to identify patients at high risk of SCD, who may be candidates for an ICD for primary prevention. The workup to identify such patients should include:[40]

- Clinical evaluation including personal history of syncope suspected to be arrhythmic
- Family history in a close relative of premature HCM-related sudden death, cardiac arrest, or sustained ventricular arrhythmias
- 48-hour ambulatory ECG for NSVT episodes
- TTE (or CMR in the case of poor echo windows)—maximal LV wall thickness, EF, LV apical aneurysm, and LGE
- A symptom-limited exercise test

TABLE 3: Comparison between ACC/AHA and ESC strategies for risk assessment.

Variables	AHA/ACC	ESC
Strategy	"Major risk marker"	"Risk score"
ICD decisions based on	≥1 major risk marker	Objective HCM risk score
Shared decision-making	Recommended	Only in low-risk patients
Sensitivity	95%	33%
Specificity	78%	92%
Flexibility	More	Less (objective score)
Tested prospectively	Yes	No
Risk markers used:		
• Unexplained syncope	Yes	Yes
• Family history of SCD	Yes	Yes
• NSVT runs	Yes	Yes
• Massive LVH	Yes	Yes
• LV systolic function	Yes	Yes
• LGE on CMRI	Yes	No*
• Left atrial diameter	No	Yes
• LV outflow gradient	No	Yes
• Age	Yes**	Yes
• LV apical aneurysm	Yes	No

* Not included as a variable in the risk score, but the ESC 2023 guidelines recommend use in low-risk patients (Class IIb).

**Not included as a major risk marker but given weightage as a variable that might impact decision-making.

Cardiac MRI is recommended for all HCM patients not identified as high-risk for SCD based on the above evaluation to assess for maximum LV wall thickness, EF, LV apical aneurysm, and extent of myocardial fibrosis with LGE.

A predefined set of variables is then used to estimate the 5-year risk of SCD using one of the validated risk prediction scores. It is important to note that clinical evaluation for SCD risk is a continuous process with periodic reevaluations every 1–2 years.

Flowchart 2 summarizes sudden death risk assessment.

RISK PREDICTION SCORES

The various validated risk prediction scores and models for adults and pediatric patients with HCM are as follows:

Risk Score for Adults with Hypertrophic Cardiomyopathy

HCM Risk-SCD Score (Table 4)[10]

This score estimates the risk of SCD at 5 years. It should not be used in pediatric patients (<16 years), elite or competitive athletes, HCM associated with metabolic diseases and syndromes, or HCM patients eligible for secondary prevention ICD. The score provides modest discriminatory ability in identifying HCM patients at high risk of sudden death (c-statistic-0.70).[41]

According to the ESC Guidelines, in patients with a 5-year risk of SCD < 4%, an ICD is generally not indicated, in patients

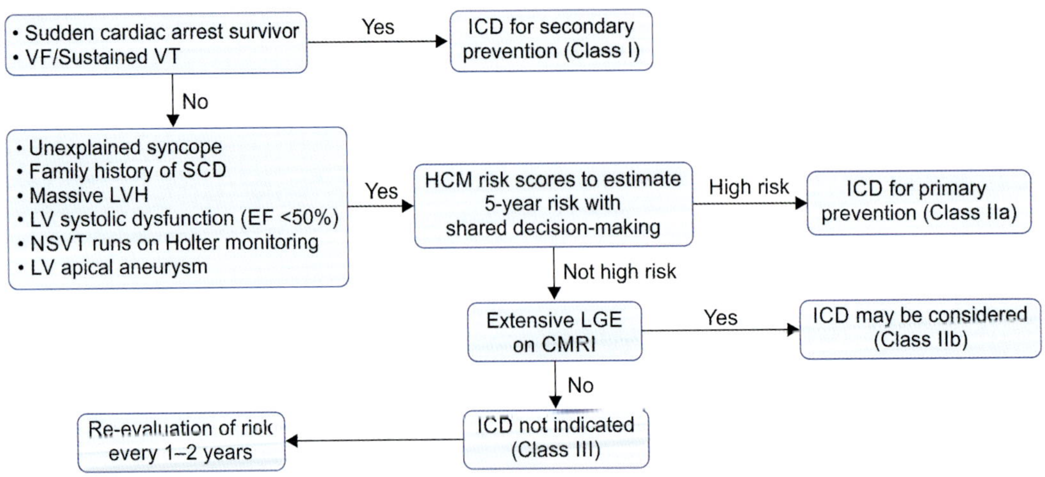

FLOWCHART 2: Summary of sudden death risk assessment and indication for ICDs.

TABLE 4: HCM risk scores.

Adult risk score	Pediatric risk scores	
HCM risk-SCD score	HCM Risk-Kids score	PRIMACY score
Age (16–80 years)	Age (1–16 years)	Age (0–18 years)
Maximum LV wall thickness	Maximum LV wall thickness z-score	Maximum IVS thickness diameter Maximum LV posterior wall diameter
Left atrial size	Left atrial diameter z-score	Left atrial diameter
LVOT gradient	LVOT gradient	LVOT gradient
Family history of SCD	–	–
NSVT	NSVT	History of NSVT in prior 6 months
Unexplained syncope	Unexplained syncope	Unexplained syncope in prior 6 months
	Gender	–
	Weight	Weight
		Height
		Genotype status

with a risk of 4–6%, an ICD may be considered and in patients with a 5-year risk ≥ 6%, an ICD should be considered.[20]

Risk Scores for Pediatric Patients with Hypertrophic Cardiomyopathy

It is now being increasingly recognized that pediatric HCM behaves differently than adult HCM, with a preponderance of syndromic and metabolic causes in infancy, a lower prevalence of HCM compared to adults, a higher sudden death risk, and different weightages of risk factors for sudden death. Adult models applied to pediatric HCM cohorts have been found to underestimate the risk with limited discriminatory power.[16] Added to this is a higher risk of device-related complications in children which necessitates separate risk stratification tools for pediatric HCM.

Among the various risk factors for sudden death, a family history of sudden death is not predictive of risk in the pediatric population and therefore is excluded from most pediatric risk scores.[42] LVOT gradient has been either found not to be associated or inversely associated with sudden death risk in some studies, making it a less useful variable in the pediatric population.[16,43] Genotype status is predictive of sudden death in the pediatric population and therefore, it has been included in some pediatric risk scores (PRIMACY risk score).[36]

HCM Risk-Kids Score (Table 4)[16]

This score is not validated for patients <1 year of age or >16 years of age, patients with a secondary prevention ICD indication, syndromic HCM, and HCM associated with inborn errors of metabolism.

PRIMACY Score (Table 4)[15]

Refer to **Table 4**.

IMPLANTABLE CARDIOVERTER DEFIBRILLATOR EXPERIENCE IN HYPERTROPHIC CARDIOMYOPATHY

The overall rate of appropriate device therapy in HCM patients with an ICD is 3.3–4.8% per year with a corresponding inappropriate device therapy rate of 4.8–4.9% per year and an annualized ICD-related complication rate of 3.4–3.8%.[44,45] For HCM patients with an ICD for secondary prevention, the rate of appropriate device therapy has been reported to be >10% per year in various studies.[46] The number of ICDs to treat and save one life ranges between 6.6 and 7.2.[39] The unpredictable course of HCM as a disorder is exemplified by the fact that 65% of initial appropriate ICD shocks occur 5 years or more after ICD implantation.[18]

CAVEATS IN THE EXISTING LITERATURE

There are still gaps in the evidence regarding sudden death in HCM. The role of provocable LVOT gradients and their impact on prognosis is still unknown. Also, the impact of alcohol septal ablation and surgical myectomy on reducing sudden death risk is still unclear despite proven efficacy in reducing LVOT gradients.

FUTURE DIRECTIONS

Subcutaneous ICDs with their attendant lower lead-related complications might overcome the barrier associated with ICD implantation, especially in pediatric patients. However, data on long-term safety and efficacy are still required.

Experimental disease-modifying therapies include N-acetyl cysteine (NAC), statins, and ranolazine. Future developments might include personalized approaches to drug therapy as per the genotype status and approaches to prevent disease onset in mutation carriers.[47]

CONCLUSION

Hypertrophic cardiomyopathy is a heterogeneous disorder with an unpredictable course and prognosis. Contemporary therapies, especially ICDs, have reduced HCM-related cardiac mortality considerably. However, it is important to appropriately select patients who might derive the greatest benefit from ICDs and reduce overtreatment at the same time.

Sudden death risk assessment in HCM entails a trade-off between preventing sudden deaths with ICD therapy and device-related complications with shared decision-making with the patient, considering various clinical variables.

ONLINE REFERENCES

Please scan the QR code provided at the end of the table of contents for References of this chapter.

CHAPTER

77

Hypertrophic Cardiomyopathy and Its Mimics: From Diagnosis to New Therapeutics

Jagdish Chander Mohan, Vinayak Agrawal, Madhu Shukla

ABSTRACT

Concentric symmetrical or asymmetric regional ventricular hypertrophy predominantly involving the left ventricle and often secondary to genetic mutation of sarcomeric proteins is the hallmark of hypertrophic cardiomyopathy (HCM). Hypertrophy preferentially affects the basal septum and anterior wall, although its morphological patterns and severity are extremely variable. There are several phenocopies of HCM seen in clinical practice which may have subtle morpho-functional distinguishing features or distinct genotypes. Biochemical, imaging, hemodynamic, and genetic markers may help in differential diagnosis. This review describes some of the HCM mimics and their impact of therapy. New therapeutic strategies are targeting myosin motor to reduce hypercontractility and hence subsequent apoptosis and fibrosis.

Keywords: Hypertrophy, hemodynamic

INTRODUCTION

Myocardial hypertrophy is an abnormal enlargement of cardiomyocytes and/or extracellular matrix. Maladaptive or noncompensatory pathological hypertrophy without increase in afterload is an important cause of heart failure, arrhythmias, and sudden death.[1] Its etiopathogenesis is incompletely understood but cellular hypertrophy, impaired myocardial energetics, calcium mishandling, and microvascular dysfunction are the common threads. This entity called hypertrophic cardiomyopathy (HCM) or sarcomeric HCM has been extensively studies in last 70 years with emphasis on genes and signaling pathways regulating hypertrophy. Dozens of genes regulating sarcomeric proteins have been identified and related phenotypes described in detail. More than a thousand point mutations have been reported in over a dozen genes in inherited forms of HCM.[1] Genotype-phenotype relationship still remains partly unresolved. Almost 50% of patients with HCM show no known genetic abnormality. Molecular discoveries have led to cell-level dysfunction and then to organ-level dysfunction in HCM. With ever-growing genomic datasets, biological phenomics are lagging behind. Major area of interest has been myosin nano-motor proteins. The ventricles are hypercontractile due to hypertrophied cardiomyocytes whose trajectories may be antianatomical (myofiber disarray). There are several closely mimicking phenotypes which need to be differentiated so that appropriate therapy can be initiated at the earliest.

VENTRICULAR HYPERTROPHY AT THE CORE

Faced with an increase in afterload, the left ventricle maintains stroke volume by increasing pressure-generating contractile units called sarcomeres in the cardiomyocytes which are laid parallel to each other resulting in thickening of the myocytes and consequently of the myocardium. This is adaptive or compensatory hypertrophy. In HCM, the same phenomenon of increased contractile protein synthesis occurs without any known stimulus and laying of sarcomeres is not necessarily parallel to each other **(Fig. 1)**. This disarray is at all level—sarcomeres, myocytes, and muscle bundles as well. In addition, it may have segmental or regional preponderance under genetic influence. Abnormalities of sarcomere function in HCM increase the energy cost of force production and result in an energy-deficient state, which is exacerbated by abnormal oxygen delivery to the thick cardiac muscle due to microvascular ischemia. This is the major source of symptoms. Collectively, phenotypical patterns of HCM are by and large distinct **(Figs. 2A to D)**. It is the most common inherited cardiomyopathy with a prevalence of at least 0.5% in the population with dynamic intraventricular obstruction in about two-thirds of the cases.[2]

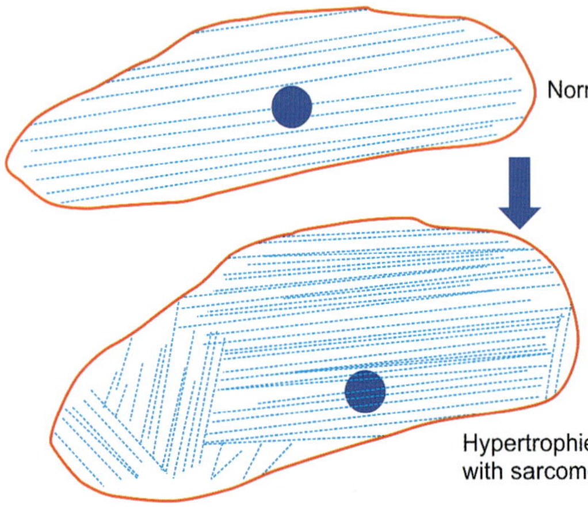

FIG. 1: Cartoon showing normal pattern of sarcomeric pattern in upper panel and sarcomeric disarray of HCM in the lower panel.

MIMICS OF HCM

Myocardial thickening in one or more segments without any known cause is the hallmark of HCM. Guidelines advocate using a diastolic wall thickness cut-off of 15 mm in one or more myocardial segments, measured by any imaging technique to diagnose HCM.[3] It needs to be differentiated from the athlete's heart, infiltrative or metabolic disorders, and neoplastic infiltration.[4] Differential diagnosis among the phenotypic expressions of HCM and other causes of myocardial thickening may be challenging. Tissue characterization, which is limited with echocardiography, could provide additional diagnostic information. The tissue characterization capabilities of cardiac magnetic resonance imaging (MRI) may help to differentiate HCM from other causes of myocardial thickening and to suggest an appropriate therapy. Clues to exact diagnosis may be given by pattern and site of hypertrophy but these are not definitive.

PHENOTYPES OF HCM

In HCM, myocardial thickening can be regional or diffuse. Specific patterns such as subaortic stenosis, mid-cavity, and

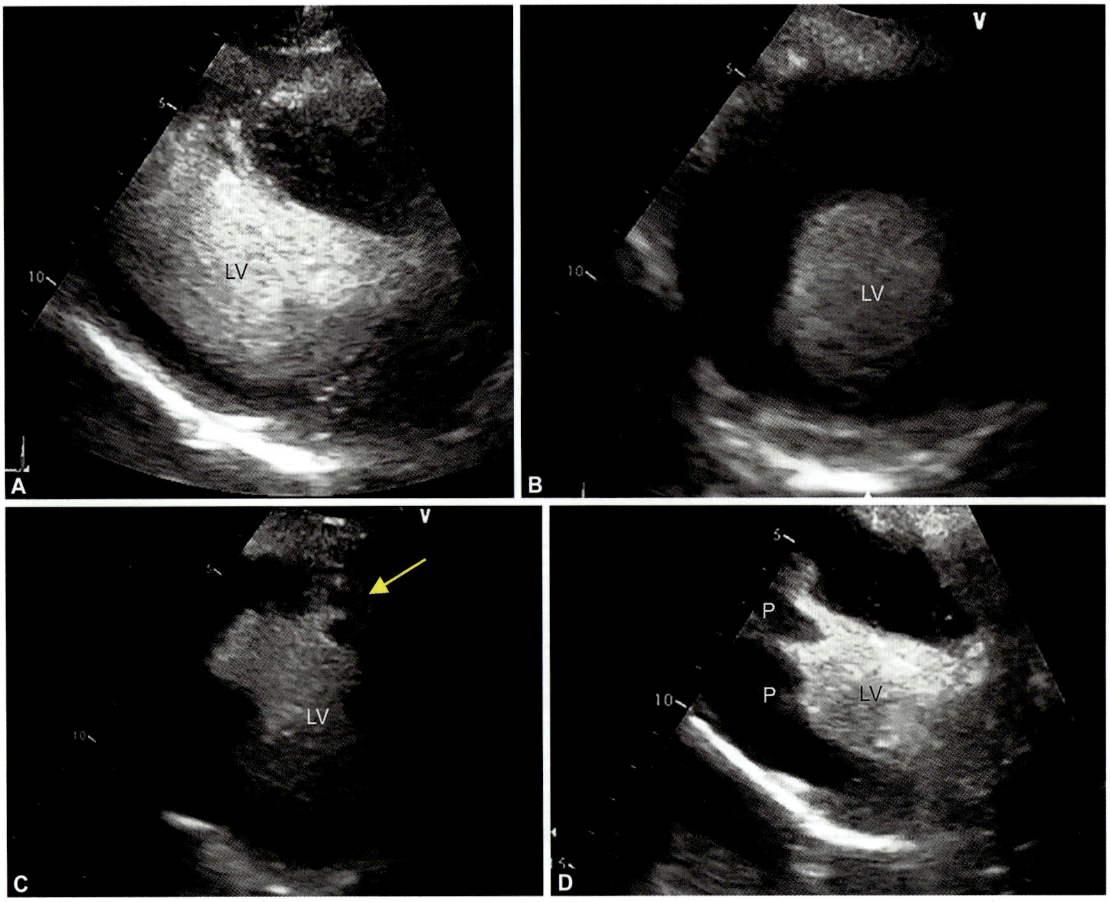

FIG. 2A TO D: Contrast-enhanced parasternal transthoracic 2D-echocardiographic long axis views (A and D) and short axis views (B and C). Note asymmetric septal hypertrophy with normal inferolateral wall. (C) Anteriorly placed papillary muscle (yellow arrow).

apical HCM etc., are well described. The hypertrophy can be concentric or asymmetric, obstructive or nonobstructive, with or without mitral valve abnormalities and may have accompaniments such as abnormal location of papillary muscles, prominent trabeculae, and myocardial crypts **(Figs. 3 to 6)**. Mitral valve abnormalities as a phenotypic

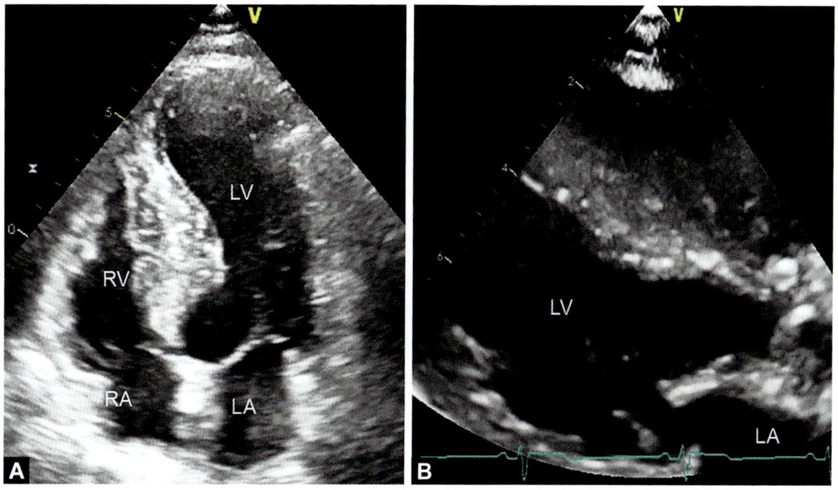

FIGS. 3A AND B: Two HCM phenotypes with isolated septal hypertrophy. (A) Reverse curvature and (B) neutral curvature of the interventricular septum. Note thickened anterior mitral leaflet in Figure B.

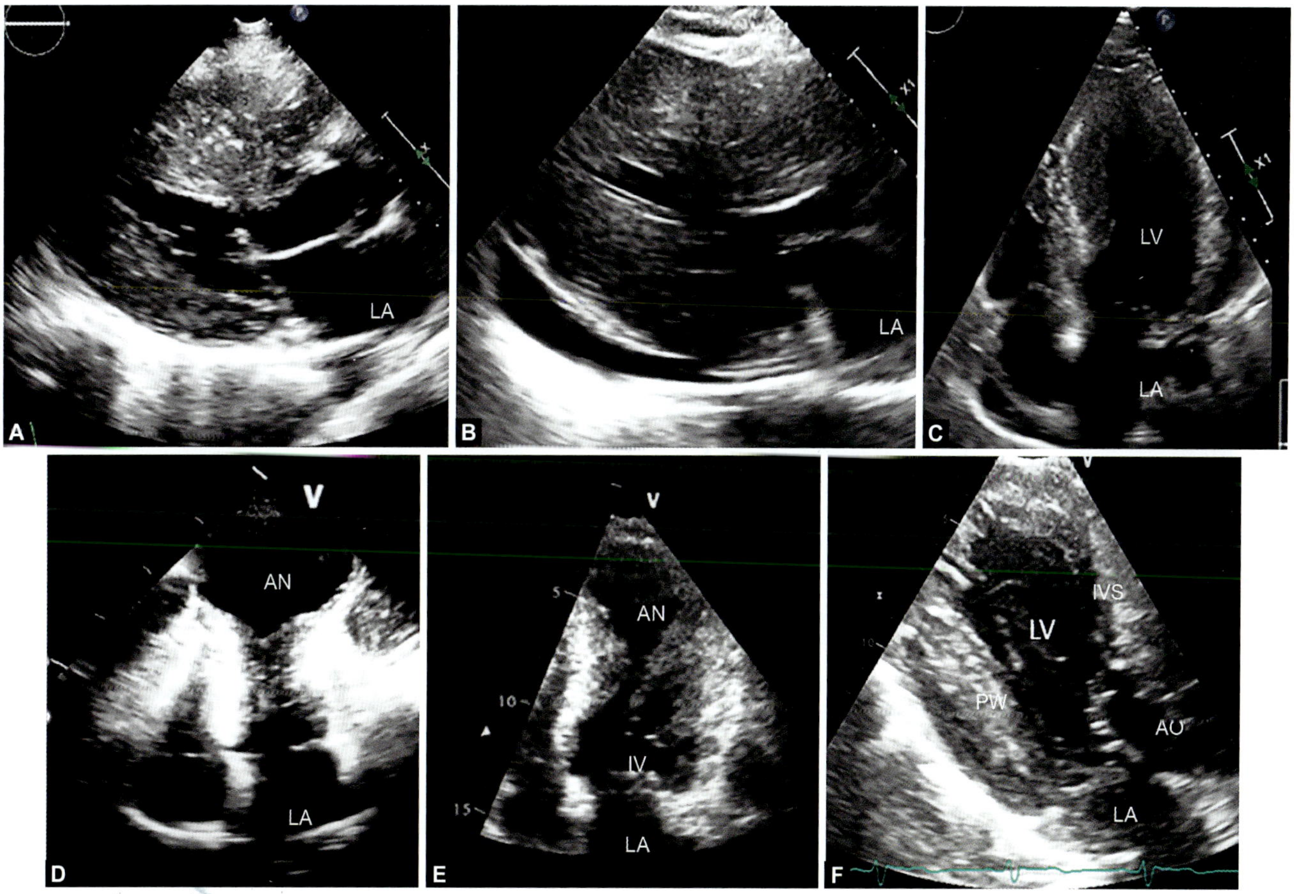

FIGS. 4A TO F: Phenotypes of HCM. (A) Classic HCM with asymmetric septal hypertrophy, systolic anterior motion of the anterior mitral leaflet and elongated leaflet. (B) Severe concentric hypertrophy. (C) typical apical HCM. (D and E) Mid-cavity obstruction with apical aneurysm (AN). (F) Unusual variety of HCM characterized by hypertrophy of inferolateral wall with elongated mitral valve leaflets and myocardial crypts.

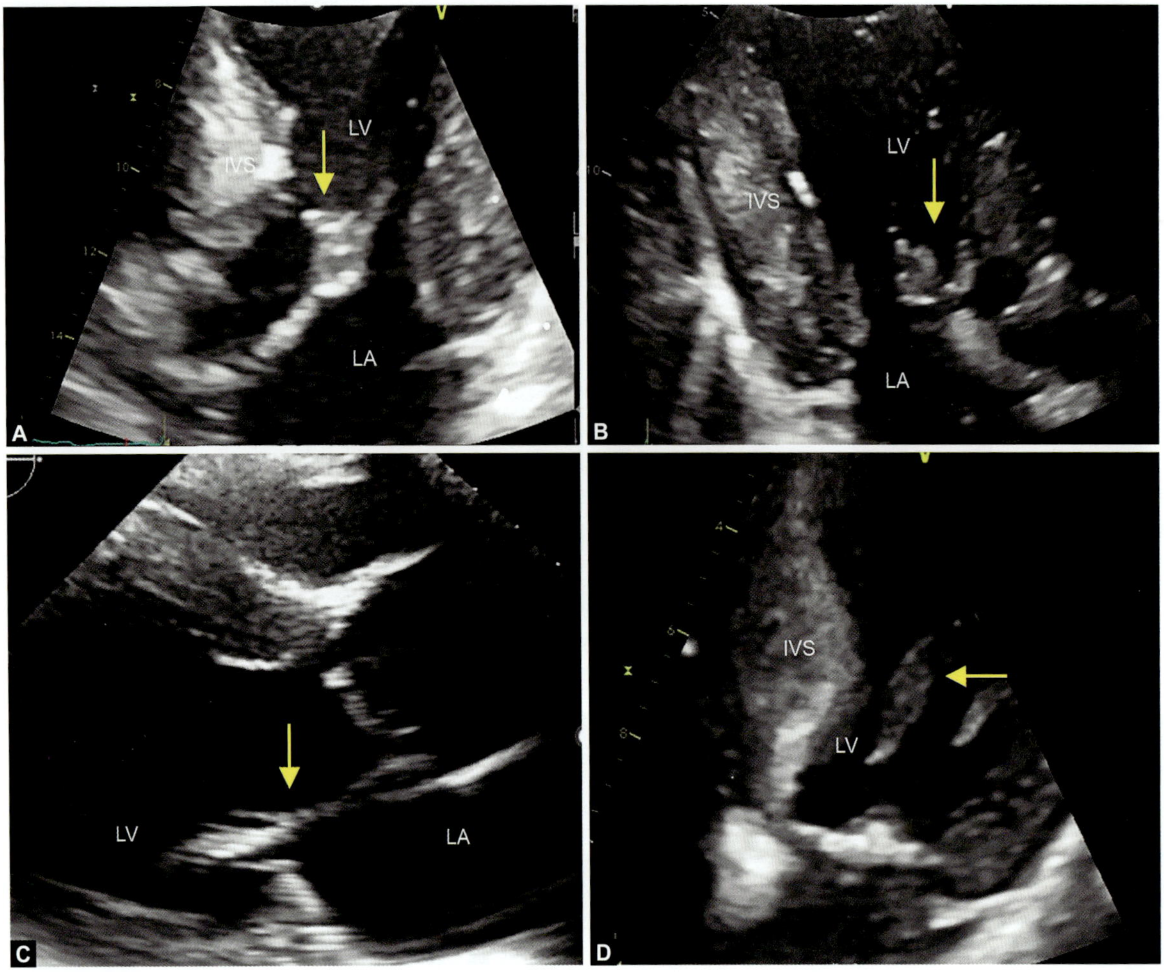

FIGS. 5A TO D: Distinctive mitral valve abnormalities in HCM. (A) Thickened anterior mitral leaflet; (B) Anomalous attachment of anterior leaflet to the septum; (C) Elongated leaflet; (D) Abnormally placed papillary muscle.

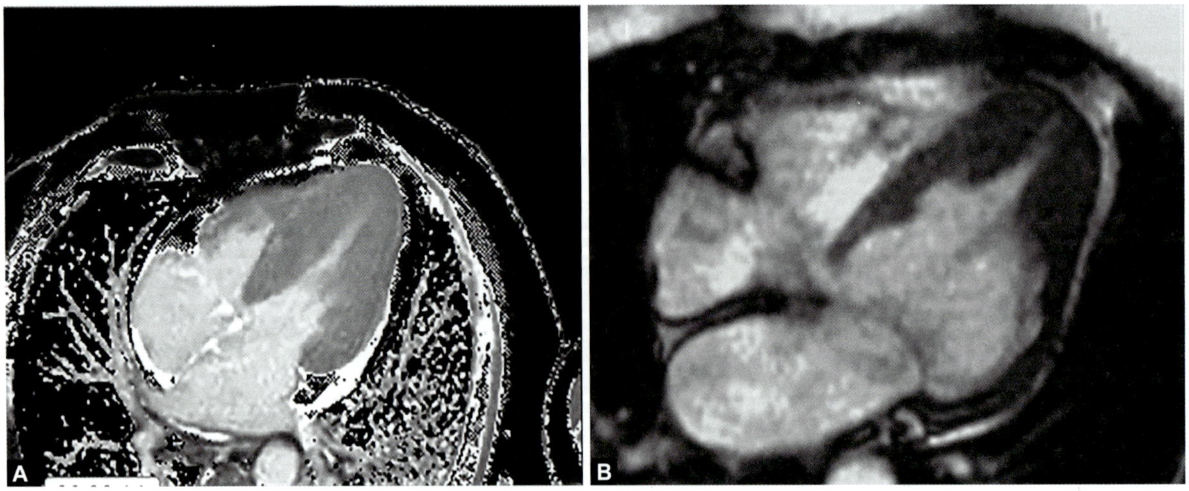

FIGS. 6A AND B: Cine magnetic resonance imaging showing (A) concentric hypertrophy and (B) typical apical HCM. Also note dilated atria.

expression of HCM are found in 50% cases.[5] Elongated mitral valve leaflets, anterior mitral tenting by displaced, hypertrophied papillary muscles, thickened leaflets, annular calcification, retracted secondary chordae, and reduced outflow size due to accessory papillary muscle-like LV muscle bundles are frequent.

Athlete's Heart

Physiological hypertrophy seen in the athlete's heart must be distinguished from pathological hypertrophy because the latter may be associated with sudden death in the young. In the athlete's heart, LV wall hypertrophy is symmetric, usually mild (≤ 15 mm in male and ≤ 13 mm in female athletes) and is associated with increase in volume of both ventricles.[6] Relative wall thickness (RWT) is <0.42 and detraining effect can be seen **(Figs. 7 to 9 and Box 1)**. A cut-off for the LV end-diastolic wall thickness (LVEDWT) related to LV end-diastolic volume (LVEDV) of <0.15 (LVEDWT/LVEDV < 0.15)[6] and an LVEDV related to LV end-diastolic mass (LVEDM) of >2.25 (LVEDV/LVEDM > 2.25) in athlete's heart can help distinguish physiological hypertrophy from HCM.[7]

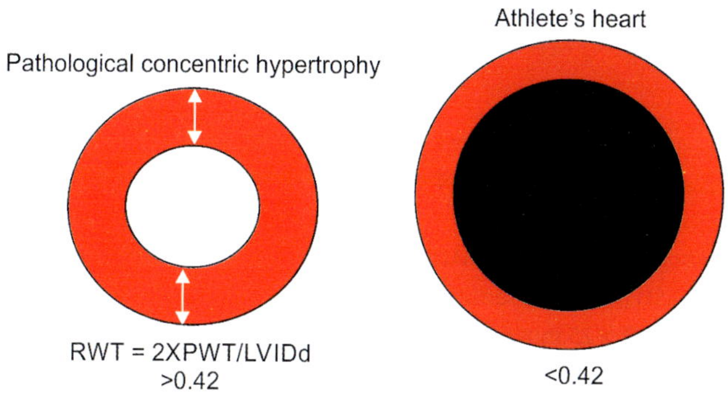

FIG. 7: Schematic depiction of pathological versus physiological left ventricular hypertrophy in an athlete.

(LVIDd: left ventricular end-diastolic diameter; PWT: posterior wall thickness; RWT: relative wall thickness)

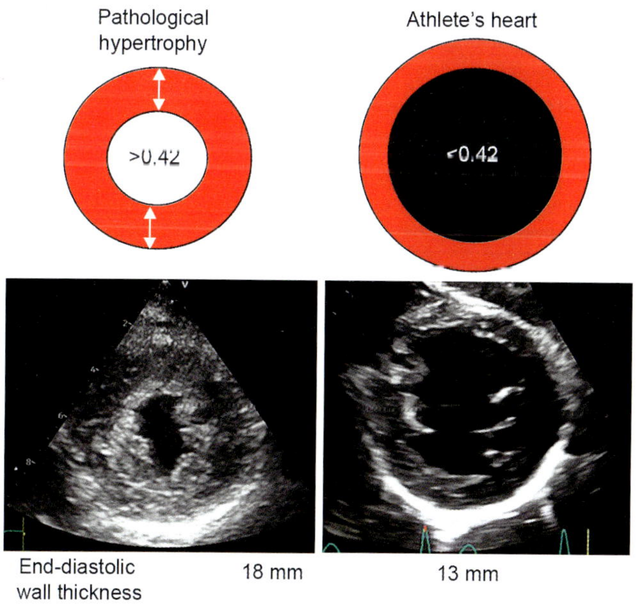

FIGS. 8A AND B: Transthoracic short axis views depicting pathological hypertrophy (A) compared to that seen in an athlete (B). Upper panels show schematic depiction with relative wall thickness in figures.

Although concentric symmetrical hypertrophy, ellipsoid geometry and favoring detraining effect suggest the presence of athlete's heart, both may coexist and cause confusion.

Hypertensive Left Ventricular Hypertrophy

Hypertension is a common vascular disorder and frequently coexists with HCM in the adults. Hypertensive left ventricular hypertrophy (LVH) can mimic nongenetic HCM more so in elderly females who may have severe LVH with mitral annular calcification. Uncommonly, asymmetric septal hypertrophy, hypertrabeculation, myocardial crypts, and systolic anterior motion of the mitral valve have been reported in hypertensive LVH. However, regional hypertrophy and isolated apical hypertrophy is not seen in the hypertensive hearts **(Box 2)**. Severe reduction in longitudinal strain and diastolic function by tissue Doppler imaging and paradoxically positive septal systolic strain usually points toward HCM with good sensitivity and specificity.[8,9]

NONCOMPACTION OR VENTRICULAR HYPERTRABECULATION

Left ventricular (LV) noncompaction is defined by an increase of trabeculations in the LV endomyocardium and is currently considered to be an acquired trait due to altered loading conditions and a rare genetic cardiomyopathy. It results in apparently thick LV walls if wall thickness is measured with inclusion of trabeculae. Hypertrabeculation is common in HCM as well in athletes and during pregnancy. About 25% of the myocardium in HCM is composed of hypertrabeculated mass.[10] It is more in females, in nonobstructive cardiomyopathy and in those with neutral septal curvature and systolic dysfunction. Hypertrabeculation is a part of HCM phenotype but can also occur in other conditions of altered hemodynamic load **(Figs. 10A to D)**.

CARDIAC AMYLOIDOSIS

Cardiac amyloidosis (CA) results from extracellular deposition of amyloidotic light chain immunoglobulins. Diffuse increase in LV wall thickness often with ground glass appearance, preserved LV ejection fraction (EF), small LV volumes, and restrictive flow pattern are characteristic features on transthoracic echocardiography.[11,12] Both types of CA (AL and aTTR) can mimic HCM. CA and HCM are characterized by increased ventricular wall thickness and mass **(Figs. 11A and B)**. Although several echocardiographic features can distinguish the two entities, these are neither sensitive nor specific **(Box 3)**. Asymmetric septal thickening, apical sparing, right ventricular (RV) hypertrophy, biatrial dilatation, pericardial effusion, and restrictive transmitral flow patterns are well described in conditions other than

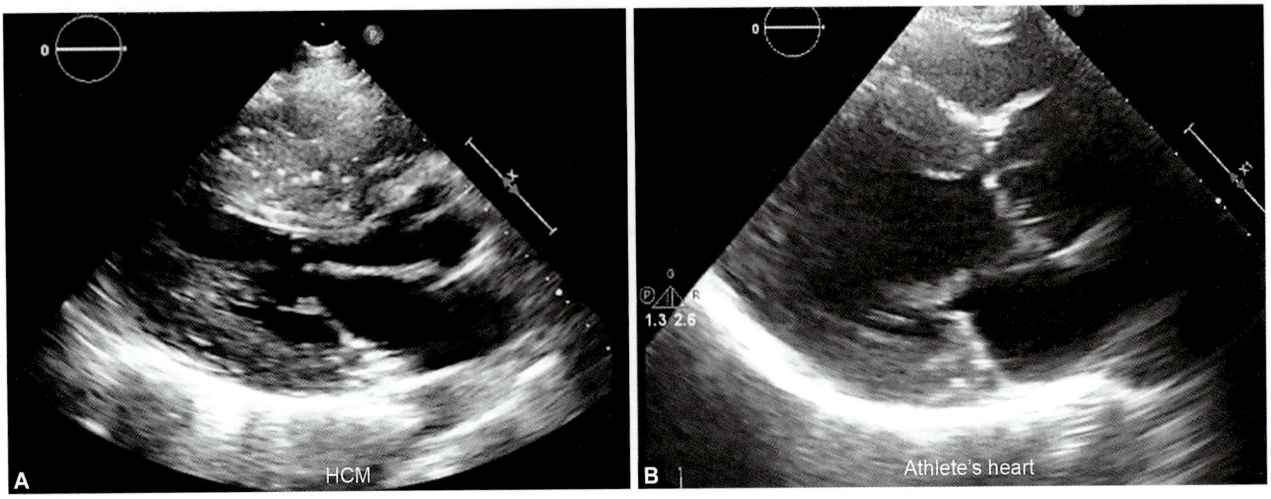

FIGS. 9A AND B: Transthoracic parasternal long axis views depicting pathological hypertrophy (A) compared to that seen in an athlete (B). (HCM: hypertrophic cardiomyopathy)

BOX 1 Distinctive features of athlete's heart.

HCM versus athlete's heart:
- In athlete's heart, relative wall thickness is <0.42
- LV end-diastolic diameter is usually > 55 mm in the athletes
- In HCM, there may be asymmetric or regional hypertrophy which is not present in athlete's heart
- Systolic anterior motion of mitral valve and mitral valve abnormalities are not seen in athlete's heart
- Diastolic function is almost always abnormal HCM while it can be normal or supernormal in athletes
- Intraventricular pressure gradients are not observed in athletes
- Left ventricular global longitudinal strain is normal or nearly normal in athletes
- Late gadolinium enhancement is a feature of HCM
- On cardiac MRI, T1 values are abnormal and extracellular matrix expands in HCM. Athletes have reduced extracellular volume
- Detraining for 3 months can cause regression of hypertrophy in athletes and this does not happen in HCM

BOX 2 Characteristic features of HCM which are usually not present in hypertensive heart disease.

Imaging features in HCM to differentiate from hypertensive heart:
- ASH (>1.3,80% sensitivity)
- LVWT > 25 mm
- Dynamic LVOT obstruction
- Elongated mitral leaflets
- Abnormal pap muscles
- Apicoseptal muscle bundles
- Myocardial crypts
- Apical aneurysms
- Paradoxical longitudianl strain, more pronounced in septum
- IVS hypokinesis
- *SAM (98% specificity)* in early systole
- Right ventricular hypertrophy

(ASH: asymmetric septal hypertrophy; HCM: hypertrophic cardiomyopathy; IVS: interventricular septum; SAM: systolic anterior motion of the mitral valve)

the two entities.[11] In rare instances, CA can mimic HCM.[13-16] Mostly CA resembling obstructive HCM is found in the senile transthyretin type, but a few cases of the AL type CA presenting as obstructive HCM are described.[17] In a recent series of 153 patients with HCM, eight patients were found to have transthyretin amyloidosis but none had obstruction.[12] On the other hand, in a consecutive series of AL amyloidosis studied over 2 years, 4% patients had typical dynamic LV outflow obstruction with systolic motion of the anterior mitral valve leaflet **(Figs. 12 to 14)**.[17]

The QRS amplitude on ECG is a useful discriminator in infiltrative versus HCM, since voltages are usually increased in muscular hypertrophy and diminished in the infiltrative myopathies.[12] Cardiac MRI demonstrates late gadolinium enhancement (LGE)—global subendocardial enhancement, an endocardial-epicardial signal intensity gradient typical for amyloidosis, with the early gadolinium clearance from the blood pool **(Figs. 14A and B)**. This pattern of gadolinium distribution suggests CA.

RASOPATHIES AND HCM

Two common malformation syndromes associated with HCM are Noonan syndrome and LEOPARD syndrome.[18] Noonan syndrome is an autosomal dominant disorder characterized by unusual facies, short height, skeletal dysmorphosis, cutaneous fragility, pulmonary or aortic stenosis, atrioventricular septal defects, and nonobstructive HCM **(Figs. 15A to D)**.

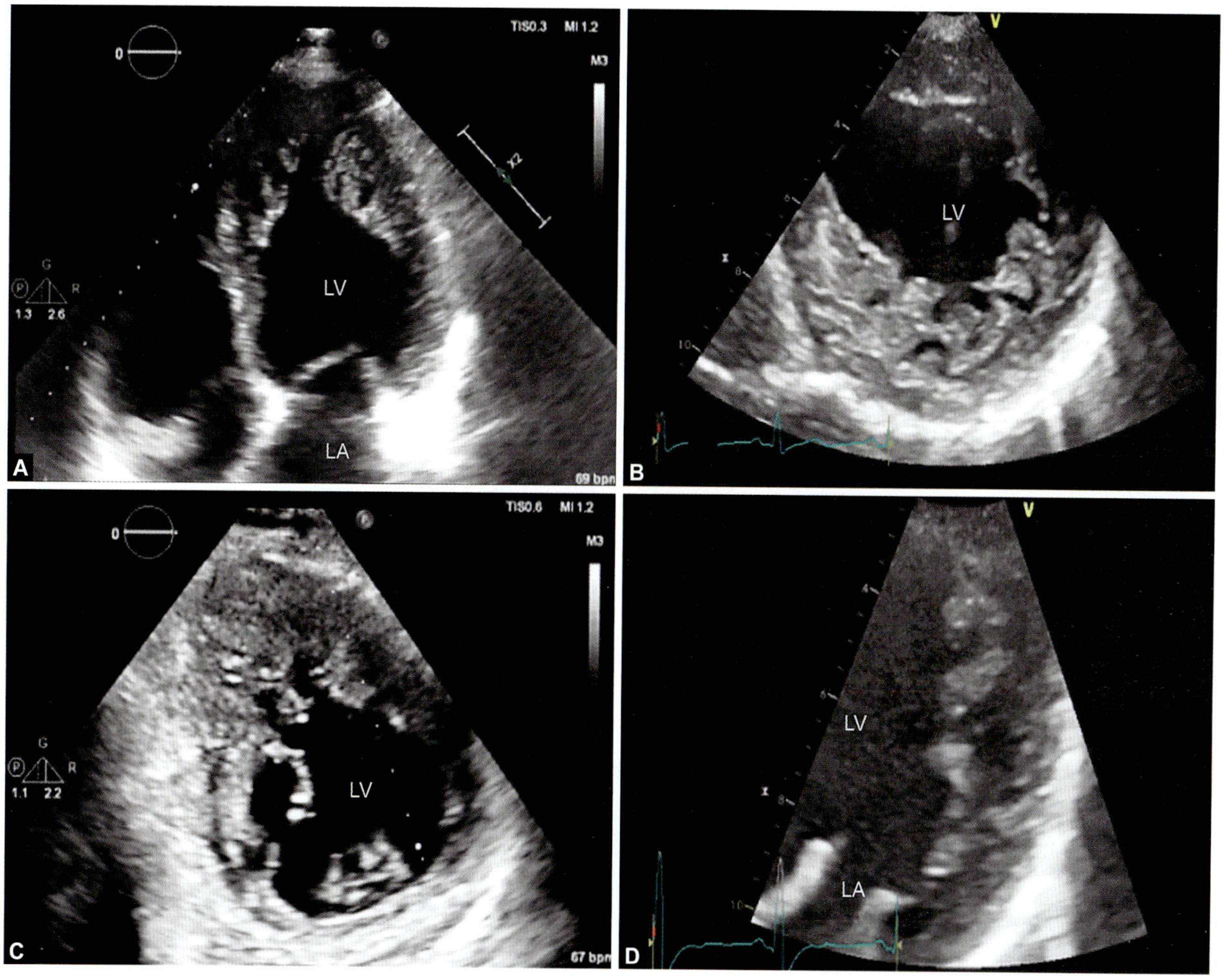

FIGS. 10A TO D: Left ventricular hypertrabeculation mimicking HCM in various disease states. (A) Apical four-chamber view in a patient on maintenance hemodialysis. (B) Short axis view in a 2-month-old child with heart failure. (C) Hypertrabeculation in an asymptomatic person. (D) Hypertrabeculated left ventricular free wall in a case of dilated cardiomyopathy.

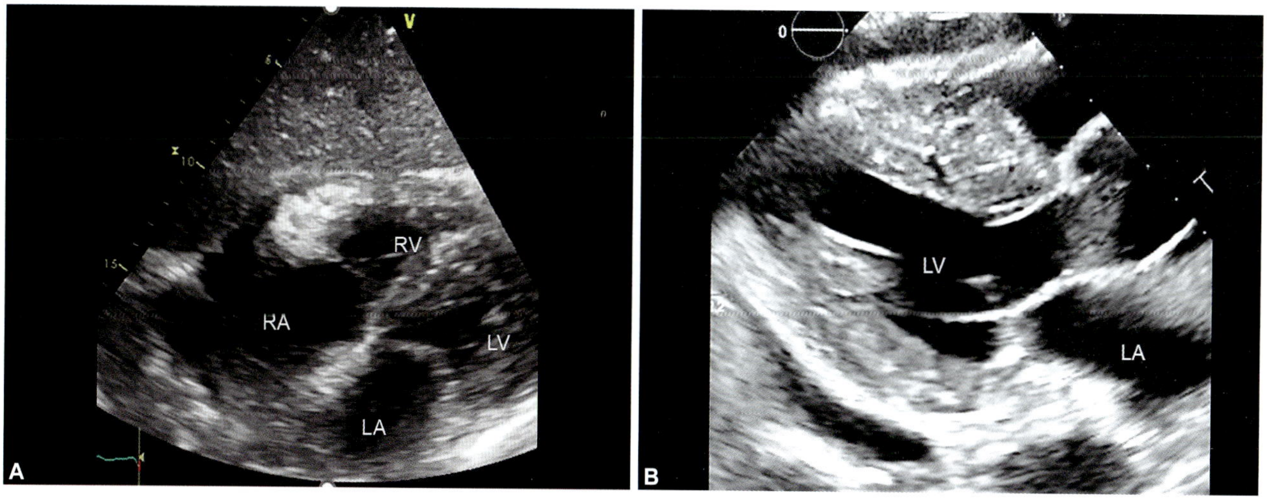

FIGS. 11A AND B: A 90-year-old man with transthyretin amyloidosis. (A) Modified apical four-chamber view showing biventricular hypertrophy with thickened atrial septum. (B) Transthoracic parasternal long axis view showing granular appearance of myocardial walls, asymmetric septal hypertrophy, and pericardial effusion.

LEOPARD syndrome is an allelic variant of Noonan syndrome characterized by lentigines, electrocardiographic abnormalities, ocular hypertelorism, retarded male genitalia growth, etc. Other syndromic variants of Noonan syndrome are rarely reported **(Figs. 16A to D)**.

BOX 3 Typical features of cardiac amyloidosis. These provide red flags but neither are sensitive or specific enough.[11]

Typical echo features of cardiac amyloidosis:

- Thick-walled LV, RV, and RA
- Granular appearance of myocardium
- 79% have asymmetric septal hypertrophy and 25% reverse septal curvature like obstructive HCM
- Restrictive or hypokinetic nondilated cardiomyopathy
- Markedly reduced global longitudinal strain (>–10%)
- Apical sparing on acoustic speckle tracking
- A dichotomy between LVEF and GLS
- Severely depressed left atrial reservoir Function
- 5-5-5 sign
- Pericardial effusion

ENDOCRINOPATHIES MIMICKING HCM

Acromegalic cardiomyopathy secondary to pituitary adenoma can present as biventricular or isolated LVH with slightly reduced longitudinal strain.[19] However, skeletal features and other endocrinal abnormalities may point to the correct etiology. Similarly pheochromocytoma as a result of adrenal adenoma can also present with episodic hypertension and severe LVH. Herein electrocardiographic changes like prolonged QT interval and ventricular ectopic activity may also be present.[20] Besides LVH, there can be transient segmental wall motion abnormalities such as seen on Takotsubo syndrome. However tissue Doppler and strain parameters are usually unaffected in pheochromocytoma **(Figs. 17A to D)**.

ONCOLOGIC PHENOCOPIES OF HCM

Both primary and secondary cardiac tumors can rarely resemble echocardiographic appearance of HCM. In fact, the first description of HCM described it as a benign cardiac

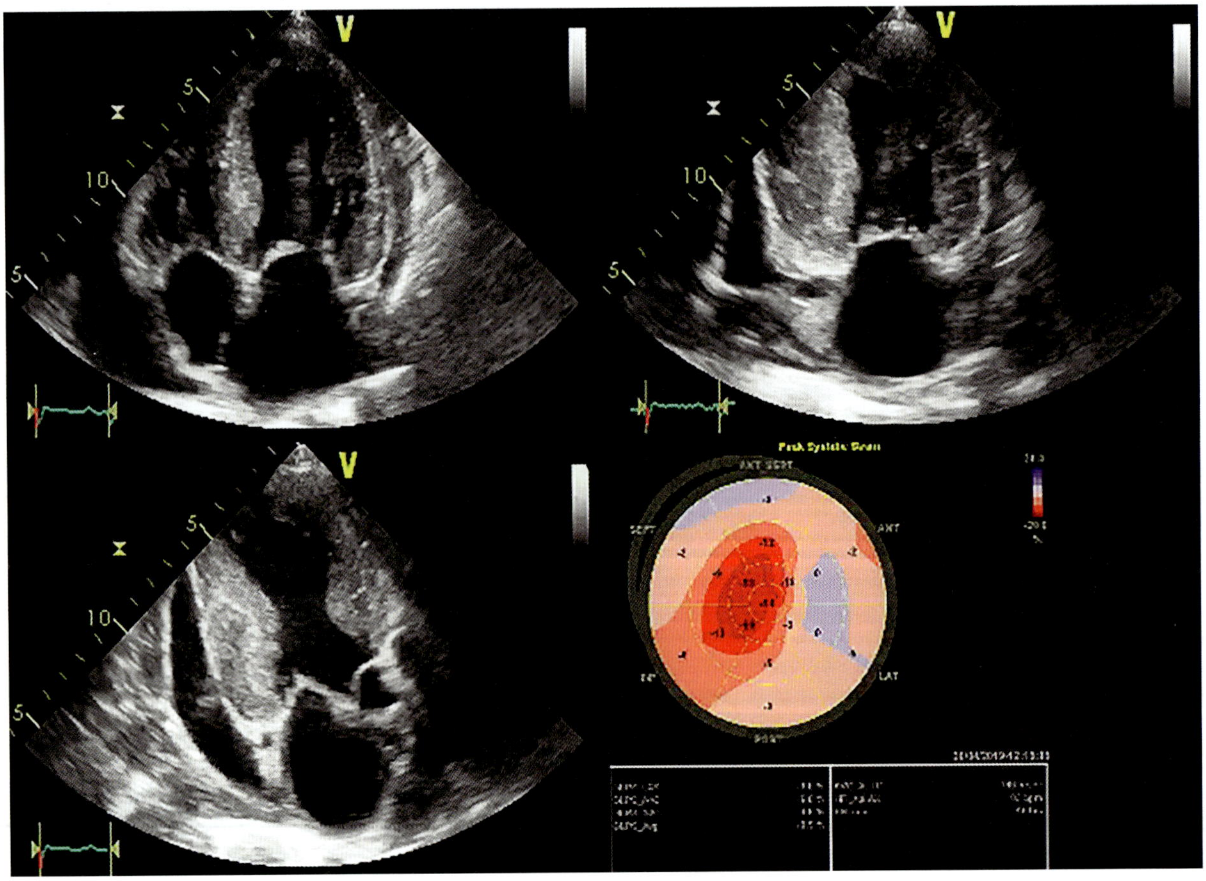

FIG. 12: A 47-year-old female with AL amyloidosis. Note increased left ventricular wall thickness in all the apical views with pronounced regional hypertrophy. Right Lower panel shows apical sparing in a Bull's eye map of the longitudinal strain derived by acoustic speckle tracking. Also note pericardial effusion which is much more common in amyloidosis than in HCM.

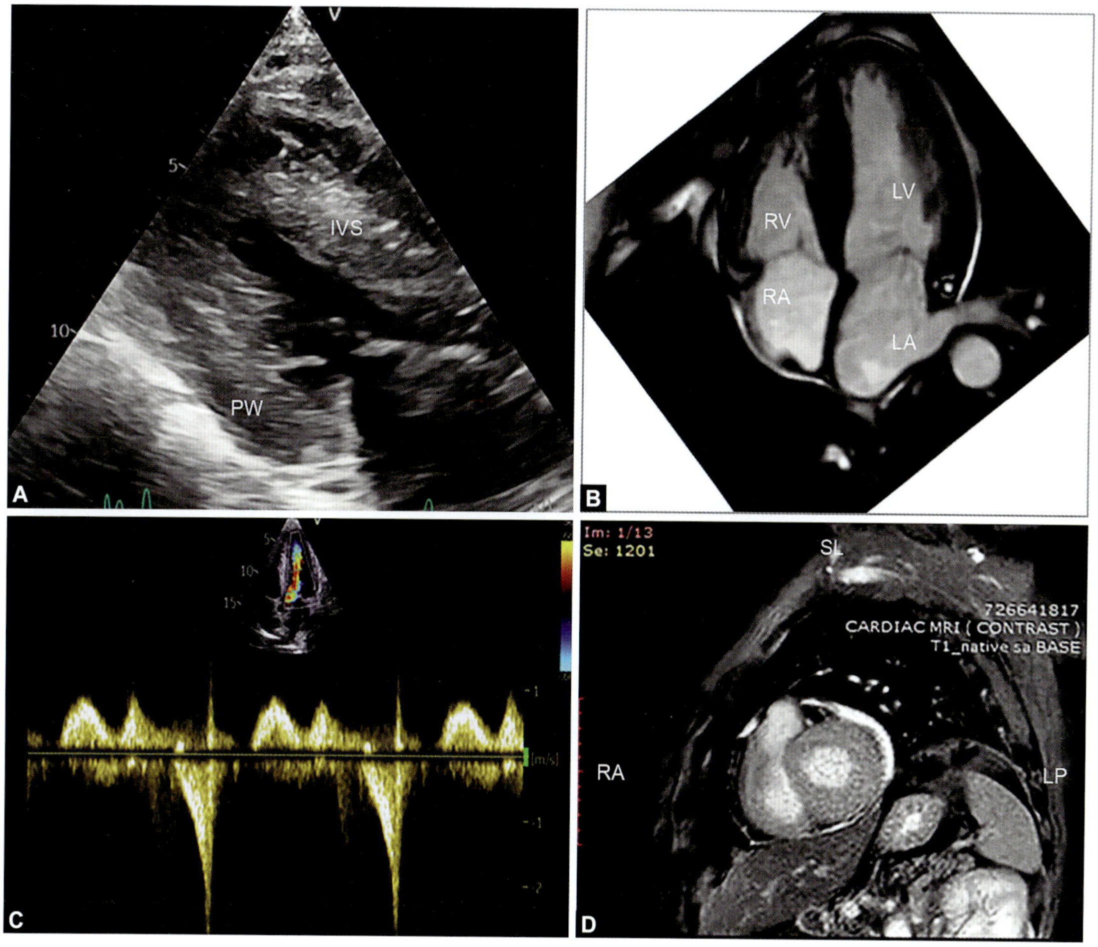

FIGS. 13A TO D: A 59-year-old male with kappa-chain AL amyloidosis presenting with syncope. (A) Left ventricular hypertrophy in modified parasternal long axis view. (B) Cine MRI four-chamber view showing left ventricular hypertrophy with more septal thickness. (C) A dynamic left ventricular peak systolic gradient of 37 mm Hg on continuous-wave Doppler examination. (D) Inability to null the myocardium on native T1 imaging in cardiac MRI due to markedly increased T1 values.

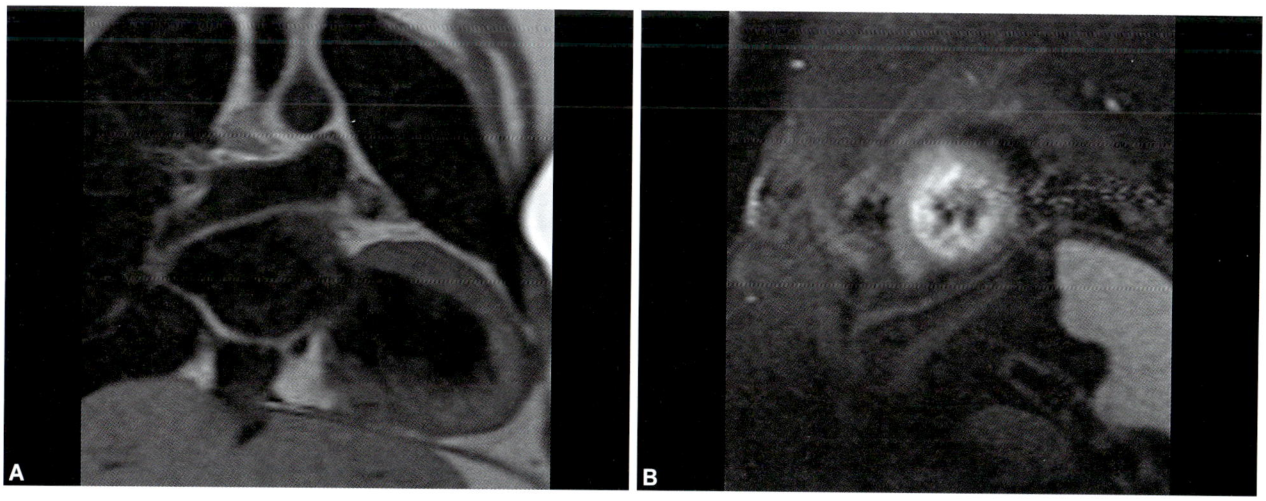

FIGS. 14A AND B: The same case as in Figure 13. (A) Left ventricular hypertrophy on black blood pool imaging (cardiac MRI) while (B) intense global subendocardial gadolinium uptake by the deposited amyloid.

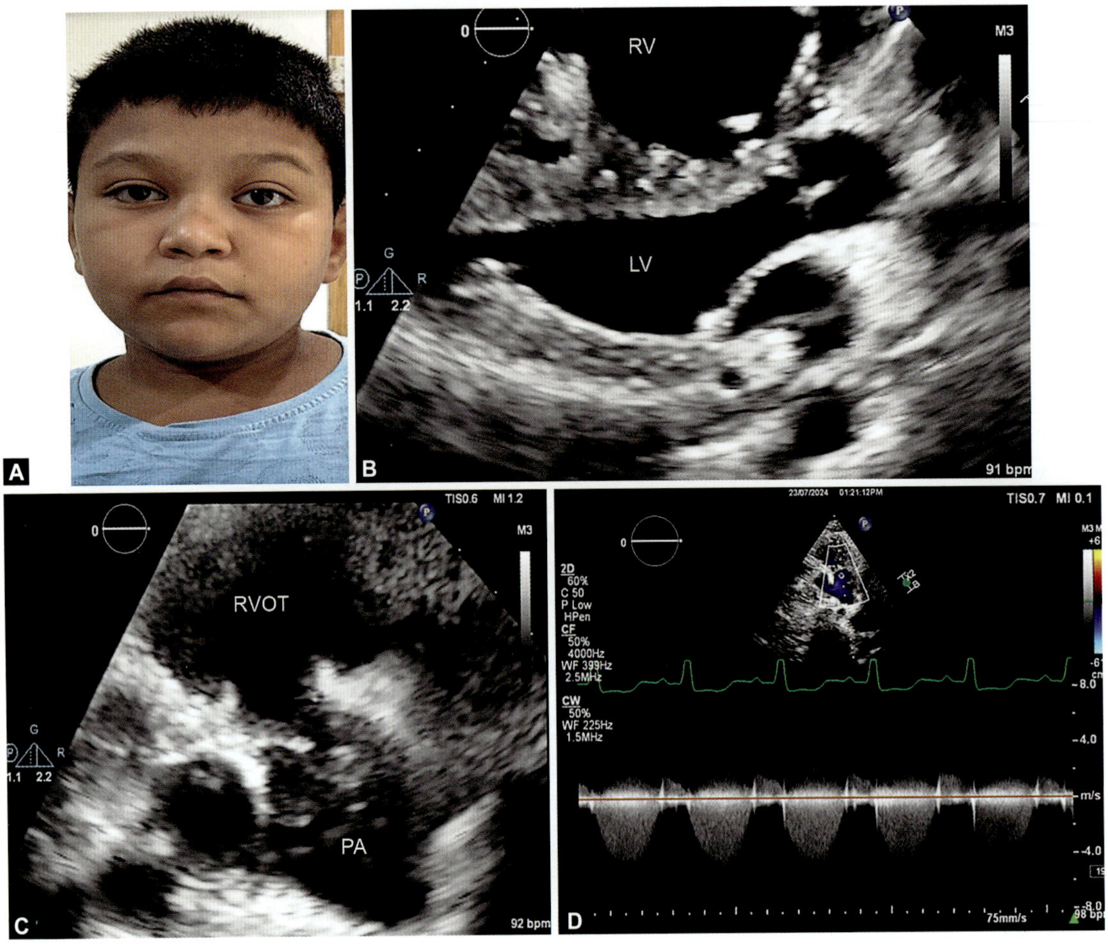

FIGS. 15A TO D: A 14-year-old boy with short stature and unusual facies with broad nostrils, epicanthic folds, and widely spaced eyes (A). (B) Dilated right ventricular (RV) outflow tract and thick walled left ventricle (LV) in parasternal long axis view. (C) Short axis view shows dysplastic pulmonary valve with a peak systolic gradient of 64 mm Hg (D).

tumor presenting as the LV outflow obstruction.[21] Cardiac tumors are underappreciated phenocopies of HCM with significant therapeutic and prognostic implications. The spectrum of neoplastic phenocopies includes lipomatous hypertrophy of interventricular septum, benign tumors such as hamartoma and fibroma rhabdomyoma, and diffuse B-cell lymphomas, metastasis from melanoma.[4] Exact diagnosis is made by a second imaging technique such as cardiac magnetic resonance or PET-CT scans. The red flags on echocardiography are pericardial effusion, asymmetric wall thickening, nonisoechoic appearance, patchy calcification, thickening of atrial walls, and interatrial septum **(Figs. 18A and B)**. A comprehensive study for the characterization of suspected myocardial hypertrophy should include T1 and T2 short-tau inversion recovery (STIR) fat-suppressed images, parametric sequences for native T1 and extracellular volume (ECV) calculation, first pass perfusion imaging, and LGE sequences **(Figs. 19A and B)**. CMR can be complemented by other imaging techniques; these include PET-CT and 18-FDG PET for documenting presence or absence of metabolically active tissue.[22]

METABOLIC STORAGE DISORDERS

Rare metabolic phenocopies are Danon disease, Pompe disease, PRKAG2, and Forbes disease.[4] Dannon disease is X-linked dominantly inherited disorder due to lysosome-associated membrane protein-2 deficiency leading to intracellular glycogen accumulation. It is characterized by HCM, proximal myopathy, and intellectual deficiency. Onset is in adolescence, disease is severer in males, and prognosis is poor. The electrocardiogram is usually characterized by short PR interval with very large QRS voltages. PRKAG2 cardiomyopathy resembles Danon disease but is autosomal dominant due to gene mutation of adenosine monophosphate-related protein kinase. Pompe disease is autosomal recessive glycogen storage disease due to acid maltase deficiency. It is characterized by muscular

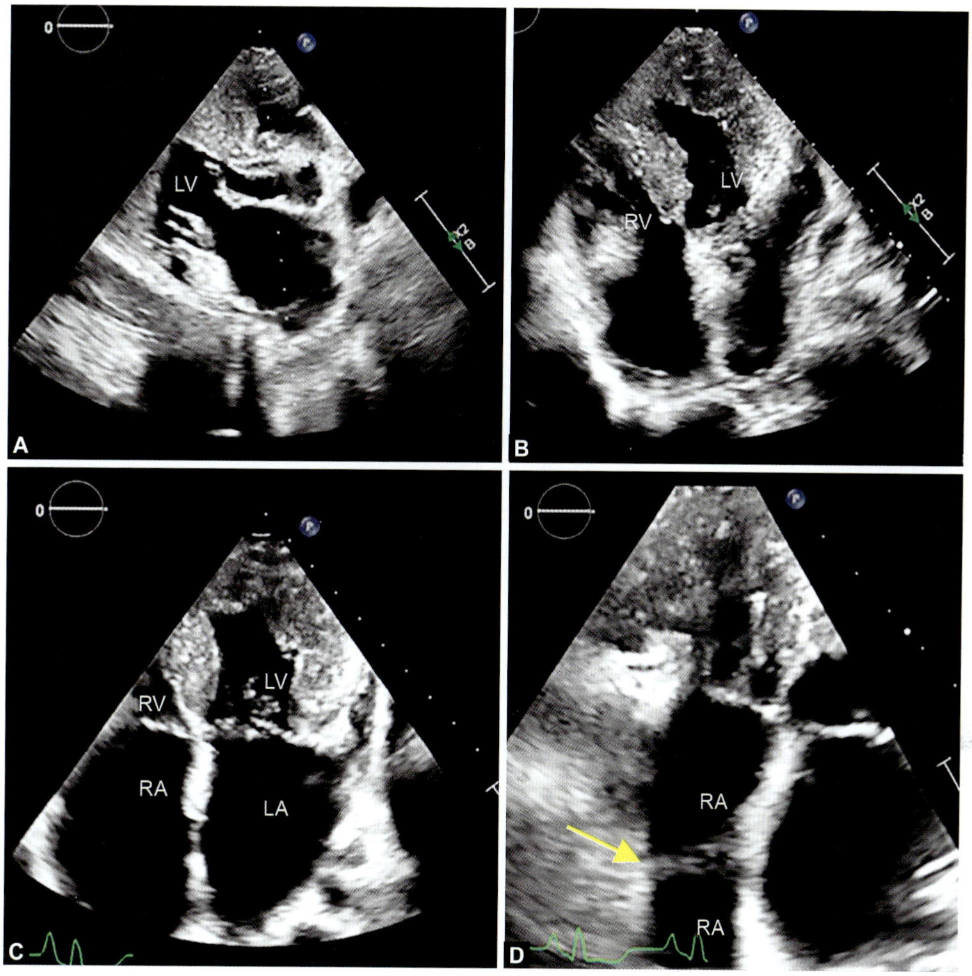

FIG. 16A TO D: A 13-year-old boy with biventricular hypertrophy (A and B) with tricuspid valve hypoplasia, dilated atria (C) and cor triatriatum dexter (D, arrow).

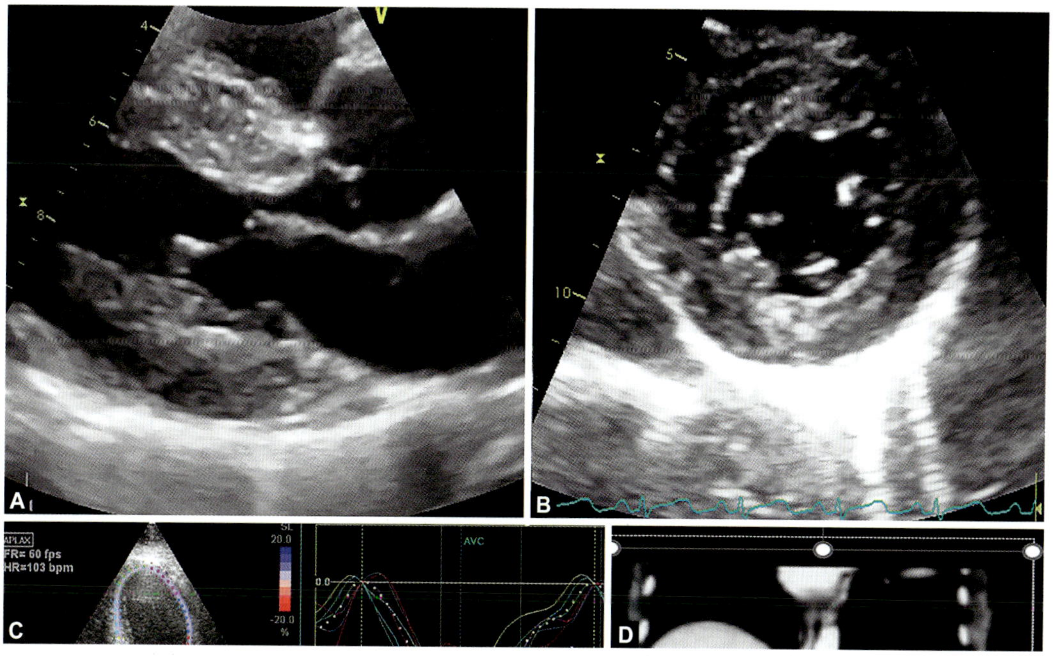

FIGS. 17A TO D: A 45-year-old female presenting with episodic palpitation. (A and B) Concentric LVH. (C) normal left ventricular longitudinal strain in four-chamber view. (D) points to a suprarenal adrenal mass.

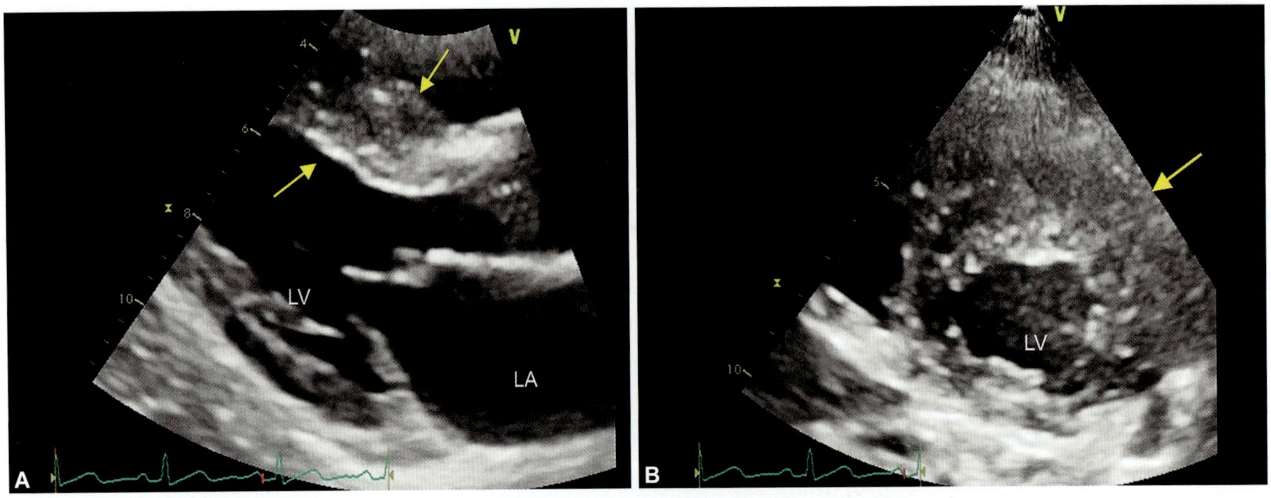

FIGS. 18A AND B: Echocardiographic phenocopy of HCM in a 52-year-old physician presenting with chest pain and finally diagnosed to have non-Hodgkin lymphoma. (A) Asymmetric septal hypertrophy in parasternal long axis (yellow arrows) and (B) shows unusual hypertrophy of the anterior and lateral wall in short axis (yellow arrow).

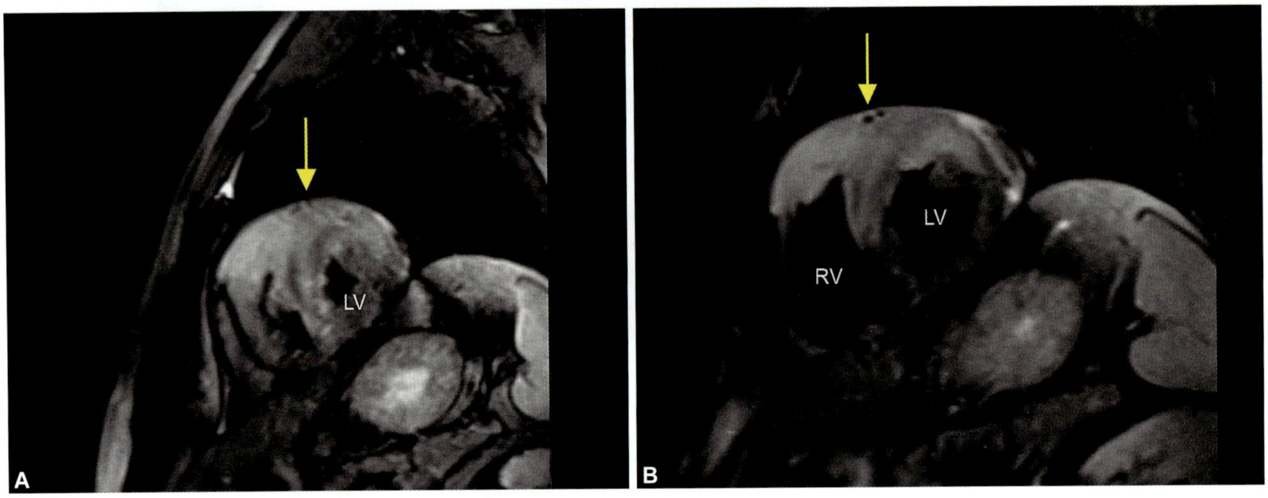

FIGS. 19A AND B: Late gadolinium enhancement on cardiac magnetic resonance imaging in the above patient. (A and B) Regional wall thickening and late gadolinium enhancement of the affected regions with subendocardial sparing.

hypotonia, macroglossia, and excessive LVH leading to dilated cardiomyopathy with early age onset. Forbes disease is an autosomal recessive glycogen storage disease due to genetic deficiency of 1,6 alpha-glucosidase deficiency and resembles other glycogenopathies in clinical picture.

ANDERSON–FABRY DISEASE

Fabry disease is an X-linked disorder due to genetic deficiency of alpha-galactosidase enzyme that results in accumulation of glycosphingolipids in various tissue. 50% of these patients present such as HCM phenocopy. Age of presentation is variable depending upon the severity of enzyme deficiency. Cutaneous angiokeratoma, hypohidrosis, acroparesthesiae, gastrointestinal disturbances, and corneal dystrophy are the usual clinical presentations with family history. Glycosphingolipid accumulation in tissues may result in LVH with dysfunction, nephropathy with proteinuria, and stroke. Characteristic features on cardiac MRI are concentric LVH with scar in basal inferolateral wall on LGE **(Figs. 20A to F)**.

NEW THERAPEUTICS IN HCM

Increased myocardial mass, arteriolar remodeling, and microvascular dysfunction associated with higher oxygen demand make HCM patients particularly vulnerable to ischemia and arrhythmias. Disabling symptoms in HCM are attributed to resting or provoked intraventricular pressure gradients. Over time, therapeutic advances have been more

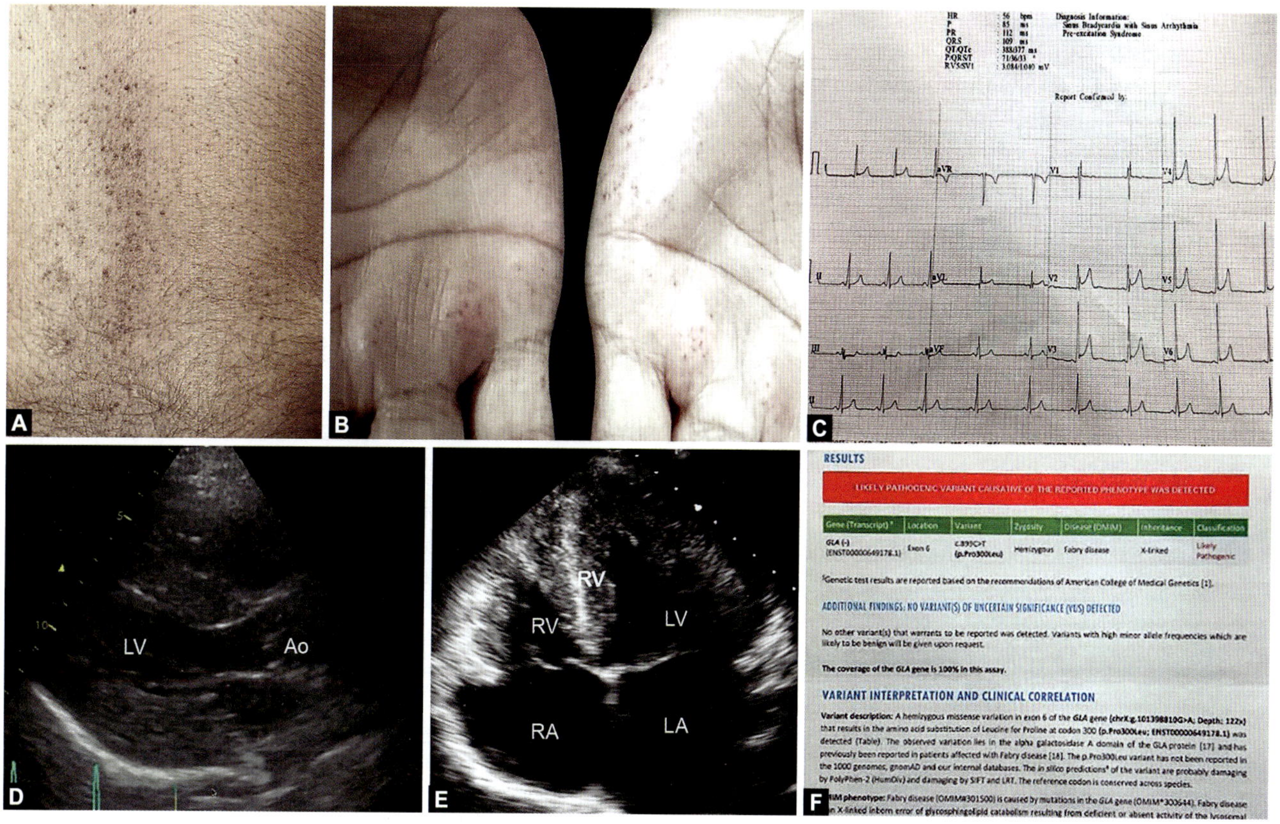

FIGS. 20A TO F: A 16-year-old boy (Anderson–Fabry disease) with angiokeratoma at the back (A), and on medial sides of both palms (B). (C) A 12-lead electrocardiogram showing left ventricular hypertrophy, short PR interval, incomplete right bundle branch block and repolarization abnormality. (D and E) biventricular hypertrophy. (F) Genetic report with a missense variation in exon-6 location of the *GLA* gene. His younger brother had similar clinical presentation.

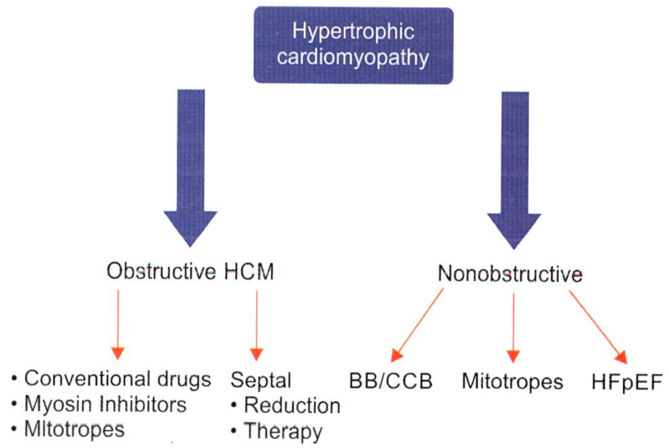

FLOWCHART 1: Treatment algorithm for HCM.

(BB: beta-blockers, CCB: calcium channel blockers; HCM: hypertrophic cardiomyopathy; HFpEF: heart failure with preserved EF)

with regard to obstructive HCM. Relief of obstruction is the major therapeutic target. Anatomical abnormalities have been targeted surgically while old and newer negative inotropic agents have been used to relieve obstruction by attenuating hypercontractility **(Flowchart 1)**.

Treatment options which can substantially improve patients' symptoms and outcome (β-adrenergic receptor blockers, disopyramide, and septal reduction therapy) are less effective in nonobstructive patients. Hypercontractility plays a major role regardless of anatomical substrate for obstruction. Drugs reducing hypercontractility do not address the core pathophysiology but provide symptomatic relief only. Conventional old drugs used for this purpose are β-adrenergic receptor antagonists, nondihydropyridine, calcium channel blockers and disopyramide (all class I therapy in 2020 guidelines).[23] β-adrenergic blockers reduce the provoked gradients only. Nondihydropyridine calcium channel blockers such as verapamil and diltiazem can be used in place of BB but may not be so well tolerated. Disopyramide, a sodium channel blocker is often used in conjunction with BB and is capable of relieving symptoms in half of the cases.[24] These conventional drugs act as weak negative inotropes and are often insufficient to control symptoms. In addition, these agents are commonly associated with side effects and chronotropic incompetence. Management of severely symptomatic nonobstructive HCM patients with normal EF is difficult as symptoms are due to diastolic dysfunction and there is no effective lusitropic agent as of now. BB and calcium channel blockers are preferable and if exertional dyspnea persists, oral diuretic can be used. For those nonobstructive patients who develop systolic dysfunction (EF < 50%), traditional heart failure drug therapy should be considered. Late sodium channel blockers like ranolazine have been tried but with no significant benefits. Current guidelines[23] recommend septal reduction therapies with either surgical septal myectomy or catheter-based alcohol or radiofrequency septal ablation in those with residual outflow pressure gradient exceeding 50 mm Hg. The proportion of patients needing these interventions may be significantly reduced with introduction of myotropes.[25]

MYOTROPES AND HCM

Ultimate aim of therapy in HCM is to retard progression of systolic and diastolic dysfunction and prevent hypertrophy and cardiac fibrosis. Myocardial contraction depends on the activity of cardiac myosin heavy chain protein isoforms. Myosin content and function is augmented in HCM. Myosin modulation has been the object of randomized clinical trials using mavacamten and aficamten. These novel allosteric inhibitors of myosin have the potential to modify fundamental pathophysiology of obstructive HCM.[25,26] These drugs reduce myosin-actin cross bridges, hypercontractility and energy requirement resulting in better ventricular compliance and favorable energetics. By reducing excessive contractility, these drugs reduce dynamic LVOT obstruction and improve lusitropic ventricular properties, which contribute to symptoms in HCM patients.[27] Double-blind, placebo-controlled, multicenter randomized trials have suggested that addition of mavacamten to maximally tolerated medical therapy could allow deferral of septal reduction therapy in severely symptomatic obstructive HCM patients. Mavacamten treatment has been shown to induce reverse cardiac remodeling, reducing LV mass index, left atrial volume, and maximum LV wall thickness along with reduction in cardiac biomarkers.[28] However, based on this mechanism of action, LV systolic dysfunction is a real possibility that requires careful monitoring for patient safety **(Flowchart 2)**.

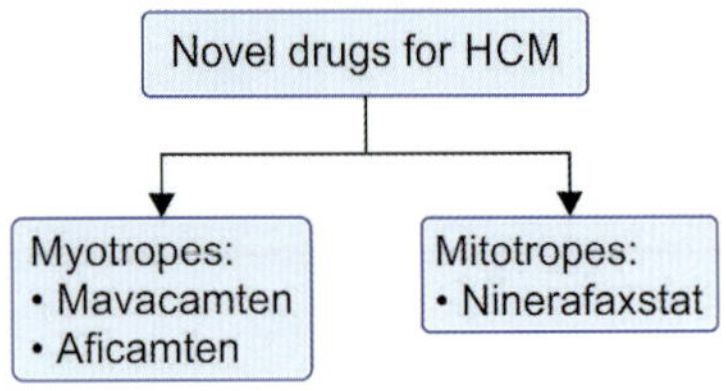

FLOWCHART 2: Novel drugs currently being explored for treatment of hypertrophic cardiomyopathy (HCM).

MITOTROPES OR METABOLIC MODULATORS

Impaired myocardial energetics and higher ATP consumption to generate equivalent force are the other hallmarks of HCM. Attempts have been made to improve energy efficiency by pharmacological agents. Basic purpose is to shift metabolism from using free fatty acids to glucose and ketones whose oxidation produces more ATP per oxygen molecule consumed.[24,25] This metabolic shift enhances cardiac efficiency by increasing recoupling of glucose oxidation and greater energy generation. Drugs such as perhexiline and trimetazidine have been tried but without much benefit. Ninerafaxstat is a novel cardiac mitotrope designed to restore myocardial energy homeostasis.[29] The primary mechanism of action is partial inhibition of fatty acid oxidation via direct competitive inhibition of 3-KAT, the last enzyme in the mitochondrial long-chain fatty acid β-oxidation pathway. The capability of ninerafaxstat to optimize cardiac energy efficiency may result in improved exercise function by enhancing myocardial relaxation, filling, and stroke volume during exertion.[29] Recent results have been modestly encouraging.[25]

CONCLUSION

We have learnt a great deal about mimics of HCM in last two decades. Red flags must be investigated to rule out mimics of this common condition. New pharmacotherapeutic options are emerging which might limit the role of septal reduction therapy and its associated morbidity.

ONLINE REFERENCES

Please scan the QR code provided at the end of the table of contents for References of this chapter.

CHAPTER

78

Cardiovascular Complications during Cancer Chemotherapy: Prevention, Monitoring, and Management

Sankar Chandra Mandal, Ferooz Ahmad Banday, Nilesh Giri, Bidyut Roy

ABSTRACT

Survival of the cancer patients has dramatically improved with the advent of cancer treatment including chemotherapy, radiation therapy, and targeted therapy. However, this comes at the cost of multiorgan side effects, of which the most notable is the effect on the cardiovascular system as, with regard to some cancers, the risk of dying from cardiovascular disease may exceed the risk of dying from cancer.

First described in 1966 in patients receiving anthracyclines,[1] the effects often are underappreciated as the side effects may go unnoticed for years or even decades. How cancer therapy causes and which patients are at a higher risk are the subjects of research.

Keywords: Cancer chemotherapy, cardiovascular complications, prevention, management

INTRODUCTION

With the widely available armamentarium of treatment modalities available for cancer treatment, ranging from antimetabolites and cell cycle inhibitors to targeted and immune therapies, the spectrum of CV effects has expanded, which includes either direct structural and functional effects of cancer therapy on CV system or accelerated progression of already-existing CV disease in the presence of traditional risk factors.[2] Cancer therapy–related CV toxicity (CTR-CVT) risk is a dynamic variable, and the risk changes throughout the pathway of care depending on type, dose, duration, and frequency of treatment **(Fig. 1)**.

This chapter focuses on some of the well-studied adverse effects of cancer therapy, including hypertension, asymptomatic and symptomatic LV dysfunction, arrhythmias, and thromboembolism.

HEART FAILURE

Among CV effects, the heart failure (both asymptomatic and symptomatic LV dysfunction) is the most disquieting complication leading to increase in morbidity and mortality. With variation in presentation (acute or chronic), onset (early or delayed), the extent of damage, and frequent interactions of different chemotherapeutic agents, it is often challenging to predict the long-term consequences of cancer treatment.[3] Some of the commonly used chemotherapeutic agents and their effects on myocardial function are discussed here **(Table 1)**.

Anthracyclines

Anthracyclines are one of the most effective class of anti-cancer drugs available, used to treat cancers of the breast, stomach, lungs, blood, etc. These work by inhibiting the enzyme topoisomerase II after interspersing into the nuclear DNA. Cardiotoxicity results from apoptosis due to growth arrest of myocytes as inhibition of proapoptotic cascade and activation of antiapoptotic cascade has been seen to result in reduced cardiotoxicity in animal models. The other mechanism of cardiotoxicity is generation of excessive reactive oxygen species, which leads to oxidative damage as it has been studied in mice models which overexpress superoxide dismutase (SOD) an important antioxidant defence is protective against the anthracycline-induced cardiotoxicity.[4]

Acute Heart Failure

Usually seen in children, acute heart failure is an uncommon but severe manifestation of cardiotoxicity. Wojnowski et al. found AHF in 0.2% of patients treated for non-Hodgkin's lymphoma.[5]

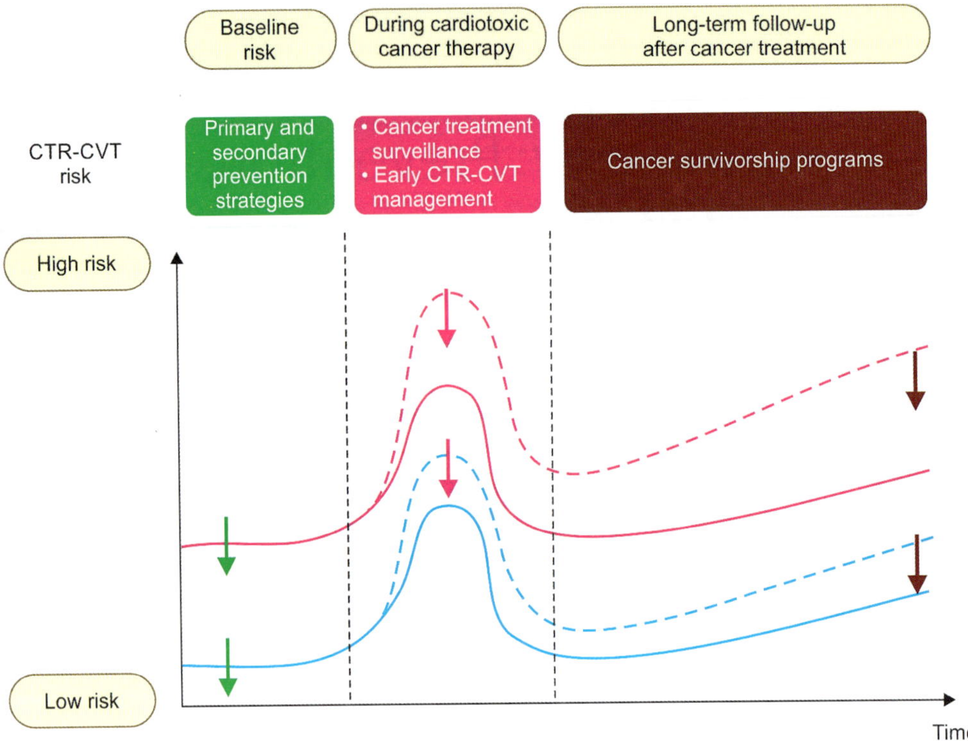

FIG. 1: Central illustration: dynamics of cardiovascular toxicity risk of patients with cancer over their therapy continuum (ESC 2022 guidelines).

TABLE 1: Classification of CTRCD.

Class	Severity	Criteria
Symptomatic CTRCD (HF)	Very severe	HF requiring inotropic support, mechanical circulatory support, or consideration of transplantation
	Severe	HF hospitalization
	Moderate	Need for outpatient intensification of diuretic and HF therapy
	Mild	Mild HF symptoms, no intensification of therapy required
Asymptomatic CTRCD	Severe	New LVEF reduction to <40%
	Moderate	New LVEF reduction by ≥10% points to an LVEF of 40–49% Or New LVEF reduction by <10% points to an LVEF of 40–49% *and* either new relative decline in GLS by >15% from baseline *or* new rise in cardiac biomarkers
	Mild	LVEF ≥ 50% *And* new relative decline in GLS by >15% from baseline *And/or* new rise in cardiac biomarkers

Chronic Heart Failure

Chronic heart failure is the progressive, usually dose-dependent, both systolic and diastolic LV dysfunction. There is an interindividual variability regarding threshold of doses causing LV dysfunction. Horan et al. in 2006 reported that the diastolic dysfunction occurred after a cumulative dose of 200 mg/m^2 of doxorubicin and systolic dysfunction occurred after a cumulative dose of 400–600 mg/m^2.[6]

Alkylating Agents

This class of drugs includes cyclophosphamide, ifosfamide, 5-FU, paclitaxel, etc. When used in isolation, these agents have lower cardiotoxicity potential as compared to anthracyclines. But when given in combination or as a sequential therapy with anthracyclines and other agents, these increase the cardiotoxicity of anthracite anthracyclines manifold. Tan-Chiu et al. in 2005, in their study on chemotherapy of breast cancer patients, found that the sequential combination of anthracyclines and cyclophosphamide followed by paclitaxel and trastuzumab resulted in 3-year incidence of heart failure or CV death of 4.1% compared to 0.8% in patients receiving anthracyclines and cyclophosphamide only.[7]

Tyrosine Kinase Inhibitors

Tyrosine kinase inhibitors are the targeted therapies of cancer treatment. By inhibiting the tyrosine kinase of cancer cell, the agents inhibit cell signaling, growth, and division. They are divided into small-molecule tyrosine kinase inhibitors and monoclonal antibodies.

Small-molecule Tyrosine Kinase Inhibitor

With widely expanding indications of the use of TKI, the CV effects, particularly LV dysfunction, are increasingly being recognized. The severity of the TKI-induced heart failure can be graded by using National Cancer Institute Common Terminology Criteria for Adverse Events (NCICTCAE) as follows:

- *Grade 1*: Asymptomatic with lab (increased BNP) or cardiac imaging abnormalities
- *Grade 2*: Symptoms with mild-to-moderate exertion on activity
- *Grade 3*: Severe, with symptoms at rest or with minimal activity (intervention needed)
- *Grade 4*: Life-threatening consequences where urgent intervention is needed, e.g., continuous IV therapy or mechanical hemodynamic support
- *Grade 5*: Death[8]

Trastuzumab (Monoclonal Antibody)

In contrast to anthracyclines which cause ultrastructural damage and hence myocyte loss, the CV toxicity of trastuzumab is often transient and simple withdrawal of trastuzumab results in recovery (even complete) of LVEF decline and it has been also observed that readministration inconsistently leads to recurrence of LV dysfunction.

A study by Ewer et al. in 2005 on reversibility of trastuzumab-related cardiotoxicity showed that recovery of LV dysfunction occurred within 1–3 months of discontinuation of trastuzumab and also only 3 out of 25 patients in whom trastuzumab was readministered developed heart failure. Heart failure is more common when combined with anthracyclines.[9]

ARRHYTHMIAS

A baseline ECG should be obtained from all patients who are planned to be subjected to chemotherapy, as arrythmias and other conduction system disturbances are well recognized although poorly studied adverse effects of many chemotherapeutic agents. These may range from asymptomatic QTc prolongation, supraventricular and ventricular ectopics, and AF to life-threatening ventricular tachycardias including torsade de pointes (TDF). It is often challenging to establish a causal relationship between a chemotherapeutic agent and an arrythmia as cancer itself can lead to arrythmias and also quite often drugs are given in combination.

Anthracyclines

In contrast to cardiomyopathy, the ECG changes induced by anthracyclines are usually dose independent. Most of the arrhythmias are secondary to cardiomyopathy. However, it is not uncommon to observe some ventricular arrhythmias occurring even when LV dysfunction has yet not ensued.[11] QTc prolongation, one of the common ECG manifestations, can be graded as follows:

- *Grade 1*: 450–480 ms
- *Grade 2*: 480–500 ms
- *Grade 3*: ≥501 ms on at least two separate ECGs
- *Grade 4*: >501 or >60 ms change from baseline and TDP or signs and symptoms of serious arrhythmia

A study by Mazur et al.[10] found that the frequency of NSVT/AF and sustained VT/VF in 73.9%, 56.6%, and 30.4% of patients with anthracycline-induced cardiomyopathy who had implanted ICDS.

Alkylating Agents

Cyclophosphamide, busulfan, and melphalan cause a broad range of arrhythmias; for example, busulfan has been associated with AF with an incidence of 6.4% when used in combination with cyclophosphamide.[12]

Antimetabolites

- *5-Fluorouracil*: After angina (due to its vasospastic effects), arrhythmia is the second most common cardiotoxicity of 5-FU. It can cause increase in P-wave duration, ST-T changes, decreased QRS voltage, and QTc prolongation. It has also been seen to cause bradyarrhythmia,[13] AV block, and IVCD.[14]
- Gemcitabine is strongly associated with AF and AF can occur even after the first dose of gemcitabine.[15]
- *Taxanes*: They cause sinus bradycardia, RBBB, LBBB,[16] VT, and SCD.[17]

- *Platinum-based agents*: Cisplatin causes hypomagnesemia which can induce TDP, PVT, asystole, or AF even when used locally like in serous cavities.[18]
- *TKIs*: The main concern with the use of TKI is the QTc prolongation and SCD in addition to other benign rhythm disturbances like sinus bradycardia, SVT, and NSVT.

THROMBOEMBOLIC COMPLICATIONS

As cancer is a known cause of thrombotic disease, treatment with chemotherapeutic agents puts the patients on an additional risk of thromboembolic complications. Platinum-based chemotherapy and anthracyclines are mostly associated with prothrombotic effect (cisplatin more than oxaliplatin); the other agents are also commonly associated with thrombotic risk, e.g., gemcitabine and 5-FU.

Platelet aggregation and endothelial damage are some of the pathophysiological mechanisms studied in this regard. The *PROTECHT* study has identified chemotherapy as an independent risk factor for thromboembolism and has stratified the patients as per the type of chemotherapy and also highlighted the benefit of thromboprophylaxis.[19]

HYPERTENSION

See **Table 2**.

CORONARY ARTERY DISEASE

Acute Coronary Syndrome

Cancer treatments that predispose to acute coronary syndromes are given in **Table 3**.

Chronic Coronary Syndromes

5-FU, capecitabine, and platinum-based chemotherapy can precipitate angina. TKIs like nilotinib can lead to accelerated atherosclerosis and angina.

MONITORING OF CARDIOVASCULAR EFFECTS OF CHEMOTHERAPY

It is of utmost importance to identify at-risk patients and to regularly monitor these subgroups for possible CV effects both during and following completion of treatment with chemotherapeutic agent. In this regard, multisocietal recommendations have been made to screen and monitor for cardiotoxic effects of various chemotherapeutic agents with more robust emphasis on anthracyclines and monoclonal antibodies.

PATIENTS AT HIGHER RISK OF CHEMOTHERAPY-INDUCED CARDIOTOXICITY[20]

- High-dose anthracycline (e.g., doxorubicin > 250 mg/m^2, epirubicin > 600 mg/m^2)
- High-dose radiotherapy (>30 Gy) where the heart is in the treatment field
- Lower-dose anthracyclines (e.g., doxorubicin < 250 mg/m^2, epirubicin < 600 mg/m^2), or HERis or VEGFis or proteosomes or BCR-ABL$_I$ and presence of any of the following factors:
  - Age > 60 years
  - Lower-dose radiotherapy (<30 Gy) where the heart is in the treatment field

TABLE 2: Hypertension.

	Criteria
Treatment threshold for hypertension before, during, and after therapy	*In patients with high CV risk* ≥ 130 mm Hg systolic and/or ≥80 mm Hg diastolic *Otherwise*: ≥140 mm Hg systolic and/or ≥90 mm Hg diastolic
Cancer therapy holding threshold	≥180 mm Hg systolic and/or ≥110 mm Hg diastolic
Hypertensive emergency	(Very high) BP elevation associated with acute hypertension-mediated organ damage (heart, retina, brain, kidneys, and large arteries), requiring immediate BP reduction to limit extension or promote regression of target organ damage

TABLE 3: Pathophysiology of ACS and offending drugs.

Mechanism	Drugs responsible
Accelerated atherosclerosis and plaque rupture	ADT (GnRH agonists), ICI, nilotinib, ponatinib, radiation therapy, VEGFi
Vasospasm	Bleomycin, fluoropyrimidines, taxanes, VEGFi, Vinca alkaloids
Coronary thrombosis	Alkylating agents (cisplatin, cyclophosphamide), erlotinib, ICI, IMiD (lenalidomide, thalidomide), monoclonal antibodies (VEGFi, anti-CD20), nilotinib, platinum chemotherapy, PI, ponatinib, VEGFi

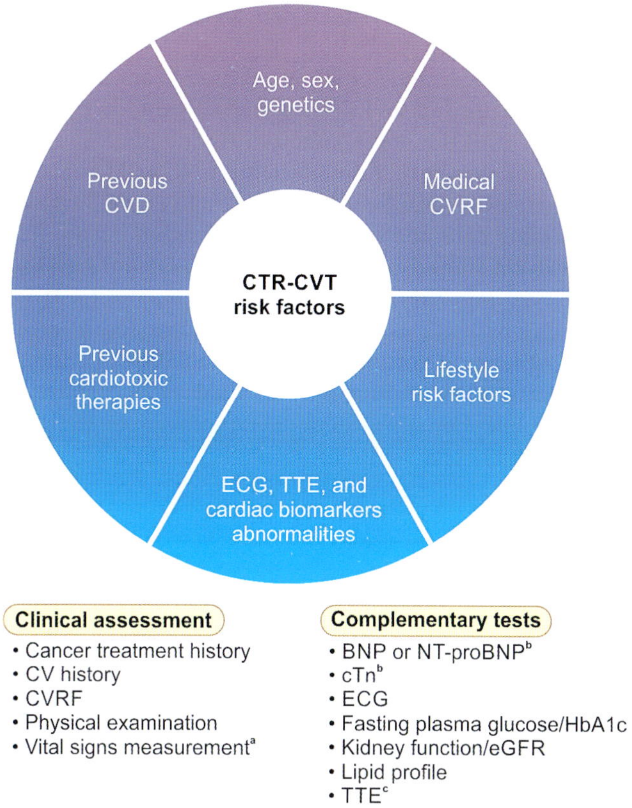

[a] Including blood pressure, heart rate, height, weight, and body mass index.
[b] Cardiac biomarkers (troponin and NP) should be measured in patients at risk of CTRCD where available and results should be interpreted according to the patient clinical status, type of cancer treatment, and kidney function.
[c] Consider other CV complementary tests in selected patients: Cardiac magnetic resonance, coronary computed tomography angiography, CPET [in selected patients for pre-operative (lung, colon, and rectal cancers) risk stratification].

FIG. 2: Baseline cardiovascular toxicity risk assessment checklist (ESC 2022 guidelines).

- >2 risk factors, including smoking, hypertension, diabetes mellitus, dyslipidemia, chronic renal insufficiency, and obesity
- Previous heart disease
- Elevated cardiac biomarkers before initiation of cancer therapy

Risk assessment should include history, physical assessment, and baseline cardiac functional measurements **(Fig. 2)**.

MONITORING OF LEFT VENTRICULAR DYSFUNCTION

Echocardiography

Echocardiography is the method of choice for screening and follow-up monitoring of LV function because of its safety (lack of radiation and contrast), easy availability, cost-effectiveness, reproducibility, and ability to detect subclinical changes in LV function. Chemotherapy-induced cardiomyopathy is defined as a decrease in LVEF of >10% to the value below the lower limit of normal and global longitudinal strain (GLS) >15% reduction from baseline.[20] Hence, it is recommended to obtain a baseline echocardiography of all patients planning to subject to chemotherapy, and to avoid discrepancies, the same imaging modality should be used for comparison throughout the treatment course.

The limitation of 2D echocardiography is its poor image acquisition, particularly in patients who have undergone thoracic surgery and chest irradiation. In these cases, the addition of contrast agents and using 3D echocardiography can improve the accuracy and reproducibility of echocardiography.

Cardiac MRI

Having higher accuracy and reproducibility, *CMR* is considered gold standard among the noninvasive testing of LVEF and other functional and structural aspects of LV. The other advantages are no risk of radiation and no contrast required for LVEF measurement which ensures rapid assessment of RV and LV functions within 10–20 minutes.[21] *CMR* is typically used when echocardiography is not diagnostic and gives borderline LVEF values.[20] Limitations are its limited availability, cost, and patient-related factors like claustrophobia, breath holding, and acquisition times.

Nuclear Imaging

Multigated acquisition (MUGA) is a highly reproducible image modality using Tc-99m MUGA, I-123 MIBG scintigraphy, and I-123 BMIPP scintigraphy for early myocardial dysfunction. It defines chemotherapy-induced myopathy as >10% points decrease in LVEF with a value of <50%.[22] Its use is limited by cumulative radiation exposure and limited structural and functional information on other cardiac structures.

Biomarkers

Cardiac troponin, BNP, and myeloperoxidase (MPO) assessment before and during treatment is safe and cost-effective way to detect early and subclinical cardiotoxicity. Among these, cardiac troponins and BNP have the most evidence in support to use.[23] Studies suggest that the normal troponin values throughout the chemotherapy are associated with no drop in LVEF and a low incidence of cardiac events, and also prompt treatment with cardioprotective drugs like ACEis on noticing abnormal troponin values may prevent overt cardiomyopathy.[24,25] The other advantages are accuracy, reproducibility, high sensitivity, and wide availability.

MONITORING FOR ARRHYTHMIAS

Obtain a baseline 12-lead ECG for rate and rhythm.

Monitor QTc, particularly in patients receiving other QTc-prolonging drugs, and electrolyte abnormalities.

Consider treatment discontinuation if QTc is >500 or >60 ms increase from baseline.

MANAGEMENT OF CARDIOTOXICITY

Once the diagnosis of cardiotoxicity is established, the cardio-oncology collaboration should discuss the further course of action considering the risk–benefit ratio of continuing and discontinuing the chemotherapy. Due to lack of specific recommendations guiding the chemotherapy-induced cardiotoxicity, it is important to manage the individual cardiotoxicity as per the existing guidelines for different diseases.

Left Ventricular Dysfunction

RAAS activation has been suggested to play a key role in chemotherapy-induced cardiotoxic effects, particularly anthracyclines, and hence RAAS blockage using ACEis and ARBs forms the cornerstone of management of cardiotoxic effects of chemotherapy.[26,27]

In one Danish study of advanced breast cancer patients where a decline of LVEF on serial measurements was analyzed, ACEi therapy resulted in rescue of LVEF in all the patients. In another double-blind trial, ACEi enalapril demonstrated a significant change in LVESWS.[28] Based on available data, the current recommendations are that ACEi can be started once the fall in LVEF from baseline is observed and the same can be extrapolated to ARBs. Regarding patients with significant baseline reduction in LVEF < 40%, any use of anthracyclines should be discouraged and heart failure should be managed as per available guidance and alternative chemotherapy should be explored **(Flowchart 1)**.

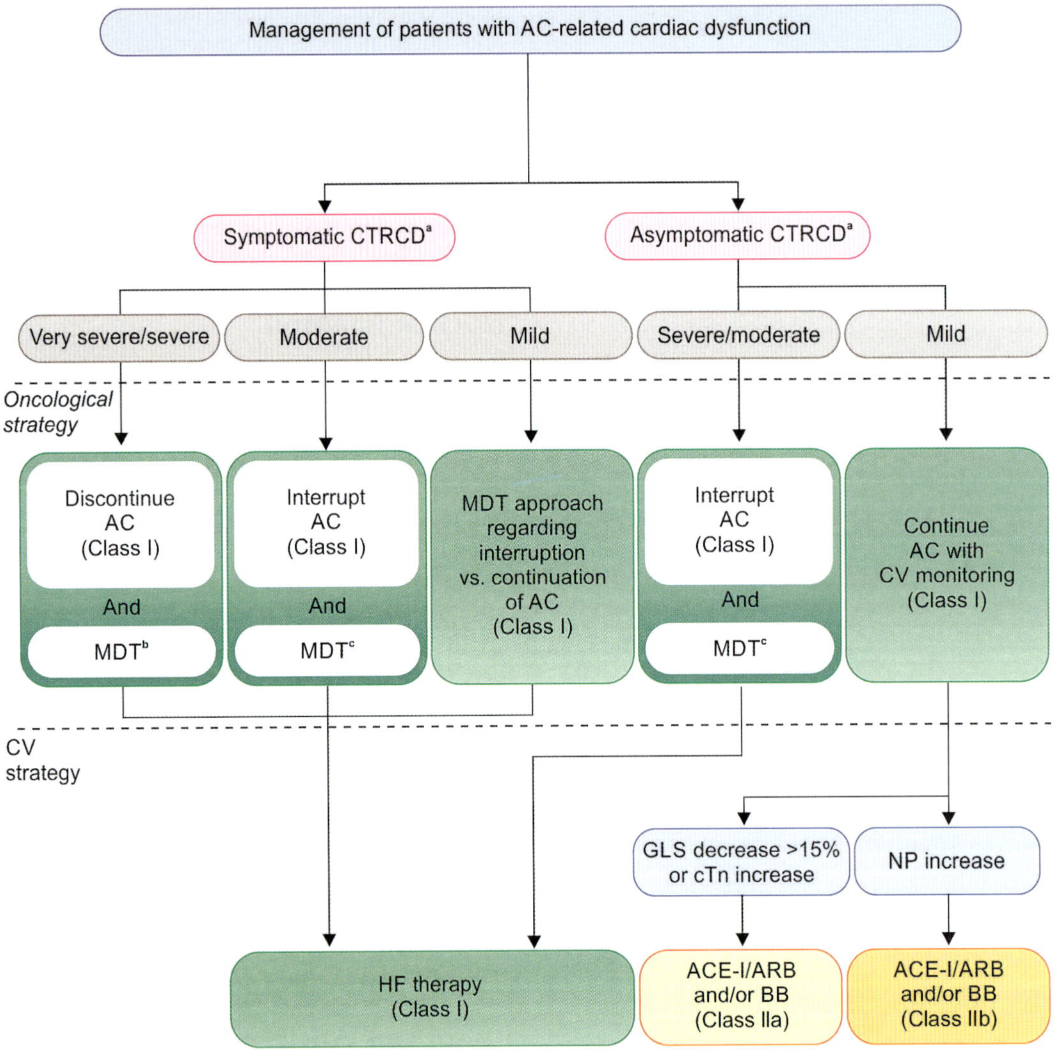

[a] Refer to **Table 1**.
[b] In rare exceptions, anthracycline chemotherapy may be restarted after recovery of LV function with optimal HF therapy.
[c] A MDT (Multidisciplinary team) discussion is recommended before restarting anthracycline chemotherapy after recovery of LV function.

FLOWCHART 1: Recommendations for the management of anthracycline-related cardiac dysfunction (ESC 2022 guidelines).

Arrythmias

As stated earlier, QTc prolongation is one of the common ECG manifestations of chemotherapy-induced cardiotoxicity. It is a risk factor for TDP. When QTc prolongation > 500 ms is observed any time during the chemotherapy, it is recommended to temporarily interrupt the chemotherapy and evaluation of consecutive etiologies should be prompted. For management of TDP, the usual care with $MgSO_4$ is considered under specialist care and if hemodynamic instability occurs, defibrillation is recommended **(Flowchart 2)**.[29]

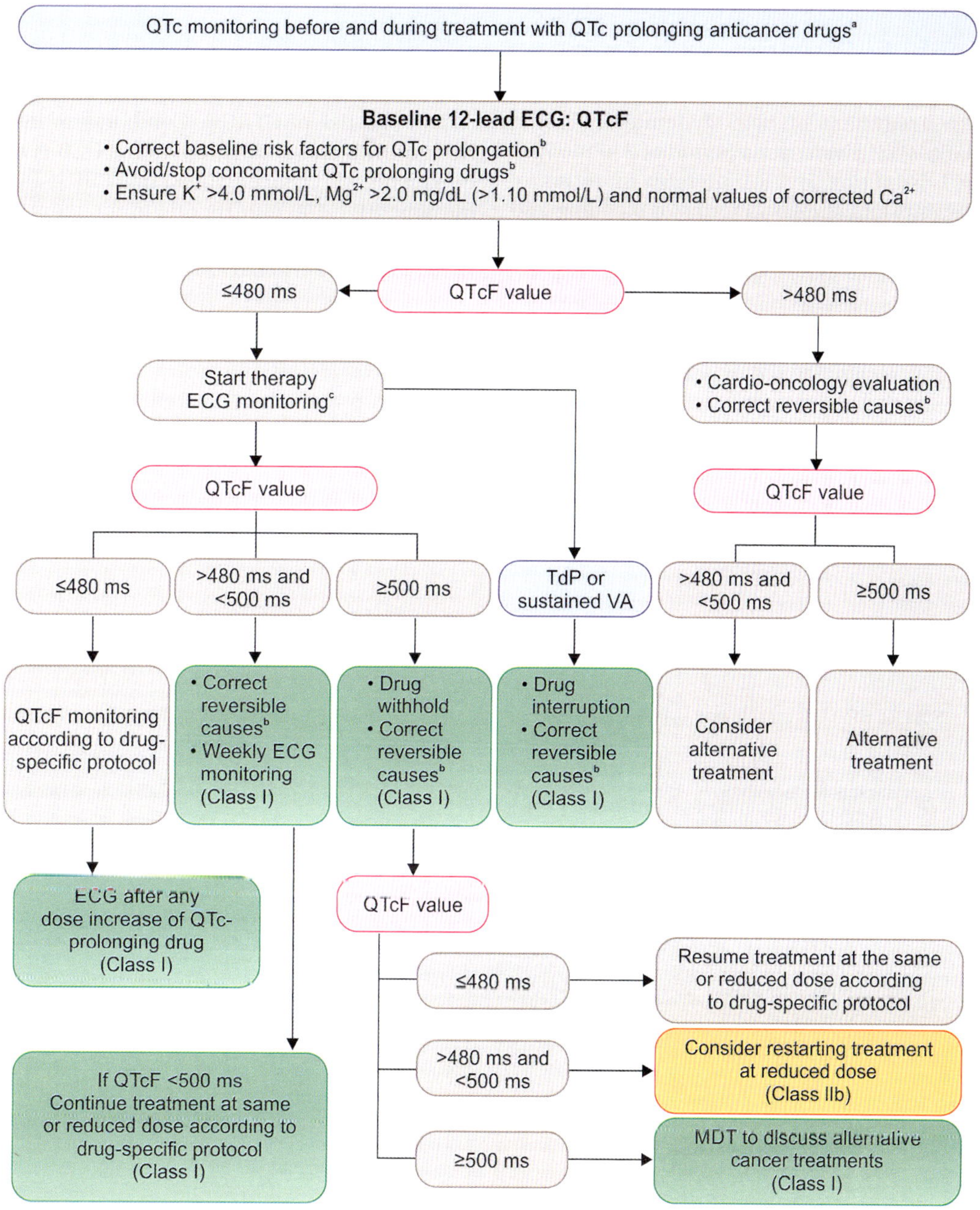

[a] Aclarubicin, arsenic trioxide, glasdegib, nilotinib, oxaliplatin, pazopanib, ribociclib, sunitinib, toremifene, vandetanib, abarelix, belinostat, brigantinib, carbozantinib, ceritinib, crizotinib, dovitinib, entrectinib, eribulin, gilteritinib, ivosidenib, lapatinib, lenvatinib, osimertinib, panobinostat, rucaparib, selpercatinib, sorafenib, tipiracil/trifluridine, vemurafenib.

[b] QT-prolonging drugs, antiarrhythmics, antibiotics, antidepressants, antifungals, antiemetics, antihistamines, antipsychotics, loop diuretics, opioids (methadone), bradyarrhythmia, electrolyte imbalance/abnormalities, hypokalemia (≤3.5 mEq/L), hypomagnesemia (≤1.6 mEq/L), hypocalcemia (≤8.5 mEq/L), inadequate dose adjustment of renal or hepatic cleared QT-prolonging drugs.

[c] ECG monitoring at baseline, once steady-state anticancer drug levels have been achieved, after each dose modification, or any treatment interruption >2 weeks; monthly for the first 3 months, and then periodically during treatment depending on patient-specific risk factors and cancer treatment.

FLOWCHART 2: Algorithm for QTc monitoring and management of QTc prolongation (ESC 2022 guidelines).

Regarding management of AF, it follows the same recommendation as in noncancer patients with the rate and rhythm control individualized with due consideration to reduction of embolic ischemic events. For anticoagulation, NOACs (Class IIa, LOE B) are preferred over LMWH and VKAs (excluding mechanical heart valves and moderate-to-severe MS) for stroke prevention.

Thromboembolic Diseases

Much of the emphasis on this subject is regarding thromboprophylaxis. Treatment of hemodynamically stable VTE consists of LMWH given over a period of 3–6 months. This strategy is superior to VKA therapy in terms of reduced VTE events and similar in terms of bleeding and mortality.[22]

Thrombolysis in PTE may also be considered.

Coronary Artery Disease

Invasive strategy is recommended in patients with STEMI and high-risk NSTEMI with life expectancy > 6 months (ESC 2022 guidelines, Class I, LOE B).

Conservative therapy is recommended in those with <6-month life expectancy and those with high bleeding risk (Class IIa, LOE C).

Short DAPT is recommended in those with high bleeding risk and treated with PCI (Class IIa, LOE C).

Hypertension

Untreated hypertension is a confirmed risk factor of HF during cancer treatment. Treatment of hypertension with ACEi or ARBs as a first-line therapy is recommended to reduce the risk of CTRCD. Combination therapy with an ACEi or ARB and a dihydropyridine CCB is recommended in patients with cancer with systolic BP ≥ 160 mm Hg and diastolic BP ≥ 100 mm Hg due to the more rapid onset of BP control with the combination compared with ACEi/ARB monotherapy **(Flowchart 3)**.

PREVENTION

Thorough pretreatment screening forms the cornerstone of prevention of cancer treatment-related cardiotoxicity.

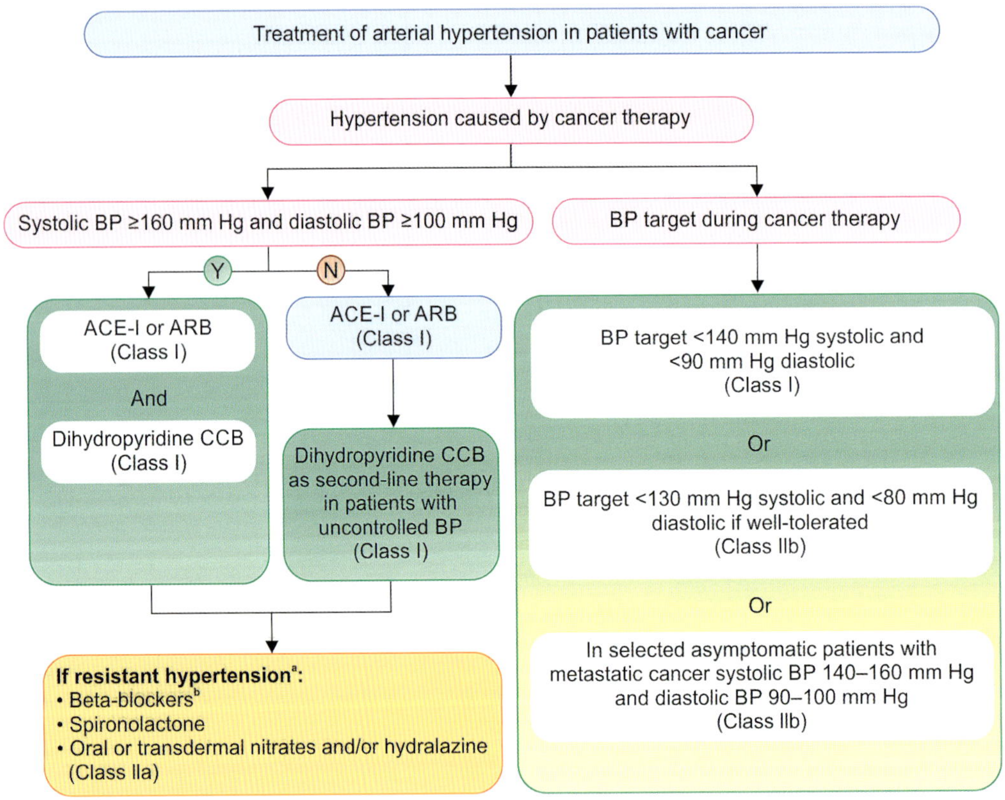

[a] Resistant hypertension is defined as BP being uncontrolled despite treatment with optimal or best-tolerated doses of three or more drugs including a diuretic, and confirmed by ambulatory and home BP monitoring.

[b] Consider beta-blockers (nebivolol or carvedilol are preferred in patients on VEGFi) at any treatment step, when there is a specific indication for their use, e.g., HF, angina, post MI, or AF.

FLOWCHART 3: Algorithm for management of hypertension during cancer chemotherapy (ESC 2022 guidelines).

It includes patient-related high-risk factors, particularly underlying CV risk factors and diseases, chemotherapeutic agent, dose, and duration of therapy. Any deviation from the normal baseline parameter should prompt cardioprotective strategies.

General Preventive Measures[22]

- Treat underlying CV diseases like hypertension, CAD, and heart failure
- Avoid QT-prolonging drugs
- Correct dyselectrolytemia
- Limit the cumulative dose of individual drugs
- Use alternative agents like dexrazoxane
- Altered delivery system, e.g., liposome and doxorubicin or continuous infusion
- Use ACEIs/ARBs and statins
- Prophylactic anticoagulation in high-risk patients like nonambulatory and hospitalized patients

CONCLUSION

With the continued advances being made in cancer care and CV risk becoming increasingly the point of concern, we need to engage all the stakeholders, i.e., cardio-oncology, to increase the awareness regarding CV health in cancer survivors. The goal of cardio-oncology specialty is to give the best cancer care to the patients and minimize CTR-CVT across the entire continuum of care and at the same time identify the patients at high risk with a proper preventive and surveillance plan for early identification and appropriate management of potential CV complications.

ONLINE REFERENCES

Please scan the QR code provided at the end of the table of contents for References of this chapter.

CHAPTER

79

Viral Myocarditis in India: Diagnosis, Treatment Options, and Current Controversies

Tanuja Makhani, Prashant Panda, Yash Paul Sharma

ABSTRACT

Viral myocarditis is one of the common causes of dilated cardiomyopathy and sudden cardiac death. The clinical spectrum of viral myocarditis varies from asymptomatic infection to clinical features of heart failure, arrhythmias and sudden cardiac arrest. Advances in cardiac MRI, and molecular detection of organism by endomyocardial biopsy have improved our ability to diagnose myocarditis. However currently there are few treatment options available for acute and chronic myocarditis. Majority of case reports have demonstrated benefit of immunosuppressive treatment but larger RCT are further needed to demonstrate its efficacy. In this review, we describe epidemiology, clinical presentation, diagnosis and treatment modalities of myocarditis.

Keywords: Viral myocarditis, Dallas criteria, anti-viral therapies, immunomodulatory therapy, COVID-19 myocarditis

INTRODUCTION

According to the WHO, myocarditis is defined as an inflammatory disease of the myocardium diagnosed by histological, immunological, and immunohistochemical criteria. Viral myocarditis is the most common cause of myocarditis. It is one of the causes of sudden cardiac death in young population. Causes of myocarditis are listed in **Table 1**.

EPIDEMIOLOGY

The true incidence of myocarditis in India is underestimated because of its underdiagnosis, and endomyocardial biopsy, which is the gold standard test, is not routinely done. Based on various autopsy studies,[1-4] the incidence of myocarditis ranges from 0.05 to 1.5% of the general population. Despite the growing understanding of coronavirus disease 2019 (COVID-19) myocardial involvement, cases of COVID-19 myocarditis are likely underreported. One recent study showed the prevalence of clinically confirmed COVID-19 myocarditis across a large multinational registry to be 0.01% (256 patients), with an associated increased mortality, highlighting the importance of diagnosing patients with myocarditis in the early phase.[5] The average age of patients ranges from 20 to 50 years, and it is more common in males

TABLE 1: Myocarditis.

Causes of myocarditis	
Viral myocarditis	• *RNA viruses*: Coxsackie virus type A and B, influenza, dengue virus, yellow fever, mumps, hepatitis C virus, HIV, measles virus, SARS-CoV-2 • *DNA viruses*: Adenovirus, herpes simplex, varicella zoster virus, parvovirus B19, cytomegalovirus, and Epstein–Barr virus
Other causes	
Infectious causes	• *Bacterial*: Rickettsial fever, tuberculosis, diphtheria, legionella, *Mycoplasma*, *Staphylococcus aureus* • *Parasites*: Toxoplasmosis, malaria, and Chagas disease • *Fungal*: Histoplasmosis, aspergillosis, mucormycosis
Immune mediated	Rheumatoid arthritis, SLE, sarcoidosis, Kawasaki disease, giant cell myocarditis
Drugs	Clozapine, carbamazepine, methyldopa, dobutamine, immune checkpoint inhibitors
Toxins	Alcohol, heavy metal poisoning (copper, lead, and iron), arsenic toxicity

than females. The most common causes of viral myocarditis are parvovirus B19 and human herpesvirus 6. Autopsy studies found that myocarditis is the cause of sudden cardiac death in patients under 40 years of age in 12%[6] and is a cause of DCMP in 9%.[7] Most of the patients recover spontaneously, but approximately 4% of cases progress to heart failure.[8] Myocarditis is one of the causes of INOCA.

PATHOPHYSIOLOGY

Viral myocarditis occurs in three phases **(Fig. 1)**:

1. *Acute phase*: This phase occurs over a period of 1 week. In this phase, the virus enters myocyte through endothelial receptor, undergoes replication, and causes direct cytotoxicity of myocytes.
2. *Subacute immune phase*: In this phase, activation of B cells, T cells, and NK cells leads to the production of cytokines and antibodies, resulting in a virus-induced cytokine storm leading to multiorgan dysfunction. This phase lasts for 1–4 weeks.
3. *Chronic phase*: This phase occurs over a period of months to years. Most of patients recover without any sequelae, but some patients develop a dilated cardiomyopathy-like phenotype due to long-standing inflammatory response and persistence of viral genome in myocytes.

CLINICAL PRESENTATION

Clinical features of myocarditis are variable, ranging from nonspecific symptoms like fatigue to life-threatening conditions such as arrhythmias and heart failure. These symptoms are preceded by a viral prodrome of respiratory or gastrointestinal symptoms. Viral myocarditis has three clinical profiles:

1. Acute coronary syndrome-like presentation with chest pain, elevated biomarkers, and ST-T changes
2. New onset of heart failure (<3 months) in the absence of CAD with impaired right or left ventricular dysfunction
3. Life-threatening condition in the absence of CAD, such as arrhythmias, cardiogenic shock, and severely impaired left ventricular dysfunction

EVALUATION

Clinical diagnosis of myocarditis should be suspected in young patients with new-onset heart failure, arrhythmias, and acute coronary syndrome-like presentation without any risk factors.

NONINVASIVE TESTS

Blood tests: These include complete blood picture and renal and liver function tests. The presence of eosinophilia indicates drug-induced myocarditis.

Biomarkers: Troponin T, I, BNP levels, ESR, and CRP will be elevated, but levels do not correlate with prognosis. Negative biomarker levels do not exclude the diagnosis.

Anticardiac antibodies: Anticardiac antibodies (directed against laminin and myosin) are elevated in 50% patients with myocarditis.[9] In acute myocarditis, the presence of antibodies indicates a risk of death and need for heart transplantation, and in chronic myocarditis, it indicates an increased risk of progression to DCM phenotype.[10]

ECG: May be normal or show nonspecific ST-T changes, or arrhythmias in the form of supraventricular tachycardia and ventricular tachycardia. Intraventricular conduction delay and prolonged QT interval are associated with poor prognosis.

2D echo: May be normal or show regional wall motion abnormalities (mainly in inferior and inferolateral walls) or global hypokinesia with left ventricular dysfunction with valvular abnormalities in the form of mitral and aortic incompetence. Left ventricular thickness may be increased due to myocardial edema. Right ventricular dysfunction is seen in 18% of patients, and pericardial effusion in 26% of patients. It also helps in ruling out other causes of heart failure such as valvular abnormalities.

Cardiac MRI: It is a noninvasive imaging modality that provides functional and morphological assessment of cardiac tissues. It helps in visualizing myocardial edema (T2W), hyperemia and capillary leak (T1W), and late gadolinium

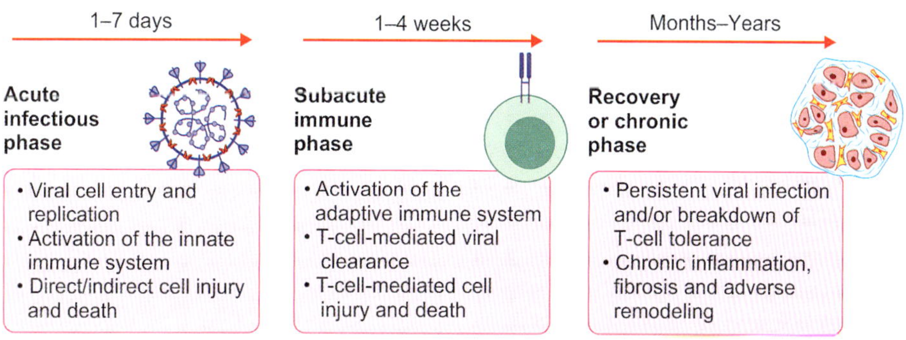

FIG. 1: Phases of viral myocarditis.

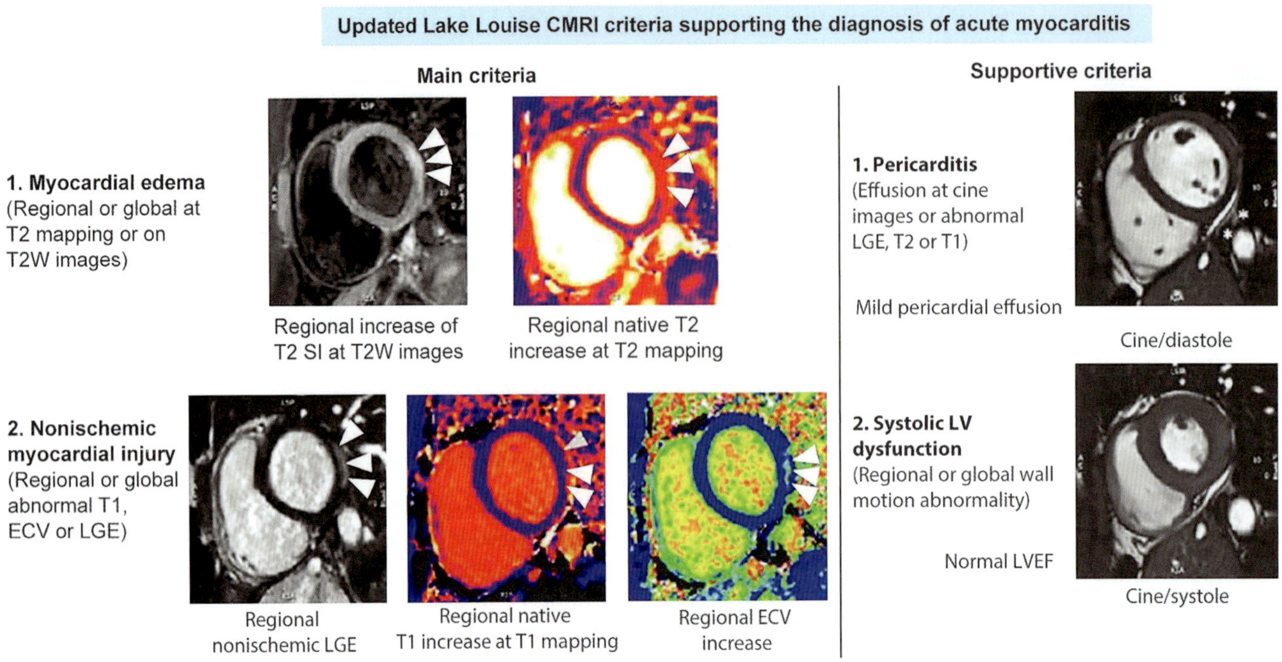

FIG. 2: MRI criteria for diagnosis of viral myocarditis.

enhancement. Diagnosis of myocarditis through MRI relies on Lake Louise criteria 2018, which has higher sensitivity than the original criteria (87.5 vs. 72%)[11] (shown in **Fig. 2**). *Limitations*: Difficult to perform in hemodynamically unstable patients, on mechanical ventilators, and claustrophobic patients **(Fig. 2)**.

microRNAs (miRNAs): These are small noncoding RNA molecules. They are epigenetic regulators of cardiac function and are involved in etiology and pathogenesis of myocarditis. miRNAs play an important role in virus upregulation, replication, myocardial inflammation, and fibrosis. miR-155, miR-221/222, miR-21, and miRNA-Chr8:96 are elevated during myocarditis and can aid in prognostication, diagnosis, and treatment[12] **(Fig. 3)**.

Viral serology: Virus-specific antibodies (IgM type) are elevated in 20–30% of patients. When combined with clinical signs, echocardiographic results, and CMR findings, a fourfold increase in the antibody titer collected 3 weeks apart is used to diagnose probable viral myocarditis. Routine viral serology testing is not recommended. With this technique, we may identify alterations in myocyte tissues before histological changes manifest. Research has demonstrated a correlation between inflammation and the expression level of tenascin C, indicating the potential utility of tenascin C as a marker for evaluating disease activity.[13]

Endomyocardial biopsy: Biopsy is considered the gold standard test for diagnosis, but it has variable sensitivity and specificity. Although the use of biopsy has declined in recent years, it should be considered for patients with life-threatening symptoms who do not respond to medical treatment. According to the Dallas criteria, acute myocarditis is defined by lymphocytic infiltrates associated with myocyte necrosis.[14] Borderline myocarditis is characterized by inflammatory infiltrates without the presence of myocyte necrosis. Endomyocardial biopsies from different parts of the right ventricle and at different time points show spatial and temporal variability. In PCR-proven viral myocarditis, Dallas criteria were absent in 50% of cases.[15] So, the sensitivity of Dallas criteria to diagnose myocarditis is low because of sampling errors and interobserver variability.

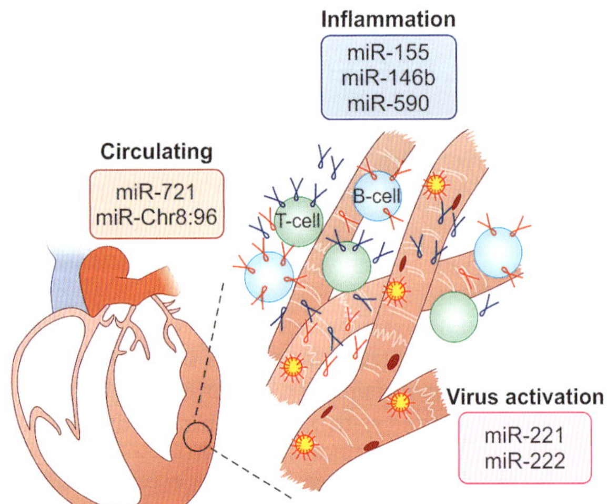

FIG. 3: MicroRNAs elevated during the acute phase of myocarditis.

Immunostaining: With this technique, we may identify alterations in myocyte tissues before histological changes manifest. Immunostaining for CD3, CD68, major basic protein (MBP), and tenascin C is useful for histological diagnosis. Research has demonstrated a correlation between inflammation and the expression level of tenascin C, indicating the potential utility of tenascin C as a marker for evaluating disease activity.[13]

DIAGNOSIS OF CLINICALLY SUSPECTED MYOCARDITIS (BOX 1)

Myocarditis should be suspected in the presence of:

- One or more of the clinical presentations with or without ancillary features
- And one or more of the diagnostic criteria from different categories
- Or when the patient is asymptomatic, two or more diagnostic criteria from different categories

Ancillary features which support the clinical suspicion of myocarditis include:

- Fever ≥38°C at presentation or within the preceding 30 days with or without evidence of a respiratory or gastrointestinal infection
- Peripartum period
- Previous clinically suspected or definite myocarditis
- Personal and/or family history of allergic asthma, other types of allergy, extra-cardiac autoimmune disease, toxic agents
- Family history of DCM, myocarditis

BOX 1 Diagnosis of clinically suspected myocarditis.

- *Clinical presentation*:
  - Acute chest pain, pericarditis, or pseudo-ischemic
  - New-onset (days up to 3 months) or worsening of: Dyspnea at rest or exercise, and/or fatigue, with or without left and/or right heart failure signs
  - Subacute/chronic (>3 months) or worsening of: Dyspnea at rest or exercise, and/or fatigue, with or without left and/or right heart failure signs; palpitation, and/or unexplained arrhythmia symptoms and/or syncope, and/or aborted sudden cardiac death
  - Unexplained cardiogenic shock
- *Diagnostic criteria*:
  - ECG/Holter: Abnormal 12-lead ECG in the form of first degree atrioventricular block to complete heart block, or bundle branch block, ST/T wave change (ST-elevation or non-ST-elevation, T wave inversion), sinus arrest, ventricular tachycardia or fibrillation and asystole, atrial fibrillation
  - Elevated markers: Elevated TnT/TnI
  - Functional and structural abnormalities on cardiac imaging (echo/angio/CMR): Regional wall motion or global systolic or diastolic function abnormality, with or without ventricular dilatation, with or without increased wall thickness, with or without pericardial effusion, and with or without endocavitary thrombi. Tissue characterization by CMR: Edema and/or LGE of classical myocarditis pattern

TREATMENT

Treatment of myocarditis includes supportive care with guideline-directed treatment of heart failure and arrhythmias. In patients of myocarditis with reduced ejection fraction, treatment includes diuretics, beta blockers, and renin–angiotensin–aldosterone blockers along with SGLT-2 inhibitors. Reverse remodeling drugs should be continued for at least 6 months after normalization of ejection fraction. In hemodynamically unstable patients, inotropes are administered. In patients with refractory cardiogenic shock, mechanical circulatory support such as IABP, ECMO, and IMPELLA are used as a bridge to recovery or heart transplantation. Abstinence from competitive sports is recommended for at least 6 months after myocarditis to decrease the risk of remodeling and sudden cardiac death.

ARRHYTHMIAS

In the acute phase of myocarditis, brady- and tachyarrhythmias are common. In cases of AV nodal block, a temporary pacemaker is inserted as most of AV blocks are transient and recover within 1 week of treatment. In patients with persistent AV nodal block, a permanent pacemaker is inserted. Tachyarrhythmias are treated with antiarrhythmic drugs in the acute phase. In chronic myocarditis, if there is no improvement in ejection fraction even after 3–6 months of treatment, an ICD is indicated for primary prevention of sudden cardiac death.

IMMUNOMODULATORY THERAPY

To date, no specific evidence-based treatment is available for viral myocarditis.

ANTIVIRAL THERAPY

Currently, there is no approved antiviral therapy for myocarditis. IFN-β and IFN-α decreased myocardial viral replication and damage, but clinical trials have found IFN-β to be more effective in clearing viral load than α.[16] Persistence of viral genome in myocardium is associated with DCMP phenotype. In the BICC study, IFN therapy was found to be effective in enterovirus- and adenovirus-associated myocarditis, but showed no efficacy in parvovirus- and herpesvirus-associated myocarditis. Large randomized controlled trials (RCTs) are required in order to prove its efficacy.

INTRAVENOUS IMMUNOGLOBULINS

Intravenous immunoglobulin (IVIG) possesses anti-inflammatory and antiviral properties. Immunoglobulins should be used in myocarditis with low ejection fraction where left ventricular function is not improving despite medical therapy. There are multiple RCTs, which showed mixed results. Till date, only two RCTs have been conducted. Intravenous immune globulin did not significantly enhance overall mortality or left ventricular function in a trial by McNamara et al.[17] in patients with myocarditis or recent-onset idiopathic DCM compared to the placebo group.[18] According to Kishimoto et al.,[19] IVIG improved the ejection fraction.

Until further studies demonstrate the benefit of IVIG in myocarditis, treatment of IVIG in viral myocarditis remains uncertain.

IMMUNOADSORPTION

The basic principle of immunoadsorption is to remove anticardiac antibodies from plasma by plasmapheresis. Some studies have shown improvement in systemic vascular resistance, cardiac output, and ejection fraction in dilated cardiomyopathy phenotype. Although promising, current guidelines do not recommend it due to the lack of RCTs.

PROGNOSIS

The clinical course of acute myocarditis ranges from spontaneous recovery to acute fulminant myocarditis, arrhythmias, death, and long-term progression to DCM phenotype. Among patients who present with left ventricular dysfunction, 50% will have complete resolution, 25% will have persistent left ventricle dysfunction, and 25% will progress toward an end-stage cardiomyopathy, resulting in transplantation or death.[16] Long-term prognosis is good with a 3–5-year survival ranging from 50% to 80%. Patients with acute fulminant myocarditis, once they survive the acute episode, have an excellent long-term prognosis of 93% at 11 years. In patients with acute myocarditis, a mortality rate of 20% at 1 year has been reported, which gradually stabilizes after 3 years. Therefore, we advise a follow-up of at least 3 years after presentation or longer since myocarditis may recur after the initial event.

COVID-19 MYOCARDITIS

Myocarditis is a significant complication of COVID-19, a condition caused by the severe acute respiratory syndrome coronavirus 2 (SARS-CoV-2) virus. The virus has spread rapidly across the globe, and on March 11, 2020, the WHO has declared COVID-19 as a global pandemic. India has recorded the second highest number of cases (45,041,192) with 533,623 deaths. Coronavirus causes myocarditis either by direct myocardial injury or through infection of endothelial cells. The administration of COVID-19 mRNA vaccines (both Pfizer and Moderna) is associated with the development of myocarditis. Evidence suggest that myocarditis rates are around 12.6 cases per million administrations of the second dose of mRNA vaccines, more common in young males.[20] Treatment includes antiviral agents (remdesivir), steroids, IVIG, and IL-6 inhibitors (tocilizumab).

CONTROVERSIES

Although the pathogenesis of viral myocarditis has been described in mice models and is supported by pathological data from humans, whether the process is fully recapitulated in humans is unclear. Genetic factors play an important role in predilection or protection to myocardial injury, so identifying the molecular basis for differences in genetic susceptibility could open a new therapeutic window for treatment or prevention. There are no specific evidence-based treatments for myocarditis. The role of immunomodulation, immunoadsorption, and miRNA has been tested only in few case reports and small studies, but large RCTs are needed to prove their efficacy.

CONCLUSION

Viral infections are the most common cause of myocarditis. The absence of specific pathognomonic features in conjunction with the wide spectrum of clinical manifestations that range from subclinical cases to sudden cardiac death (SCD) makes myocarditis diagnosis particularly challenging. Treatment of myocarditis is mainly supportive. Immunosuppressive therapy can be beneficial in patients with giant-cell myocarditis and sarcoidosis; however, its role in chronic myocarditis, although promising, requires further clarification. The use of immunomodulatory and antiviral therapy remains largely investigational at this time. Large, randomized, controlled trials are needed to determine their role.

ONLINE REFERENCES

Please scan the QR code provided at the end of the table of contents for References of this chapter.

CHAPTER

80

Cardiac Amyloidosis: When to Suspect, Newer Therapeutics

Goutam Datta, Anirban Das

ABSTRACT

Cardiac amyloidosis (CA) is a form of infiltrative cardiomyopathy characterized by interstitial deposition of misfolded amyloid proteins in different organs, leading to organ dysfunction. While numerous forms of CA exist, two subtypes dominate clinical prevalence: Transthyretin amyloidosis (ATTR) and immunoglobulin light-chain amyloidosis (AL). The clinical presentation of CA is diverse, ranging from heart failure with preserved ejection fraction (HFpEF) to different kinds of arrhythmias to conduction abnormalities and heart block. Apart from these, there are various extracardiac manifestations as well, most commonly being neuropathy and renal involvement. As the disease is relentlessly progressive and carries high mortality in advanced stages, early diagnosis and specific treatment are of immense value. The high degree of clinical suspicion backed with ECG, echocardiography, and strain imaging along with cardiac mitral regurgitation (MR) play a valuable role in detecting CA. On the other hand, genetic testing, tomographic scintigraphy, light-chain assay, and tissue biopsy are indispensable for disease-specific diagnosis. Although various chemotherapeutic agents have been used for decades for immunoglobulin light chain (AL) amyloid, management of ATTR amyloidosis was largely symptomatic until the approval of tafamidis, a TTR-tetramer stabilizing agent. Since then, various other therapeutic avenues have been explored and a number of novel agents are undergoing late-stage clinical trials. This chapter delineates the current standard of care for CA therapy.

Keywords: Amyloidosis, ATTR, heart failure, light chain, infiltrative cardiomyopathy, multiple myeloma, tafamidis, transthyretin

INTRODUCTION

Amyloid was first described by Rudolf Virchow in 1853. It refers to the extracellular deposition of a variety of low-molecular-weight serum proteins that are misfolded and form beta-pleated sheet structures. They can deposit any organ in the body leading to organ dysfunction. Advanced age, male sex, black ethnicity, genetic predisposition, and presence of chronic infection are some of the established risk factors. Although nine different types of cardiac amyloidosis (CA) have been described, most cases correspond to monoclonal immunoglobulin light-chain amyloidosis (AL) or transthyretin amyloidosis (ATTR), either in its hereditary (ATTRv) or acquired (ATTRwt) form. The ATTRwt form, which is associated with aging, is currently considered the most common form of CA worldwide. The heart is affected in 50–70% of cases of AL disease. Rarer forms of CA are *AA amyloidosis* (acquired in a background of the chronic inflammatory or infectious process), *ApoA-IV amyloidosis* (due to apolipoprotein 4 mutation), and *isolated atrial amyloidosis* (*IAA*; resulting from overproduction of atrial natriuretic peptide). The worldwide prevalence of CA is not known. Nowadays, heart failure with preserved ejection fraction (HFpEF) accounts for 50% of total heart failure-related hospitalizations. In a recent study on hospitalized HFpEF patients, an endomyocardial biopsy revealed that 14% had actually CA (AL, ATTR, and AA diseases).[1] Therefore, CA is not a rare disease. If remain untreated, the median survival of AL, ATTRh, and ATTRwt cardiomyopathy is 1.5, 2.5, and 3.5 years, respectively.[2] However, with the advent of novel therapies, the natural history of this disease is rapidly improving.

WHEN TO SUSPECT

Clinical recognition of CA at an early stage of the disease is critical, as it offers an affected individual the widest array of treatment options that have a favorable impact on survival. Unfortunately, 35–45% of patients with ATTR-CA do not receive a timely diagnosis within 6 months of symptom onset.[3] Overlap with other more "common" diseases and the noncardiac constellation of clinical findings like musculoskeletal, neurologic, gastrointestinal (GI), and renal manifestations hinders arriving at a correct diagnosis **(Fig. 1)**.

Not only this, the cardiac manifestations are also nonspecific. The increased left ventricular wall thickness may be mistaken for hypertensive heart disease, concentric hypertrophy from aortic stenosis (AS), hypertrophic cardiomyopathy (HCM), or other infiltrative cardiomyopathies like Fabry disease. To overcome these issues and to ease the diagnosis of CA accurately, both ACC[4] and ESC[5] proposed some algorithms in 2023 to help practicing cardiologists. The first clue to suspect CA is the presence of both cardiac and extracardiac presentation. ESC 2023 has suggested a screening criterion, as shown in **Table 1**. All cardiologists must be aware of some clues ("red flags") that are associated with CA phenotype as well as serve as diagnostic tools that assist in identifying the disease. A high degree of suspicion is a must for diagnosis; otherwise, diagnosis cannot be established based on routine testing alone.

The clinical clues or "*red flags*" in CA are broadly divided into cardiac and extracardiac manifestations **(Table 1)**. Among the extracardiac manifestations, a history of carpal

TABLE 1: 2023 ESC recommended screening criteria for cardiac amyloidosis.

Essential criteria		≥1 "red flag" signs
Left ventricular wall thickness ≥ 12 mm	Plus	Heart failure in ≥65 years
		Aortic stenosis in ≥65 years
		↓BP/hypotension in a hypertensive patient
		AD/sensory neuropathy
		Peripheral polyneuropathy
		Severe proteinuria
		Spontaneous skin bruising
		Ruptured biceps-tendon
		Bilateral carpal tunnel syndrome
		↓ QRS voltage-to-mass ratio
		Pseudo-Q-waves in ECG
		AV conduction disease
		↓Longitudinal strain + apical sparing
		LGE or increased ECV in CMR
		Possible family history of ATTR
		Chronically increased cTn
		Known patient of MM or MGUS

(AD: autonomic dysfunction; ECV: extracellular volume; LGE: late gadolinium enhancement)

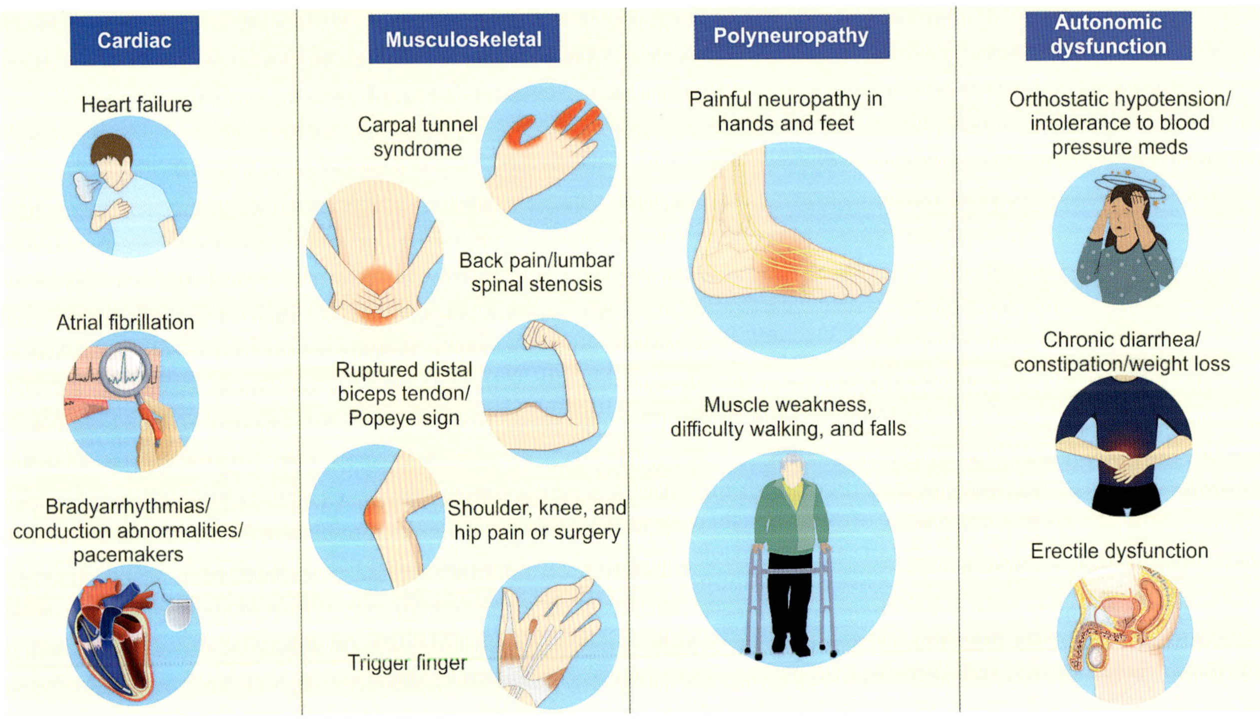

FIG. 1: Various clinical manifestations of ATTR amyloidosis.

Source: Nativi-Nicolau J, Karam C, Khella S, et al. Screening for ATTR amyloidosis in the clinic: overlapping disorders, misdiagnosis, and multiorgan awareness. Heart Fail Rev. 2022;27(3):78593.

tunnel syndrome, spinal stenosis, hip or knee replacement surgery, prior shoulder surgery, proteinuria, or peripheral/ autonomic neuropathy provide major clues. There are some pathognomonic extracardiac manifestations of AL amyloidosis like macroglossia/submandibular gland enlargement from soft-tissue involvement and periorbital purpura from capillary fragility and acquired factor X deficiency. On the other hand, musculoskeletal manifestations, such as spontaneous biceps tendon rupture and spinal stenosis, are unique to ATTR amyloidosis.[4]

Cardiac amyloidosis can be diagnosed by using invasive and noninvasive diagnostic criteria. Invasive diagnostic criteria apply to all forms of CA, whereas noninvasive criteria are applicable to ATTR only.[5] *Invasive criteria* include demonstration of amyloid fibrils within cardiac tissue or, alternatively, demonstration of amyloid deposits in extracardiac biopsy plus characteristic features of CA on echocardiography or CMR. *Noninvasive criteria* include typical echocardiographic/CMR findings combined with grade 2 or 3 myocardial radiotracer uptake in tomographic scintigraphy (SPECT) and exclusion of a clonal dyscrasia (by serum free light-chain assay, serum and urine protein electrophoresis with immunofixation).

Tomographic scintigraphy should be considered in order to reduce the number of misclassifications. *False-negative scans* are rarely found in certain ATTRv genotypes; in such situations where clinical suspicion is high but the scan is negative/equivocal, biopsy should be considered. *False-positive scans* may be due to AL disease, recent myocardial infarction, or long-term chloroquine use. DPD/ PYP/HMDP scan cannot distinguish between ATTRwt and ATTRv. TTR genetic testing is therefore recommended for all patients with ATTR cardiomyopathy. Characteristic ECG, echocardiographic, CMR, and scintigraphy findings are summarized in **Table 2**.

Diagnostic Workup

Both the 2023 ACC expert consensus GL on CA and 2023 ESC GL for cardiomyopathy have proposed diagnostic workup strategies for CA with subtle differences. Whereas the 2023 ESC GL suggested hematological assays (to rule out

TABLE 2: Characteristic features of different diagnostic modalities in AL and ATTR-CA.[6,28]

	AL amyloidosis	ATTR amyloidosis
ECG	Low voltage-to-mass ratio	
	Pseudo-infarct pattern	
	Low QRS voltage (late-phase phenomenon, not sensitive but specific). Low voltage is more common in AL variety, because of the presence of toxic light chains	
		Conduction disease
		LVH is found in 15% of cases
Echocardiography	Left ventricular wall thickness > 12 mm	
	Low tissue Doppler velocities	
	Restrictive filling pattern	
	Atrial septal thickening	
	Apical sparing in strain-echo ("cherry on top" appearance)	
	LV wall thickness is usually <15 mm	LV wall thickness is usually >15 mm
		Concomitant aortic stenosis
Cardiac MR	Late gadolinium enhancement (in any pattern)	
	Elevated native T1 and extracellular volume	
	Extracellular volume is higher in AL than in ATTR	Native T1 is lower in ATTR than AL
Tissue biopsy or endomyocardial biopsy	Positive Congo red staining	
	Apple-green birefringence under polarized light	
	Fat pad biopsy positive > 50%	Fat pad biopsy positive < 50%
	Renal involvement	Lumbar spine and median nerve involvement at carpal tunnel (CTS)
	Median nerve involvement (CTS)	
Serum biomarkers	Elevated cTn and NT-proBNP based on the stage of disease	
	Abnormal free light-chain ratio	Normal free light-chain ratio
	Monoclonal protein present on immunofixation	No monoclonal protein was found on immunofixation

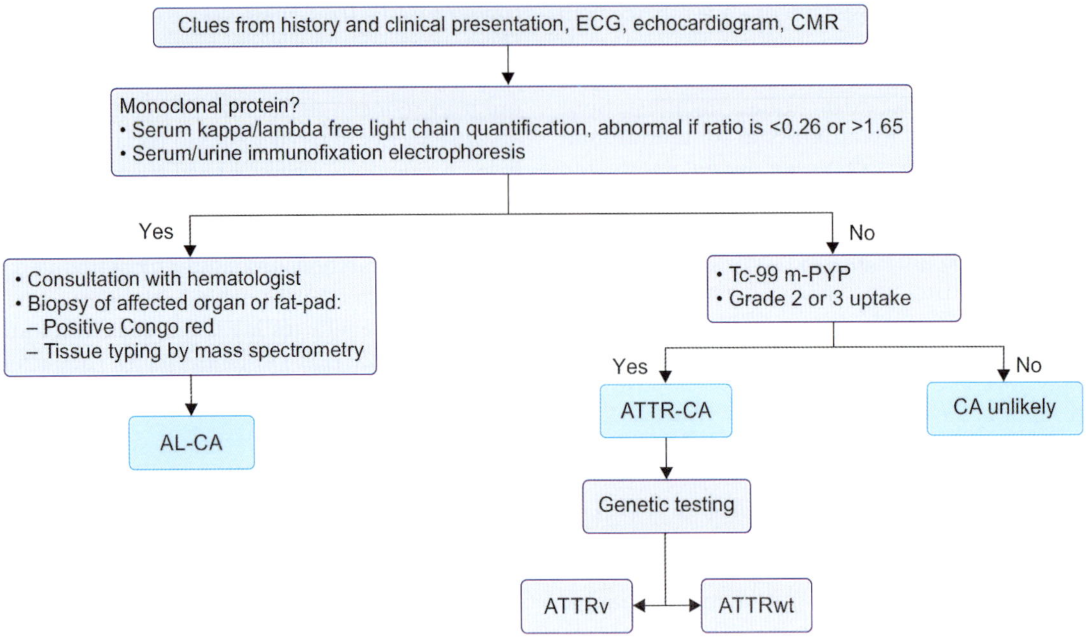

FLOWCHART 1: 2023 ACC expert consensus diagnostic algorithm of CA.

AL disease) and cardiac scintigraphy simultaneously at the very beginning, the 2023 ACC expert consensus proposed a step-wise approach that seems to be cost-effective and more applicable in a resource-limited country like ours **(Flowchart 1)**.

NEWER THERAPEUTICS

Treatment of CA depends on the type (ATTR vs. AL) and clinical symptoms. **Figure 2** shows an overview of general measures of CA management applicable to both variants. Antiplasma cell therapy has been used as a specific treatment of AL amyloidosis for decades, while ATTR amyloidosis was only treated symptomatically until recent years when a bunch of targeted therapies emerged and have shown to improve heart failure symptoms, reduce complications, and delay the progression of ATTR-related disease.

MANAGEMENT OF CARDIAC AMYLOIDOSIS: GENERAL PRINCIPLES

Management of Heart Failure

Apart from *diuretics* and *mineralocorticoid receptor antagonists* (MRAs), other standard HF drugs are not well tolerated in CA. Angiotensin-converting enzyme (ACE) inhibitors and angiotensin-II receptor blockers (ARBs) often precipitate hypotension and beta blockers lead to symptomatic bradycardia. However, *low-dose beta-blockers* were associated with a lower risk of mortality in patients with HFrEF. No significant mortality benefits were observed in patients with LVEF > 40%.[7] In a recent multicenter, longitudinal, observational study conducted on patients with ATTR CM ($n = 2{,}356$), it has been found that *SGLT-2 inhibitors* were not only well tolerated but also effective in reducing heart failure symptoms, renal function, and diuretic use. It was also associated with lower risks of HFRH, cardiovascular mortality, and all-cause mortality across varying ejection fractions.[8] Treating the psychological aspect of HF is often a neglected component of therapy. The prevalence of anxiety and depression is much higher in CA patients compared to the general population.[9] Progressive HF goes hand in hand with impaired quality of life (QoL), which ultimately leads to social isolation and worsening depression. Early psychotherapy programs and coping strategies are therefore beneficial in improving QoL and relieving symptoms of HF.[5]

Arrhythmias, Conduction Abnormalities, and Device Therapy

Atrial fibrillation (AF) is the most common arrhythmia found in CA. Controlling heart rate without compromising the cardiac output poses a real challenge to the treating physician. While low-dose beta-blockers and amiodarone appear to be well tolerated in CA, nondihydropyridine CCBs should be avoided as they may precipitate cardiogenic shock as per some older case reports in patients with CA.[10] Despite some controversy, digoxin at a time can be very useful in AF-rate control in selected patients of CA.[11] The role of catheter ablation in these patients is poor with high rates of AF recurrence.[12] *Ventricular arrhythmias* is the second most common arrhythmia in CA which carries a high risk of

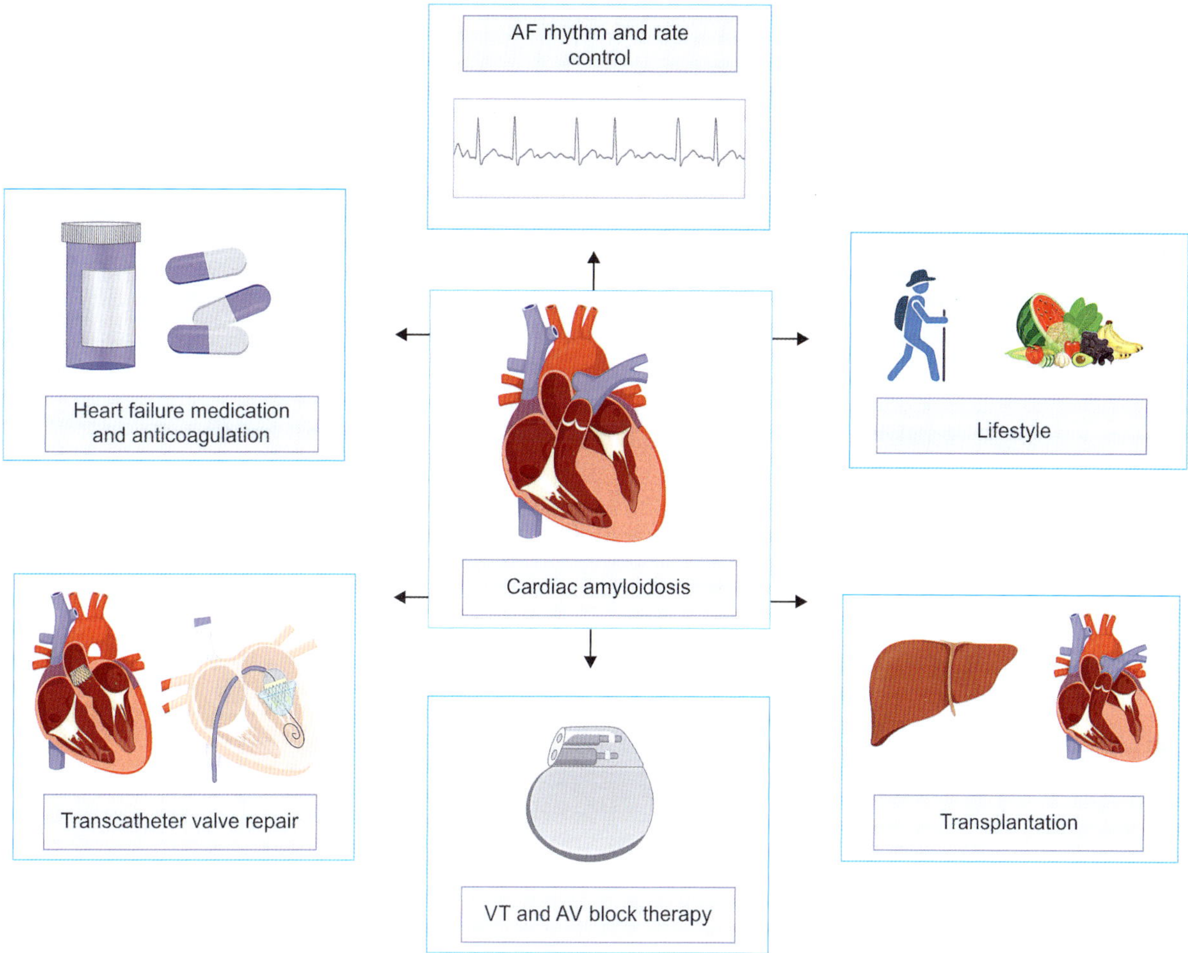

FIG. 2: General measures of management of cardiac amyloidosis. © Creative Commons Attribution 4.0 International License.
Source: Vogel J, Carpinteiro A, Luedike P, et al. Current therapies and future horizons in cardiac amyloidosis treatment. Curr Heart Fail Rep. 2024;21:305-21.

SCD. ICD implantation as a mode of primary prevention is controversial given the lack of survival benefits. ICD is useful as a measure of secondary prevention. However, its role is undefined in AL amyloidosis with background multiple myeloma and is currently a field of active research. CA patients with *symptomatic conduction block* are treated with pacemaker implantation as per standard recommendation.

Anticoagulation Strategy

Cardiac amyloidosis patients have a higher propensity to develop intracardiac thrombi, even in sinus rhythm,[13] compared to age- and sex-matched controls. Therefore, anticoagulation is preferred irrespective of CHA_2DS_2-VASc score who develop AF to attenuate the risk of stroke.[14] Either DOAC or VKA can be used, and no difference was found in terms of efficacy and major bleeding in this population.[15]

Transplantation

Cardiac amyloidosis patients who present with ACC/AHA stage-D heart failure pose a unique challenge to more advanced HF therapies like the use of LV-assist devices due to marked LVH, small LV cavity size, and concomitant RV dysfunction.[16] In this subset of the population, cardiac transplantation may be a valuable option. As the liver is the production site for TTR tetramers, therefore hepatic transplantation was the treatment of choice for ATTRh amyloidosis in the past. With the advent of highly effective therapy, it is however considered rare in present days.[17] Patients with multiple myeloma are not eligible for heart transplantation.[18]

Interventions

Aortic stenosis, mitral regurgitation (MR), and tricuspid regurgitation (TR) are quite common in amyloid heart due to architectural distortion of heart valves secondary to the deposition of amyloid fibrils. At the same time, patients with CA are frequently old and have prohibitive surgical risks. The safety and efficacy studies of minimally invasive procedures like TAVR for AS[19] and transcatheter edge-to-edge repair (TEER) for MR[20] and TR[21] have already been completed,[22] and they are well-established therapies for high-risk CA populations nowadays.

SPECIFIC THERAPY FOR ATTR AMYLOIDOSIS

Transthyretin (TTR) is a tetrameric protein produced in the liver. The tetrameric structure binds and transports thyroxin (T4). When TTR dissociates into monomers, it becomes more prone to misfolding leading to amyloid formation. At present, three groups of therapy are used for the management of ATTR amyloidosis: (1) Agents that suppress the production of TTR protein (*silencers*), (2) agents that stabilize the TTR tetramer (*stabilizers*), and (3) agents that disrupt the TTR-amyloid fibrils. The pathogenesis of CA and the mechanism of action of different amyloid-specific agents are illustrated in the central illustration **(Fig. 3)**.

Stabilizers

Stabilizers work by binding to the TTR protein, preventing its dissociation into monomers and thereby decreasing

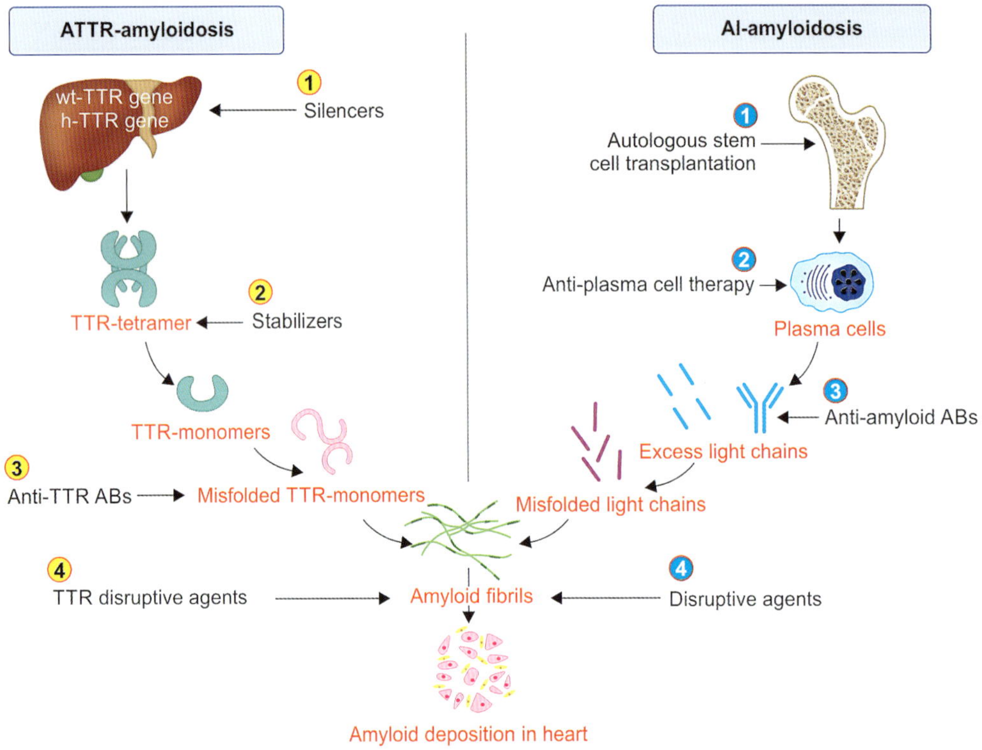

Amyloid specific therapeutic agents and their site of action	
1 Silencer • siRNA: Patisiran, vutrisiran • ASO: Inotersen, eplontersen • CRISPR-Cas9 gene editer: NTLA-2001	**1 ASCT**
2 Stabilizers • Tafamidis • Acoramidis (AG10) • Diflunisal	**2 Antiplasma cell therapy** • Bortezomib • Daratumumab
3 Anti-TTR ABs • NI006 • PRX004	**3 Antiamyloid ABs** • Birtamimab • CAEL-101 • AT-02, AT-03
4 TTR disruptive agents • Doxycycline • TUDCA	**4 Disruptive agents** • Doxycycline • EGCG

FIG. 3: Central illustration: Pathogenesis of cardiac amyloidosis and mechanism of action of different amyloid-specific therapeutic agents. (ABs: antibodies; ASCT: autologous stem cell transplantation; ASO: antisense oligonucleotide; CRISPR: clustered regulatory interspaced palindromic repeats; EGCG: epigallocatechin gallate; h-TTR: hereditary transthyretin; siRNA: small interfering RNA; TUDCA: tauroursodeoxycholic acid; Wt-TTR: wild type transthyretin)

their misfolding and attenuating the progression of ATTR amyloidosis.

- *Tafamidis:* At present, tafamidis is the only approved drug for cardiac ATTR amyloidosis, which binds with high-affinity thyroxine-binding site on TTR and stabilizes the tetrameric structure. It is extremely well tolerated and devoid of any side effects. Tafamidis (20 or 80 mg) was tested against a placebo in a randomized controlled *ATTR-ACT trial* which showed that tafamidis is associated with a doubling of life expectancy compared to standard therapy,[23] 30% reduction hazard in all-cause mortality and a 32% reduction hazard in cardiovascular-related hospitalization. Tafamidis also retards the progression of ATTRv polyneuropathy.[24]
- *Acoramidis (AG10):* This is another agent that mimics the structural influence of the protective *Thr119Met* mutation, leading to the natural stabilization of TTR tetramer. The *attribute-CM trial*, a multinational, randomized, double-blind, placebo-controlled phase-III trial, investigated the effect of Acoramidis in CA. The study demonstrated a favorable safety profile, along with lower mortality and cardiovascular hospitalization over a period of 15 months.[25]
- *Diflunisal:* This is a nonsteroidal anti-inflammatory drug (NSAID), which binds to the T4-binding site of TTR and stabilizes the tetramer. Diflunisal at the dose of 250 mg twice a day improves survival in ATTRwt CA.[26] GI and renal side effects are typical as expected from NSAIDs.
- *Epigallocatechin-3-Gallate (EGCG):* This is a green tea extract which at the dose of 600 mg/day has been shown to reduce myocardial mass in CMR. Further studies are required to demonstrate its efficacy in amyloid cardiomyopathy.[27]

Silencers

Transthyretin silencers target the hepatic synthesis of TTR proteins. They utilize RNA interference (RNAi) to target the messenger RNA (mRNA) responsible for producing TTR.

- *Patisiran* acts as small interfering RNA (siRNA) in hepatocytes and blocks the production of TTR protein by inducing splitting of TTR-mRNA. In the *APOLLO-B* trial, Patisiran showed improvement in the 6MWT and Kansas City Cardiomyopathy Questionnaire overall summary at 12 months but failed to show any significant advantage over the established therapy.[29] Other agents that are undergoing phase-III clinical trials at present are summarized in **Table 3**.
- *CRISPR-Cas9 in vivo gene editing and NTLA-2001:* Apart from inducing siRNA, other pathways of gene silencing like modulating the CRISP-Cas9 pathway have been explored recently in a phase-I clinical trial (*NCT04601051*) in a small group of patients ($n = 6$) with ATTRv. In this trial, *NTLA-2001*, a novel and first-in-the-class in vivo gene editing agent, was tested in patients with ATTRv and polyneuropathy with or without cardiomyopathy. After 28 days of infusion, there was an 87% mean reduction of TTR level with only mild adverse events. Further studies are expected for this targeted treatment of CA.[34]

Antibodies

Immunotherapy with monoclonal antibodies (mABs) is emerging as a novel therapy of ATTR cardiomyopathy. These antibodies get attached to misfolded TTR monomers in the heart and stimulate macrophages and giant cell-mediated phagocytosis, thereby fostering recovery of organ function.

TABLE 3: Phase III clinical trials of "silencers" in ATTR CM.

Trial name	Intervention	End-points	Study progress
HELIOS-B NCT04153149[30]	Vutrisiran (siRNA)	• Primary end point was a composite of death from any cause and recurrent cardiovascular events at 36 months • Secondary end points was death from any cause, any change in 6MWT, and any change in Kansas City Cardiomyopathy Questionnaire–Overall Summary (KCCQ-OS) score	Treatment with vutrisiran led to a lower risk of death from any cause, reduced cardiovascular events and improved functional capacity and quality of life
NEURO-TTR NCT01737398[31]	Inotersen (ASO)	Changes in echocardiographic parameters in ATTR-polyneuropathy patients ($n = 172$) with and without cardiomyopathy	No significant differences in echocardiographic parameters between the two groups
CARDIO-TTRansform NCT04136171[32]	Eplontersen (ASO)	• Composite of CV mortality and recurrent • CV clinical events in NYHA class I–III patients up to 140 weeks	Enrolment completed mid-2022. Results are expected to be available in 2025
ENDEAVOUR NCT02319005[33]	Revusiran (siRNA)	Composite of all-cause mortality	Stopped prematurely due to increased mortality (13% in the revusiran group vs. 3% in the placebo group). However, no clear cause of death was identified

(ASO: antisense oligonucleotide; siRNA: small interfering RNA)

Two potential mABs, namely *NI006* and *PRX004*, are under investigation for treatment of ATTR cardiomyopathy. Both of them completed phase-I clinical trial without any drug-related serious adverse events. *NI006* was associated with a reduction in cardiac biomarkers (NT-proBNP and cTn-T) and improvement in cardiac imaging parameters (decreased cardiac tracer uptake in scintigraphy and decreased ECV in cardiac MRI) at 12 months, indicating potential therapeutic efficacy.[35] *PRX004* (*Prothena*) was associated with an increase in global longitudinal strain and significant improvement in neuropathic pain (*NCT03336580*).

Amyloid Fibril Disruption

Transthyretin disruptive therapy aims to remove amyloid fibrils from tissues after their deposition. A combination of *doxycycline* and *tauroursodeoxycholic acid* (TUDCA) was used in a small study with 53 patients with ATTR cardiomyopathy and showed improvements in left ventricular global longitudinal strain (–12 to –17%) and reduction in troponin-T levels.[36]

KEY DIFFERENCES IN THE MANAGEMENT OF ATTR-CA IN USA AND EUROPE

Recommended-based management strategy, differences in prevalence, and diagnosis of transthyretin CA as per practice update from AHA/ESC are summarized in **Table 4**.

SPECIFIC THERAPY FOR AL-AMYLOIDOSIS

Clonal proliferation of plasma cells in the bone marrow is the source of free light chains that deposit as amyloid in AL amyloidosis. Before initiation of treatment, patients are categorized into low-, intermediate-, or high-risk groups depending upon their age, blood biomarkers (e.g., NT-proBNP, troponin), and functional class (NYHA class or ECOG grade), and therapy is decided accordingly. The cardiac Mayo classifications from 2004 and 2012 were established to assess the severity of the disease.

Autologous Stem Cell Transplantation

Myeloablative chemotherapy with ASCT was introduced for the treatment of amyloidosis in 1985. Stem cell transplantation in patients with CA carries a mortality rate as high as 10%, which is quite unacceptable in the modern era, particularly when alternative drugs are available.[38] However with proper patient selection using Mayo criteria **(Box 1)**, transplant-related mortality can be brought down to 2.5%, hematological response rate to 66%, and cardiac response rate (≥30% reduction of baseline NT-proBNP) to 41%. This therapy option is now used only in selected cases as part of first-line therapy.[39]

Antiplasma Cell Therapy

For patients who are not eligible for ASCT, *Bortezomib-based* chemotherapy is presently the standard of care. One such regimen is the combination of cyclophosphamide + bortezomib + dexamethasone (CyBorD), where a hematological response rate of 60%, a cardiac response rate of 17%, and a renal response rate of 25% were achieved.[40] *Daratumumab*, which is the anti-CD-38 monoclonal antibody, is highly effective in the management of AL amyloidosis. As per the *Andromeda* study, the complete response rate was 53% versus 18% and the cardiac response rate was 42% versus 22% favoring daratumumab.[41] In another multicenter retrospective study on advanced AL-amyloidosis patients, a clear benefit was shown by adding daratumumab to the antiplasma cell therapy.[42]

BOX 1 Mayo eligibility criteria for ASCT.

- "Physiologic" age < 70 years
- Performance score ≥ 2
- Systolic blood pressure > 90 mm Hg
- Trop-T < 0.06 ng/mL or hs trop-T < 75 ng/mL
- Creatinine clearance ≥ 30 mL/min
- New York Heart Association Class I/II

Source: Eli Muchtar, Dispenzieri A, Gertz MA, et al. Treatment of AL amyloidosis: Mayo stratification of myeloma and risk-adapted therapy (mSMART) consensus statement 2020 update. Mayo Clin Proc. 2021;96(6):1546-77.

TABLE 4: Differences in the management of ATTR-CA in USA and Europe.[37]

Parameters	USA	Europe
wtATTR percentage	48%	25%
Tracers used for nuclear scintigraphy	Pyrophosphate (PYP)	3,3-diphosphono-1,2-propandicarboxylic acid (DPD) Hydroxymethylene diphosphonate (HMDP)
Recommended therapy	Tafamidis	Tafamidis
Alternative/adjunct therapy	• Diflunisal (off-label) • Patisiran (vATTR with neuropathy) • Inotersen (vATTR with neuropathy)	Diflunisal (off-label)

Antiamyloid Antibodies

Presently, three antifibril antibodies are under investigation for the treatment of cardiac AL-amyloidosis.

- *Birtamimab* is a monoclonal antibody that binds to immunoglobulin (Ig) light chains and thereby promotes phagocytosis of amyloid deposits by macrophages and neutrophils.[43] As of October 2023, the FDA has granted birtamimab orphan drug status and fast-track designation for the treatment of AL amyloidosis. However, it is still considered an investigational agent and is not yet approved by any regulatory authority.
- *CAEL-101* is a chimeric monoclonal antibody that binds to a cryptic epitope when amyloid Ig light chains are misfolded. In phase-I and II studies, patients treated with CAEL-101 showed therapeutic response in CA by improved NT-proBNP and imaging modalities.[44] Two randomized trials with *CAEL-101* are ongoing (*NCT04504825* and *NCT04512235*) in patients with advanced AL amyloidosis.
- *AT-02* and *AT-03* are two monoclonal antibodies that bind to different forms of amyloid proteins and support the removal of amyloid deposits.[45]

Amyloid Fibril Disruption

Doxycycline and *epigallocatechin gallate (EGCG),* a green tea extract, have nonspecific activity against amyloid fibrils, and therefore they exhibit a comparable effect in ATTR and AL amyloidosis. A phase-IV study compared doxycycline therapy plus CyBorD with CyBorD monotherapy and failed to exhibit any improvement in progression-free survival by adding doxycycline on top of chemotherapy.[46] Impact of EGCG in AL amyloidosis in two phase-II trials have already been completed (*NCT02015312* and *NCT01511263*), and results are awaited.

CONCLUSION

Often considered a rare disease, CA is increasingly recognized nowadays due to the aging of the population and the integration of highly sensitive noninvasive imaging modalities like nuclear scintigraphy into the armamentarium of diagnostic algorithms. For ATTR amyloidosis, only tafamidis is currently approved by different international

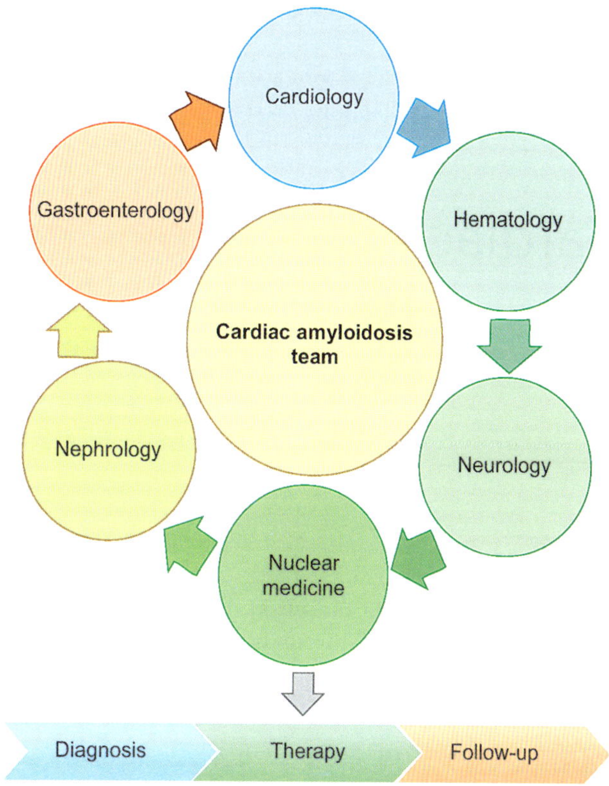

FIG. 4: Concept of amyloidosis team: Integration of different subspecialties is the present norm of standard care for the management of cardiac amyloidosis to achieve the best result.

bodies. However, several other drugs are in the pipeline and waiting for approval. Treatment of AL amyloidosis includes anti-plasma-cell therapies with a highly potent combination regimen. Exploring different pathophysiologic pathways and manipulating different genetic components to discover novel therapeutic agents is a field of active clinical research. With future approvals, treatment options will become more complex, which will require expertise and often multidisciplinary cooperation. The concept of the CA team is depicted in **Figure 4**. In addition to disease-specific therapy, supportive care like taking care of the mental health of the patient, treatment of heart failure, arrhythmias, conduction disturbances, thromboembolism, and aortic stenosis; also plays a vital role. This again emphasizes the establishment of a specific "amyloidosis care center."

ONLINE REFERENCES

Please scan the QR code provided at the end of the table of contents for References of this chapter.

CHAPTER

81

Cardiac Amyloidosis in India

Ashish Kumar Jain, Vivek BS, Rajiv Passey, Rajneesh Jain

ABSTRACT

Deposition of amyloid protein in the heart results in anatomical and functional myocardial dysfunction. This form of infiltrative cardiomyopathy is the most frequent and prognostically most important organ involvement in systemic amyloidosis. Unfortunately, this not so rare entity is often missed mainly because of lack of suspicion amongst physicians which in turn leads to unfortunate delay in diagnosis and management of an otherwise fatal disease.

Keywords: CA, microvascular, ATTR

INTRODUCTION

Cardiac amyloidosis (CA) is an infiltrative cardiomyopathy which develops due to deposition of abnormal amyloid protein in cardiac interstitium leading to cardiac structural and functional impairment.[1] Over 35 amyloidogenic proteins have been identified to cause systemic amyloidosis; however, CA is mainly caused by either of two amyloid proteins—(1) AL or (2) ATTR.[2] Certain conformational changes in these proteins renders them resistant to natural proteolytic enzymes. Deposition of amyloid protein in cardiac interstitium leads to toxicoinfiltrative cardiomyopathy causing diastolic dysfunction in early stage, systolic dysfunction in later stage, conduction abnormalities, or angina due to microvascular dysfunction.[3]

AL CARDIAC AMYLOIDOSIS

AL-CA occurs due to deposition of abnormal light chain immunoglobulin in cardiac interstitium, majority being of lambda type. Approximately 75% of AL cases have cardiac involvement.[4]

ATTR CARDIAC AMYLOIDOSIS

ATTR-CA occurs due to deposition of misfolded transthyretin (TTR) protein (also known as prealbumin). Normally, it is synthesized in liver and used for transport of thyroid hormone and retinol. TTR is composed of four subunits, which can dissociate, misfold, and aggregate into amyloid fibrils. Deposition of these fibrils in the heart cause structural and functional damage.

There are two types of ATTR-CA:

1. *Hereditary ATTR (variant type)*: This is an autosomal dominant condition occurring due to single-nucleotide polymorphisms (SNP) in *TTR* gene (chromosome 18).
2. *Wild ATTR (senile type)*: This is a sporadic condition in which misfolding of proteins is due to an unknown cause, described more commonly in males and elderly population.[5]

EPIDEMIOLOGY OF CARDIAC AMYLOIDOSIS IN INDIA

Cardiac amyloidosis is a rare disease with an estimated incidence of 0.2–0.4/100,000/year. AL form of CA was reported to be more common earlier. However, with availability of better noninvasive diagnostic modalities, a large number of patients with ATTR-CA are increasingly being identified.[6] Exact epidemiology of CA in India is not known because of paucity of studies, lack of awareness, under diagnosis, and under representation.[7]

A retrospective clinicopathological study was conducted by Seth et al.,[8] focusing on the presentation, diagnosis, and prognosis of CA in Indian patients. The study included 40 patients with CA, all diagnosed using endomyocardial biopsy (EMB). Patients in this study could not be subcategorized into AL or ATTR-CA. Median age of the patients was 51 years with male predominance (65%). Majority of the patients had heart failure symptoms (42% in NYHA II). On ECG, 81% of the patients had low voltages and 9.5% had a pseudoinfarct pattern. Bradyarrhythmia was observed in 19% of the patients. Echo showed left ventricular hypertrophy (LVH) in 90%, LV dysfunction in 35%, and interatrial septal thickening in 10% of the patients.

The biopsy findings showed that all patients had amyloid deposits. The study also provided survival data for a subset of patients. The age range of patients who died was 46–52 years. Median survival was 25 months from the time of diagnosis. The study concluded that CA presents with heart failure with preserved ejection fraction (HFpEF) and unexplained LVH, diagnosis being made through EMB with patient showing a poor prognosis (median survival of 2 years).

Another study by Jain et al.[9] analyzed data from 31 patients with CA and aimed to study the clinical characteristics, diagnostic approach, and types of CA. ATTR-CA was found in 13 (41.2%) patients and AL CA in 10 (32.2%) patients. Majority of the patients were males (51.6%), with a mean age of 64.5 years. HPpEF (41.9%) was the most common presentation. Arrhythmias, particularly atrial fibrillation (AF), was present in almost half of the patients. Extracardiac manifestations of amyloidosis were seen in 71% of patients, including renal and gastrointestinal involvement, peripheral polyneuropathy, and macroglossia. ECG abnormalities were seen in 67.7% of cases—most common being arrhythmias (AF), pseudoinfarct pattern, low voltage complexes, and bundle branch blocks. The echocardiographic study showed that 87% had LVH, 12.9% had isolated RVH and almost one-third had biventricular hypertrophy. Left and right ventricular systolic dysfunction was seen in 32.2% and 17.1%, respectively, with biatrial enlargement being observed in 41.3% patients. Abnormal global longitudinal strain (GLS < –15%) with apical sparing (cherry on top appearance) was evident in 87.5% of the patients. Rectal, pericardial, lingual, and gastric biopsies confirmed the diagnosis in one-fifth of patients.

Another study by Mohan et al.[7] included 13 patients with CA (eight patients with AL amyloidosis). The median age was 65 years (range 29–85) with male preponderance (male-to-female ratio of 9:4). Majority 69% patients presented with symptomatic heart failure. The median LVEF was 45% with a median GLS of –9.4%. LVH and left atrial enlargement were present in all patients. Cardiac MRI confirmed late gadolinium enhancement (LGE) and LVH in four patients. 46% of patients died within the follow-up period. The median survival was 15 months. 30% died within 6 months of diagnosis and among survivors, 71% continued to have NYHA grade III/IV symptoms.

In another retrospective analysis of data of six patients of CA diagnosed; the mean age of patients was 51 years with slight male preponderance. HFpEF was the most common manifestation. Atrial arrhythmias were seen in 33%. A speckled interventricular septum (66%) or thickened interatrial septum (16%) on echocardiography strongly favored CA. LGE on CMR was characteristic of CA. Plasma cell dyscrasia confirmed light chain amyloidosis. Abdominal fat pad and rectal biopsy confirmed the diagnosis. Chemotherapy for plasma cell dyscrasia was administered in 50% of patients.[10]

A study by Vivek et al.[11] retrospectively analyzed six patients with ALCA who had been admitted with various noncardiac diagnoses. The age range was 54–72 years. All the patients presented with signs and symptoms of heart failure. Echocardiogram showed concentric LVH, speckled appearance, reduced GLS, and relative apical sparing in all patients. CMR done in three of these patients showed typical features of amyloidosis including subendocardial LGE and absence of nulling. All the patients in this study were being treated for other noncardiac ailments. Lack of suspicion in all these patients led to an avoidable delay in appropriate treatment. During the short follow-up of 6 months, two patients died **(Table 1)**.

DIAGNOSIS OF CA

First and foremost, diagnosis of CA requires a high index of suspicion because it can be easily missed due to perceived rarity of disease, wide variety of symptoms or being mistaken for other common disease such as hypertrophic cardiomyopathy or isolated aortic stenosis. Specific laboratory and imaging tests are required and may not be ordered without an appropriate index of suspicion **(Fig. 1)**.[12]

Electrocardiogram

Usual features on electrocardiogram (ECG) are low voltage QRS complexes in limb leads and inferior or anterior pseudoinfarct pattern. Disproportionate low voltage on ECG and LVH on Echo is quite specific for this disease. LVH and LBBB pattern can be seen in minority of ATTR patients. Prevalence of AF increases with age. Ventricular arrhythmias and various degrees of AV block and can be found **(Fig. 2)**.[12]

Echocardiography

Conventional ECHO has limited sensitivity and specificity for CA but serves as a useful and economical noninvasive screening tool. The most common findings include ventricular hypertrophy, IAS thickening, diastolic dysfunction, and biatrial enlargement.[14] GLS is significantly reduced in CA, and reliably picks up abnormalities of systolic function even when ejection fraction is normal.[15] Relative apical sparing (cherry on top) is another specific parameter for CA. A study demonstrated a sensitivity of 93% and specificity of 82% in a small cohort with ventricular hypertrophy.[16] The sensitivity values for EF/GLS ratio (a cut off value of 4.95) and SA/SB ratio (a cut off 2.10) are 93% and 80%, respectively **(Fig. 3)**.[17]

Cardiac Magnetic Resonance Imaging

Cardiac magnetic resonance (CMR) features suggestive CA are global subendocardial LGE, myocardial nulling before

TABLE 1: Summary of Indian studies of CA (excluding case reports).

Study	Seth et al.[8]	Jain et al.[9]	Mohan et al.[7]	Raut et al.[10]	Vivek et al.[11]
Year	2021	2023	2022	2019	2023
Duration	1987–2019	2015–2022	2018–2022	2008–2015	2021–2023
n	40	31	13	6	6
Differentiation into AL and ATTR amyloidosis	No	Yes	No	No	Yes
Median age	51	64.5	65	51	65
Common presenting symptoms	• HF symptoms (100%) • Periorbital ecchymosis (7.5%) • Macroglossia (10%)	• HFpEF (42%) • HFrEF (25%) • Arrhythmia (48.4%) • GI symptoms (29%) • Peripheral neuropathy (6.5%) • Macroglossia (2.5%)	• Symptomatic HF (69%) • Nephrotic syndrome (15.3%) • Gastrointestinal (7.6%)	• Heart failure • Atrial arrhythmia (33%)	• Heart failure • Syncope • Macroglossia (in two patients)
NYHA class	• NYHA II—42.8% • NYHA III—19%	–	–	–	NYHA II (83.3%)
ECG	• Low voltage complexes (66.6%) • Poor R wave progression (9.5%) • LBBB (4.7%)	• Low voltage (16.1%) • Pseudo infarct pattern (16.1%) • AF (32.3%) • LBBB (16.1%)	–	–	Low voltage complex Poor R wave progression (100%)
Echo	• Isolated LVH (55%) • Isolated RVH (10%) • BVH (35%) • Biatrial enlargement (10%) • GLS (not known)	• Isolated LVH (48.3%) • Isolated RVH (12.9%) • BVH (29%) • Reduced GLS with apical sparing (87.5%)	• Mean LVEF 45% • Mean GLS –9.48%	• LVH Biatrial enlargement • Speckled IVS (66%) • Thickened IAS (16%)	• LVH (100%) • Speckled myocardial appearance (66.6%) • Reduced GLS with apical sparing (100%) • Biatrial enlargement (100%)
Bone Scintigraphy	–	• Available for 22% • Grade II uptake (31.8%) with ATTR • Grade III uptake (36.6%) with ATTR	–	–	–
Cardiac MRI	–	• Available for 13 patients showing concentric LVH • Subendocardial LGE in LV, RV in 38.4%	Available for 4 patients showing LVH and LGE	LGE	• Available in three patients • Sub-endocardial LGE (100%)
Survival data	Median OS 25 months (Range, 5–49)	NA	30% patients dead within 6 months, overall 46% mortality, median OS 15 months	Only one patient alive at 1 year	Two patients died within 6 months

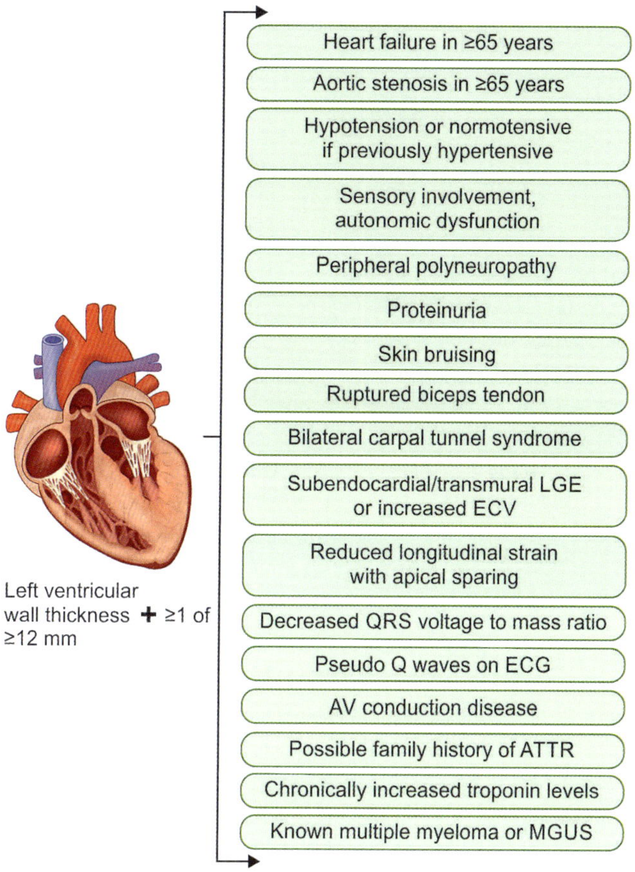

FIG. 1: Screening for cardiac amyloidosis.[13]

blood, increased extracellular volume > 40% along with LVH, biatrial enlargement, and thickened IAS.[18] This has a very high sensitivity for detecting CA and ruling out its mimickers.

Tc99 Scintigraphy

Technetium-labeled pyrophosphates (Tc99-PYP) localizes to TTR fibrils, giving a highly specific method of diagnosing TTR-CA on imaging. Myocardial uptake is graded from zero to three based on relative uptake in the ribs **(Fig. 4)**. Diagnostic

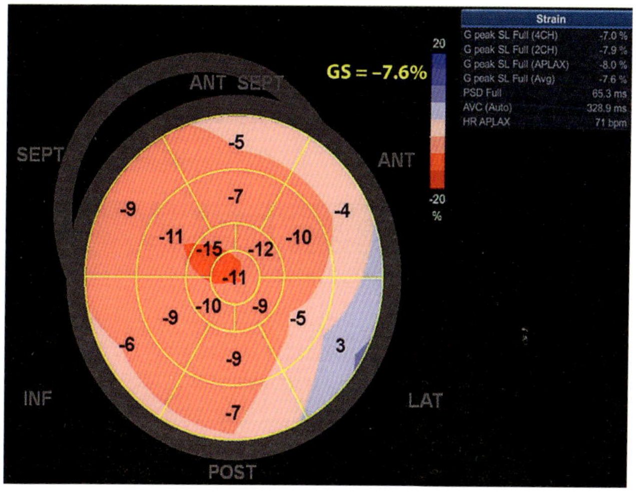

FIG. 3: Speckle tracking derived longitudinal strain from three apical views shows typical bulls eye pattern with sparing of apical segments.

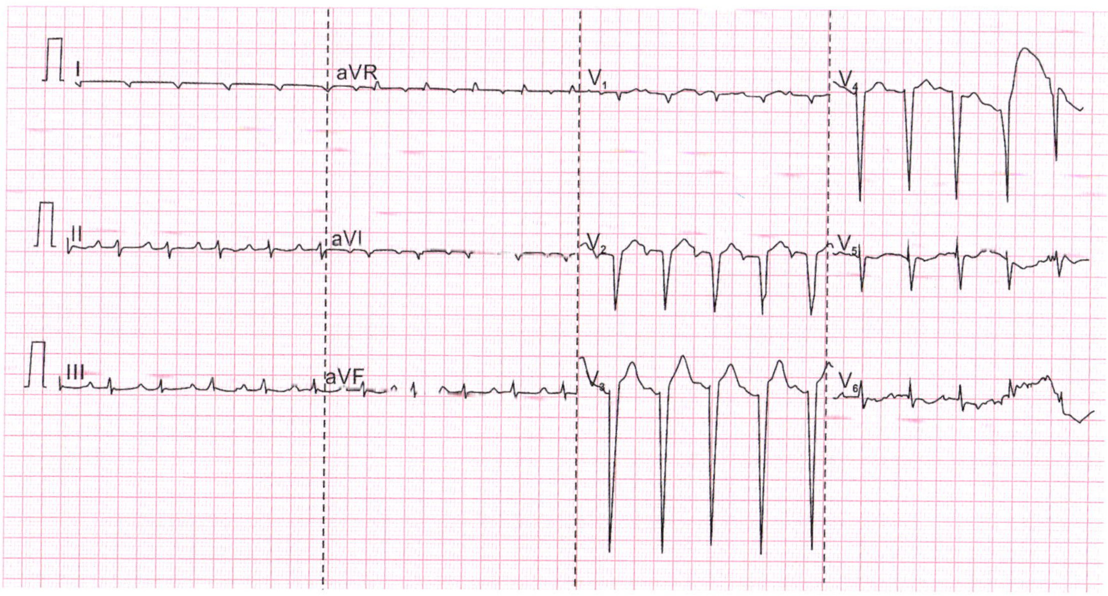

FIG. 2: Electrocardiogram of patient showing sinus rhythm with pseudoinfarction pattern in chest leads.

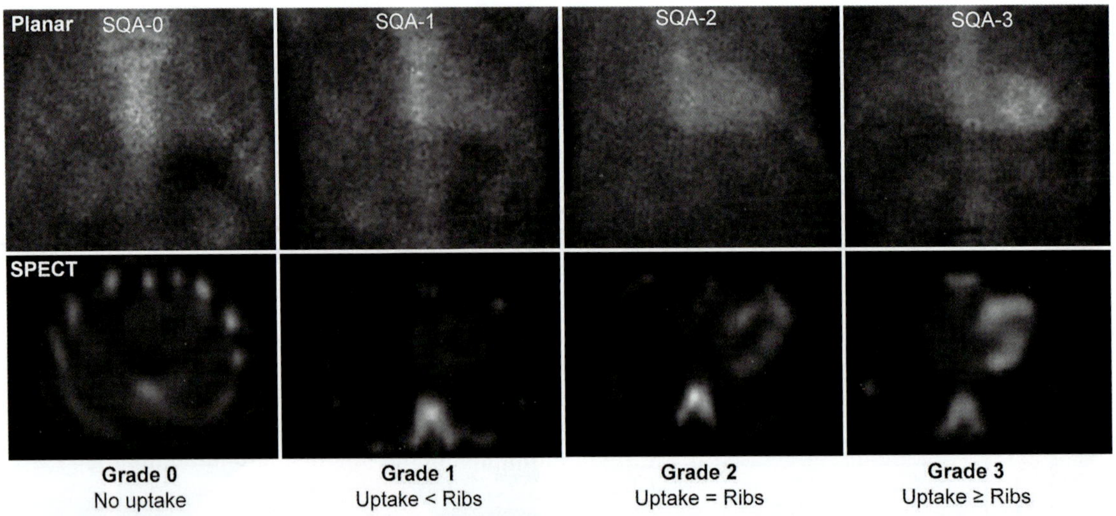

Grade	Myocardial Tc-99m PYP uptake
Grade 0	No uptake and normal bone uptake
Grade 1	Uptake less than rib uptake
Grade 2	Uptake equal to rib uptake
Grade 3	Uptake greater than rib uptake with mild/absent rib uptake

FIG. 4: PYP scan reporting.

performance of Tc99 scans depends on grade of uptake, with increasing positive predictive value (88–100%) from grades 1 to 3.[19] Up to 20–30% of patients with AL amyloidosis may have false positive Tc99 scans, and the positive predictive value and specificity of Tc99 scanning reach almost 100% once AL amyloidosis is excluded by testing for paraprotein.[20]

HISTOPATHOLOGICAL DIAGNOSIS

Histopathology is required for confirmation of diagnosis especially for AL-CA and performing subtyping. EMB is considered the gold standard, offering 100% specificity for CA. With improvements in imaging techniques, the indications for EMB are reducing, but it is still recommended when a Tc99 scan is nondiagnostic or unavailable, or biopsy from noncardiac tissue is noncontributory.[15] Abdominal fat pad biopsy is simple and inexpensive but is associated with high rates of false negatives. It has a sensitivity of approximately 70% for AL amyloid but <20% for wtTTR. Congo red staining is used for demonstration of amyloid protein and under polarized microscope amyloid protein shows apple green birefringence **(Fig. 5)**.[21]

TREATMENT

The treatment of CA revolves around two main principles—(1) the management of symptoms associated with cardiac failure and (2) the implementation of disease-modifying therapy.

Treatment of Heart Failure

The CA patients have a narrow therapeutic window in regard to the optimal diuretic dose because of small, stiff ventricles with reduced cardiac output. Loop diuretics remain the cornerstone of treatment in CA patients symptomatic with heart failure. Mineralocorticoid receptor antagonist has shown to provide symptomatic relief. Guideline-directed medical therapy often does not apply to CA as it is largely excluded from randomized controlled trials. RAAS blockers and beta-blockers are poorly tolerated.[12] Beta-blockers may be used with caution in patients with an EF < 40%.

Atrial fibrillation is common during the course of the disease. Amiodarone is usually the antiarrhythmic of choice. Anticoagulation is advocated irrespective of CHA_2DS_2VASc score due to heightened risk of thromboembolic

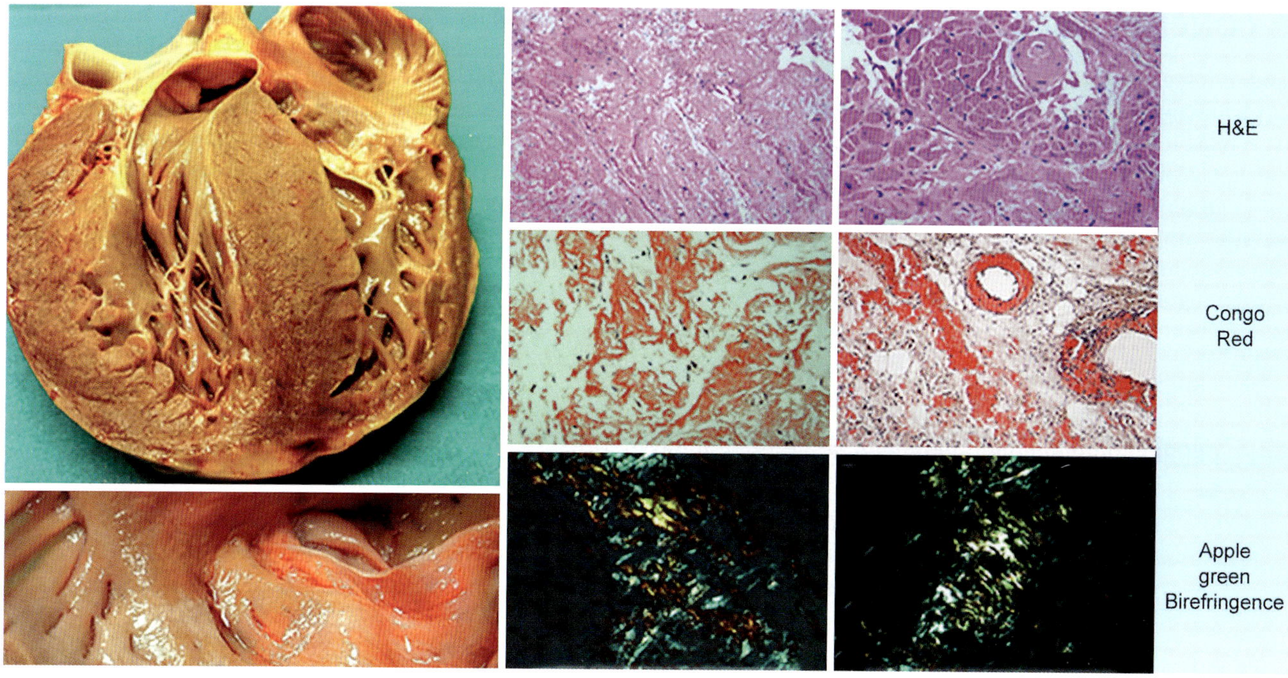

FIG. 5: Histopathology of CA.

complications. There are no trials suggesting preference of NOACs or VKA.[22]

Disease-specific Therapy

AL Amyloidosis

For AL-CA, the primary objective is to suppress the plasma cell clone, thereby impeding the ongoing synthesis of light chains, and is measured by a reduction in FLC levels and absolute value of involved light chain (iFLC). The use of bortezomib-based triplet combinations (cyclophosphamide/bortezomib/dexamethasone) has shown good response addition of daratumumab (monoclonal anti-CD38 antibody) to the above regimen augments overall hematologic response. Cardiac response, defined as a 30% reduction in NT-proBNP, was noted in 53% of patients.[23] Despite the efficacy, current costs of daratumumab-based combinations in India cannot be afforded by most in a country like India.

ATTR Amyloidosis

Transthyretin Expression Silencer

Expression of TTR can be reduced by silencing synthesis of TTR protein. Inotersen is an antisense oligonucleotide which blocks target mRNA and inhibits production of TTR. Its dosage is 300 mg subcutaneously once in a week. It stabilizes cardiac symptoms in ATTRv amyloidosis. It also improves neurological symptoms. Main side effects are thrombocytopenia and glomerulonephritis.[24]

Patisiran is a siRNA drug which inhibits RNA encoding for TTR. In APOLLO study on 225 patients with familial ATTR with polyneuropathy and NYHA Class I–II, patisiran (0.3 mg/kg every 3 weeks) was found to be superior. Furthermore, in a predefined group of 126 patients with CA, patisiran reduced left ventricular wall thickness, GLS, and NT-proBNP values. A posthoc analysis showed a 46% reduction in hospitalization and all-cause mortality in patients randomized to patisiran compared with those on placebo.[25]

Transthyretin Stabilizer Drugs

These drugs stabilize the tetrameric TTR protein complex, thereby preventing its dissociation into amyloidogenic TTR monomers and oligomers.

Tafamidis is an oral drug that acts by binding with high affinity and selectivity to thyroxine sites on both wild-type and variant TTR preventing dissociation. In the ATTR-ACT trial, 441 subjects affected by cardiac TTR amyloidosis (wild-type and familial) were randomized to 80 or 20 mg of tafamidis or placebo for 30 months. The trial showed that treatment with tafamidis, especially at a dose of 80 mg/day, compared with placebo, was associated with stabilization of TTR in almost all patients, with a significant reduction in all-cause mortality and reduction in hospitalizations for cardiovascular causes.[26] This is the only drug for wild-type ATTR which has been approved by US FDA till date. Acoramidis is another such stabilizer which has proved to be beneficial in a large RCT (ATTRibute-CM). However, extremely high costs are prohibitory for most patients even in developed nations.

CONCLUSION

Epidemiological data about CA is scarce in India. Lack of suspicion and subsequent failure to recognize the red flags of CA plays a big role in the unfortunate delay in its diagnosis and management, especially in a developing nation like India. The combined total of published clinical data on CA in India includes around 100 patients, a significant epidemiologic, diagnostic, and prognostic lacuna is evident. Exact prevalence and demography cannot be determined. However, CA is not as uncommon as it was perceived earlier. Timely diagnosis of this otherwise progressively deteriorating disease will go a long way in reducing the associated morbidity and mortality. Early initiation of novice treatment options holds an exciting promise of favorably modifying this otherwise lethal condition. Low index of suspicion leads to delayed diagnosis and poor outcomes particularly in low resource setting with survival of <1 year after the onset of symptoms. Use of novel parameters on strain Echo can effectively identify candidates for further confirmatory testing. Effective disease-modifying therapy are now available and improve survival if instituted early. Survival is further expected to improve with lowering costs of therapy for myeloma and possible availability of TTR stabilizing therapy in India in the near future.

ONLINE REFERENCES

Please scan the QR code provided at the end of the table of contents for References of this chapter.

CHAPTER

82

Heart Transplant: Pre- and Postmanagement

Devesh Kumar, Sandeep Seth

ABSTRACT

Cardiac transplant is currently the cornerstone in the management of advanced heart failure. Limited donors, high cost, high incidence of rejection, and post-transplant complications form major obstacles in widespread adaptation of cardiac transplant. However, over the last decade there has been relaxation of donor selection criteria to expand the donor pool, decrement in the financial burden, newer strategies to decrease rejection rates, and more advanced peri- and postoperative care which has led to an increase in the transplants worldwide and a 12-year median survival posttransplant. In this review, we discuss the contemporary practices of pretransplant and posttransplant care and the posttransplant complications.

Keywords: Advanced heart failure, cardiac transplant, donor selection, rejection, coronary artery vasculopathy, primary graft dysfunction

INTRODUCTION

Heart failure is a modern day epidemic which affects 1–2% of the total population.[1] With advances in medical therapy and the implementation of the four pillars of guideline-directed medical therapy, there has been a dramatic 75% relative reduction in mortality.[2] However, advanced heart failure has emerged as a raging problem with very high cost of recurrent hospitalizations, a 1-year survival with medical therapy of only 40% and limited therapeutic options.[3] The true worldwide prevalence of advanced heart failure continues to be an enigma, however, studies have estimated it to be 1–10% of all heart failure patients and the numbers have continued to rise in the last two decades.[4] The gold standard treatment strategy for advanced heart failure is cardiac transplant. However, heart transplant is plagued with the perennial problems of a limited donor pool, limited transplant centers, high cost, and posttransplant complications.[3] In this chapter, we briefly review the indications, and aim to discuss the pretransplant and posttransplant management of heart transplant patients.

INDICATIONS

The most common patient subgroups needing cardiac transplant are patients with advanced heart failure, patients with refractory cardiogenic shock supported on IV vasopressors or mechanical assist devices, end-stage heart failure due to congenital heart disease, patients with refractory angina without any remaining therapeutic options, and patients with recurrent life-threatening ventricular arrythmias despite all therapy.[5]

SURGICAL CONSIDERATIONS

The two most common surgical approaches for the implantation of the heart are biatrial and bicaval approaches. The bicaval approach is the more commonly accepted approach worldwide and involves five anastomosis—(1) left atrium, (2) pulmonary artery, (3) aorta, (4) inferior vena cava, and (5) superior vena cava. The bicaval approach decreases the need of permanent pacemaker implantation. It was introduced with the intent to reduce right atrial size, minimize distortion of the recipient heart, preserve atrial conduction pathways, and decrease tricuspid regurgitation.[6,7]

DONOR SELECTION

Cardiac transplant is plagued by the perennial shortage of suitable donor hearts. The short preservation time tolerated by the heart (ischemia time of 4–5 hours), further worsens the problem as the procurement distances are limited, thus limiting donor availability. Potential heart donors must meet brain death criteria and be free of any cardiac pathology. It is imperative to obtain a complete medical history from the donor, including any relevant cardiovascular disorders before brain death. All donors are screened for communicable disorders such as hepatitis and HIV infection. Donors must be screened for presence or absence of thoracic trauma, disseminated cancer, donor hemodynamic instability, pressor and inotropic requirements, duration of cardiac arrest, and need for cardiac pulmonary resuscitation. 2D transthoracic echocardiography is required for all donors and angiography is needed for donors older than 50 years of age, depending on other risk factors. The final decision, however, to accept a heart for transplantation is made at the time of harvesting, after direct examination of the heart for coronary calcification, LV hypertrophy, or dilation.[8]

In recent times, steps have been taken to overcome the obstacle of limited donor supply by allowing more donors to donate after circulatory death, by removing geographic constraints with the use of ex vivo perfusion platforms and finally by allowing more equitable donation using the revised heart transplantation allocation policy. The ex vivo heart perfusion platform maintains the donor heart in a warm, beating state for transplantation. In donation after circulatory death (DCD), retrieval of organs for the purpose of transplantation occurs from patients (those with severe and irreparable brain injury but who do not meet brain death criteria) whose death is declared and confirmed using cardiorespiratory criteria as life support is withdrawn. Asystole must be confirmed for at least 5 minutes for declaration of death. The heart is then removed and resuscitated through the use of ex vivo heart perfusion as described above. A major challenge with DCD heart donation is the assessment of myocardial viability as the heart is exposed to an unavoidable period of severe, warm ischemia. The challenge for transplant using DCD donors is the minimization of ischemic injury of the donor organs **(Flowchart 1)**.[9]

However, recently ISHLT guidelines for heart transplant have been relaxed deliberately to increase the donor pool **(Table 1)**.

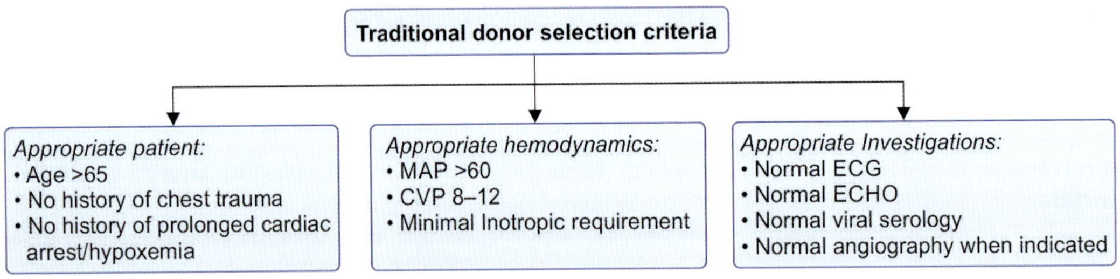

FLOWCHART 1: The traditional donor selection criteria.[10]

TABLE 1: The latest recommendations for donor selection in special circumstances.

Donor quality	Special comments
Donor age	• Age < 45 years: Have sufficient reserves to withstand the rigors of heart transplant (HT) even in settings of prolonged ischemic time, recipient comorbidities, and multiple previous recipient operations with hemodynamically destabilizing bleeding • Age 45–55 years: Use when the ischemic time is 4 hours and recipient does not have comorbidities or surgical issues • Age > 55 years: Only used if the survival benefit of HT for a recipient unequivocally exceeds the decrement in early survival due to transplantation of a heart with limited myocardial reserves
Donor infections	• Donors with risk factors for acute HIV, hepatitis B, and hepatitis C infection are safe for transplantation, recipients should be monitored and treated in according to guidelines • Donors with known bacteremia can be used if donor has received 24–48 hours targeted antimicrobial therapy, left ventricular function is normal and there is no evidence of endocarditis upon direct inspection of the donor heart • Donors with bacterial meningitis may be used provided the donor has received 24–48 hours of targeted antimicrobial therapy and the recipient receives an appropriate course of targeted therapy following transplantation • Hearts from donors with positive hepatitis C viremia may be used provided the recipient is monitored and treated in accordance with established guidance
Drug use	• Donors with history of alcohol abuse, active or past use of cocaine, and drug over-dose can be considered • Use of hearts from donors who have died of carbon monoxide intoxication can be recommended with caution

Continued

Continued

Donor quality	Special comments
Donor heart function	• A donor heart should not be used in the presence of intractable ventricular arrhythmias, the need for excessive inotropic support (dopamine at a dose of 20 mg/kg/min or similar doses of other adrenergic agents despite aggressive optimization of preload and afterload), discreet wall motion abnormalities or LVEF < 40% • Higher risk donor hearts with obstructive disease in any major coronary artery should be avoided unless the heart is being considered for coronary bypass surgery for a recipient who is marginal, older or at risk of death • Donor organs with LV septal or posterior wall thickness >13 mm should be used with caution, especially in conjunction with other high-risk characteristics such as age 55 years and an allograft ischemic time > 4 hours
Ischemia time	• The ischemic time should be <4 hours. However, donor hearts with ischemic times longer than 4 hours may be utilized when other risk-compounding factors are ideal including: favorable age and size matching; normal cardiac function; and absence of significant inotropic and vasopressor support • Donation after circulatory death (DCD) is reasonable at centers with: experience using marginal donor hearts, familiarity with the use of ex situ organ perfusion devices for preservation and transportation, and experience instituting perioperative mechanical support and its after-care for possible primary graft dysfunction

PRETRANSPLANT WORK-UP

The benchmark for the consideration of cardiac transplantation is marked reduction in functional capacity despite maximum implementation of conventional therapies. Functional capacity is best demonstrated by measuring exercise capacity using cardiopulmonary exercise testing or a 6-minute walk test. A peak oxygen consumption of <10 mL/kg/min is a marker of very poor functional capacity and is considered an indication of cardiac transplant. Similarly, a 6-minute walk distance of <300 m is considered an indication of markedly decreased functional capacity. All these patients with advanced heart failure and severe functional impairment have to be seen for any absolute contraindication for cardiac transplant and if absent should be listed for transplant and worked up with investigations for transplant **(Flowcharts 2 and 3)**.[11]

POSTOPERATIVE CARE

Like any cardiac surgery, a posttransplant patient requires utmost care and diligence for optimizing prognosis. Several issues such as cardiac denervation, allograft dysfunction, management of arrhythmias, rejection, immunosuppression, and infectious complications are very specific to the transplant patient.

Immediate Postoperative Care

Once hemodynamic and physiologic conditions are adequate, the patient is separated from cardiopulmonary bypass, temporary pacing wires are placed, hemostasis is achieved, the chest is closed, and preparations for transportation to the ICU commence.

On admission to ICU, patients generally require inotropic support, patients with elevated pulmonary vascular resistance require beta-agonists (e.g., dobutamine, low-dose epinephrine and phosphodiesterase inhibitors (milrinone) to increase right ventricular function without increasing pulmonary vascular resistance. Patients generally require inotropes till 3–5 days posttransplant and should be weaned off from day 3. It is advised that perioperative monitoring of heart transplant recipients include continuous ECG monitoring; postoperative12-lead ECG; invasive arterial pressure monitoring; direct measurement of right atrial pressure or central venous pressure; measurement of left atrial or pulmonary artery wedge pressure; intermittent measurement of cardiac output (CO); intermittent measurement of systemic vascular resistance; continuous measurement of arterial oxygen saturation; intermittent measurement of mixed venous saturation; intraoperative transesophageal echocardiogram (TEE); and continuous assessment of urinary output **(Table 2)**.[12]

POSTOPERATIVE PHARMACOTHERAPY[12-15]

Postoperative medications are given for three major purposes to prevent any surgical site infection by administering broad antibiotic coverage (day 0), immunosuppression (day 1) to prevent graft rejection and oral antibiotic prophylaxis (day1) to prevent opportunistic infections.

Intravenous (IV) antibiotics are given starting from day 0 of the transplant to offer patients a wide spectrum coverage against both typical and atypical bacterial infections. Most patients receive a third-generation cephalosporin (Gram-ve) along with teicoplanin (gram + coverage) and levofloxacin to cover for atypical organisms. Patients are also administered 500 mg methylprednisolone for three doses over 24 hours just after coming off bypass and followed by switch to oral prednisolone.

From day 1 of surgery, the patient is administered triple immunosuppression comprising steroids, calcineurin

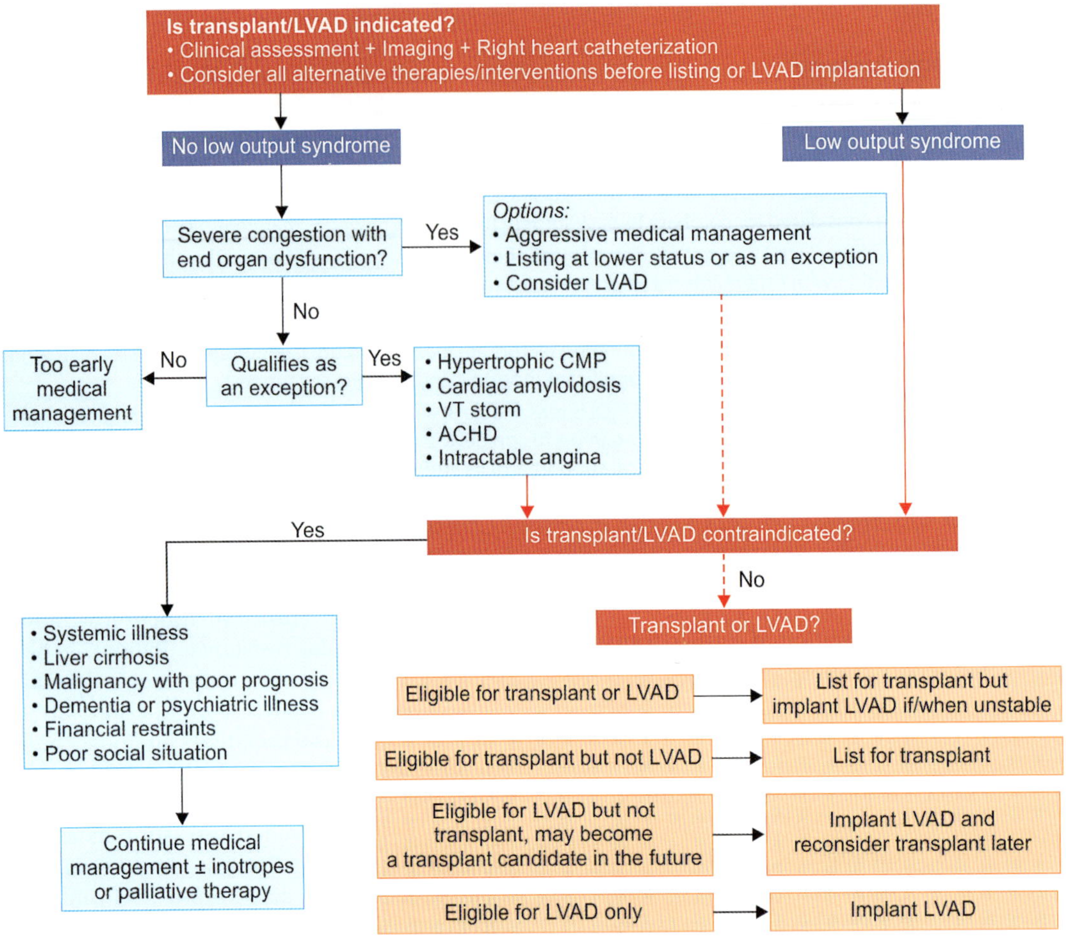

FLOWCHART 2: Algorithm for management of patients with advanced heart failure.

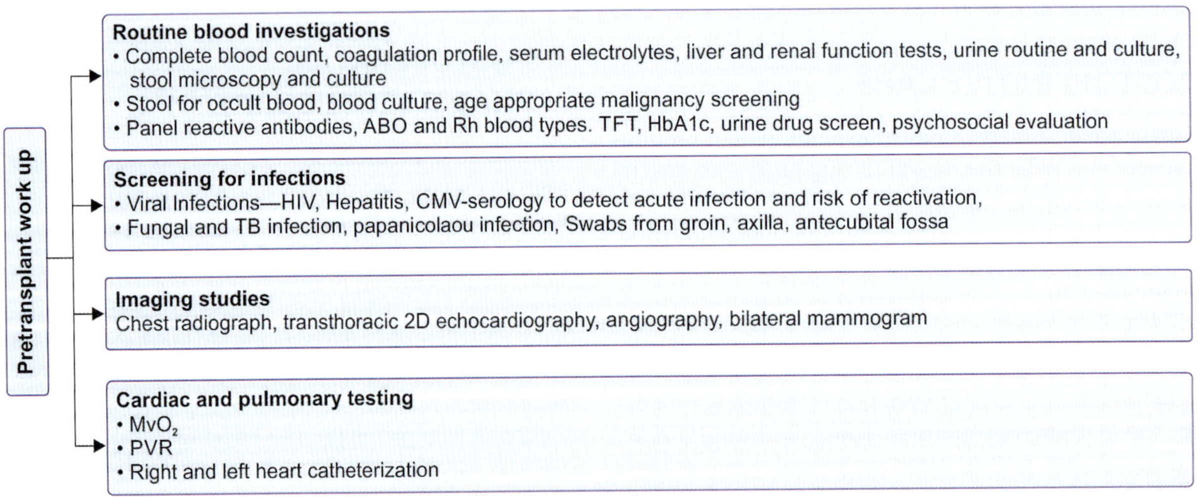

FLOWCHART 3: Showing the essential pretransplant work up for heart transplant candidates.

TABLE 2: Demonstrating the important monitoring parameters in the first week after transplant.

Day 0	Day 1	Day 2	Day 3–6
Hemodynamic stabilization: • MAP: > 90 mm Hg • RAP: 810 mm Hg	Echocardiography and Ultrasonography	Monitor for bleeding	Watch for bleeding
Antibiotic prophylaxis: • Ceftazidime 1 g IV TDS • Teicoplanin 400 mg IV OD • Levofloxacin 500 mg IV OD	Hemodynamic monitoring—continue inotropes	USG lung and echocardiography	Chest X-ray
Analgesia and ulcer prophylaxis: • Antacid: Injection pantoprazole 40 mg IV OD • Analgesic: Injection paracetamol 1 g IV QID and Injection tramadol 50 mg IV OD	*Immunosuppression*: Tablet cyclosporine, tablet mycophenolate mofetil	Weaning of inotropes	USG lung and echocardiography
• *Monitoring*: Observe chest tube drainage for first 4 hours, chest X-ray 8 hourly • Start weaning from ventilator	*Antibiotic prophylaxis*: • Tablet valganciclovir 450 mg OD • Tablet septran DS 1 tablet OD • Tablet voriconazole 200 mg PO OD	Chest X-ray—12 hourly	*Investigations*: HMG, RFT
	Chest X-ray—8 hourly	*Sepsis screening*: • Cultures: Blood, ET, urine, skin swab and drain fluid	*Sepsis screening*: • Cultures: Blood, ET, urine skin swab, and drain fluid
	Investigations: CBC, RFT, LFT, PT/INR	Surgical wound inspection and dressing	Surgical wound inspection and dressing
	Sepsis screening: Blood, ET aspirate, urine, skin swab, and drain fluid wound inspection	Incentive spirometry and chest physiotherapy	Incentive spirometry and chest physiotherapy

inhibitor (cyclosporine or tacrolimus) and an antimetabolite (azathioprine or mycophenolate mofetil). The triple combination regime is the norm for all patients and is continued for a prolonged duration of time, thus chronic side effects of these drugs are important for clinicians as most patients report side effects due to use of these drugs. Amongst the calcineurin inhibitors, tacrolimus has lesser metabolic side effects and is thus preferred to cyclosporine. Tacrolimus has more of dysglycemia and neurological side effects than cyclosporine but lesser incidence of accelerated hypertension, renal failure, gum hyperplasia, and hypertrichosis. This makes tacrolimus a more favored cyclophilin inhibitor than tacrolimus. Amongst the antimetabolite, mycophenolate mofetil is preferred due to its better tolerability than azathioprine.

The third arm of pharmacotherapy that is very relevant clinically are drugs to prevent opportunistic infections in a transplant patient with a compromised immune system. All patients routinely get valganciclovir, voriconazole, and septran to prevent them from opportunistic fungal and viral infections.

POSTTRANSPLANT COMPLICATIONS

Cardiac transplant is a procedure that warrants diligent post operative care to tide over postoperative complications. However, frequently it is plagued with both acute and chronic complications.

Tricuspid Regurgitation

Incidence of tricuspid regurgitation posttransplant is estimated to be at 19–84% in postcardiac transplant patients. Intraoperative and postoperative monitoring is required in patients with regurgitation posttransplant. Most patients with moderate to severe disease are asymptomatic and in symptomatic patients most do well with IV diuretics.[16] However rarely some patients with torrential TR leading to symptomatic right heart failure may warrant surgical repair with De Vega annuloplasty.[17]

Right Ventricular Dysfunction

Right ventricular dysfunction accounts for 50% of all complications and 20% of all deaths following cardiac transplant.[18] Many plausible mechanisms have been described like ischemia—reperfusion injury, mechanical trauma during harvest, air embolism in the right coronary artery, and less preservation of the right ventricle as compared to left ventricle and high PVR pretransplant.[19] Right ventricular dysfunction is generally managed conservative with IV diuretics and IV inotropes in the posttransplant patients and recovery of RV function is associated with better prognosis.[20]

Arrythmias

Posttransplant sinus node dysfunction is common with a prevalence of up to 44%. Sympathetic denervation, biatrial technique, ischemic injury to the sinus node, graft ischemia, and drug effects are the major mechanisms. In most patients the dysfunction recovers with time and only 10–15% require pacemaker implantation.[21]

Primary Graft Dysfunction

In an international survey of 47 centers treating almost 10,000 patients, a primary graft dysfunction rate of 7.4% was established with a 30 day mortality of 30%. The donor heart is subject to a series of insults during the transplantation process, including brain death and its sequelae in the donor, hypothermic ischemia during transport, warm ischemia during implantation, and reperfusion injury after release of the aortic cross-clamp in the recipient.[22] Additionally, systemic factors in the recipient may create a hostile milieu that further compromises donor heart function after reperfusion. There are no biomarkers for PGD, and treatment is supportive. Many of the risk factors for PGD are not modifiable, such as age, diabetes, and need for inotropic support. However, the length of cold ischemia time could be improved with an ex vivo heart perfusion platform and this perhaps is one of the most modifiable factors that could protect from primary graft dysfunction **(Flowchart 4)**.[23]

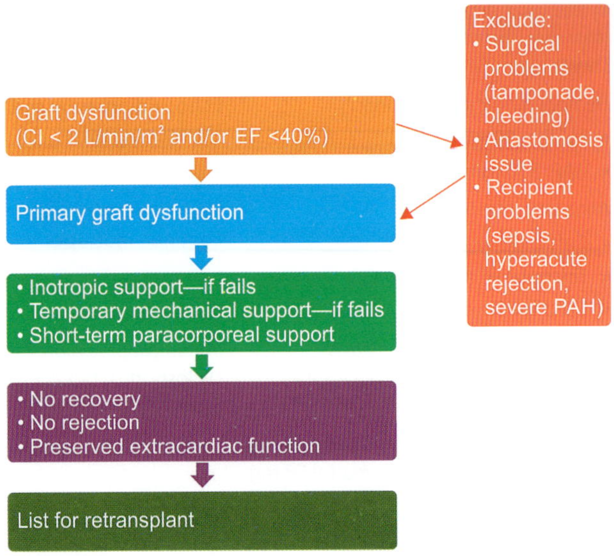

FLOWCHART 4: A schematic representation of patients with primary graft dysfunction.

Cardiometabolic Problems

Hypertension is seen in the vast majority (90%) of transplant patients at 5 years after transplant. This is predominantly due to the use of cyclosporin/tacrolimus and the associated renal insufficiency. Most patients generally require multiple drugs as the hypertension is difficult to control with a single antihypertensive drug.[24] New-onset diabetes is found in up to 30% of patients by 5 years posttransplantation and is caused by the compounding effect of both corticosteroids and CNIs. Risk factors for new-onset diabetes besides the conventional risk factors involve African American race and use of high-dose steroids, tacrolimus in particular.[25] Total cholesterol, LDL cholesterol, and triglycerides increase after 3 months and then generally fall after the first year. Lipid-lowering therapy with any statin was strongly associated with a marked improvement in 1-year survival in the heart transplant lipid registry.[26] The incidence of renal failure after heart transplant is 10–15% by 5 years. Acute kidney injury complicates the early postoperative course in as many as 40–70% of patients. Cyclosporine use, new onset of diabetes and hypertension, and recurrent urinary infections all have a complimentary role in causing renal insufficiency.[27]

Malignant Neoplasia

Malignancies are commonly seen in patients postcardiac transplant on triple immunosuppression. Skin and lung and posttransplant lymphoproliferative disorders cancers are most common.[28]

Coronary Allograft Vasculopathy

It is the most common reason for late graft failure of cardiac transplant patients. It occurs at a rate of 5–10% per year posttransplant and is seen in 40–50% of patients at 5 years follow-up after transplant. Coronary allograft vasculopathy (CAV) occurring early after transplant is a form of chronic graft rejection with severe concentric myointimal hyperplasia and cellular infiltration, diffuse disease, and distal pruning.[29] It is seen more frequently in patients with more number of rejections, longer duration of rejections, CMV positive donors, and patients having typical risk factors for CAD (diabetics, hypertensives, and smoker). Angiography and computed tomography coronary angiography (CTCA) fail to diagnose CAV, as the remodeling is concentric and is diffuse and is seen first in more distal vessels. Therefore, IVUS is the gold standard investigation for most patients as it has the ability to pick up disease much earlier. An increment of intimal thickness of >0.5 mm on serial IVUS scans is diagnostic of CAV. CAV can be managed with percutaneous coronary intervention (PCI) with drug-eluting stents (DES) and in cases with diffuse disease involving multiple vessels can be managed with coronary artery bypass grafting (CABG).[30]

The last resort for management of CAV once severely symptomatic with systolic dysfunction is retransplant and hence in the light of the limited donor pool, prevention of CAV is of paramount significance.[31] Many studies have showed that statins, vitamin C, vitamin E, and everolimus offer some protection from CAV.[32]

Infections

With more potent immunosuppression the incidence of rejection has decreased but opportunistic infections remain an important risk. Posttransplant infections are common given the immunosuppressed state of transplant patients and are the most common cause of death (20%) in the first year after cardiac transplant.[33] The most common infections are caused by bacteria and virus. Bacterial infections are most common at surgical sites as well as urinary and chest infections. Among the viral infection CMV is the most common and the risk is especially high when the recipient is negative and the donor is CMV positive.[34] Fungal infections are generally caused by *Candida* and *Aspergillus*. Mortality is highest for fungal infections followed by protozoa, bacterial, and viral infections. PCP, herpes, and oral candidiasis require prophylactic regimes to be used during the first 6–12 months after transplant. Prophylactic oral ganciclovir is given for variable periods in CMV seronegative recipients of a transplant from a CMV positive donor.[35]

Rejection

With the current immunosuppressive regimens the incidence of rejection has dramatically decreased. Rejection after transplant involves either cell or antibody-mediated cardiac injury resulting from recognition of the cardiac allograft as nonself **(Table 3)**. Rejection irrespective of its type can lead to graft failure and needs both pretransplant screening for possible risk factors and posttransplant immunosuppression for prevention of rejection.[36] Risk factors for rejection include black race, female donor, female recipient, young donors, CMV positive donors, HLA mismatch, and poor compliance with immunosuppressive drugs.[37]

While endomyocardial biopsy remains the gold standard for diagnosis of rejection posttransplant, newer modalities have come up in a big way. Peripheral blood gene expression (ALLOMAP) has come up in a big way which utilizes an 11-gene expression signature derived from peripheral blood mononuclear cells as a noninvasive test for acute cellular rejection. However this cannot be used to diagnose antibody mediated rejection.[38] Another innovative technique uses cardiac MRI T2 sequence and ECV expansion to diagnose rejection early.[39] Lastly, the cell-free DNA has emerged as a newer technique to noninvasively diagnose rejection. Cell-free donor derived DNA is present in urine and blood of most transplant recipients. This cell-free DNA in blood and urine released from donor graft can be quantitatively measured to detect both cellular and antibody rejection.[40]

Identification and quantification of anti-HLA antibodies are most commonly performed using solid-phase assays. Quantification is important because antibodies of greater intensity in vitro are considered potentially more cytotoxic in vivo. The presence of high levels of anti-HLA antibodies (usually above 3,000–5,000 median fluorescent intensity) is considered potentially cytotoxic.[41] The ability of donor-specific antibodies to fix complement is a better marker of their cytotoxic caliber. Activation of the classical complement pathway by antibodies begins with their binding of C1q, the first component of the pathway.[42] Once activated by C1q, the classic pathway leads to the formation of the membrane attack complex and ultimately results in cell lysis and death. Detection. Knowledge of anti-HLA antibodies prior to transplantation is important as one could avoid donors who have HLA corresponding to high-level anti-HLA antibodies in the potential recipient, as this would be a risk for hyperacute rejection.[43,44] With the virtual crossmatch, HLA corresponding to high-level anti-HLA antibodies in the transplantation candidate are listed as "avoids" in the United Network of Organ Sharing database, and thus, potential donors with such HLA are not considered.[45] The identity and intensity of anti-HLA antibodies is useful

TABLE 3: Types of rejection posttransplant.

Type of rejection	Time of presentation	Immune reaction	Clinical presentation
Hyperacute rejection	Within minutes to hours after circulation is established	Preexisting antibodies to antigens on the vascular endothelial cells of the donor	Rapid occlusion of the vascular graft with intravascular thrombosis
Acute cellular rejection	First week to several years after transplant (Mostly within first year of Surgery)	Helper T-cells and cytotoxic T cells	Graft dysfunction with cellular rejection on biopsy
Acute humoral rejection	Days to months after transplant	Antibodies against donor HLA or endothelial cell antigens	Graft dysfunction without cellular rejection on biopsy
Chronic rejection	Months to years after transplant	Progressive graft loss mediated through ischemia vasculopathy by occlusion of graft vasculature	Coronary allograft vasculopathy

not only in safely finding a donor organ for a sensitized recipient but also in deciding on which sensitized patients require desensitization.[46] Centers often use a threshold of the calculated PRA (cPRA) to decide on treatment of the sensitized patient. The cPRA is the frequency of unacceptable HLA in the donor population. Antibodies will impact the ability to find a suitable donor heart more than others.[47] If the cPRA is above 50–70%, therapies to reduce antibody levels prior to transplantation may be used if a HTx candidate had high-level antibodies relative to that of common HLA, the cPRA may be 90%, and thus, only 10% of all potential donors would be compatible. cPRA highlights the fact that some high-level anti-HLA antibodies will impact the ability to find a suitable donor heart more than others.[47] Management of the sensitized patient involves protocols to target antibodies by inactivation [IV injection of immunoglobulin (Ig)], removal (plasmapheresis), and decreased production rituximab[48] and bortezomib.[48,49] If the protocol of IVIg and rituximab is ineffective in reducing the cPRA below 50%, or if a patient requires rapid desensitization (i.e., they are listed as status 1A), then bortezomib, a proteasome inhibitor against plasma cells, may be used.[49] To increase effectiveness, bortezomib may be combined with plasmapheresis.[49]

CONCLUSION

As we continue to expand the boundaries of HTx to higher risk patients who are older and who require mechanical circulatory support and antibody sensitization, the goal must be to maintain superior outcomes with this scarce resource. Challenges remain in the management of HTx recipients, including the scarce supply and equitable distribution of donor hearts, prevention of primary graft dysfunction, diagnosis of rejection, and management of sensitization. The future holds promise to improve the posttransplant survival and morbidity of patients living with advanced heart failure.

ONLINE REFERENCES

Please scan the QR code provided at the end of the table of contents for References of this chapter.

SECTION 8

Cardio-Obstetrics

Section Outline

CHAPTER

83

Cardiovascular Diseases in Women: Challenges and Differences

Mohit M Bhagwati, Roopa Salwan

ABSTRACT

Cardiovascular disease (CVD) is a leading cause of mortality and morbidity in women, but historical perceptions have resulted in it being underrecognized and undertreated. This chapter explores the complexity of CVD in women, highlighting the biological, social, and cultural factors that contribute to disparities in its presentation and consequences compared to men. Menopause is emerging as a critical period of cardiometabolic transition, increasing the risk of various forms of coronary heart disease. The analysis identifies both traditional risk factors, such as hypertension and diabetes, and unique factors specific to women, including gestational hypertension and autoimmune diseases, that increase cardiovascular risk. The clinical spectrum of ischemic heart disease in women often manifests itself differently, which leads to problems in diagnosis and treatment. A paradigm shift is necessary to better understand and recognize CVD in women and support more aggressive prevention and intervention efforts.

Keywords: Cardiovascular disease, women, ischemic heart disease, coronary microvascular dysfunction, menopause, risk factors, spontaneous coronary artery dissection, myocardial infarction

INTRODUCTION

Cardiovascular disease (CVD) remains a leading cause of mortality and a significant cause of morbidity in women.[1] Historically, women were believed to be protected and at low risk of heart disease, and as a result, they were underdiagnosed and inadequately treated. Women were also underrepresented in the trials. This was called "Yentl syndrome." In the 1990s, this gap was recognized and over the past three decades, significant progress has been made in understanding the spectrum of heart disease in women. Biological differences between the sexes, influenced by genetic, epigenetic, and sex-hormone-mediated factors, are complex and not fully understood.[2] In addition, social and cultural (gender) factors contribute to differences in the prevalence, presentation, and natural history of CVD in women.[3]

Menopause represents an important cardiometabolic transition, increasing the risk of CVD in women, sometimes even in the fourth decade of life. Ischemic heart disease (IHD) in women encompasses a wide spectrum, including atherosclerotic obstructive coronary artery disease, coronary microvascular dysfunction (CMD), endothelial dysfunction, vasomotor abnormalities, spontaneous coronary artery dissection (SCAD), stress-related cardiomyopathy, and myocardial infarction with nonobstructive coronary artery disease (MINOCA).[4] Women with IHD show a higher prevalence of angina pectoris, a lower burden of obstructive coronary artery disease, and a worse prognosis compared to men.[5] Advances in the understanding of sex-specific presentations, recognition of conventional and novel risk factors, and pathophysiology of coronary heart disease have led to improved clinical outcomes in women.[6]

PATHOPHYSIOLOGY OF ISCHEMIC HEART DISEASE IN WOMEN

Women have smaller coronary arteries per 100 g of left ventricular mass and increased arterial stiffness. Plaque rupture, characterized by a disrupted thin-cap fibroatheroma and large necrotic cores with macrophages, is more common in men and older women, while plaque erosion is more common in younger women.[7] Plaque erosion is characterized by thrombus overlying smooth muscle cells in a proteoglycan/collagen-rich matrix, intimal

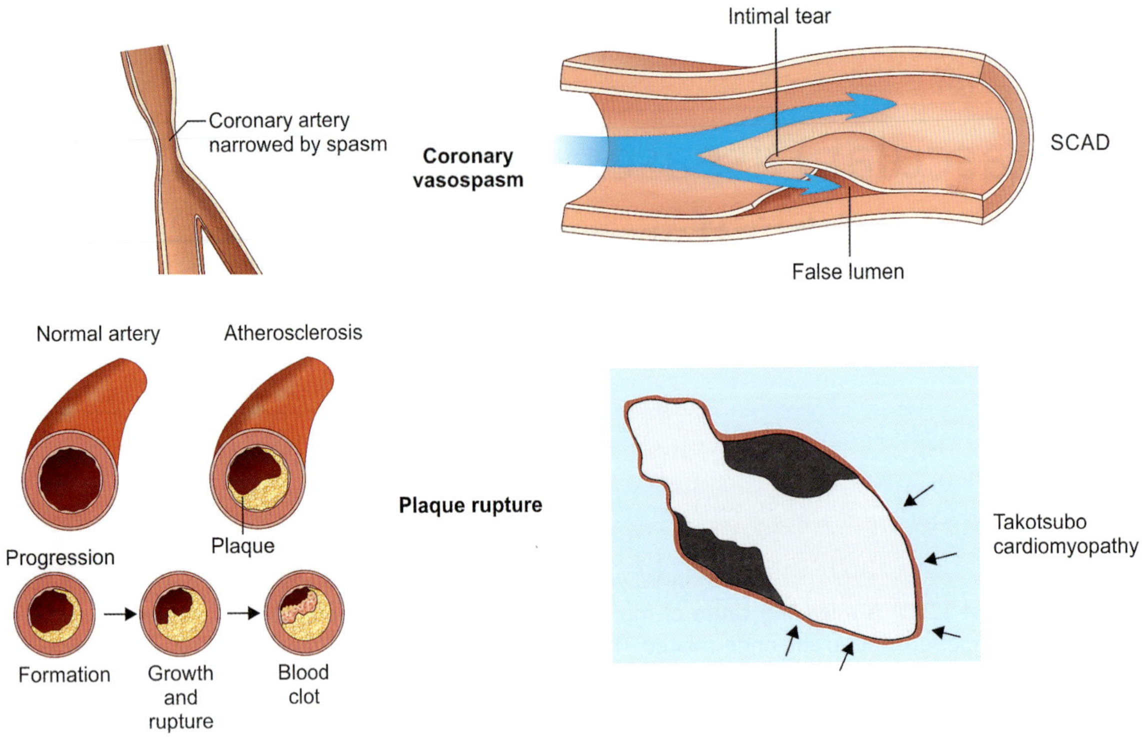

FIG. 1: Pathophysiology of ACS in women.

thickening and luminal endothelial apoptosis, and absence of inflammatory cells and lipid core. This leads to increased distal microembolization from platelet-rich debris **(Fig. 1)**.[8] A calcified nodule is a lesion with nodular calcification with disruption of the fibrous cap, overlying fibrin thrombus, and absence of endothelial cells. It is more common in elderly patients with underlying diabetes and/or chronic kidney disease.

Microvascular coronary dysfunction (MCD) and endothelial dysfunction are major contributors to heart disease in women. Intramural arterioles < 100 µm regulate coronary blood flow in response to metabolic demands, prearteriolar vessels of 100–150 µm respond to changes in pressure, and those of 150–500 µm respond to flow. An attenuated coronary dilation response to adenosine of <2.5-fold is a marker of MCD.[9] Endothelial cells regulate vasomotor activity by producing nitric oxide and endothelin and are central to platelet adhesion, leukocyte migration, and thrombosis. In the presence of left ventricular hypertrophy, structural abnormalities in the form of intimal and medial thickening causing luminal narrowing, perivascular fibrosis, and capillary rarefaction are seen.

Cardiovascular Risk Factors in Women

Classic CVD risk factors are similar in men and women, but there are differences in prevalence and unique factors between women. Hypertension, diabetes mellitus (DM), and smoking are stronger risk factors for myocardial infarction (MI) in women. Nontraditional risk factors that are unique to women include early menopause or menarche, gestational DM, hypertension, preeclampsia and eclampsia during pregnancy, and systemic inflammatory disorders.[10,11]

Traditional Risk Factors (Table 1)

Women have a higher prevalence of traditional risk factors, and often have suboptimal control leading to an increased cumulative risk.

Age

The prevalence of CVD increases with age, affecting one in eight women aged 45–64 years and one in three women over 65 years.[12]

Hypertension

After menopause, there is an increase in the prevalence of hypertension, especially isolated systolic hypertension reflecting aortic stiffness. Hypertensive women have a higher prevalence of atrial fibrillation, stroke, and heart failure (HF) with preserved ejection fraction. Hypertension increases twofold to threefold in women using oral contraceptives.[13]

Diabetes

The relative risk of CVD is 44% higher in women with DM than in similarly affected men. The risk of mortality is 3.5 times higher in diabetic women compared to nondiabetic women or men with diabetes. Diabetic women also have a higher risk of developing HF, stroke, and peripheral vascular disease compared to diabetic men.[12]

TABLE 1: Risk factors for cardiovascular disease in women.

Risk factor	Description
Age	Increased prevalence with age; significant risk after menopause
Hypertension	Higher prevalence and poorer control in older women
Diabetes	Higher relative risk and mortality in women compared to men
Smoking	Synergistic risk with oral contraceptive use
Dyslipidemia	Adverse changes in lipid profile postmenopause
Family history	Premature coronary event in first-degree relative is a significant risk factor
Physical inactivity	Strongly predicts all-cause mortality; more common in women
Metabolic syndrome	Higher prevalence and associated risk in women
Autoimmune disease	Accelerated CVD risk in conditions like RA and SLE
Gestational hypertension	Increases long-term CVD risk
Polycystic ovarian syndrome	Linked with increased risk of coronary atherosclerosis and adverse events
Breast cancer therapy	Increased risk of IHD postradiotherapy
Hysterectomy	Increased CVD risk, especially with oophorectomy
Psychosocial factors	Significant association with AMI and other CVD events

Smoking

Although women smoke less than men, it can be more harmful. The prevalence of smoking is increasing among younger women. The combination of smoking with the use of oral contraceptives significantly increases the risk of acute myocardial infarction (AMI), stroke, and venous thromboembolism.[13]

Dyslipidemia

Metabolic changes with menopause lead to an increase in LDL cholesterol and triglycerides, and a decrease in HDL with an increase in the risk of CVD. Dyslipidemia has the highest population-adjusted risk in women, at 47.1%, compared with all other known risk factors for CVD. Pharmacological therapy for secondary prevention of dyslipidemia has been shown to be equally effective in reducing recurrence in women and men. Statin rather than menopause hormone therapy is the preferred therapy for dyslipidemia in women with CVD.

Family History

Premature IHD in a first-degree female relative is a relatively stronger risk factor for family history than in a male relative.[14]

Physical Activity and Fitness

Women are more likely to be sedentary and inactivity increases with age. Physical inactivity is associated with higher blood pressure, worse cholesterol, poorer glucose metabolism, poor mental health, and obesity. Exercise capacity strongly and independently predicts all-cause mortality in women.[15]

NEW RISK FACTORS SPECIFIC FOR WOMEN

Metabolic Syndrome

Metabolic syndrome and obesity are more common in women, increasing the relative risk of developing CVD by 2.6 times. In the Framingham Heart Study, obesity increased the relative risk of IHD by 64% in women compared to 46% in men.[15] Obesity during pregnancy can contribute to the development of hypertension and gestational diabetes.

Autoimmune Diseases

Women are more likely to develop rheumatoid arthritis and systemic lupus erythematosus (SLE). Autoimmune diseases lead to an inflammatory state with endothelial dysfunction and accelerated atherosclerosis. Steroids used for treatment can worsen hypertension, diabetes, and dyslipidemia. Patients with rheumatoid arthritis have a twofold to threefold increased risk of MI and a 50% higher risk of stroke. Young women with SLE are 2.27 times more likely to be hospitalized for an AMI, 3.8 times more likely to develop congestive HF, and 2.05 times more likely to develop a stroke.[16-18]

Gestational Hypertension

Pregnancy is a stress test for future cardiovascular events.[19] Any form of gestational hypertension increases the risk of hypertension, chronic kidney disease, diabetes, stroke, and CVD. Women with preeclampsia have approximately twice the risk of subsequent IHD, stroke, and venous thromboembolic events.

Polycystic Ovary Syndrome

Disruption of the ovulatory cycle due to estrogen deficiency, androgen excess, and insulin resistance in premenopausal women is associated with an increased risk of coronary atherosclerosis and adverse cardiovascular events. Polycystic ovary syndrome (PCOS) is prevalent in 10–13% of women and is associated with an increased risk of diabetes and hypertension during pregnancy.[20]

Breast Cancer Treatment

Women who have survived breast cancer have an increased risk of developing CVD. Exposure of the heart to ionizing radiation during breast cancer radiotherapy increases the rate of IHD development. The risk is proportional to the mean radiation dose to the heart, with a 7.4% increase in CVD per 1 Gy of radiation. Newer techniques have been developed to minimize the dose to the heart to <3 Gy. The risk of IHD begins within a few years of exposure and lasts for 20 years. The absolute risk is highest in women with preexisting CVD risk factors.[21]

Hysterectomy

Hysterectomy is the most common nonobstetric procedure performed on women. Ovarian failure can develop after hysterectomy from a reduction in vascular supply. Data from the Swedish Hospital Discharge Register on 184,441 women who underwent hysterectomy between 1973 and 2003 showed that hysterectomy in women aged 50 years or younger substantially increases the risk of CVD later in life. Oophorectomy further increases the risk of both IHD and stroke.[22]

Psychosocial Factors

In the INTERHEART study, aggregate exposure to psychosocial risk factors, including depression, perceived home/work stress, low locus of control, and major life events, was significantly associated with AMI. In women with MI or other forms of coronary heart disease, depression is associated with an approximately threefold increased risk of death or subsequent cardiac events, independent of depression severity. Persons with higher social support experience a better quality of life and fewer symptoms of depression at 12 months.[23]

CLINICAL SPECTRUM OF ISCHEMIC HEART DISEASE

The Framingham study previously suggested that the development of CHD in women lags behind men by approximately 10 years; however, current data show that women are susceptible to IHD at a much younger age. The mean age of women in the Kerala ACS Registry was 64.4 ± 11.7 years; they were 5 years older than men (mean age for men 59.3 ± 11.9 years; $p < 0.001$).[24] Most patients have chest pain, but women are more likely to report numerous associated symptoms such as back, neck, and jaw pain, shortness of breath, paroxysmal nocturnal dyspnea, nausea, indigestion, and fatigue. Women are more likely to have NSTEMI and nonobstructive coronary heart disease.[5]

Women more often delay seeking care and more often suffer from diabetes, hypertension, and HF with preserved ventricular systolic function. Mechanical complications and HF with reduced ejection fraction are more likely to develop in women, while ventricular arrhythmias occur similarly in both sexes after AMI. Women with acute coronary syndrome (ACS) are treated less aggressively, with fewer catheterization interventions, thrombolytic therapy, and bypass surgery, resulting in less favorable clinical outcomes with higher mortality and lower health-related quality of life. Compared to men, women with ACS and after coronary revascularization have longer hospitalizations, higher in-hospital mortality, more bleeding complications, and up to 30% more rehospitalizations within 30 days after the index hospitalization. Regardless of age, more women than men die within 1 year of their first AMI (26% of women and 19% of men); more women than men (47% of women and 36% of men) die, develop HF, or have a stroke within 5 years of their first AMI. Studies consistently report a high risk of mortality after AMI in younger women. The mechanisms, probably multifactorial, contributing to excess risk and poorer health in young women remain unclear.[5]

Ischemia with Nonobstructive Coronary Arteries

Cardiac ischemia without obstructive CAD is caused by CMD and coronary spasm, which cause a mismatch between blood supply and myocardial oxygen demand. Ischemia with nonobstructive coronary arteries (INOCA) is more common in women aged 45–55 years with a prevalence of 34.4–62%. Early diagnosis and treatment are essential due to the increased risk of major adverse cardiac events (MACE).[9]

Myocardial Infarction with Nonobstructive Coronary Arteries

MINOCA accounts for up to 2–6% of all AMIs and is diagnosed more often in women, especially younger women. Conventional risk factors such as hyperlipidemia and diabetes are less common, but a higher prevalence of hypertension is observed. It is caused by plaque erosion, distal embolization, and endothelial and microvascular dysfunction that exacerbates the consequences of a spastic or thrombotic event. MINOCA patients have an increased risk of CVD with an overall in-hospital mortality of 0.9%, a 2% risk of death or reinfarction within 6 months, a 15% readmission rate within 6 months, and a 12-month mortality of 4.7%. Up to 25% of MINOCA patients report persistent angina after MI and experience similar rates of HF, hospitalizations, and repeat tests due to angina as their counterparts with obstructive CAD. After 10 years, death from CVD or MI occurred in 6.7% of patients without overt angiographic CAD and in 12.8% of patients with nonobstructive CAD.[25]

Spontaneous Coronary Artery Dissection

In the last decade, SCAD has been recognized as a nonatherosclerotic, nontraumatic cause of ACS and sudden cardiac death. SCAD is characterized by the presence of blood that enters the layers of the coronary artery wall and separates them to form a false lumen, causing compression of the true coronary lumen, limiting coronary blood flow and leading to myocardial ischemia.[26]

Women account for 87–95% of SCAD cases, with a mean age of presentation between 44 and 53 years. Single-center studies have estimated the prevalence of SCAD in up to 4% of patients with ACS and as the underlying cause of up to 35% of all cases of ACS in women aged ≤ 50 years, with 20–25% of cases occurring in the peripartum period. The classic presentation is a young healthy woman without traditional ASCVD risk factors and sudden-onset ACS.[26]

Spontaneous coronary artery dissection can be associated with multifocal fibromuscular dysplasia (FMD), which can affect almost any arterial course and manifest as arterial stenosis, aneurysm, tortuosity, or dissection. Intracranial aneurysm can be observed in 12.9% of patients. Screening for extracoronary arteriopathy by imaging between the brain and the pelvis is recommended.[27]

Patients with SCAD are usually diagnosed late. A high index of clinical suspicion is therefore required in women with typical chest pain and abnormalities of either electrocardiogram (ECG) or cardiac biomarkers, even where conventional cardiac risk factors are absent.

Spontaneous coronary artery dissection can be identified angiographically in most cases **(Figs. 2A to E)** with confirmation by intracoronary imaging if there is uncertainty. Unfortunately, the diagnosis is often missed, in part because of the persistent incorrect expectation that a false lumen in SCAD will usually be apparent angiographically. The left anterior descending artery is often affected, with middle to distal segments primarily affected. Conservative treatment is preferred in stable SCAD patients with preserved distal coronary flow. PCI for SCAD is associated with a lower technical success rate and higher complications and should be reserved for patients with ongoing acute ischemia.[26] Revascularization outcomes are poorer in SCAD than in atherosclerotic disease and are often complicated by hematoma propagation, which requires long lengths of stenting to restore coronary architecture and flow. With conservative management, most SCAD dissections heal with no residual detectable abnormalities on follow-up imaging. Coronary artery bypass grafting is used in some patients where PCI has failed. Dissected arteries are fragile and unlikely to hold a suture. Most grafts occlude on follow-up because the healing of the native arteries causes competing flow.[28]

Treatment is therefore aimed at alleviating symptoms with optimal medical therapy, including single antiplatelet therapy, blood pressure control, antianginals, and analgesics. Statins are associated with recurrent SCAD and should be used with caution.[26]

Patients are advised to engage in regular moderate exercise while avoiding extreme endurance training, exercise to exhaustion, high-level competitive sports, vigorous exertion in extreme temperatures, and heavy lifting that requires exertion or prolonged Valsalva. The postdischarge MACE rate is 2.7% at 30 days, with a high recurrence rate of 17% in women only, a 10-year mortality rate of 7.7%, and a high MACE rate of 47.4%.[28]

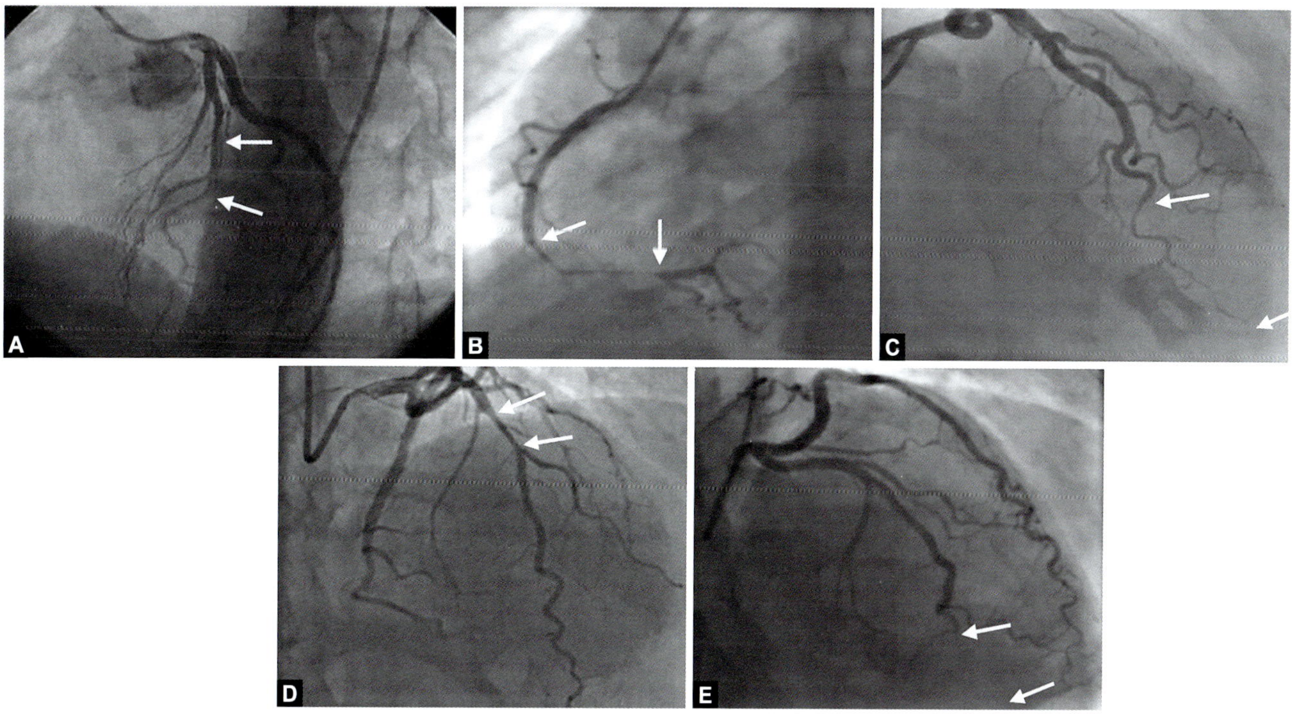

FIGS. 2A TO E: Types of SCAD: (A) Type 1, false lumen is visible; (B) Type 2a, long narrowing with no visible false lumen and normal distal vessel; (C) Type 2b, no visible false lumen or distal vessel; (D) Type 3, mimics atherosclerosis and requires intracoronary imaging for distinction; and (E) Type 4, distal occlusion with subsequent confirmed healing and no identified embolic source.

Takotsubo Cardiomyopathy

Takotsubo cardiomyopathy, also known as stress-induced cardiomyopathy or "broken heart syndrome," is characterized by transient left ventricular dysfunction that mimics ACS but without significant coronary artery obstruction. It mainly affects women after menopause, often after strong emotional or physical stress.[29]

Pathophysiology

The exact mechanism of Takotsubo cardiomyopathy is not well understood but is thought to involve catecholamine-induced myocardial stunning, coronary artery spasm, and microvascular dysfunction. High levels of circulating catecholamines such as adrenaline can have a direct toxic effect on the myocardium, leading to the characteristic left ventricular apical ballooning seen in this condition **(Flowchart 1)**.[30]

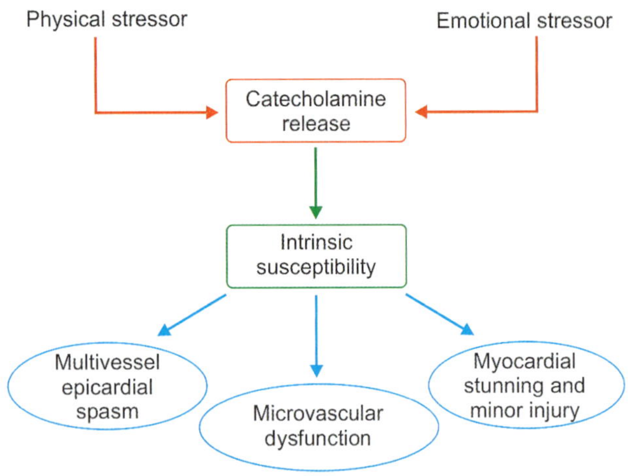

FLOWCHART 1: Pathophysiology of Takotsubo cardiomyopathy.

Clinical Picture

Patients with Takotsubo cardiomyopathy typically present with chest pain and dyspnea like ACS. ECGs often show ST-segment elevation, and cardiac biomarkers may be mildly elevated. However, coronary angiography usually does not reveal any significant obstructive coronary artery disease, and left-sided ventriculography or echocardiography demonstrates the characteristic apical balloon pattern **(Table 2)**.[31]

TABLE 2: Diagnostic criteria for Takotsubo cardiomyopathy.

Criteria	Description
Acute onset	Sudden onset of chest pain or shortness of breath, typically following stress
ECG changes	ST-segment elevation or T-wave inversion
Absence of obstructive CAD	Coronary angiography showing no significant blockages
Left ventricular dysfunction	Apical ballooning pattern on imaging (echocardiography or ventriculography)
Recovery	Reversible myocardial dysfunction within a few weeks to months

Diagnosis and Treatment

The diagnosis of Takotsubo cardiomyopathy is based on the clinical presentation, imaging findings, and the exclusion of obstructive coronary heart disease. Treatment includes supportive care, similar to ACS, with an emphasis on beta-blockers and ACE inhibitors or ARBs to manage cardiac function. Most patients recover fully within weeks to months, although complications such as HF, arrhythmias, and thromboembolism may occur.[29]

CONCLUSION

Cardiovascular disease is the leading cause of death in women. The traditional training of cardiologists to equate IHD with angiographically defined obstructive CAD has contributed to less aggressive preventive and therapeutic interventions in women compared with men. A paradigm shift beyond the mere anatomical description of obstructive CAD is necessary for earlier detection of CAD risk and treatment in women. Education is essential for women, including young women, to recognize the vulnerability of the female heart to coronary heart disease and the potential for risk recognition and interventions to delay or prevent coronary events. A holistic approach to prevention and treatment will improve clinical outcomes for patients.

ACKNOWLEDGMENT

One of the authors, Roopa Salwan, is a Principal Investigator for the SCAD International Registry from India. Please contact roopa.salwan@maxhealthcare.com to report your cases for this registry.

ONLINE REFERENCES

Please scan the QR code provided at the end of the table of contents for References of this chapter.

CHAPTER 84

Pregnancy and Valvular Heart Disease

Shibba Takkar Chhabra, Abhishek Garg

ABSTRACT

India is undergoing a significant shift in obstetric care, with cardiac ailments now accounting for a considerable proportion of maternal mortality. Valvular heart disease (VHD) is often first diagnosed during pregnancy, and obstructive lesions can particularly worsen during the second trimester and labor. The management of prosthetic valves faces challenges due to the need for anticoagulant therapy and monitoring, especially in resource-limited regions such as India. Additionally, administering diuretics, antiarrhythmic drugs, ACE inhibitors (ACEIs), and angiotensin receptor blockers (ARBs) requires caution, particularly during the first trimester when organogenesis occurs. For patients experiencing decompensation, procedures such as transcatheter aortic valve implantation (TAVI), valve repair, and valve replacement should be tailored to ensure fetal and maternal well-being.

Keywords: Valvular heart disease, rheumatic, pregnancy, India

INTRODUCTION

India is currently experiencing a transition in maternal mortality patterns. Maternal deaths are no longer predominantly due to primary obstetrics or infectious causes; instead, cardiovascular diseases now account for a significant proportion of maternal mortalities. Valvular heart disease (VHD) is common during pregnancy. With an increasing number of women with underlying valvular and congenital heart diseases surviving into adulthood, particularly those who have undergone corrective interventions, the landscape of maternal health is undergoing significant changes. Among the VHDs, rheumatic heart disease (RHD), especially mitral stenosis (MS) with regurgitation, as well as aortic stenosis (AS) and aortic regurgitation, are the most frequently observed conditions, each requiring specific evaluation and management and carrying potential complications. Moreover, prosthetic valves need anticoagulation, necessitating careful consideration of maternal and fetal risks and benefits. Preconceptional management through the postpartum period should involve maternal-fetal medicine specialists, cardiologists, obstetricians, and anesthesiologists, employing a multidisciplinary approach to address these issues.

EPIDEMIOLOGY

Maternal heart disease affects approximately 4% of pregnancies,[1] yet it contributes a significant proportion of 10–25% of maternal mortality.[2-4] Kumari et al.[5] revealed that the most common etiology of VHD during pregnancy was rheumatic—87.3%, followed by mitral valve prolapse. In the M-PAC registry, encompassing 1,029 consecutive pregnancies, a significant proportion of pregnant patients (60.5%) were newly diagnosed with heart disease during their pregnancy.[6] RHD emerged as the most prevalent condition, affecting 42% of the cohort, while pulmonary hypertension was identified in one-third of the cases. Besides its high prevalence, RHD in developing countries is distinguished by the occurrence of severe VHD at a younger age compared to developed nations.[5] Shrestha et al.[7] showed the overall prevalence of heart disease among pregnant women was found to be 1.46%. The incidence of preterm labor and delivery in pregnant women with heart disease was 17.63%. Furthermore, the maternal and fetal mortality rates were 26.14 and 50.48 per 1,000 pregnant women with heart disease, respectively.

RISK STRATIFICATION

Valvular heart disease can arise from either congenital factors or acquired conditions. While (some lesions present low risks to both maternal and fetal health, others pose significant challenges) **(Table 1)**.[8]

In India, where VHD is highly prevalent, risk stratification tools for pregnant patients created in high-income countries and mainly for congenital heart disease cases may not be as relevant. The M-PAC registry revealed that the statistics of the WHO classification **(Table 2)** for predicting maternal cardiac events and death were 0.794 (95% CI 0.763–0.826) and 0.796 (95% CI 0.732–0.860), respectively.[6] For pregnant patients with VHD, the DEVI score demonstrated better concordance between predicted probabilities and observed outcomes compared to the CAPREG II score, with an area under the receiver-operating characteristic curve of 0.884 (95% CI 0.844–0.923) for the DEVI score and 0.808 (95% CI 0.753–0.863) for the CARPREG-II models **(Table 3)**.[6] Therefore, valve lesion-specific scores such as the DEVI score may be more effective in identifying patients at risk of adverse cardiac outcomes in India, where RHD is common.[6]

Siu et al. found four predictors for maternal complications, a prior cardiac event, a prepregnancy NYHA greater than II, a left heart stenotic lesion with moderate-to-severe grade, and a left ventricular ejection fraction of < 40%.[9]

TABLE 1: Classification of valvular heart diseases in pregnancy risks according to maternal and fetal risk.

Low maternal and fetal risks	High maternal and fetal risks	High maternal risk
Asymptomatic aortic stenosis with a low mean outflow gradient (< 50 mm Hg); normal LV systolic function	Severe aortic stenosis with or without symptoms	Ejection fraction < 40%
Aortic regurgitation, NYHA Class I or II with normal LV function	Aortic regurgitation, NYHA Class III or IV	Previous heart failure
Mitral regurgitation, NYHA Class I or II, with normal LV function	Mitral stenosis, NYHA Class II, III, or IV	Previous stroke or transient ischemic attack
Mitral valve prolapse with none to moderate mitral regurgitation, normal LV function	Mitral regurgitation, NYHA Class III or IV	
Mild-to-moderate mitral stenosis, no pulmonary hypertension	Aortic or mitral valve disease with pulmonary hypertension	
Mild-to-moderate pulmonary valve stenosis	• Maternal cyanosis • Reduced functional status, NYHA Class III or IV	
Aortic or mitral valve disease with LV dysfunction		

(LV: left ventricle; NYHA: New York Heart Association)

TABLE 2: The WHO risk stratification for valvular heart disease in pregnancy.

WHO class	Description	Risk level	Follow-up
I	• Mild or uncomplicated pulmonary stenosis • Mitral valve prolapse	Patients can be considered very low risk, with no increased mortality and/or mild increase in morbidity	A patient's follow-up with a cardiologist can be limited to one or two visits during pregnancy
II	• Mild or uncomplicated uncorrected ASD or VSD • Tetralogy of Fallot (repaired) arrhythmias	Patients can be considered at low-to-moderate risk with a mild increase in maternal mortality and a moderate increase in morbidity	The patient's follow-up with a cardiologist should be every trimester
III	• Mechanical valve • Aortic dilatation 40–45 mm (in Marfan syndrome or bicuspid aortic valve)	Patients can be considered high risk with significantly increased morbidity and mortality	Patients should be cared for by an expert multidisciplinary interdisciplinary team. Monthly or bimonthly cardiac and obstetric monitoring if pregnancy is pursued
IV	• Severe mitral stenosis • Severe symptomatic aortic stenosis • Marfan syndrome with aorta dilated > 45 mm or aortic dilatation > 50 mm with bicuspid aortic valve	Patients should be considered extremely high risk and pregnancy contraindicated secondary to high risk of maternal mortality and severe morbidity	If pregnancy does occur, close monthly or bimonthly follow-up is necessary

TABLE 3: Various scores for risk stratification of valvular heart disease.

CARPEG-II score—general risk stratification tool		
Risk factor	**Score**	**Risk of cardiac complications**
Prior cardiac event or arrhythmia	+3	
Baseline NYHA II–IV or cyanosis	+3	
Mechanical heart valve	+3	
Ventricular dysfunction	+2	
High-risk left valve disease/LV outflow tract obstruction	+2	
Pulmonary hypertension	+2	Score: % risk
Coronary heart disease	+2	0: 5%
High-risk aortopathy	+2	1: 27%
No prior cardiac intervention	+1	>2: 75%
Late pregnancy assessment	+1	
Prior cardiac event or arrhythmia	+3	
Baseline NYHA II–IV or cyanosis	+3	
Mechanical heart valve	+3	
DEVI score—valvular heart disease-specific tool		
Factors	**Score**	
Prior cardiovascular event	+4	
Pulmonary hypertension	+4	
Severe mitral stenosis	+4	
Moderate mitral stenosis	+2	
Prosthetic heart valve	+2	
Mild mitral stenosis	+1	
Taking cardiac medications	–1	

Note: In pregnancy with valvular heart diseases—the DEVI score better predicts patients at risk of adverse cardiac outcomes.

Lesniak-Sobelga et al.[10] reported that maternal mortality varies based on the type and location of the lesion, as well as the presence of myocardial dysfunction.

In the M-PAC registry,[6] maternal mortality was found to be 1.9%, with the highest rates observed in patients with prosthetic heart valves.

REVIEW OF CARDIAC PHYSIOLOGY IN PREGNANCY

Four major physiological changes during pregnancy[3] **(Fig. 1)** are increased intravascular volume, decreased systemic vascular resistance, increased hypercoagulability, and fluctuations in cardiac output (CO).

Around 5 weeks of gestation, compensatory mechanisms enhance oxygen delivery to maternal and fetal tissues.[10] Systemic vascular resistance decreases by 20% by 24 weeks due to progesterone. By 28 weeks, CO increases by 30–50%, heart rate by 10–15 beats/min, and stroke volume by 20–30%.[10] Uterine contractions cause an autotransfusion of about 500 mL of blood into the maternal circulation. Postpartum, CO, and stroke volume increase by 50% and 60–70%, respectively, 1 hour after delivery due to autotransfusion of remaining uteroplacental blood as the uterus involutes. Cardiac status gradually returns to baseline within 2–6 weeks postpartum.[10]

VALVULAR HEART DISEASE

Mitral Stenosis

Mitral stenosis is the most common VHD encountered during pregnancy.[11] It is almost always a consequence of rheumatic fever.[12] This condition often remains asymptomatic until pregnancy, when physiological changes can reveal its presence.

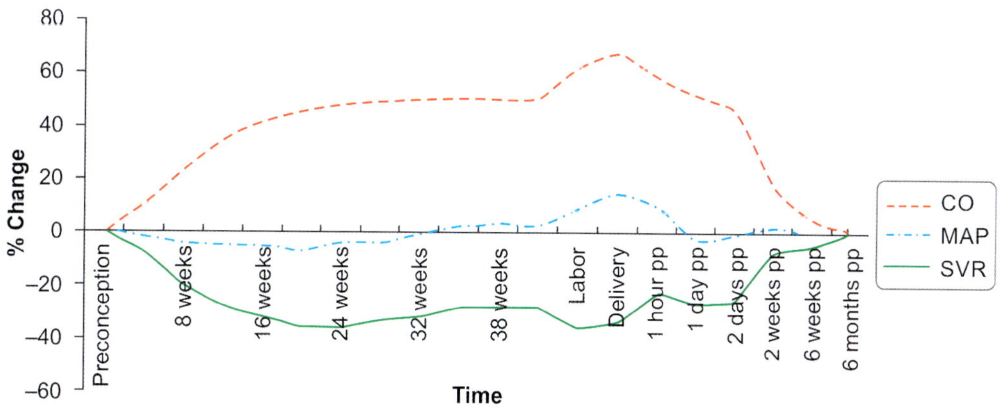

FIG. 1: Hemodynamic changes in pregnancy, during labor, and postpartum.

Long-term elevated blood volumes in the left atrium (LA) can cause LA dilation atrial arrhythmias.[10] The patient can present with orthopnea, paroxysmal nocturnal dyspnea, dyspnea on exertion, and pulmonary edema. Mostly, these symptoms become prominent in the second trimester of pregnancy. Echocardiographic imaging can reveal classic features of rheumatic mitral valve disease, including fibrous thickening and calcification of the valve leaflets, fusion of the commissures, and thickening/shortening of the chordae tendineae.[13]

Management

Heart rate management is the utmost clinical aspect for patients with MS. A rapid heart rate reduces diastolic time, increases left atrial and pulmonary venous pressures, and leads to symptoms of pulmonary venous hypertension.[14] Controlling heart rate significantly alleviates these symptoms. If tachycardia has a reversible cause, it should be addressed before considering rate-controlling agents.[14] Various drugs are used to control heart rate during pregnancy and are considered relatively safe. Beta-blockers, previously classified as Food and Drug Administration (FDA) drug classes B and C, can be used but may cause intrauterine growth retardation and fetal bradycardia. Verapamil, diltiazem, and digoxin, labeled FDA category C, may also be used if the benefits outweigh the risks. The FDA drug classification system is now being replaced with the Pregnancy and Lactation Labeling Rule (PLLR).[14]

Therapeutic options for patients diagnosed with MS encompass a range of medical, surgical, and catheter-based interventions, depending upon the severity of stenosis and the patient's symptomatic presentation.[13] Severe cases of MS, classified as high risk according to the WHO class IV, often necessitate percutaneous balloon mitral valvuloplasty (BMV) for symptomatic relief when medical intervention and bed rest prove inadequate.[13] Numerous research studies conducted in India have demonstrated that BMV is both a secure and effective treatment for patients with symptomatic MS, achieving a success rate of approximately 98%. It is recommended to perform this procedure after 20 weeks and in the second trimester of pregnancy for optimal results.[15]

For patients presenting with atrial fibrillation, left atrial thrombus, or a history of embolism, therapeutic anticoagulation is imperative.[13] In instances where pregnant patients experience severe symptoms and/or pulmonary artery pressure exceeds 50 mm Hg despite medical management, open mitral valve replacement surgery may offer a viable solution if percutaneous valvuloplasty is not feasible.[13] However, fetal well-being poses a significant concern in open surgery scenarios.[13]

All patients, regardless of symptomatology, with moderate or severe MS should be advised against pregnancy, and intervention should be pursued before conception, with valvuloplasty being the preferred approach.[13]

In obstetric management, vaginal delivery is recommended for patients with mild MS, as well as for those with moderate or severe stenosis who exhibit NYHA Class I–II symptoms without pulmonary hypertension.[13] Cesarean section may be warranted for patients experiencing Class III–IV symptoms.[13]

Mitral Regurgitation

Mitral regurgitation (MR) in RHD is commonly associated with MS, while isolated MR is less prevalent. MR can also be related to primary mitral valve disease, known as mitral valve prolapse, which may occur in isolation, be inherited as an autosomal dominant disorder, or be associated with Marfan syndrome or Ehlers–Danlos syndrome.[16]

Pathophysiology

Mitral regurgitation is typically well tolerated during pregnancy with favorable outcomes.[9] As systemic vascular resistance decreases in pregnancy, the balance between backward flow to the atrium and forward flow to the aorta improves, increasing blood flow to the systemic circulation.[10] Heart failure (HF) occurs in 20–25% of women with moderate-to-severe MR, without a higher risk of obstetric complications.[10] Fetal issues include intrauterine growth restriction in 5–10% of cases and other complications in < 5% of females with moderate-to-severe MR.[10]

Management

Mitral regurgitation in patients with normal left ventricular systolic function typically requires only regular observation and monitoring. However, in patients with decreased systolic function, medical management becomes necessary, and surgery may be considered if symptoms pose a risk to fetal health **(Table 4)**.[13] These patients require a comprehensive management plan, including appropriate medications to optimize heart function and close monitoring throughout pregnancy.

Aortic Stenosis

In developed countries, aortic valve disease is most frequently caused by a congenital bicuspid aortic valve (BAV), which can occur in an isolated form. In developing countries, aortic valve disease commonly occurs in association with mitral valve disease due to RHD.[13]

When AS is diagnosed early and is managed with appropriate follow-up, patients with mild-to-moderate obstruction (aortic valve area > 1.0 cm^2) can generally tolerate pregnancy well.[13] Recent studies indicate that even in cases of severe AS, the overall maternal mortality rate is < 1%.[13] However, the risk of complications for both the fetus and mother increases significantly as the severity of AS intensifies. For instance, about one-third of pregnant women with an aortic valve

TABLE 4: Medical management of heart failure in pregnancy.[17]

Drugs	Purpose	Previous FDA class
Diuretics		
Furosemide	• Pulmonary edema • Contraindicated in uteroplacental hypoperfusion	Class C
Vasodilators		
ACE inhibitors/ ARB	Contraindicated throughout pregnancy due to teratogenic effects	• Class C for the first trimester • Class D for second and third trimester
Amlodipine	Alternative to ACE inhibitors in pregnancy	Class C
Nitrates	May be used to treat decompensated heart failure	Class C
Beta-blockers		
Carvedilol, metoprolol, bisoprolol	• Generally safe and effective in pregnancy • Beta-blockers should be continued throughout pregnancy	Class C
Aldosterone antagonists		
Spironolactone, eplerenone	No data support safety in pregnancy	Class D
Anticoagulants		
Warfarin		Class X
Heparin	Can be used in pregnancy and especially after the 36th week of gestation	
LMWH	Can be used in pregnancy till the 36th week of gestation	

area of < 1.5 cm² require hospitalization, and these patients are also at higher risk for adverse fetal outcomes such as growth restriction, preterm birth, respiratory distress, and low birth weight.[13] Although studies on this patient group have been limited in size, estimates suggest that HF affects approximately 7–17% of pregnant women with severe AS, while arrhythmias are observed in 3–33% of cases.[13] This underscores the importance of preconception counseling and rigorous monitoring throughout pregnancy for this patient population.[13] Interestingly, some women with severe AS can maintain a successful pregnancy, especially if they remain asymptomatic during exercise testing before conception.[13]

While no definitive medical treatment exists for AS, patients may benefit from activity restriction and preload reduction using diuretics, administered cautiously in symptomatic cases.[13] For those unresponsive to medical therapy, options include early pregnancy termination, catheter-based valvuloplasty, and surgical valve replacement, contingent upon clinical status and resource availability.[18] Symptomatic severe AS patients should undergo surgery before pregnancy.[13] Even asymptomatic with severe AS with left ventricular dysfunction, ejection fraction below 50%, or exercise-induced symptoms, face higher risks of adverse outcomes and should be considered for prepregnancy surgery. In severe symptomatic AS, cesarean delivery is generally recommended. For mild-to-moderate AS, vaginal delivery is preferred, avoiding epidural anesthesia due to the significant decrease in peripheral vascular resistance.[13]

Aortic Regurgitation

Aortic insufficiency in women of childbearing age can arise from various pathological conditions, including endocarditis or RHD, BAV, and aortic annular dilatation associated with ascending aortic dilatation.[13] The placental circulation reduces systemic vascular resistance, thereby decreasing afterload and positively influencing the hemodynamics of aortic insufficiency.[13] In the absence of significant left ventricular dysfunction, chronic left-sided valvular insufficiency can be well tolerated during pregnancy. A thorough evaluation should be performed before pregnancy. For those with moderate or severe regurgitation, exercise testing is recommended before pregnancy.[13]

In cases of left ventricular dysfunction, the increased volume load of pregnancy may precipitate symptoms of pulmonary congestion, necessitating activity restriction, dietary sodium reduction, and medical management of HF, including diuretics, beta-blockers, and/or vasodilators **(Table 4)**.[13] Vasodilators should be used cautiously in pregnant women to avoid uteroplacental hypoperfusion. Commonly used for afterload reduction, such as angiotensin-converting enzyme inhibitors and angiotensin receptor blockers, are contraindicated during pregnancy due to their teratogenic effects.[13] Preload and afterload reduction can be safely achieved during pregnancy with a combination of hydralazine and nitrates. Other medications that have proven effective in treating hypertension during pregnancy include methyldopa, labetalol, and amlodipine.[13]

Women without severe regurgitation, who have normal left ventricular systolic function and no symptoms, are at low risk for complications. Those with severe regurgitation and symptoms, or with decreased left ventricular function, are referred for valve surgery before pregnancy, with a preference for repair.[13] Surgical intervention for severe valvular regurgitation during pregnancy is rarely indicated, except in cases of life-threatening infective endocarditis. In patients with severe symptomatic regurgitation or AS, valve surgery can be performed in conjunction with a cesarean section once fetal maturity is achieved. Vaginal delivery is preferred for women with severe regurgitant valve disease, utilizing an epidural and a shortened second stage of labor.[13]

Patients with BAV disease frequently present with associated aortopathy, such as aortic coarctation, dilatation, or aneurysms. Hence, all women with BAV should have imaging of the ascending and proximal descending aorta performed before pregnancy as part of their prepregnancy risk assessment.[13] Women with unrepaired native coarctation, residual coarctation, aneurysms, and/or persistent hypertension are at increased risk for aortic dissection, rupture, or cerebral aneurysm rupture. Aortic surgery should be considered before pregnancy if the ascending aorta measures over 50 mm (or 27.5 mm/m^2).[13]

Right-sided Heart Valvular Heart Disease

Tricuspid regurgitation (TR) is typically functional, resulting from annular dilatation due to right ventricular pressure or volume overload, often in conjunction with mitral valve disease, previous endocarditis, or RHD. Isolated TR, in the absence of right ventricular dysfunction, rarely leads to clinical sequelae during pregnancy, labor, or delivery, and usually does not require correction before pregnancy.[13]

Pulmonic stenosis (PS) is mostly due to the congenital and typically valvular, though subvalvular or supravalvular forms may also occur. Homograft deterioration following a Ross procedure can result in PS or pulmonic regurgitation (PR). Even severe PS is generally well tolerated during pregnancy.[19] Severe PS can lead to right ventricular strain, failure, and arrhythmias. Ideally, PS should be relieved before pregnancy using balloon valvuloplasty, which is recommended when the peak forward flow gradient exceeds 64 mm Hg.[13] Mild or moderate PS is considered low risk.

Balloon valvuloplasty during pregnancy is rarely indicated and is reserved for patients unresponsive to medical management and bed rest. Untreated severe PS is associated with significant fetal complications, including a 17% incidence of preterm birth and a 4.8% offspring mortality rate.[19] Vaginal delivery is usually possible and preferable for patients with mild or moderate PS, as well as for those with severe PS who exhibit class I or II symptoms. Females with severe PS and class III/IV symptoms, for whom percutaneous intervention has failed or is not feasible, should undergo delivery via cesarean section. However, even in patients with severe PS vaginal delivery is most commonly the preferred method.[13]

Severe PR can result from previous balloon valvuloplasty for PS or repaired tetralogy of Fallot. Severe PR is an independent predictor of maternal complications, especially in patients with impaired right ventricular function.[13] Pregnancy can lead to progressive right ventricular failure, which may persist postpartum. In symptomatic patients with severe PR and reduced right ventricular function and/or dilatation, pulmonic valve replacement should be considered before pregnancy.[13]

Prosthetic Valve and Anticoagulation

Pregnant patients with prosthetic heart valves pose unique challenges throughout pregnancy. Outside of pregnancy, warfarin generally is the preferred anticoagulant for patients with mechanical heart valves.[19] In a study by Ng et al.,[20] the presence of a prosthetic valve increased the risk of major adverse cardiovascular events by 22 times and also led to longer hospital stays and higher costs. There was no significant difference in maternal outcomes between patients with mechanical or bioprosthetic valves. Similar fetal complications were more likely in females with prosthetic valves, but the risk remained comparable between the two types of valves. In pregnancies with bileaflet valve prostheses and single-tilting discs, maternal mortality, and thromboembolic complications were reduced when using vitamin K antagonists (VKAs) with an international normalized ratio (INR) target of 2.5–3.5, compared to low-molecular-weight heparin (LMWH).[21] Women who use VKAs throughout pregnancy face a 2% risk of anticoagulant-related adverse events affecting the fetus or neonate.[21] While sequential treatment removes the risk of anticoagulant-related embryopathy, it still carries a risk of anticoagulant-related fetopathy. On the other hand, women on LMWH do not encounter drug-related fetal adverse events because heparins do not cross the placenta.[21]

Vitamin K antagonists are advised for women with mechanical heart valves in the second and third trimesters and may be considered in the first trimester if a daily dose of ≤5 mg achieves therapeutic INR.[21] This approach is reasonable but has several considerations. Firstly, data on live births and fetal adverse events, categorized by warfarin doses above 5 mg/day versus ≤5 mg/day, should be cautiously interpreted.[21] Despite live births being twice as high and fetal adverse events being five times lower with warfarin doses ≤5 mg/day, recent data from the Registry of Pregnancy and Cardiac Disease (ROPAC) did not indicate reduced fetal loss with low first-trimester doses of VKAs (warfarin ≤5 mg/day, acenocoumarol ≤2 mg/day).[21] Furthermore, many studies fail to distinguish between anticoagulant-related and unrelated adverse events and do not address fetopathy, resulting in an underestimation of anticoagulant-related fetal adverse events.[21] These studies usually focus on the first-trimester dose of warfarin, which may not represent the doses used later in pregnancy, when warfarin fetopathy can still develop.[21] Additionally, women with stable INRs in the 3 months before pregnancy may need higher doses of VKAs during pregnancy.[21] Hence, although fetal adverse events seem to rise with warfarin doses above 5 mg/day, fetal loss and adverse events can still happen with doses ≤5 mg/day. The safety of first-trimester VKA doses ≤5 mg/day requires further validation and should be thoroughly discussed with the patient.[21] If females on LMWH intensive anti-Xa monitoring are to be done with target anti-Xa activity of 1.0–1.2 units/mL for the mitral valve and 0.8–1.0 units/mL for the aortic valve at post-dose, trough level >00.6 IU/mL, followed by dose adjustment.[21]

During childbirth, special care is required for patients with prosthetic valves, especially those on anticoagulation therapy. Enoxaparin should be stopped 24 hours before an epidural to prevent the risk of an epidural hematoma. Women on unfractionated heparin should have a normal activated partial thromboplastin time before an epidural is placed.[10] Due to LMWH's longer half-life, patients are usually switched to unfractionated heparin at 36 weeks of gestation, which is then stopped at least 4–6 hours before delivery. Depending on delivery circumstances, unfractionated heparin or LMWH can be resumed as soon as 6 hours postpartum.[10] Warfarin can be restarted once there is no significant bleeding risk, with LMWH or unfractionated heparin continued until the INR is within the therapeutic range of 2.5–3.5.[10]

MODE AND TIMING OF DELIVERY

Vaginal delivery is generally preferred for women with cardiovascular conditions due to its association with reduced blood loss, lower infection risk, and fewer venous thromboembolic events.[13] Cesarean section is typically recommended for patients with NYHA III/IV, pulmonary hypertension, severe AS, Eisenmenger syndrome, or those on oral anticoagulants during labor.[13]

Patients with cardiovascular disease under cardio-obstetric care should reach full term. Labor induction at 40 weeks is advised to avoid emergency cesarean sections and stillbirths. Immediate delivery should be considered for women with HF and hemodynamic instability, regardless of gestational age.[13]

KEY STEPS FOR POSITIVE OUTCOMES: MATERNAL AND FETAL WELL-BEING

Key steps for positive outcomes—maternal and fetal well-being—are shown in **Table 5** and **Box 1**.

TABLE 5: European guidelines for management of valvular heart disease in pregnancy.[22]

Recommendations	Class
Prepregnancy evaluation with echocardiography and counseling is recommended for any women with known or suspected valvular disease	I
If cardiac surgery is to be performed after 24 weeks and before 37 weeks of gestation, then corticosteroids are recommended for the mother	I
Fetal echocardiography by experienced specialists is recommended when there is an elevated risk of fetal abnormalities	I
Mitral stenosis	
Restricted activities, and beta-1 selective blockers are recommended	I
Diuretics are recommended when congestive symptoms persist despite beta-blockers	
Therapeutic anticoagulation using heparin, and VKA is recommended in case of AF	
Interventions should be considered before pregnancy in patients with severe MS area < 1 cm^2	
Aortic stenosis	
Intervention Is recommended before pregnancy in patients with severe aortic stenosis if: • Are symptomatic • LVEF < 50% • Develop symptoms during exercise testing	I
Chronic regurgitant lesions	
Surgical treatment is recommended before pregnancy in patients with severe aortic or mitral regurgitation with symptoms of impaired ventricular functions	I
Medical therapy is recommended in pregnant women with regurgitant lesions when symptoms occur	

BOX 1 Key steps for positive outcomes of valvular heart disease in pregnancy.

Preconception planning and evaluation:
- Thorough history including palpitations and physical exams
- ECG to be done prepregnancy
- Echocardiography for etiology and hemodynamics of valvular lesions
- Effective contraception until pregnancy is desired
- Consider valve repair or replacement if symptomatic before conception
- Genetics referral for patients with hereditary cardiac lesions

Continued

Continued

Assessment during pregnancy:
- History and physical examination at least once per trimester
- Changes in functions class
- Serial echocardiography for any changes in symptoms
- For mild to moderate stenosis or regurgitation can be followed up once every trimester and before delivery, while monthly follow-up during the second trimester, is a safe option
- Valvuloplasty if necessary and appropriate

Management during labor and delivery:
- Short vaginal delivery with shortened of the second stage of labor
- Left lateral decubitus position
- Cesarean section as per obstetric indications
- Medical therapy for loading conditions
- Treatment of pulmonary edema

Postpartum concerns:
- Treat anemia
- Medical therapy of pulmonary edema
- Valve repair or replacement
- Contraception

CONCLUSION

In conclusion, navigating pregnancy with VHD in India requires careful consideration of both maternal and fetal well-being. With a growing awareness and access to medical advancements, early detection, timely interventions, and multidisciplinary care are essential for ensuring optimal outcomes. While challenges exist, a proactive approach, including preconception counseling, close monitoring, and tailored management strategies, can significantly reduce the risks and enable women with VHD to experience safe pregnancies and deliveries.

ONLINE REFERENCES

Please scan the QR code provided at the end of the table of contents for References of this chapter.

CHAPTER

85

Management of Cardiac Emergencies in Pregnancy

Preeti Gupta, Abhinav Aggarwal

ABSTRACT

Cardiac emergencies during pregnancy present unique clinical challenges due to the physiological changes in the cardiovascular system and the need to balance maternal and fetal well-being. This chapter provides a comprehensive overview of the management strategies for various cardiac emergencies that can occur in pregnant women, including arrhythmias, heart failure, acute coronary syndrome, venous thromboembolism, aortic dissection, stuck mechanical valves, cardiac arrest, and pulmonary hypertension. The chapter also addresses the role of multidisciplinary teams, the use of diagnostic imaging, and the selection of pharmacological and nonpharmacological interventions that minimize risks to both mother and fetus. Additionally, it explores the implications of delivery timing and mode, as well as postpartum care for patients with cardiac conditions.

Keywords: Pregnancy, cardiac arrest, spontaneous coronary artery dissection, mechanical valve, cardiac emergency

INTRODUCTION

There are multiple hemodynamic changes in response to pregnancy due to the need for increased metabolism. These changes are physiological and help in accommodating the needs of the developing fetus but can also exacerbate preexisting cardiac conditions or reveal undiagnosed cardiac issues. Sometimes, the patients may directly present with a cardiac emergency, which can be life-threatening if not recognized and managed appropriately in time.

PHYSIOLOGIC CHANGES IN PREGNANCY

It is important to know the physiological changes during pregnancy in order to understand the pathophysiology of common cardiac emergencies during pregnancy. **Table 1** summarizes the important cardiovascular adaptations during pregnancy.

TABLE 1: Cardiovascular adaptations in pregnancy.

Adaptation	Change	Clinical Implications
Cardiac output	Increases	This supports increased metabolic demands but may exacerbate heart failure in women with preexisting conditions
Systemic vascular resistance	Decreases	It can lead to hypotension; important in conditions like aortic stenosis
Heart rate	Increases	It may worsen tachyarrhythmias or precipitate new arrhythmias
Plasma volume	Increases	It helps meet the increased oxygen and nutrient demands
Red blood cell (RBC) mass	Increases. However, the increase in plasma volume is much more than increased RBC mass	It leads to dilutional anemia
Autonomic nervous system changes	Enhanced sympathetic activity	It helps in maintenance of blood pressure despite the vasodilatory effects of pregnancy

DIFFERENT CONDITIONS PRESENTING AS CARDIAC EMERGENCIES DURING PREGNANCY

Heart Failure in Pregnancy

It can be attributed to several factors, including preexisting cardiomyopathies, valvular heart disease, ischemic heart disease, and peripartum cardiomyopathy (PPCM). The majority of heart failure (HF) diagnoses are made in the postpartum period, with a considerable number of cases occurring as late as 5–12 months after delivery.[1] The PPCM is characterized by left ventricular (LV) systolic dysfunction during the last month of pregnancy or in the first 5 months after delivery in the absence of any obvious cause and known preexisting heart disease.

It is crucial to distinguish between HF and normal pregnancy symptoms that mimic HF. Echocardiography remains the gold standard for assessing cardiac function, while biomarkers like NT-proBNP can aid in diagnosis.

The management of HF during pregnancy is challenging due to the limited safety profile of many cardiovascular drugs and the need to balance maternal and fetal well-being. The management is summarized in **Table 2**.

Mode of delivery: Vaginal delivery is generally preferred, but cesarean section may be necessary in cases of significant hemodynamic instability.

Mitral stenosis (MS) due to rheumatic heart disease (RHD) is an important cause of acute pulmonary edema during pregnancy. Patients with known RHD may present with exacerbation of dyspnea during pregnancy or sometimes, the disease may be diagnosed for the first time during pregnancy. Moderate-to-severe MS is poorly tolerated during pregnancy. An increase in heart rate reduces diastolic filling time, resulting in elevated pulmonary hypertension (PH) and pulmonary venous congestion.

Percutaneous transvenous mitral commissurotomy (PTMC) is a safe and effective treatment for rheumatic MS during pregnancy and is generally recommended to be performed after 20 weeks of gestation **(Figs. 1A and B)**.

Cardiac Arrest in Pregnancy

Same principles of resuscitation are to be followed for cardiac arrest as in nonpregnant patients. There are a few special points that need to be considered and have been mentioned as follows:

- In women in the later stages of pregnancy, an emergency cesarean section, also known as perimortem cesarean delivery (PMCD) should be considered within 4 minutes of maternal collapse if there is no return of spontaneous circulation (ROSC). Fetus should be delivered ideally within 5 minutes. It has been shown to improve both maternal and fetal survival.
- Airway management is more challenging during pregnancy due to increased vascularity, which leads to upper airway edema.
- Ventilation volumes may need adjustment because of higher position of the diaphragm.
- Chest compressions should be done at a relatively higher level on the sternum if the uterus is enlarged.
- The uterus can compress the inferior vena cava (IVC), potentially disrupting maternal hemodynamics and complicating resuscitation efforts. An effective technique is to place a wedge under the pregnant patient's side to laterally displace the uterus, thereby reducing compression on both the aorta and IVC.
- *Role of left uterine displacement (LUD):* Manually displacing the uterus to the left also increases preload by relieving pressure on the IVC.
- A broad range of potential causes for the cardiac arrest should be considered and underlying cause should be treated.

TABLE 2: Management of heart failure in pregnancy.

Treatment	Indications	Considerations
Diuretics (e.g., furosemide)	Fluid overload and pulmonary congestion	Safe in pregnancy; monitor for electrolyte imbalance
Beta-blockers (e.g., metoprolol)	Rate control and hypertension	Safe; caution in bradycardia or asthma
ACE Inhibitors/ARBs	Not recommended	Contraindicated due to teratogenic effects
Vasodilators	To reduce preload and afterload	Nitroglycerin can be used cautiously
Bromocriptine	In peripartum cardiomyopathy	Useful as an adjunctive treatment—data from small studies
Hydralazine	To decrease afterload	Can be used in heart failure until delivery
Spironolactone	Should be avoided	Potential to cause masculinization of female fetuses
Inotropes	Reserved for cases of severe decompensation	Caution is required due to the potential for arrhythmias
Mechanical circulatory support: Intra-aortic balloon pumps or left ventricular assist devices	Can be used in refractory cases	Typically used as a bridge to definitive therapy or delivery

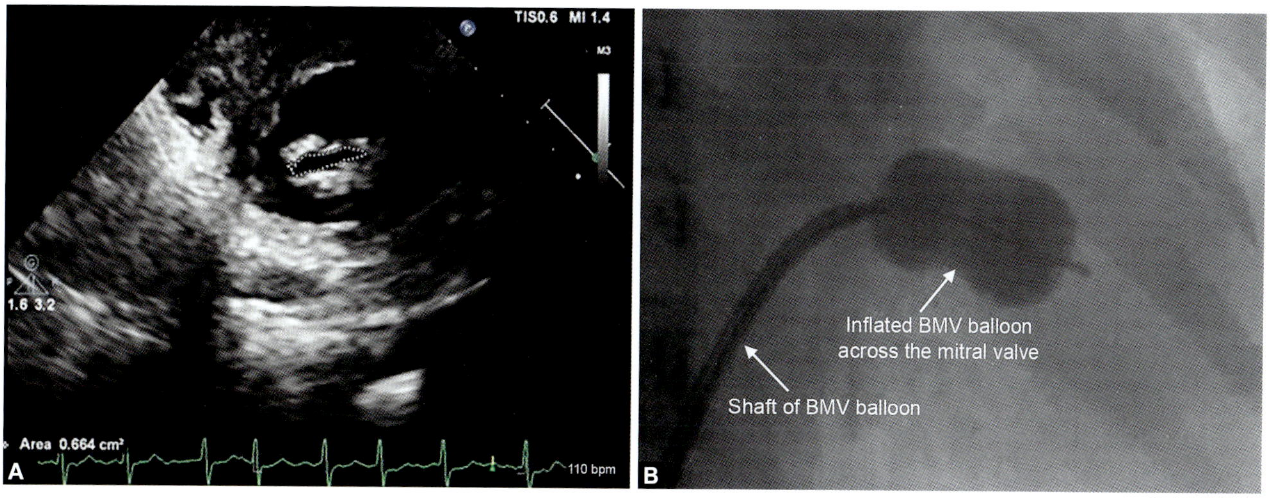

FIGS. 1A AND B: Severe mitral stenosis presenting with pulmonary edema during pregnancy, which was treated with emergency percutaneous transvenous mitral commissurotomy (PTMC).

Arrhythmias in Pregnancy

Arrhythmias are relatively common in pregnancy due to the increased sympathetic activity and altered hemodynamics. Supraventricular tachycardia (SVT) is the most frequently encountered arrhythmia, but ventricular tachycardia (VT) can also occur, particularly in women with structural heart disease.

Hemodynamically Stable Arrhythmias

Vagal maneuvers, adenosine, or beta-blockers are used for arrhythmias dependent on the AV node.

In case where recurrence rate is high, such as rheumatic MS with atrial fibrillation, rate control may be achieved with a beta-blocker, verapamil, or in rare cases, digoxin.

- *Beta-blockers*: Safe and effective for rate control
- *Calcium channel blockers*: Can be used in cases of SVT
- *Antiarrhythmics*: Amiodarone should be avoided due to potential fetal thyroid dysfunction.
- *Catheter ablation*: Can be considered after the first trimester in refractory cases

Hemodynamically Unstable Arrhythmias

Immediate cardioversion: Electric cardioversion is safe and should be performed without delay in cases of life-threatening arrhythmias during pregnancy irrespective of the period of gestation.

During cardioversion, continuous fetal monitoring should be done.

Ablation of the arrhythmia substrate can be used in refractory cases **(Fig. 2)**.

Acute Coronary Syndromes in Pregnancy

Acute coronary syndromes (ACS) occur relatively rarely in pregnancy but can have devastating outcomes and can lead to a rapidly worsening clinical condition, posing risk of heart failure, cardiogenic shock, and malignant arrhythmias.

The pathophysiology often differs from nonpregnant populations, with a higher incidence of spontaneous coronary artery dissection (SCAD) and thromboembolism. Pregnancy-associated spontaneous coronary artery dissection (P-SCAD) can happen during or after pregnancy, with a significant majority of cases (over 70%) occurring postpartum, most frequently within the 1st week after delivery.[2]

This timing suggests that the physiological changes associated with pregnancy, delivery, and the postpartum period might contribute to the vulnerability of the coronary arteries. These changes can include hormonal fluctuations, increased blood volume, and the physical stress of labor, all of which can impact the cardiovascular system.

However, SCAD can happen as early as 2 weeks into pregnancy. It usually affects the left coronary artery territory but can occasionally involve multiple vessels.

Compared to SCAD unrelated to pregnancy, SCAD in pregnancy presents more severely, with impaired left ventricular function, shock, and a higher incidence of left main and multivessel dissections.[3]

Salient features of ACS management in pregnancy:

- Aortic dissection or pulmonary embolism (PE) should be ruled out in pregnant patients with suspected ACS.
- Unfractionated heparin and aspirin can be safely given to the pregnant patient.
- Management of SCAD is similar to that of nonpregnant patients. Decreasing the vessel stress by decreasing the heart rate and blood pressure is of utmost importance. Heparin should be avoided in cases of SCAD. Given the potential for worsening the condition, medications like glycoprotein IIb/IIIa inhibitors and fibrinolytics are contraindicated.

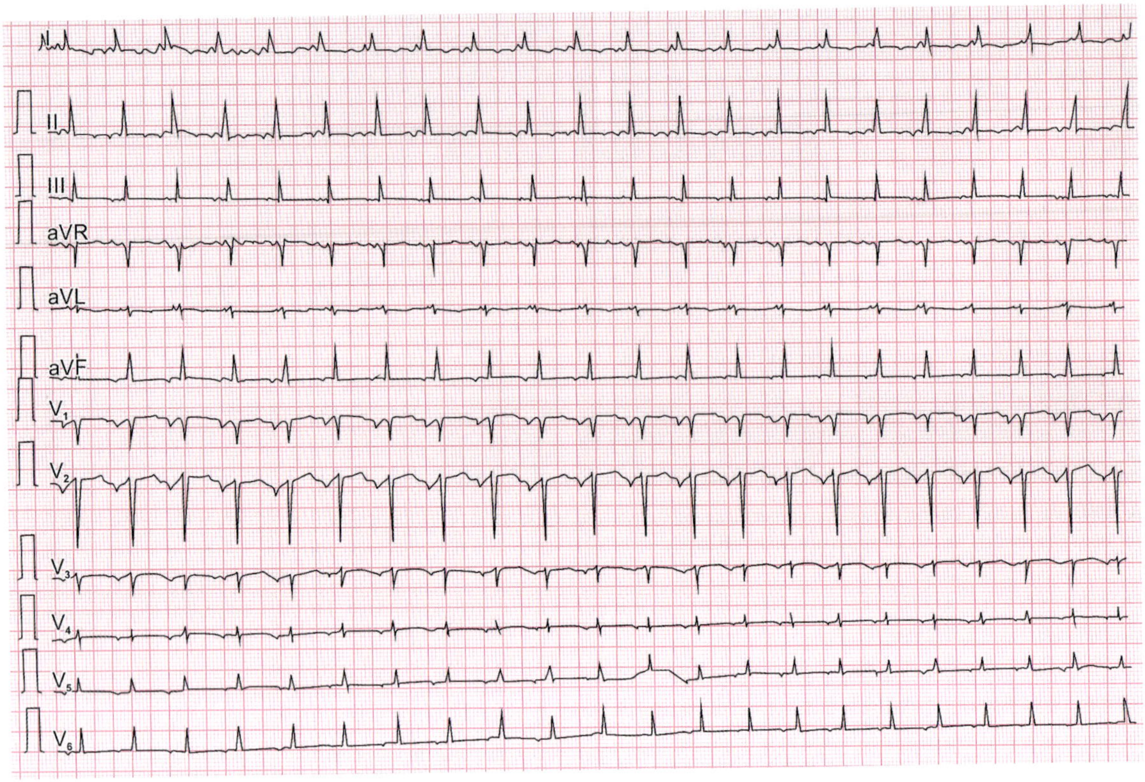

FIG. 2: ECG showing narrow complex tachycardia with P waves that were inverted in V_1–V_3 with late precordial transition and positive P waves in inferior leads suggestive of ectopic atrial tachycardia with likely origin from superior tricuspid annulus. This patient presented with tachycardia-induced cardiomyopathy and incessant tachycardia leading to intrauterine death of the fetus. Successful ablation led to the resolution of symptoms.

- Most cases of stable SCAD heal on their own, favoring a conservative approach. Surgical consultation may be rarely necessary.
- In cases where two antiplatelets are needed, clopidogrel is regarded as safe but should be used for the shortest duration possible.
- Safety and efficacy data on other antiplatelets such as bivalirudin, prasugrel, ticagrelor, and glycoprotein IIb/IIIa inhibitors is limited. Hence, they should not be used.
- Beta-blockers are safe, though some effects on fetal growth have been observed.
- Thrombolysis is relatively contraindicated during pregnancy. Thrombolysis is generally not advised if SCAD is suspected, due to the heightened risk of hemorrhage and potential progression of the dissection.
- Thrombolysis is also contraindicated in patients with placenta previa or those nearing term. However, successful treatment of hemodynamically-significant PE has been reported when administered well before delivery.
- Percutaneous coronary intervention (PCI) is indicated for ongoing ischemia or hemodynamic instability; minimizing radiation exposure is important.
- In SCAD, stenting is typically considered only if the symptoms are refractory to medical treatment or if the patient is hemodynamically unstable due to a flow-limiting lesion. Aggressive manipulation in the presence of a dissection can lead to progression of the dissection. Continuous monitoring is essential during interventions.

Aortic Dissections in Pregnancy

The increased hemodynamic stress of pregnancy, especially during the third trimester, can precipitate dissection, particularly in women with connective tissue disorders like Marfan syndrome, uncontrolled hypertension, and women with bicuspid aortic valve. Maximum risk is in the third trimester and the peripartum period.

In patients who present with severe chest or back pain, differential blood pressure between arms, pericardial effusion, aortic regurgitation, and stroke are important diagnostic clues to the presence of dissection.

Urgent CT angiography with abdominal shielding or echocardiography (in some cases where dissection flap is clearly visible) is needed for diagnosis.

- *Type A dissection:* Requires emergency surgical repair
- *Type B dissection:* Managed conservatively unless complications develop; thoracic endovascular aortic repair can be done in selected cases **(Fig. 3)**.
- *Blood pressure control:* Beta-blockers are first line to reduce aortic wall stress.

Cesarean section may be preferred to reduce hemodynamic stress.

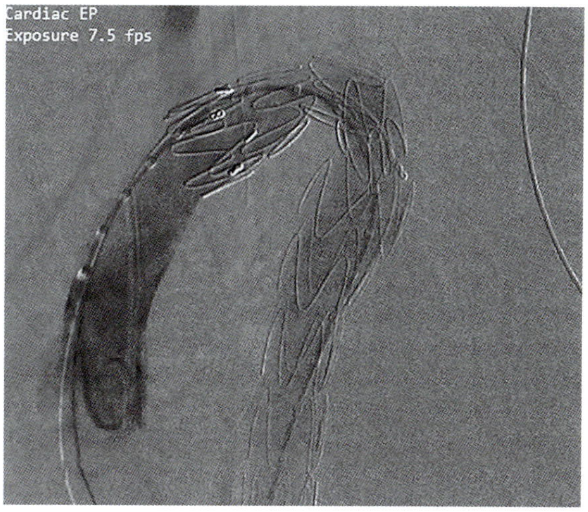

FIG. 3: Emergency thoracic endovascular aortic repair (TEVAR) for a patient presenting with aortic dissection during pregnancy.

Venous Thromboembolism in Pregnancy

There is an increased risk of venous thromboembolism (VTE) during pregnancy. Peak incidence is seen in the peripartum period.

It should be suspected when patient presents with unilateral leg swelling, pain, and redness (for DVT); or with dyspnea and chest pain (for PE).

- *D-dimer testing:* Elevated levels are expected in pregnancy; used primarily to rule out VTE. It has a high negative predictive value but low positive predictive value.
- *Imaging:* Ultrasound for DVT and CT pulmonary angiography (CTPA) for suspected PE is done, with appropriate shielding to minimize fetal radiation exposure.
- *Management:*
    - *Anticoagulation:* Low molecular weight heparin (LMWH) is the preferred anticoagulant due to its safety profile during pregnancy (class 1).
    - Direct oral anticoagulants are not recommended in pregnancy (class 3).
    - *Thrombolysis:* It is considered in life-threatening PE with hemodynamic instability but is used cautiously due to the risk of bleeding. Thrombolytic therapy carries a considerable risk of placental hemorrhage and fetal mortality, despite the fact that alteplase does not cross the placenta. As a result, it is typically reserved for severe cases involving hemodynamic instability.
    - After delivery, consider transitioning LMWH to warfarin or direct oral anticoagulants (DOACs) depending on breastfeeding status and patient preference. Warfarin can be used during breastfeeding while there is no evidence about the use of DOACs during breastfeeding.
    - In high-risk women, LMWH should be converted to unfractionated heparin (UFH) at least 36 hours prior to delivery and UFH infusion should be stopped 4–6 hours before anticipated delivery.
    - Induction or cesarean section should be performed 24 hours after the last dose of LMWH in low-risk women on LMWH.
    - Planned delivery around 39 weeks should be considered to avoid the risk of spontaneous labor while fully anticoagulated.

Management of Prosthetic Heart Valves

Women with mechanical heart valves need continuous anticoagulation and are at risk for valve thrombosis or hemorrhage. Thromboembolism in mother, acute prosthetic valve dysfunction, and acute bleeding in the mother or fetus may occur.

Vitamin K antagonists (VKAs) carry risks such as miscarriage or embryopathy when exposed during the first trimester.

Different Strategies for Pregnant Women with Prosthetic Heart Valves on Vitamin K Antagonists[4]

- Women with prosthetic heart valves (PMHV) and low-dose VKA (warfarin <5 mg/day or acenocoumarol <2 mg/day)
    - *Pre-pregnancy:* Continue VKA until pregnancy is confirmed.
    - *First trimester:*
        - *Option 1:* Continue VKA with monitoring of INR at least every 14 days (class 2A).
        - *Option 2:* Switch to iUFH IV UFH with aPTT >2× control (class 2B).
        - *Option 3:* Switch to LMWH twice daily with close monitoring (class 2B).
    - *Second and third trimesters:*
        - Continue VKA with INR monitoring (class 2A).
        - For those on heparin, switch back to VKA, monitoring INR at least every 2 weeks (class 2A).
    - *At 36 weeks:* Switch to IV UFH or LMWH with close monitoring.
    - *36 hours before planned delivery:* Switch to IV UFH (aPTT >2× control).
    - *Delivery:* Stop UFH 4–6 hours before delivery and restart 4–6 hours after delivery if there is no bleeding.
- *Women with PMHV and high-dose VKA (Warfarin >5 mg/day or acenocoumarol >2 mg/day):*
  Continue VKA antagonist until pregnancy is confirmed.
    - *First trimester:*
        - *Option 1:* Continue VKA with INR monitoring at least every 14 days (class 2B).
        - *Option 2:* Switch to IV UFH with aPTT >2× control (class 2A).
        - *Option 3:* Switch to LMWH twice daily with close monitoring (class 2A).
    - *Second and third trimesters:*
        - Continue VKA with INR monitoring (class 2A).

- For those on heparin, switch back to VKA (with INR monitoring every 2 weeks) (class 2A). OR continue LMWH twice daily with close monitoring (class 2B)
  - *At 36 weeks:* Switch to IV UFH or LMWH with close monitoring.
  - *36 hours before planned delivery:* Switch to IV UFH (aPTT > 2× control).
  - *Delivery:* Stop UFH 4–6 hours before delivery and restart 4–6 hours after delivery if there is no bleeding.

Cesarean section may be recommended for women with mechanical heart valves to minimize the risk of hemorrhage.

Anti-Xa levels should be monitored for LMWH and INR should be monitored for warfarin to avoid complications.

Management of Patients with Prosthetic Heart Valve Thrombosis

Increased transvalvular gradient across the valves during pregnancy may simply be due to the increased cardiac output and does not necessarily indicate valve thrombosis.

Advanced imaging, such as transesophageal echocardiography (TOE), should be considered when necessary. In cases where the diagnosis is uncertain, fluoroscopy to visualize valve leaflet motion can be used. The radiation dose is low, and it is relatively safe during pregnancy.

Treatment: Perform an emergency cesarean section followed by valve surgery if the fetus is viable, or proceed with high-risk surgery without terminating the pregnancy.

Thrombolysis is typically reserved for women with prohibitive surgical risks. Placental hemorrhage, systemic bleeding, embolization of thrombus, and failure of therapy may occur.

Pulmonary Hypertension in Pregnancy

Pulmonary hypertension is poorly tolerated in pregnancy, with deterioration often occurring in the second trimester. Symptoms such as fatigue, dyspnea, syncope, and chest pain usually arise during this time, corresponding to the physiological increase in cardiac output and blood volume. It is associated with a high maternal and fetal mortality and pregnancy is contraindicated in PH due to any cause.

Termination of pregnancy should be considered if any woman with PH becomes pregnant. In women who decide to continue the pregnancy, management is complex, and the following points summarize the management:

- Echocardiography is safe for serially assessing the right ventricular (RV) function.
- *Anticoagulation:* LMWH or unfractionated heparin is recommended for idiopathic and hereditary pulmonary arterial hypertension (PAH) and chronic thromboembolic pulmonary hypertension (CTEPH).
- Low-dose aspirin may be considered to reduce the risk of preeclampsia.
- Calcium channel blockers for patients with a positive vasodilator test are generally well-tolerated during pregnancy and are not linked to teratogenic risks.
- During pregnancy, only prostacyclins and phosphodiesterase type-5 inhibitors are considered safe, endothelin receptor antagonists and guanylate cyclase stimulators are teratogenic.
- Prostaglandins are recommended for patients in WHO functional class III or IV with reduced RV function due to their vasodilator effect, as they may improve RV function.
- Parenteral prostaglandins are recommended for pregnant women with WHO functional class IV and severe RV dysfunction.
- Inhaled iloprost and intravenous treprostinil combined with sildenafil are possible options during pregnancy.
- *Elective delivery* is recommended around 34–36 weeks of pregnancy, with cesarean section being the preferred mode of delivery.
- Vaginal delivery may be safe for some patients with PH associated with congenital heart disease (CHD) and for those in functional class I or II who are well-controlled.
- Routine pulmonary artery (PA) monitoring is not generally recommended during delivery.
- Oxytocin, used to prevent postpartum hemorrhage, may trigger a pulmonary hypertensive crisis, leading to significant systemic hypotension.

CONCLUSION

The management of cardiac emergencies in pregnancy requires a delicate balance between ensuring maternal cardiovascular stability and safeguarding fetal health. This chapter has underscored the complexities involved in diagnosing and treating cardiac conditions in pregnant women, emphasizing the importance of early recognition and prompt intervention. Key to successful outcomes is the integration of a multidisciplinary approach, involving obstetricians, cardiologists, anesthesiologists, and neonatologists, to provide comprehensive care tailored to the unique needs of both mother and fetus.

Pharmacological therapies and surgical interventions must be carefully selected, considering the altered physiological state of pregnancy and potential teratogenic effects. The use of diagnostic tools, while crucial, must be judicious to minimize fetal exposure to ionizing radiation. Continued research and education in this area are essential to further refine management strategies and improve maternal–fetal health.

ONLINE REFERENCES

Please scan the QR code provided at the end of the table of contents for References of this chapter.

CHAPTER

86

Paracardiac Fat, Coronary Calcification, and Postmenopausal Women

Meenakshi Kadiyala, R Rameshwar, SR Sharath Shanmugam

ABSTRACT

Cardiovascular disease (CVD) is a leading cause of morbidity and mortality in women. Gender-related differences are observed in the etiology, symptomatology, outcome, and management of coronary artery disease (CAD). Angina is more common in women than men; women have a lower incidence of obstructive CAD, less eccentric plaques, smaller coronary arteries, more coronary microvascular disease, and endothelial dysfunction. They present later to the doctor than men, undergo less invasive procedures, and have an overall worse prognosis than men. CVD prevalence in women increases after the fifth–sixth decade, indicating the loss of a protective factor after the fifth decade when they attain menopause and lose the beneficial effect of the estrogen, namely, estradiol (E2). This is supported by epidemiological studies where an increased risk of CVD occurs even in women with early-onset menopause, irrespective of the cause. Additional markers are therefore required to redefine cardiac risk-stratification in postmenopausal women.

Keywords: Paracardiac fat, epicardial fat, coronary artery calcification

INTRODUCTION

Early detection of subclinical atherosclerosis is mandatory to prevent the progression of cardiovascular disease (CVD). Important surrogate markers of coronary atherosclerosis are coronary artery calcification (CAC) and heart fat.[1] Several studies, including the MESA and the Framingham Heart Study, have reported that increased cardiac fat deposition is a predictor for CVD in women independent of conventional risk factors. There have been many studies relating body fat with CVD, but its role in postmenopausal women has been sparsely studied.[1,2]

THE CARDIAC FAT DEPOSITS

There are two cardiac fat depots: (1) Epicardial adipose tissue (EAT), which lies within the pericardial sac and closely covers the heart, and (2) the paracardiac adipose tissue (PAT), which lies external to the pericardial sac **(Figs. 1 and 2)**. EAT and PAT have different embryological origins, blood supply, and metabolic activities, and are distinct from each other.[3] EAT originates from the splanchnopleuric mesoderm

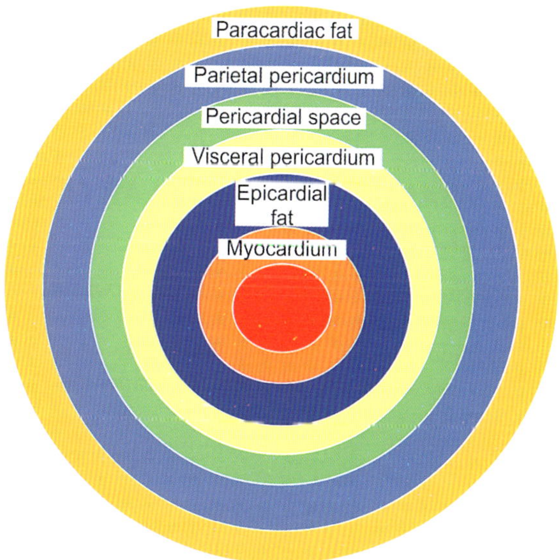

FIG. 1: Diagrammatic representation of the epicardial and paracardiac fat deposits and their relation to the pericardium and myocardium.

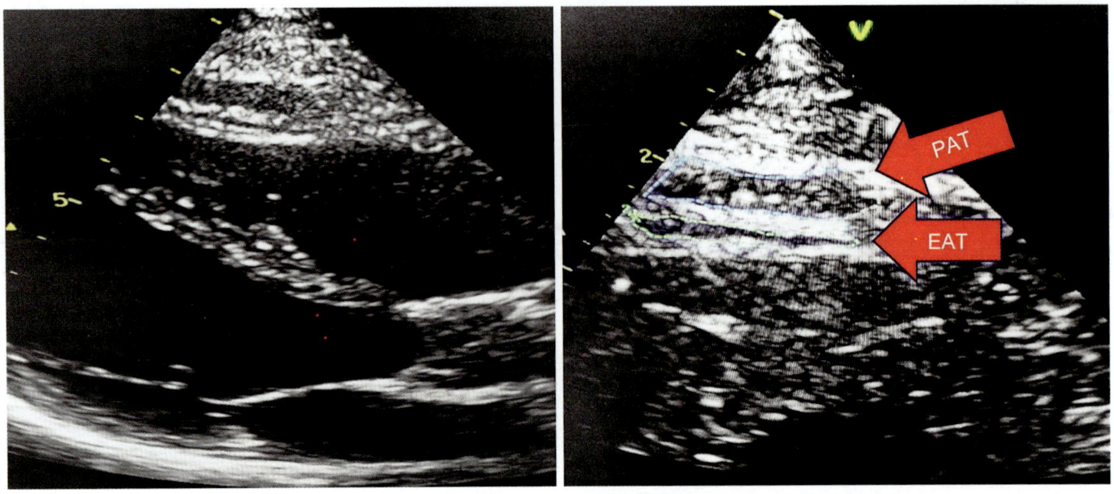

FIG. 2: Parasternal long axis showing the epicardial and paracardiac fat.

and derives its blood supply from the coronary circulation, is metabolically active, and is an energy source for the heart. PAT, on the other hand, has its origin in the primitive thoracic mesenchyme and derives its blood supply from the pericardiophrenic artery.[4]

Heart fat has been thought to be responsible for the pathogenesis of coronary artery disease (CAD) by virtue of its contiguity to the heart and because it secretes anti- and proinflammatory adipokines which are normally in balance, but a tilt in this balance to a proinflammatory milieu can occur when the fat deposit expands.[5]

Greater paracardiac volume results in increased risk of atherosclerosis. Postmenopausal women have larger PAT deposits than premenopausal women probably due to dwindling estrogen levels, raising the speculation whether the cardiac fat deposits could be reduced by exogenous estrogen.[3]

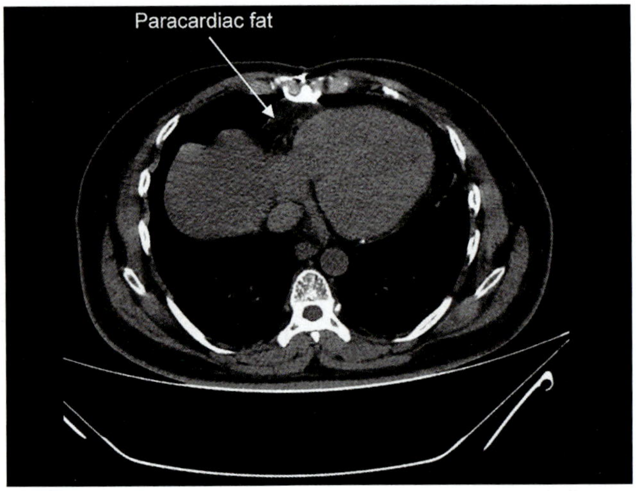

FIG. 3: Computed tomography—arrow showing the paracardiac fat.

THE SWAN CARDIOVASCULAR FAT ANCILLARY STUDY

The SWAN cardiovascular fat ancillary study was designed to assess the relationship between each heart fat depot and CAC in women in midlife and to determine whether this association was altered by menopausal transition and the lower estrogen levels.[4]

Coronary calcification was quantified using the C-150 ultrafast CT scanner, and electron beam CT was used to quantify EAT and PAT **(Figs. 3 and 4)**.

Patients were classified based on frequency and regularity of menstrual bleeding as premenopause, early perimenopause, late perimenopause, and postmenopause.[4]

A 1-SD unit PAT increase was associated with the presence of CAC, which was 80% higher in postmenopausal women compared with pre- or early perimenopausal women. The increase in PAT in postmenopausal women

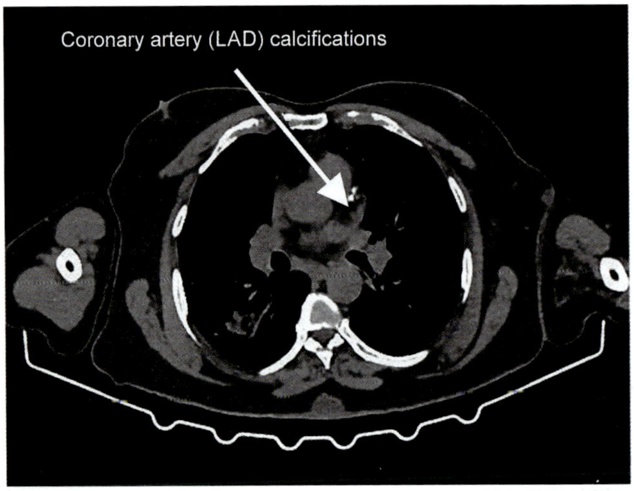

FIG. 4: Computed tomography—arrow showing calcified left anterior descending artery.

was independent of study covariates like age, race, and other CVD risk factors, but was dependent on estrogen levels.[4] PAT was greater and was more pronounced in women with the lowest E2 levels. 20% higher PAT volumes than EAT volumes were found in late peri- and postmenopausal women compared with pre- and early perimenopausal women.[4] Thus, PAT can be considered as a menopause-specific CAD risk marker in women during midlife.

THE ESTROGEN EFFECT

In premenopausal women, estrogen production occurs in the ovaries. After menopause, estrogen is produced in extragonadal organs such as the liver, adipose tissue, brain, and skin.[6] The three main forms of physiological estrogen synthesized are estrone (E1), estradiol [(E2) or 17β-estradiol], and estriol (E3). Estradiol is the most potent estrogen and is the main estrogen in premenopausal women, whereas estrone is the estrogen in postmenopausal women and is three times less potent than E2.[6]

Paracardiac adipose tissue and EAT are distinct fat deposits, and the former but not the latter is influenced by E2 levels. ERα and ERβ are estrogen receptors in human mature white adipocytes, which generally mediate E2 effects.[1,3] ERα is in more abundance than ERβ and plays a vital role in regulating adipose tissue function and protecting it from damage due to inflammation. The function of ERα depends on circulating E2 levels and in the setting of low E2, ERα could bind to other adipocyte function-specific factors, resulting in detrimental metabolic effects and expansion of adipose tissue.[2,3] ERα, is more expressed in PAT than in EAT, and there by any change in levels of E2 can cause changes in PAT rather than EAT volumes.[4]

THE KRONOS EARLY ESTROGEN PREVENTION STUDY

The KEEPS (Kronos Early Estrogen Prevention Study) multicenter, randomized, placebo-controlled trial studied the 48-month progression of subclinical atherosclerosis among 727 early menopausal women, to determine the effects of estrogen on heart fat and indirectly on coronary calcium using 0.45 mg/day oral conjugated equine estrogens in one arm or 50 μg/day transdermal 17β-estradiol in the other arm when compared to placebo.[3] Both arms receiving estrogen also received progesterone. Participants had heart fat and CAC measured at both baseline and after 48 months. Heart fat in CT has a threshold of –190 to –30 Hounsfield units distinguishing it from other heart tissue. CAC was determined by Agatston score as a hyperattenuating lesion >130 Hounsfield units. The total calcification score was the sum of two sequential scans in four major coronary arteries. A baseline CAC score of 0 which increased at 48 months to a CAC score of >0 or a baseline CAC score of >0 but <100 which increased to ≥10 was defined as CAC progression.[3] Oral conjugated equine estrogens had no effect on EAT or PAT accumulation, whereas EAT increased with placebo. Transdermal 17β-estradiol had no effect on EAT but increased progression of CAC associated with an increase in PAT accumulation.[3] This study highlights that exogenous estrogen effects could vary depending on the specific estrogen, dose, and route of administration. The transdermal estrogen used in this trial contains only 17b-estradiol, whereas the oral form consists of 10 natural estrogens including ring B unsaturated estrogens (equilin and equilenin) which are strong antioxidants which were probably responsible for the favorable effect on EAT accumulation. When the preparation has a weak antioxidant effect, there is overexpression of oxidative stress leading to adiposity and its complications.[3] One thinking is that in this trial, transdermal E2 did not raise estrogens adequately to prevent CAC progression and PAT accumulation.[3]

THE NORTH AMERICAN MENOPAUSE SOCIETY

The North American Menopause Society has also reported dissimilarities in estrogen effects based on dose, duration of use, route of administration, timing of initiation, and whether a progestogen is used or not.[3]

HORMONE THERAPY

There are not many clinical trials on the effects of exogenous estrogen on heart fat accumulations in postmenopausal women. On the contrary, there are several clinical trials to evaluate the effects of different hormone therapies (HTs) on CVD with inconsistent reports.

The cardiovascular benefits of HT have been promoted for years. That coronary events in women without previous CVD could be reduced by HT was reported by the Nurse's Health Study.[7] HERS study however reported an increase in nonfatal venous thromboembolism (VTE), myocardial infarction, and ischemic heart disease (IHD) death in the first year and a smaller increase for 3–5 years thereafter when compared to placebo after HT.[7] The SMART study showed significant benefits at 12 months. 22 published studies, mostly in menopausal women over 60 years from the 2017 Cochrane Review found that women on combination HT had an increased risk of IHD, VTE, stroke, breast cancer, biliary disease, and death from lung cancer. Estrogen-only HT was associated with decreased risk of breast cancer and bone fracture with no increased risk of IHD.[7] Exogenous effects of estrogens are most apparent only when the underlying vessel is normal or minimally diseased and its effect is less in more pronounced atherosclerosis.[7] Therefore, from these and a plethora of other studies, no definite conclusion could be drawn on HT for the prevention of CVD.

CACTI STUDY

Coronary artery calcium and incident CVD are more prevalent in type 1 diabetes than adults without T1DM and in diabetic women than men. Women with diabetes have nine times higher CVD risk than nondiabetic women in contrast to diabetic men who have four times higher risk than nondiabetic men.[8]

The CACTI study is the first trial comparing the association of subclinical atherosclerosis in women with and without type 1 diabetes during menopausal transition. The trial concluded that type 1 diabetic women at all ages have higher PAT and CAC compared to women without type 1 diabetes, but this difference was greater after menopause and was not influenced by CVD risk factors.[8]

CONCLUSION

Significant sexual dimorphism in adipose tissue deposition and distribution is seen in postmenopausal women. After menopause, there is redistribution in the adipose tissue to the visceral sites, probably due to the changes in sex hormone concentrations.

Epicardial adipose tissue thickness and volume have been reported to be associated with subclinical atherosclerosis in middle-aged perimenopausal women but are not affected by menopause or E2 levels. PAT volumes and the consequent coronary calcification, on the other hand, increase with menopause, probably due to decreasing E2 levels. Thus, PAT can be considered a menopause-specific CAD risk marker in women during midlife. Further research is however mandatory to confirm this hypothesis. CAC is also a surrogate for subclinical atherosclerosis, and although it may not reflect the extent of soft plaque, it has been shown to be a proxy for future cardiovascular events particularly associated with the expansion of PAT in postmenopausal women. Strategies to reduce heart fat and in particular PAT in women during the menopausal transition can reduce CVD risk. Results with exogeneous HT have not been consistent and are associated with a variety of adverse reactions. Currently, the only indication for HT is to treat menopausal symptoms in early menopause and for the shortest duration and not to protect against CVD. The mist that shrouds the utility of HT mandates the identification of other preventive strategies to reduce PAT expansion and its accomplice CAC in order to reduce CVD risk postmenopause.

ONLINE REFERENCES

Please scan the QR code provided at the end of the table of contents for References of this chapter.

CHAPTER 87

Cardio-Obstetrics as a Subspecialty: How to Start the Program

Justin Paul Gnanaraj, Anne Princy Steaphen, Anish Keepanasseril

ABSTRACT

Cardio-obstetrics is a multidisciplinary approach to care for pregnant women at high risk of cardiovascular disease. This team includes experts from maternal–fetal medicine, cardiology, obstetric anesthesiology, neonatology, nursing, social work, and pharmacy. The goal is to optimize pregnancy outcomes and prevent complications during delivery. The field is crucial to reduce maternal morbidity and mortality and can be incorporated into medical curriculums and programs.

Keywords: Cardio-obstetrics, pregnant women, high risk, complications

INTRODUCTION

Cardio-obstetrics (CO) refers to caring for pregnant women with established or at high risk of cardiovascular (CV) disease in pregnancy under a multidisciplinary, collaborative team to optimize their pregnancy outcomes.[1] This multidisciplinary team (MDT) comprises experts from maternal–fetal medicine or obstetrics, cardiology or internal medicine, obstetric anesthesiology, neonatology, nursing, social work, and pharmacy.[2] The goal is to ensure comprehensive care for these women throughout the pregnancy and postpartum, including planning the delivery to avoid complications for the mother and child. This dedicated team of health professionals is often called the cardio-obstetric team, maternal cardiology team, or pregnancy and heart team.[3]

WHY DO WE NEED CARDIO-OBSTETRICS PROGRAMS?

Improvements in the diagnosis and management of heart disease (HD) in infancy and early childhood increase the burden of preexisting CV disease during pregnancy. In addition, pregnancy can exacerbate an already existing CV illness or can unmask a previously unrecognized disease, adding to this burden. The increasing prevalence of unhealthy lifestyle habits, along with delayed marriages and late conceptions, also contribute to the rising incidence of CV diseases developing during pregnancy and postpartum. CV diseases are a leading cause of indirect cause of maternal mortality, especially in high-income countries.[4,5]

With a reduction in maternal deaths from direct causes following various strategies under the Millennium and Sustainable Developmental Goals (MDG and SDG), low- to middle-income countries are experiencing a gradual shift through the stages of obstetric transition, with an increase in the contribution of CV disease to maternal mortality.[6] Pregnant women with HD are at risk of adverse cardiac events, including mortality. Studies have shown that as much as two-thirds of maternal deaths due to HD could have been prevented by changes in care.[7,8] The presence of metallic prosthetic heart valves, pulmonary hypertension, and heart failure during pregnancy, the three conditions identified by the MPAC registry, to be associated with high risk of maternal mortality in India, need multidisciplinary care to improve pregnancy outcomes.[9]

Further, with improving healthcare in most nations, there is a changing epidemiology of the spectrum of HD in pregnancy, with an increasing proportion of nonrheumatic HDs during pregnancy. Therefore, healthcare systems must improve their expertise and develop the MDT needed to manage complex HDs during pregnancy, with which they were unfamiliar. Hence, nations such as India need to focus on developing CO programs, with all specialists needed for the care of a PWWHD under one umbrella, and enabling them to work together to reduce maternal morbidity and to avoid mortality from HDs. This will contribute toward our nation achieving the SDG 3.1 of maternal mortality ratio of <70 per 100,000 live births.

HOW TO START A CARDIO-OBSTETRIC PROGRAM?

Before venturing into starting a CO program, evaluating human resources and the infrastructure availability in the institution/hospital is essential. The key component of any CO program is the availability of a team with expertise in managing the various stages of pregnancy and optimizing the cardiac condition to avoid developing adverse cardiac events. The complexity of a condition determines the specialties needed to manage a PWWHD, which may comprise a cardiologist, maternal–fetal medicine specialist, obstetrician, intensivist, neonatologist, or obstetric–anesthesiologist. Each team member's participation level and the frequency of prenatal visits can be individualized on a case-to-case basis.

Step 1: Evaluation of the Availability of Health Human Resources to Form a Cardio-Obstetrics Team

Developing a successful CO service relies heavily on multidisciplinary care. First, it is prudent to determine which level of care the hospital or institution belongs to. A CO team can be formed with available specialists or healthcare providers based on their interest in CO. Every team member must understand the team's purpose and functionality. The team can plan the timing and mode of transfer of PWWHD's care to a higher care center if deemed necessary.

Medical Colleges or Tertiary Care Setting

In tertiary care centers, the CO team can include cardiologists and obstetricians with interest and expertise in CO, obstetric anesthetists, intensivists, nursing specialists, neonatologists/pediatricians, cardiothoracic surgeons, etc. Specialists need to be chosen to be a part of the team based on the complexity of the HD in the patients, and they ought to supplement each other in the planning of their care.

Human Resource-limited Healthcare Setting

In settings where all specialists are unavailable, the CO team can be formed with a cardiologist, an obstetrician, an anesthetist, and a pediatrician. In the absence of a cardiologist, an internist with a special interest or expertise in managing pregnant women with cardiac lesions can be part of the team along with others. Remote support from a cardiologist is an important addition to this setting.

Step 2: Development of Necessary Infrastructure for the Functioning of the Cardio-Obstetrics Team

The obstetrics and cardiology departments should develop infrastructure to manage high-risk deliveries and antennal intervention when necessary. The proximity of the two departments can aid in reducing the transfer in time in case of emergencies. CO special clinics or high-risk pregnancy clinics should be conducted where the specialists sit together periodically and as needed to plan management for complex HD. The provision of ECG and echocardiography facilities in the high-risk labor ward, obstetric ICU, and obstetric theater helps improve care. In addition, the institution should ensure the availability of all pharmaceutical agents and investigations to manage high-risk HD during pregnancy. In the absence of CO clinics, periodic MDT meetings with experts can be called for or should be conducted on an on-call basis, based on the admission of a pregnant lady with complex HD. In the absence of a particular infrastructure, the risk assessments of the patients should be conducted at an earlier visit, and a timely referral to an institution nearby for a shared care approach with inputs from the CO team may aid in optimizing the outcomes.

Step 3: Enabling Interdisciplinary Collaboration

Ensure good communication and coordination exists between CO team members of the different disciplines. The creation of online CO communities/social media groups involving the CO team coordinator of the institution enables ease of communication between the specialists. This can be a shared closed group platform to discuss the management of patients. This could be used to plan the antepartum cardiac optimization and delivery, as well as intra- and postpartum monitoring. In addition, regular CO grand rounds or case discussions can help to enhance professional skills and team building in CO. The state governments can play a proactive role by mandating formation of CO teams in all tertiary care hospitals in the state, managing high-risk pregnancies, to instruct for formation of CO team in all its institutions and to enable interdisciplinary collaboration. The Government of Tamil Nadu showed the way by instructing all Government Medical Colleges in the state to form CO team.[10]

Step 4: Identification of the Roles and Responsibilities Involved in the Management of PWWHD

The CO team members have to understand the role they fulfill in patient care from preconception counseling through the postpartum period, not limited to the following:

Preconception

- Risk stratification for women with known cardiac disease before
- Optimize the patient's cardiac condition through appropriate medical, surgical, or interventional therapies.
- Evaluate and discontinue unsafe medications for women planning pregnancy, if any.
- Engage in discussions with the patient to understand her reproductive goals and provide tailored counseling.

- Educate the patient about her cardiac condition and make her aware of potential warning signs.
- Counsel the woman about what to expect during pregnancy and the best place for pregnancy care.
- Provide advice on suitable contraception methods during the prepregnancy and interconception periods.

Postconception

- Continue risk stratification and counseling after conception.
- Prescribe the timing and frequency of antenatal visits.
- Offer guidance on medical termination of pregnancy, if necessary.
- Advise on appropriate management for HD during pregnancy.
- Provide counseling and management for newly diagnosed or developed HD during pregnancy.
- Create a delivery plan, including the mode and timing of delivery, anesthesia, and analgesia.
- Anticipate and address cardiac complications that may arise during pregnancy.

Post-termination of Pregnancy

- Provide advice on lactation while optimizing cardiac drug usage
- Offer guidance on suitable contraception methods.
- Deliver counseling and lifestyle recommendations to optimize long-term CV health for women who have experienced adverse pregnancy outcomes (APOs).

General Responsibilities

- Review of medications by the various specialists is critical because each specialty can balance the risks and benefits of treatments during pregnancy and lactation.
- For patients living far away from a center with a CO team, detailed antepartum care and delivery plans must be developed to avoid unplanned delivery at a hospital with fewer resources and for timely referral.
- Organize weekly clinics, interdisciplinary case-based discussions, and maternal death audits, which can achieve better comprehensive coordination among the team members.
- Organize periodic review of potential metrics for quality assessment and improvement like rate of adverse cardiac events, maternal deaths attributed to cardiac lesions, and perinatal losses or complications among mothers with HD.

Step 5: Development of Standard Operating Procedures, Management Guidelines, and Risk Stratification Tools

The currently available guidelines to manage PWWHD are from high-income countries, which do not consider the limited resources setting in countries such as India.[11,12] Based on its infrastructure and HR facility, each institution can develop its own SOP, managing various HDs until a national or state protocol is developed and made available. A national evidence-based, resource-sensitive, culturally appropriate, easily adaptable protocol needs to be developed.

Prioritizing the patient's care using standardized risk stratification instruments is essential. This would include the modified World Health Organization risk stratification, the CARPREG scores, and other indigenous risk stratification tools such as the MPAC and DEVI scores.[13] The care can be tailored according to the patient's needs which the CO team can decide.

Step 6: Encouraging Research in the Field of Cardio-Obstetrics

There is an increasing need to conduct research focusing on PWWHD, addressing pathogenic factors, implementing initiatives for quality improvement, and discovering viable treatments in Indian settings. In addition, a multicenter registry is needed to collect CVD management data before, during, and after pregnancy. The creation of registries can be a source of quality improvement initiatives that can identify and address disparities in maternal and postpartum morbidity and mortality, as well as long-term outcomes and help understand the profile and outcomes of pregnancies in women with various HDs, risk stratification tools, and management protocols. Funding agencies should encourage research studies and registries in CO.

Step 7: Improving Training and Education

Cardiology, obstetrics, and anesthesia training programs should include mandatory CO teaching hours. Learning objectives and teaching content should be prepared, and an exclusive curriculum for fellowships in CO should be developed. Davis et al. have identified three levels of training in CO for cardiology fellows in training (FIT).[14] Level I training aims to gain basic exposure and understanding of CO and is a must for all FIT. It should be included as a part of the routine cardiology curriculum. Level II training aims to provide about 3–6 months of practical clinical experience and practical knowledge. Level III training is more advanced and provides 6–12 months of practical training and leads to CO fellowships. Expected core competencies have been identified for each level of training. This must be modified appropriately and integrated into our academic and clinical settings. Similar training levels and core competencies must be identified and prepared for linked disciplines of obstetrics, anesthesia, and maternal-fetal medicine.

Multidisciplinary grand rounds in CO should be encouraged. Collaborative sessions during national societal meetings and workshops on CO should be organized to share knowledge and aid team building. Forums for complex case presentations involving the management of PWWHD, highlighting the challenges faced, should be set up. Continued medical education and training should be provided to the CO team members, including nurses and paramedics involved in the care of PWWHD. The training should include education on the guidelines and protocols involved in the management of PWWHD, risk stratification, triaging, and follow-up of the PWWHD.

Step 8: Advocacy and Professional Societies Partnerships

Medical, paramedical, nursing personnel, councils, medical universities, health administrators, political leaders, news and print media, and the general public must be made aware about the need to develop CO as a subspecialty in India. Governmental agencies and central and state health societies should render all possible support in developing this field. The formation of patient support groups and identification of patient ambassadors in this field should be encouraged. Organizations, societies and associations of cardiology, and obstetrics and obstetric anesthesia can be more involved in formulating policies, creating educational initiatives, and facilitating the widespread dissemination of knowledge and expertise in CO.

Enhancing institutional support for expectant mothers through health policy is necessary to improve CO care. Cardiologists and obstetricians with expertise and interest in CO should focus on developing collaborations with each other, and together, they should seek support from professional societies, patient support groups, healthcare institutions, and health policymakers for the cause of CO in our nation. Social media platforms can be utilized to spread research articles, recommendations, best practices, and awareness in CO.

Enhancing the CV health and well-being of mothers throughout and after pregnancy is a responsibility that should be reflected in our clinical practices, policies, and systems. Even while the requirements mentioned above may be easier to establish in a medical college or tertiary care setting, they would continue to be challenging in a limited resource setting. The processes for establishing a cardio-obstetric unit can be tailored to the infrastructure and the available human resources, which should define the scope of CO care offered in such settings and should have a policy of a timely referral or remote support from a specialized CO team.

CONCLUSION

The growing frequency of HDs during pregnancy makes it imperative that we advance the field of cardiac obstetrics to lower maternal morbidity/mortality from these conditions by increasing medical professionals' understanding of this subject. This can be achieved by incorporating CO into the curriculum and motivating medical students to perform research in this field to expand their knowledge. A CO program can be established in any setting if the members are committed and interested in this field to provide dedicated care to pregnant women with HD.

ONLINE REFERENCES

Please scan the QR code provided at the end of the table of contents for References of this chapter.

SECTION 9

Congenital Heart Disease

Section Outline

CHAPTER

88

Cardiovascular Symptom Assessment and Interpretation

SK Dwivedi, Ayush Shukla, Umesh Tripathi

ABSTRACT

History taking is the first and most important step in cardiovascular evaluation of a patient with suspected cardiac disease. Chest pain, breathlessness, fatigue, palpitation, edema, and syncope are common presenting symptoms, in isolation or in combination. Their systematic evaluation may give an insight into underlying cardiovascular etiology, pathophysiology, severity, functional limitation, prognosis, and course of treatment. An analysis of symptoms at each step of management results in comprehensive care of patients for the best outcome.

Keywords: Symptoms, interpretation, angina, dyspnea, palpitations, syncope, fatigue, edema, NYHA class, hemodynamics, pathophysiology

"Listen to your patient. He is telling you the diagnosis."

—William Osler

INTRODUCTION

In a patient with a known or suspected cardiovascular disease, a detailed history is invaluable, the depth and duration of which depends on the clinical context and severity. Personal face-to-face interaction is superior to online sessions in developing trust between physician and patient, which is integral for comprehensive care. Current cardiology practice is shifting toward symptom-centric investigations for rapid assessment, but it can never surpass the importance and relevance of a good skillfully taken detailed history. A good history, if assessed with the clinical context, can help decipher underlying cardiac pathophysiology, etiopathogenesis, course of treatment, and prognosis. Interpretation of cardiac symptoms is also very useful in triaging and quick management of patients coming to the emergency room, which can be lifesaving.

Symptoms in clinical cardiology can be broadly divided into those that occur frequently and have a dynamic course or some uncommon symptoms that do have importance but are not very specific. Major cardinal symptoms are chest discomfort, dyspnea, fatigue, edema, palpitations, and syncope.[1] This chapter describes these cardinal symptoms, how to assess them, and their interpretations.

CHEST DISCOMFORT

Chest discomfort or chest pain is one of the most frequent reasons for a patient to visit the emergency department for suspected acute coronary syndrome (ACS), but on evaluation, only 5–15% of patients actually have ACS.[1] The most serious cause of chest pain is myocardial ischemia or infarction, and physicians should always aim not to miss this diagnosis. Ischemic chest pain or angina pectoris is described as heaviness, pressure, squeezing, burning sensation, difficulty in breathing, and a sense of impending doom with or without excessive diaphoresis. This may be an isolated symptom or in combination with other symptoms. Location, duration, radiation, character, aggravating and relieving factors, reproducibility, and gesture at the presentation are important while assessing the symptoms. Anginal pain often radiates to the left shoulder, neck, and mostly the ulnar aspect of the left arm, below the jawline, or at the epigastrium. Pain originating above the jawline or predominantly in the abdomen is unlikely to be angina. Intensity is crescendo over 1–2 minutes and can be triggered by emotional or physical stress, usually decreasing after a few minutes. Pain lasting for a few hours or a few seconds indicates nonischemic etiology. Anginal pain is diffuse rather than being localized, worsened by exertion and relieved by rest and/or sublingual nitroglycerin. Pain that is localized and pinpointing is nonanginal. Past history of angina, if present, is important as subsequent ischemic pain presents with similar pain characteristics. Repetitive chest pain with shifting location is unlikely to be cardiac in origin.

Patients may not present as classical angina but "angina equivalent" with isolated shoulder or jaw pain, or stress-induced breathlessness or fatigue, or profuse diaphoresis. There may be atypical presentations with gastrointestinal symptoms such as nausea and vomiting, epigastric discomfort, flatulence, dyspepsia, or bloating. These atypical presentations are more common in the elderly, females, and diabetics.

Angina pectoris can be classified as follows:[2]

- *Stable angina*: Angina precipitated on exertion and relieved at rest or with nitrates. These patients are hemodynamically stable most of the time. Angina is generally not very severe.
- *Unstable angina*: It is a nonhomogeneous group based on variable presentation: (1) Angina at rest, (2) recent onset (<2 months) angina, and (3) crescendo pattern with more severity, precipitated by less exertion, longer duration, and more frequent than previous episodes.
- *Prinzmetal angina*: Usually occurs at rest in a cyclical pattern at night, due to coronary spasm.[3]
- *Nocturnal angina*: Angina occurring at night is usually seen in aortic regurgitation or may suggest a critical narrowing of the coronary artery supplying a very large area, for example, ostial LAD or left main.[4]
- *Postprandial angina*: Symptoms occurring after taking food may suggest severe left main artery disease or major vessel ostial disease.[5]
- *Angina mimickers*: These are a variety of chest pains that are nonischemic, and it is imperative to distinguish them from ischemic pain. Various causes and their differentiating features are mentioned in **Table 1**.[6]

Assessment of Severity of Angina

After relevant information is obtained from history, it is essential to categorize it into functional classes based on exercise intensity. Although no threshold of minimum extent of ischemic myocardium for angina is defined, the severity of coronary narrowing in large epicardial coronary vessels often directly correlates with the level of exertion precipitating cardiac ischemia. There are various classification systems described in literature,[7-9] but none is perfect. They are based on subjective or objective level of exertion, resulting

TABLE 1: Differential diagnosis of chest discomfort.

System involved	Syndrome	Clinical features	Distinguishing features
Vascular	• Aortic dissection • Pulmonary embolism	• Sudden onset of severe ripping pain starting from chest, along course of aortic vessels, often radiating to the back • Sudden onset (predominantly) of dyspnea with pleuritic pain	• Usually occurs in the setting of hypertension or Marfan syndrome • Signs of right-sided heart failure present
Pulmonary	• Pleuritis or pneumonitis • Spontaneous pneumothorax	• Pleuritic pain, usually brief over the involved area • Abrupt onset of rapidly increasing dyspnea	• Pain varying with respiratory cycle • Associated with pain in the lateral chest wall
Gastrointestinal	• Esophageal reflux • Peptic ulcer • Gall bladder disease • Pancreatitis	• Burning substernal and epigastric discomfort, 10–60 minutes duration • Prolonged epigastric burning • Prolonged right upper quadrant pain • Prolonged, intense epigastric and substernal pain	• More prominent on lying down after meals • Relieved by antacid or food • May be limited only to abdomen • May be limited to abdomen and back mostly due to alcoholism or gallstones
Musculoskeletal	• Costochondritis • Cervical disc disease • Trauma or strain	• Sudden onset of intense fleeting pain • Sudden onset of fleeting pain • Constant pain	• Localized pain, may be reproduced by pressure over the affected costochondral joint • Reproduced with movements of the neck • Reproduced by palpation or movement of the chest wall or arms
Infectious	Herpes zoster	Prolonged burning pain in a dermatomal distribution	Typical skin changes and hypersensitivity seen
Psychological	Panic disorder	Chest tightness and dyspnea for 30 minutes or more, unrelated to exertion or movement	Patients may have other emotional disorders

TABLE 2: A comparison of various functional classifications.

Class	NYHA classification*	CCS classification†	Specific activity scale‡
I	• Ordinary physical activity does not produce symptoms • No limitation of activity • Comfortable at rest	• Ordinary physical activity does not cause angina • Strenuous activity produces angina	Physical activity of >7 METs does not cause symptoms
II	• Ordinary physical activity produces symptoms • Slight limitation of activity • Comfortable at rest	• Walking >2 blocks or climbing >1 flight of stairs produce angina • Slight limitation of ordinary activity	Patient can perform activities of >5 METS but cannot perform to complete activities of >7 METs
III	• Less than ordinary activities cause symptoms • Marked limitation of activity • Comfortable at rest	• Walking 1–2 blocks or climbing 1 flight of stairs can produce symptoms • Marked limitation on ordinary activity	Patient can perform activities of >2.5 METS but cannot perform to complete activities of >5 METs
IV	• Any physical activity may produce symptoms • Marked limitation of activities • Symptoms may be present at rest	• Inability to carry out activities without discomfort • Symptoms may be present at rest	Patients cannot perform to complete activities requiring >2 METs

*NYHA classification for angina, dyspnea, palpitation, and fatigue.
†Canadian Cardiovascular Society classification for angina only.
‡Specific activity scale outlines activities of different MET equivalents in classification.

in angina, but exact comparative quantification is lacking. The New York Heart Association (NYHA) scale **(Table 2)** is the most widely used. It is a very subjective classification and depends upon the activity level or fitness of the patient, but due to its limitations (categorization of walk-through angina or variable threshold angina) and lack of objectivity, the Canadian Cardiovascular Society scale[8] is preferred for angina classification.

Interpreting Angina

Angina as primary presentation in an elderly invariably indicates an underlying atherosclerotic narrowing in the coronary artery. In young individuals, besides atherosclerotic lesions, it may indicate underlying structural heart disease (commonly valvular disease), hypercoagulable state, abnormal origin of coronary arteries, or spontaneous dissection and microvascular angina, etc. Typical effort angina appears when diameter narrowing is >70%. Increasing severity of narrowing results in angina at lesser exertion. Angina appearing at minimal exertion may indicate an underlying narrowing of >90%. Long-standing severe narrowing (>90%) stimulates the development of collaterals. The presence of collaterals may reduce the infarct size but is not sufficient to fulfill oxygen demand at peak stress in an ischemic zone. History of prior angina in ACS may indicate preexisting significant narrowing if angiography reveals a single-vessel disease. The onset of angina often underlines the duration of total occlusion seen at the angiogram.

In valvular heart disease, the presence of typical effort angina indicates left-sided outflow obstruction. The history of nocturnal angina may indicate aortic regurgitation. Ventricular hypertrophy may also lead to myocardial ischemia due to demand-supply imbalance, but chest pain in these situations is nonclassical generally.

The presence of other cardinal symptoms is extremely helpful in limiting the diagnostic probabilities. Angina associated with breathlessness may be due to coronary ischemia with preexisting left ventricular dysfunction or may indicate a large area of ischemia if there is no history of prior ACS.

Resting chest pain followed by syncope can be a sign of ACS, particularly ST-segment elevation MI or aortic dissection. Exertional chest pain, followed by syncope, is typically associated with valvular or subvalvular left ventricular outflow obstruction. However, it may rarely be a presentation of severe proximal coronary artery narrowing.

DYSPNEA

Dyspnea is defined by the American Thoracic Society as a "subjective experience of breathing discomfort that consists of qualitatively distinct sensations that may vary in intensity."[10] In simple terms, it is shortness of breath or uncomfortable awareness of one's own breathing. A patient presenting with dyspnea can have varied etiology as it represents both cardiac and pulmonary origin. Common causes of dyspnea have been enumerated in **Table 3**. Dyspnea is a subjective feeling, and its manifestation is dependent on prior conditioning. Walking two flights of stairs may cause dyspnea in a normal person with no cardiac or pulmonary disease but not in a conditioned athlete.

Formal Measurement of Dyspnea

There are many scales for quantification of dyspnea such as the modified Borg scale, MMRC, NYHA scale, or WHO scale.[11,12] The NYHA scale is most commonly used for dyspnea of heart failure origin but has various shortcomings. The modified Borg scale is a reliable assessment tool for

TABLE 3: Common causes of dyspnea.

System	Causes
Cardiac:	
• Cardiomyopathy	Dilated cardiomyopathy, HCM, RCMP, peripartum cardiomyopathy, ischemic LV dysfunction
• Heart failure	HFrEF, HFpEF, acute decompensated heart failure
• Valvular	Mitral stenosis, aortic stenosis, mitral and aortic regurgitation
• Pericardial	Constrictive pericarditis, cardiac tamponade
• Vascular	Acute pulmonary embolism, CTEPH
• Congenital	ASD/VSD/PDA/AVCD/CCHD
Respiratory	COPD, ARDS, pleural effusion, lung fibrosis, ILD
Neuromuscular	Myasthenia gravis, poliomyelitis, Guillain–Barré syndrome
Musculoskeletal	Scoliosis, kyphosis
Physiological	Anemia, exercise, fever, pregnancy, psychogenic

dyspnea. It is a point score system where a patient rates his degree of discomfort during a specified physical activity, for example, 6-minute walk test. A score above 5 denotes severe breathlessness. Visual analog scale (VAS) consists of a line, usually 100 mm in length, placed either horizontally or vertically upon a page, with anchors to indicate extremes of a sensation, from "not breathless at all" to "extremely breathless."[13] Scoring is accomplished by measuring the distance from the lowest end of the scale. The reliability and validity of the VAS as a measure of dyspnea have been reported to be superior to the Borg scale as it involves subjective assessments.[14]

Differentiating Cardiac and Respiratory Dyspnea

Since breathlessness is predominantly caused either by cardiac or by respiratory lesions, it is paramount to differentiate the likely etiology in the beginning. The following historical features may help in this regard:

- Rapid breathing with a sense of suffocation may indicate congestive heart failure (CHF) while tightness of the chest with heavy breathing and incomplete exhalation may indicate asthma. Shallow breathing indicates restrictive lung disease.
- Look for the associated symptoms. Respiratory origin dyspnea is usually preceded by a cough with thick sputum and is different from the pink frothy sputum of pulmonary edema where dyspnea precedes cough. Dyspnea due to heart failure may be associated with sweating and chest pain with or without cyanosis.
- Prior history may differentiate respiratory (prior asthma or COPD) from cardiac (prior MI or known cardiac disease) etiology. Other historical features like profuse diaphoresis or paroxysmal nocturnal dyspnea (PND) may indicate cardiac origin.
- A history of relief of dyspnea by bronchodilators and corticosteroids (inhaled or oral) suggests bronchospasm, whereas relief by rest and diuretics is suggestive of heart failure.

TYPES OF DYSPNEA

- *Paroxysmal nocturnal dyspnea*: Nocturnal breathlessness developing after 2–3 hours of sleep, where patients rise from sleep for a gasp of air. In the majority, it is cardiac in origin. It may be a manifestation of nocturnal asthma, particularly in children.
- *Orthopnea*: Breathlessness occurring or worsening on lying-down position, relieved by sitting or standing, almost always indicates severe cardiac condition.
- *Trepopnea*: Breathlessness occurring while lying on one side and not on another. This is predominantly caused by respiratory diseases. However, it may be a manifestation of right-sided pleural effusion in patients with CHF.[15]
- *Platypnea*: Breathlessness while standing which is relieved in recumbent position. This is due to hypoxia produced by shunting of desaturated blood in intracardiac or intrapulmonary shunts.[16]
- *Bendopnea*: Dyspnea occurring on bending forward is a manifestation of raised PCW.[17]

Interpreting Dyspnea

Primary presentation of breathlessness in a cardiac patient indicates an underlying raised pulmonary capillary wedge pressure. Breathlessness on exercise indicates a rise in capillary wedge pressure only at exertion, being normal at rest. With advancing cardiac dysfunction, breathlessness appears at lesser exertion. In patients with a history of prior ACS, it generally indicates a resting LVEF of <40%. In patients without a known coronary artery disease (CAD), it may also be a manifestation of diastolic heart failure, also known as HFpEF, with a typical phenotype of obesity, hypertension, and female sex. In valvular heart disease, the appearance of dyspnea indicates a severe underlying disease with impending left ventricular dysfunction and is an indication for intervention, except in mitral stenosis (MS), where it may appear in moderate MS also. Orthopnea or breathlessness at rest indicates an underlying PCW of >25 mm Hg and resting LV dysfunction. PND may be a relatively earlier presentation of left ventricular dysfunction than orthopnea. A history of PND in a suspected valvular disease classically indicates an underlying MS, generally moderate in severity. However, in the absence of MS, it indicates underlying left ventricular dysfunction. The appearance of breathlessness in the natural history of valvular lesions portends a grave prognosis if unintervened. However, clinicians should always be cautious to rule out intercurrent infection, anemia, arrhythmia, or acute rheumatic fever in a relatively stable course of illness.

Chronology of breathlessness may also indicate underlying lesions. Sudden-onset and rapidly progressive dyspnea indicates acute left ventricular dysfunction due to ischemia with severe CAD or acutely developing MR or AR or RSOV. In patients without structural heart disease or ischemia, it may also be due to acute diastolic heart failure. A short history of dyspnea may indicate an inflammatory or infective etiology while a long history indicates a chronic ongoing process. A long-standing history of nonprogressive dyspnea is not consistent with natural history of isolated severe left-sided valvular stenosis or regurgitation, except aortic regurgitation.

Association of other cardinal symptoms is also important. Breathlessness, followed by pedal edema, indicates a left-sided pathology leading to right heart failure. Presentation with exertional palpitations along with breathlessness favors a regurgitant lesion in patients with valve disease. Temporal association of chest pain and dyspnea generally indicates ischemic heart disease with LV dysfunction. In valvular heart disease, history of associated chest pain is generally nonspecific because of coronary demand-supply imbalance due to chamber hypertrophy. History of associated classical effort anginal pain indicates LV outflow narrowing, most commonly valvular aortic stenosis, while nocturnal angina indicates aortic regurgitation. In patients with a history of rheumatic fever, primary presentation with PND almost always indicates underlying MS. Appearance of fatigue on exertion indicates reduced cardiac output due to underlying heart disease, left-sided if associated with breathlessness or right-sided associated with pedal edema alone.

PALPITATIONS

Palpitation is defined as an uncomfortable awareness of one's own heartbeat. This is a subjective feeling that is perceived by a patient due to changes in rate, rhythm, or the volume of pulse. It is usually described as a feeling of skipped or missed beat and sometimes as a pounding sensation in the chest. Terminologies described are also crucial as flip-flopping in the chest is suggestive of atrial or ventricular ectopic, fluttering is suggestive of AF or VT, and neck vibrations or bulging with prominent rapid venous pulsations are suggestive of AVNRT known as "frog sign." Patients should be encouraged to describe palpitations by tapping their finger on the table describing the rate and rhythm. Persistent palpitations, even at rest, are usually due to noncardiac causes such as thyrotoxicosis, anemia, and anxiety but may be present in severe regurgitant valvular lesions. Episodic and irregular palpitations may indicate atrial fibrillation or frequent ventricular or atrial premature beats. Drug intake such as beta-agonists, cocaine, alcohol, and caffeine can cause palpitations.

Approach to Palpitations

Historical evaluation of palpitation episode should assess duration, onset, termination, slow or rapid, regular/irregular, activity-related, posture-related (AVNRT initiated by standing posture from bending over), and associated symptoms like giddiness, syncope (VT), angina (tachycardia-related supply mismatch) or dyspnea (dilated/ischemic cardiomyopathy, hypertrophic obstructive cardiomyopathy). Episodic palpitations changing into persistent palpitations may be a hallmark of atrial fibrillation. Exercise-induced palpitations can be arrhythmic, due to catecholamine-induced ventricular tachycardia or due to vagal-induced atrial fibrillation but can occur in severe regurgitant lesions. If the episode of palpitation is associated with syncope, it may indicate ventricular tachycardia and rarely supraventricular tachycardia. Bradyarrhythmias like complete AV block, sick sinus syndrome, and tachy-brady syndrome can cause slow-rate palpitations with syncope. A history of AV node-modifying drug or QT-prolonging drug intake may be crucial for diagnosis.

FATIGUE

Fatigue, also expressed as effort intolerance, is often least understood and difficult to express. These patients usually seek consultation with a complaint of getting easily tired with physical activity. Like dyspnea, this too is a subjective feeling and is often expressed interchangeably by patients. Easy fatigability even at rest is more of a sign of anxiety and nutritional deficiencies. It is a nonspecific symptom in the majority if this is the only symptom. However, in the elderly, it is a very important symptom of ischemia and is considered as an anginal equivalent.

In cardiac patients, fatigue is a manifestation of low cardiac output state and it is due to inadequate oxygen delivery to muscles. Skeletal muscle myopathy due to decreased oxygen delivery and inflammation is the primary cause. Fatigue can also be due to overdiuresis in patients with heart failure leading to potassium depletion. Patients with advanced heart failure may become cachexic, which is an adverse sign.

EDEMA

Edema is classically described as diffuse swelling at the extremities, and patients complain of pitting in the feet extending up to the shin or tightening of slippers. Edema is due to excessive fluid accumulation and is generally a late sign of heart failure. In ambulant patients, edema occurs in the legs in daytime and diminishes at night. In bedridden patients, edema develops in the sacral region and therefore must be looked for. In patients with CHF, at least 2 kg of weight gain is present before edema is manifest. In patients with left ventricular failure, dyspnea manifests earlier than edema in natural history. On the other hand, the appearance of edema first indicates primarily right heart involvement or constrictive pericarditis.

SYNCOPE

Nowhere in clinical cardiology is history as important as in the assessment of syncope in isolating the underlying cause. It is defined as abrupt, transient, complete loss of consciousness associated with the inability to maintain postural tone with rapid and spontaneous recovery. The mechanism described is usually cerebral hypoperfusion. It is very important to differentiate various other conditions that can present with loss of consciousness and mimic syncope. Assessment of syncope is important as it can be the only warning sign before sudden cardiac death. **Box 1** lists the various causes of syncope.

Approach to Syncope

Eliciting a good history is important to differentiate various causes of syncope. Rapid onset and offset always suggest a vasomotor reflex mediated or cardiac syncope, while metabolic causes like hypoglycemia have a gradual onset. Altered sensorium due to perceived CNS causes is never transient, except for seizure disorder. Elderly patients usually do not remember the episode of fall in true syncope; therefore, detailed accounts from the onlookers should also be assessed particularly to differentiate it from seizure. Specific questions regarding postictal confusion, oral trauma, incontinence, and myalgias should be asked to rule out in seizure disorders. Position at the time of presentation and precipitating factors should be examined. Syncope after prolonged standing suggests vasovagal syncope, while arrhythmic syncope has no relation to the posture. Precipitating factors can include sight of blood, sleep or food deprivation, alcohol, painful strong emotions or occurring within 2 minutes of standing suggesting orthostatic hypotension. A history of prodrome of sweating, nausea, and blurring of vision just prior to syncope may indicate vasomotor syncope. Exercise-induced syncope is seen with structural abnormalities like HOCM, AS, PS, PAH, and in severe CAD as well as some primary arrhythmic conditions like long QT syndrome and idiopathic VT in children like CMVT. Syncope at nighttime is usually seen in QT prolongation. VT remains the first possibility in arrhythmic syncope as SVT and AF generally do not cause syncope in isolation unless associated with underlying poor left ventricular function, except in very elderly patients.

Higher risk cardiac syncope is strongly suspected in elderly >60 years of age, male sex, in the presence of an underlying structural heart disease, or in the background of exertional fainting or family history. Nonlife-threatening syncope is usually recurrent like vasomotor syncope and has a prolonged history, often over decades, while life-threatening syncope is usually nonrecurrent and has a short history.

BOX 1 Causes of syncope.

- *Vascular causes*:
  - *Anatomic:*
    - Vascular steal syndromes (subclavian steal syndrome)
  - *Orthostatic:*
    - Autonomic insufficiency idiopathic
    - Volume depletion
    - Drug and alcohol induced
  - *Reflex mediated:*
    - Carotid sinus hypersensitivity
    - Neurally mediated syncope (common faint, vasodepressor, neurocardiogenic, vasovagal)
    - Glossopharyngeal syncope
    - Situational (acute hemorrhage, cough, defecation, laugh, micturition, sneeze, swallow, postprandial)
- *Cardiac causes*:
  - *Anatomic:*
    - Obstructive cardiac valve disease
    - Aortic dissection
    - Atrial myxoma
    - Pericardial disease (e.g., cardiac tamponade, hypertrophic obstructive cardiomyopathy)
    - Myocardial ischemia, infarction
    - Pulmonary embolism
    - Pulmonary hypertension
  - *Arrhythmias:*
    - Bradyarrhythmias
      - Atrioventricular block
      - Sinus node dysfunction, bradycardia
    - Tachyarrhythmias
      - Supraventricular tachycardia
      - Atrial fibrillation
      - Paroxysmal supraventricular tachycardia (AVNRT, WPW)
      - Ventricular tachycardia
    - Structural heart disease
    - Inherited syndromes (ARVD, HCM, Brugada syndrome, long-QT syndrome)
    - Drug-induced proarrhythmia
    - Implanted pacemaker or ICD malfunction

History of prior fainting, dizziness, or lightheadedness occurs in nearly 70% of patients who experience true syncope. Presyncope involves similar symptoms, but loss of consciousness does not occur. History of drugs, particularly antihypertensives, beta-blockers, nitrates, and diuretics, should be obtained.

OTHER SYMPTOMS

While evaluating cardiac patients, other symptoms, particularly cognitive and behavioral patterns, should also be assessed as they may indirectly reflect the severity of disease;

for example, a patient with advanced decompensated heart failure may behave irrelevantly due to hypoxia or patients with bradycardia after MI patient hypotension may go into a state of hypoxic-ischemic encephalopathy. It is also important to differentiate functional disorders from actual cardiac illness, particularly in the female population in India due to various socioeconomics, educational, and geopolitical factors. They may not only hide their symptoms but at times may present with atypical symptoms.

CONCLUSION

History taking is a fast disappearing art. An elaborate history sets the foundation of an intricate relationship between patient and treating physician. Cardiovascular pathologies present with a myriad of symptoms. Their assessment and interpretation remain a challenge. Combination of symptoms markedly narrows down the probability. Assessing symptoms together can indicate ongoing hemodynamic alterations and chronology of symptoms may indicate the changes in underlying pathophysiology over time. An astute clinician always assesses the chronology to ascertain whether it fits in the natural history of suspected disease or not. It is an ongoing process throughout the course of illness that not only leads to diagnosis but also gives insight into the course of illness, line of management, response to therapy, and prognosis.

"To cure sometimes, to relieve often, and to comfort always."

—Hippocrates

ONLINE REFERENCES

Please scan the QR code provided at the end of the table of contents for References of this chapter.

CHAPTER

89

Electrocardiography in Congenital Heart Diseases

Neeraj Awasthy, Sudeep Verma

ABSTRACT

Electrocardiography (ECG) is an easy available invaluable tool in the basic evaluation of heart disease in children. Some of the ECGs are quite specific for the given case scenario/heart disease but alone ECG is not sufficient enough for diagnosing majority of congenital heart disease (CHD). Yet its importance cannot be undermined and it should be interpreted along with clinical details and available radiologic data in any CHD to arrive at plausible diagnosis.

Keywords: Electrocardiography, tool, heart disease, children

INTRODUCTION

Rhythmic contraction of the heart appears first in bulboventricular portion of the primitive, unlooped heart tube. Sinus node get first morphologically identified in the human embryo just after looping (5 weeks of gestational age). It occupies a subepicardial position at the lateral junction of superior vena cava and right atrium. Malposition of the sinus node generally occurs in conditions, in which normal atrial arrangement is lacking such as:

- *Isomerism of right atrial appendage (right heterotaxy)*: Bilateral sinus nodes are formed.
- *Isomerism of left atrial appendage (left heterotaxy)*: Sinus node may not be identifiable, ectopic atrial rhythm
- *Juxtaposed atrial appendage*: Anterior displacement of sinus node—ectopic atrial rhythm/atrial tachycardia/flutter is seen. It is seen with complete transposition of the great arteries, tricuspid atresia, dextro-mesocardia, and hypoplastic right ventricle.

After origin of cardiac impulse from sinus node, there is preferential conduction of cardiac impulse through the atrium to the atrioventricular node. The atrioventricular conduction consists of the atrioventricular node, bundle of His, and the specialized conduction system of ventricle (right and left bundle branches).

STEPS OF ECG EVALUATION

It is imperative to follow steps for better ECG evaluation which are as under:

- *Step 1*: Getting vital data like age, gender, clinical details including location of cardiac mass, saturation, and blood pressure. There may be significant variation as per the age of the patient **(Table 1)**.

TABLE 1: Peculiarities of neonates and changes in ECG occurs with increasing age.

Peculiarities of neonates and infants	Changes occurs with increasing age
• Low QRS voltage in precordial and limb leads • Low T wave changes • RV dominance • Right axis deviation up to 180° • Upright T waves in right precordial leads in first week of life • Preterm: Smaller complex, LV dominator, more variability	• HR decreases • All duration and Interval increases • RV dominance gradually changes to LV dominance • QRS axis less RV shift • R wave on RPLs decreases and in LPLs increases. This is reverse for S wave • By 3 years QRS axis approaches the adult mean level of + 50 • Gentle upward slope - J depression - normal in adolescent age

TABLE 2: P wave assessment of ECG.

AVR	AVL	II, III, AVF (inferior leads)	P-axis	
Negative	Positive	Positive	LLQ (0-90)	Sinus rhythm
Positive	Negative	Positive	RLQ (90-180)	• EAT • Atrial situs inversus
Positive	Positive	Negative	Superior	• Coronary sinus rhythm (left heterotaxy) • EAT

- *Step 2*: Technical consideration: leads information, paper speed, standardization
- *Step 3*: Heart rate, rhythm (including P-axis) and conduction including 1:1 conduction and PR interval **(Table 2)**
- *Step 4*: Assessment of atrial enlargement
- *Step 5*: Assessment of ventricular enlargement
- *Step 6*: QRS axis determination
- *Step 7*: Arrhythmia assessment
- *Step 8*: Assessment of conduction disturbances
- *Step 9*: Amalgamation of all available information—plausible interpretation and diagnosis

Once the above basic steps of ECG assessment are implemented, the specific ECG in congenital heart diseases (CHDs) may be assessed as under.

ECG IN SPECIFIC CONGENITAL HEART DEFECTS

ECG in CHD generally reflects the deranged hemodynamics resulting from the heart defect. Some subtle ECG variation can, however, occur which could serve as "pointer" to one morphological subset. Because of its low sensitivity, ECG is often not considered as first-line investigation for diagnosing CHD. But even in present era, its importance cannot be undermined and ECG served as an important part of clinical cardiology for complete evaluation of CHD. Some specific role of ECG includes:

- Assessment of hemodynamics in making decision for operability in left-to-right shunts
- Assessment of rhythm disturbances specific to heart lesion (e.g., prolonged PR in ASD/AVSD/DORV, WPW in Ebstein's, heart block in CCTGA)
- Follow-up of postoperative cardiac patients (QRS duration and RBBB in TOF, heart block after device closure of ASD/VSD repair of AVCD, atrial flutter/atrial tachycardia/sinus nodal dysfunction after TAPVC repair)

ACYANOTIC HEART DISEASE (LEFT-TO-RIGHT SHUNTS)

Pretricuspid Left-to-Right Shunts

Left-to-right shunts occurring at the atrial level (atrial septal defect, anomalous pulmonary venous drainage) produce volume overload of the right atrium and right ventricle. ECG changes seen as follows:

- Prominent P wave suggestive of dilated RA
- Abnormal P axis seen with sinus venosus ASD (less than +30) and common atrium
- Advanced first degree heart block occurs commonly in familial ASD **(Fig. 1)**. 10% of secundum ASD showed prolonged PR. With Holt-Oram syndrome, PR prolongation, ectopic atrial rhythm, and sinus bradycardia are reactively common. 50% of primum type ASD has first degree heart block.
- Right axis deviation (RAD) or a normal axis will suggest atrial septal defect in the fossa ovalis or sinus venosus defect or partial anomalous pulmonary venous connection **(Fig. 2)**. Presence of left axis deviation (LAD) of –30° to –60° will suggest ostium primum atrial septal defect **(Fig. 3)**.
- RSR, Rsr, rsr, or RsR, patterns in right-sided chest leads (V_4R, V_1) referred as incomplete right bundle branch block (RBBB) pattern **(Figs. 2 and 4)**. It occurs due to late activation of dilated RVOT in the depolarization sequence producing distinct pattern of QRS in right lead particularly V_1.
- Crochetage refers to notched QRS in inferior leads **(Figs. 2 and 4)**. Exact reason for crochetage is not known exactly but its presence along with lead V_1 changes is more suggestive of presence of ASD.
- In presence of "significant" right ventricular hypertrophy (RVH) with pretricuspid shunt, one should suspect associated pulmonary arterial hypertension (PAH) or pulmonic stenosis (PS). It is, however, very difficult to diagnose right ventricular hypertrophy in the presence of preexisting RBBB **(Fig. 5)**.
- Common atrium is actually an admixture lesion presented with cyanosis. ECG features are peaked P, prolonged PR, counterclockwise loop, and RAD **(Fig. 6)**.
- Flutter and fibrillation are more common in the fourth decade of life due to long-standing atrial enlargement **(Fig. 7)**. Sinus arrhythmia is not seen with large ASD. It is due to minimal change in right heart volume with breathing with already overloaded right heart.

Post-tricuspid Left-to-Right Shunts

The left-to-right shunts in this group can occur at the level of either the ventricle (ventricular septal defect,

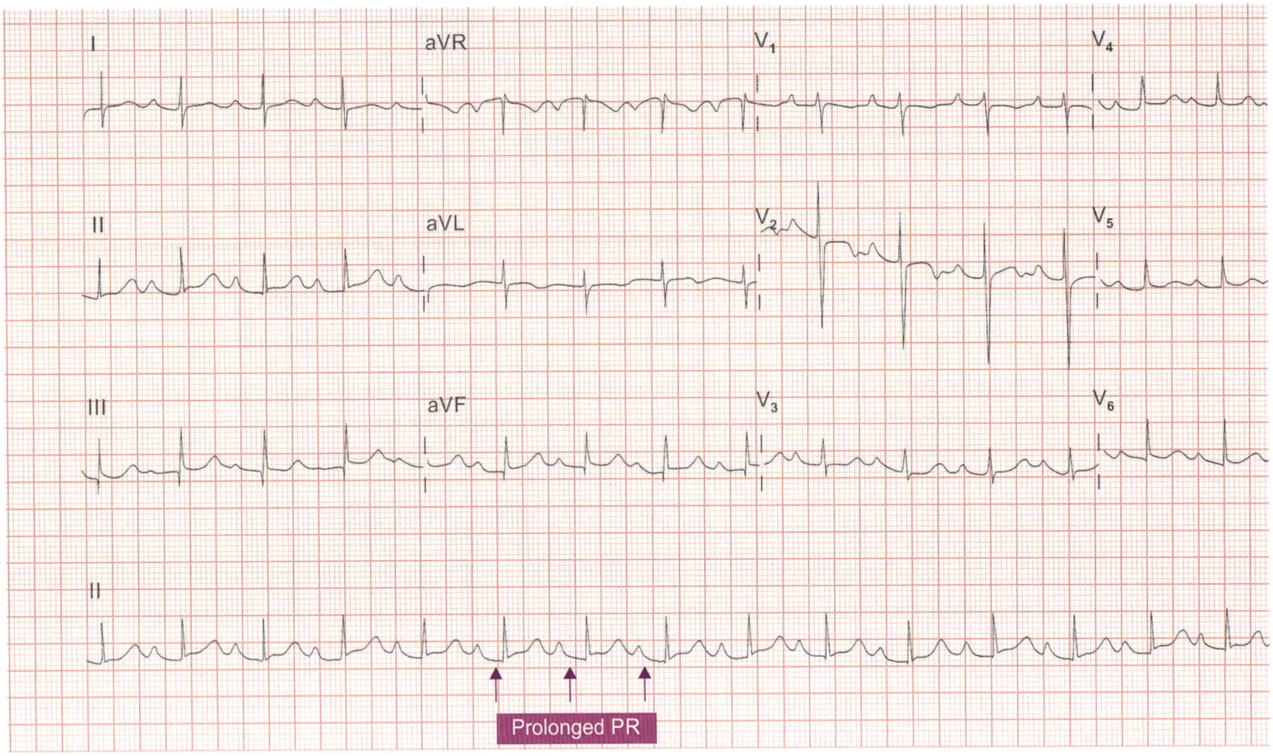

FIG. 1: A 6-year-old patient with OS ASD showing RAD and prolonged PR.

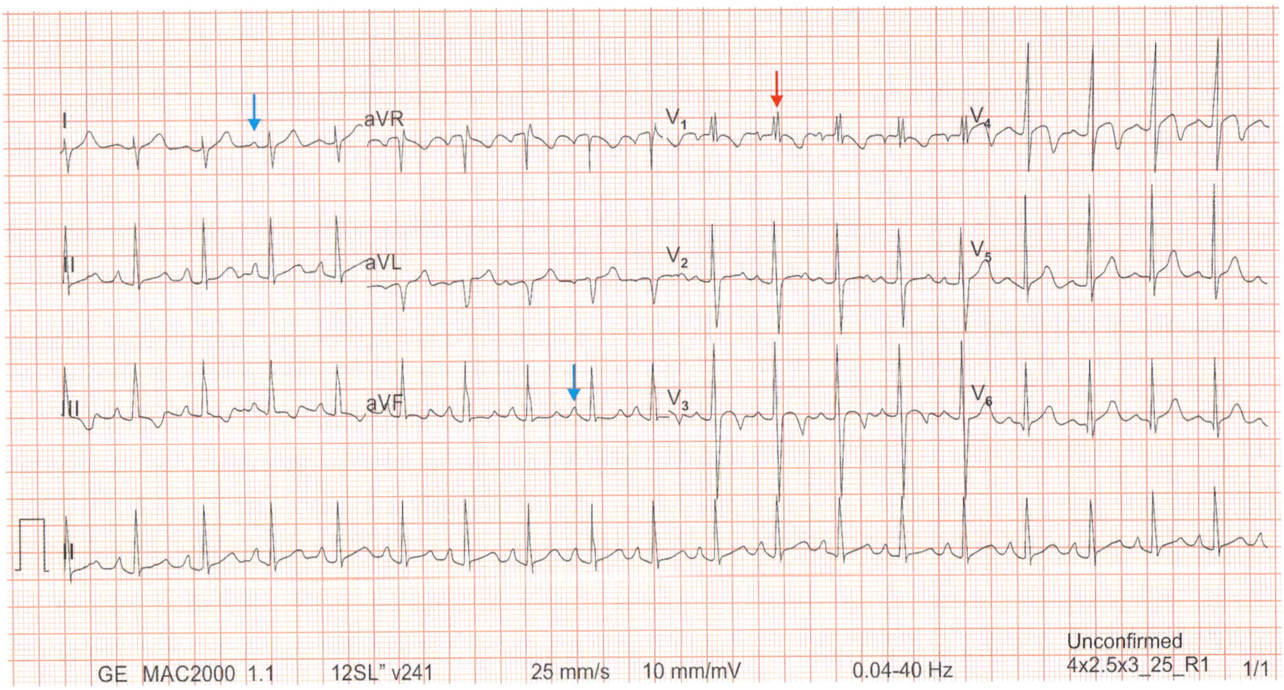

FIG. 2: Typical ECG of ostium secundum ASD showing normal P axis, prominent P, RAD, clockwise loop, RSR, in V_1 and crochetage in inferior leads.

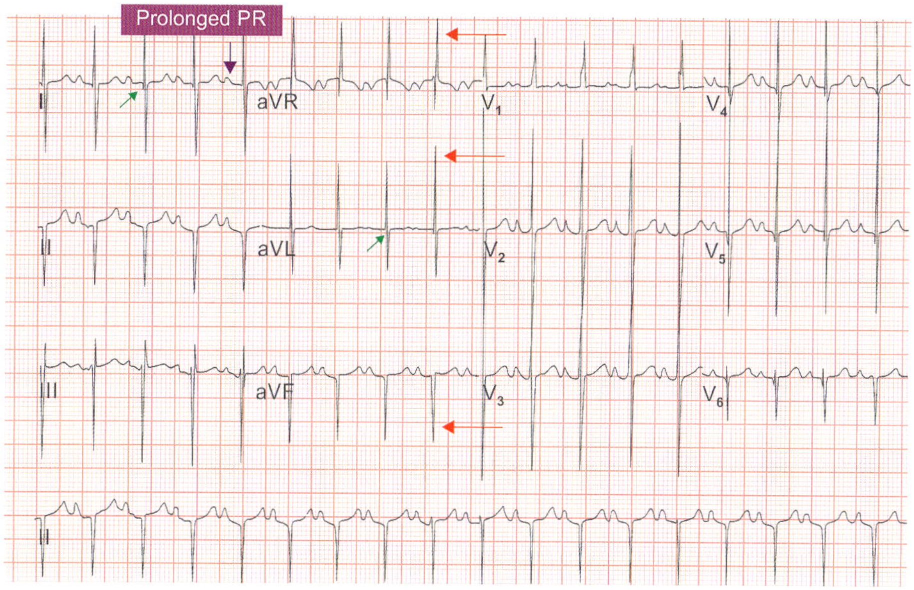

FIG. 3: ECG in a 5-month-old with large OP ASD and small VSD (transitional AVCD) showing normal P axis, prolonged PR, superior QRS axis, Q wave in I and aVL, biventricular forces and rR′ in V_1.

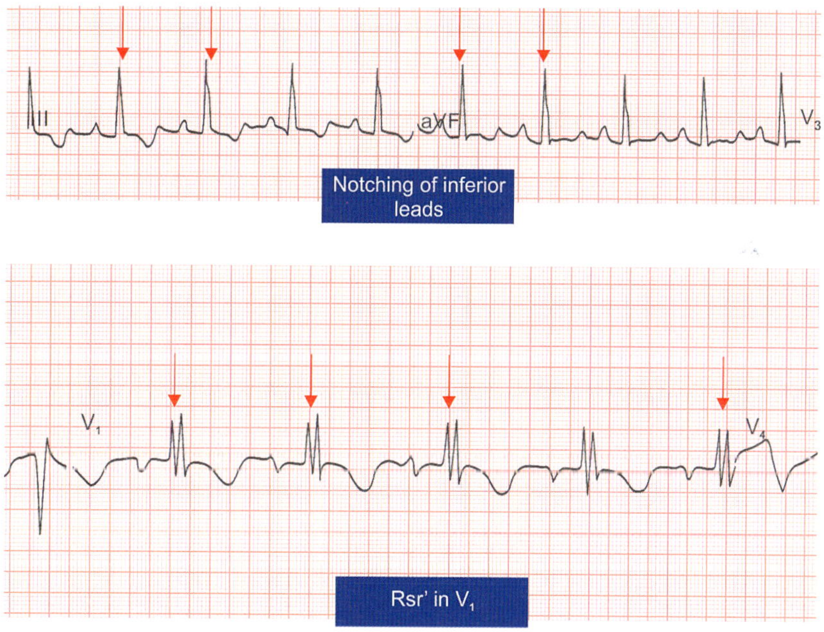

FIG. 4: Zoomed view of lead V_1 and inferior limb leads (AVF and III) to show incomplete RBBB and crochetage.

double outlet right ventricle without pulmonary stenosis with normally related great vessels) or the great vessels (patent ductus arteriosus or aortopulmonary window). The common feature of all these defects is volume overloading of the left ventricle and left atrium if the defect is significant. Large defects cause equalization of right and left ventricular pressures and this is reflected in the ECG in the right ventricular leads early in the natural history of the disease. The following ranges of ECG changes can thus be encountered depending upon the volume of shunt:

- *Normal ECG*: A small patent ductus arteriosus (PDA) or ventricular septal defect (VSD) with small shunt because the volume overload is not severe enough to produce ECG changes. The QRS axis in patients with small to moderate defects remains normal.

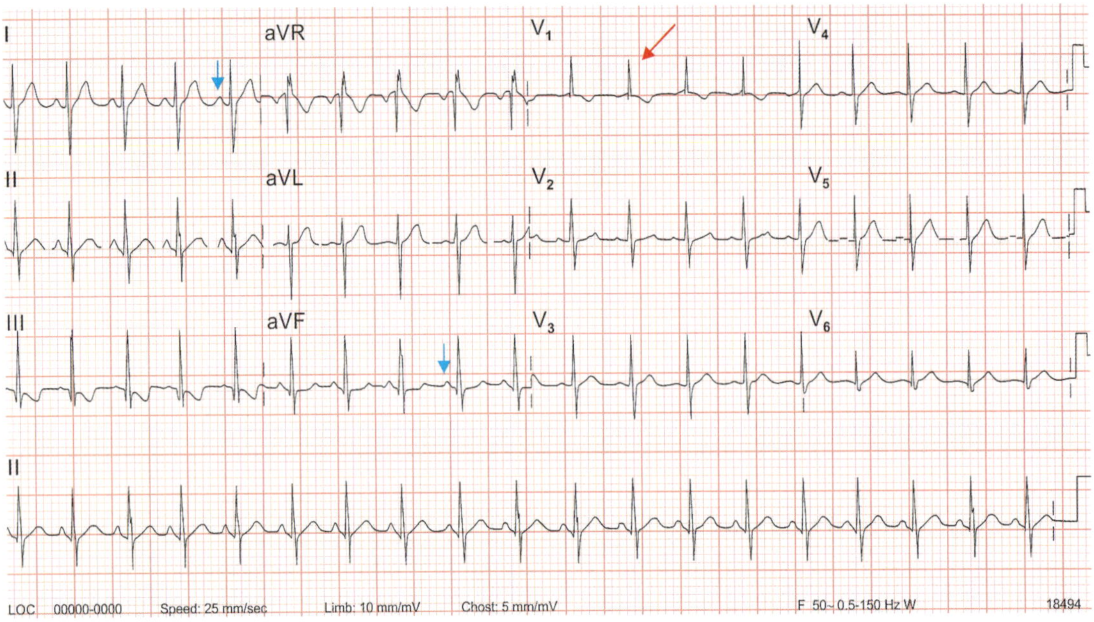

FIG. 5: ECG from 2-years-old child with fossa ovalis ASD, severe pulmonary stenosis. ECG shows normal sinus rhythm, normal "P" wave axis, right axis deviation (QRS +140°), and RVH.

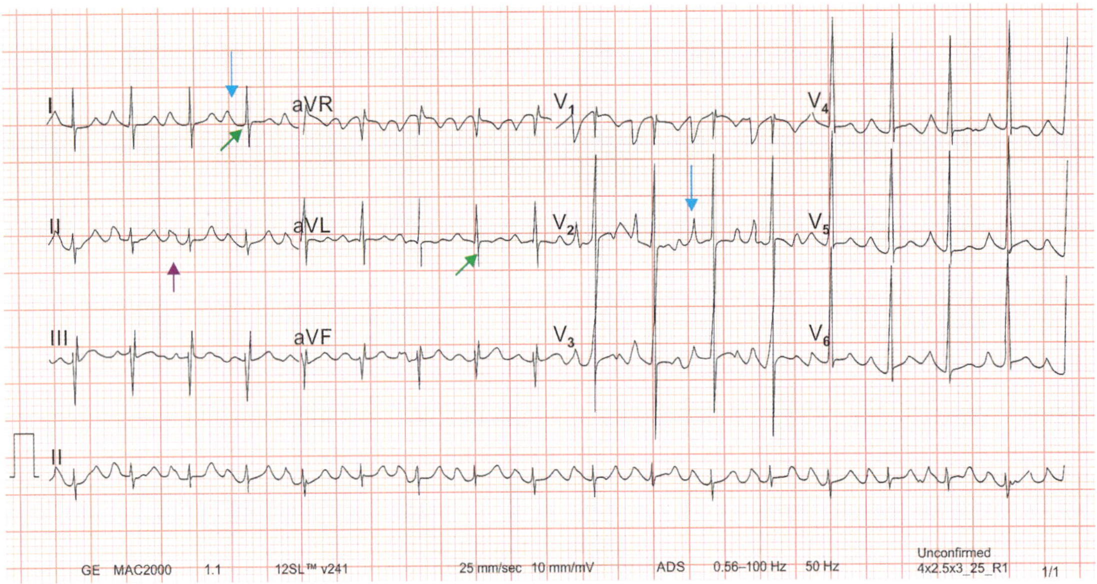

FIG. 6: A 7-years-old with common atrium showing normal p axis, peaked P, prolonged PR interval, superior QRS axis and counterclockwise loop.

- *Left ventricular and left atrial volume overload patterns in the ECG*: Seen with larger shunts in the absence of severe pulmonary arterial hypertension. Represented by tall R and T waves with prominent Q waves in left precordial leads. Left atrial volume overload is shown as prolonged or biphasic P wave **(Fig. 8)**.
- *Biventricular hypertrophy*: Is a feature of large defects with severe PAH. In Infants its usual to have biventricular forces owing to dominant RV (feature of an infant heart) with additionally, associated large shunt causing prominent left forces **(Fig. 9)**. But left-to-right shunt is, however, still dominating. In older children and grown up with large shunt, biventricular forces can be reflected as Katz-Wachtel phenomenon. It is referred as large diphasic complexes over 50 mm in either leads V_2, V_3, V_4 (mid precordial leads) **(Fig. 10)**. In a patient with doubtful

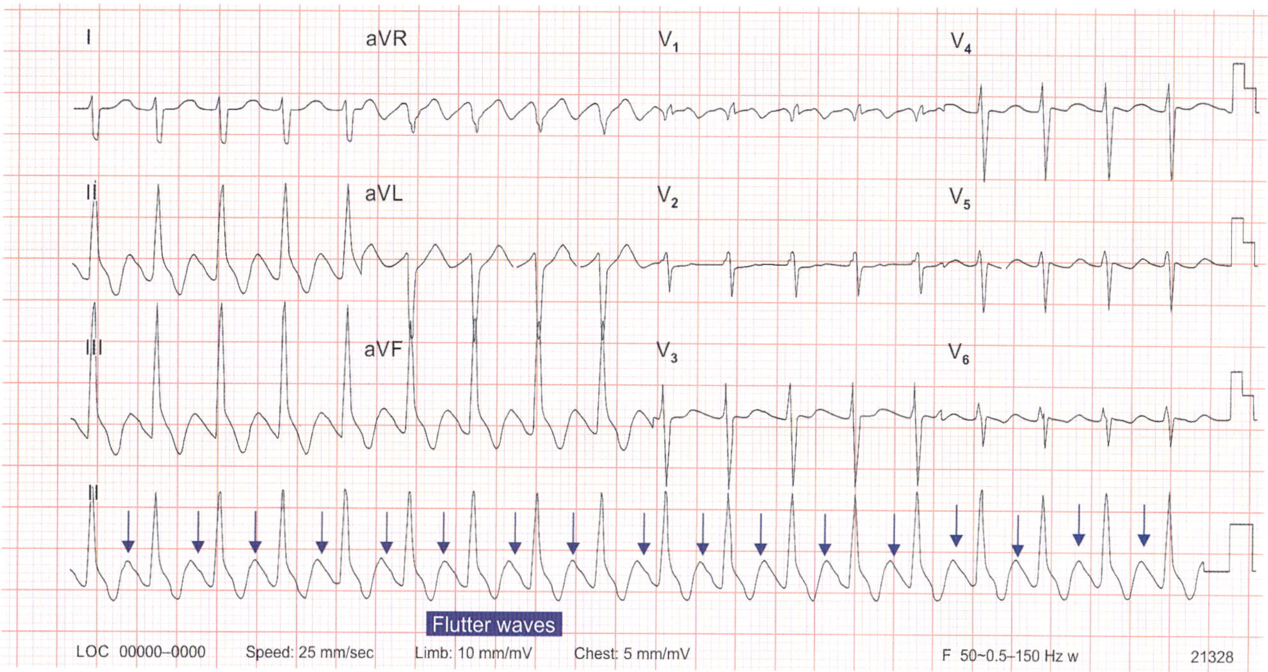

FIG. 7: A 29-year-old known case of large fossa ovalis defect showing atrial flutter with ventricular rate of 115/min.

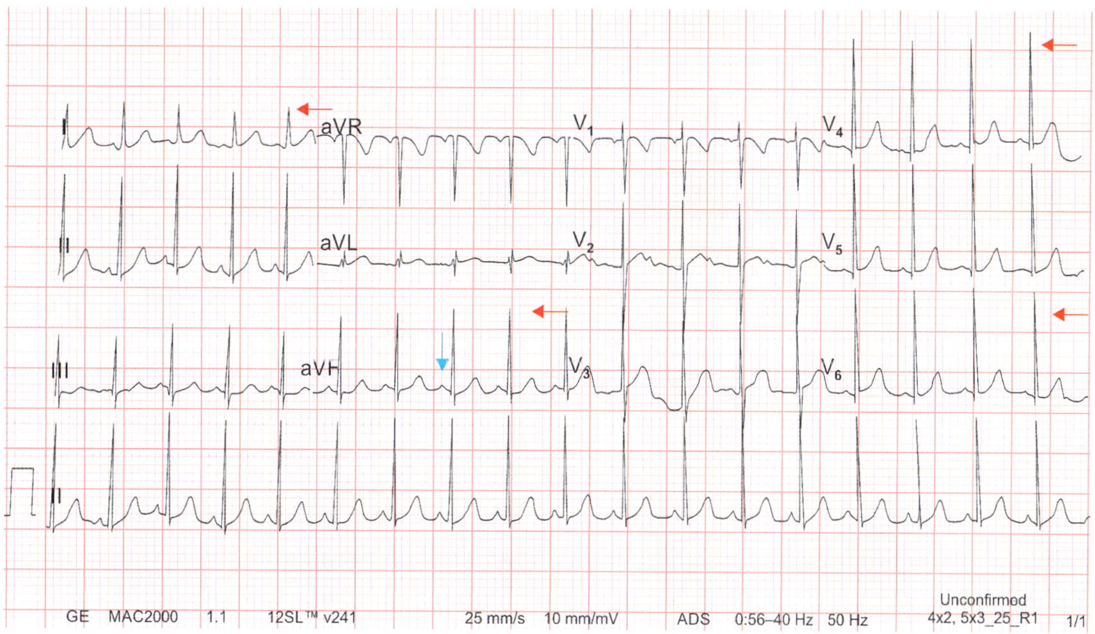

FIG. 8: A 6-month-old with large VSD showing HR of 120 beats/min, normal P axis, QRS axis of 60 (LLQ) with volume overloading pattern in left leads (prominent Q with prominent R wave). Biphasic RS complexes in mid precordial leads.

operability, presence of KW phenomenon is indicative of pre-Eisenmenger phase (in absence of other contributory factors like AV valve regurgitation or anemia).

- *Dominant right ventricular hypertrophy*: In untreated large defects as pulmonary vascular disease progresses, the left ventricular forces start diminishing and in advanced stages of disease only right ventricular hypertrophy is seen. This is sign of development of Eisenmenger phenomenon suggestive of inoperability of the given lesion. Features of RVH can also be seen if

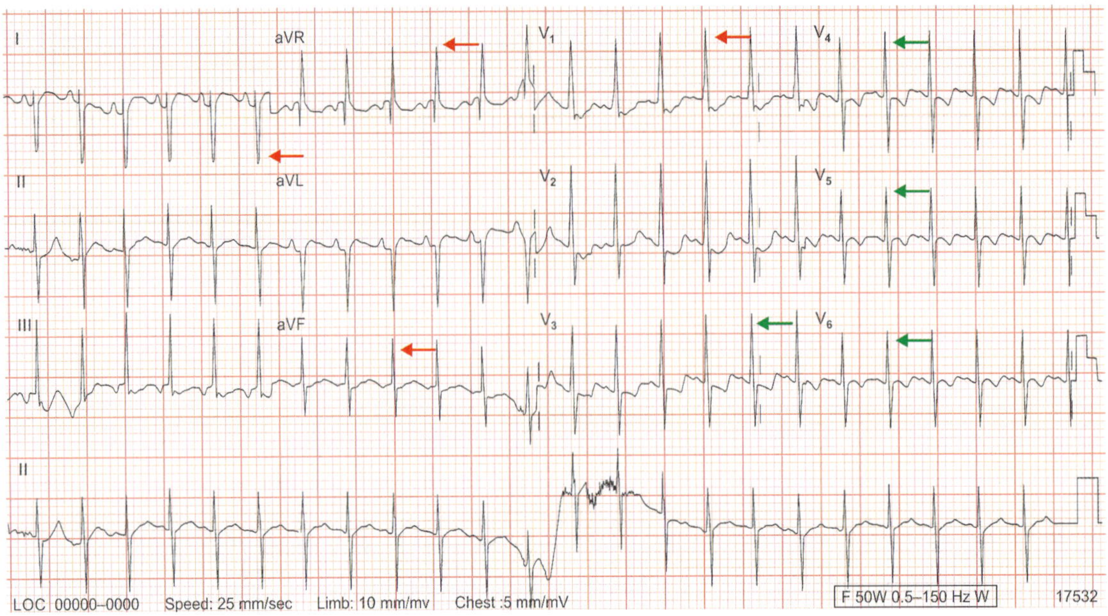

FIG. 9: ECG from 6-month-old child with nonrestrictive perimembranous ventricular septal defect showing normal 'P' wave axis, sinus tachycardia (HR: 150 beats/min), right axis deviation (QRS +160°), biventricular hypertrophy (chest leads in ½ voltage).

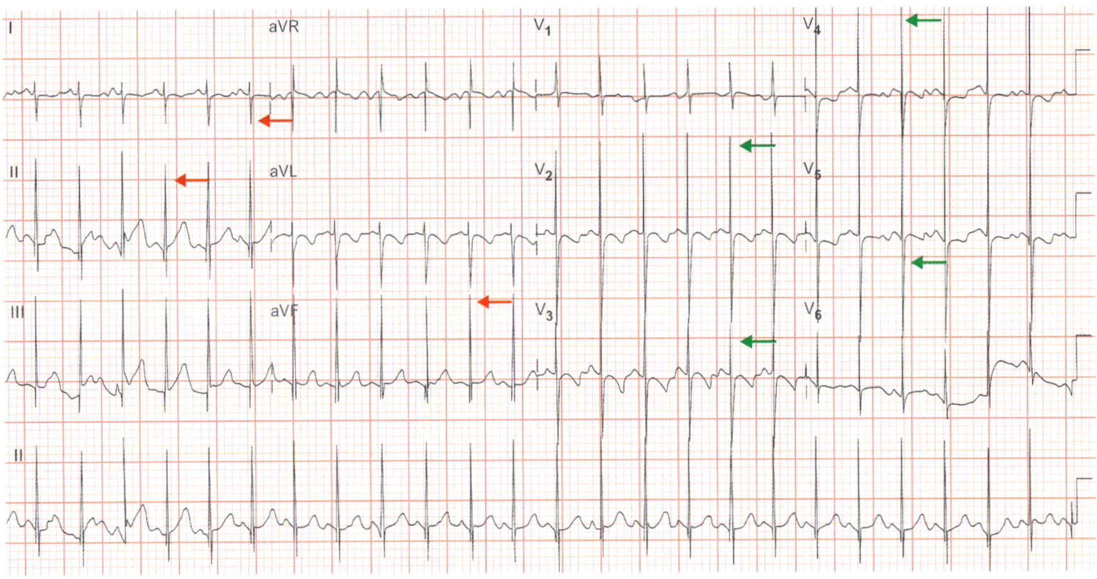

FIG. 10: A 6-year-old with large perimembranous VSD with severe PAH presented for assessing operability. Tachycardia is present (HR: 150 beats/min), normal P axis, clockwise vector loop, RAD, biventricular hypertrophy with preserved Q waves in left leads. Mid precordial leads are showing RS complexes more than 50 mm suggestive of biventricular hypertrophy.

pulmonary stenosis develops progressively. It can be seen as monophasic R in V_1 and deep S in V_6. Development of pulmonary vascular disease or pulmonary stenosis progresses the QRS axis changes to right **(Fig. 11)**.

- Left axis deviation in this group of patients will suggest atrioventricular septal defect/inlet VSD **(Fig. 12)**. Rarely multiple muscular defects/VSD with criss-cross heart/perimembranous VSD with MSA can present with left axis deviation **(Fig. 13)**. Superior axis can be seen in syndromic PDA with Rubella.
- 10–20% of PDA is associated with prolonged PR. PR prolongation can also be seen with inlet VSD or with AVCD.
- Obligatory shunts like LV to RA jet show additional right atrial P wave/RSR' suggestive of right heart volume overload along with signs of left side volume overload

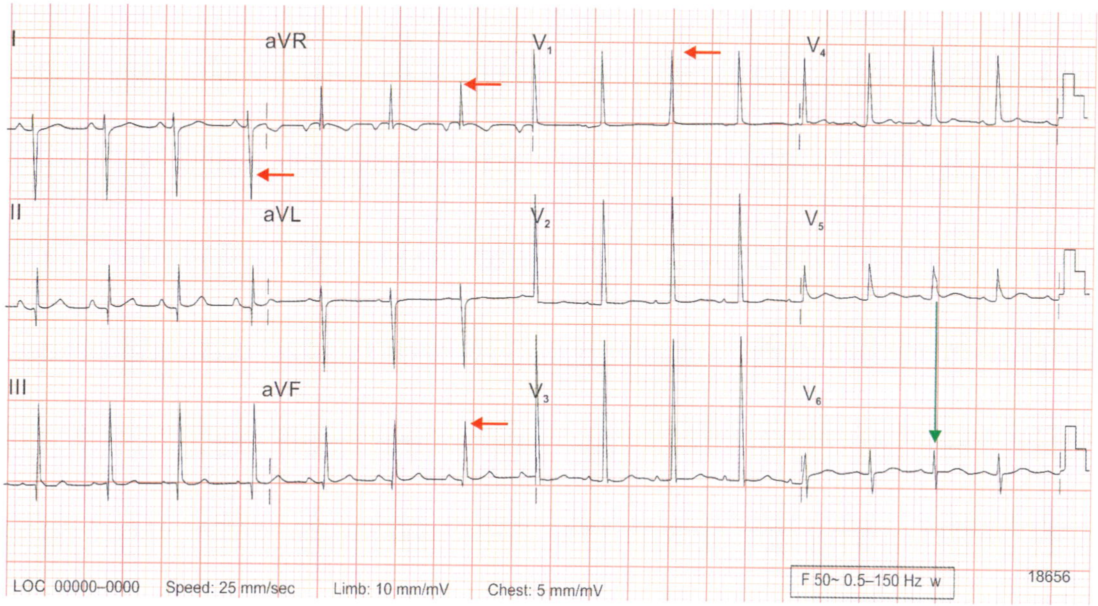

FIG. 11: ECG from a 6-years-old child with small muscular VSD, severe pulmonary stenosis (RVOT gradient—110 mm Hg). To start with this child had nonrestrictive muscular VSD and mild pulmonary stenosis. On follow-up, VSD became smaller and pulmonary stenosis progressed. ECG showed normal sinus rhythm (HR: 75 beats/min), right axis deviation (QRS +140°), severe RVH (chest leads in ½ voltage), delayed transition (in lead V_6).

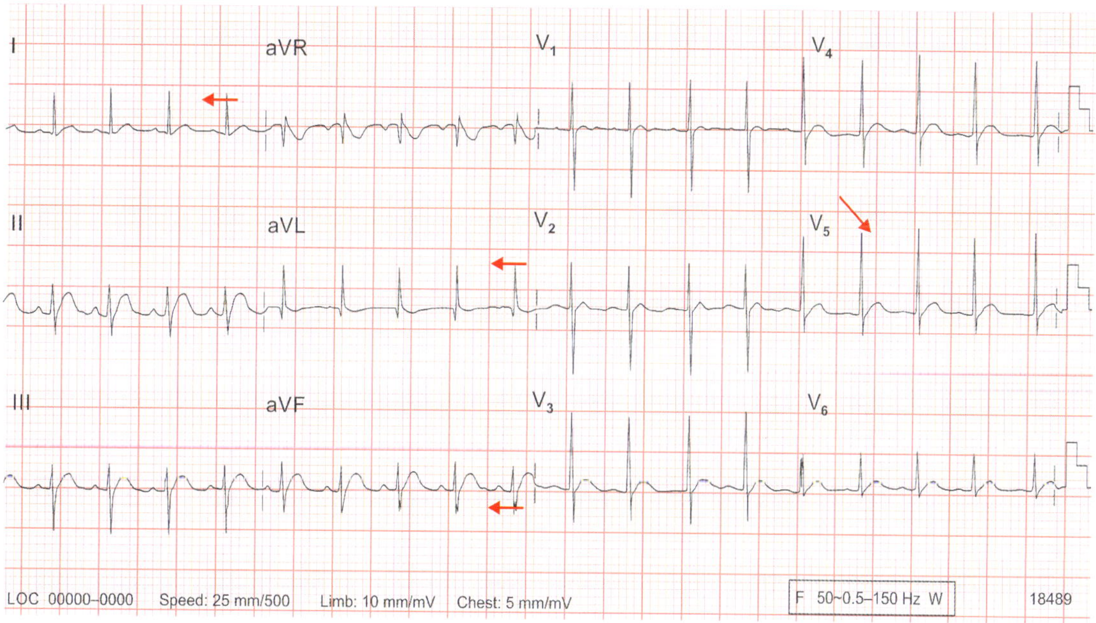

FIG. 12: ECG from 5-month-old child with nonrestrictive inlet VSD, PAH showing sinus rhythm (HR: 120 beats/min), normal "P" wave axis, left axis deviation (QRS axis –20°), biventricular hypertrophy (chest leads in ½ voltage).

as described above. Similarly, CAVF shows features of volume overloading as per the site of drainage (RA/CS—prominent P wave, RV/PA/LA/LV—dilated P wave), biventricular forces with fistula draining into RA or body of RV. LV hypertrophy is seen with fibula to RV outflow, LA or LV **(Fig. 14)**.

- Ischemic pattern in presence of coronary steal seen with CAVF particularly with shunt involving LCA system.

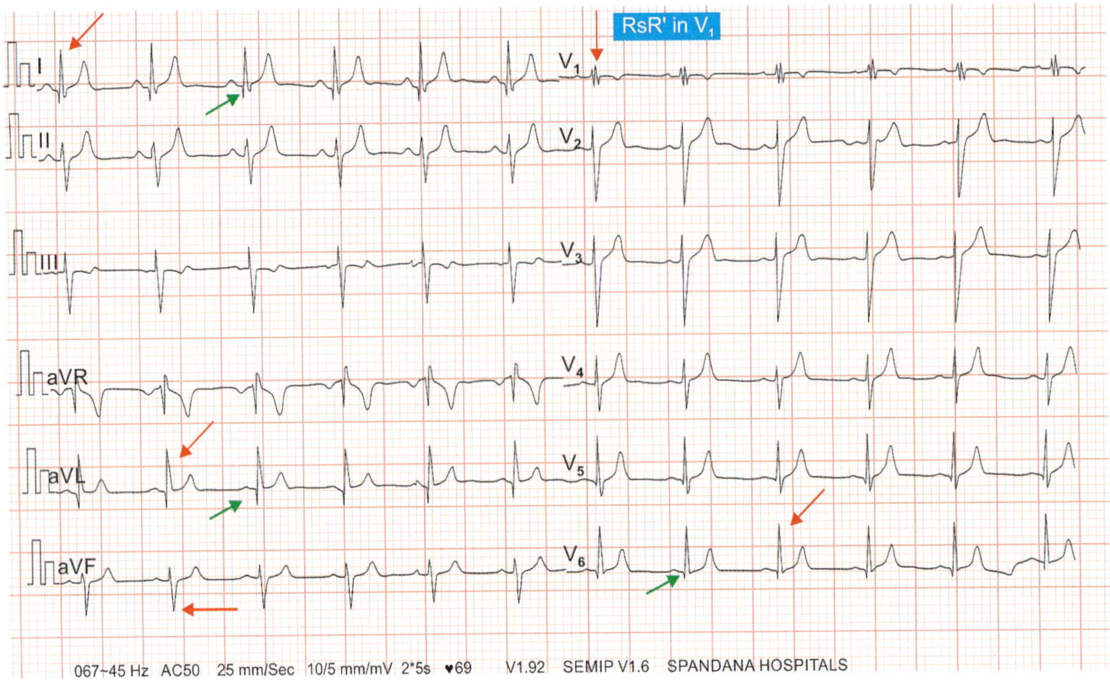

FIG. 13: An 18-year-old with perimembranous inlet muscular VSD and large MSA with large LV to RA jet. ECG is showing normal P axis with counterclockwise loop and left axis deviation. Along with this left leads showing volume overload pattern. Right heart dilatation is also present as depicted by RsR, in V_1 (chest leads in half voltage).

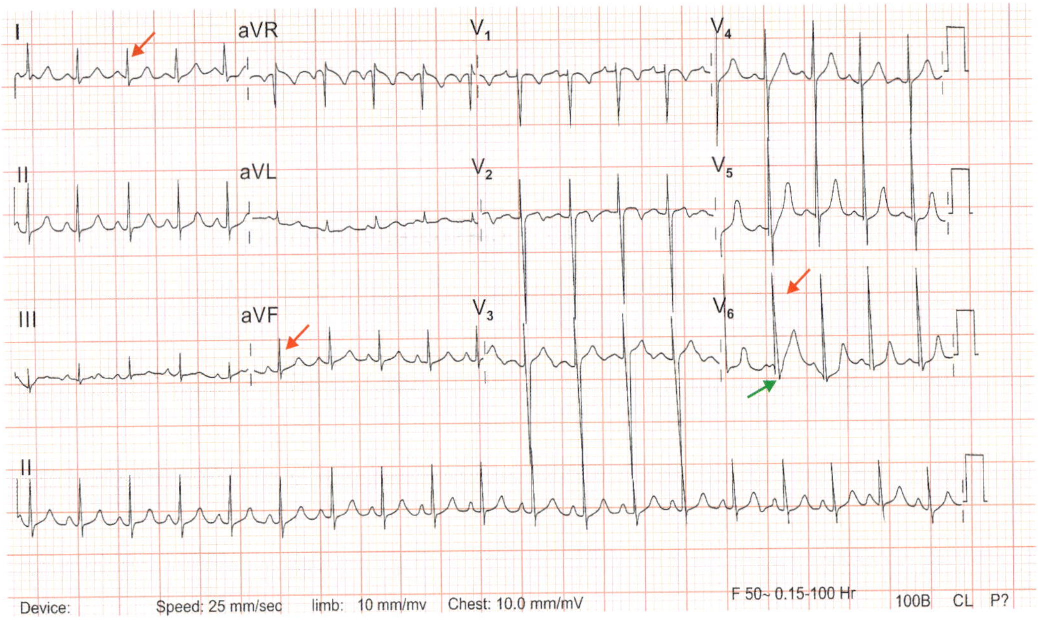

FIG. 14: An 11-year-old with CAVF to RV showing prominent P, normal P axis, RAD, volume overloading pattern on left preordain leads.

ACYANOTIC HEART DISEASE: OBSTRUCTIVE LESIONS

ECG shows prominent RV forces with RVOTO and prominent LV forces with LVOTO. With right-sided obstruction, ECG correlation with severity of stenosis is more sensitive and specific than left-sided obstructive lesions and ECG has been found to be a useful predictor of its severity. Electrocardiographic prediction of severity of aortic stenosis (AS) is not as accurate as in pulmonary stenosis.

Right Ventricular Outflow Obstruction

Specific ECG pattern can be seen with increasing severity of PS. With severity, P wave becomes more prominent:

- *Mild pulmonary stenosis*: ECG may be normal. Persistence of upright T wave in right chest leads may be the only ECG findings in infants and children.
- *Moderate PS*: Normal ECG is uncommon (10%). Mean QRS axis is usually between +90° and +120. rR or RS complexes (with R/S more than 4) are seen in V1 and R in V1 may be up to 20 mm in amplitude.
- *With severe PS* **(Fig. 15)**: Right atrial P wave is seen, QRS axis of +110° to +150° or more, pure R or qR in V1 with R wave of 20 mm or more, delayed transition of R waves in precordial leads, later the delay more severe the stenosis is. Deeply inverted T waves in 2, 3 and AVF is suggestive of strain pattern **(Fig. 15)**.

The height of the pure R wave in V_1 or VR correlates well with the right ventricular systolic pressure in pure valvular pulmonary stenosis. "R" wave magnitude in mm in V_1 or VR multiplied by 5 or R wave in mm multiplied by 3+47 indicates the approximate right ventricular systolic pressure. Children tend to generate higher R waves amplitude in V_1 as compared to adults with similar degree of obstruction.

The ECG in any right-sided obstruction like infundibular pulmonary stenosis, obstructing anomalous muscle bundles of right ventricle, supravalvular pulmonary stenosis, or peripheral pulmonary stenosis is essentially similar to those in valvular pulmonary stenosis. In obstructing muscle bundles of RV, an upright T wave in V_3 R may be the only evidence of RVH in up to 40% of the patients. Infants with critical pulmonary stenosis and hypoplastic right ventricle may show RAD with LVH in the ECG **(Fig. 16)**.

Not surprisingly similar ECG changes may also be seen in the group of patients with large VSD with pulmonary stenosis (see tetralogy of Fallot below). Attempts to differentiate ECG changes in isolated severe right-sided obstruction where the right ventricular pressures can exceed the left ventricular pressure (suprasystemic) from the group of lesion with large ventricular septal defect and pulmonary stenosis where the right ventricular pressure cannot exceed left ventricular pressure (delayed transition of QRS complex) have met with high specificity but very limited sensitivity.

Left Ventricular Outflow Obstruction

The ECG will show varying grades of left ventricular hypertrophy (LVH) depending upon the severity of obstruction. Electrocardiographic prediction of severity of aortic stenosis (AS) is not as accurate as in pulmonary stenosis.

- Left ventricular hypertrophy with deeply inverted T waves with ST depression in left-sided leads indicates severe aortic stenosis, though their absence does not exclude severe aortic stenosis. T wave usually points in direction opposite to QRS complexes **(Fig. 17)**. In some cases, ECG may be normal even in severe aortic stenosis. Supravalvular and discrete subvalvular aortic stenosis are electrocardiographically indistinguishable from valvular aortic stenosis. In supravalvar stenosis, presence of coronary ostial obstruction is reflected by feature of ischemia.

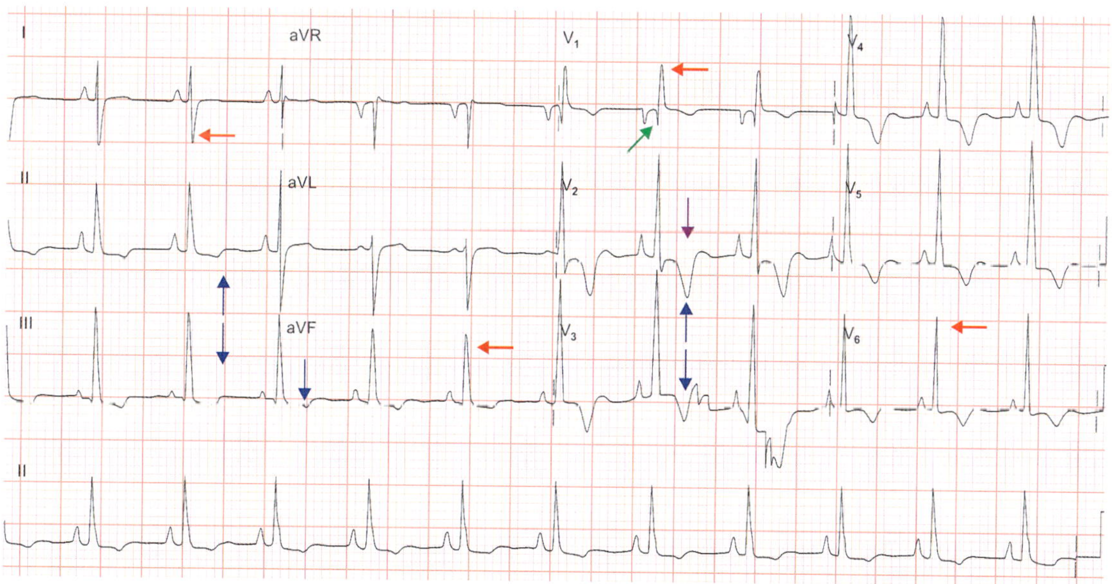

FIG. 15: ECG from 12-year-old child with severe valvar pulmonary stenosis (suprasystemic RV pressure) with intact interventricular septum. ECG shows normal sinus rhythm, normal "P" wave axis, RA enlargement (tall "P" wave), right axis deviation (frontal QRS axis +100°), RVH, presence of RV strain pattern (q wave in lead V_1, T wave inversion in V_1–V_6), absence of transition.

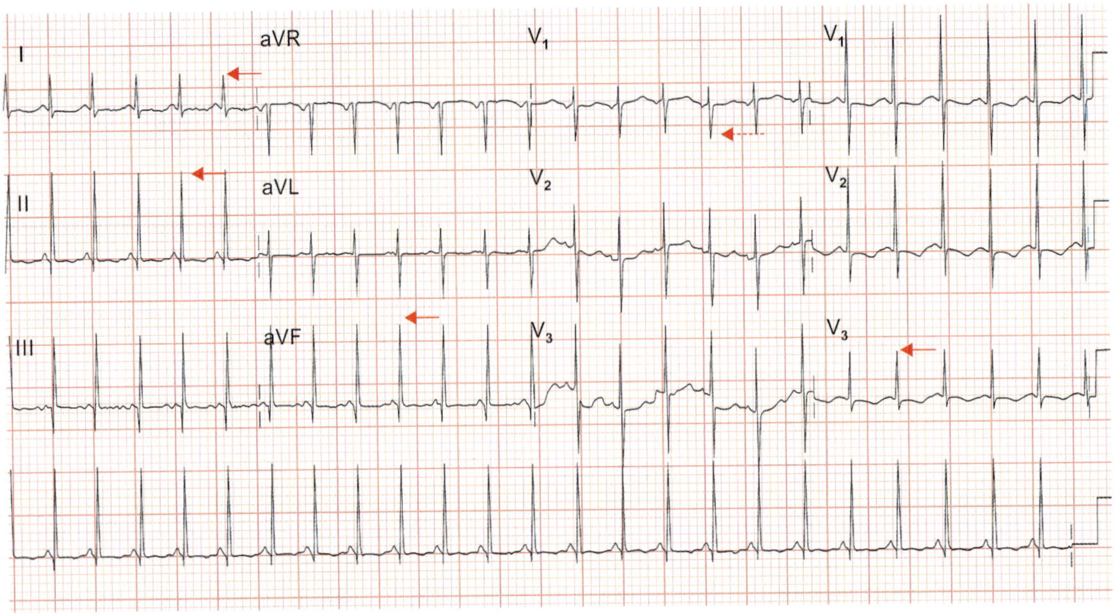

FIG. 16: ECG in severe valve PS showing RAD with superior axis. Strain pattern is seen in right precordial leads (prominent R with ST changes). V_1 shows qR pattern suggestive of hypertensive RV.

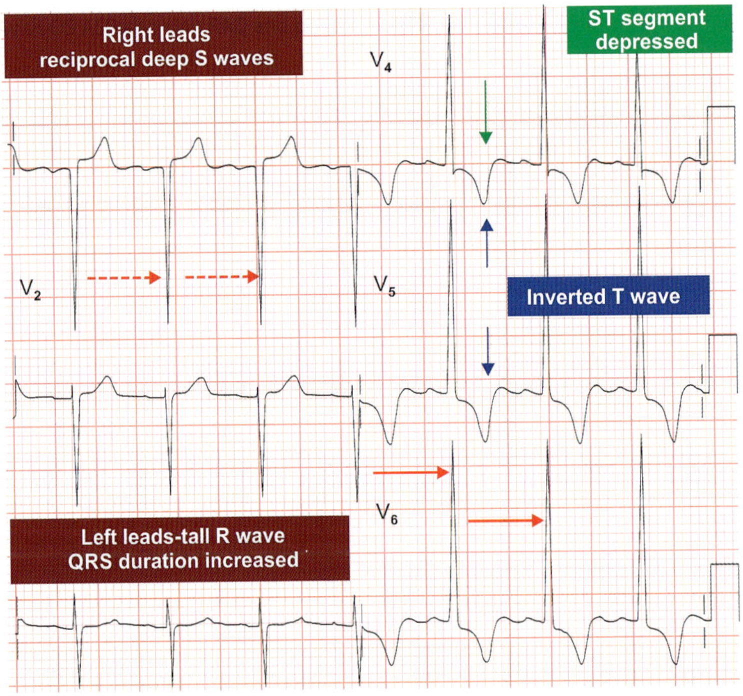

FIG. 17: Left precordial leads showing strain pattern in presence of severe LVOTO. Tall R waves with depressed ST segment and inverted T waves are suggestive of hypertrophy with strain. QRS-T angle is also increased. Reciprocal deep S waves are seen in right leads.

- Coexisting BAV with COA is reflected in as coved ST segment depression with ST segment depression. Prominent Q waves in left leads suggest AR causing volume overdosing due to bicuspid aortic valve **(Fig. 18)**.
- *Right ventricular hypertrophy*:
    - Supravalvular aortic stenosis and associated peripheral PS as with William syndrome may produce RVH in the ECG.

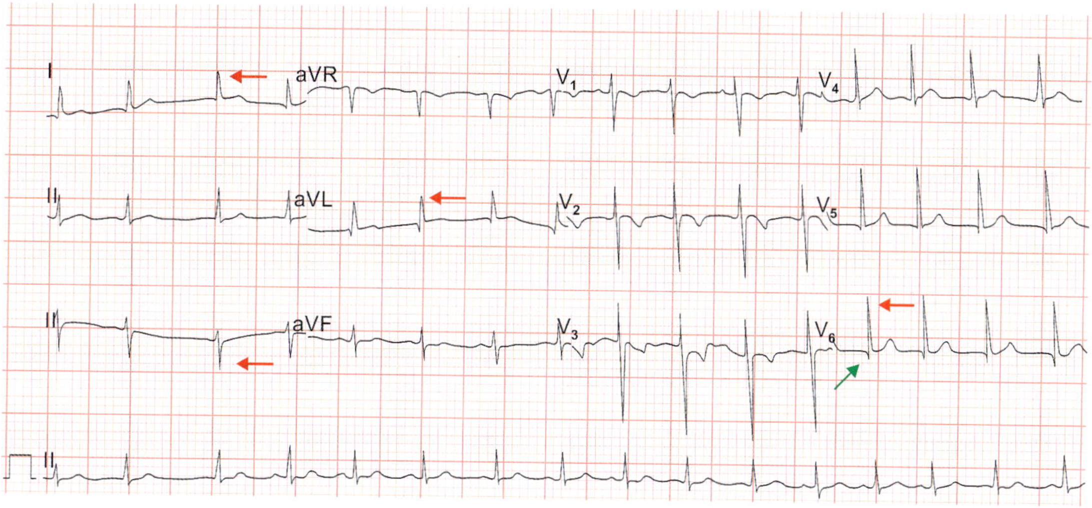

FIG. 18: ECG of a 10-year-old case of bicuspid valve with moderate AS and severe AR. LAD is seen, with prominent LV volume overloading forces in left precordial leads. All leads are half standardized.

- ○ RVH is reserved for neonates with pinpoint AS, pulmonary hypertension, small LV cavity and a left-to-right shunt across PFO.
- The ECG in coarctation of aorta in infants may show RVH often with a strain pattern in V_1 or V_3R without any evidence of left ventricular forces. LVH develops in most patients with hemodynamically significant aortic coarctation by 2 years of age. Strain pattern (ST depression and T inversion) in left-sided leads is rare in uncomplicated coarctation of aorta and suggests associated endocardial fibroelastosis, severe aortic stenosis, or mitral regurgitation.
- Broad notched P wave if present indicates significant coexisting MR or seen with LVOTO in adults with LVH. P wave prominence is seen with symptomatic infants with COA/LVOTO

CYANOTIC HEART DISEASES

Basically, it includes two main group of lesions—decreased pulmonary blood flow (known as VSD-PS or TOF physiology) and cyanosis with increased blood flow (known as admixture lesion).

TETRALOGY OF FALLOT PHYSIOLOGY

Tetralogy of Fallot (TOF) or VSD-PS physiology includes spectrum of following lesions:

- Classical tetralogy of Fallot
- Double outlet right ventricle with PS
- Complete transposition of great arteries (dTGA) with ventricular septal defect, and pulmonary stenosis
- Corrected transposition of great arteries (L-TGA) with ventricular septal defect and pulmonary stenosis
- Atrioventricular canal defect (AVCD) with pulmonary stenosis
- Tricuspid atresia with pulmonary stenosis
- Single ventricle with pulmonary stenosis

Distinctive pattern of ECG features are seen in this group:

- *RVH with RAD*: This is classical pattern seen with prototype of VSD-PS physiology. Most of this group has prominent RV forces due to RVH **(Fig. 19)**. One of the typical feature is abrupt transition from monophonic R in V_1 to rS in V_2. Although the exact reason for this feature is unknown, it is believed to be secondary to catching of LV forces though VSD over the lead V_2 placed at the septal level. QRS axis usually lies between 120 and 150°. With TGA, VSD-PS and VSD-PA axis may lie between 150 and 180° **(Fig. 20)**. Typical VSD-PS patient shows normal P wave amplitude and of duration due to normal force of contraction of RA and reactively small LA. Presence of Q waves in left leads along with its depth in left leads gives goon indicator of PBF and LV filling. Restrictive VSD in TOF presents with right heart failure and suprasystemic RV visible as prominent P, RAD, monophonic R in V_1 with poor progression of R wave (like severe PS).
- *DORV VSD-PS*: The ECG may show RAD beyond +180° (abnormal quadrant axis). When the QRS axis lies beyond 180 (north west quadrant), it has to be differentiated from extreme left axis deviation. This is possible by looking at the activation sequence (loop) of the QRS complex. One of the important features is counter-clockwise loop as depicted by Q waves in 1 and aVL. Sometimes, PR interval is prolonged.
- *RVH with LAD*: Seen with complete atrioventricular septal defect with pulmonary stenosis, DORV, restrictive VSD **(Fig. 21)**. Here, RVH in present owing to severe PS but LAD is related to abnormal activation or abnormal severe LVOTO as with restrictive VSD

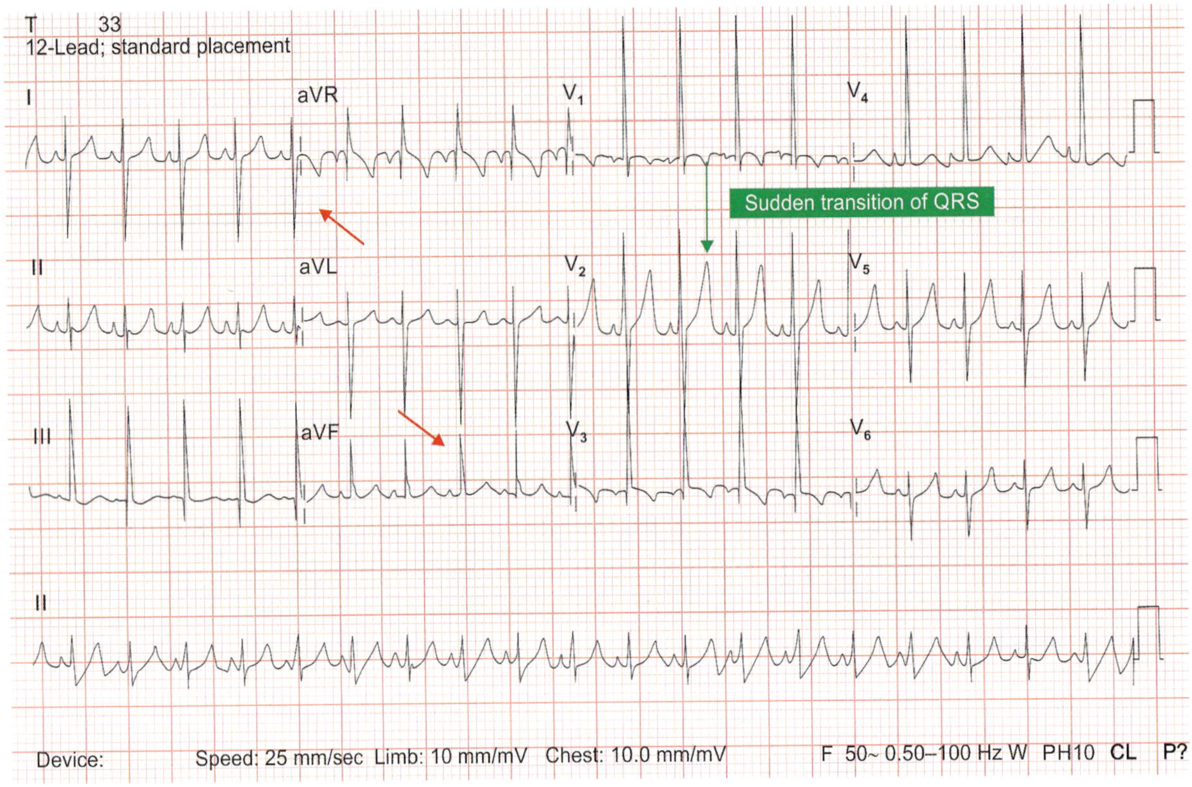

FIG. 19: ECG in typical TOF showing RAD with features of RVH. Sudden transition of monophasic R wave from V_1 to negative and equiphasic to V_2-V_3.

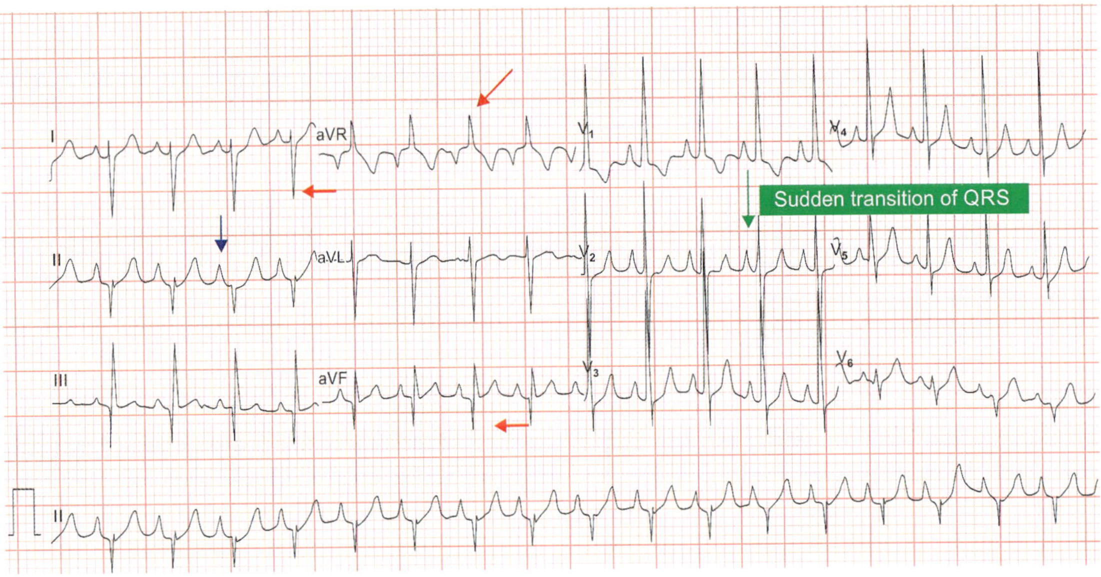

FIG. 20: ECG is VSD-PA showing peaked P wave, RAD with QRS axis > 150, clockwise vector loop and sudden transition like typical TOF from V_1 to V_2-V_3.

- *LVH with LAD*: Tricuspid atresia with pulmonary stenosis, pulmonary atresia intact IVS
Clinically indistinguishable but striking ECG features are seen in a group of lesion associated with right ventricular hypoplasia. The ECG then shows complete absence of right ventricular forces (rS pattern in V_1 and dominant R in V6) which in a cyanotic heart disease stands out as most unusual. These lesions are

mentioned below and may be differentiated from each other:

- *Tricuspid atresia*: In this condition, the frontal plane QRS axis is left-sided Himalayan P wave common especially in lead 2 **(Fig. 22)**
- Isolated RV hypoplasia with or without PS. In these cases, the cyanosis is related to right to left shunting at atrial level. The frontal plane QRS axis is usually normal.

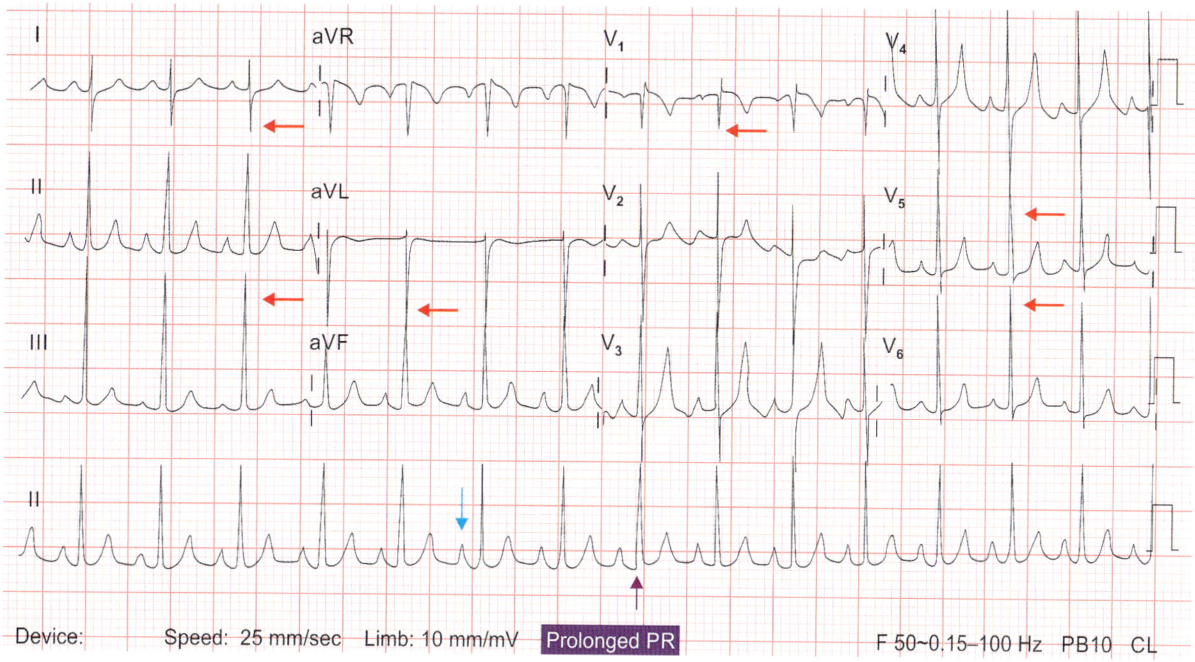

FIG. 21: 15-year-old showing peaked P with vertical axis. Precordial leads showing prominent LV forces which is not usual from typical TOF. Thus patient diagnosed to have DORV, severe PS with VSD restriction causing LVH.

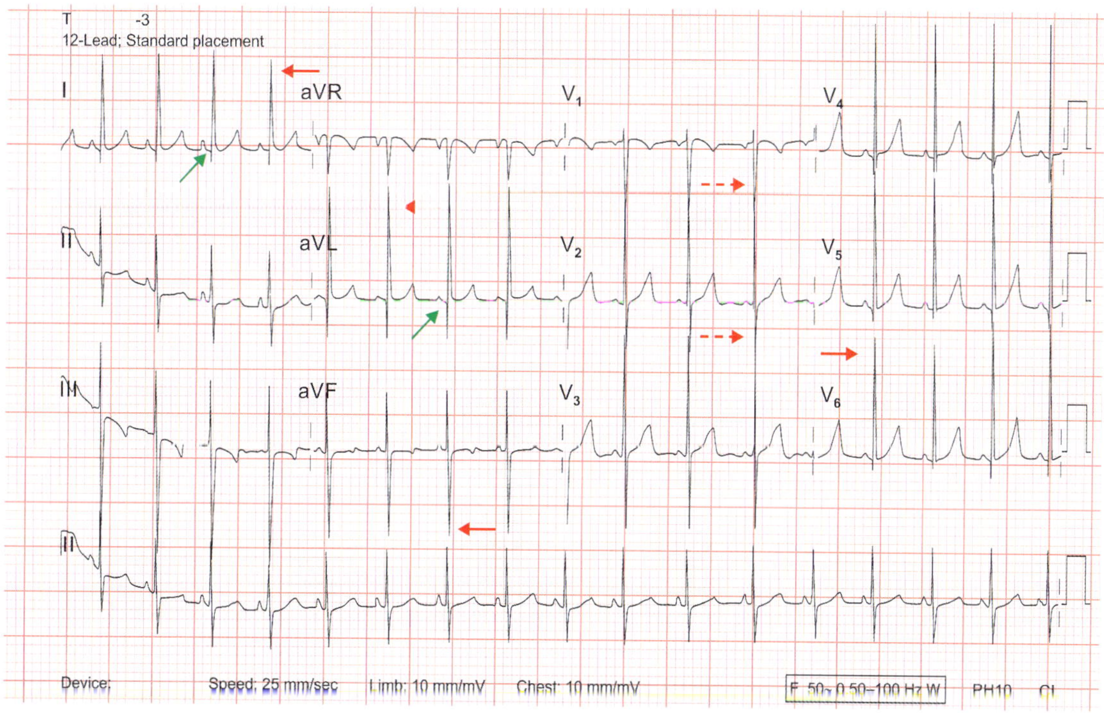

FIG. 22: 1-month-old cyanotic showing LAD, super axis, counterclockwise loop and prominent LV forces with diminutive RV forces. Diagnosed to have tricuspid atresia 1B. Similar pattern can be seemed with PA intact IVS with small RV and DILV or rarely with DORV restrictive VSD.

  - Straddling/overriding of tricuspid valve leading to RV hypoplasia in patients with transposition of great vessels or double outlet right ventricle with pulmonary stenosis. In these cases, the frontal plane QRS axis is right.
  - Pulmonary atresia with intact septum: The frontal plane QRS axis is right.
  - Single ventricle: The frontal QRS axis can be right or left.
- Discordance between QRS axis and ventricular hypertrophy (RAD with LVH or LAD with RVH) or presence of monomorphic QRS complexes favors the diagnosis of single ventricle with PS **(Fig. 23)**.
- *CCTGA VSD-PS*: Two AV nodes are found in CCTGA—regular AV node does not make contact with infranodal right and left bundle branches. Instead, an anomalous anterior AV node with long bundle penetrated the AV fibrous annulus which with increasing age replaced with fibrous tissue responsible for AV block. 75% of CCTGA patients exhibit varying degree of heart block when all ages are included. Overall incidence of complete heart block is 30%.

Left axis deviation is also a feature of corrected transposition of great arteries (L-TGA). This rare condition is, however, differentiated by looking at the activation sequence of the of the QRS complex in the horizontal leads. Presence of Q waves in V_1 and V1R and their absence in aVL, V_6, and I deep Q wave in III and aVF suggest ventricular inversion. ECG features of corrected transposition of great arteries vary depending upon the associated heart defects as ventricular septal defect, pulmonary stenosis, AV valve abnormalities. Corrected transposition of great arteries can be associated with varying degrees of atrioventricular block. ECG features of ventricular inversion are a less constant feature when corrected transposition is associated with dextrocardia. Also, heart block is rare with CCTGA with situs inversus **(Fig. 24)**.

TOF APV: Although included in TOF but its ECG features are different from classical pattern. Tall T wave extends up to adjacent chest leads (c/f TOF and VSD-PA). Prominent P is usual than exception.

Pink TOF: It is a loose term used for the patients of TOF with preserved anterograde flow in spite of severe RVOTO. Hemodynamically it behaves like moderate VSD. ECG shows featured of LV volume overload with good RV forces. Sudden transition of monophasic V_1 to biphasic/prominent negative in V_2 rarely noted.

VSD-PA: It behaves like TOF but in presence of significant collaterals, axis remained normal with preserved or prominent LV forces **(Fig. 25)**.

ADMIXTURE LESIONS (CYANOTIC HEART DISEASE WITH INCREASED PULMONARY BLOOD FLOW)

Admixture lesions are class of CHDs characterized by cyanosis, increased pulmonary blood flow and congestive heart failure in infancy. Here, the mixing occurs in one

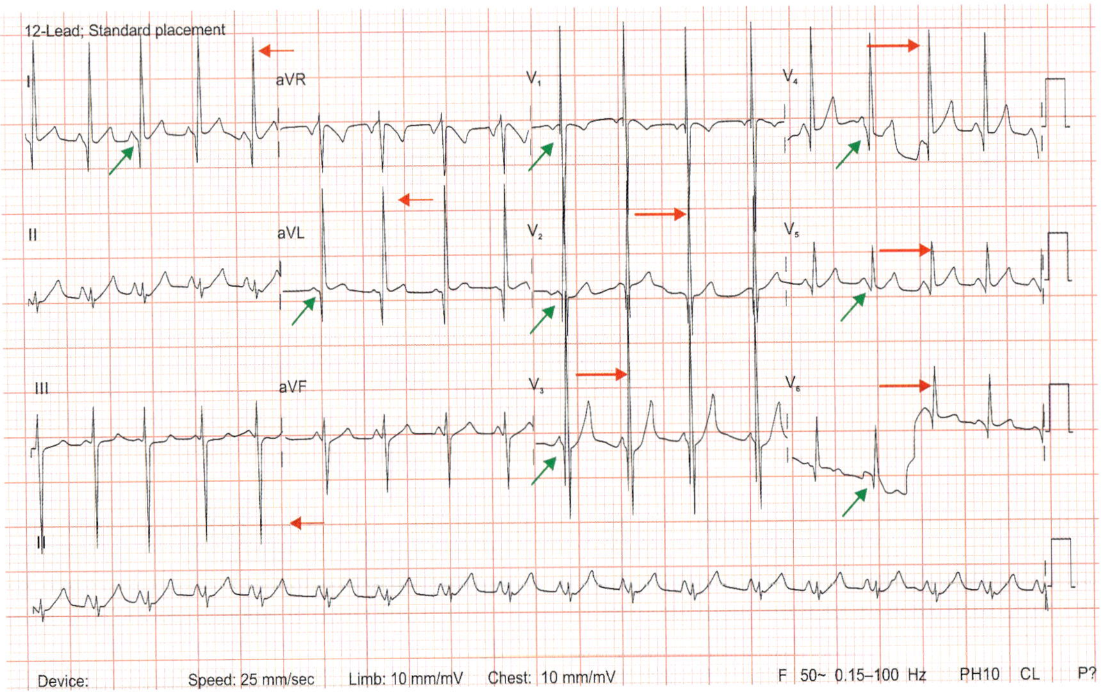

FIG. 23: Three months cyanotic child diagnosed to have DILV, DORV, severe PS, and significant AS. ECG is showing LAD, counterclockwise loop, similar type OS complexes with varied voltage in precordial leads.

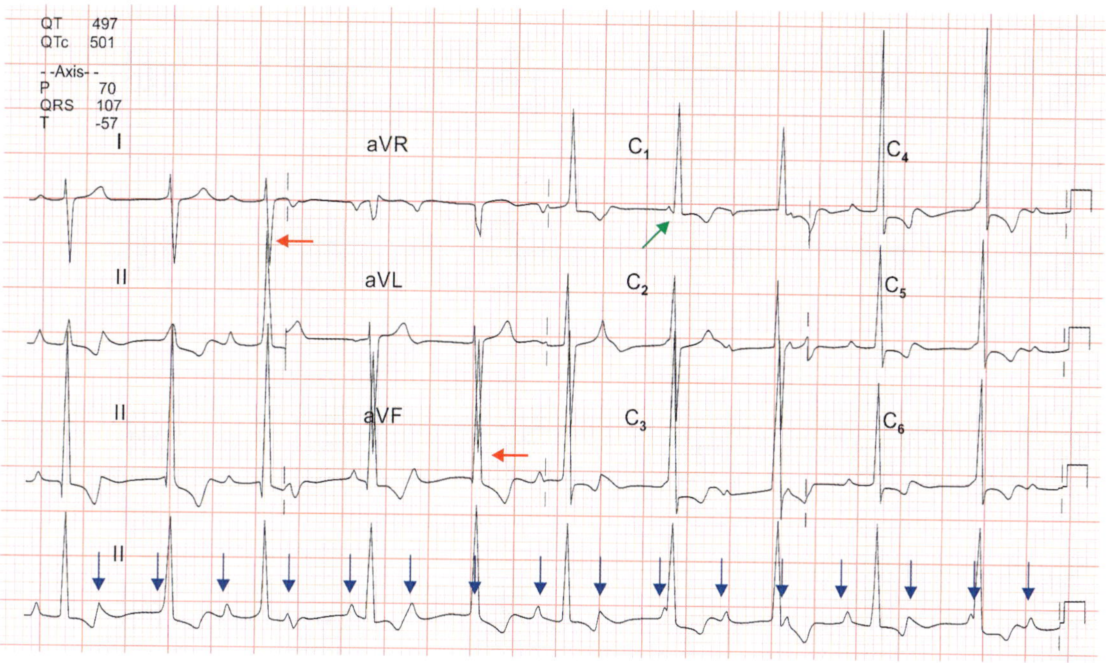

FIG. 24: ECG from 11-year-old child with corrected transposition (L-TGA) of great vessels, nonrestrictive VSD, severe pulmonary stenosis. ECG shows HR: 60 beats/min, complete AV dissociation, absence of Q wave in left-sided leads, right axis deviation (frontal QRS +110°), biventricular hypertrophy.

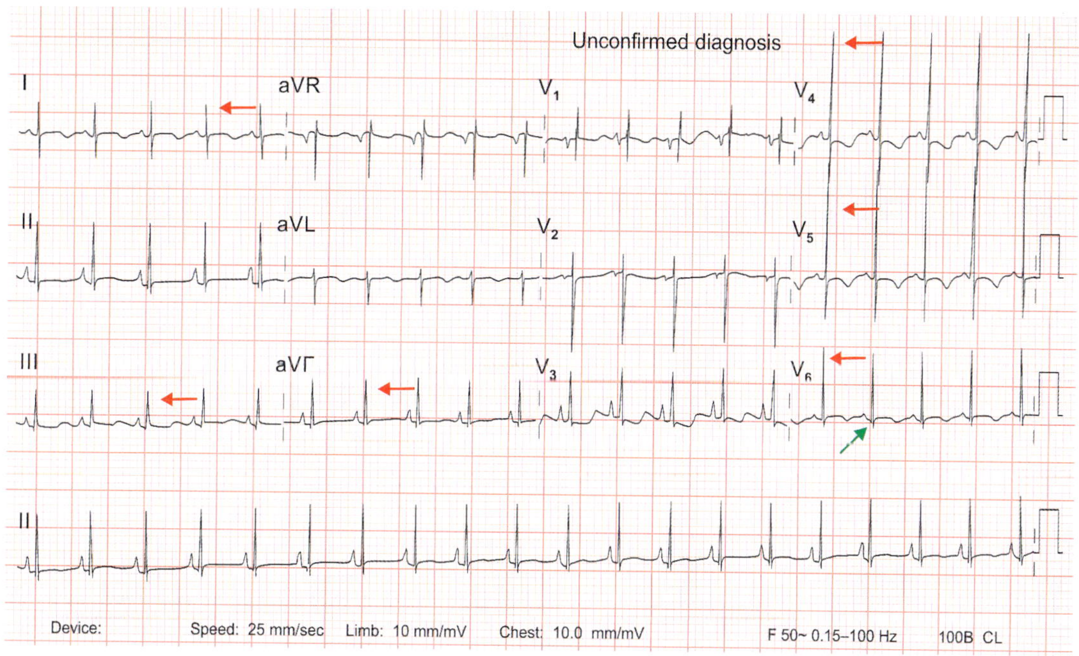

FIG. 25: A 5-month-old with diagnosis of VSD PA and large collaterals. ECG showing RAD with left ventricle volume overloading pattern along with transition pattern between V_1 to V_2.

chamber and then distributed to whole body. Mixing at atrial level seen with common atrium. TAPVC, mixing at ventricular level seen with DORV with VSD, single ventricle, tricuspid atresia, and mixing at great vessel level occur with persistent truncus arteriosus. Incomplete mixing occurs with TGA and it depends on ASD/VD/PDA to maintain adequate flow.

DORV-VSD, TGA, and truncus with high pulmonary blood flow are the lesions that usually shows hemodynamics similar a large VSD due to volume overloading of left ventricle. The right ventricle is also under systemic pressure. Thus, ECG will show biventricular enlargement and right side frontal plane QRS axis. The group of patients with tricuspid atresia and single ventricle show left axis deviation and left ventricular forces. Hypoplastic left heart syndrome shows RAD and RVH with absence of LV forces.

DOUBLE OUTLET RIGHT VENTRICLE WITHOUT PULMONARY STENOSIS

It behaves like large VSD. ECG changes vary with type of VSD and great vessels relation. With transposed great vessels, ECG shows prolonged PR and counter-clockwise loop (Q wave in 1 and aVL). LAD is important featured of DORV subaortic VSD along with large RS complexes in midprecordial lead and by tall waves in left precordial leads. In DORV subpulmonic VSD (Taussig-Bing), PR interval prolongation is less frequent, QRS axis is vertical/rightward with clockwise depolarization resembling of TGA **(Fig. 26)**.

TRANSPOSITION OF GREAT ARTERIES

ECG is normal in initial days of life. Tall peaked P wave is seen due to increased mean RA pressure related to CCF or due to increase in volume. Left atrial P wave is seen with large ASD with increased pulmonary blood flow. RAD is variable as per pulmonary blood flow with degree of pulmonary flow obstruction.

TGA, VSD without PS: RAD in moderate or absent, LV volume overload is seen. Biventricular hypertrophy is seen due to low PVR and volume and pressure overloading of LV. In spite of high LV volume, Q waves are absent in left leads and precordial R waves are small in left leads. Right leads show taller T waves as compared to left leads.

TGA with ASD and increased PBF: RAD is most striking, pure RVH is seen

TGA, VSD, with PS/PVOD—obstruction to PBF: Here, decrease in LV volume and concomitant increase in right ventricle volume is seen due to hypervolemic systemic circulation. It is seen as pure RVH on ECG **(Fig. 27)**.

Truncus Arteriosus

In absence of any pulmonary flow obstruction, QRS axis can be normal/leftwards owing to LV volume overload. Precordial leads show biventricular forces with volume overloading pattern in left leads, and equiphasic QRS in midprecordial leads. With PS, QRS axis is rightwards with clockwise loop.

Total anomalous pulmonary venous connection shows ECG features similar to large pretricuspid shunt like atrial septal defect with prominent P wave, RAD, and RVH.

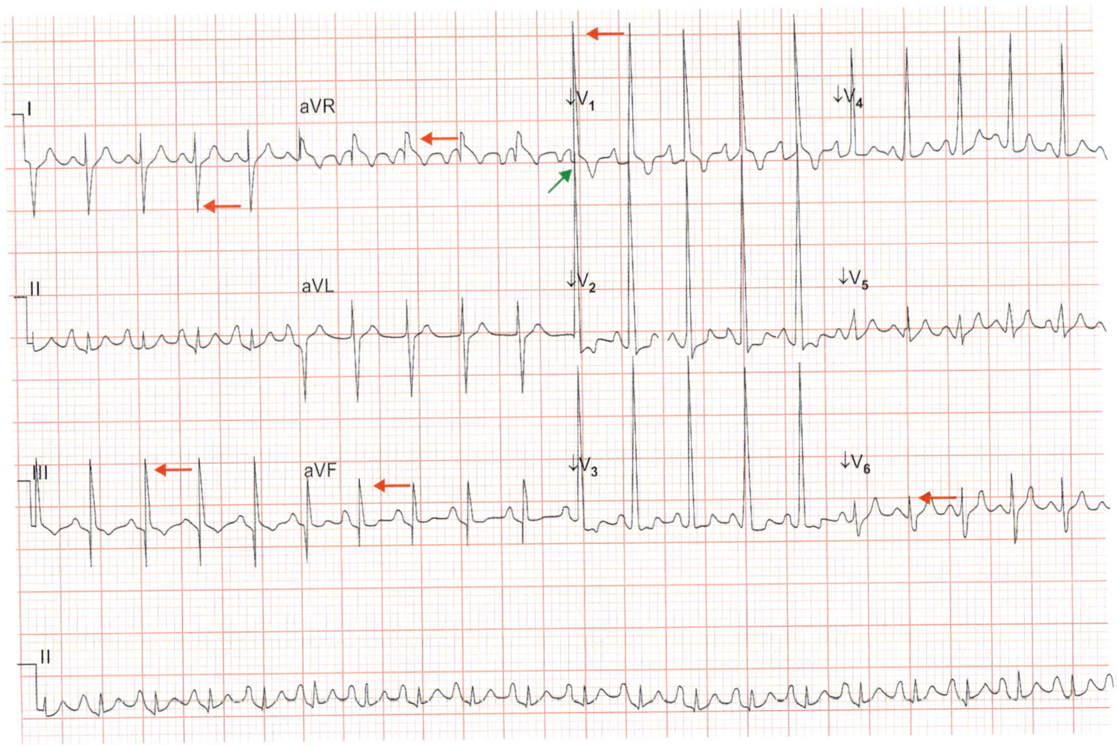

FIG. 26: ECG in an infant with DORV VSD PAH showing biatrial enlargement, RAD and monophasic R wave in with regression pattern toward left leads.

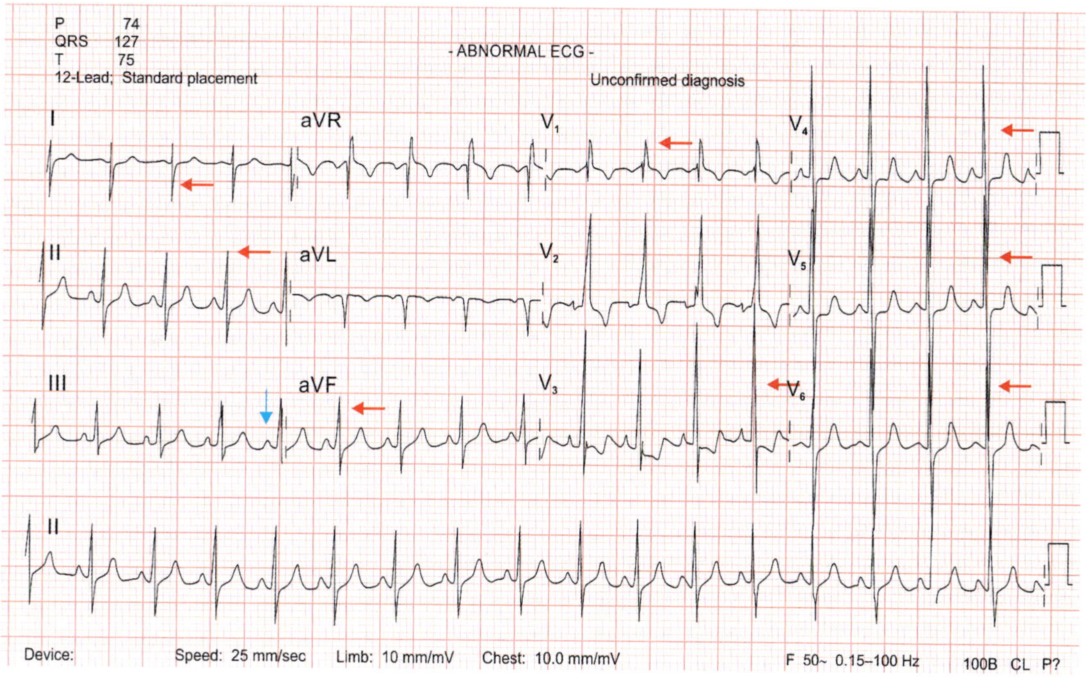

FIG. 27: A 26-year-old case of TGA-ASD-Eisenmenger syndrome showing normal P axis, right atrial enlargement, RAD, RSr′ in V_1, R wave in V_2–V_3, and equiphasic QRS complexes in left leads. Reciprocal S waves due to RVH are seen in left leads.

SINGLE VENTRICLE

Single ventricle shows variety of pattern owing to varied ventricular morphology, great artery relationship and increased or decreased pulmonary blood flow. With increased blood flow, left atrial P waves are seen while with PS right atrial P waves are seen.

Single ventricle with morphological LV: More common as compared to morphological RV. With morphological LV, ECG features differ with location of outflow chamber.

Morphological LV with inverted outflow chamber shows QRS axis inferior and to the right (away from outflow chamber and towards main mass), PR is prolonged with occasionally CCHB, clockwise depolarization (Q waves in 2, 3, AVF), Q waves in right precordial leads, dominant r in V1 and RS equiphasic complexes in mid leads.

Morphological LV with noninverted outlet chamber shows left and superior axis, counterclockwise loop (Q in 1 and avL), small Q waves in left precordial leads and stereotyped QRS in precordial leads.

Single ventricle with morphological RV shows normal PR, usually right axis deviation with occasional left and superior axis, tall stereotyped precordial R.

SPECIAL SITUATION AND SPECIFIC ECG PATTERN

As emphasized before, it is very rare to reach a morphological diagnosis by the ECG in CHD. There are however some lesions which produce "classic" ECG patterns.

ANOMALOUS LEFT CORONARY ARTERY FROM PULMONARY ARTERY

Characteristic ECG pattern in this condition is one of anterolateral myocardial infarction with deep Q waves in 1, aVL, and V_4–V_6 with ST segment elevation and T wave inversion. As the child grows older, if he survives with development of collaterals, ST and T wave changes may disappear and Q waves diminish in size. ECG features of LVH and LAD are common especially in older patients. This represents true cardiac hypertrophy especially of the posterobasal portion of the left ventricle **(Fig. 28)**. Left atrial overload pattern may also be present due to high LV filling pressure or associated ischemic MR. Other congenital abnormality like coronary origin stenosis can also present with similar pattern.

EBSTEIN'S ANOMALY

ECG is rarely normal in Ebstein's even with mild disease. Classical features of Ebstein's anomaly are right atrial overload and presence of large (Himalayan) P waves dwarfing the small right sided (V_1) leads **(Fig. 29)**. It is due to prolonged conduction in hugely dilated right atrium. Prolonged PR also attributed to prolonged conduction in the large right atrium. QRS shows right ventricular conduction delay of RBBB pattern present in 75–95% cases. Distinctive second QRS complex (originate from atrialized RV) is attached to preceding normal complex. Splintered QRS complexes are seen making difficulty in determining QRS axis but usually it is inferior axis **(Fig. 29)**. Deep Q waves are seen in inferior

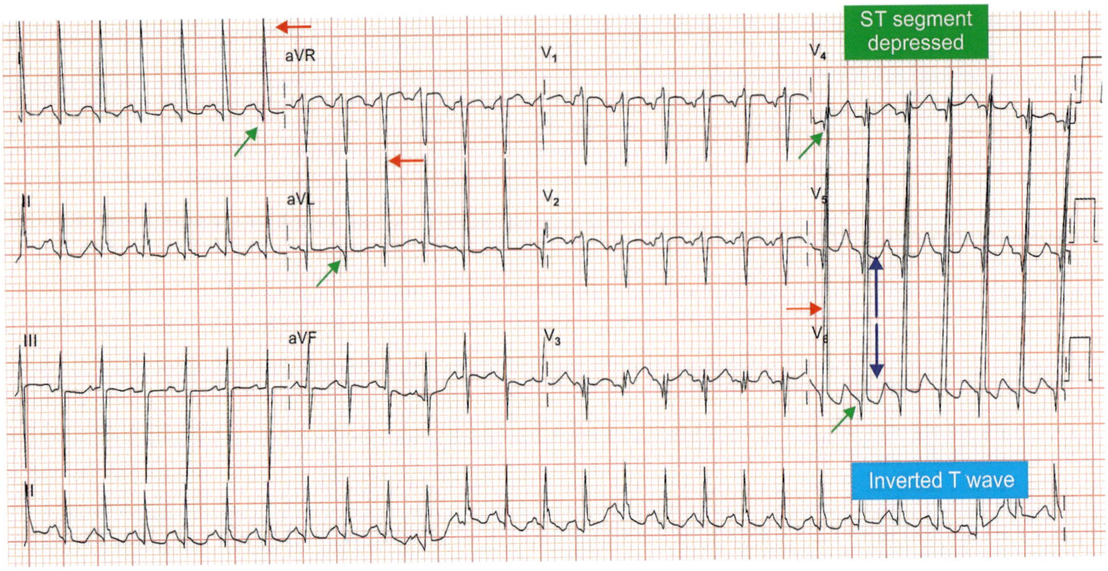

FIG. 28: A 12-year-old presented with severe MR with preserved LV function diagnose to have ALCAPA. ECG is showing tachycardia, broad and bifid P wave, LAD with ischemic pattern in left precordial and limb leads (deep Q, ST depression, T inversion) suggestive of coronary steal seen with ALCAPA.

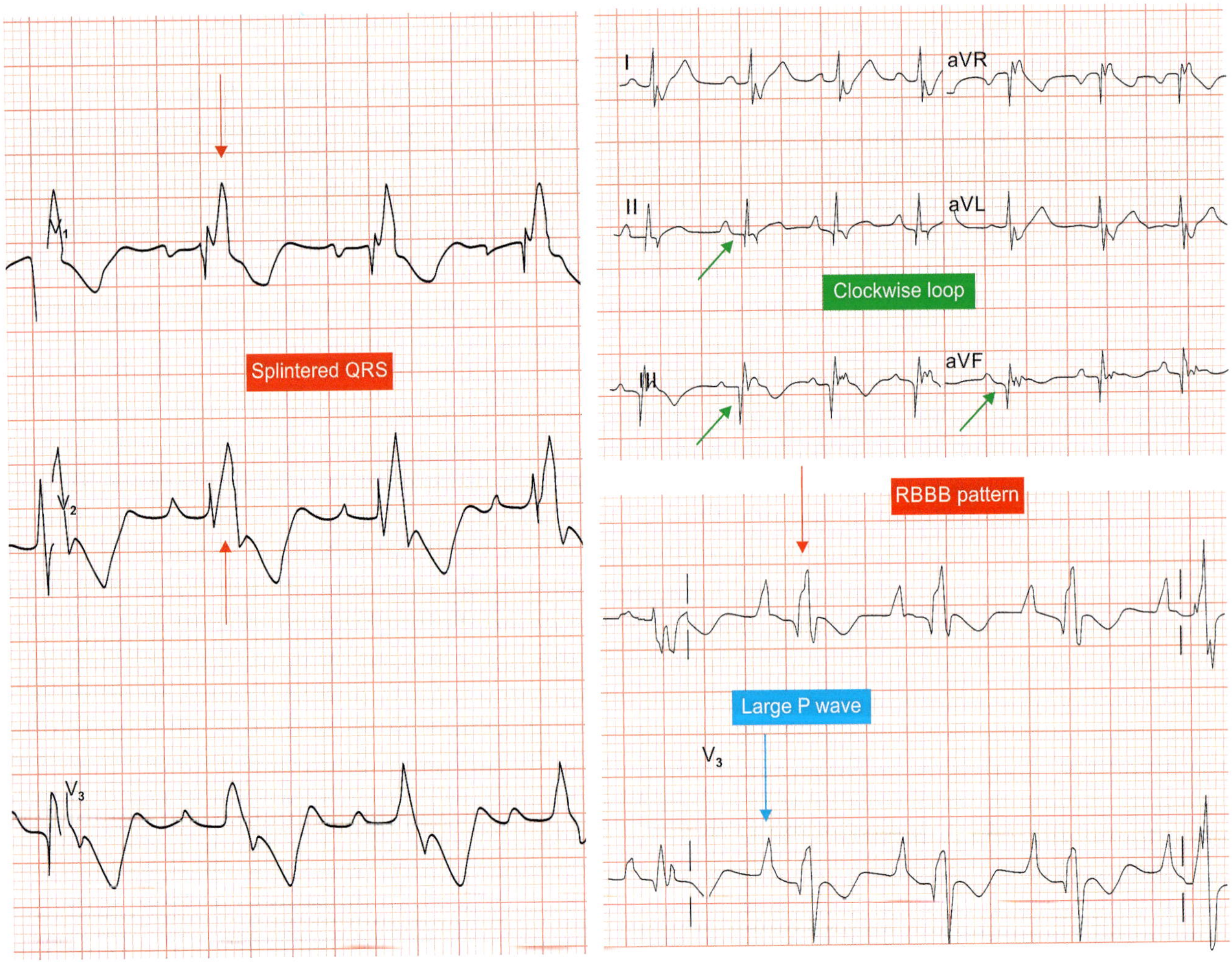

FIG. 29: Typical ECG findings seen with Ebstein's anomaly. Splintered QRS, clockwise loop and very large Himalayan P wave.

leads and most importantly in V_1 or V_1–V_4 due to recording of RV intracavitory potential by precordial leads unusually far leftwards due to large size of atrium **(Fig. 29)**.

Rhythm disturbances in the form of SVT, atrial flutter, and AF are present in 25–30% cases. Type B WPW is seen in 5–25% cases making it only cyanotic CHD associated with preexcitation. It causes left superior axis.

DEXTROCARDIA

In dextrocardia, the ECG helps to identify the atrial and ventricular positions. The abnormal position of heart in the routine ECG may be suspected by the presence of progressive decrease in QRS amplitudes toward V6 **(Fig. 30)**. With cardiac position in right hemithorax, situs can be solitus, inversus, or isomerism (left or right). Complex heart defects are more likely to occur when dextrocardia occurs with situs solitus or with isomerism.

Dextrocardia with situs inversus (mirror image dextrocardia): In dextrocardia with situs inversus, the cardiac anatomy, the position of cardiac chambers, sinus node and the conduction system are all a mirror image of the normal (mirror image dextrocardia). P waves are negative in lead I and aVL and positive in aVR. The P wave axis is shifted to right inferior (atrial inversion) quadrant. Lead aVR resembles aVL and lead III resembles lead II of the normal ECG. The Q waves normally seen in leads V_5, V_6, I, and aVL are seen in V_5 R, V_6R, and aVR. The left-sided chest leads V_1–V_6 show RS complexes of diminishing voltages.

Dextrocardia with situs solitus (isolated dextrocardia): In dextrocardia with normal visceroatrial sinus and D-loop ventricle (atrioventricular concordance), the left ventricle is relatively anterior and the right ventricle lies to the right. V_1 and V_2 reflect left ventricular forces and V_5R and V_6R reflect right ventricular forces. The initial septal depolarization is normal hence the Q waves are present in V_1 and V_2 and RS complexes in V_5R and V_6R leads. As the atria are in normal position, the P wave morphology and axis is normal. In the presence of L-Loop ventricles (atrioventricular discordance) in this condition, the Q waves appear on the right-sided chest leads (V_5R, V_6R), reflecting inverted pattern of septal depolarization. However, one should remember that the ECG in patients with dextrocardia would show additional changes according to the associated defects.

Dextrocardia with isomerism ***(Flowchart 1)***: Usually have associated complex heart defects, univentricular atrioventricular connection, so ECG does not show any consistent finding. It reflects the findings of associated lesions.

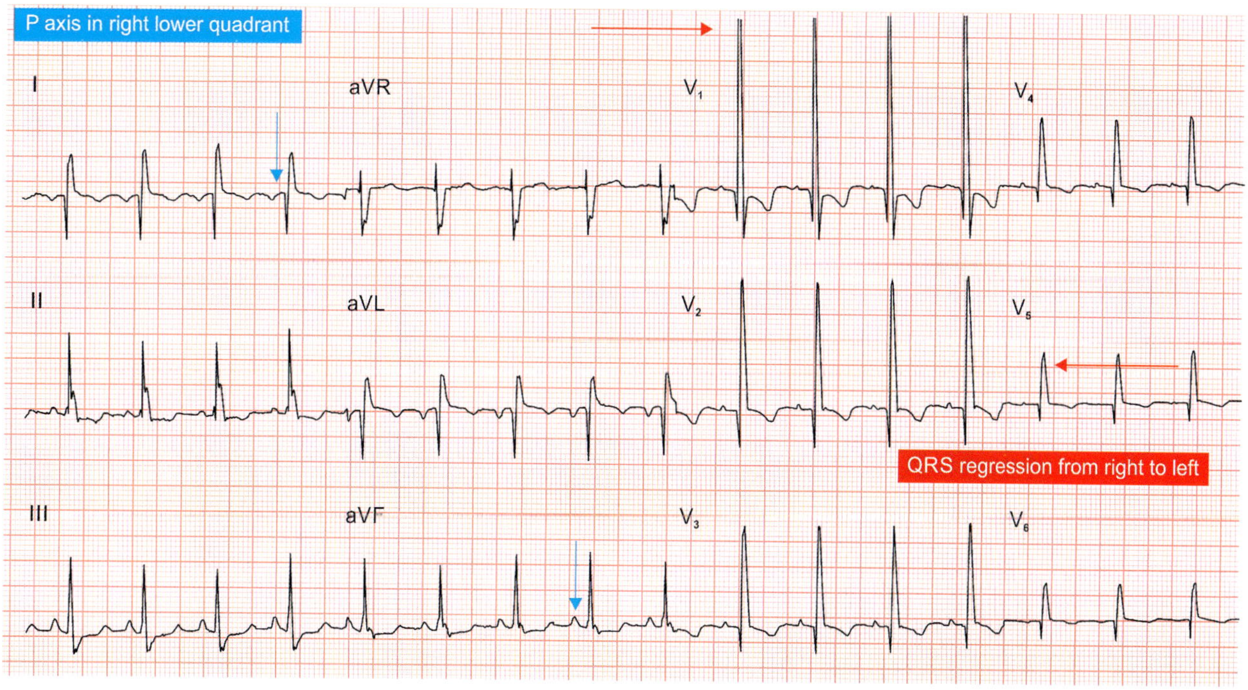

FIG. 30: ECG with normally placed leads from a 4-year-old child with situs inversus, dextrocardia, atrioventricular and ventriculoarterial concordance, VSD, PS. ECG shows atrial situs inversus ("P" wave negative in aVL, I, positive in aVR, II, III, aVF), frontal QRS axis +90°, regression in QRS voltages from right to left.

CONCLUSION

ECG gives insight to the hemodynamics about the particular group of legions. Its yield increases with consideration of age, saturation, and chest radiograph. With an algorithmic approach the diagnosis can be narrowed down to a specific physiological subgroup **(Flowcharts 1A to C)**. Subtle clues can then be sought in the ECG like the frontal plane QRS axis in trying to further narrow down the differential diagnosis. Only rarely there are some lesions, which show classic ECG findings which help in reaching specific diagnosis. It is important to remember normal variations in ECG, criteria for ventricular/atrial enlargement, ability to calculate frontal QRS axis accurately.

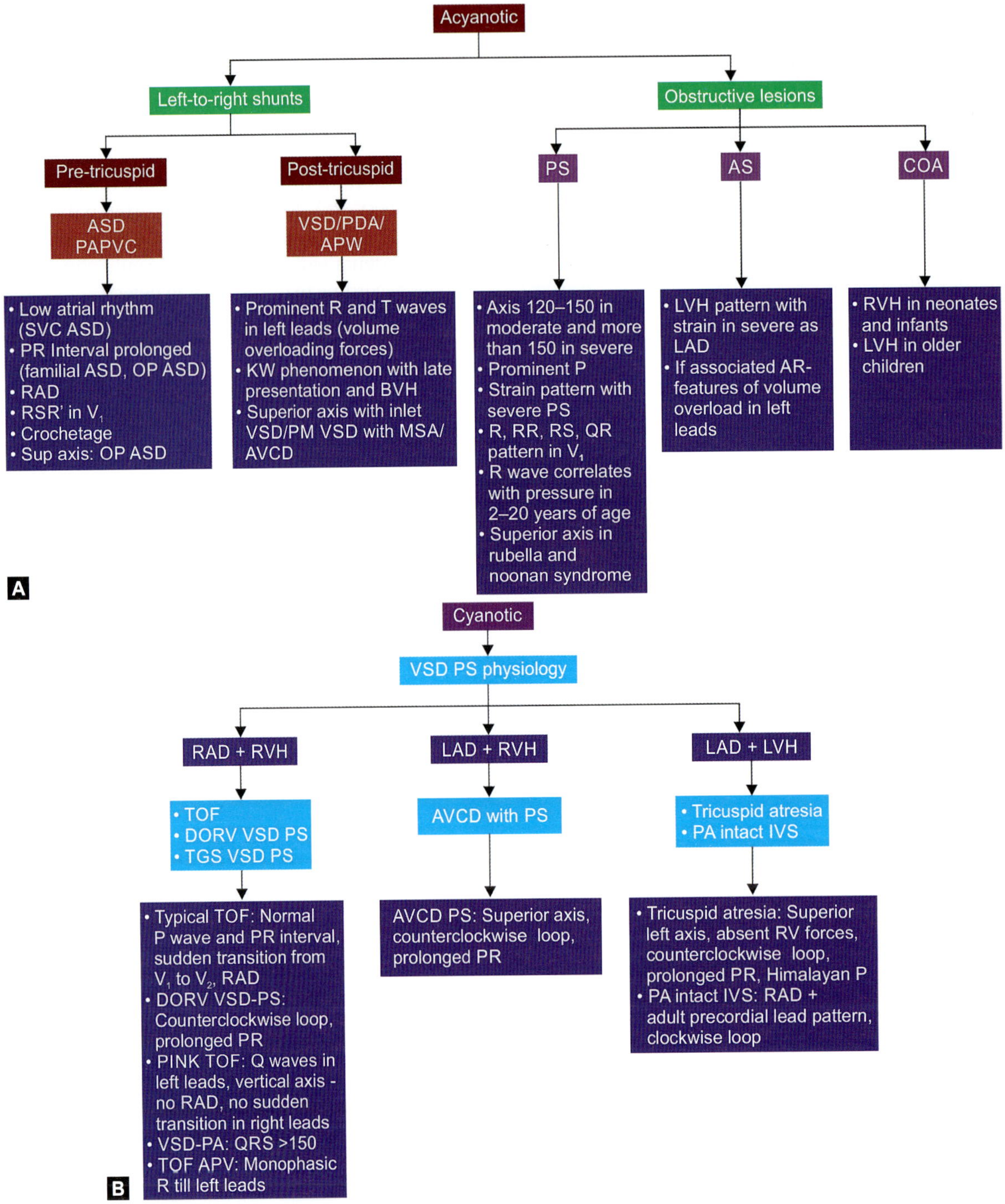

FLOWCHARTS 1A TO C: *Continued*

Continued

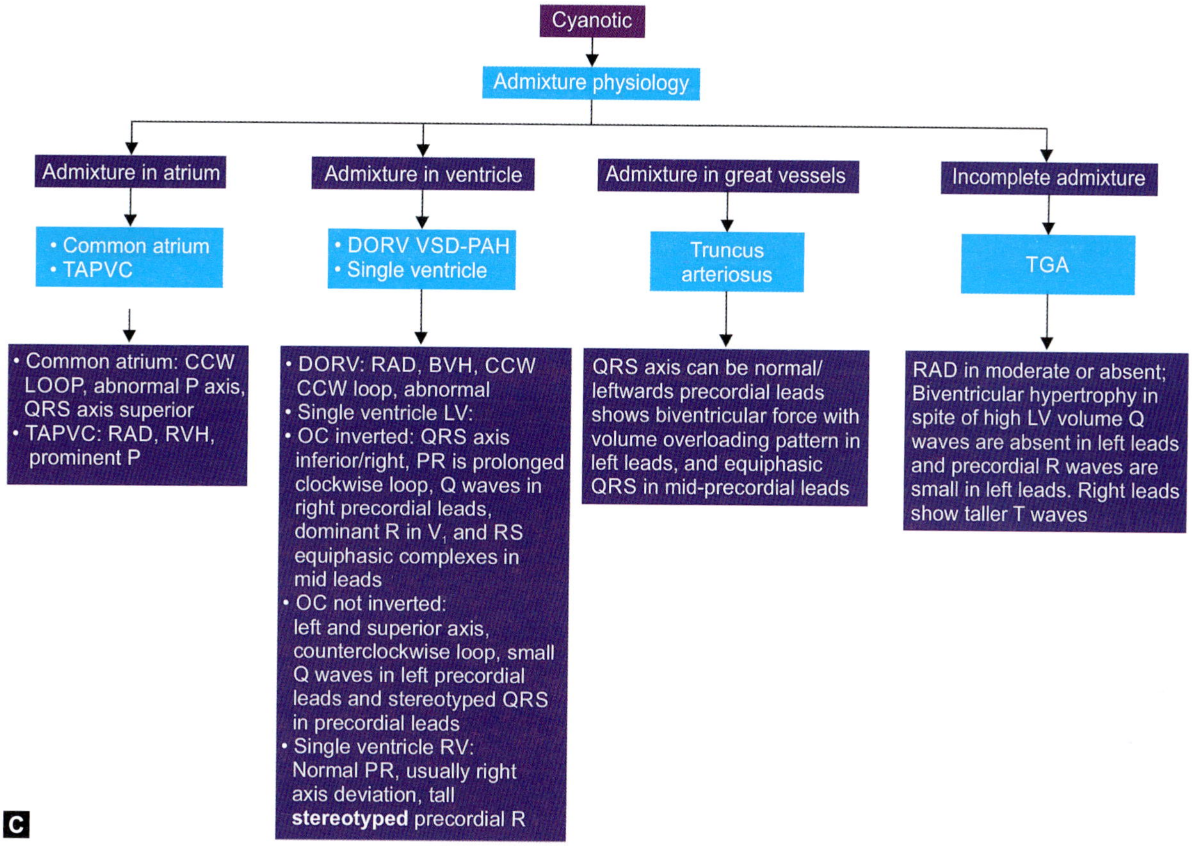

C

FLOWCHARTS 1A TO C: Simplified approach for ECG changed found in congenital heart disease.

ONLINE REFERENCES

Please scan the QR code provided at the end of the table of contents for References of this chapter.

CHAPTER

90

Chest X-ray in Congenital Heart Disease

Ankur Handa, Praveen Arumugam, Nirmal Ghati

ABSTRACT

Imaging is one of the most indispensable investigational modalities in the diagnosis and management of cardiovascular diseases. Innovations of newer technologies and better understanding of conventional imaging have made our lives easy by delineating the anatomy and physiologic basis of cardiovascular diseases of all ages. However, in this era of advancements, we should not ignore simple, inexpensive but highly informative imaging tools such as chest X-ray. A systematic and thoughtful interpretation of chest X-rays can decode lots of information regarding both simple and complex congenital heart diseases. It not only helps to narrow down differentials but also complements other investigations such as echocardiography, cardiac tomography, and magnetic resonance imaging. This chapter provides a guide to the systematic interpretation of a chest radiograph and a review of the classic radiological signs of congenital heart diseases.

Keywords: Chest X-ray, congenital heart disease, transposition of great arteries (TGA), tetralogy of fallot (TOF)

INTRODUCTION

Chest X-ray gives a lot of information in cardiovascular patients, especially with congenital heart disease (CHD). It is an inexpensive and easily available investigation that not only helps in diagnosis but is also, useful in tracking disease course in follow-up. The information we get from the image includes the situs, cardiac size, specific chamber enlargement, pulmonary arterial and venous enlargement, pulmonary hypertensive changes, lungs, and soft-tissue abnormalities. Like any other imaging modalities, they should be interpreted with basic information such as the patient's age, symptoms, and presence of cyanosis. A stepwise thoughtful approach helps in improving the clinical diagnosis.

SITUS

Determination of visceroatrial situs should be the first step while assessing chest X-rays of patients with suspected CHD. Certain abnormalities of abdominal and thoracic visceral situs increase the probability of complex CHD and heterotaxy syndromes.[1] Thoracic or tracheobronchial situs depends on the relation of the bronchus to the pulmonary artery. The right bronchus is wider, shorter, and course vertically above the right pulmonary artery (i.e., eparterial) whereas the left bronchus is longer and runs more horizontally below the left pulmonary artery (i.e., hyparterial). Tracheobronchial situs corresponds better with atrial situs than abdominal situs. Abdominal situs can be identified by the occupation of liver and stomach gas shadow in the abdominal compartment **(Fig. 1A)**. Situs solitus totalis denotes the normal arrangement of organs where the right lung is trilobed, the left lung is bilobed, the morphologic right atrium is at the right side of the morphologic left atrium, the spleen and stomach on the left side, and the liver on right side of the abdomen. Situs inversus totalis denotes the exact mirror imaging pattern **(Fig. 1B)**. Situs ambiguous does not fit in either solitus and is often associated with isomerism or heterotaxy syndrome. The liver may occupy the central transverse position, and there may be malrotation of bowels, absence of gallbladder, and duplication of right or left-sided structures. They may be also associated with asplenia or polysplenia syndromes **(Figs. 2B and C)**.

The next step is the determination of cardiac apex. The cardiac apex usually points toward the left side (levocardia). In dextrocardia, the cardiac apex is toward the right side, and in mesocardia **(Fig. 2A)**, the heart occupies the central position. Situs solitus with levocardia is the most common

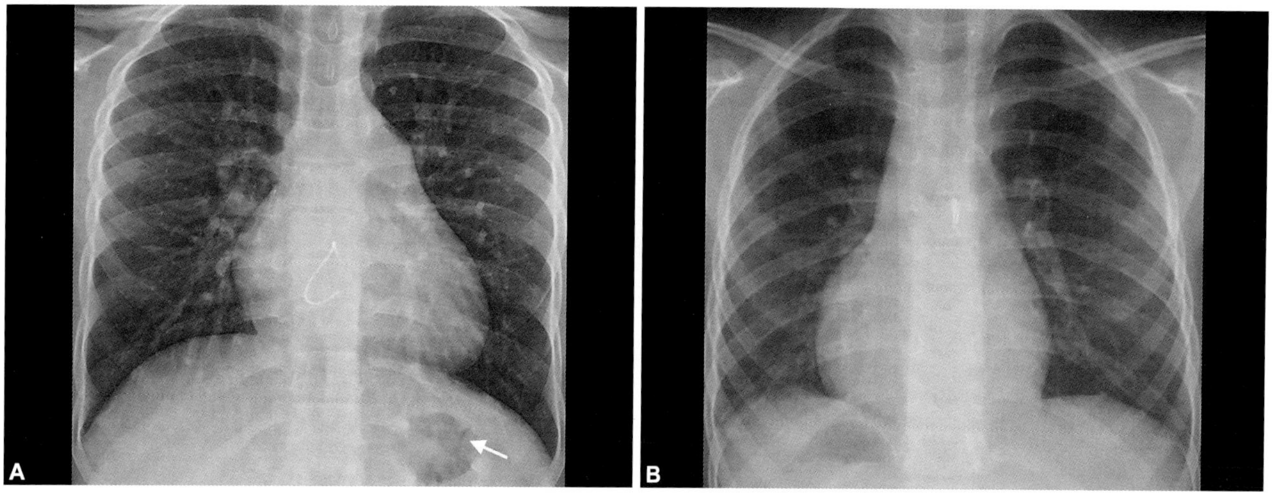

FIGS. 1A AND B: (A) X-ray of patient with situs solitus and levocardia. The gastric shadow is on left (arrow). Right bronchus is short and wide whereas left bronchus is horizontal and long compared to right one. Artefact is seen in the middle; (B) X-ray of patient with situs inversus dextrocardia. The bronchial pattern is mirror image of situs solitus.

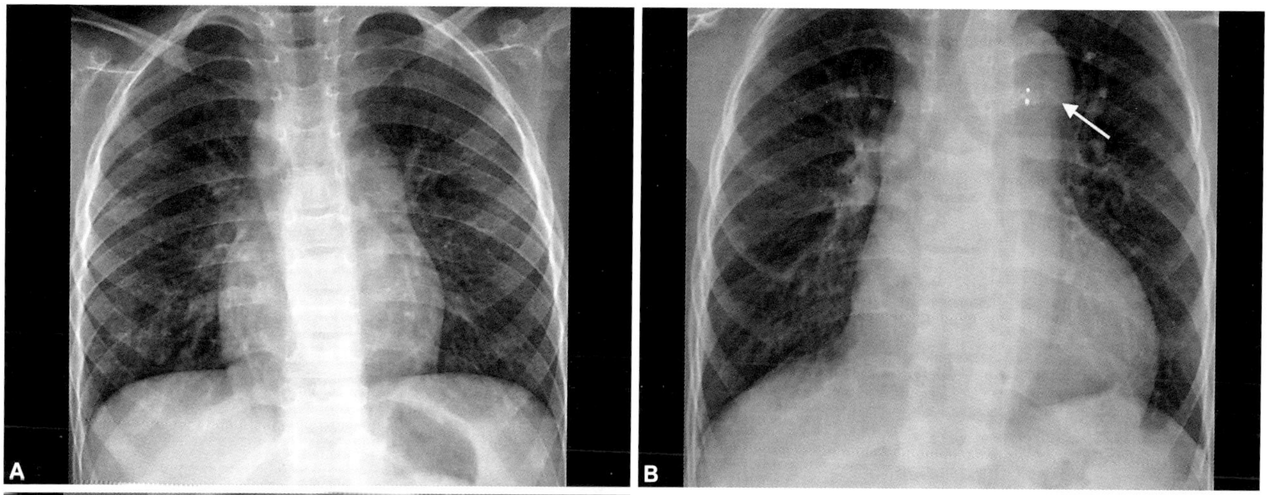

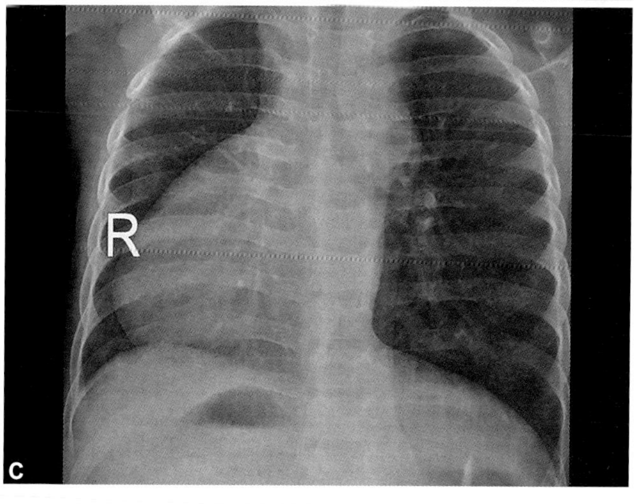

FIGS. 2A TO C: (A) Patient with mesocardia and TGA. (B) X-ray showing left bronchial isomerism. Patient had associated polysplenia and PDA. ECG was suggestive of ectopic atrial rhythm. PDA device is also seen (arrow). (C) Patient with situs inversus, dextrocardia, and right isomerism. One can see right bronchus morphology on both sides.

(ECG: electrocardiograph; PDA: patent ductus arteriosus; TGA: transposition of the great arteries)

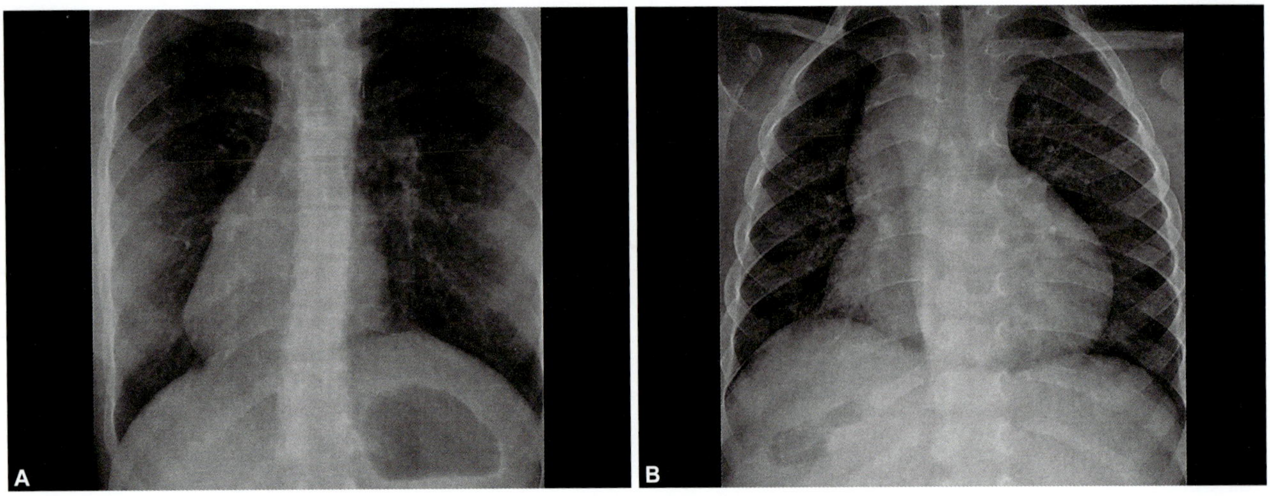

FIGS. 3A AND B: (A) Patient with situs solitus and dextrocardia with DORV, VSD and PS; (B) Patient with situs inversus levocardia. This patient had associated corrected TGA, DORV, VSD and PS with left isomerism.

(DORV: double outlet right ventricle; PS: polysplenia syndrome; TGA: transposition of the great arteries; VSD: ventricular septal defect)

anatomic variation with the least incidence of CHD (~0.8%). The incidence of CHD is 3–5% in the mirror image variation, i.e., situs inversus with dextrocardia. Patients having situs solitus with dextrocardia and situs inversus with levocardia have a high incidence (>90%) of complex CHD **(Figs. 3A and B)**. These patients usually have cyanotic CHD such as congenitally corrected transposition of great arteries (cc-TGA), double-outlet right ventricle (DORV), pulmonary atresia, and venous anomalies. Discordance between thoracic and abdominal situs is rare and also associated with a high incidence of CHD.

CARDIAC SIZE AND CHAMBER ENLARGEMENT

A cardiothoracic ratio of >60% in neonates and 55% in infants defines cardiomegaly.[2] One should be aware of whether the film was taken in the inspiratory or expiratory phase and anteroposterior (AP) or posteroanterior (PA) view. Expiratory film and AP films may have apparent cardiomegaly. The thymic shadow may give the appearance of cardiomegaly in infants. The cardiomegaly in the majority of patients is due to ventricular enlargement; however, it can be due to atrial enlargement or pericardial effusion. In mild-to-moderate ventricular enlargement, the right ventricular has an upturned apex over the left hemidiaphragm and left ventricular enlargement has a broader apex dipping into the diaphragm. The ventricular enlargement may be due to volume overload (left-to-right shunts, valvular regurgitation) or a failing ventricle. They are also enlarged in anemia, hyperthyroidism, and systemic arteriovenous malformations.

In right atrial (RA) enlargement, the right atrium occupies at least three intercostal spaces, and the height of the right heart border from diaphragm to superior vena cava—right atrium (SVC-RA) junction is larger than that of SVC-RA junction to arch. In adults, the right atrial margin >5.5 cm from the midline denotes RA enlargement.[3] RA enlargement may be due to left-to-right shunt at an atrial level as in atrial septal defect (ASD) **(Fig 4)**, Gerbode defect, isolated tricuspid regurgitation with pulmonary stenosis/atresia, Ebstein anomaly, tricuspid stenosis or atresia, and total anomalous pulmonary venous connection (TAPVC). In patients with left atrial (LA) enlargement, there is straightening of the left heart border due to left atrial appendage enlargement. There is elevation of the left bronchus and there may be a double atrial shadow along the right heart border. LA enlargement happens in left-to-right shunts such as ventricular septal defect (VSD), patent ductus arteriosus (PDA), atrioventricular

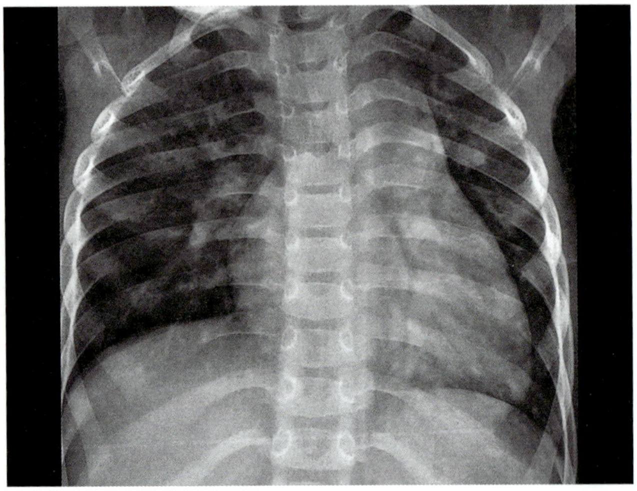

FIG. 4: X-ray of ASD patient showing right atrial enlargement and prominent PA conus.

(ASD: atrial septal defect; PA: pulmonary artery)

septal defect (AVSD), aortopulmonary (AP) window, mitral stenosis/atresia, and hypoplastic left heart syndrome (HLHS). Left-side obstructive lesions have pulmonary venous hypertension without cardiomegaly, except in failing ventricles and HLHS.

GREAT VESSELS

Main Pulmonary Artery

The main pulmonary artery gives clues regarding the relation of great vessels. The pulmonary area in the left heart border is formed by the main pulmonary artery and part of the left pulmonary artery. The absence of normal pulmonary shadow in its position indicates transposition of great arteries (TGA) or decreased pulmonary blood flow as in pulmonary atresia and tetralogy of Fallot (TOF). The pulmonary artery segment is prominent when there is increased blood flow as in ASD, VSD, PDA, AVSD, severe pulmonary artery hypertension, or pulmonary artery aneurysm. They are also enlarged in pulmonary stenosis due to poststenotic dilatation.

Aorta

The aortic arch may be right or left-sided. The isolated right aortic arch is not uncommon in patients without CHD. However, the patients with right side aortic arch with suspected CHD almost always have associated VSD.[4] The right-sided aortic arch also has increased incidence in specific heart diseases such as common arterial trunk (CAT), VSD with pulmonary atresia, and TOF. The sidedness of the arch can be identified by the presence of indentation over the tracheal shadow. The left aortic arch has indentation on the left side of the trachea as the arch courses through. The right aortic arch has indentation over the right side of the trachea.

Pulmonary Vasculature

The pulmonary vasculature gives an idea about increased or decreased blood flow and pulmonary venous hypertension. The normal pulmonary artery vasculature is seen well in the medial one third of the hemithorax. The pulmonary vessels are also visible in the middle third but lesser than the medial one-third. Very few vessels can also be seen in the outer third but are less prominent. Pulmonary oligemia is present when pulmonary vessels in the middle one-third and lateral one third are markedly attenuated. The pulmonary plethora is present when there is a prominent right descending pulmonary artery (RDPA) or significant end-on vessels in lung fields. The transverse diameter of the RDPA ≥ 16 mm or more than the size of the trachea is considered significant.[5] The end-on vessels are compared to the accompanying bronchus to say it is prominent and are significant when there are ≥3 end-on vessels on either side or ≥5 end-on vessels in total.[6] They are prominent when there is a left-to-right shunt and increased blood flow physiology in CHD.

TABLE 1: Grading of pulmonary venous hypertension.[7]

Grades of PVH	Mean PCWP (mm Hg)	CXR features
Grade 1	14–19	Cephalization of blood flow
Grade 2	20–25	Interstitial pulmonary edema Kerley B lines
Grade 3	>25	Alveolar edema

(CXR: chest X-ray; PCWP: pulmonary capillary wedge pressure; PVH: pulmonary venous hypertension)

Pulmonary veins are usually not prominent in the upper zone of the lungs. They become prominent when there is pulmonary venous hypertension (PVH) due to left-side obstruction (AS, MS, CoA, cor triatriatum), pulmonary vein stenosis, and obstructed TAPVC. The findings vary depending on the degree of hypertension **(Table 1)**. Mild obstruction causes prominence of the pulmonary venous system in the upper zone due to redistribution (Antler sign). Further increase in pressures causes interstitial and interlobular edema manifesting as Kerley lines.[7] Severe obstruction leads to white-out lungs with pulmonary edema. This is important in patients with obstructed TAPVC where there is no cardiomegaly and can mimic hyaline membrane disease.

ACYANOTIC HEART DISEASE: LEFT-TO-RIGHT SHUNTS

Atrial Septal Defect

A significant shunt at the atrial level causes volume overload of the right atrium and ventricle along with dilated pulmonary artery. X-ray shows a dilated right atrium along with an enlarged pulmonary shadow **(Fig. 5)**. There is evidence of pulmonary plethora.[4] LA enlargement is usually reserved for adult patients with atrial fibrillation. Patients with sinus venosus ASD may have local dilatation of SVC at the site proximal to the attachment to the right atrium. In Scimitar syndrome, anomalous partial pulmonary venous connection to the inferior vena cava forms a distinct parallel shadow to the right cardiac silhouette. The heart is shifted to the right due to right lung hypoplasia.

Ventricular Septal Defect

The shunt at the ventricular level causes both volume overload and pressure overload to the pulmonary artery depending on the size of VSD. There is a volume overload of the left atrium and ventricles which will be evidenced in X-ray as cardiomegaly along with LA enlargement and apex of LV type **(Fig. 6)**. Like ASD, there is evidence for increased pulmonary blood flow. The patient with a small VSD may have an X-ray like a normal heart. Patients with AVSD will have X-ray features such as large VSD.

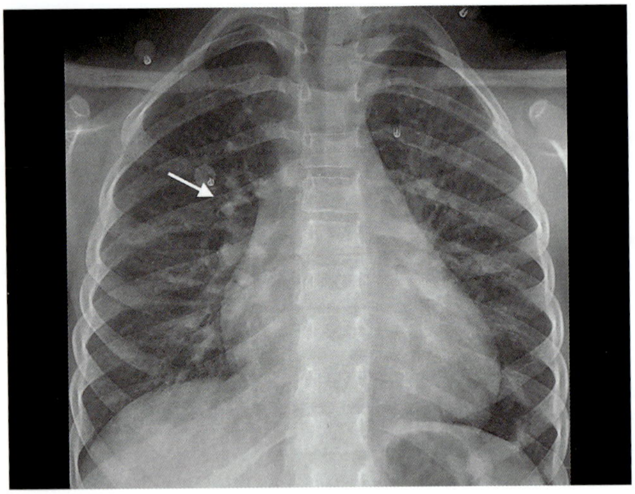

FIG. 5: X-ray of patient with atrial septal defect showing right atrial enlargement and increased pulmonary blood flow. Arrow showing prominent end on vessels.

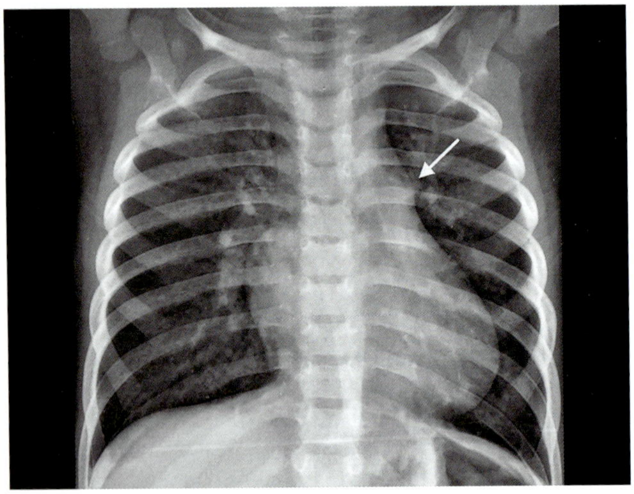

FIG. 6: Patient with large ventricular septal defect showing cardiomegaly with increased pulmonary blood flow features. There is also prominent pulmonary conus (arrow).

Patent Ductus Arteriosus and Aortopulmonary Window

Patent ductus arteriosus and AP windows will also cause left-side volume overload such as VSD. In addition to the features present in VSD, patients with PDA and AP windows will have dilated aorta. The aorta is inconspicuous at birth but becomes dilated once the circulation through the aorta increases. Sometimes, PDA may be seen in frontal X-rays as a small convex shadow between the aorta and pulmonary artery.[8]

ACYANOTIC HEART DISEASE: OBSTRUCTIVE LESIONS

Pulmonary Stenosis

Pulmonary stenosis unless associated with a shunt at the atrial or ventricular level does not cause cyanosis. The X-ray may look normal, except for pulmonary oligemia in the initial stages. There will be associated cardiomegaly once ventricular dysfunction and or tricuspid regurgitation develops. The main pulmonary artery may be dilated **(Fig. 7)** due to poststenotic dilatation; however, they may be normal in patients with dysplastic pulmonary valve.

Aortic Stenosis and Left Heart Disease

X-rays of patients with aortic stenosis may be normal, except for dilated ascending aorta which is common in patients with bicuspid aortic valve (BAV). The ascending aorta may be dilated even without stenosis in patients with BAV. There is cardiomegaly once ventricular dysfunction develops **(Figs. 8A and B)**. Neonates with critical aortic stenosis and coarctation of the aorta (CoA) may have huge cardiomegaly due to biventricular dysfunction. Old patients with CoA can have rib notching due to collateral formation through intercostal arteries. There may be a "3" sign at the site of coarctation with prominent upper and lower segments **(Fig. 9)**. Left atrial enlargement is a sign of severity. The aortic arch may be small in an associated hypoplastic arch.

The obstruction at mitral level in congenital MS will have evidence of LA enlargement with features of PVH. LA enlargement will be absent if the obstruction is due to cor-triatriatum or pulmonary vein stenosis.

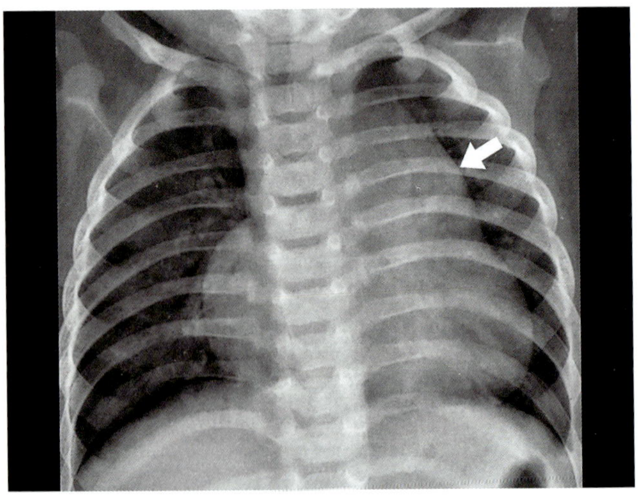

FIG. 7: X-ray of a patient with severe pulmonary stenosis. There is hugely dilated main pulmonary artery (arrow) with decreased pulmonary blood flow.

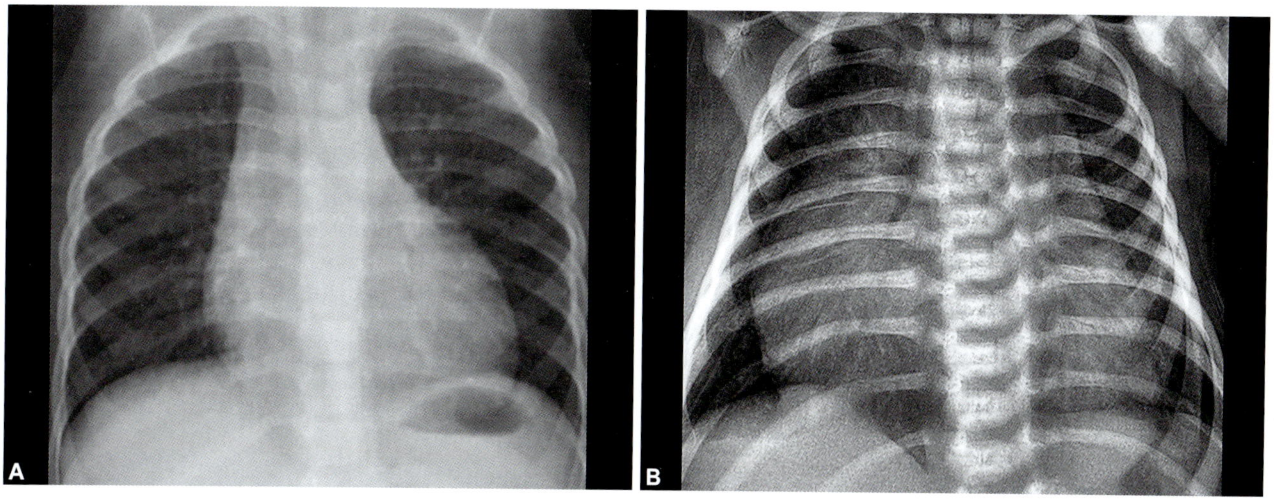

FIGS. 8A AND B: (A) Neonatal presentation of severe valvular AS presenting with LV dysfunction. There is cardiomegaly with enlarged left heart border. (B) Neonatal CoA with severe biventricular dysfunction. There is huge cardiomegaly with enlargement of right-side structures also.

(AS: aortic stenosis; CoA: coarctation of the aorta; LV: left ventricular)

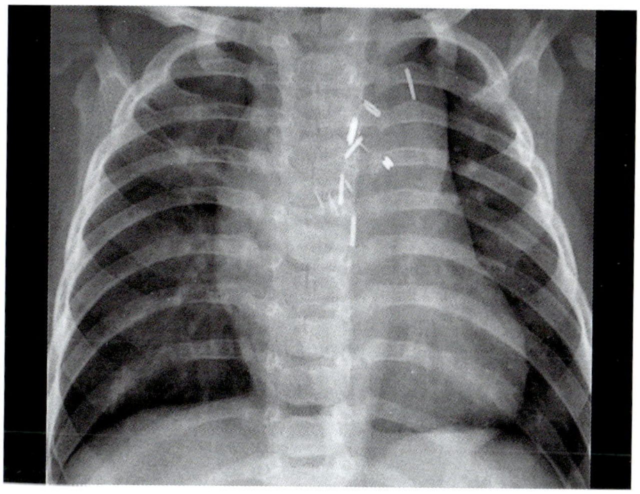

FIG. 9: Postoperative X-ray of patient with coarctation of aorta. There is a dilated ascending aorta proximal to repaired segment. Surgical clips are present.

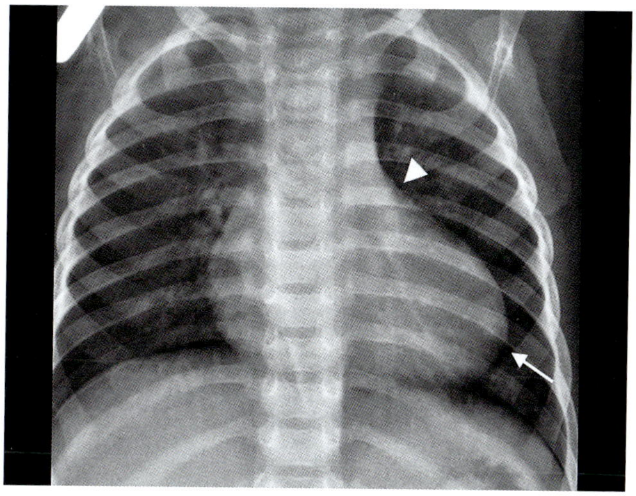

FIG. 10: Classic TOF with boot-shaped heart. There is evidence of RV enlargement with upturned apex (arrow). There is pulmonary oligemia with absent pulmonary bay (arrowhead).

(TOF: tetralogy of Fallot; RV: right ventricular)

CYANOTIC HEART DISEASE

Tetralogy of Fallot and its Physiology

Any lesion with VSD and associated PS has TOF physiology of which classical TOF is more common. The boot-shaped heart (Cœur en Sabot) is the classical X-ray appearance in TOF **(Fig. 10)**. It results from the combination of a small underfilled left ventricle that lies above a horizontal ventricular septum, inferior to which is a hypertrophied nondilated right ventricle. One can see this manifestation as an upturned apex. Other findings are pulmonary oligemia, empty pulmonary bay, and dilated aorta.

Tetralogy of Fallot with absent pulmonary valves have features of TOF except for the hugely dilated main pulmonary artery **(Fig. 11)**. In addition, there may be compression of bronchi due to dilated PAs.

Ventricular septal defect with pulmonary atresia may have decreased or increased pulmonary blood flow depending on collateral supply. Increased pulmonary blood supply due to large collaterals may cause cardiomegaly and the increased blood supply will appear as reticular shadows due to collaterals.

Total Anomalous Pulmonary Venous Connection

Total anomalous pulmonary venous connection without obstruction has cardiomegaly with evidence of increased pulmonary blood flow. There is right atrial and ventricular enlargement. The "snowman sign" or "figure of eight sign" is usually seen in patients with supracardiac TAPVC due to dilatation of the vertical vein and is seen commonly after infancy **(Fig. 12A)**. Patients with obstruction do not have cardiomegaly. They usually have evidence of PVH, sometimes which may even produce a white-out lung **(Fig. 12B)** due to pulmonary edema.

Transposition of Great Arteries

In the dextro-transposition of great arteries (d-TGA), the cardiac shadow looks like an "egg-on-side" appearance. There is cardiomegaly, pulmonary plethora, and a narrow base **(Fig. 13)**. The narrow pedicle is due to the AP arrangement

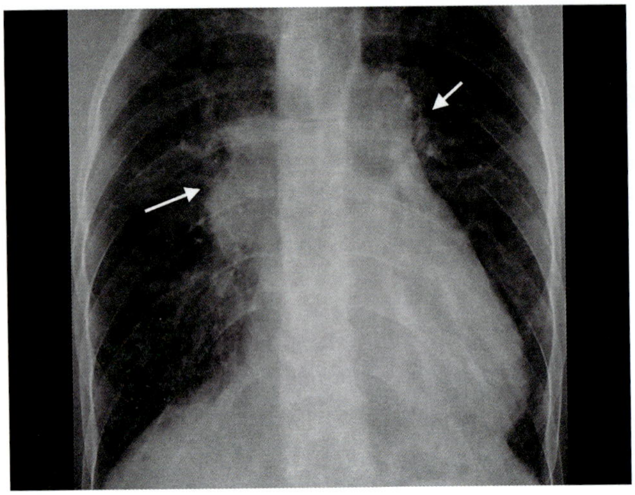

FIG. 11: Tetralogy of Fallot with absent pulmonary valve. One can note hugely dilated pulmonary arteries (arrows) with peripheral pulmonary oligemia.

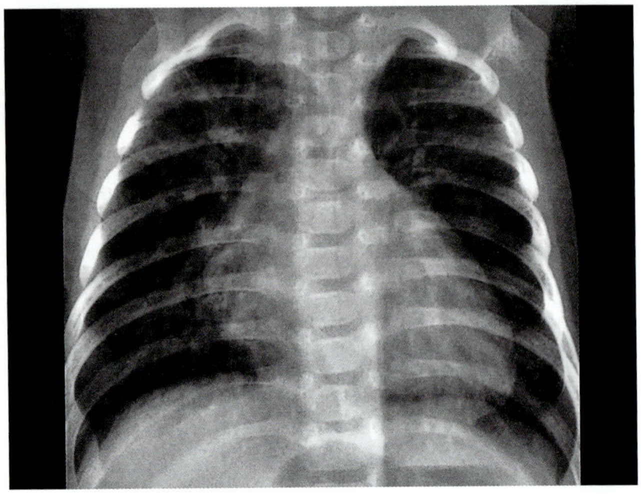

FIG. 13: Chest X-ray of patient with dextro-transposition of the great arteries and intact ventricular septum. There is egg-on-side appearance due to enlarged right atrium on right side and left ventricle border on left. The pedicle is narrow due to anteroposterior great vessel arrangement and absent thymic shadow.

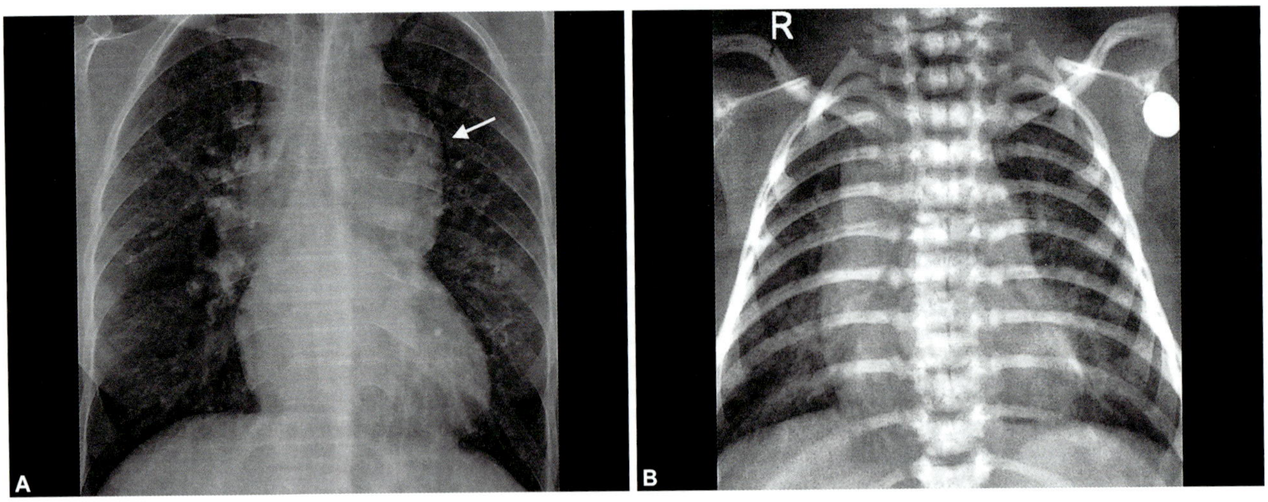

FIGS. 12A AND B: (A) 24-year-old women with supracardiac TAPVC. The vertical vein is dilated (arrow) giving the appearance of snow man. (B) Obstructed supracardiac TAPVC of a 4-day-old neonate. Vertical vein was crossing to right and was draining into SVC innominate vein junction with obstruction at draining site. There is evidence of pulmonary venous hypertension with no cardiomegaly and prominent right upper border formed by vertical vein.

(SVC: superior vena cava; TAPVC: total anomalous pulmonary venous connection)

of great vessels and the absence of thymic shadow. TGA with VSD or PDA and restrictive ASD will have features of pulmonary venous hypertension. The left heart border is straight when there are juxtaposed atrial appendages.

Tricuspid Atresia

The right heart silhouette is more prominent due to RA dilatation and relatively straight IVC because of hypoplastic RV. The apex is formed by the left ventricle. Tricuspid atresia with pulmonary stenosis has decreased blood flow. In both normally related great vessels and transposition, the left atrium is enlarged when pulmonary blood flow is unrestrictive.

Common Arterial Trunk

Increased pulmonary blood flow causes pulmonary plethora and cardiomegaly. The main pulmonary trunk when present as in Van Praagh type A1, arises higher than normal position. The main pulmonary segment is absent in type A2 patients where there is a separate origin of pulmonary arteries **(Fig. 14A)**. The left pulmonary artery is usually more prominent than the right. Pulmonary arteries are very prominent in patients with pulmonary vascular disease. CAT patients may have an absence of either pulmonary artery and are manifested as oligemic lung fields and smaller hemithorax **(Fig. 14B)**. The pulmonary arteries are absent commonly on the same side as the aortic arch in contrast to TOF where they are absent on the contralateral side to that of the arch. Cardiomegaly may be absent when pulmonary blood flow is restricted because of stenosis and the patient will be cyanotic. However, cardiomegaly is present even in cyanotic patients when truncal regurgitation is significant. The right aortic arch is commonly associated with CAT and their incidence increases if the patient has 22q11 mutation.

Eisenmenger Syndrome

Patients with long-standing left-to-right shunt in acyanotic heart disease and increased pulmonary blood in cyanotic patients develop pulmonary vascular disease. The time of developing pulmonary vascular disease depends on the magnitude of the shunt and duration. There will be peripheral pruning of pulmonary vessels, where the descending order of pulmonary branch size is >50% lesser than previous order branches. There is pulmonary oligemia where one can find black-out lung fields beyond the hilar region. The pulmonary conus becomes prominent. In patients with VSD, PDA, and AP window, the cardiac size becomes normalized due to a decrease in shunting. This may not be the case in ASD, and X-ray may not give clue, except for oligemia and peripheral pruning **(Fig. 15A)**. AVSD with Eisenmenger behaves like a large VSD, except in cases with significant atrioventricular valve regurgitation where one can find cardiomegaly. The differentiating feature of TOF with Eisenmenger syndrome is that there will be the absence of signs of increased pulmonary blood flow and the aorta will be larger in TOF. The exception will be the PDA and AP window where the aorta may be prominent as they are enlarged to start with **(Fig. 15B)**.

Ebstein Anomaly

The cardiac silhouette varies from normal to massive enlargement depending on the severity of the anomaly. Even in an otherwise normal-sized heart, the right heart border is

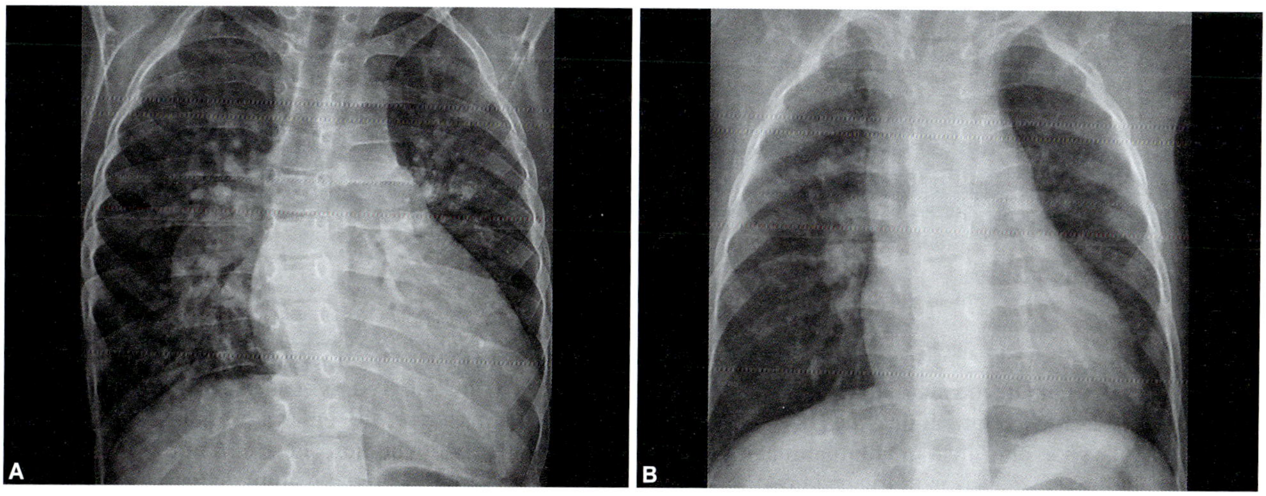

FIGS. 14A AND B: (A) Patient with type A2 Truncus (Van praagh). Pulmonary artery is prominent with high origin. There is cardiomegaly. (B) Truncus type A3 (Van praagh). The right-side pulmonary artery is prominent and left side pulmonary blood flow is reduced. PDA is reforming LPA and supplying left lung.

(LPA: left pulmonary artery; PDA: patent ductus arteriosus)

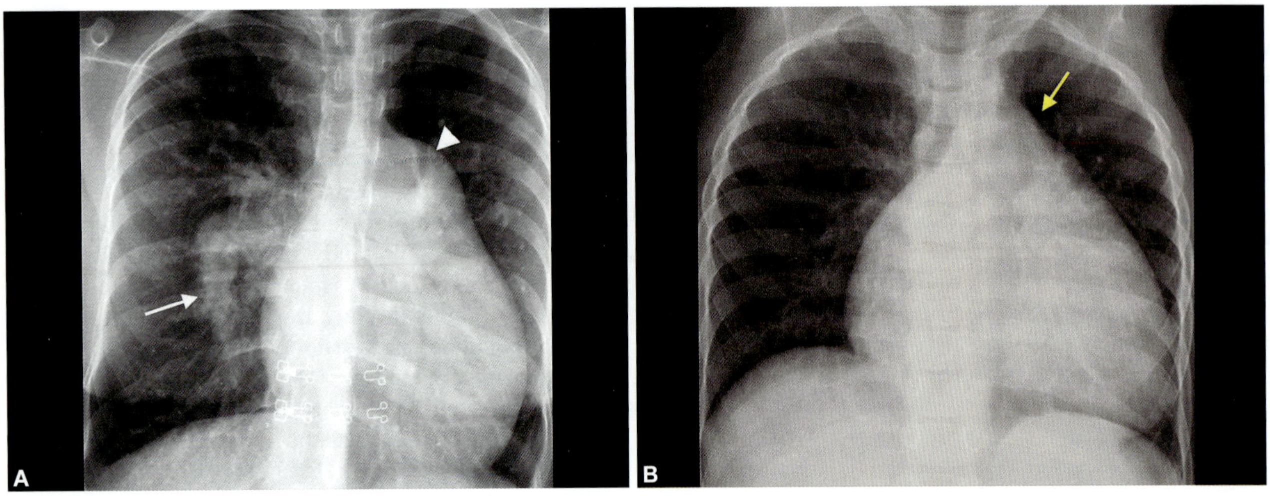

FIGS. 15A AND B: (A) 45-year-old women with ASD and Eisenmenger syndrome. There is prominent right descending PA (arrow) and pruning of peripheral pulmonary arteries with pulmonary oligemia. The cardiomegaly is present and pulmonary conus is prominent (arrowhead). (B) Patient with PDA and Eisenmenger syndrome. The aorta is prominent (yellow arrow) with dilated pulmonary artery. Cardiomegaly is present due to associated ASD and LV dysfunction. Peripheral pulmonary artery pruning and oligemia present in both lung fields.

(ASD: atrial septal defect; LV: left ventricular; PDA: patent ductus arteriosus)

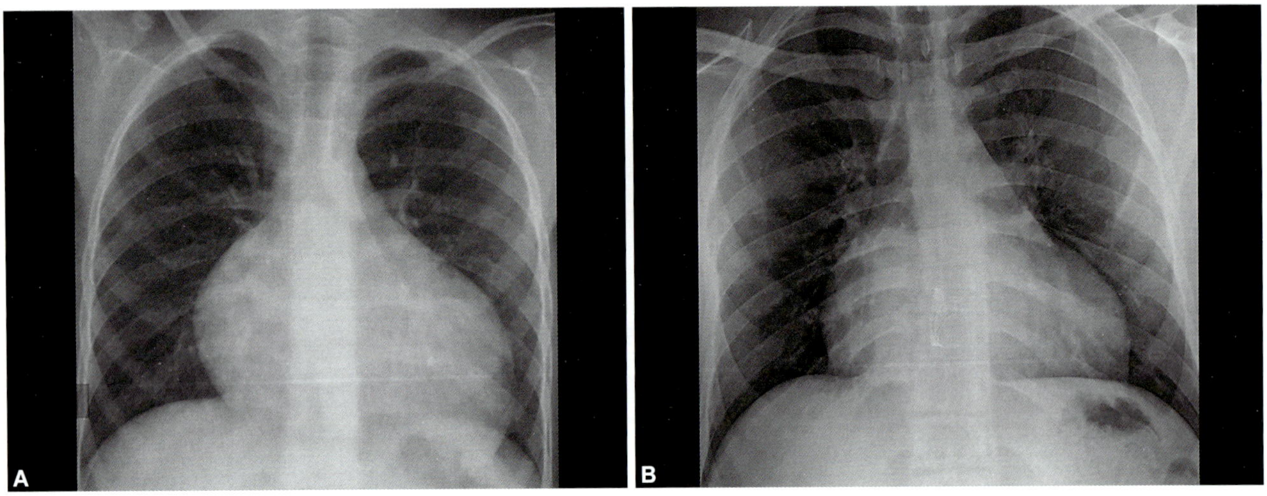

FIGS. 16A AND B: (A) X-ray of patient with Ebstein anomaly. The heart is box shaped. RA border is dilated and there is narrow pedicle. Pulmonary blood flow is decreased. The differential diagnosis would be pulmonary atresia or stenosis with severe TR. (B) Patient with Ebstein anomaly who underwent bioprosthetic tricuspid valve replacement.

(RA: right atrium; TR: tricuspid regurgitation)

seldom normal and is enlarged. The right atrium is hugely enlarged in severe anomaly and there is decreased pulmonary vascularity with cyanosis. Sometimes, they can occupy the entire thoracic cavity. The close differential diagnosis will be critical pulmonary stenosis with tricuspid regurgitation, where the pulmonary artery segment may be prominent. One can differentiate it through ECG as pulmonary stenosis patients will have strong RV forces. Marked rightward convexity of the enlarged right atrium together with marked leftward convexity of the enlarged infundibulum account for a box-like configuration **(Figs. 16A and B)**. The vascular pedicle is narrow because the pulmonary trunk is not border forming and the ascending aortic shadow is inconspicuous or absent.

Congenitally Corrected Transposition of the Great Arteries

The usual borders formed by ascending aorta on the right side and aortic knuckle with pulmonary artery on the left side are completely lost in corrected TGA. The aorta is left and anteriorly placed while the pulmonary artery is right and posteriorly placed. The ascending aorta shadow on the left base may be absent, straight, slightly concave or convex-shaped. The dilated pulmonary artery may cause a prominent upper right border by displacing SVC. The prominent features of the morphologically right ventricle are a hump-shaped appearance caused by the infundibulum and septal notch which is a small indentation corresponding to the apical position of the interventricular grove **(Fig. 17)**.

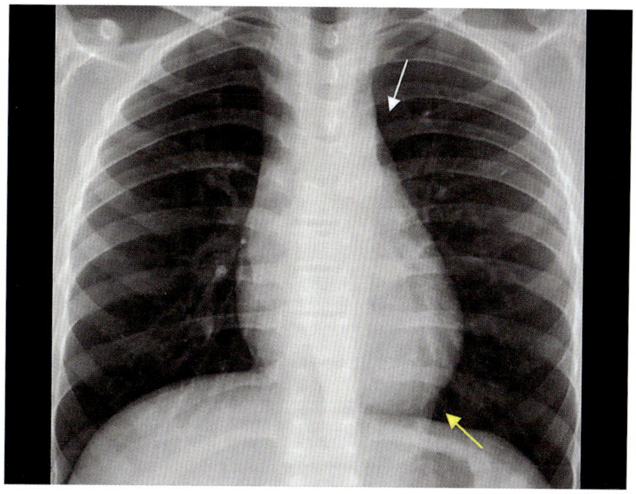

FIG. 17: X-ray of patient with congenitally corrected TGA. There is L-posed aorta (arrow). Yellow arrow showing the septal notch.
(TGA: transposition of the great arteries)

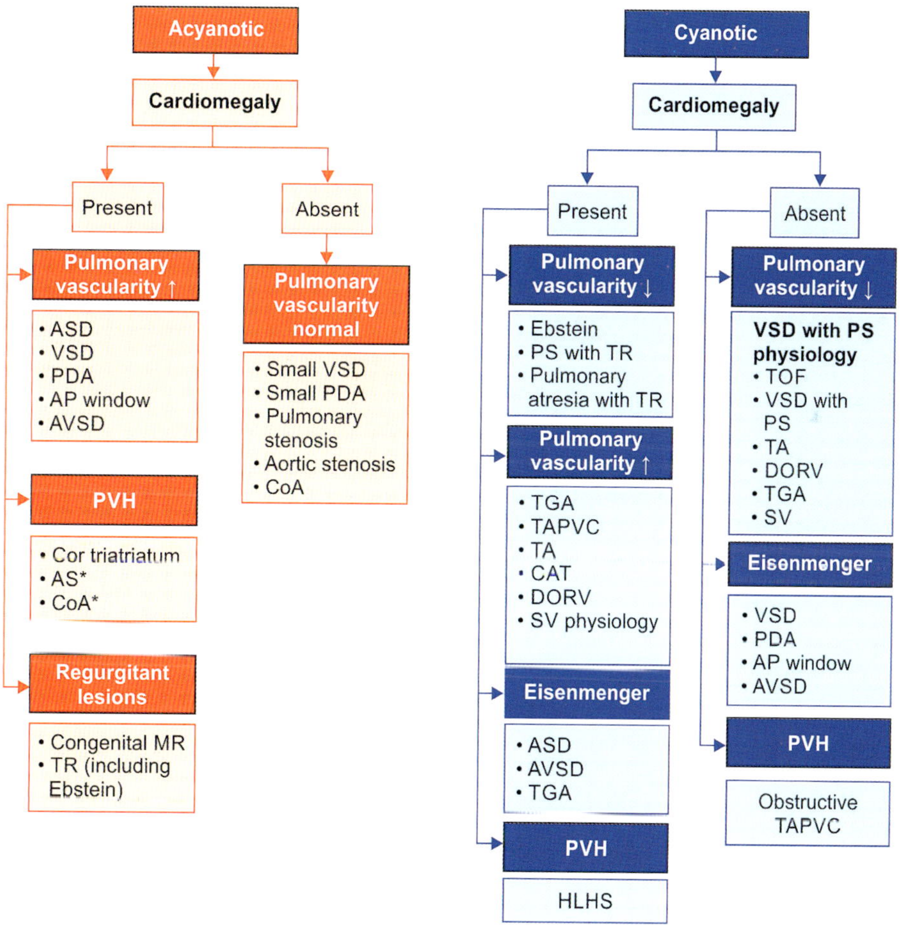

*With LV failure.

FLOWCHART 1: Systematic assessment of chest X-ray in patients with CHD.
(AP window: aortopulmonary window; AS: aortic stenosis; ASD: atrial septal defect; AVSD: artrioventricular septal defect; CAT: common atrial trunk; CHD: congenital heart disease; CoA: coarctation of the aorta; DORV: double-outlet right ventricle; HLHS: hypoplastic left heart syndrome; MR: mitral regurgitation; PDA: patent ductus arteriosus; PS: pulmonary stenosis; SV: single ventricle; TA: tricuspid atresia; TAPVC: total anomalous pulmonary venous connection; TGA: transposition of the great arteries; TOF: tetralogy of Fallot; TR: tricuspid regurgitation; VSD: ventricular septal defect)

CONCLUSION

Chest radiography and its interpretation has become a lost art in the modern era of advanced imaging techniques even though it can confer unique and valuable information in patients with CHD. The differential diagnosis of CHD can be narrowed down based on the presence of cardiomegaly and pulmonary vasculature in chest X-ray **(Flowchart 1)**. Being a simple, quick, and cheap test that yields useful diagnostic information, chest X-ray should be considered as one of the essential basic investigations in every patient with CHD.

ONLINE REFERENCES

Please scan the QR code provided at the end of the table of contents for References of this chapter.

CHAPTER

91

Computed Tomography in Congenital Heart Disease

Krishnamoorthy KM, Gopalakrishnan A, Valakkada J

ABSTRACT

In congenital heart disease (CHD), computed tomography (CT) is a useful tool in the diagnosis and surgical or interventional management as well as follow-up. This chapter reviews the indications, techniques, and dose reduction in CT imaging in CHD. Illustrations of common forms of CHD evaluated by CT are discussed.

Keywords: CHD, CT, management, techniques

INTRODUCTION

Computed tomography (CT) is a noninvasive, complementary imaging modality in the evaluation of congenital heart diseases (CHD). Despite the risk of radiation exposure, CT plays increasing role in management both before and after surgical or percutaneous intervention. Cardiac and extracardiac anatomy, coronary arteries, and vascular structures can be assessed. We discuss the basics of CT, radiation awareness, techniques, some illustrative examples.

INDICATIONS OF CARDIAC CT

Cardiac computed tomography (CT) is done when echocardiography (echo) is inadequate to provide complete anatomical information or when clinical assessment is inconsistent with another diagnostic test. CT is also done as an alternative to catheterization in sick patients. It is also used in postoperative assessment and for 3D printing in preoperative planning of complex congenital heart disease (CHD). CT is the primary modality for evaluating vascular ring or sling, aortopulmonary collateral arteries, and coronary artery anomalies. Patients with pacemakers, cochlear implants, defibrillators, or intrathoracic metal in whom MRI is contraindicated are also served well by cardiac CT. Appropriate-use criteria for cardiac CT have been laid down.[1]

Invasive catheterization has a higher risk and greater radiation exposure, requiring a larger volume of intravascular contrast and often anesthesia. CT use in CHD has increased with a decrease in cardiac catheterizations.[2] CT is superior to transthoracic echo for vascular imaging and complex anatomy.[3] It is less operator dependent than echo.[4] With advancements in technology, newer scanners can image faster with higher quality 2D reformation and 3D reconstruction, making it easier to demonstrate anomalies and analyze complex cardiovascular anatomic features before surgery and to demonstrate post-treatment complications.

PHYSICS AND PREPARATION

It is recommended to do CT with a 64-slice MDCT scanner or higher with a gantry rotation time of <400 ms. Additionally, it is advised to employ adaptive multisegmented reconstruction, dual-source CT, ECG gating capabilities, and a dual-head contrast injector for better image quality. Clear instructions about the gantry environment, strict immobilization, and breath-holding should be provided to children, particularly older ones. Acquiring details about previous surgical procedures is vital, and ensuring the removal of all metallic objects and establishing a secure IV line are imperative.

Prior to administering iodinated contrast for pediatric thoracic CT angiography, it is important to confirm the absence of contraindications. Leg vein is recommended for contrast administration, as contrast into an upper limb vein may lead to streak artifacts in the superior vena cava, potentially obstructing the mediastinal vasculature, particularly the right pulmonary artery (PA) and vein. A 24G cannula is recommended for children under 2 years of age, while a 22G cannula is advised for older children. It is imperative to avoid air injection to prevent systemic embolism. Sedation is often necessary, with oral sedation for children aged 6 months to 5 years and alternative methods for older children. The use of low-osmolar or iso-osmolar intravascular iodinated contrast agents (300 mg iodine/mL or greater) at a dosage of 2 mL/kg body weight, followed by a 5–10 mL saline chaser, is recommended. In complex CHD cases, a smaller volume of saline chase may be considered to ensure adequate contrast opacification of both ventricles.

A dual-head power injector gives consistent and uniform intravascular enhancement. This involves a split-bolus injection followed by a saline chaser. Proper positioning of the patient, along with ECG gating if necessary, is essential to ensure optimal image quality. A low-dose frontal scout topogram is acquired and in certain cases, a noncontrast-enhanced CT is conducted to minimize radiation exposure. Commonly used methods for timing CT image acquisition with IV contrast injection include test dose injection, fixed delay, and automated bolus detection methods, each with its advantages and disadvantages. Test dose injection entails a small test dose followed by repeated image acquisition to calculate the contrast arrival time. Fixed delay utilizes an empirical delay post initiation of the contrast injection. Automated bolus detection methods involve real-time contrast bolus tracking with premonitoring, monitoring, and angio scan phases. The scan range is determined based on the indication, with whole thoracic coverage typically being adequate.

While a non-ECG-gated study is generally sufficient for most cases, an ECG-gated study is recommended for coronary artery assessment. Nonetheless, a nongated study may be adequate for specific questions about the proximal coronary artery. During a gated study, for heart rates exceeding 100 bpm, beta-blockers should be considered (especially in lesser advanced scanners). It is important to refrain from using beta-blockers to reduce the heart rate in critically ill young children with severe heart disease, as it may diminish coronary blood flow and blood pressure.

SPECIFIC LESIONS

Acyanotic Congenital Heart Diseases

Coronary Arteries

Anomalies in the origin of coronary arteries is a cause of sudden death. CT can show ostia, dominance, and angulation from the aortic root. Malignant interarterial course of coronary artery can cause compression resulting in sudden death **(Figs. 1A to C)**.

A coronary arteriovenous fistula can be diagnosed and followed up **(Fig. 2A)**. Screening of coronary lesions after coronary manipulation surgeries like arterial switch or Nikaidoh procedure will need CT for follow-up. Along with evaluation of coronary arteries after Ross operation, dilatation of the autograft causing aortic regurgitation and homograft pulmonic valve stenosis can be assessed.

Kawasaki disease has diagnostic and prognostic information from CT.[5] Sequelae like coronary artery aneurysm, ectasia, thrombosis, stenosis or occlusion, and coronary artery bypass graft status can be assessed. CT is as accurate as conventional angiography for evaluation of postoperative coronary artery abnormalities and assessing stenosis, stretching, kinking, or compression.[6] CT is good for imaging of small caliber vessels, proximal and mid coronaries, and intramural course **(Fig. 2B)**.[7,8]

Arch Anomalies

Coarctation of the aorta: Sensitivity of CT for coarctation is 100% versus 87.5% by echo.[9] Measurement can be

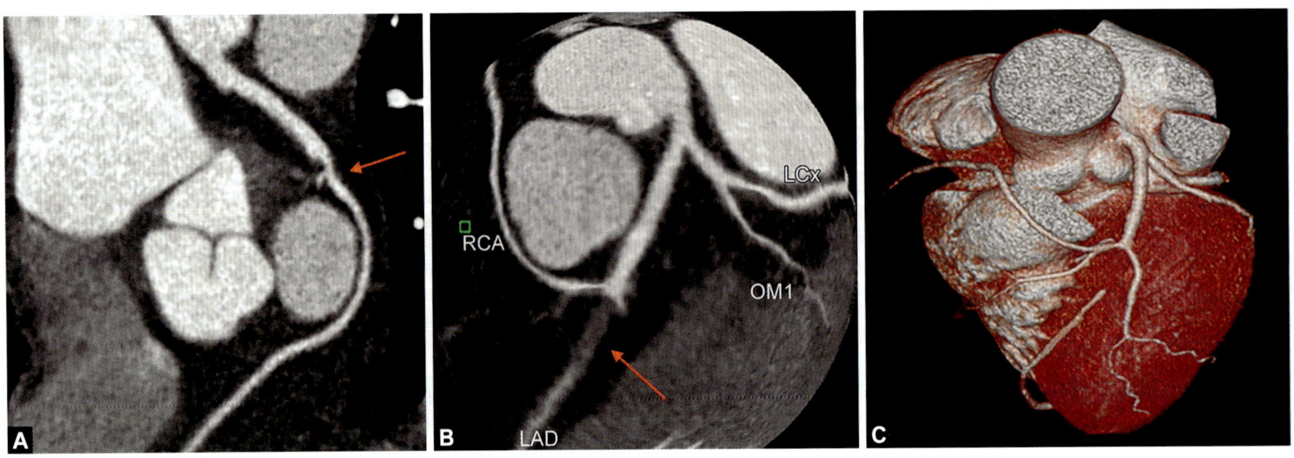

FIGS. 1A TO C: Anomalous origin of coronary artery: (A and C) Anomalous origin of RCA from LAD with prepulmonary course; (B) Mid-LAD occlusion.

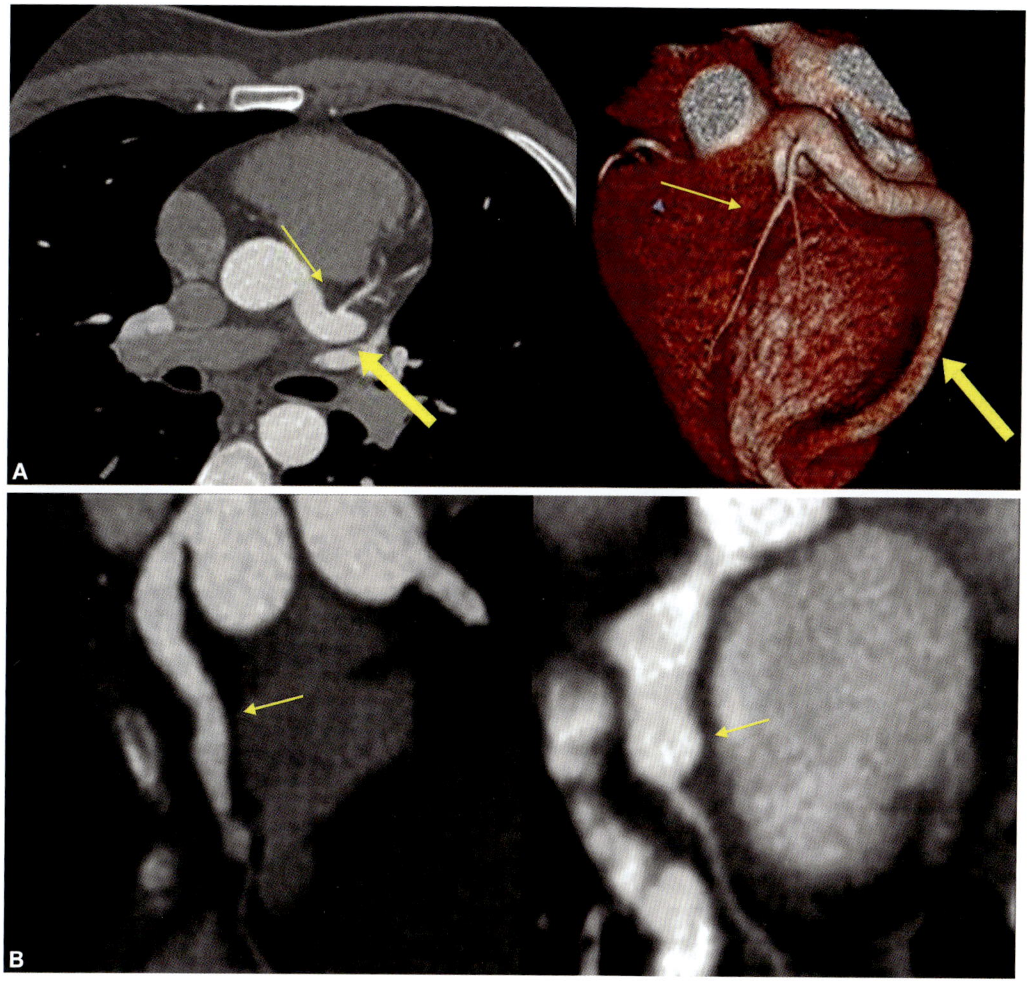

FIGS. 2A AND B: (A) Coronary arteriovenous fistula and (B) Kawasaki disease.

made in truly orthogonal planes. 3D reconstruction helps visualization of arch hypoplasia, poststenotic dilations, and aneurysms. For patients suspected to have aortic arch hypoplasia, CT provides information about the exact location, shape, and length of the hypoplastic segment, as well as the course of the collateral vessels. In complex arch anomalies, CT helps to identify the anomaly and the relationship between the trachea and esophagus **(Figs. 3A to F)**. **Figs. 4A to C** show interrupted arch.

Vascular rings: These abnormalities encircle the trachea and esophagus producing airway compromise or dysphagia. Any atretic segments represented by ligamentum will not be shown by CT. Local mass effect (dynamic if using ECG gating) and tenting or traction effect on the aorta, subclavian, or pulmonary arteries can be seen as indirect markers. Double-aortic arch can present as trachea-esophageal compression which can be better seen in CT angiography **(Figs. 5A to E)**.[10] The dominance of the arches is important for the surgeon to divide the smaller arch. Kommerell's diverticulum must be suspected if the second arch is not visualized.

Absent PA is another indication for CT. PA sling where left PA originates from the right PA can show tracheal narrowing with ring cartilage **(Figs. 6A and B)**. Stenosis of the bronchus may be seen with chronic left-to-right shunts resulting in bronchomalacia. Compression of bronchus by a dilated PA can be seen **(Figs. 7A to D)**.

Pulmonary veins: Anomalous pulmonary venous return can be in supracardiac, cardiac, or infracardiac locations. Sites of obstruction can be delineated, especially infracardiac and mixed types **(Figs. 8 and 9)**. Postoperative restenosis can be identified. In scimitar syndrome, CT scan is particularly useful in delineating the entry of the inferior pulmonary vein location to IVC, large aortic collaterals to lung and in depicting the degree of lung hypoplasia **(Figs. 9A to D)**.

Supravalvular aortic stenosis: In supravalvular aortic stenosis, CT demonstrates the extent of stenosis and determine the permeability of the coronary ostia, as in Williams syndrome **(Fig. 10)**. In these patients, invasive coronary angiography carries a high risk.

Abernathy malformation: In this anomaly, splanchnic blood drains directly into the inferior vena cava. It may be complete (type 1) or partial (type 2). Hepatic encephalopathy, pulmonary hypertension, pulmonary arteriovenous fistula, hepatopulmonary syndrome, and hepatic neoplasms can occur. Surgical or innovative transcatheter occlusion has

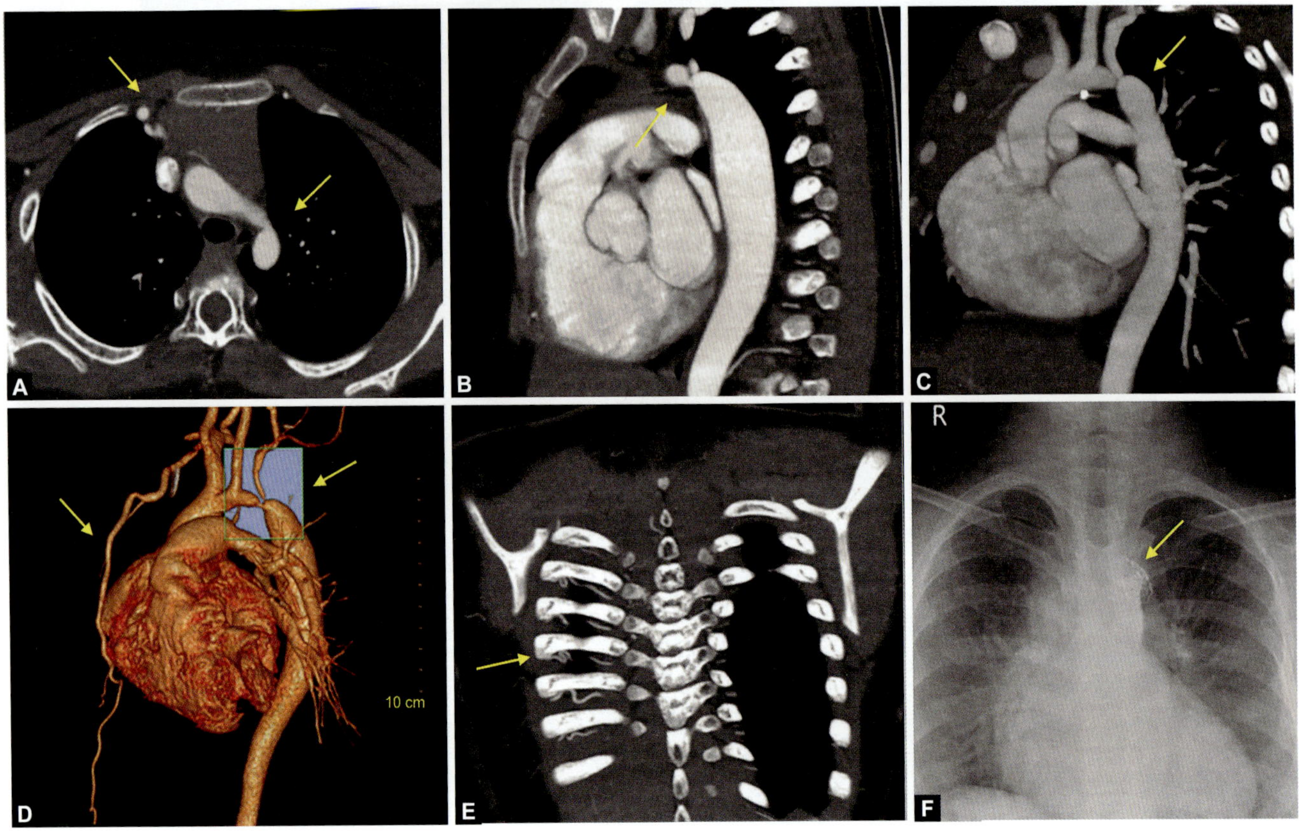

FIGS. 3A TO F: Coarctation of the aorta: Short segment re-coarctation (length of 7 mm, minimal diameter of 3 mm), located 8 mm distal to left CCA origin (A to C). Focal tight stenosis at LSCA origin (D). Hypertrophy of intercostal arteries (E) and right IMA (A and D) and right lateral thoracic artery noted. Poststenting follow-up chest radiograph showing aortic stent (F).

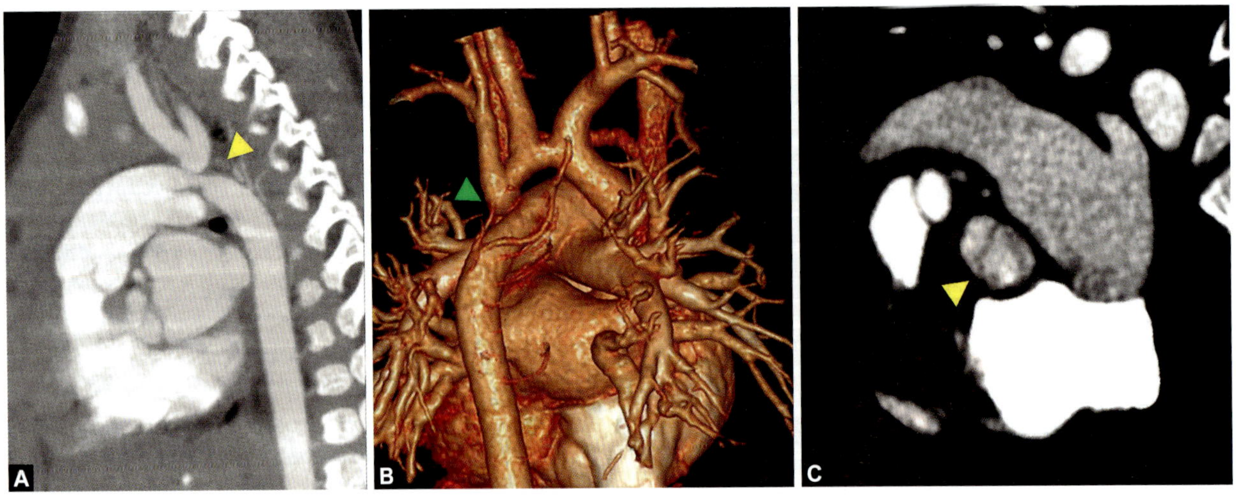

FIGS. 4A TO C: Interrupted aortic arch: Complete anatomical and luminal discontinuity distal to the left subclavian artery with normal origin of the right subclavian artery: Interrupted aortic arch (Type A, subtype 1) (A and B); Bicuspid aortic valve (C).

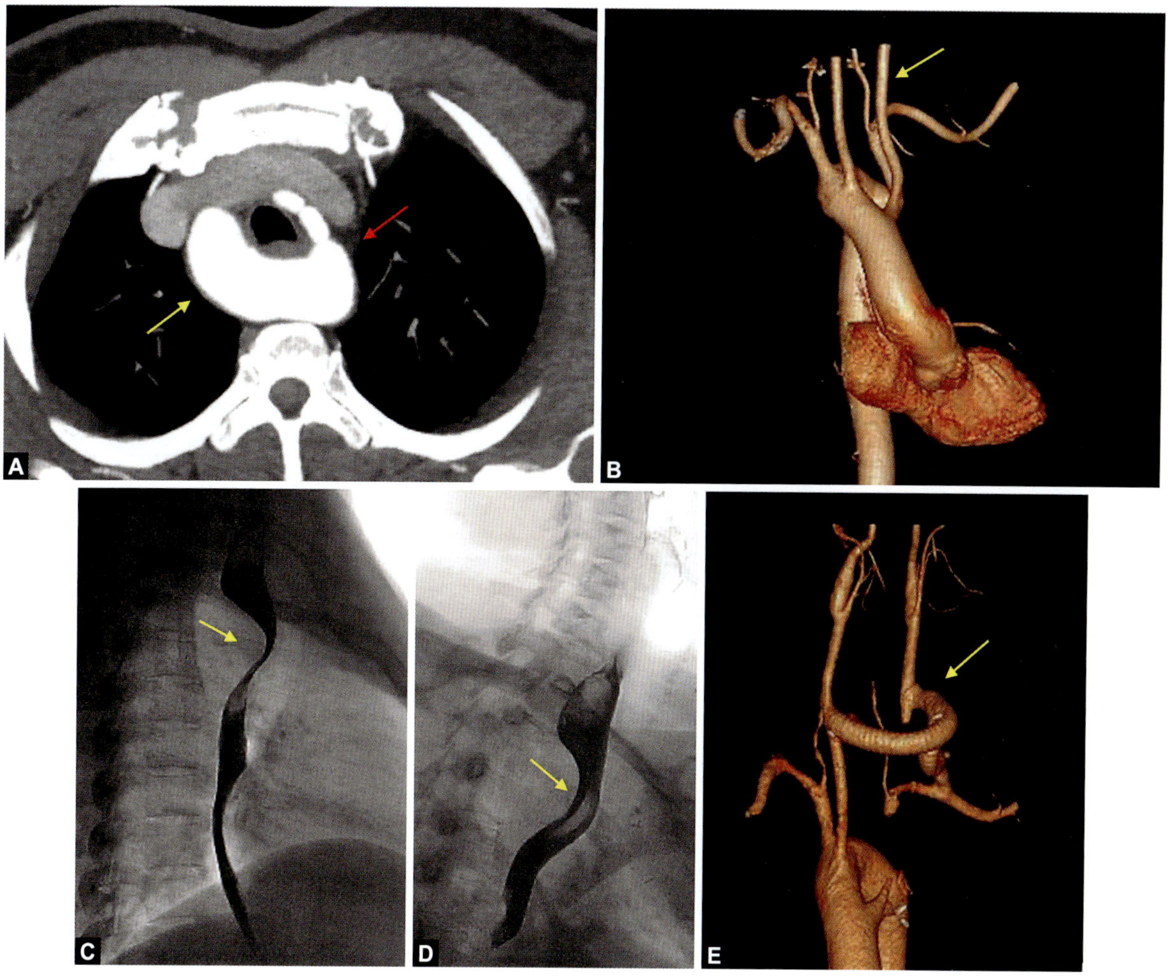

FIGS. 5A TO E: Double aortic arch: Superior right aortic arch (yellow arrow in A) with right subclavian and common carotid arteries noted. Inferior left aortic arch (red arrow in A) with left subclavian and common carotid arteries. The vascular ring encircles the trachea and esophagus with tracheal and esophageal compression. Arch vessels appear normal (B). Barium esophagogram shows persistent esophageal compression (C and D). (E) Status after right-to-left carotid–carotid bypass + carotid-left subclavian bypass and left subclavian artery ligation.

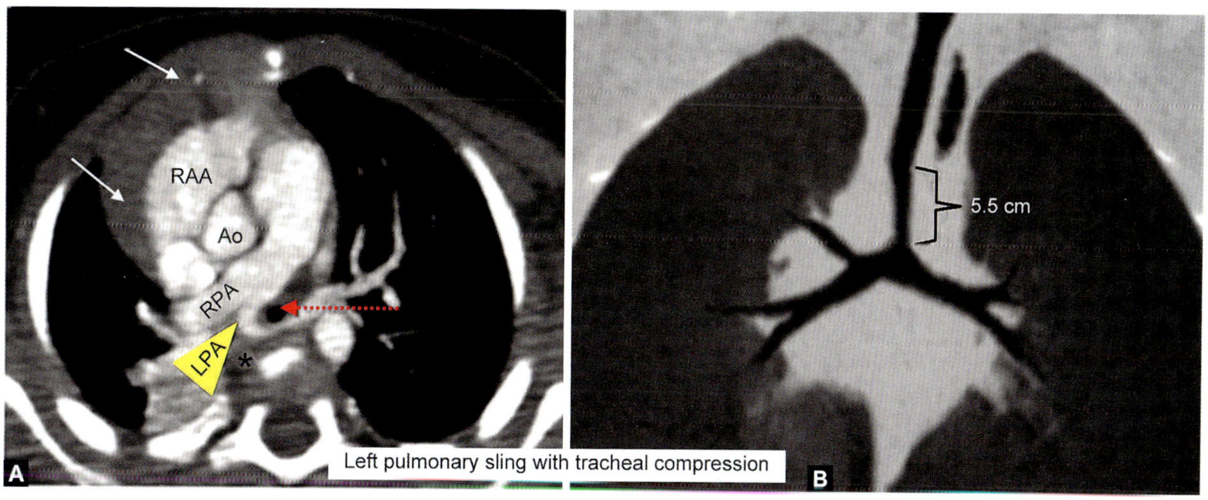

FIGS. 6A AND B: Pulmonary artery sling.

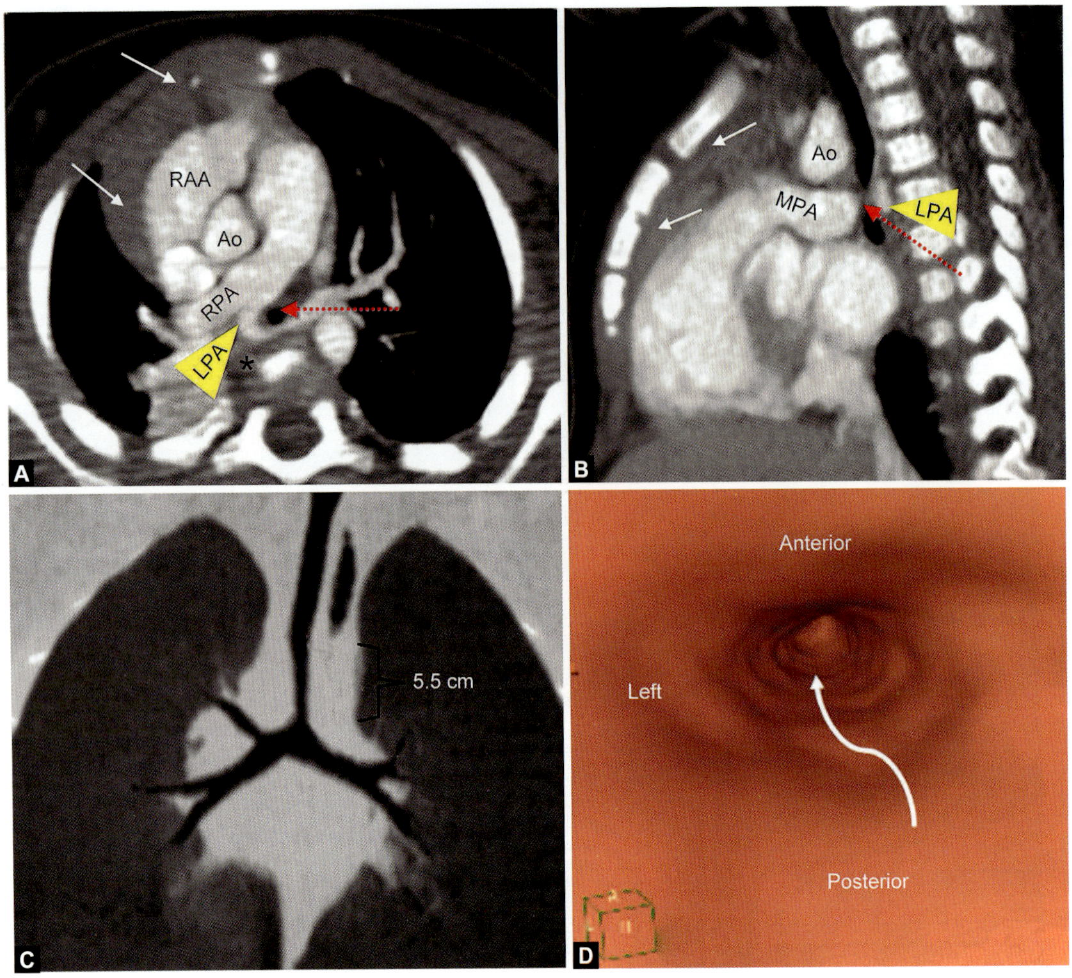

FIGS. 7A TO D: Compression of bronchus by dilated PA: (A and B) Posterior tracheal impression and narrowing (red dotted arrow) by left PA (yellow arrowhead in A). Position of esophagus is denoted by asterisk (*). Enlarged thymus is noted anterior and lateral to the right atrial appendage, in the retrosternal location (white arrows in A and B) which is responsible for the prominent right heart border in Figure 1A. (C) Coronal reconstruction demonstrates distal tracheal stenosis (black bracket). (D) Virtual bronchoscopy image reveals concave posterior margin and mucosal indentations of complete tracheal rings as ribbings (curved white arrow).

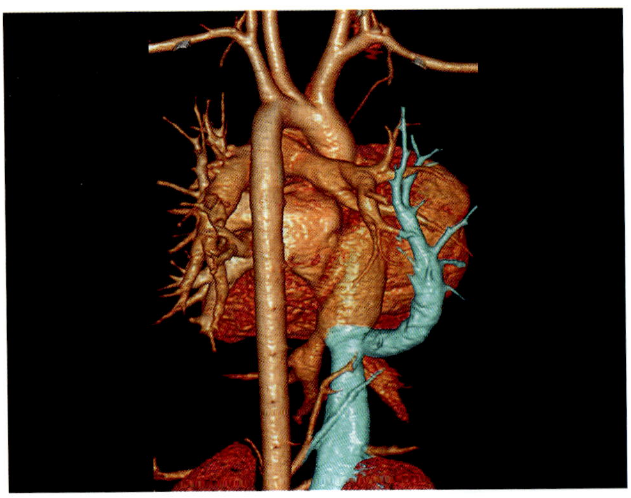

FIG. 8: Right lower pulmonary vein to inferior vena cava.

been performed in type II malformation. CT will help in preoperative delineation of the anatomy, integrity of portal veins, and postprocedure follow-up **(Fig. 11)**.

Left-to-right shunts: These can be demonstrated with associated malformations **(Figs. 12A to D)**.

Sinus venosus atrial septal defect: A covered stent is being deployed to close selected patients with this defect. CT is useful to assess the diameter, length, and number of stents to be planned **(Figs. 13A to D)**. Delineating pulmonary venous drainage is crucial.

Aortopulmonary window: One-third of patients may not have complete diagnosis with noninvasive evaluation with echo.[11] CT can show the size and the location and its relationship with the origin of the coronary arteries **(Figs. 14A to D)**.

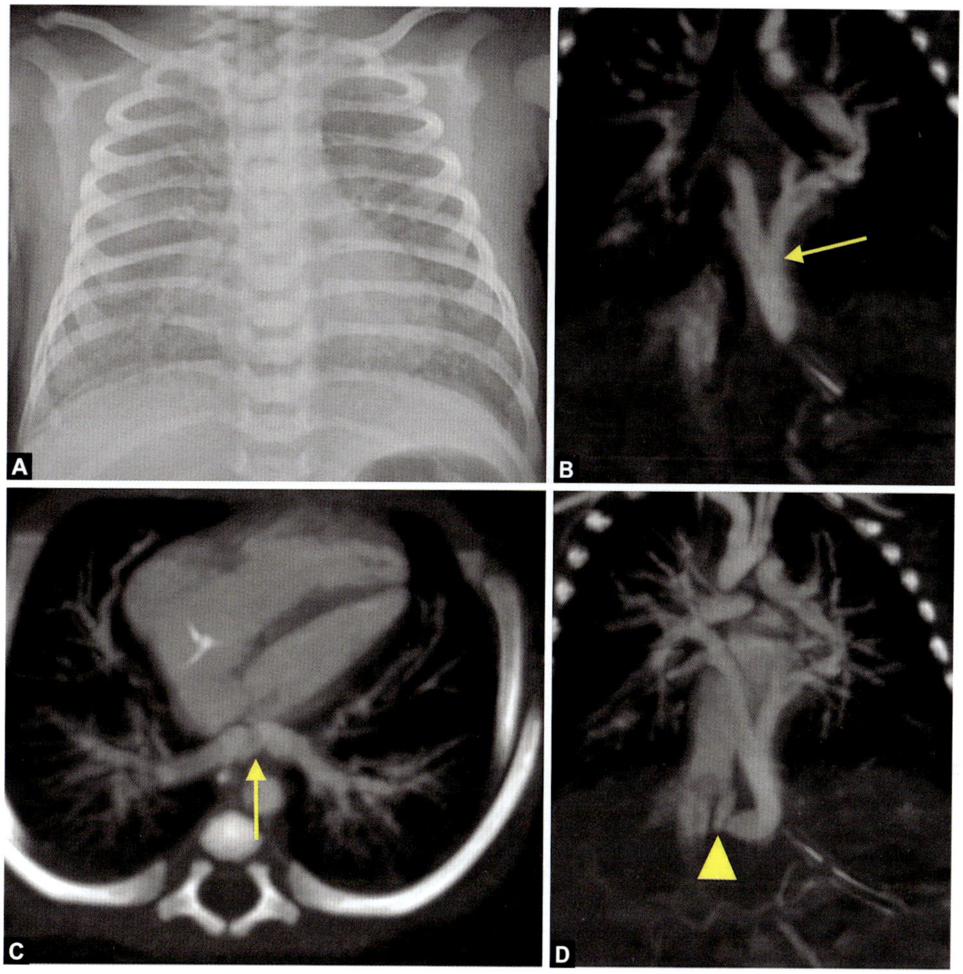

FIGS. 9A TO D: Infracardiac TAPVC: (A) Frontal chest radiography showing a normal cardiothoracic ratio with congestive changes in lung; (B) Joining of four pulmonary veins and forming a common channel (arrow); (C) Common channel posterior to left atrium (arrow); (D) Draining of common descending vein inferiorly through the diaphragm into IVC via ductus venosus. Severe stenosis is noted at the opening site of descending common pulmonary vein into ductus venosus (arrowhead).

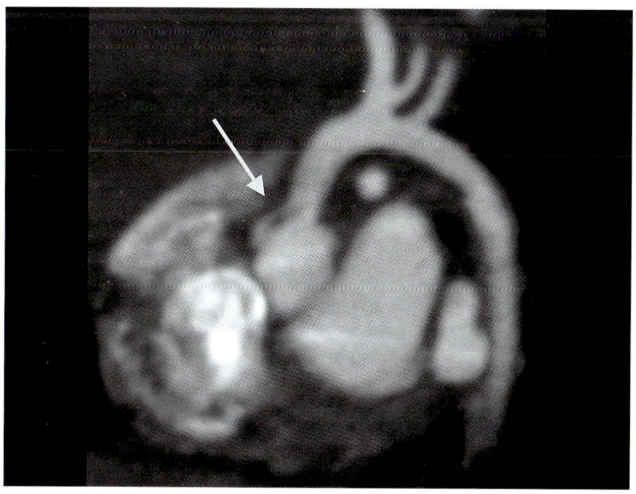

FIG. 10: Supravalvular aortic stenosis.

CYANOTIC CONGENITAL HEART DISEASES

Tetralogy of Fallot (TOF) (Figs. 15A to C)

Preoperative

Preoperative role includes:

- Level and extent of right ventricular outflow tract (RVOT) obstruction and the size, location, and number of ventricular septal defects
- PA anatomy **(Figs. 16A and B)**
- *Coronary artery anatomy*: Look of prominent vessel that crosses RVOT. When LAD arises from RCA and crosses RVOT, there is risk of coronary arterial injury during intracardiac repair.
- *Additional sources of pulmonary blood flow*: From aortopulmonary collateral or PDA

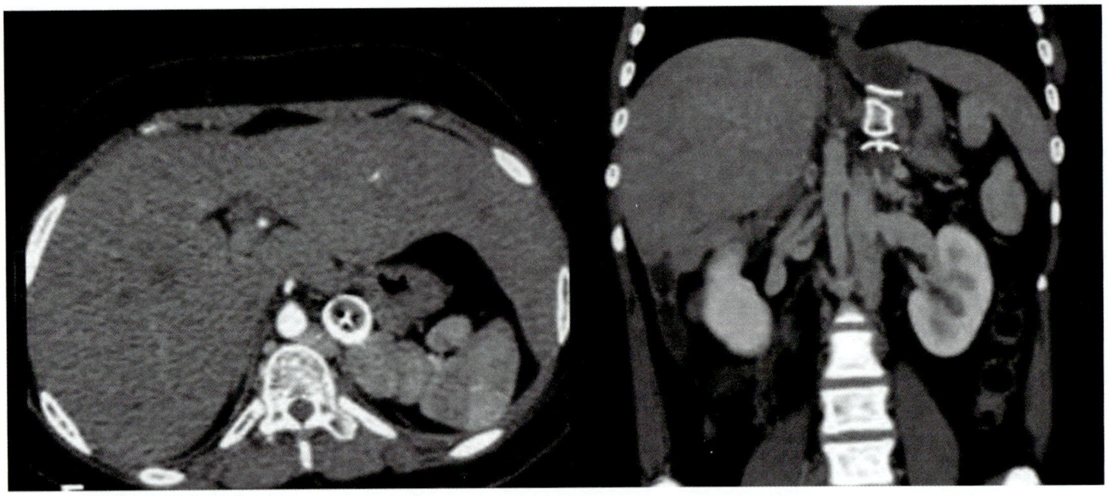

FIG. 11: Abernethy malformation.

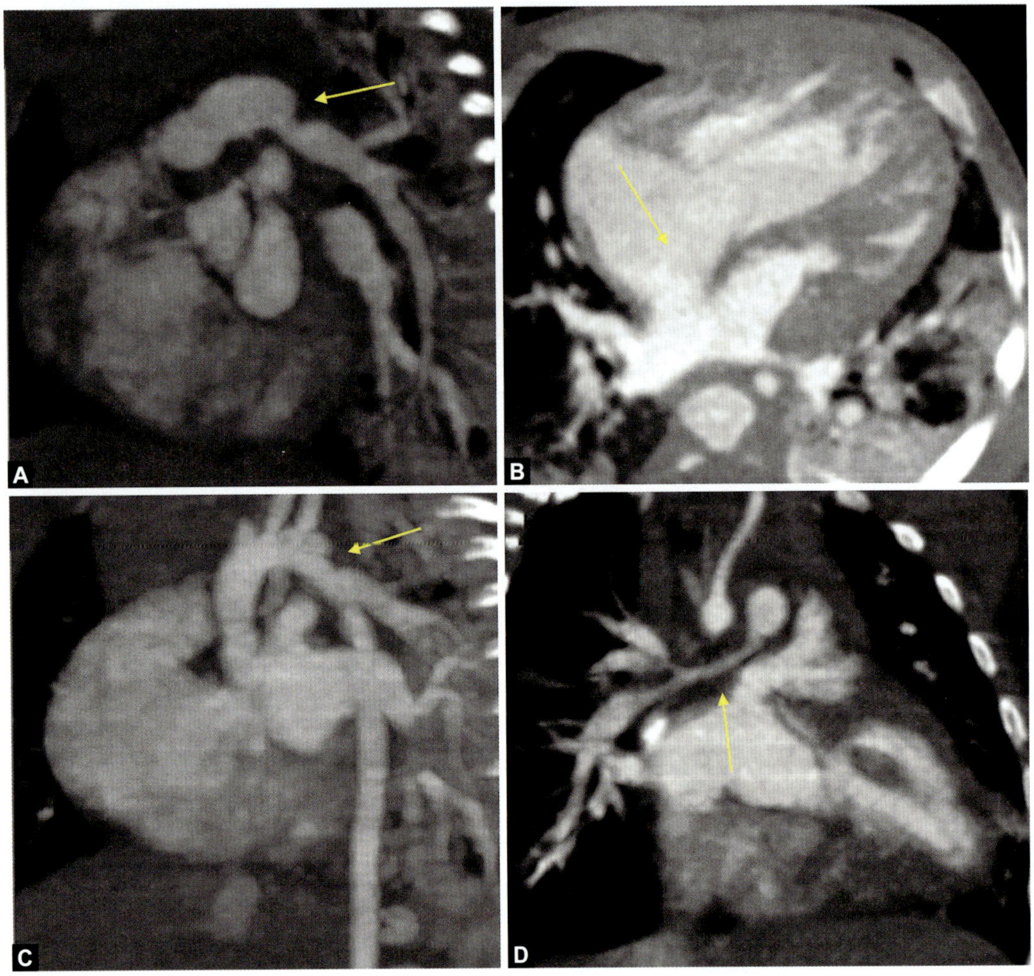

FIGS. 12A TO D: Atrial septal defect (ASD) with hypoplastic right PA: (A) Focal stenosis of RPA; (B) ASD with dilated RA and RV; (C) Mild narrowing of aortic isthmus; (D) Diffuse hypoplasia of RPA.

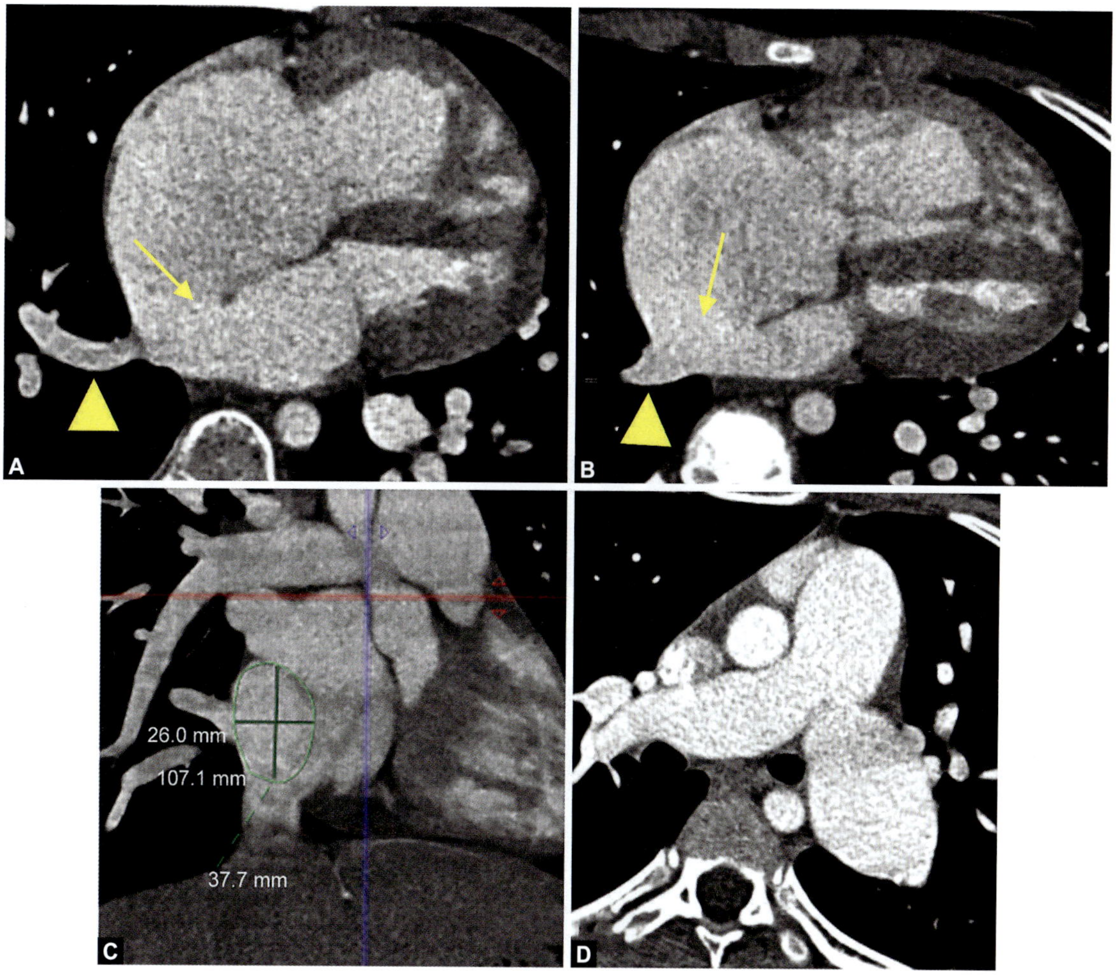

FIGS. 13A TO D: Sinus venosus ASD: (A and B) ASD (arrow) in the inferior aspect of septum along with anomalous drainage of right lower lobe pulmonary vein into right-sided atrium (arrowhead); (C) Defect size; (D) Pulmonary artery hypertension features with dilated main, right and left pulmonary arteries. Sinus venosus ASD—inferior type.

- Anatomy of the PDA to plan PDA stenting
- Aorta-related information: Aortopathy, side of aortic arch

Postoperative

Imaging postpalliative interventions or surgery include the following:

- Delineating PA anatomy after right ventricular outflow tract stenting, PDA stenting, and surgical aortopulmonary shunts. CT is also useful in delineating the pathology in suspected shunt obstruction.
- *Imaging postintracardiac repair*: Defining the RVOT and PA dimensions in pulmonary regurgitation when pulmonary valve replacement is indicated by clinical evaluation and right heart volume assessment by MRI. CT is also useful in defining aortic dimensions in progressive aortic root dilatation in aortopathy associated with TOF.

Absent pulmonary valves can dilate the pulmonary vessels producing bronchial compression resulting in dyspnea and bronchomalacia which can be seen in CT **(Figs. 17A to C)**.

Tetralogy of Fallot with Pulmonary Atresia (Figs. 18A to D)

Preoperative

Delineate the anatomy of PA and sources of pulmonary blood flow. The parameters assessed on CT include:

- Length of the atretic segment
- Presence of PA confluence
- Diameter of main PA and right and left PA at the origin and the hilum
- Branch PA stenosis

- Sources of pulmonary blood flow to each lung and lung segment—single/multiple
- Number of bronchopulmonary segments supplied by native pulmonary arteries
- Anatomy of MAPCAs—origin, course, size, territory supplied, communicating or noncommunicating

Some of the parameters calculated after CT in TOF with pulmonary atresia include McGoon ratio, Nakata index, and

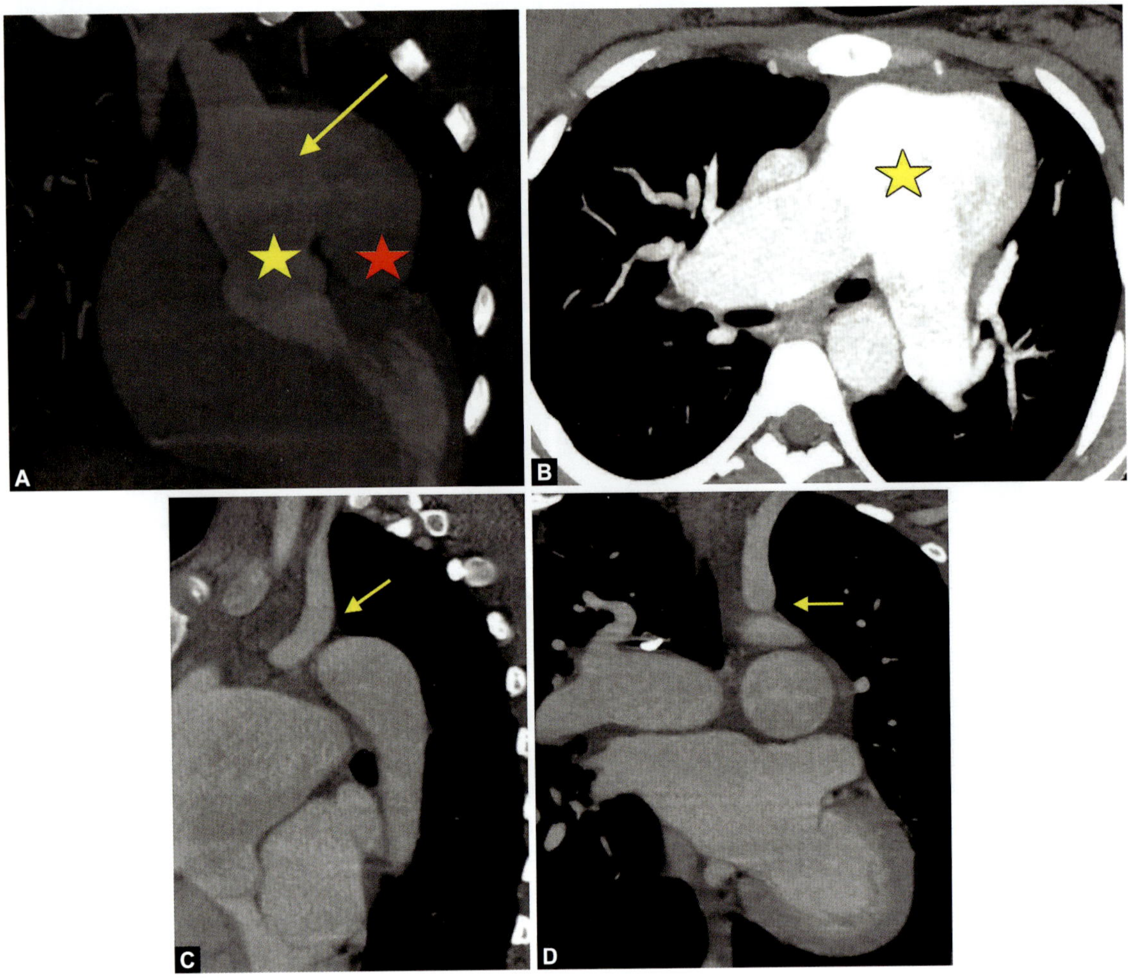

FIGS. 14A TO D: Aortopulmonary window: A communication (yellow arrow in A and star in B) between the aorta and PA (proximal and distal) just above the valvular plane suggestive of type III aortopulmonary window, well-defined aortic (yellow star in A) and pulmonary valve apparatuses (red star in A) is noted. Type A interrupted aortic arch (yellow arrow in C and D).

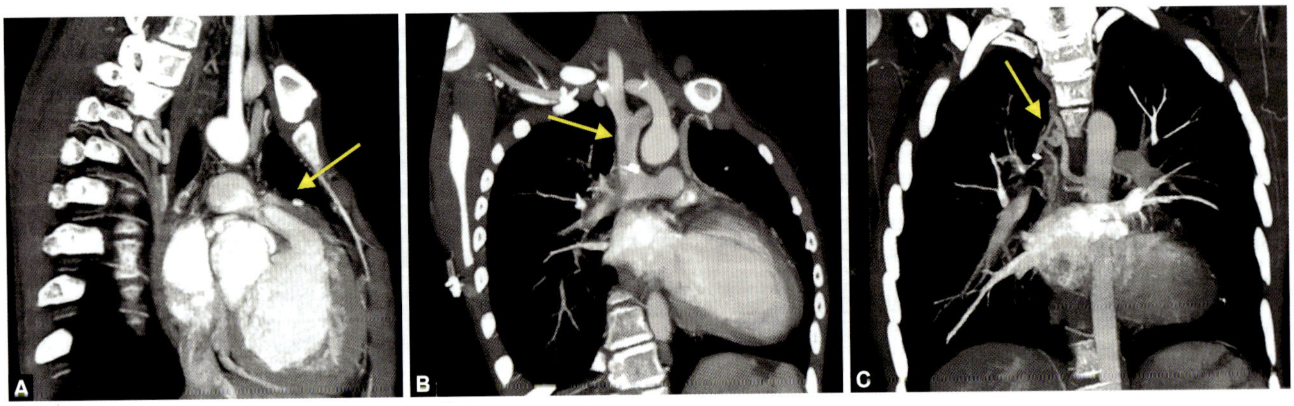

FIGS. 15A TO C: Tetralogy of Fallot: Right ventricular outflow tract obstruction and collaterals.

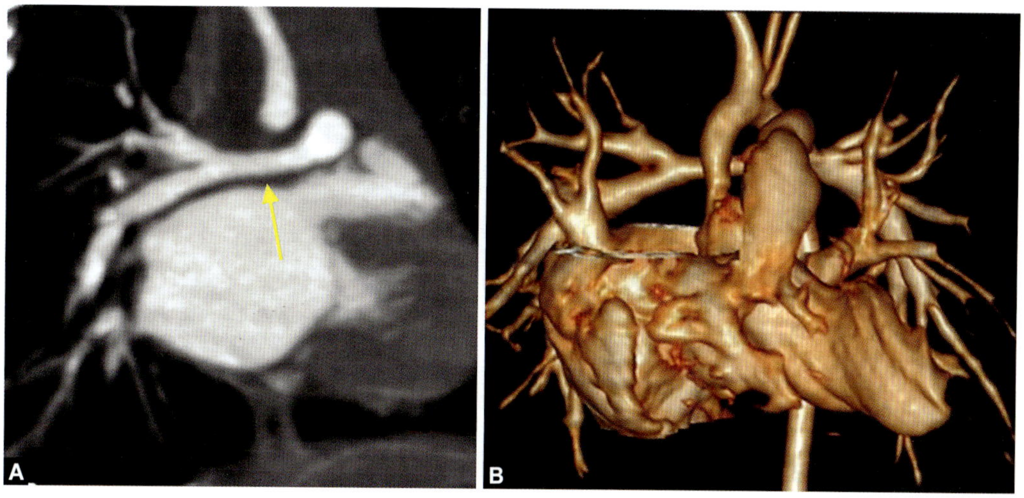

FIGS. 16A AND B: Long-segment hypoplasia of RPA and origin of LPA.

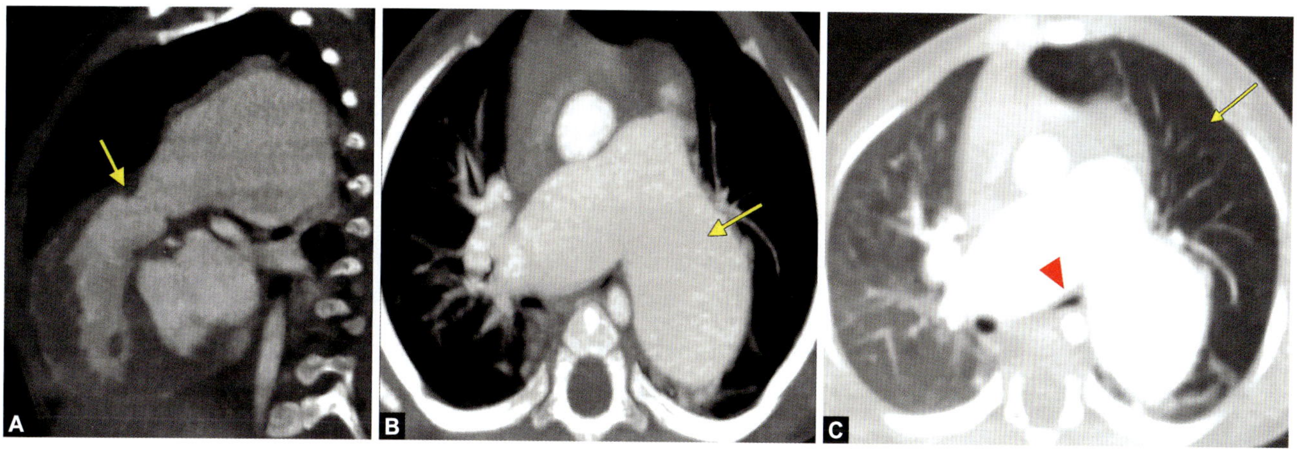

FIGS. 17A TO C: Tetralogy of Fallot with absent pulmonary valve: Absent pulmonary valve with pulmonary annulus measuring 10.5 mm (A) with postannulus aneurysmal dilation of MPA, RPA, and LPA (B); severe compression of the left main bronchus (red arrowhead in C) due to the dilated RPA resulting in hyperinflation of the entire left upper lobe (yellow arrow in C).

total neopulmonary artery index (TNPAI). McGoon ratio > 1.2, Nakata index > 150 mm^2/m^2, and TNPAI > 200 mm^2/m^2 are factors associated with low postoperative RV/LV pressure ratio and acceptable postoperative hemodynamics for complete primary repair.[12] CT is crucial to decide on single-stage versus multistage repair in pulmonary atresia, the need for unifocalization versus ligation of MAPCA, and the need for an aortopulmonary shunt for rehabilitation of PA or a combined approach.[13]

Postoperative

Define conduit calcification and substernal anatomy to plan conduit revision or pulmonary valve replacement, evaluation of focal pathology like confluence stenosis, conduit aneurysm, and aortopulmonary collaterals for coil embolization.

Ebstein's Anomaly (Fig. 19)

Occasionally, CT is useful in the evaluation of Ebstein's anomaly with pulmonary atresia in the newborn period. Cardiac magnetic resonance imaging has replaced CT due to the advantage of combined anatomical and functional information without radiation exposure.

Univentricular Heart

Preoperative (Figs. 20 and 21)

Computed tomography is rarely required in preoperative evaluation of second or third stage of univentricular palliation along the Fontan pathway.[14] The role of CT in planning for total cavopulmonary connection includes:

- *Assessment of previous palliative surgery or intervention*: Aortopulmonary shunt, ductal stent, bidirectional Glenn shunt

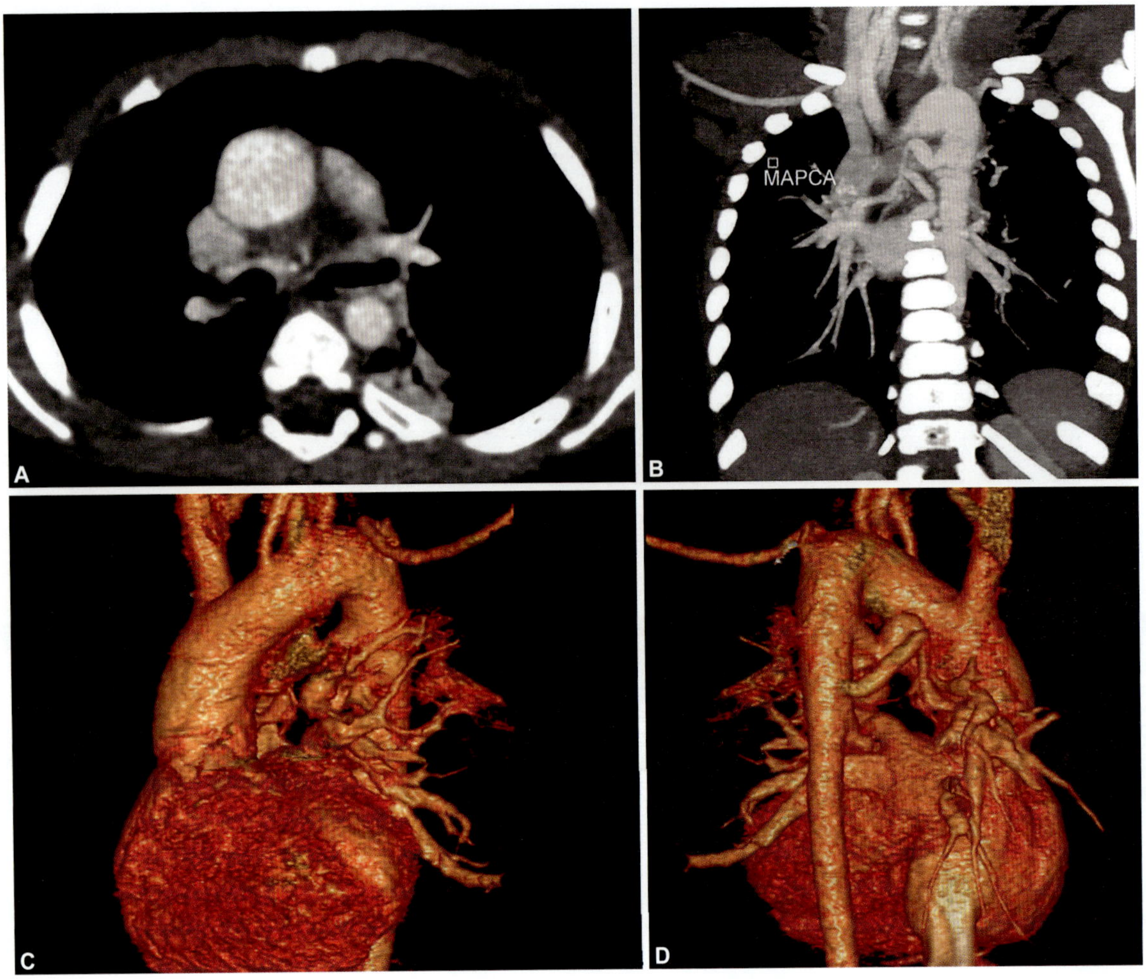

FIGS. 18A TO D: Pulmonary atresia with VSD with MAPCA-dependent circulation.

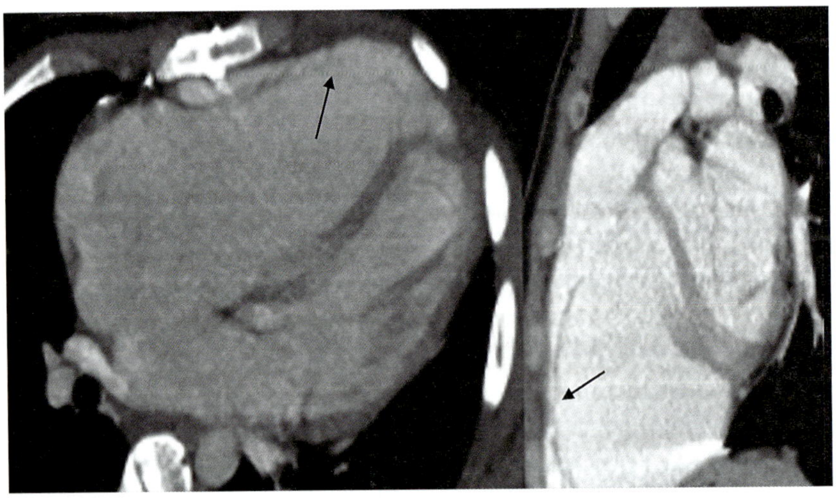

FIG. 19: Ebstein's anomaly.

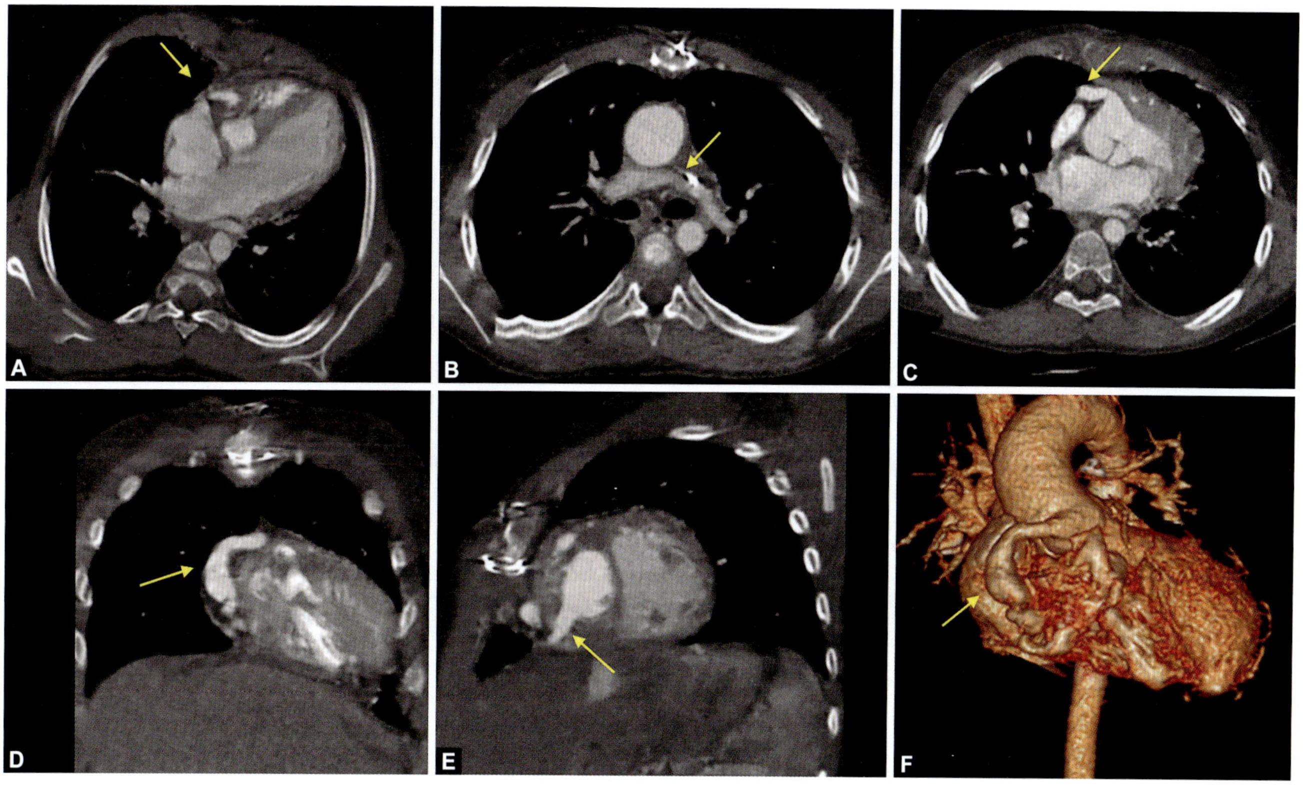

FIGS. 20A TO F: Tricuspid atresia: (A) Tricuspid atresia with hypoplastic RV and intact ventricular septum; (B) Long segment pulmonary atresia with LPA origin stenosis; (C to E) VRT image (F) showing dilated RCA with a tortuous course and distal RCA communicating with RV cavity (E).

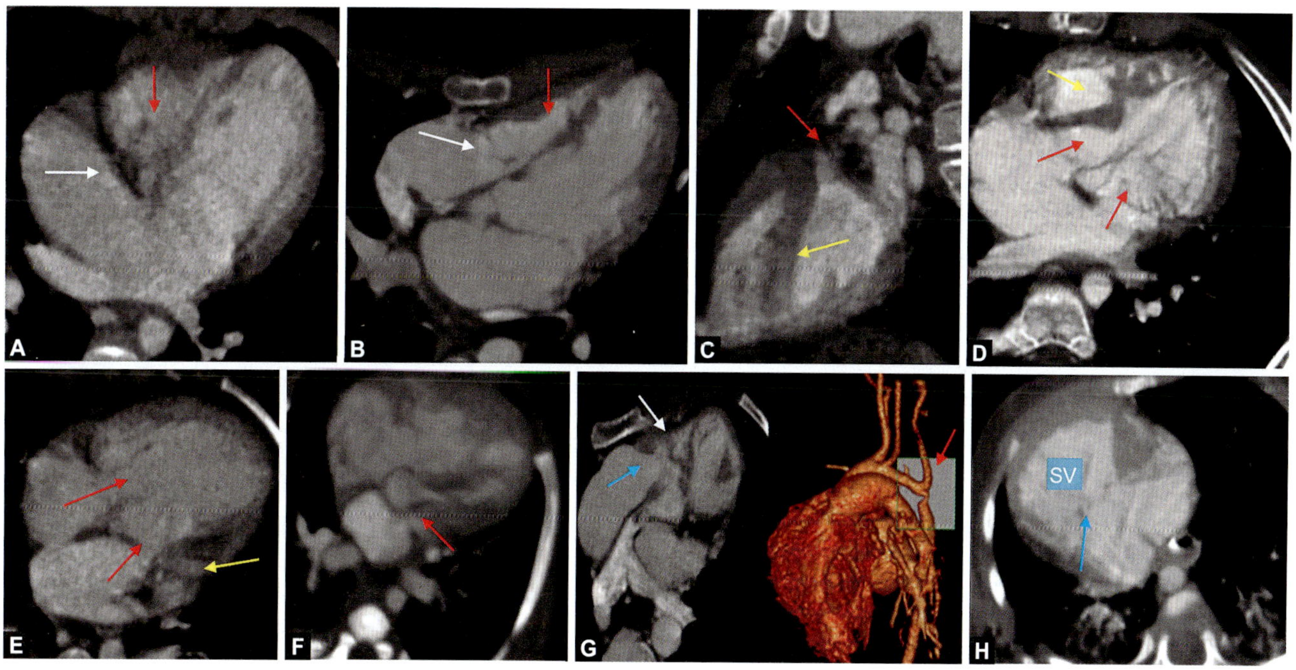

FIGS. 21A TO H: Univentricular heart: (A) Tricuspid atresia (white arrow) with hypoplastic right ventricle (red arrow); (B) RV hypoplasia (red arrow) and tricuspid valve hypoplasia (white arrow); (C) Pulmonary atresia (red arrow) with intact ventricular septum (yellow arrow); (D) Double-inlet left ventricle (red arrows showing direction of blood flow into the left ventricle) with rudimentary RV (yellow arrow); (E) Double-inlet right ventricle (red arrows showing direction of blood flow into the right ventricle) with rudimentary LV (yellow arrow); (F) DORV with mitral atresia (red arrow); (G) HLHS (blue arrow—mitral hypoplasia, white arrow—left ventricle hypoplasia, box—arch hypoplasia, red arrow—coarctation of aorta); (H) AVCD (blue arrow) with hypoplastic ventricle.

- *Assessment of systemic veins*: Superior cavopulmonary anastomosis, drainage of the inferior caval vein, screening for drainage of hepatic veins into the inferior caval vein versus directly into the atrium, apicocaval juxtaposition
- *Assessment of pulmonary venous anatomy*: Intracardiac or abnormal drainage, any obstruction in the pathway to the atrium
- *Assessment of PA anatomy*: Central and branch PA, distal arborization
- *Delineation of accessory sources of pulmonary blood flow*: Evaluation of the need for coiling or ligation of major aortopulmonary collaterals.
- *Ruling out systemic outflow tract obstruction*: Subvalvar, valvar, aortic arch anatomy
- Demonstration of the anatomy of venovenous collaterals and pulmonary arteriovenous malformations
- *Evaluation of relevant coronary artery pathology*: Right ventricle to coronary artery communications and RV-dependent coronary circulation in pulmonary atresia with intact ventricular septum
- *Relevant extracardiac pathology*: Lung hypoplasia, sequestration, diaphragmatic palsy, eventration, heterotaxy syndromes, kyphoscoliosis and related thoracic cage issues, portosystemic communications, assessment of retrosternal anatomy

Postoperative (Figs. 22A to F)

The role of CT in evaluating patients after Fontan completion, in addition to the preoperative list, includes:

- Evaluation of Fontan pathway for anatomic narrowing/distortion/stenosis
- Evaluation of the position of Fontan fenestration

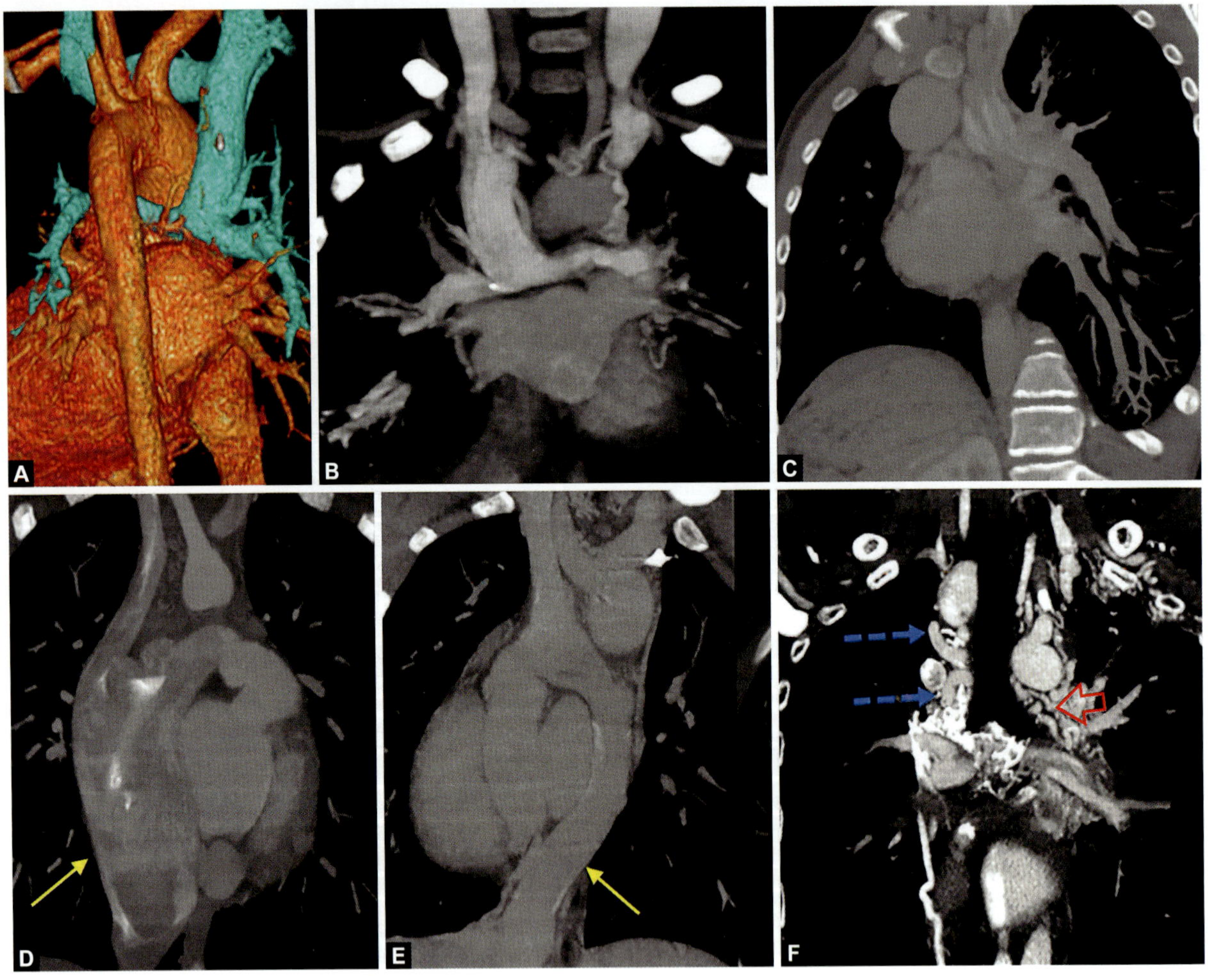

FIGS. 22A TO F: Univentricular heart postoperative: (A) BDG; (B) BDG with venovenous collateral; (C) BDG with pulmonary AVF; (D) Atriopulmonary Fontan; (E) Extracardiac Fontan; (F) MAPCA.

- Evaluation of pulmonary thromboemboli
- Evaluation for heart transplantation

Double-outlet Right Ventricle (DORV)

Preoperative

3D reconstruction and 3D printing tools are useful in characterizing complex anatomy. The role of CT in DORV includes:

- Defining the morphology of the ventricles and confirmation of the diagnosis, atrioventricular relationship, and ventriculoarterial relationship
- Delineation of the location of the VSD and its relationship to the semilunar valves
- Assessment of the routability of VSD for intracardiac tunneling by characterizing the size of the VSD in relation to the annular dimensions of the aorta and PA, distance between the VSD and the aorta/PA, atrioventricular valve straddling and/or overriding, and any other tissue in the path of proposed ventricular tunnel to the aorta.
- Characterization of the anatomy to assess for biventricular versus univentricular repair
- Screening for associated cardiac pathologies like abnormal venous drainage, juxtaposition of the atrial appendages, aortic arch sidedness, and heterotaxy
- Defining coronary artery anatomy and its implications in planning surgical repair

Postoperative

Computed tomography can serve as an adjunct to echocardiography and/or MRI to delineate postoperative complications like residual VSD, ventricular outflow tract obstruction, homograft calcification/stenosis, and coronary artery abnormalities following arterial switch operation.

Transposition of Great Arteries (TGA)

Preoperative

Delineate coronary anatomy if it is not clear by echocardiography. In addition, CT can demonstrate the anatomy of the semilunar valves, ascending aorta, PA, aortic arch, and the atrioventricular valves to plan definitive repair. Identification of aortopulmonary collaterals, size and location of the VSD, and assessment of routability in TGA with VSD are also possible with CT imaging. **Figures 23A and B** show corrected transposition of great arteries.

Postoperative

Computed tomography is used to evaluate coronary artery abnormalities, neoaortic and neopulmonary artery stenoses, and branch PA distortion after arterial switch operation. It can also characterize pulmonary and systemic baffle obstruction and leaks after Senning repair. However, MRI offers better spatial resolution and better delineation of intracardiac anatomy in these situations besides information on ventricular function.

RADIATION

Drawbacks are exposure to radiation and contrast-induced renal dysfunction. Approximately 1.5–2% of cancers are attributed to CT radiation.[15] Thoracic CT dose ranges from

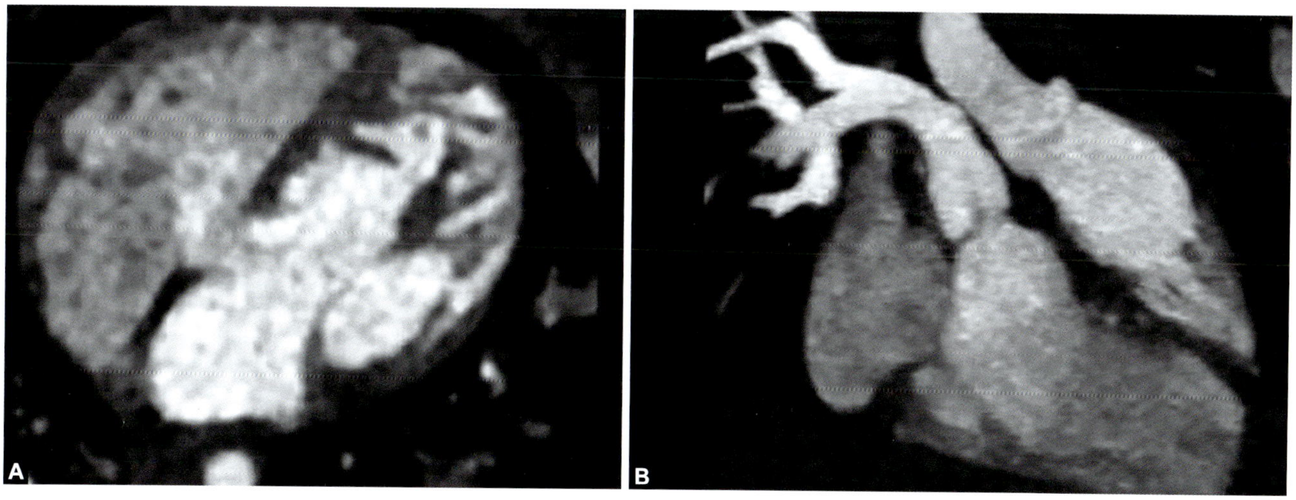

FIGS. 23A AND B: (A) Atrioventricular and (B) ventriculoarterial discordance in corrected transposition of great arteries. Aorta is L-posed.

1 to 10 mSv. Better scanners and reconstruction algorithms and dual-energy and photon-counting CT have reduced the dose to 0.5 mSv.[16] Limited hemodynamic information is provided by CT. Techniques to reduce exposure include reducing tube current and potential, increasing pitch and table speed, avoiding multiphasic imaging, and minimizing scan coverage. Rotational tube current modulation and reducing kilovoltage to 80 kVp decrease dose. It is important to select the appropriate kilovoltage based on patient's weight and adjust the current based on vessel size. The use of automatic dose modulation mode is recommended to ensure the appropriate amount of mAs.[17]

CONCLUSION

Cardiac CT is used for detailed, rapid imaging without sedation. Caregivers should discuss the risks and benefits compared to other modalities. Understanding cardiac CT parameters and implementing a dose management program are crucial for high-quality images with minimal radiation exposure.

ONLINE REFERENCES

Please scan the QR code provided at the end of the table of contents for References of this chapter.

CHAPTER

92

Hemodynamics Interpretation in Congenital Heart Disease

Anuja Gadre, Manojkumar Rohit

ABSTRACT

Collection and interpretation of hemodynamic data is one of the crucial elements for the diagnosis and treatment of various congenital heart diseases (CHD). It requires thorough knowledge of the normal cardiac physiology, pressure, resistance, flow and oximetry parameters, and their alterations in various pathological conditions. It is the gold standard investigation for correct diagnosis and deciding operability especially when clinical and other noninvasive tests have provided contradictory results. This chapter aims to cover the basic understanding of various hemodynamic data and their clinical implications for the management of various CHD, including recent advances in the field of cardiac magnetic resonance imaging (CMRI) and its role in hemodynamic evaluation.

Keywords: Congenital heart disease, cardiac magnetic resonance imaging, hemodynamics, intracardiac shunts, oximetry, vascular resistance

INTRODUCTION

Hemodynamics is an integral part of any cardiac catheterization and its interpretation is vital for understanding various physiologic and pathologic conditions, especially congenital heart diseases (CHD). It involves basic understanding of normal pressure waveforms and oxygen saturation, and measurements of blood flow, cardiac output, and vascular resistance. These measurements are required for detection, quantification, and deciding operability in shunt lesions, and the measurement of stenotic valve orifice area, especially when noninvasive tests such as echocardiography and computed tomography have not proven adequate. Thus, basic knowledge of the hemodynamics in CHD is a must for every cardiologist.

DISCUSSION

Normal Pressure Waveforms

Any pressure waveform has two components: absolute value and contour. Abnormalities in these components can be diagnostic of a specific pathology. The normal pressure values of the various cardiac chambers and great vessels are given in **Table 1**,[1] and their waveforms/contours are as shown in **Figure 1**.[1]

Pullback pressure tracings can help us diagnose the exact location of stenosis and magnitude of the gradients across it. The pressure gradients at various levels which are considered

TABLE 1: Normal pressures of cardiac chambers and major vessels.

	Average (mm Hg)	Range (mm Hg)
Right atrium (RA)	a6, v5	a2–7, v2–7
RA mean	3	1–5
Right ventricle (RV)	25/4	15–30/1–7
Pulmonary artery (PA)	25/9	15–30/4–12
PA mean	15	9–19
Pulmonary capillary wedge pressure (PCWP)	9	4–12
Left atrium (LA)	a10, v12	a4–16, v6–21
LA mean	8	2–12
Left ventricle (LV) (peak systolic/LVEDP)	130/8	90–140/5–12
Central aorta (peak systolic/end-diastolic/mean)	130/70/85	90–140/60–90/70–105

(LVEDP: left ventricular end-diastolic pressure)

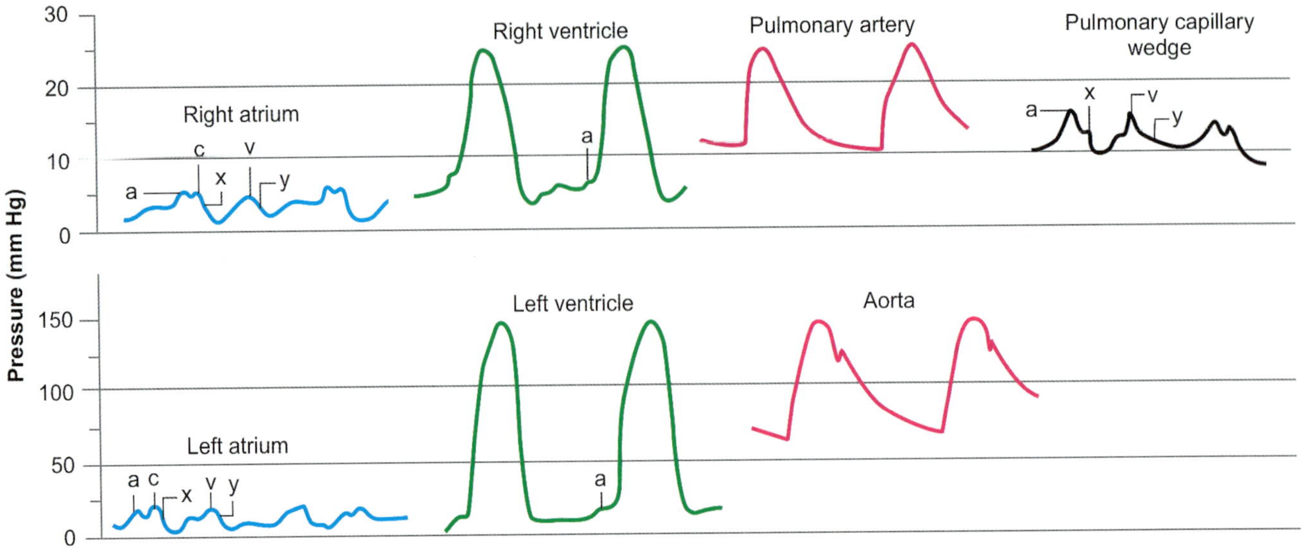

FIG. 1: Normal pressure waveforms in cardiac chambers and major vessels.

abnormal are given in **Table 2.**[2] Pressure gradients measured by direct cardiac catheterization measure peak-to-peak gradients, whereas echocardiography measures instantaneous gradients, hence catheterization gradients are lower than that of echocardiography.

TABLE 2: Abnormal pressure gradients at various levels.

Level	Peak/End (mm Hg)	Mean (mm Hg)
Mitral	Any	5
Tricuspid	1.9	2
Aortic	25	–
Pulmonary	25	–
Peripheral PS	20	–
Coarctation of aorta	20	–

Cardiac Output Measurement

Three different methods used to calculate cardiac output in the catheterization laboratory are:

1. Thermodilution method
2. Fick method
3. Ventriculographic method

Fick method is the most commonly used method in the catheterization laboratory for all practical purposes. Fick's principle calculates cardiac output based on the arteriovenous oxygen difference across the lungs and the rate of oxygen uptake from lungs, assuming that systemic blood flow (Q_s) is equal to pulmonary blood flow (Q_p) in the absence of an intracardiac shunt.[3]

$$\text{Fick cardiac output (L/min)} = \frac{\text{Oxygen consumption (mL/min)}}{\text{Hb} \times 1.36 \times 10 \times (\text{A–V})\ O_2}$$

Where, Hb is hemoglobin concentration, 1.36 is the constant to adjust for oxygen carrying capacity of hemoglobin, and (A–V) O_2 is the arteriovenous oxygen saturation difference.

To account for dissolved oxygen, a correction of 0.03 × pO_2 should be added to hemoglobin bound oxygen to calculate total oxygen content, which is not so significant in room air, but can introduce reasonable error in patients on supplemental oxygen.

Vascular Resistance Measurement

As per Ohm's law, vascular resistance is the ratio of change in pressure across a vascular segment to the flow across it.

$$\text{Systemic vascular resistance (SVR)} = \frac{\text{Mean aortic pressure – mean right atrial pressure}}{\text{Cardiac output}}$$

$$\text{Pulmonary vascular resistance (PVR)} = \frac{\text{Mean pulmonary artery pressure – mean left atrial or pulmonary capillary wedge pressure (PCWP)}}{\text{Cardiac output}}$$

The SVR and PVR divided by the body surface area give the systemic vascular resistance index (SVRI) and the pulmonary vascular resistance index (PVRI), respectively.

The normal values of vascular resistance are as given in **Table 3.**[2]

TABLE 3: Normal vascular resistance of major vessels.

	Vascular resistance (Mean ± standard deviation, in dyn·s/cm⁵)	Wood units (Range)
PVR	67 ± 30	1–3
SVR	1,170 ± 270	15–30
PVRI	123 ± 54	-
SVRI	2,130 ± 450	-

(PVR: pulmonary vascular resistance; PVRI: pulmonary vascular resistance index; SVR: systemic vascular resistance; SVRI: systemic vascular resistance index)

The decision regarding operability of CHD is often based on PVR, and various criteria have been proposed for the same. In general, PVRI/SVRI ratio <0.3 and PVRI <6 Wood units/m^2 (WU/m^2) are considered to be signs of operability, whereas PVRI/SVRI ratio of 0.3–0.5 and PVRI of 6–8 WU/m^2 need reversibility testing, and PVRI/SVRI >0.5 and PVRI >8 WU/m^2 are considered as inoperable.[4,5]

CLINICAL IMPLICATIONS

Cardiac catheterization, including both oximetry and pressure data, is crucial for the diagnosis of various CHD, deciding their operability, and monitoring the response to therapy.

Shunt Lesions

Shunt Detection and Quantification

The normal values of oxygen saturation in various cardiac chambers are as given in **Table 4**.[6] Any systemic arterial desaturation (<95%) should raise a suspicion for right to left shunt, while unexpectedly high pulmonary artery (PA) saturation (>80%) should raise a suspicion for left-to-right intracardiac shunt. The exact location of the shunt can then be evaluated with a detailed oximetry run to asses in which chamber the step-up or step-down is occurring. It is recommended to obtain samples from the following areas:

- Left or right pulmonary artery
- Main pulmonary artery
- Right ventricle (RV)—outflow, mid-cavity, and inflow
- Right atrium (RA)—low, mid, and high
- Superior vena cava (SVC)—low and high
- Inferior vena cava (IVC)—low and high
- Left ventricle (LV)
- Aorta (distal to ductus)
- Left atrium (LA) and pulmonary vein, if possible

The criteria for significant step-up at various levels and the common causes are as listed in **Table 5**.[6-8] A step-down of 2% is significant at any level and the causes for desaturation at various levels are given in **Table 6**. A very low mixed venous oxygen saturation indicates a low cardiac output and large

TABLE 4: Normal oxygen saturation of cardiac chambers and major vessels.

	Normal neonate (<1 week age)	Normal child/ adult
Superior vena cava (SVC)	60%	74%
Right atrium (RA)	65%	75%
Right ventricle (RV)	65%	75%
Pulmonary artery (PA)	65%	75%
Pulmonary vein (PV)	99%	99%
Left atrium (LA)	99%	98%
Left ventricle (LV)	99%	98%
Aorta	99%	97%

arteriovenous oxygen saturation difference, indicating that patient's general condition is poor and patient is quite sick.

The pulmonary blood flow (Q_p) and systemic blood flow (Q_s) are calculated using Fick equation.

$$Q_p = \frac{\text{Oxygen consumption (mL/min)}}{\text{Pulmonary venous oxygen content } (PvO_2) - \text{Pulmonary artery oxygen content } (PaO_2)}$$

$$Q_s = \frac{\text{Oxygen consumption (mL/min)}}{\text{Systemic artery oxygen content } (SaO_2) - \text{Mixed venous oxygen content } (MVO_2)}$$

The mixed venous oxygen saturation (MVO_2) is calculated by the Flamm's formula.[9]

$$MVO_2 = \frac{3\ SVC\ O_2 + 1\ IVC\ O_2}{4}$$

Thus, in unidirectional shunt,

$$\text{Left-to-right shunt} = Q_p - Q_s$$

$$\text{Right-to-left shunt} = Q_s - Q_p$$

In cases of bidirectional shunt, effective pulmonary blood flow (Q_{ep}) and effective systemic blood flow (Q_{es}) needs to be calculated. Q_{ep} is the deoxygenated blood reaching the pulmonary capillary bed for oxygenation, and Q_{es} is the oxygenated blood reaching the systemic circulation. Thus, effective blood flow (Q_{eff}) is a hypothetical entity that gives the flow that would exist in the absence of any shunt.

$$Q_{eff} = Q_{ep} = Q_{es} = \text{Oxygen consumption (mL/min)}$$

Pulmonary venous oxygen content (PVO_2) - Mixed venous oxygen content (MVO_2)

Here, left-to-right shunt = $Q_p - Q_{ep}$, and right-to-left shunt = $Q_s - Q_{es}$

TABLE 5: Significant step-up at various levels and their causes.

Level	Q_p:Q_s	Mean step-up	Highest step-up	Causes
Atrial (SVC/IVC-RA)	>1.5–1.9	7%	11%	ASD, PAPVC, RSOV to RA, coronary cameral fistula, VSD with TR, LV-RA shunt (Gerbode defect)
Ventricular (RA-RV)	>1.3–1.5	5%	10%	VSD, ostium primum ASD, PDA with PR, RSOV to RV, coronary cameral fistula
Great vessel (RV-PA)	>1.3	5%	5%	PDA, aortopulmonary window, outlet VSD, RSOV to PA, coronary cameral fistula
Any level (SVC-PA)	>1.5	7%	8%	All of the above

(ASD: atrial septal defect; PAPVC: partial anomalous pulmonary venous connection; LV: left ventricle; PA: pulmonary artery; PDA: patent ductus arteriosus; PR: pulmonary regurgitation; RA: right atrium; RSOV: ruptured sinus of Valsalva; RV: right ventricle; SVC: superior vena cava; VSD: ventricular septal defect; TR: tricuspid regurgitation)

TABLE 6: Causes for desaturation at various levels.

Level of desaturation or R→L shunt	Causes
Pulmonary vein	Lung disease, hypoventilation, pulmonary edema, and pulmonary AV fistula
Left atrium	Ebstein's anomaly, tricuspid atresia, severe PS with TR, unroofed coronary sinus, large ASD, ASD with PS/PAH, RPA to LA fistula
Left ventricle/ ascending aorta	TOF, Eisenmenger VSD
Descending aorta	Eisenmenger PDA, PDA with coarctation of aorta or interrupted aortic arch

(ASD: atrial septal defect; LA: left atrium; PAH: pulmonary artery hypertension; PDA: patent ductus arteriosus; PS: pulmonary stenosis; RPA: right pulmonary artery; VSD: ventricular septal defect; TR: tricuspid regurgitation; TOF: tetralogy of Fallot)

The flow ratio Q_p:Q_s gives important physiologic information about the significance of shunt, and can be calculated without knowledge of oxygen consumption.

$$Q_p{:}Q_s = \frac{SAO_2 - MVO_2}{PVO_2 - PAO_2}$$

Ideally, Q_p:Q_s ratio should be 1 for optimal oxygen delivery to tissues. A Q_p:Q_s ratio of >2 indicates significant left-to-right shunt, and is an indication for closure of the defect, while a Q_p:Q_s ratio of <1.5 is suggestive of a small left-to-right shunt that is not hemodynamically significant enough to warrant closure, and may be left alone. Flow ratios between 1.5 and 2 are intermediate and surgical closure may be considered if operative risk is low. A flow ratio of <1.0 is suggestive of net right-to-left shunt, and irreversible pulmonary vascular disease.[1,2]

To minimize errors in calculation using oximetry, blood samples from various sites should be obtained rapidly, and mean of all values in a particular chamber should be considered instead of highest value. The calculation of MVO_2 is important because, for the same level of systemic oxygen saturation, any change in cardiac output or arteriovenous oxygen saturation difference, produces a significant change in Q_p:Q_s ratio.

The magnitude of shunt flow depends upon size of the defect as well as PVR. The size of the defect is a more important factor for a restrictive defect, whereas outflow obstruction is more important contributing factor when defect is large and unrestrictive. In unrestrictive defects, there is equalization of systolic pressures between the two communicating chambers.

Correlation of clinical and hemodynamic data is important for arriving at correct diagnosis and planning management. For example, a small atrial septal defect (ASD) is less likely to cause severe pulmonary hypertension and so other causes of pulmonary hypertension must be sought as ASD may only be a bystander, and closing it may not be beneficial. A small restrictive ventricular septal defect (VSD) (<1 cm^2/m^2), is unlikely to cause left ventricular volume overload, so other features like associated aortic regurgitation must be sought in case of significant left ventricular volume overload in the presence of small VSD.

Reversibility Testing

Long-standing left-to-right shunt leads to progressive increase in pulmonary vascular resistance, the propensity for which increases with patient age, size of the defect, and post-tricuspid shunts compared to pretricuspid. Cardiac catheterization is important to differentiate flow-related pulmonary hypertension (which is usually reversible with intervention), from permanent pulmonary hypertension due to irreversible remodeling of the pulmonary vascular bed. Reversibility of pulmonary hypertension can be tested with pulmonary vasodilator agents; intravenous (prostacyclins, endothelin antagonists, and adenosine) or inhaled (nitric oxide). The definition of a positive response is fall in mean PA pressure by 10 mm Hg to an absolute value of <40 mm Hg, without fall in cardiac output.[10] An acute reduction of PVRI to <6 WU and a PVRI/SVRI ratio below 0.3 can be considered reliable indicators for acute tolerance of shunt closure.[10] Transcatheter temporary occlusion of the defect with a balloon can be used to predict whether defect closure will be effective and tolerated, in case of high risk lesions with borderline pulmonary hypertension. In cases where reversibility is still questionable, partial closure of the defect with a fenestrated patch or device can be done to partially close the communication and decrease shunt volume, while still allowing some mixing to decompress the high pressure chamber.

Obstructive Lesions

Evaluation of Valvular Stenosis

Cardiac catheterization plays an important role in evaluation of severity of valvular stenosis based on pressure gradient across the valve and the stenotic orifice area, especially when there is discordance between the clinical examination and noninvasive evaluation.

According to hydraulic principles, area of an orifice is equal to the flow across it divided by the velocity of flow. The flow velocity is proportional to the square root of the pressure gradient across the orifice. Thus, the valve area is calculated by using Gorlin's formula,[11] as follows:

$$\text{Valve area} = \frac{\text{Flow (mL/sec)}}{C \times 44.5\ (\text{Pressure gradient across orifice})^{1/2}}$$

Where, C is the orifice constant.

$$\text{Thus, aortic valve area (AVA) (cm}^2) = \frac{\text{Cardiac output/(systolic ejection period} \times \text{heart rate)}}{44.3 \times (\text{mean transaortic gradient})^{1/2}}$$

And,

$$\text{Mitral valve area (MVA) (cm}^2) = \frac{\text{Cardiac output/(diastolic filling period} \times \text{heart rate)}}{37.7 \times (\text{mean transmitral gradient})^{1/2}}$$

The normal AVA is around 2.6–3.5 cm^2, and the normal MVA is 4–6 cm^2.[1]

Accurate measurement of cardiac output and pressure gradients is crucial to avoid errors in valve area estimation. The pressure gradients may be erroneously low in patients with low cardiac output, thus overestimating valve area. In such patients, the Fick method should be used. In patients with mixed stenotic and regurgitant lesions of the same valve, both thermodilution and Fick method lead to underestimation of valve area. In patients with pure aortic or mitral regurgitation, left ventriculography is the method of choice for cardiac output estimation.

Cyanotic Congenital Heart Disease

Just as hemodynamic evaluation is important for shunt detection and quantification, interpretation of pressure tracings and oximetry gives valuable information for diagnosis and surgical planning of various complex cyanotic congenital heart disease (CCHD) as well. In CCHD, if saturation <80%, Q_s is more than Q_p, and if saturation is >85%, Q_s is less than Q_p. In case of balanced shunt, saturation is in the range of 80–85%, except in case of transposition of great arteries (d-TGA) and unfavorable streaming.

TETRALOGY OF FALLOT PHYSIOLOGY

In tetralogy of Fallot (TOF) physiology, large unrestrictive VSD causes equalization of systolic pressures in LV and RV, whereas PA pressures are low. Degree of cyanosis depends on severity of pulmonary outflow obstruction, as well as degree of mixing of blood, which depends upon the size and site of defect as well as presence of collaterals. Right heart catheterization can help in diagnosing level of obstruction (infundibular, valvular, or supravalvular), and whether VSD is restrictive or nonrestrictive, thus guiding for procedural planning in addition to cineangiography for chamber and vessel anatomy. For example, classical TOF with unrestrictive VSD will have equal pressures in both ventricles, whereas TOF with restrictive VSD has features of right ventricular hypertrophy, and double outlet right ventricle (DORV) with restrictive VSD has left ventricular hypertrophy.

Further, in TOF, Q_p is equal to Q_{ep}, (as there is no net left to right shunt), whereas in admixture lesions, Q_p is equal to sum of Q_{ep} and left-to-right shunt. So, for the same Q_p, Q_{ep} is higher for TOF than admixture lesion, and the least for TGA. Thus, for identical cyanosis, TOF has the least cardiac size, admixture lesions like single ventricle with pulmonary stenosis (PS) has mild cardiomegaly, and TGA with VSD and PS has maximum cardiomegaly.

TRANSPOSITION PHYSIOLOGY

In TGA physiology, the normal blood flow, which is in series, is altered, and there is mixing of systemic and pulmonary venous return at either atrial or ventricular or great artery level, leading to systemic desaturation, early heart failure and pulmonary hypertension. In TGA physiology, the systemic oxygen saturation is always lower than that of the PA. The degree of cyanosis depends upon the degree of mixing, the obstruction to Q_p, either due to PS or pulmonary hypertension, and the effect of streaming of blood, which may or may not be favorable.

Some of the difficulties in using standard formulas and calculations in transposition physiology are inability to calculate mixed venous oxygen saturation accurately when one of the pulmonary veins joins SVC/IVC, unless sample is taken just before the entry of pulmonary vein. There is error in Q_s calculation in cases of coarctation of aorta and patent ductus arteriosus (PDA) with right-to-left shunt, as the proportion of flow in ascending aorta and descending aorta are not known. One pulmonary vein may not be representative of all pulmonary veins, hence, left atrial sample should be taken for mixed pulmonary venous saturation, unless there is right-to-left shunt at the atrial level. There may be difference in the saturation between both branches of the PA, in case of PDA, collaterals, and aortopulmonary shunt. As the bronchial collateral flow is not accounted for, Q_p is often overestimated, and PVR is underestimated.

ADMIXTURE PHYSIOLOGY

Resting Q_p can vary from very low to very high depending upon magnitude of the shunt, but resting Q_s maintains a close range of values. Thus, in case of admixture lesions, change in Q_p has a curvilinear relationship with the systemic saturation, assuming a constant Q_s. Thus, with intervention to reduce Q_p, large decrease in flow causes proportionately only little fall in systemic saturation, which can be well tolerated. Similarly, with aortopulmonary shunts, large increase in Q_p, increases systemic saturation marginally, but to an acceptable level, without causing ventricular volume overload.

Effect of Streaming

Streaming is selective flow of blood in a particular direction. Streaming is said to be favorable if deoxygenated blood selectively flows toward the PA, and oxygenated blood flows toward the aorta. In such cases, cyanosis may be missed unless there is severe decrease in Q_p. Thus, pulmonary vascular disease may be underestimated, and DORV with large shunt may be mistaken for VSD. Similarly, when there is unfavorable streaming with deoxygenated blood flowing toward aorta, and oxygenated blood flowing toward PA, Q_p is underestimated, and pulmonary vascular disease is overestimated. For example, DORV with subaortic VSD has favorable streaming with less cyanosis, whereas DORV with subpulmonic VSD, also known as the Taussig–Bing anomaly, has unfavorable streaming, and presents with severe cyanosis, and may be mistaken for TGA.

TOTAL ANOMALOUS PULMONARY VENOUS CONNECTION

In total anomalous pulmonary venous connection (TAPVC), all the pulmonary veins drain into the right atrium, and an intraatrial communication is required for survival. The left atrial pressure is always lower than the right, with a wave more prominent than the v wave. The PA pressure may be very high in case of obstructed TAPVC. Errors in Q_p and Q_s calculation can occur due to inability to obtain accurate mixed venous oxygen saturation, difficulty in obtaining pulmonary venous saturation in obstructed TAPVC, and the very low arteriovenous oxygen difference in case of unobstructed TAPVC. The saturation in all four cardiac chambers is same, so additional post-tricuspid shunt cannot be detected by oximetry. SVC type TAPVC has unfavorable streaming, whereas IVC type TAPVC has favorable streaming.

TRUNCUS ARTERIOSUS

There is a common arterial trunk supplying the systemic, pulmonary, and coronary circulations. Perfusion pressure is equal in both great vessels, but Q_p:Q_s and systemic saturation depend on relative resistance. Early development of pulmonary hypertension usually occurs. However, assessment of pulmonary vascular resistance may be difficult in case of severe stenosis of one PA. Vasoreactivity testing is not reliable as both pulmonary and systemic pressures fall with vasodilator.

TRICUSPID ATRESIA

There is admixture at the level of LA and LV, and Q_p depends on size of VSD and severity of right ventricular outflow tract obstruction (RVOTO). Tricuspid atresia with large VSD without severe RVOTO has early development of pulmonary vascular disease.

SINGLE VENTRICLE

One ventricle is rudimentary or absent, and there is complete mixing of systemic and pulmonary circulation. Interatrial communication may be large or restrictive. Clinical presentation and management depends on degree of mixing, streaming, and systemic or pulmonary outflow tract obstruction. Assessment of PA pressures, pulmonary vascular resistance, and ventricular end-diastolic pressures are some of the important parameters that need to be assessed prior to selecting patients for single ventricle palliation, or the total cavopulmonary connection (the Fontan pathway). For an ideal Fontan candidate, PVRI should not exceed 4 WU/m^2.[12]

RECENT ADVANCES

Role of Cardiac Magnetic Resonance Imaging

Cardiac magnetic resonance imaging (CMRI) plays an important role is evaluation of cardiac anatomy and function. Evaluation of CHD requires quantification of blood flow and volumes, which is done by acquisition of multiple 2D phase contrast and bright blood cine steady state free precession (SSFP) planes. However, as 2D acquisition encodes velocity in only one direction, errors can occur due to underestimation of flow if acquisition plane is not orthogonal to the flow.

Four dimensional (4D) flow MRI is emerging as simpler, faster, and more accurate technique than 2D phase contrast

MRI[13] for comprehensive assessment of CHD.[14,15] The 4D flow consists of a volumetric time-resolved acquisition that is gated to the cardiac cycle, providing a time-varying vector field of blood flow as well as registered anatomic images. Retrospective multiplanar navigation enables flexible retrospective flow quantification through any plane across the volume with good precision. The various flow parameters that can be assessed include peak velocity, stroke volume, regurgitant fraction, shunt volumes as well as wall shear stress, and pressure gradients can be derived from velocity data. Real-time beat-to-beat respirophasic variations in flow can also be quantified.[16] Another advantage of CMRI is visualization and quantification of fibrotic myocardial remodeling by late gadolinium enhancement (LGE) or parametric T1 mapping, and indicates worse outcomes in patients with CHD.

The CMRI acquisition and interpretation in the pediatric population is even more challenging due to smaller size, higher heart rates, and inability to perform long breath-holds, thus may need to be performed under general anesthesia.

CLINICAL APPLICATIONS

Shunt Lesions

Though not commonly used for this purpose, CMRI can provide an accurate assessment of shunt location, size of the defect as well as the Q_p:Q_s and ventricular volume overload to determine significance of shunt and postoperative complications.

Tetralogy of Fallot

After surgical repair of TOF, pulmonary valve regurgitation, right ventricular dysfunction, and arrhythmias are important causes of morbidity and mortality and may require reintervention. Assessment of pulmonary regurgitant fraction and right ventricular volumes by CMRI are important factors to decide need for pulmonary valve replacement. Contrast-enhanced MRI can be used to assess fibrosis based on LGE.

Transposition of Great Arteries

The CMRI can be used to assess ventricular and valvular function with SSFP gradient echo sequences. Neoaortic dilatation and regurgitation, branch PA stenosis, baffle leaks, and obstruction can be assessed after surgical correction. LGE images can help in detecting systemic right ventricular failure after atrial switch repair.

Coarctation of Aorta

The CMRI is useful for assessing location as well as severity of coarctation by measurement of peak flow velocity. Collateral flow can also be assessed by quantifying flow just proximal to the coarctation and in the descending aorta at the level of the hiatus. Associated aortic arch hypoplasia, aortic valve stenosis, and left ventricular hypertrophy can also be visualized with SSFP cine sequences.

CONCLUSION

Hemodynamic interpretation of CHD requires knowledge of the cardiac physiology, correct use of the recording apparatus in the catheterization laboratory to minimize errors, and use of appropriate invasive and noninvasive ways to collect and interpret data for diagnostic, prognostic, and therapeutic purposes so as to ensure maximum benefit to the patient.

ONLINE REFERENCES

Please scan the QR code provided at the end of the table of contents for References of this chapter.

CHAPTER

93

Timing of Surgery/Intervention for Congenital Heart Diseases: Indian Perspective

Snehal Kulkarni, Ronak Sheth

ABSTRACT

Uncorrected congenital heart defects account for one of the major causes of early childhood mortality as well as significant morbidity in adolescence/adulthood. Early identification and timely repair/intervention and long-term surveillance are essential for ensuring a good outcome. The essence is to operate/palliate before irreversible cardiovascular, pulmonary vascular, or systemic ill effects set in.

Keywords: Congenital heart disease, timing of intervention

INTRODUCTION

Congenital heart defects are the most common congenital anomalies.[1] Critical congenital heart defects account for one of the major proportions of infant and under-5 mortality in India.[2-4] At the same time, uncorrected congenital heart defects account for the major proportion of morbidity in older children, adolescents, and adults.[5] Although prompt identification and timely palliation/repair are essential, concerted efforts to mitigate the ill effects of malnutrition and infections also play a pivotal role in deciding the outcome in congenital heart diseases (CHDs).[6,7] A wide variety of morphological lesions and complex interplay of multiple pathophysiological factors affect the manifestations, as also the need, timing, and type of intervention.[8,9]

ACYANOTIC HEART DEFECTS WITH LEFT-TO-RIGHT SHUNTS

Atrial Septal Defect

Indications and Contraindications

Isolated atrial septal defects causing right ventricular volume overload merit closure **(Table 1)**. Patients with significant pulmonary hypertension or right heart hypoplasia need

TABLE 1: Recommendations for closure of ASD depending upon the anatomy.

ASD	Symptoms	Age group and recommendation
Secundum ASD	Asymptomatic	• Between 2 and 4 years of age (class I) • *Beyond 4 years of age*: Elective closure is recommended in all patients with a significant shunt and right heart volume overload and operable pulmonary vascular resistance
Sinus venosus ASD	Asymptomatic	Between 4 and 5 years of age (class IIA)
ASD	Early symptomatic in infancy with CHF or regurgitation or AV valves, PAH	Early ASD closure is recommended (class I) (rule out other associated lesions causing heart failure)
PFO/ASD ± atrial septal aneurysm	Symptomatic with sequelae of paradoxical emboli—stroke/TIA	Elective closure (class IIA)

careful evaluation and may be unsuitable for complete closure of the atrial shunt.

Method/Mode of Intervention

Surgical repair of atrial septal defect is an established modality (class I); however, transcatheter device closure of atrial septal defects with adequate surrounding rims is the treatment of choice for secundum atrial septal defects (class I) except when contraindicated.

Contraindications for transcatheter closure of the defect are as follows:

- Primum or sinus venosus or coronary sinus form of atrial septal defects
- Secundum defects which are unsuitable for device placement due to small child (<15 kg), deficient rims (<5 mm), large defects (>20 mm/m^2 body surface area), and multiple defects which cannot be closed with finite devices

Sinus venosus atrial septal defects, especially in adults, can be evaluated for feasibility of transcatheter closure using a covered stent.[10]

Ventricular Septal Defect

Indications and Contraindications

Most of the large VSDs need closure in infancy to prevent the development of pulmonary vascular disease **(Tables 2 and 3)**. Closure of the defect is contraindicated in the presence of irreversible pulmonary vascular disease. In certain high-risk scenarios for the development of pulmonary vascular disease like trisomy 21, patients with large VSD presenting even in late infancy or beyond infancy may need assessment for operability before proceeding with surgery.

Patients with large ventricular septal defects with bidirectional shunts or resting oxygen saturation of 90% or less, or X-ray chest with no cardiomegaly with peripheral pruning will need careful evaluation and cardiac catheterization for measurement of pulmonary vascular resistance index (PVRI) and vasodilatory testing for reactivity of the pulmonary vascular bed.

Recommendation for Operability with Elevated PVRI

Cardiac catheterization for assessment of shunt severity and pulmonary vascular resistance is recommended as the outcomes depend on the severity and reversibility of pulmonary vascular disease.[11-13] Recommendations are listed in **Table 4**.

Patent Ductus Arteriosus

Indications and Contraindications

All PDAs need to be closed for the risk of heart failure, development of pulmonary vascular disease, or infective endocarditis except silent PDA.

Timing/Ideal Age

Elective closure should be done between 12 and 18 months of age. For moderate PDAs, closure should be planned between 6 months and 1 year of age. For large PDAs with significant left heart volume overload, congestive heart failure, and pulmonary hypertension, early closure should be planned by 3 months of age.

Method/Mode of Intervention

Transcatheter device closure of PDA is the standard of care in all feasible ductus morphologies in patients weighing >5 kg.

Surgical PDA ligation is recommended for children with weight < 5 kg, ductal aneurysm, ductal endarteritis, and ductus with unusual morphologies unsuitable for device closure.

TABLE 2: Recommendations for closure of VSD depending upon size.

VSD classification	Features	Symptoms	Age group and recommendation
Small VSD	Normal PA pressure, no left heart dilatation, no aortic valve distortion	Asymptomatic	• Annual cardiac review till 10 years of age; then every 2–3 years • Surgical repair indicated if patient develops an episode of endocarditis; aortic valve distortion; RVOT obstruction
Moderate VSD	Normal PA pressure, dilated left heart chambers	Asymptomatic	VSD closure by 2–5 years of age
		Controlled symptoms	VSD closure by 1–2 years of age
Large VSD	Growth failure, congestive heart failure symptoms	Controlled heart failure	VSD surgical closure by 4–6 months of age
		Poorly controlled with medications	VSD closure as soon as possible
VSD with aortic cusp prolapse	VSD-related aortic cusp prolapse leading to more than trivial aortic regurgitation	Asymptomatic or symptomatic	Surgical VSD closure ± aortic valve repair as soon as possible

TABLE 3: Modalities for closure of VSD depending upon the size and site of VSD.

VSD	Symptoms/features	Modality and recommendation
Moderate or large VSD	Standard	Surgical patch closure of VSD is recommended
	Multiple—Swiss-cheese or inaccessible VSDs *Or* Contraindications to cardiopulmonary bypass/sepsis	Pulmonary artery banding as a palliative measure (class I) followed by complete VSD closure surgery at a later date
	Borderline operability due to elevated pulmonary vascular resistance	Fenestrated VSD patch closure/flap valve patch/ fenestrated ASD patch (class IIb) may be done in experienced tertiary centers after counseling/ discussion with family
Small or moderate VSD	Midmuscular, anterior muscular, postoperative residual VSD	Elective transcatheter device closure (class I)
Weight >8 kg and significant shunt (>1.5:1)	Perimembranous VSD with good separation from the aortic valve (>4 mm)	Elective transcatheter device closure (class IIB)
	• Preexisting conduction system abnormality or LBBB • Aortic regurgitation • Associated surgical lesion • Inlet VSD • Subpulmonic VSD	• Transcatheter attempt is contraindicated (class III) • Device deployment should be aborted if device causes any significant TR/MR/AR or any conduction abnormality
	• Infant with large muscular VSD • Percutaneous transcatheter closure is difficult due to large sheath required	Hybrid approach/perventricular device closure may be considered (class IIB)

TABLE 4: Cardiac catheterization for vasoreactivity testing and recommendation for closure.

Unrepaired late-presenting left-to-right shunt lesion		
Hemodynamic assessment	**Acute vasoreactivity testing**	**Recommendation**
PVRI < 4 WU m^2 PVR/SVR < 0.3		Usually safely operable with favorable long-term outcome
PVRI 4–8 WU/m^2 PVR/SVR = 0.3–0.5	>20% fall in PVRI and PVR/SVR ratio with respective final values	*Gray zone*: "Possibly repairable" if demonstrable acute vasoreactivity; recommendation for individualized decision making in tertiary center taking into account multiple factors including age, pathophysiology, clinical features, and imaging data
PVRI > 8 WU/m^2 PVR/SVR > 0.5		Usually inoperable

Recommendations for operability in late-presenting large PDA are similar to those in VSD. Transient test occlusion of the PDA can be done to assess suitability for closure. More than 25% reduction in mPAP relative to baseline value is considered significant in favor of operability; also, a post-test balloon occlusion systolic PA/Ao pressure ratio >0.5 is considered adverse for operability and is a pointer of irreversible persistent pulmonary hypertension even after shunt closure.[14]

Preterm PDA is a distinct pathophysiological entity.

Trial of pharmacological PDA closure using paracetamol/ibuprofen/indomethacin is recommended for hemodynamically significant PDA in preterm babies.[15-17]

Hemodynamically significant preterm PDA persisting with failure of pharmacological measures needs individualized decision-making about the timing and modality of closure (surgical vs. transcatheter option).

Aortopulmonary Window

Timing/Ideal Age

Elective surgical repair should be done by 3 months of age, unless uncontrolled heart failure necessitates earlier surgery. From late infancy onward, the patient may need to be assessed for operability if there is suspicion of elevated pulmonary vascular resistance.

Method/Mode of Intervention

Surgical repair is the standard of care (class I).

In carefully selected patients with an intermediate-type aortopulmonary window, transcatheter device closure may be recommended (class IIA).

Atrioventricular Septal Defect

Timing/Ideal Age

Surgical repair—by either modified single-patch or double-patch technique—should be performed for complete AV canal defect with uncontrolled heart failure by 3 months of age. Patients may have different morphology of the atrioventricular valve and ventricular asymmetry and need to be assessed carefully for suitability of biventricular repair. Older infants > 6 months of age and especially with a background of trisomy 21 may have elevated pulmonary vascular resistance and may need operability assessment prior to operating.

Partial and Intermediate AV Canal

The ideal time of surgical repair is around 2–3 years of age. In exceptional scenarios with significant heart failure due to AV valve regurgitation, earlier repair may be considered. Long-term outcomes and prognosis are related to residual left AV valve stenosis or regurgitation, subaortic stenosis, atrial arrhythmias, and complete heart block.

There are some uncommon lesions causing left-to-right shunt which may need closure **(Table 5)**.

Left Ventricular Obstructions

Coarctation of Aorta

Indications

These include patients with mean gradient across coarctation segment of >20 mm Hg or gradient < 20 mm Hg with coexisting LV hypertrophy/dysfunction/upper limb hypertension/collateral formation, or hypertensive patients with >50% narrowing at the site relative to descending aorta at the diaphragm, irrespective of pressure gradient.

Timing/Ideal Age

Emergency repair/intervention is indicated in patients with congestive cardiac failure or those with left ventricular dysfunction or who present shock in the neonatal period **(Table 6)**. In case of upper limb hypertension, elective intervention is recommended by 3–6 months of age.

In cases with a coexisting ventricular septal defect, both defects should be corrected in the same setting by surgical repair.

TABLE 6: Method/mode of intervention—coarctation of aorta.

Features	Recommendation
Neonatal presentation	Surgical repair (class I)
Coarctation with aortic arch hypoplasia	Surgical repair (class I)
Neonate with shock-like state/severe LV dysfunction	Balloon coarctoplasty (class IIA) as bailout procedure
Infant native coarctation	• Surgery (class I) • Balloon angioplasty (class IIA)
Infant recoarctation	Balloon coarctoplasty (class IIA)
Child < 25 kg with native coarctation	• Balloon coarctoplasty (class I) • Surgery (class IIA)
Child < 25 kg with recoarctation	Balloon/stent coarctoplasty (class I)
Child > 25 kg, adults with native coarctation	Coarctation stenting (class I)
Child with age < 10 years	Elective endovascular stenting of coarctation is contraindicated

TABLE 5: Uncommon left-to-right shunt lesions.

Defect	Symptoms	Age group and recommendation
Anomalous origin of PA from aorta		Surgical repair (preferably in the neonatal period)[18,19]; risk of early development of pulmonary vascular disease, as early as 3 months of age
Coronary cameral fistula	Small- or moderate-sized distal fistula	Close follow-up with echocardiography and/or angiography to determine increase in quantum of shunt
	Small- to moderate-sized + ischemia/arrhythmia/ventricular dysfunction or endarteritis	Percutaneous/surgical closure (percutaneous approach preferable if feasible; preferably surgical approach if weight < 5 kg or complex fistula anatomy)[20-22]
	Large fistula (irrespective of symptoms)	
Anomalous origin of left coronary artery from pulmonary artery		Surgical repair is indicated as early as possible (regardless of age or symptoms) to establish a dual coronary system[23-25] (direct reimplantation, Takeuchi transpulmonary baffling, two-flap technique, subclavian left coronary anastomosis, ligation of ostium with coronary artery bypass graft) + Medical management to optimize heart failure

Cyanotic Congenital Heart Lesions with Excessive Pulmonary Blood Flow

Total Anomalous Pulmonary Venous Connection

Indications and Contraindications

All total anomalous pulmonary venous connections (TAPVCs) should be treated by surgical repair even if the patient is asymptomatic.

Timing/Ideal Age

Emergency surgical repair is indicated in obstructed TAPVCs. Even in nonobstructive TAPVCs, surgical repair is recommended as soon as feasible.

Long-term Prognosis

Residual pulmonary vein stenosis, residual PAH, pulmonary venous anastomotic stenosis, and late-onset arrhythmias are the major determinants of long-term prognosis.

Truncus Arteriosus

Indications and Contraindications

Severe pulmonary hypertension with irreversible pulmonary vascular disease is a contraindication for surgical repair.

Timing/Ideal Age

Surgical repair of truncus arteriosus should be done by 4–8 weeks of age in patients with controlled symptoms, or earlier if there is refractory heart failure. In complex scenarios/multiorgan system dysfunction/contraindications for cardiopulmonary bypass, a palliative bilateral branch PA banding may be a temporizing option.

Method/Mode of Intervention

Surgical repair with RV–PA conduit and closure of VSD is the treatment of choice in most cases. Truncal valve repair may be needed if there is significant truncal stenosis or regurgitation preoperatively. Most patients will have progressive conduit dysfunction contributed by the child's growth and conduit degeneration and require future conduit revision surgery/RVOT rehabilitation. Elder patients need evaluation for operability.

Transposition of Great Arteries

Preoperative Stabilization

Ductal patency is maintained to allow circulatory mixing: PGE1 infusion (with a dose of 0.05 μg/kg/min) may be required soon after birth if there is desaturation beyond 75% or there is significant lactic acidosis (class I). Respiratory monitoring/elective mechanical ventilation may be instituted as there is a risk of significant respiratory depression with PGE1 infusion.

Balloon atrial septostomy is indicated with significant hypoxemia despite PGE1 infusion, with restrictive interatrial communication (class I) **(Table 7)**.

Rapid two-stage arterial switch surgery involves the first step of LV retraining. This LV retraining can be achieved by (1) PA banding + aortopulmonary shunt/bidirectional Glenn shunt or also by (2) ductal stenting (class IIB). Such two-stage arterial switch in a late-presenting TGA child is inherently higher risk as compared to early ASO in a neonate.

TABLE 7: Timing/ideal age/method/mode of intervention.

TGA ± associated lesions	Age	Recommendation
TGA with intact ventricular septum	Neonate	Arterial switch operation (class I), ideally between 7 days and 3 weeks of age, but exact timing based on individual patient parameters and institutional preferences
	1–2 months of age	Arterial switch operation may be feasible depending on the degree of LV regression and availability of mechanical circulatory support (class IIA)
	2–6 months of age	• Arterial switch operation with mechanical circulatory support or • Rapid two-stage arterial switch operation or • Atrial switch surgery (class IIA)
	6 months to 2 years of age	• Atrial switch surgery (class IIA) • In selected cases, rapid two-stage arterial switch operation may be considered (class IIB)
TGA with large VSD/large PDA	Less than 6 weeks of age	Arterial switch operation + VSD closure + PDA ligation by 6 weeks of age (class I); these patients are at risk of early development of pulmonary vascular disease and may have borderline operability in late infancy
TGA with VSD with coarctation of aorta	Neonate	Arterial switch surgery + VSD closure + aortic arch repair as soon as possible (class I)

Continued

Continued

TGA ± associated lesions	Age	Recommendation
TGA with VSD with significant LVOT obstruction (pulmonary stenosis)	Resectable subvalvular obstruction only	ASO with resection of subvalvular pulmonary stenosis
	Unresectable subvalvular or pulmonary valvular obstruction	• Neonate/early infancy with significant cyanosis: Systemic to pulmonary artery shunt followed by complete repair (Rastelli/root translocation) at 2–3 years of age/weight > 10 kg • REV procedure may be considered at 4–6 months of age • Pulmonary root translocation may be considered at 6–12 months of age • Nikaidoh procedure may be considered beyond 6–9 months of age • *Older child beyond 2–3 years of age*: Rastelli/Nikaidoh/root translocation surgery • If VSD is remote or nonroutable, staged univentricular palliation to be considered

Hypoplastic Left Heart Syndrome

Indications and Timing

HLHS is a subset with a complex morphological abnormality with a poorly developed systemic ventricle and systemic great artery and ductus-dependent systemic circulation. Norwood surgery continues to be one of the highest risk-carrying congenital heart operations. The ideal timing for Norwood surgery is between the second and the seventh day of life.[26,27] In resource-limited scenarios, only comfort care may be a viable option after detailed discussion with the family members, due to the high risk and reserved long-term cardiac and neurodevelopmental outcomes in this subset.

Method/Mode of Intervention

There is a trend of preference of RV–PA Sano shunt as the source of pulmonary blood flow to offer better hemodynamics and stability in Norwood Stage I and Interstage I of palliation (Sano modification of Norwood).

In higher-risk critically ill neonates, the hybrid palliative approach may be preferred. This involves bilateral PA banding + stenting of the ductus ± atrial septostomy. This defers the neoaortic arch reconstruction step to the comprehensive second stage.

In further palliative stages, Stage II (Glenn) and Stage III (Fontan) operations are similar to other univentricular hearts and need detailed evaluation and assessment at each step (similar to univentricular hearts).

Tetralogy of Fallot and Tetralogy of Fallot–Pulmonary Atresia

Timing/Ideal Age

In asymptomatic or minimally symptomatic children with mild cyanosis, elective surgical repair should be performed by 6–12 months of age. In young infants with marked symptoms and severe cyanosis or refractory spells despite medical therapy, palliative systemic to pulmonary artery shunt (BT shunt/central shunt) or RV to PA shunt (Sano) or RVOT augmentation (Brock's procedure) or ductal stenting/ RVOT stenting is recommended. Early complete repair can be performed in symptomatic children with good anatomy.

In patients with tetralogy of Fallot (TOF)-pulmonary atresia or those with coronary artery crossing RV outflow tract where RV–PA conduit may be required for complete repair, the complete repair is ideally done at 2 years of age/10 kg weight. In patients with TOF-absent pulmonary valve, elective surgical repair is recommended around 1 year of age; additional steps such as branch pulmonary artery reduction angioplasty/LeCompte maneuver may be required to relieve airway obstruction.

Neonates with VSD with pulmonary atresia may need stabilization by PGE1 infusion. Stenting of the PDA or aortopulmonary shunt may be required to maintain adequate oxygen saturation. These patients will require early surgery by 6–12 months with closure of VSD and RV–PA conduit insertion. These patients will require frequent change of conduits as they grow.

Double-outlet Right Ventricle

Surgical repair of double-outlet right ventricle is indicated in all patients except those who have developed irreversible pulmonary vascular disease **(Table 8)**. The type of the repair depends upon the location of VSD.

Congenitally Corrected Transposition of Great Arteries

Most of these patients have associated lesions like ventricular septal defects, left ventricular outflow tract obstruction, and systemic AV valve (tricuspid valve) regurgitation.

Surgical repair should be considered in patients with severe tricuspid (systemic AV valve) regurgitation before systemic ventricular failure sets in (class IIA).

TABLE 8: Types of surgical repair for DORV depending upon the site of VSD.

DORV type	Age group and recommendation
Subaortic VSD and pulmonary hypertension (VSD type)	• Surgical closure of DORV-VSD by 6 months of age • *Beyond 6 months*: Assessment for operability (pulmonary vascular disease) followed by surgery if operable
Subaortic VSD and pulmonary stenosis (TOF subtype)	• Similar to TOF • *Significant desaturation in early infancy*: Aortopulmonary shunt • *Later infancy to older child*: Complete repair
Subpulmonary VSD with pulmonary hypertension (TGA type)	• Arterial switch operation + VSD closure by 6 weeks of age; associated coarctation/arch hypoplasia to be repaired in the same surgery • Beyond 3 months of age, may need assessment for operability
Subpulmonary VSD with pulmonary stenosis	• If resectable PS, arterial switch operation + resection of subvalvular pulmonary stenosis • In valvular/complex obstruction, may need root translocation/REV/Rastelli/Nikaidoh procedure
Remote VSD/complex associated lesions	• Complex biventricular repair with LV–aorta baffling depending on specific anatomy and in experienced pediatric cardiac centers • When this is not feasible, staged univentricular palliation is recommended

TABLE 9: Surgical repair in CCTGA depending upon the anatomical details.

CCTGA ± associated lesions	Age	Recommendation
No associated lesions	At any age	Medical follow-up to monitor systemic AV valve function, systemic ventricular function, and AV nodal conduction
With large VSD	<3 months of age	PA banding followed by double-switch operation
	3–6 months of age	• PA banding followed by double-switch operation or • Direct double-switch operation • Depending on individual scenario/institutional policy
	>6 months of age	Double-switch operation if not yet developed pulmonary vascular disease

With large VSD and pulmonary stenosis		• If no desaturation and not symptomatic, can be considered for long-term medical follow-up
		• In case of significant desaturation:
		  ○ Early infancy: Systemic to pulmonary artery shunt
		  ○ Late infancy and beyond: Double-switch operation (atrial switch + Rastelli) (class I) if biventricular repair is feasible; if not feasible, staged univentricular palliation to be offered (class IIA)

With complete heart block		Permanent dual-chamber pacemaker implantation (class I)

Anatomic repair is recommended when the left ventricle is conditioned (at systemic or near systemic pressures) and other factors are favorable for anatomic repair **(Table 9)**.

Univentricular Hearts

Subsets

Indications and Contraindications

Univentricular hearts require timely staged palliative procedures aimed at separating the pulmonary and systemic circulations at the cost of raised systemic venous pressures. The timing and nature of staged surgical palliation depend on the morphology and whether there is increased or reduced pulmonary blood flow **(Table 10)**.

Patients with significant regurgitation of systemic AV valve, severe biventricular dysfunction, and pulmonary vein stenosis are at a high risk for surgery with a poor long-term outcome. They need to be counseled regarding the risk prior to surgery.

Ebstein's Anomaly

For neonatal presentation with significant cyanosis, supplemental high-flow oxygen and sildenafil are recommended as a temporizing measure to accelerate fetal-neonatal

TABLE 10: Stages and timings of univentricular repair.

	Severe pulmonary stenosis/ pulmonary atresia	Unrestricted pulmonary blood flow	Additional remarks
Presenting in neonatal period/early infancy (up to 3 months of age)	Systemic to pulmonary artery shunt/ ductal stenting	PA banding	• *Ideal timing*: 4–6 weeks of age, preferably before 3 months of age • Additional procedures may be required to correct systemic outflow obstruction—aortic arch/coarctation repair
Later infancy to 3 years of age	Patients with pulmonary stenosis or those who have undergone PA banding in early infancy—those presenting after 4–5 months of age with saturations falling below 70% can be considered for bidirectional Glenn shunt surgery	May need detailed evaluation to assess operability—those who have a reactive pulmonary vascular bed may benefit from PA banding	• Ideal time is 6 months to 1 year of age • Additional procedures may be required at this time—atrial septectomy
4–7 years of age (weight > 12–15 kg)	Total cavopulmonary connection (Fontan completion)		Fenestrated Fontan is recommended in higher-risk cases

transition and fall in pulmonary vascular resistance. Diuretics may be used in case of significant heart failure. Surgery is recommended for those not stabilized by medical therapy. Surgical risk is very high, and the patients may be considered for heart transplant if facilities are available.

For older children and adults, surgical repair of the tricuspid valve is indicated when there are significant symptoms, exercise intolerance, desaturation < 90%, paradoxical embolism, cardiomegaly on chest X-ray (>65%), and progressive right ventricular dilatation and dysfunction.

Symptomatic patients with arrhythmias need catheter ablation therapy.

Method/Mode of Intervention

Cone repair of the tricuspid valve is the usually preferred surgical modality. It should be performed by 2 years of age. Additional bidirectional Glenn shunt (to achieve a one and half ventricle repair) is undertaken in selected scenarios. In the most challenging cases, where the tricuspid valve is not repairable, valve replacement may be offered; univentricular repair may have to be planned in young patients with significant displacement of the tricuspid valve with a very small-sized functional right ventricular cavity.

Valvular Lesions

Valve repair surgery is preferable to valve replacement surgeries. Valve replacement may be considered if repair is not feasible. Bioprosthetic valve replacement is preferable in young female patients who may plan pregnancy in future. Mechanical valve replacement can be considered in other groups of patients. The Ross procedure should be considered for severe aortic valve pathology. The need for lifelong anticoagulation with frequent monitoring of INR after mechanical valve implantation should be explained to the parents **(Table 11)**.

In patients with subvalvular obstruction, there is recurrence of obstruction even after successful surgical repair and they need close follow-up **(Table 12)**.

Method/Mode of Intervention

Transcatheter balloon valvuloplasty is the desired mode of intervention for all valvular pulmonary stenoses (class I).

Surgical intervention is recommended for subvalvular or supravalvular pulmonary stenosis, failed balloon valvuloplasty, dysplastic valve, or hypoplastic valve annulus (class I).

For peripheral pulmonary stenosis, transcatheter balloon/stent angioplasty is recommended for focal branch/ peripheral PA stenosis with >50% diameter narrowing or elevated RV systolic pressure >50 mm Hg or >50% systemic pressure or lung perfusion scan showing >20% difference in both lung perfusion or if symptomatic (class I).

Aortic Regurgitation

Indications and Timing

- All symptomatic patients with moderate to severe AR (class I)
- Asymptomatic patients with severe AR with either significant LV dilatation LVESD Z score >4 or with onset of ventricular dysfunction—LVEF < 50% (class I)

Newer surgical techniques for aortic valve repair using Ozaki aortic neocuspidization have shown promising results in children.[28-31] When repair is not feasible, aortic valve replacement using pulmonary autograft (Ross procedure) is preferred.[32-35]

TABLE 11: Aortic stenosis—types of intervention in various subsets of aortic stenosis.

Lesion	Echo features	Symptoms	Recommendation
Valvular	Neonate with severe AS with duct-dependent systemic circulation	Irrespective of symptoms	Balloon valvuloplasty/surgical valvotomy
	Infant or child with severe AS with LV dysfunction, irrespective of absolute gradient	Irrespective of symptoms	Balloon valvuloplasty/surgical valvotomy
	AS gradient (mm Hg): • >64 peak (Doppler) • >40 mean (Doppler) • >50 peak-to-peak (catheter)	Irrespective of symptoms	Elective balloon valvuloplasty
	AS gradient (mm Hg): • <64 peak (Doppler) • <40 mean (Doppler)	Asymptomatic	Intervention is not indicated
	Aortic stenosis with more than mild aortic regurgitation		Balloon valvuloplasty is contraindicated
Subvalvular	AS gradient (mm Hg) >50 peak instantaneous (Doppler)		• Surgical intervention (class I) • Balloon dilatation in selected cases of thin membranes with good separation from aortic valve (class IIB)
	AS gradient (mm Hg): <50 peak instantaneous (Doppler) + more than mild AR *Or* LV dysfunction *Or* Contemplating competitive sports or pregnancy		Surgical resection (class I)
	AS gradient 30–50 mm Hg		Surgical resection (class IIB)
	AS gradient < 30 mm Hg with up to trivial AR	Asymptomatic	Class III (intervention not indicated)
Supravalvular	*AS gradient (mm Hg)*: • >64 peak (Doppler) • >50 mean (Doppler)	Symptomatic	Surgical repair (class I)
	AS gradient <50 mean (Doppler), with low surgical risk	Asymptomatic	Surgical repair (class IIB)
	AS gradient (mm Hg): <50 mean (Doppler) + symptoms *Or* Severe LV hypertrophy *Or* LV systolic dysfunction *Or* Myocardial ischemia due to coronary ostial involvement	Symptomatic	Surgical repair (class I)

TABLE 12: Pulmonary stenosis (PS)—balloon valvuloplasty in different age groups depending upon severity.

Lesion	Echo features	Symptoms	Recommendation
Valvular	Neonate with severe PS with duct-dependent pulmonary circulation	Irrespective of symptoms	Immediate balloon valvuloplasty/surgical valvotomy (class I)
	Infant or child with severe PS with RV dysfunction, irrespective of absolute gradient	Irrespective of symptoms	Immediate balloon valvuloplasty/surgical valvotomy (class I)
	PS gradient (mm Hg): >64 peak (Doppler)	Irrespective of symptoms	Elective balloon valvuloplasty (class I) (class IIA if dysplastic valve)
	Any degree of PS	Mild RV hypoplasia with mild hypoxia	Elective balloon valvuloplasty (class IIA)

Mitral Regurgitation

Indications and Timing

- All symptomatic patients with moderate-to-severe MR with LV ejection fraction > 30% (class I); when LVEF is <30%, it is a class IIB indication.
- All asymptomatic patients with severe MR with either significant LV dilatation LVESD *Z* score > 3 or onset of ventricular dysfunction—LVEF < 50% (class IIA).
- Asymptomatic patients with moderate or severe AR undergoing cardiac surgery for another indication (class IIA).

Cardiac Pacing

General recommendations for pacing in children are as follows **(Table 13)**:[8,36]

- Permanent pacing can be achieved by implanting pacing leads either endocardially or epicardially.
- Children form a unique subset as pacing considerations need special assessment and precaution because of their growth potential and the likelihood of requiring lifelong therapy, thus needing multiple repeat procedures for replacing pacemaker pulse generator or pacing leads. Hence, implantation sites and venous channels should be cared for and conserved as much as possible.

TABLE 13: Recommendations for pacemaker in children.

Recommendation	Type of conduction abnormality	Symptoms or additional features
Class I	Advanced second-/third-degree AV nodal block	Symptomatic
	Sinus node dysfunction–related bradycardia	Symptomatic
	Postoperative advanced second-/third-degree AV conduction block	Lasting beyond 7–10 days postoperatively, not expected to spontaneously resolve
	Congenital complete AV block	• Either of the following: ○ Wide QRS escape rhythm ○ Complex ventricular ectopy ○ Ventricular dysfunction ○ Prolonged QTc ○ Long pause > 3× cycle length ○ Slow ventricular rate (Infant with CHD—HR <55; infant without CHD—HR < 70; older child with CHD—HR < 50; older child without CHD—HR < 70)
Class IIA	Sinus bradycardia	Unrepaired/complex CHD with HR < 40/min or pause >3 seconds
	Sinus bradycardia or loss of AV synchrony	CHD with significant hemodynamic impairment
	Repaired CHD complicated by transient CHB with residual fascicular block	Unexplained syncope (other causes of syncope ruled out)
Class IIB	Sinus bradycardia	Biventricular repaired CHD with HR <40/min or pause > 3 seconds
	Congenital complete AV block	• Asymptomatic • Acceptable ventricular rate • Narrow QRS complex • Normal QTc • Normal ventricular function
	Repaired CHD complicated by transient CHB with residual fascicular block	Asymptomatic
Class III (pacemaker implantation is not recommended)	Repaired CHD with transient CHB with full recovery	Asymptomatic
	Repaired CHD with bifascicular block or first-degree AV block	Asymptomatic
	Type I second-degree AV block	Asymptomatic
	Sinus bradycardia with longest pause <3 seconds and minimum HR > 40/min	Asymptomatic

- During transvenous pacing lead implantation in children, an additional loop of pacing lead should be left redundant in the right atrium to allow for lengthening with the growth of the child.

Indications for epicardial pacing include:
- Weight < 10 kg
- Unrepaired, palliated, or repaired CHD with persistent right-to-left shunt
- Congenital or acquired absence of transvenous access to the chamber to be paced (post-Glenn/Fontan palliation, venous abnormalities of the superior vena cava or innominate vein)
- Post-CHD surgery where additional future open heart surgery is anticipated
- Mechanical tricuspid valve (for ventricular pacing)

CONCLUSION

This chapter is an attempt at simplification of complex CHD pathophysiology to facilitate and guide decision-making about the timing of intervention/surgery in various CHDs. The essence is to operate/palliate before irreversible cardiovascular, pulmonary vascular, or systemic ill effects set in.

ONLINE REFERENCES

Please scan the QR code provided at the end of the table of contents for References of this chapter.

CHAPTER

94

Palliative Surgeries in Congenital Heart Diseases

Rishika Mehta, Amitabha Chattopadhyay

ABSTRACT

Palliative procedures are done in patients with congenital heart diseases (CHD) who cannot undergo definitive corrective repairs to improve the quality of life and to prepare for future definitive or further palliative procedures. Imaging plays an important role in evaluating patients with CHD, for early diagnosis and prevention of complications and assessment for subsequent procedures. Better knowledge of normal anatomy and the hemodynamics helps in planning better palliative procedures. Common complications of various palliative procedures include thrombosis, stenosis, pseudoaneurysm, infection, and congestive cardiac failure.

Keywords: Palliation, surgery, CHD, complications

INTRODUCTION

Surgeries for congenital heart diseases may be curative (i.e., restoring the normal anatomical heart structure and function along with relieving the symptoms of the disease) or palliative (i.e., operations which do not totally correct the structure but improve the abnormal heart function, and minimize the symptoms). With the advancement in anesthetic and surgical techniques along with improved quality of postoperative ICU care, early total corrective surgeries are performed in most CHDs. However, palliative procedures have found a role in children who cannot undergo total curative procedures due to their age, preterm birth, low birth weight, pneumonia, sepsis, intracerebral bleed, multiorgan failure, unstable hemodynamics, or the underlying anatomy where definitive correction either is not possible or carries a very high risk. Many palliative procedures are now obsolete, but some procedures prepare the circulation for subsequent palliative or definitive procedures and some of these procedures are a part of hybrid procedures.

Palliative procedures have been divided into five categories according to the specific goals and indications:

1. *Increasing pulmonary blood flow for pulmonary oligemia, correcting cyanosis and hypoxemia*: Shunt procedures including single-ventricle palliation.
2. *Reducing pulmonary blood flow for pulmonary overcirculation*: Pulmonary banding and Norwood procedure.
3. *Improving intracardiac admixture for systemic hypoxemia*: Different techniques of atrial septostomy.
4. Palliative procedures directed toward transposition of great arteries.
5. *Other procedures*: Congenital valvar stenosis, coarctation of aorta, palliation, and hybrid palliation for hypoplastic left heart syndrome (HLHS).

SHUNT PROCEDURES

Shunts between the systemic and pulmonary arteries are called systemic-PA shunts. They are used to normalize pulmonary blood flow and pressure in a fashion which is regulated so as to prevent heart failure and overcirculation, maintain correct right ventricle (RV) preload without causing hemodilution, maintain unobstructed systemic afterload for appropriate coronary perfusion, and relieve pulmonary venous obstruction.[1]

Indications:

- To decrease cyanosis in high-risk children with unfavorable anatomy till they undergo a complete repair in TOF patients.

- To help in growth of pulmonary arteries in pulmonary atresia, ventricular septal defect (VSD) with major aorto-pulmonary collaterals in preparation for a subsequent unifocalization.
- As a part of stage I palliation in patients with single ventricle physiology (e.g., tricuspid atresia, HLHS, pulmonary atresia with intact ventricular septum). The pulmonary and systemic vessels are small sized in neonates, and adequate pulmonary artery growth is a prerequisite for performing a Fontan procedure. So, systemic-PA shunts are done in neonates to facilitate the growth of PAs. Pulmonary arterioles multiply in number till the age of 3 years and increase in diameter till the age of 11 years. Glenn shunt and Fontan procedures are subsequently performed in a staged manner.

Various types of shunt procedures are described in the following text **(Fig. 1)**.

Classic Blalock–Taussig–Thomas Shunt

Direct end-to-side anastomosis between a transected subclavian (or brachiocephalic) artery and the ipsilateral PA is performed on the side opposite to the aortic arch to minimize kinking of the subclavian artery without using any prosthetic material. It helps to improve branch pulmonary artery size and has a growth potential.

Disadvantages:
- Extensive dissection is required.
- Ischemia of the upper limb and brain (subclavian steal)
- Injury to the phrenic nerve and the thoracic duct
- Technical difficulties during takedown
- Distortion of pulmonary arteries
- Postoperative management involves strict vigilance and control of the overflow and underflow situation.

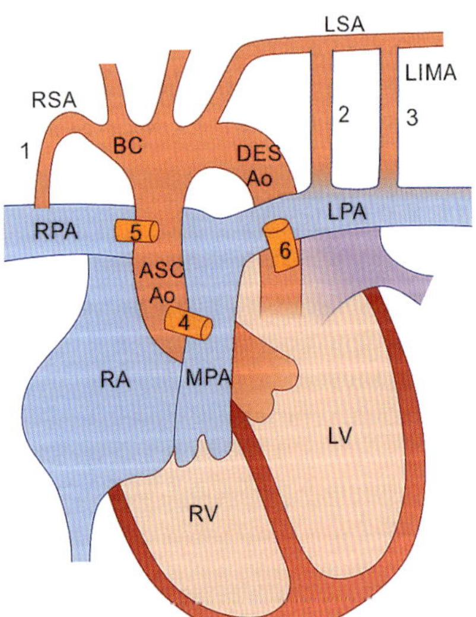

FIG. 1: Various types of systemic to PA shunts: (1) Classical BT shunt, (2) modified BT shunt, (3) LIMA to LPA shunt, (4) Davidson shunt, (5) Waterston–Cooley shunt, and (6) Potts shunt.

Modified BT Shunt

Modified BT shunt is an interposition graft [polytetrafluoroethylene (PTFE) or Gore-Tex)] between the ipsilateral subclavian and pulmonary arteries. It remains patent for a longer time and causes lower PA distortion. It does not cause any arm ischemia or subclavian steal.

Disadvantages:
- Seroma is an early complication in 4–20% of patients due to leakage from the graft.
- No growth potential
- Coronary artery steal due to decreased coronary diastolic flow caused by continuous forward flow through systemic to pulmonary circulation
- Shunt stenosis due to somatic growth, anatomic distortion, intimal proliferation, or complex morphology

Mortality of BT shunt is around 10%, particularly in lower-weight babies, and the cause of death is mostly shunt thrombosis.

Internal Mammary Artery-to-Pulmonary Artery Shunt

It is done after the failure of a previous Blalock–Taussig shunt. It provides growth and flow adaptation, without the risk of prosthetic graft infection and affecting blood flow to the arms.

Davidson, Mee, Melbourne, Waterson, Cooley, and Potts shunts are the different types of *central shunts***,** where the different segments of the aorta are connected to different segments of the main or either branch pulmonary arteries **(Fig. 2)**.

Advantages:
- Can be done in small children with small peripheral vessels
- Prevention of distortion of pulmonary arteries

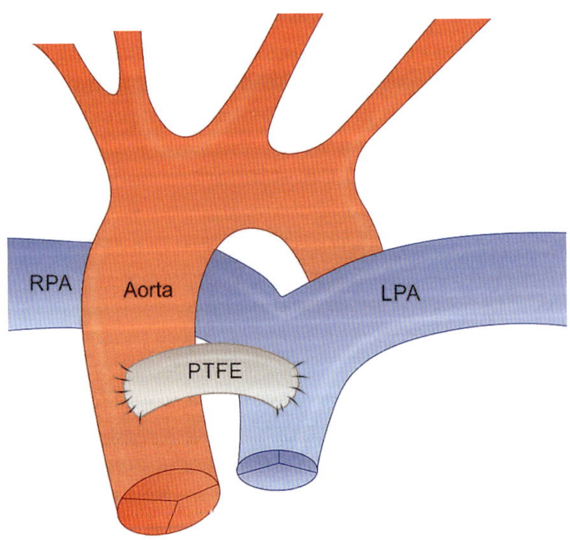

FIG. 2: Creation of central shunt using PTFE graft.

- Provides equal pulmonary blood flow to both lungs
- They have lower occlusion rates.
- No issue of subclavian artery steal
- Easy closure during corrective repair

Disadvantages:

- Waterson, Cooley, and Potts shunts cause preferential blood flow to one lung (right lung with the Waterston shunt, left lung with the Potts shunt) with hypoplasia of the contralateral PA.
- Pulmonary overcirculation
- Pulmonary hypertension
- Cardiac failure
- Thrombus
- PA aneurysm, pseudoaneurysm, or dissection due to shear stress and high-pressure pulsatile flow
- Entry into the pericardium

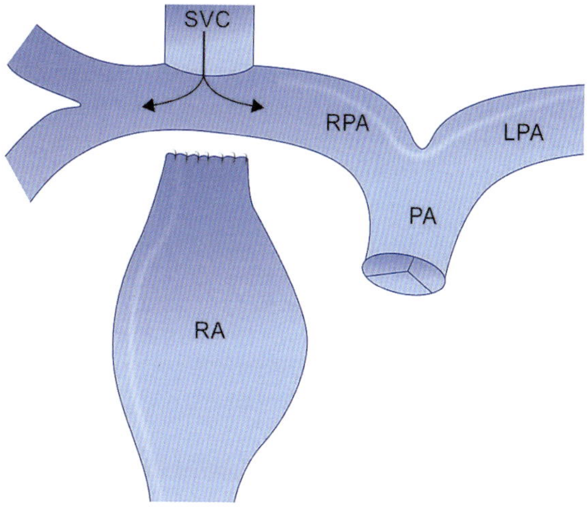

FIG. 4: Modified bidirectional Glenn shunt.

GLENN SHUNT PROCEDURE (FIGS. 3 AND 4)

A connection between the superior vena cava and the truncated right pulmonary artery is known as a classic Glenn shunt which started in the late 1950s. It improves oxygen saturation by providing venous flow to the lung fields for oxygenation, rather than an arteriovenous mixture without increasing the RV volume overload. It offloads the single ventricle. In a modified bidirectional Glenn shunt, the transected end of the lower SVC is anastomosed to the side of an undivided right PA which provides equal perfusion to both lungs. If the inferior vena cava (IVC) is interrupted with azygos continuation, all of the systemic venous blood except the hepatic veins is directed to the lungs. It is called a Kawashima procedure. Some cyanosis persists due to IVC blood coming to systemic circulation.

If the main pulmonary artery is not ligated, it is called pulsatile Glenn. It helps to increase oxygen saturation, and leads to better pulmonary artery growth, lowers pulmonary vascular resistance, and has a reduced risk of pulmonary arteriovenous malformations due to the presence of hepatic effluent flow which contains protective factors like transforming growth factor-beta (TGF-β). However, it causes a higher volume load than the classic Glenn shunt with interruption of the main pulmonary artery.

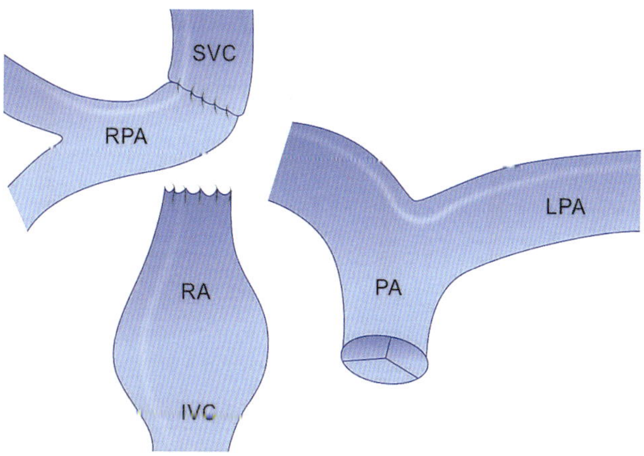

FIG. 3: Classic Glenn shunt.

Complications:

- It has a mortality rate of 2.9%.
- Desaturation in infants <4 months of age due to the decreased proportion of venous blood flow from the upper body compared to the lower body
- Venous collaterals may be seen due to elevated pulmonary venous pressure.
- Pulmonary arteriovenous malformations causing right-to-left shunt, stroke, and hypoxia especially in nonpulsatile Glenn
- Thrombus in the shunt or PA
- Occlusion or stenosis of the anastomosis
- SVC syndrome
- Other complications like bleeding, infection, dehiscence, and arrhythmias

FONTAN PROCEDURE

The Fontan procedure is the final palliative stage for a single ventricle surgery, hence the name total cavopulmonary anastomosis. The SVC flow is directed to the PA after the Glenn surgery. After the Fontan completion, the entire systemic venous blood flow is redirected to the lungs along with loss of the subpulmonary ventricular pump and separation of the systemic and pulmonary circulations causing normalization of saturations and 100% offloading of the ventricle. It is done preferably after 4 years of age. The high central venous pressure propels the blood into pulmonary circulation which becomes nonpulsatile and low pressure. Physiologically, there is suboptimal pulmonary flow, with lesser cardiac output and lower exercise capacity.[2]

Types of Fontan circuit are as follows **(Figs. 5A to C)**:

- *Classic Fontan*: Anastomosis between the right atrial appendage and the pulmonary artery, either directly or through a homograft, patch, or valved conduit. As it caused right atrium dilatation and tachyarrhythmia, leading to poor long-term outcomes of heart failure, this technique is obsolete.
- *Lateral (intra-atrial) tunnel or intracardiac Fontan*: IVC blood is directed to the PA via a baffle in the RA wall. It allows growth but atrial sutures are used.
- *Extracardiac Fontan shunt*: Conduit outside the right atrium and ventricle which directs IVC blood to the PA confluence. Though it is without the use of sutures, it has no growth potential.

Complications:

- *Cardiovascular complications* ***(Figs. 6A to C)***:
  - Heart failure: 34% of deaths in patients with a Fontan shunt are due to heart failure. It could be from either failure of the systemic ventricle or failure of the Fontan circulation due to chronic venous hypertension and low cardiac output. Morphologic RV, overloading in the first stage and low preload in the Fontan stage, increased venous pressure, atrioventricular valve regurgitation, increased pulmonary vascular resistance, and aortic obstruction are few of the causes of heart failure.
  - *Arrhythmias*: 41% of individuals after a Fontan completion experience arrhythmias at some stage. They are caused due to atrial scarring and enlargement, underlying CHD or intrinsic myocardial abnormality.
  - *Thromboembolism*: 1–33% of patients experience it. Predisposing factors are atrial dilatation, low cardiac output, nonpulsatile pulmonary flow, systemic venous stasis, arrhythmias, decreased hepatic anticoagulative factors, and polycythemia. In post-

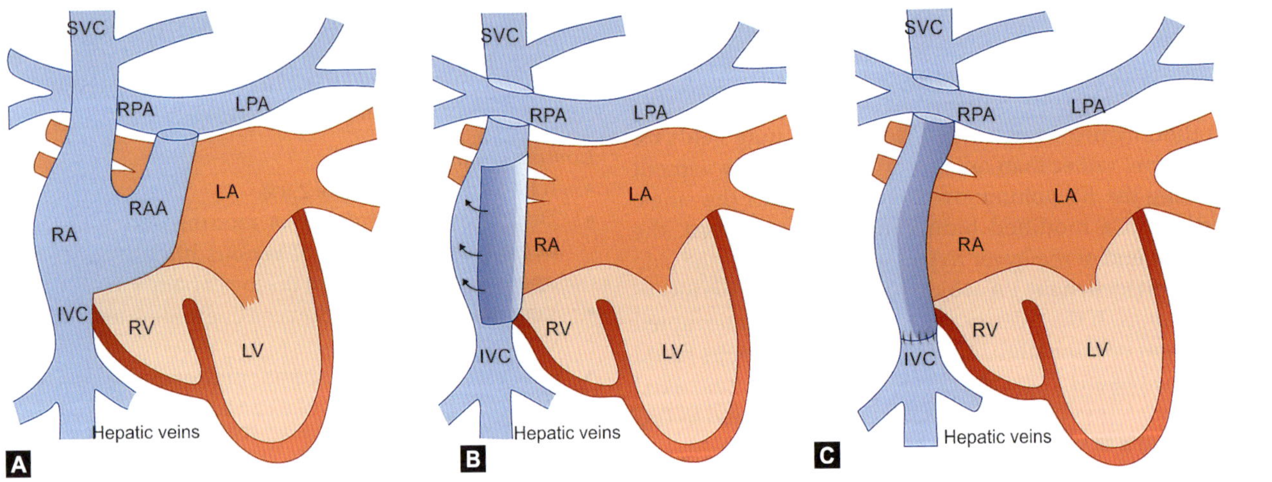

FIGS. 5A TO C: Types of Fontan procedures: (A) Atriopulmonary connection; (B) Intra-atrial rerouting/lateral tunnel Fontan; (C) Extracardiac rerouting.

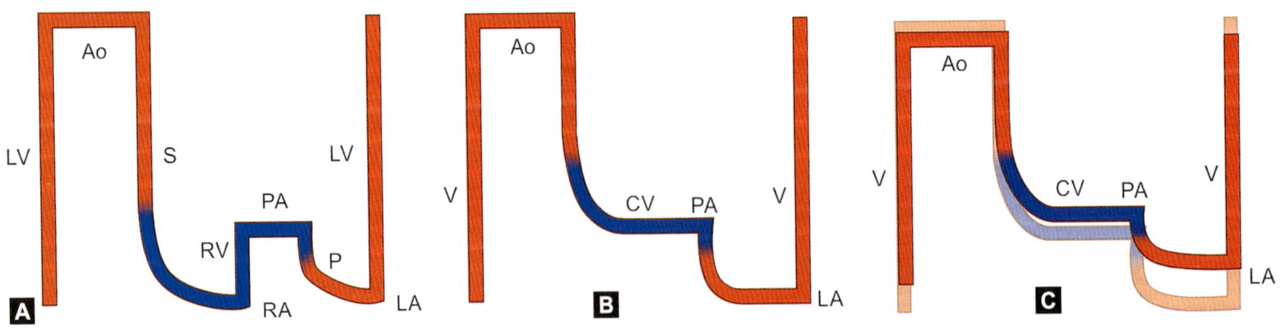

FIGS. 6A TO C: (A) Normal cardiovascular circulation where the pulmonary circulation is connected in series to the systemic circulation. Due to the compliance of the right ventricle, the right atrial pressure is lower than the left atrial pressure and provides a driving force to the blood to overcome pulmonary impedance. (B) Fontan circulation where the caval veins are directly connected to the PA and the systemic venous pressures are markedly elevated to ensure proper Fontan flow. (C) Late Fontan superimposed on early Fontan circuit: With time, the pulmonary resistance increases resulting in an increase in CV congestion but even more in reduced flow, which increases ventricular filling pressure.

Fontan patients, pulmonary embolism is the most common cause of sudden death out of hospital.
  - *Cyanosis and hypoxemia*: Caused by venovenous collaterals draining into pulmonary venous system, fenestration in the Fontan circuit, and pulmonary arteriovenous malformations
  - Other complications are pulmonary hypertension, conduit stenosis or dilatation, anastomotic site stenosis, leakage, and PA stenosis.[3]
- *Extracardiac complications*:
  - Lymphatic complications: Caused due to transmission of high SVC pressure to the thoracic duct:
    - Plastic bronchitis: 1–4% of patients with obstructive, thick, gelatinous, lymph-rich fluid in the bronchi from broncholymphatic connections
    - Protein-losing enteropathy: 5–15% of Fontan patients experience mesenteric vascular resistance and intestinal inflammation due to chronic low cardiac output.
    - Chylothorax
    - Pleural and pericardial effusion
  - *Fontan-associated liver disease (FALD)*: Seen in almost all patients with a Fontan shunt, with 43% suffering from liver fibrosis 30 years after the Fontan procedure

Fenestrated Fontan

Fenestrated Fontan consists of a 4- to 5-mm opening in the Fontan conduit connecting to the systemic atrium. It is usually done in patients with a high risk of Fontan shunts, e.g., in those with ventricular dysfunction or small PAs to relieve systemic venous pressure at the cost of arterial desaturation and higher volume load.

Next-generation Fontan

To overcome the above-mentioned complications, various methods have been obtained, especially in the era of advanced imaging. Some of these are as follows:
- Computational modeling based on patient-specific data: It can determine the best point of insertion, angulation, and offset options for placement of the Fontan conduit between the inferior cava and pulmonary arteries.
- Use of Y-shaped extracardiac conduit, based on simulations which can predict distributions of superior and inferior cava flow to the right and left lungs, respectively
- Probable use of power generator referred to as a "viscous impeller pump" to overcome the Fontan paradox[4]

Transcatheter Fontan

With increasing survival of CHD patients with single ventricle into adulthood, there are appearances of age-related different complications where there would be need for multiple sternotomies and cardioplegic arrest. In such high-risk patients, the use of transcatheter or percutaneous interventional techniques can safely achieve the goal of completing the Fontan by eliminating the need for a redo sternotomy by collaboration between cardiological, surgical, and industrial teams.

PULMONARY ARTERY BANDING

Pulmonary artery banding was described by Muller and Danimann, in 1952, as a treatment for a large VSD with pulmonary overflow by creating artificial pulmonary stenosis in a 5-month-old baby. The principle of PA band is reduction of the main pulmonary artery diameter to reduce the pulmonary blood flow (Qp) and decrease pulmonary artery pressure along with improvement of cardiac output and systemic pressure.[5]

Indications of PA band according to physiology are as follows:
- In CHD with increased pulmonary flow which requires a procedure to protect the pulmonary tree till complete two-ventricle repair or an effective single-ventricle palliation is done
- In heart diseases with LV requiring retraining for the next-stage surgery
- As a first stage of palliation in case of HLHS

It is contraindicated in subaortic obstruction as the PA band causes pressure overload over the subpulmonic ventricle and worsens the subaortic obstruction by virtue of muscular hypertrophy and worsens atrioventricular valve regurgitation as well.

Effectiveness of Pulmonary Artery Band

Pulmonary artery banding is called effective if:
- The diameter is reduced by 50%
- PA pressure decreased to half systemic pressure

For deciding the final PA diameter, Trusler formula is used:
- 20 + (1 mm/kg of body weight) in those without bidirectional mixing disorder
- 24 + (1 mm/kg of body weight) in those with bidirectional mixing disorder

Complications

- About 36% of patients do not tolerate PA band due to changes in pulmonary flow and pressure.
- Band erosion into the arterial lumen
- Band migration
- Pseudoaneurysm from a stretched PA
- Scarring and fibrosis at the band site
- Subaortic obstruction and hypertrophy of ventricles
- Thrombosis
- Pulmonary regurgitation
- Decreased ventricular compliance

NORWOOD PROCEDURE (FIGS. 7 AND 8)

Norwood procedure is the first stage of the three-stage palliation in patients with HLHS which is performed in the first week of life. During a Norwood procedure, a neosystemic circuit is created from the RV. The hypoplastic ascending aorta is attached to the main PA by a Damus-Kaye-Stansel procedure. In a DKS procedure, the distal main PA is resected and the proximal PA is anastomosed either end to side, by patch augmentation, or by a double barrel to the ascending aorta. Pulmonary blood flow is maintained by either a Sano shunt or a modified BT shunt. The aortic arch is reconstructed. Atrial septectomy is done to provide unrestricted oxygenated blood flow from the pulmonary veins to the RV.

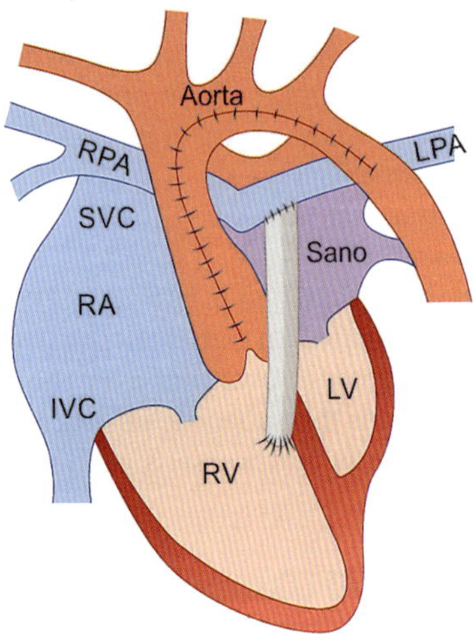

FIG. 7: Sano modification for Norwood surgery.

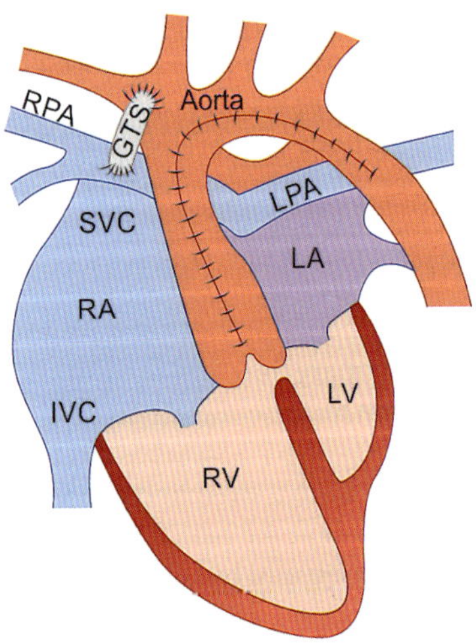

FIG. 8: Blalock–Thomas–Taussig shunt for Norwood surgery.

Sano shunt is a modification in the Norwood procedure where there is a use of the RV to pulmonary artery conduit so that blood is pumped directly to the lungs. It has better hemodynamic stability due to less coronary steal, as flow is limited to the systole and growth of the branch pulmonary arteries is better.

Complications of Sano shunt:

- Ventricular arrhythmias and dysfunction due to RV incision
- Conduit stenosis and regurgitation

Complications of Norwood procedure:

- About 22% mortality rate due to pulmonary overcirculation and low cardiac output, especially in low-birth-weight babies and those with severe tricuspid regurgitation
- Pulmonary hypertension
- Obstruction of pulmonary and systemic veins

ATRIAL SEPTAL PROCEDURES

Different procedures are used for atrial septal-level communication to improve intracardiac mixing, which are useful in various cyanotic diseases, particularly in DTGA. They are as follows:

- Blalock-Hanlon operation (atrial septectomy without cardiopulmonary bypass)
- Park procedure (balloon or blade atrial septostomy)
- Rashkind procedure (balloon catheter atrial septostomy)

ATRIAL SWITCH PROCEDURE

The atrial switch operation is a palliative surgery for DTGA and CCTGA. The two types of atrial switch operations are Senning operation and Mustard operation. The principle behind the atrial switch operation is diversion of deoxygenated systemic venous return to the left ventricle and oxygenated pulmonary venous blood to the RV by using baffles. In both the procedures, the right atrium is opened and the wall between the atria is fully removed. While in Mustard operation, baffle is made using pericardial flaps, the native atrial septum is used in the Senning surgery directing blood from the veins in the right atrium toward the left ventricle.

Complications:

- Baffle leaks usually not significant, but if large they may cause cyanosis, stroke, and paradoxical embolism
- 7–10% of patients with atrial switch surgery have systemic ventricle (morphologic RV) failure as it cannot withstand systemic pressures.
- Tricuspid valve regurgitation due to altered geometry of the tricuspid annulus
- 61% of patients who underwent atrial switch operation have RV fibrosis leading to arrhythmias and poor function.

PALLIATIVE ATRIAL/ARTERIAL SWITCH

In patients with TGA with VSD with severe pulmonary vascular obstructive disease, these palliative procedures are performed in deeply cyanotic patients without closure of the VSD, after doing cardiac catheterization if the difference between the aortic and the pulmonary saturation is at least 10%. The procedure is done to relieve hypoxemia and improve quality of life.[6]

Hybrid Palliation

Using hybrid palliation, the Norwood stage I surgery can be avoided in the neonatal period, so that patients get time for suitable LV growth if possible and can be listed for cardiac transplantation. During a hybrid procedure, various combinations can exist like bilateral pulmonary artery banding, ductus arteriosus stenting, balloon atrial septostomy, and even innominate artery-to-main pulmonary artery shunt.[7]

CONCLUSION

Though there are much less indications for palliative procedures in congenital heart defects due to early diagnosis and advancement in techniques of primary total correction of lesion, they still have an important role in high-risk patients with complex cardiac lesions. They are important in improving quality of life and life expectancy.

ONLINE REFERENCES

Please scan the QR code provided at the end of the table of contents for References of this chapter.

CHAPTER

95

Tetralogy of Fallot: Evaluation for Total Correction

Anil Sivadasan Radha, Jenu Rose Jose E

ABSTRACT

Tetralogy of Fallot (TOF) is the most common form of cyanotic congenital heart disease and one of the first to be successfully corrected. Advances in the diagnosis, perioperative and surgical treatment, and postoperative care have made those born with TOF to survive to adulthood. Here, we focus on the anatomical basis of this morphology and the various imaging modalities necessary for the best possible lifelong treatment of this congenital heart disease.

Keywords: Tetralogy of Fallot, morphology, echocardiography, imaging

INTRODUCTION

Tetralogy of Fallot (TOF) is one of the most common forms of cyanotic heart disease (CHD) and occurs in about 1 in 3,000 live births and accounts for 5–7% of all CHD. The classic morphologic tenants of the TOF, right ventricular outflow tract obstruction, right ventricular hypertrophy, ventricular septal defect, and aortic override have undergone considerable scrutiny since the seminal description of this disorder.[1] Unrepaired TOF carried a poor prognosis, with only 50% of patients reaching the age of 3 years and only a few surviving to 40 years of age.[2,3] The pioneering shunt created by Blalock, Taussig, and Thomas in 1945 to augment pulmonary blood flow was followed by Lillehei's original intracardiac repair in 1954,[4] setting the stage for dramatic improvements in survival.

Earlier and improved diagnosis (frequently prenatal) has enabled timely repair,[5-7] typically in the first half of the first year of life.[8] Intracardiac repair ideally involves relief of RVOT obstruction (with preservation of RV structure and function) and minimal disruption of pulmonary valve function.[9] Surgical techniques previously included a right ventriculotomy (for VSD closure and resection of RVOT infundibular stenosis) along with widespread use of a transannular patch.[10] It is well-recognized that a transannular patch contributes to residual PR and is associated with adult arrhythmias and pulmonary valve replacement (PVR). Nevertheless, early postoperative survival after repair exceeds 98%, and most survive into adulthood, with approximately 90% alive at 30 years.[11]

Transatrial and transpulmonary approaches have replaced ventriculotomy so that RV dysfunction and scarring are minimized.[12] Pulmonary valve-sparing strategies have been preferentially adopted in the contemporary era when feasible. An RV-pulmonary artery (PA) conduit is required in the setting of pulmonary atresia, absent pulmonary valve variant or if an anomalous coronary artery crosses the RVOT and is occasionally used to provide improved hemodynamic stability in a child who has undergone recent transannular patch repair but is struggling with severe restrictive physiology.[13]

MORPHOLOGY

The most frequent segmental anatomy of TOF is levocardia, normal atrial situs, with concordant atrioventricular and ventriculoarterial connections.[1,14] TOF in situs inversus total is uncommon (<5%). The morphological findings of TOF include pulmonary stenosis of a specific infundibular character; a nonrestrictive ventricular septal defect located between the anterior and posterior limbs of the trabecular[15] septal band; overriding of the aorta; and right ventricular hypertrophy. Right ventricular hypertrophy is progressive, reflecting the myocardial response to right ventricular outflow tract obstruction and the significant, nonrestrictive ventricular septal defect.[16,17]

The malalignment of the infundibular septum is now considered the essence of the TOF.[18] The subpulmonary infundibulum in TOF is characterized by small volume, short and thick infundibular septum, which has anterosuperior deviation.[19] Pulmonary stenosis is related to this deviation of the infundibular septum; thus, obstruction is muscular. The infundibular obstruction could be worsened by associated hypoplastic pulmonary valvular annulus, a bicuspid valve with thickened cusps and fused commissures causing valvular stenosis, anomalous muscle bundles, and by presence of varying degrees of hypoplasia of the main pulmonary trunk and its branches. Patients without outlet septum are not classical examples of TOF, despite having similar hemodynamics.[17,20,21]

Kirklin and Barratt-Boyes indicate that the overriding of aorta which is also identified in patients with TOF varies from about 30–90%. Aortic override is associated with a variable degree of clockwise rotation of the aortic root as viewed from the ventricular apex. This rotation moves the base of the noncoronary cusp rightward and superiorly onto the posterosuperior margin of the ventricular septal defect and away from the base of the anterior or aortic leaflet of the mitral valve. Other morphological variables influencing surgery include variability in pulmonary arteries and epicardial distribution of coronary arteries.[1,14,16]

Variability in PA size is common in TOF. Even tiny arteries reflect underfilling because of severe outflow tract obstruction.[10,22,23] Multiple diffuse caliber abnormalities, arterial stenoses, and arborization abnormalities can be occasionally seen in TOF and a perforate outflow tract, but these are much more common in patients with pulmonary atresia with multiple aortopulmonary collaterals. Small indirect aortopulmonary collaterals and enlarged bronchial arteries can be easily identified in older infants and children, reflecting increasing hypoxemia. Large direct aorto-pulmonary collateral vessels originating from the descending thoracic aorta are rare in patients with "uncomplicated" TOF.[13,23]

Stenosis of the left PA at the site of ductal insertion (ductal-related PA coarctation) in patients with TOF has been estimated to be as high as 25%.[23,24] The right and left pulmonary arteries may be nonconfluent with one PA, usually the left originating from the ascending aorta, or it may have a distal ductal origin.[20]

Coronary artery anomalies can complicate the repair of TOF because of their potential for interruption or damage at the time of right ventriculotomy. The most common abnormality is the origin of the left anterior descending coronary artery from the right coronary artery, seen in about 5% of patients. Here, the anterior descending coronary artery crosses the right ventricular outflow tract, at a variable distance from the pulmonary valve. An accessory anterior descending artery originating from the right coronary artery occurs in about 2.5% of patients with TOF. Other less common anomalies are a single right or left coronary artery, anomalous origin of the left coronary artery or the anterior descending coronary artery from the main pulmonary trunk, origin of both coronary arteries from the pulmonary trunk or multiple coronary arteries–cameral fistulae.[23,24]

About 75% of patients with TOF have a left aortic arch with normal branching pattern. Aberrant origin of the right subclavian should however be always excluded. 25% of patients with TOF will have a right-sided aortic arch. In right-sided aortic arch with an aberrant left subclavian artery, the anomalous subclavian artery almost always originates directly from the descending aorta, not from an aortic diverticulum.

Other anomalies include isolated left subclavian artery having origin from the left PA. After closure of the left arterial duct, the left subclavian artery will be isolated, filling from a left vertebral and causing subclavian steal. Arterial duct if present normally closes physiologically in TOF. Bilateral arterial ducts have also been described.[22,23]

Rarely coarctation of the aorta or interruption of the aortic arch have been described in the patient with TOF, confounding the general rule of fourth and sixth aortic arch reciprocity. Other associated anomalies include cervical aortic arch, double aortic arch, and vascular ring with and without bronchial compression.[17]

ECHOCARDIOGRAPHY

Echocardiography is the most important tool used in the diagnosis and following up with patients with TOF. In most patients, all of the salient features of the anatomy and physiology can be obtained from a transthoracic echocardiogram, so other imaging modalities are unnecessary. The echocardiographic features mirror the pathological features of the disease found at surgery, making echocardiography the surgeon's reference point.

Intraoperative echocardiography (either epicardial or transesophageal) is useful particularly in checking the completeness of VSD closure and relief of RVOTO.[25] In the immediate postoperative phase, echocardiography is done routinely to assess LV and RV function, atrioventricular valve function, and presence of RVOTO. In postoperative follow-up, it is useful in surveillance of late complications, particularly in patients with PR. The presence of MAPCAs is often detectable by echocardiography with color flow mapping, but additional imaging will be required to fully delineate their course and distribution.[7]

Cardiac CT and MRI has a complementary role in assessment of rare aortic arch anomalies as well as MAPCAs, hypoplastic branch pulmonary arteries in the setting of associated pulmonary atresia, and also in absent pulmonary valve syndrome.

The prominent echocardiographic features of TOF are seen from the classical long-axis and subcostal coronal views **(Figs. 1 and 2)**. A single great artery is seen to override the ventricular septal defect to a variable degree. Thus, three of the four features of tetralogy namely, ventricular septal

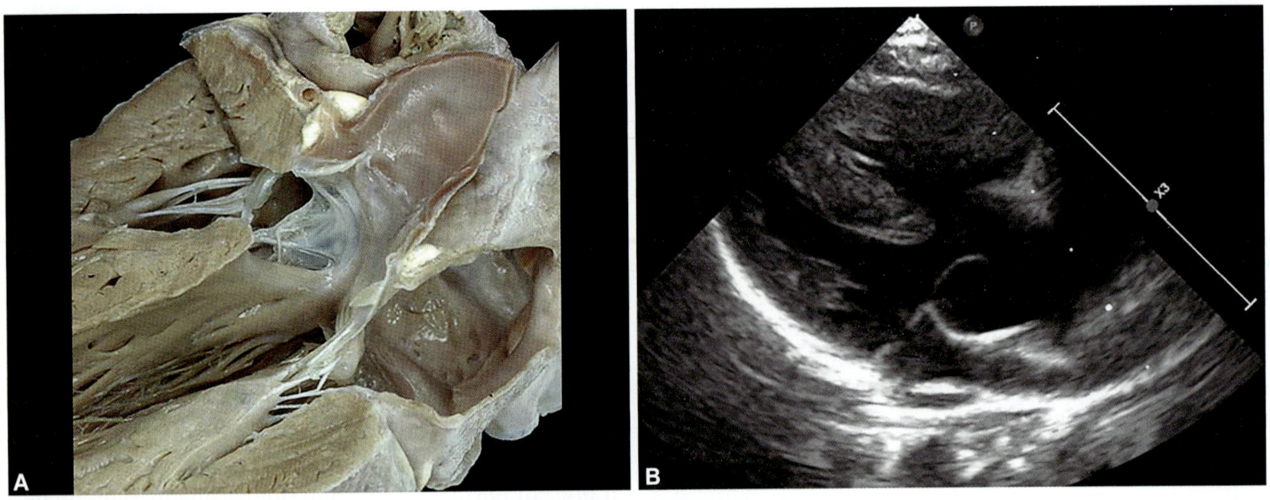

FIGS. 1A AND B: (A) Autopsy specimen shows large malaligned subaortic VSD; (B) PLAX view in echo shows nonrestrictive VSD with overriding of aorta.

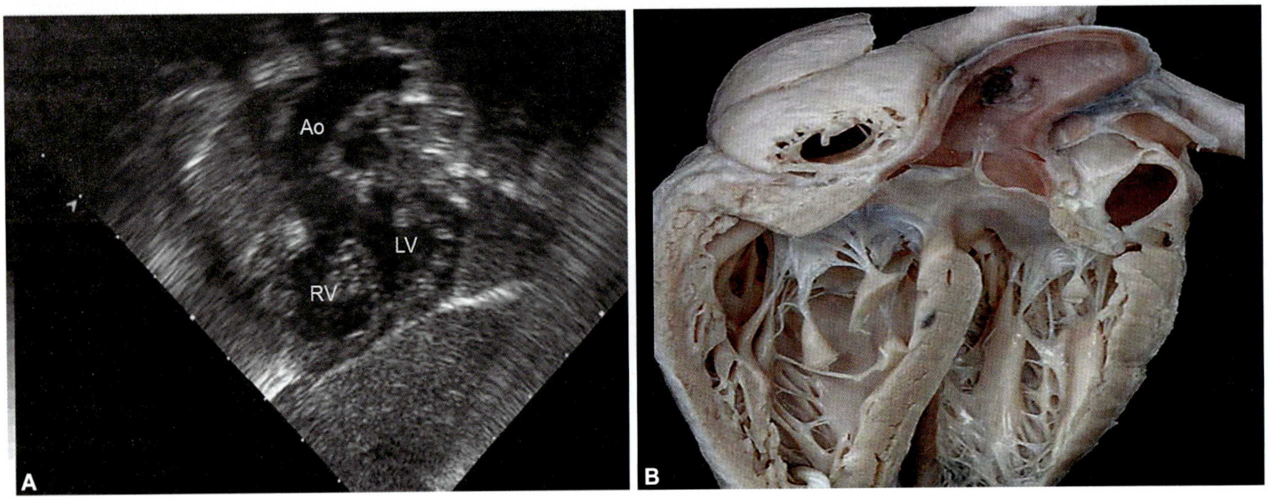

FIGS. 2A AND B: (A) Subcostal short-axis view shows large conoventricular VSD with overriding aorta; (B) Autopsy specimen showing the malaligned VSD, overriding aorta and the right ventricular hypertrophy

defect, aortic override, and right ventricular hypertrophy can be seen from these views.[26]

The last feature of the tetrad namely deviated outlet septum and infundibular hypoplasia was initially reported by Niels Stensen in 1671, and renamed by Van Praagh the "monology of Stensen". This can be demonstrated from a variety of subcostal, coronal, sagittal, and parasternal views **(Figs. 3A and B)**.

These views show the deviated outlet septum, the narrowed right ventricular outflow tract and pulmonary valvar pathology, additionally the main PA and its branches can be assessed **(Figs. 4A and B)**. Parasternal short-axis view which is used to complement the subcostal views can define ventricular size, hypertrophy, infundibular narrowing, annular size, branch pulmonary anatomy, and physiology. Continuous wave Doppler also differentiates valvar from infundibular narrowing by the different timing of the velocity curves originating at these two sites **(Fig. 4B)**.[27]

Detailed pulmonary valve anatomy is critical for surgical correction, particularly for transannular patch correction. Pulmonary annular size, valvar morphology, and branch PA narrowing are demonstrated by echocardiography. Current surgical thinking in TOF tries to spare the valve so that the degree of pulmonary valvar incompetence having long-term deleterious consequences may be minimized.

The pulmonary valve is best detected by short-axis views orientation of the probe in the appropriate plane **(Figs. 5A to C)** so that it passes through the plane of the valvar leaflets is different from its orientation when defining the normal pulmonary valve, because right ventricular enlargement will push the valve annulus higher and deeper into the chest, making the pulmonary valve lie further from the precordium and positioned in a more vertical orientation.

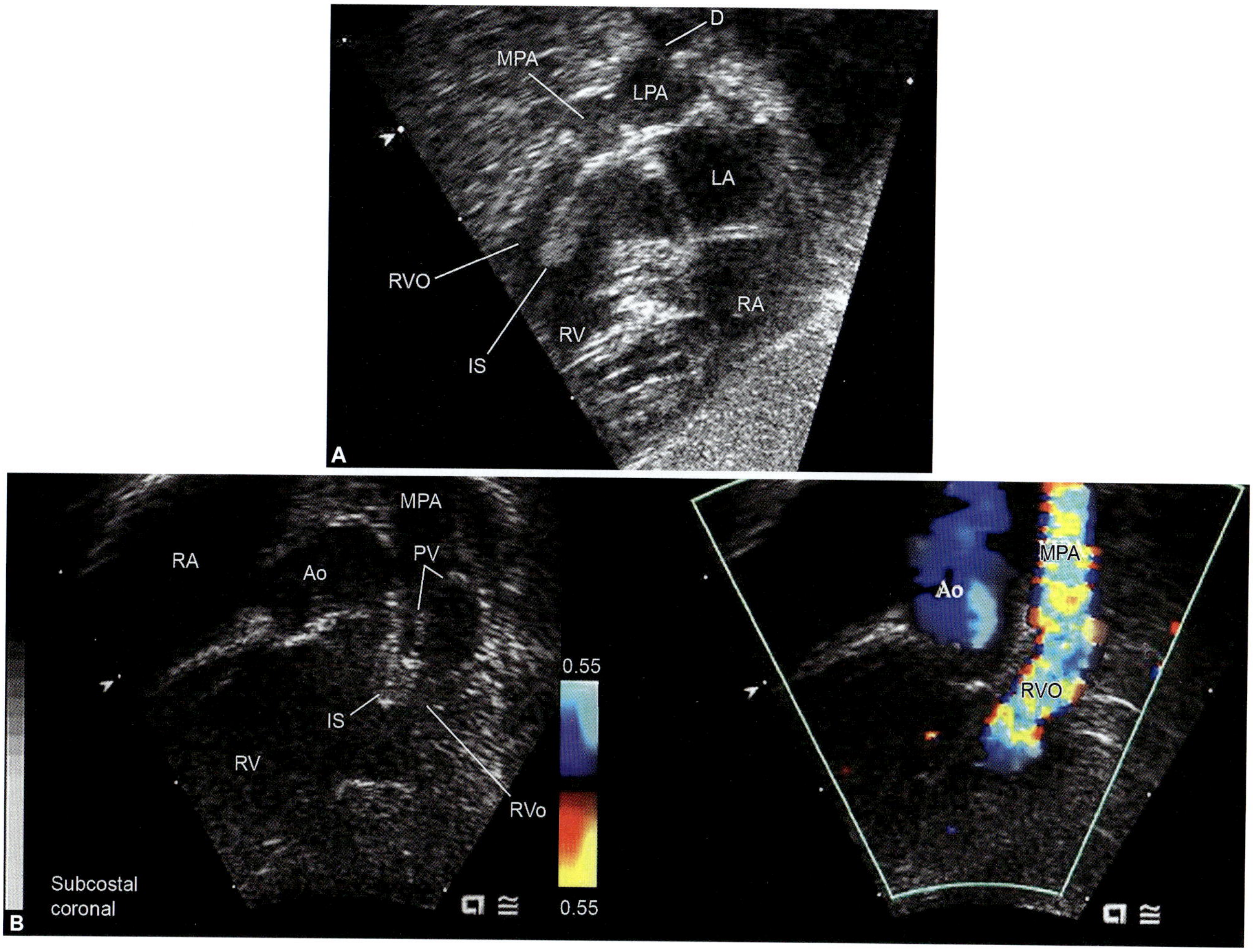

FIGS. 3A AND B: (A) Imaging of the RV outflow showing deviated outlet septum with narrowing of RVOT; (B) 2D and color flow imaging of the RV outflow tract showing infundibular and valvar pulmonary stenosis.

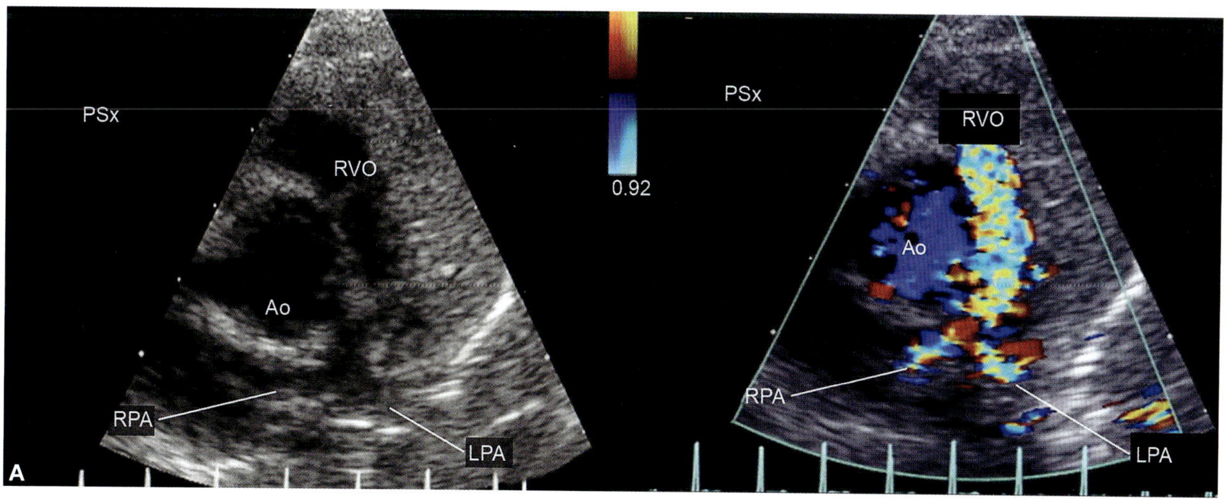

FIGS. 4A AND B: *Continued*

Continued

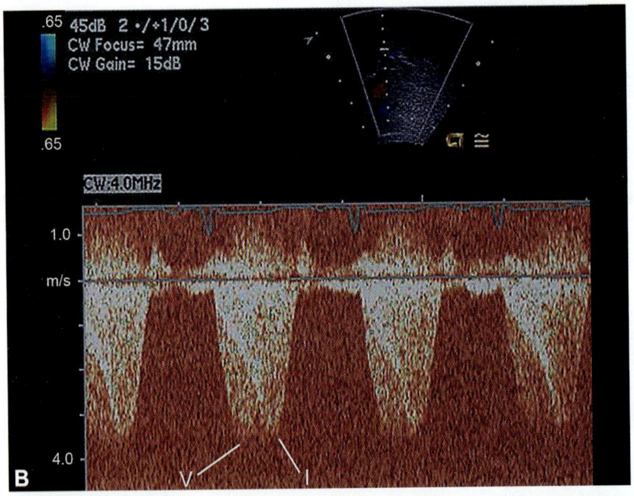

FIGS. 4A AND B: (A) Parasternal short-axis view showing the deviated outlet septum, infundibular, and valvar RV outflow obstruction with MPA and branch PA narrowing; (B) Continuous flow Doppler imaging across the RV outflow showing severe obstruction at multiple levels, across RV infundibulum (dagger shaped envelope) and pulmonary valve (symmetrical envelope).

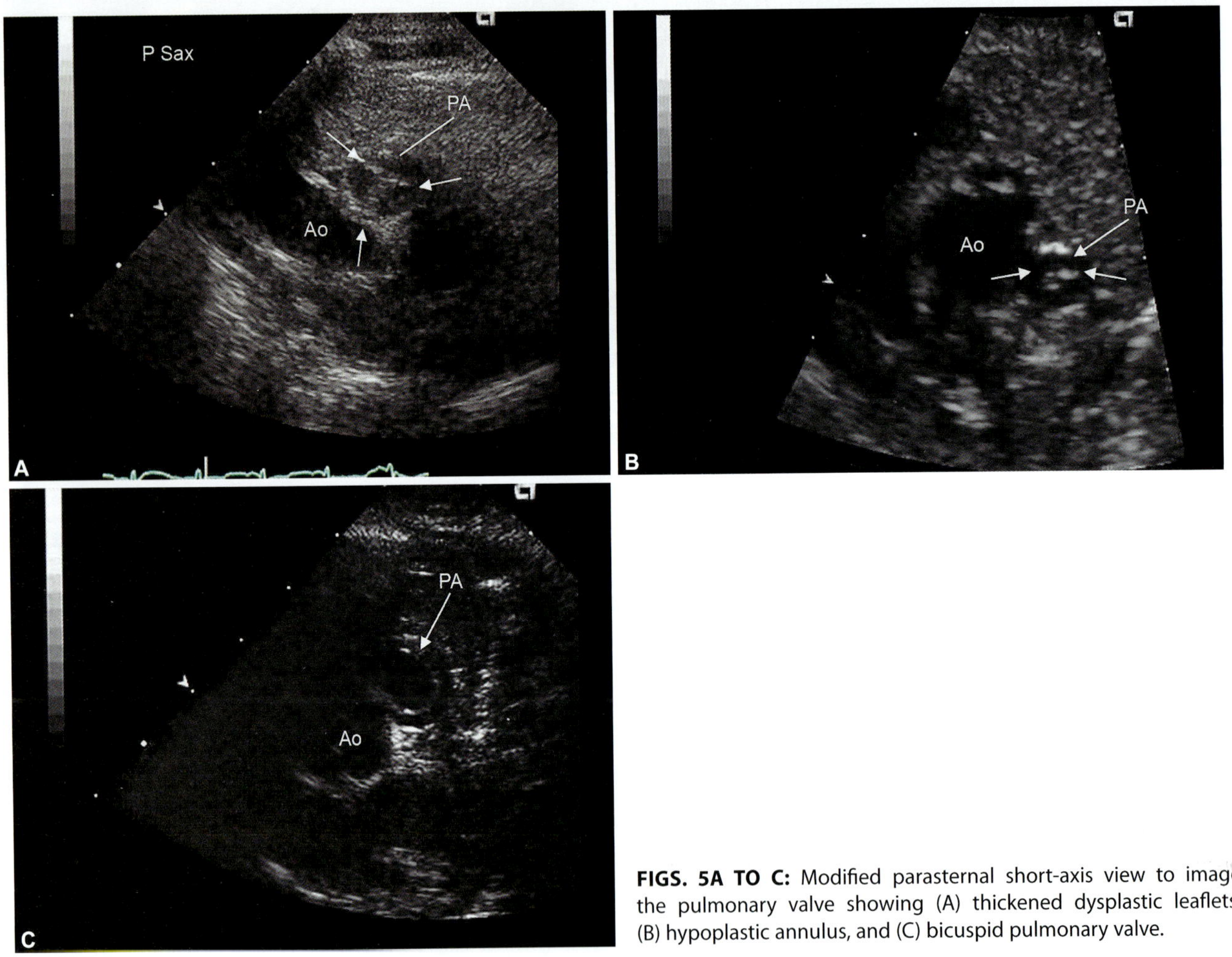

FIGS. 5A TO C: Modified parasternal short-axis view to image the pulmonary valve showing (A) thickened dysplastic leaflets, (B) hypoplastic annulus, and (C) bicuspid pulmonary valve.

To image the valve more clearly, the probe must be placed in a higher precordial position with clockwise rotation. The valve is frequently bicuspid. If the valve is tricuspid, keeping the infundibular incision between the cusps of the valve may prevent valvar destruction. In unicuspid valve, there is no option but to incise the leaflet, thereby creating greater pulmonary valvar incompetence.[20,26]

Complete delineation of the diameters of the central and branch pulmonary arteries to the hilum of each lung can be done by echocardiography. It is also possible to define stenosis at the origin of the branches and the branch size.

Another important morphologic feature in the TOF that needs definition is coronary arterial anatomy. Most commonly, the left main coronary artery runs in a proximal course behind the main PA **(Fig. 6)**. In these cases, the left anterior descending coronary artery is protected from the surgeon's knife. Coronary arteries that run across the right ventricular outflow tract are not protected, especially if buried in pericardial scarring from prior surgery. If the left anterior descending arises from the right coronary artery and runs in front of the right ventricular outflow tract, it is at risk of being cut. Although the surgeon can usually see this artery, if it is buried or running in a pericardial adhesion, it is at risk. Using a high parasternal view, the artery is easily recognizable **(Fig. 6)**. Large conus branches or dual left anterior descending coronary arteries that run across the right ventricular outflow tract are also at risk. This can usually be differentiated by identifying the left anterior descending coronary artery that runs its usual course behind the PA in these situations.

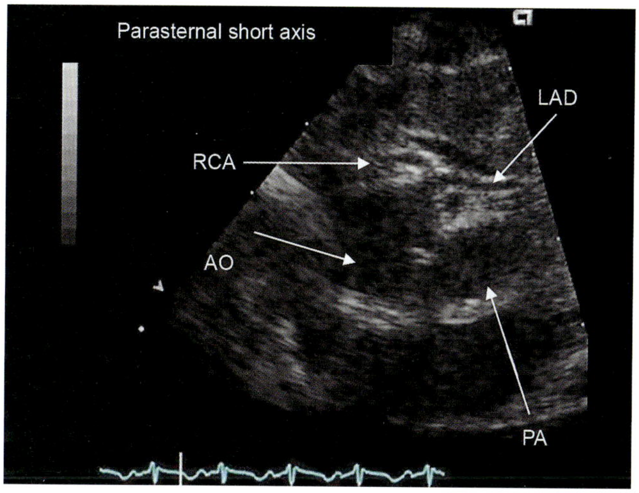

FIG. 6: High parasternal short-axis view showing LAD from RCA and coursing anterior to the RV outflow tract.

Surgical repair in patients with TOF and associated pulmonary atresia is more complicated. Here, pulmonary blood flow could arise either solely from an arterial duct **(Figs. 7A and B)** or from major aortopulmonary collateral arteries. A duct arising from the base of an innominate artery is easily identifiable from standard views. The arterial duct may also arise from the base of a right aortic arch, in which cases it is usually small, tortuous, and oriented in a vertical direction **(Figs. 7A and B)**. The major aortopulmonary collateral arteries commonly arise from the descending aorta but may also arise from the arch vessels or even from the abdominal aorta. These collaterals usually run from below to above, having a slightly cranially oriented course, while the arterial duct is usually caudally directed.[28] This course is because of the embryonic ascent of the lung and the systemic arteries that take their blood supply as the lung ascends, while the vertical orientation of the duct is due to the reversed fetal flow direction into the pulmonary arteries via the arterial duct. When the intrapulmonary pulmonary arteries anastomose with the sixth arch vessels, they usually lose contact with the major aortopulmonary collateral arteries.

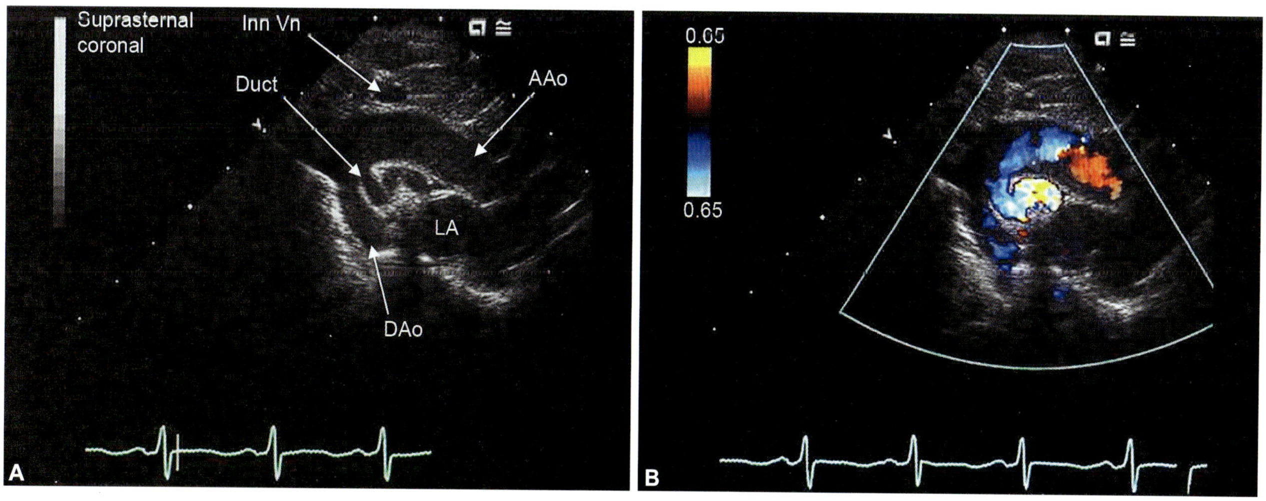

FIGS. 7A AND B: Suprasternal long-axis view, 2D and color flow imaging, shows tortuous, almost vertical duct from the base of the right aortic arch in a child with TOF and pulmonary atresia.

Complete delineation of major aortopulmonary collateral arteries requires angiography due to the complex nature of the disorder and its surgical repair.

A critical information for the surgeon is the presence of multiple ventricular septal defects. Additional defects may be missed in routine imaging techniques, including angiography because the tendency is for the blood to flow through the larger hole, as the ventricular pressures are equal on both sides. These additional defects may be identified intraoperatively by transesophageal echocardiography only after the patient comes off bypass, when the blood is forced through a smaller defect as the pressure between the ventricles assumes more normalcy.

Large defects can however be easily detected. Defects in the atrioventricular canal associated with tetralogy can also be readily seen as the ventricular septal defect is usually large and extends into the inlet septum.[29]

CARDIAC MRI

The CMR is rarely used in preoperative TOF in young patients, as echocardiography offers good imaging and is generally sufficient for surgical planning. It is usually reserved for complex anatomy, such as pulmonary atresia for delineation of the hypoplastic pulmonary branches and aortopulmonary collaterals. In older postoperative TOF patients, cardiac MRI is crucial as serial evaluations guide management with planning of surgical or interventional PVR, heavily relying on well validated CMR criteria.

CARDIAC CT

Multidetector CCT offers excellent spatial and temporal resolution and gating and heart rate control with β-blockers is required for optimal acquisition.

The protocol for CCT assessment in TOF includes visualization of PA anatomy, for size and arborization and measurement of the lumen and wall thickness of the ascending aorta since progressive root dilation is common. Biventricular end-diastolic and end-systolic volumes can be measured with reasonable accuracy comparable to the CMR.

It is extremely helpful in depicting the origin and course of coronaries, as well as RV to PA conduits and their relation to surrounding structures, thus enabling correct planning of surgical or transcatheter interventions.

Despite the good imaging quality of CCT in TOF, it should be reserved only for patients with absolute contraindications to CMR, given its ionization, the young age of the patients and the need for serial imaging throughout their lifespan.

The CCT provides superior delineation of small vessels, aortopulmonary collaterals and pulmonary arteries, as compared to cardiac MRI. Other advantages include being less affected by stainless steel artifacts and having shorter acquisition times reducing the need for sedation.[30]

CARDIAC CATHETERIZATION ANGIOGRAPHY

Cardiac catheterization angiography (CCA) is reserved for complex CHD anatomy, such as TOF with pulmonary atresia or prior aortopulmonary shunts, or during evaluation for possible transcatheter interventions. CCA is the gold standard for evaluation of intracardiac pressures, delineation of peripheral pulmonary arteries, and coronary anatomy.

CONCLUSION

Early detection and successful correction of TOF has been possible by the advances in imaging and refinements in surgical techniques and it is now possible for total correction in most children in infancy.

ONLINE REFERENCES

Please scan the QR code provided at the end of the table of contents for References of this chapter.

CHAPTER

96

Repaired Tetralogy of Fallot: An Overview

Ankit Garg, S Radhakrishnan

ABSTRACT

Tetralogy of Fallot is the most frequently encountered cyanotic congenital heart disease. Initial management strategies started with palliative surgery followed by complete intracardiac repair. Presently, only a few patients require palliation with complete repair accomplished before their first birthday. After the complete repair survival matches with general population during the initial decades only. On long-term follow-up, a multitude of plausible anatomic and physiological complications plague these patients requiring a lifelong surveillance. A multimodality imaging is essential during follow-up to anticipate, and monitor sequelae so as to intervene in time before they become clinically significant. This chapter focuses on long-term issues in this subgroup of patients and their necessary management.

Keywords: Repaired, tetralogy of Fallot, follow-up, cyanotic congenital heart disease

INTRODUCTION

Tetralogy of Fallot is the most common form of cyanotic congenital heart disease with an estimated incidence of about 3 per 10,000 live births.[1] It was first described by Niels Stenson in 1671, which was refined and published by Étienne-Louis Fallot in 1888.[2] In unrepaired tetralogy of Fallot, only half of them survive by 3 years and there is rare survival after 30 years of age.[2,3] The first palliation which was done in 1945 included a systemic to pulmonary artery shunt performed by surgeon (Alfred Blalock and Vivien Thomas) and cardiologist (Helen Taussig).[4,5] The first complete intracardiac repair of tetralogy of Fallot was reported a decade later, by Lillehei in 1954.[5,6] During the initial epoch, intracardiac repair was accomplished using either a longitudinal or a transverse right ventricle incision. This surgical technique with right ventriculotomy had long-term concerns of right ventricle scar and risks of sudden cardiac death due to arrythmia. Transatrial repair which considerably eliminated the complications of ventriculotomy was first reported in 1963 by Hudspeth et al.[7] At present transatrial-transpulmonary approach is the preferred strategy for complete repair of tetralogy of Fallot. Primary repair at the age of 6–12 months is recommended given the low mortality and length of hospital stay.[8,9] Palliative procedures are reserved for only a few presenting very early in the natural history with severe cyanosis or those with unfavorable anatomy. In the initial era of tetralogy of Fallot repair, there was a substantial mortality rate, however, with advancing surgical methods current survival rate is expected to be >90% at 30 years follow-up.[10,11] Improved survival has resulted in a constant growth of population achieving adulthood after complete repair. Nevertheless, a myriad of potential sequelae can occur in later stages warranting a lifelong follow-up in operated tetralogy of Fallot.

LATE OUTCOMES OF REPAIRED TETRALOGY OF FALLOT

Long-term survival is encouraging in the first few decades. However, it falls away from the age-matched normal population after the fourth decade with features of exercise intolerance, right or left heart failure, arrythmia, and sudden cardiac death **(Figs. 1A and B)**.[12,13] A number of potential complications of varying severity affect these patients leading to considerable morbidity and mortality. Some of the studies report an incidence of event free survival of as low as 25% at 40-year follow-up.[12,13] Patients with inherited genetic syndromes, specifically 22q11 microdeletion and

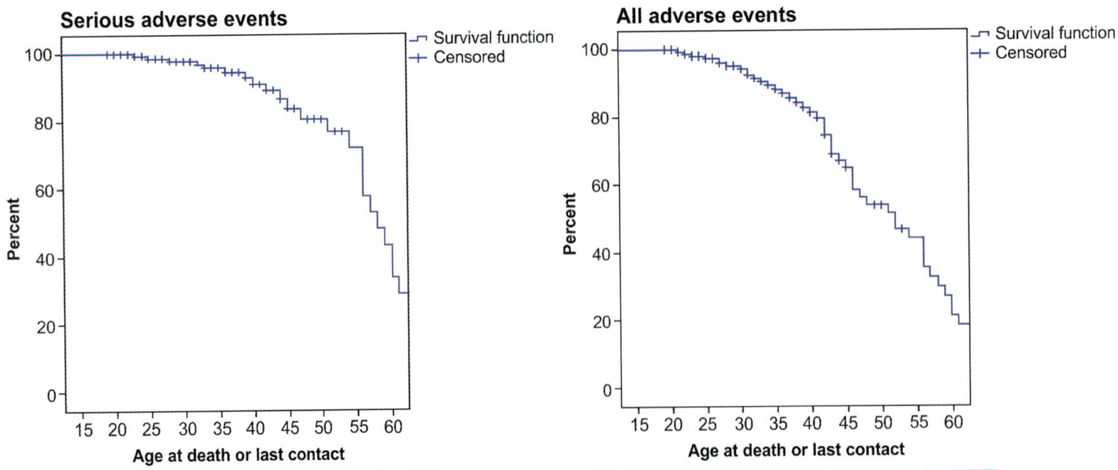

A

Age	20	30	40	50	60
Patient at risk	167	108	53	23	9

B

Age	20	30	40	50	60
Patient at risk	167	108	53	23	9

FIGS. 1A AND B: Kaplan–Meier curve demonstrating age-related cumulative incidence for (A) serious adverse events (including death, heart failure admission, ventricular arrhythmia, and cardiac transplant) in repaired tetralogy of Fallot and (B) all adverse events (including serious adverse event and endocarditis, atrial arrhythmia, defibrillator, and pacemaker implantation).

tetralogy with pulmonary atresia are at an increased risk of high and premature mortality. Long-term sequelae depend on a number of prognostic factors including right ventriculotomy technique, previous palliative surgery, presence of transannular patch, branch pulmonary artery stenosis, residual lesions, and late presenting patients.

Right Ventricle and Outflow Tract Dysfunction

Right ventricular outflow tract dysfunction in the form of pulmonary obstruction, pulmonary regurgitation, or a combination of both is the most frequent hemodynamic sequelae encountered in repaired tetralogy of Fallot **(Fig. 2)**.[2,12,14] Pulmonary regurgitation occurs due to aggressive infundibular resection or use of transannular patch for right ventricle outflow tract reconstruction. Pulmonary regurgitation is exacerbated by concomitant distal branch pulmonary artery stenosis or pulmonary artery hypertension (rare). Pulmonary regurgitation is generally well tolerated for years, however, with chronic pulmonary regurgitation begins a cascade of hemodynamic events leading to right ventricle dilatation and subsequent right ventricle dysfunction.[2,14,15] Right ventricular dilatation leads to tricuspid valve dilatation which portents progressive secondary tricuspid valve regurgitation. Right ventricle restrictive physiology defined as diastolic antegrade flow in pulmonary artery with coincident atrial systole throughout the respiratory cycle is protective for right ventricle dilatation in presence of pulmonary regurgitation.[2,14] Restrictive physiology is associated with better exercise capacity, lower cardiothoracic ratio and lower QRS duration on ECG.[2] Residual obstruction is encountered at multiple levels in right ventricular outflow tract including infundibular, annular, degenerative or progressive obstruction in replaced pulmonary valve or conduit, and distal branch pulmonary arteries. Chronic obstruction leads to progressive right ventricle hypertrophy. Mild obstruction rarely causes any symptoms albeit those with significant obstruction exhibit exercise intolerance, chest pain, or rarely syncope and require early intervention. Volume overload, pressure overload, or a combination of both cause adverse remodeling of the right ventricle leading to varying degrees of dilatation and hypertrophy, increased wall stress, interstitial fibrosis, and dyssynchrony.[2,15] This in long-term precipitates right ventricle dysfunction, ventricular arrhythmia, heart failure, and risk of sudden cardiac death. Progressive dilatation

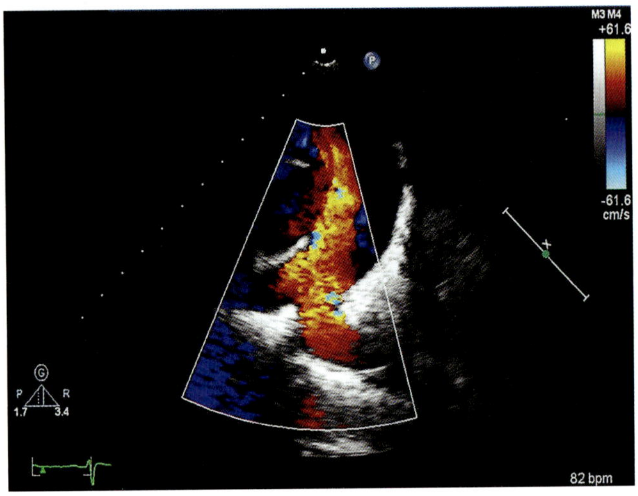

FIG. 2: Echocardiogram in parasternal short axis view with color flow mapping showing severe pulmonary regurgitation.

of right ventricle manifests as QRS prolongation which is identified as one of the important predictors of adverse outcomes after tetralogy of Fallot repair.[2] A prolonged QRS leads to electromechanical dissociation, a duration of >180 ms or a rate of increase by 6 ms per year is a marker of ventricular arrythmia or mortality.[2,16] Additional concern in repaired tetralogy of Fallot is the akinetic or aneurysmal segment of right ventricle outflow tract which may or may not be related to presence of a transannular patch. This akinetic segment is an independent risk factor for right ventricle dysfunction and a focus for ventricular tachycardia. With the recognition of right ventricle outflow tract dysfunction as the main culprit for hemodynamic derangements a pulmonary valve replacement if performed at optimal time leads to improvement in functional class, symptoms, and reduction in right ventricle volumes.[2] Distal pulmonary artery stenosis further increases the impact of pulmonary incompetence or right ventricle pressure overload (in absence of pulmonary incompetence) **(Fig. 3)**. Right pulmonary artery stenosis is typically seen in patients with prior palliative right modified BT shunt. Left pulmonary artery stenosis can have multiple causes including preexisting stenosis corrected by patch enlargement and progressive right ventricle dilatation distorting the left pulmonary artery.

Left Ventricle Dysfunction

The consequences of chronic pulmonary regurgitation are not limited to the right ventricle and it has now been well established that the left ventricle is also affected in corrected tetralogy of Fallot due to reverse Bernheim effect.[2,14,17] The definite cause of this deterioration in left ventricle function on follow-up has been incompletely understood. As both the right and left ventricles are anatomically integrated through the subepicardial layer, share a common interventricular septum and both being enclosed in the same pericardial cavity; it may explain the adverse interventricular interactions.[2,17] Additional plausible factors include long-standing cyanosis in late presenting cases, inadequate myocardial protection during repair, volume overload from long-standing palliative shunts, residual ventricular septal defect, compression of left coronary artery while intracardiac repair and aortic regurgitation. A decrease in left ventricle circumferential strain and to some extent longitudinal (left ventricle) strain due to reduced left ventricle apical rotation has been well demonstrated both with right ventricle volume and pressure overload.[15,17] There is a linear correlation between the right and left ventricle function on late follow-up.[2,17] Left ventricular function is one of the strongest predictors of risk of arrhythmia and long-term survival in corrected tetralogy of Fallot.[13,17]

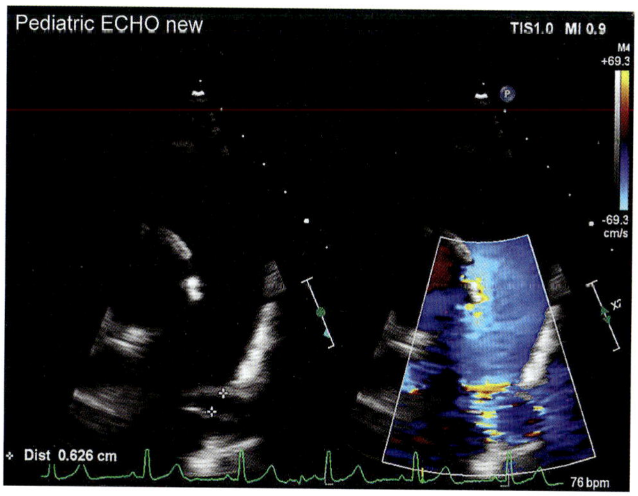

FIG. 3: Echocardiogram in parasternal short axis view showing severe left pulmonary artery stenosis.

Aortopathy

Aortic root enlargement is frequently seen in patients with tetralogy of Fallot which is attributed to both increased right-to-left shunt and intrinsic histological abnormalities of the aortic medial wall (cystic medial necrosis).[2,15] The prevalence varies from 30 to 50%.[18] Male gender, tetralogy of Fallot with pulmonary atresia, and long interval between palliative and complete repair are more prone for having aortic root enlargement. A progressive aortic root enlargement predisposes these patients to aortic regurgitation, aortic aneurysm, and very rarely aortic dissection. The relative risk of aortic dissection is slightly higher than the general population, however, it is less than in connective tissue disorders such as Marfan syndrome. However, there is no consensus on the optimal timing of intervention, an aortic root size of >55 mm or early in the presence of aortic regurgitation is considered as a cutoff for aortic surgery.[2,18]

Arrythmia and Risk of Sudden Cardiac Death

Late-onset arrythmia and the risk of sudden cardiac death are the major causes of morbidity and mortality in repaired tetralogy of Fallot. The predisposition to arrythmia is attributed to the hemodynamic perturbations and the presence of surgical scars after total correction. A prevalence of atrial and ventricular arrhythmia is estimated to be 20% and 15%, respectively.[18-20] Substantial increase is noticed after the age of 45 years.[18-20] The most frequent atrial tachycardia is reentrant/reentry arrythmia involving either the cavotricuspid isthmus or lateral right atrial wall followed by focal atrial arrythmia. The risk factors are dilated right atrium, multiple surgeries, and the presence of at least moderate tricuspid regurgitation.[19,20] The prevalence of atrial fibrillation increases after 40 years of age, the factor associated being dilated left atrium, left ventricle dysfunction, and hypertension. Rhythm control strategy is preferred over rate control in treatment in atrial arrythmias.[19,20]

Sudden cardiac arrest remains the leading cause of mortality amongst adults with an annual risk ranging from 0.9 to 3% per year.[20-22] Ventricular tachycardia is the most prevailing cause of this increased risk; monomorphic ventricular tachycardia being the dominant variant. Predisposing variables increasing the probability of sudden death are an older age at repair, presence of a transannular patch, systolic or diastolic ventricular dysfunction, prolonged QRS duration, QRS fragmentation, nonsustained ventricular tachycardia, and ventricular scarring **(Fig. 4)**.[20-22] The predictive value of a QRS duration > 180 ms for risk of ventricular tachycardia is higher in older cohorts and those who underwent transventricular repair.[20] Recently QRS fragmentation has been identified as superior to QRS duration in predicting myocardial fibrosis, risk of ventricular tachycardia, and sudden cardiac death.[22] The predominant mechanism of ventricular tachycardia is macroreentry facilitated by slow conduction due to progressive fibrosis across various well-defined anatomical isthmus.[20] These anatomic isthmuses which are targets for electrophysiology interventions are bordered by well-defined inexcitable regions including patch material, valve annulus, and post-surgical dense scar. The role of programmed stimulation for inducible ventricular tachycardia is limited to symptomatic or high-risk patients.[20,22,23] Implantable cardioverter-defibrillator as primary prevention is restricted only to patients with multiple risk factors for risk of sudden cardiac death, whereas survivors of cardiac arrest and spontaneous sustained ventricular tachycardia are offered secondary prevention.[22,23]

REINTERVENTION

Reintervention is common after repair of tetralogy of Fallot and is usually aimed at addressing right ventricle outflow tract insufficiency or obstruction. Other indications for reoperation include residual ventricular septal defect, severe tricuspid regurgitation, and branch pulmonary stenosis. Pulmonary regurgitation is the most common residual defect after repair of tetralogy, more frequent with transannular patch repair, leading to progressive right ventricle dilatation and serves as an important determinant for late complications.[14,15] Progressive right ventricle dilatation is often accompanied by increasing QRS duration, dyssynchrony, and myocardial fibrosis, culminating into right ventricle dysfunction.[2,14] Restoring pulmonary valve competence is imperative to halt the adverse remodeling of right ventricle before irreversible right ventricle dysfunction occurs. Pulmonary valve replacement is effective in reducing right ventricle volume, increasing left ventricle function, decreasing QRS duration, and improving exercise capacity. The prognostic value of pulmonary valve replacement in severely dilated right ventricle and right ventricle dysfunction is well established whereas in patients without severe right ventricle dilatation or preserved function this prognostic benefit is lacking.[24] The optimal timing of pulmonary valve replacement is thus contentious. An early replacement in view of the limited longevity of the prosthetic valve predisposes to multiple interventions and risk of endocarditis whereas waiting for too long may induce irreversible damage and risk of sudden cardiac death. Contemporary clinical

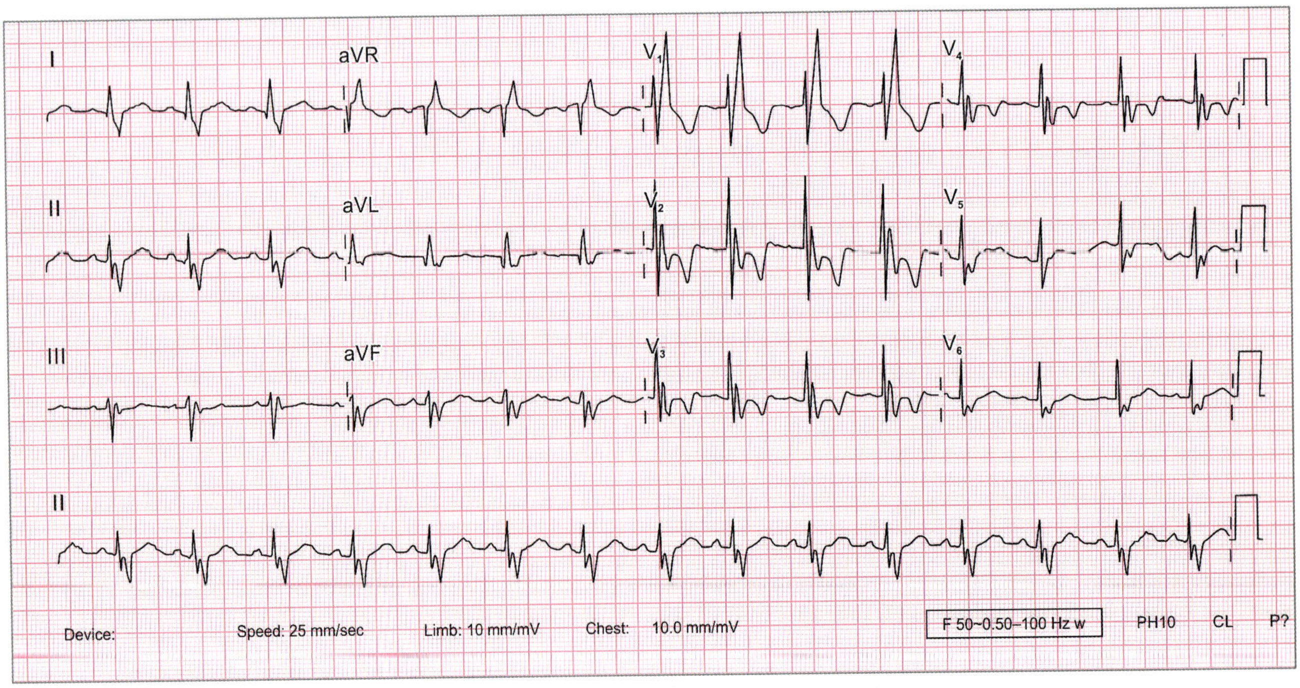

FIG. 4: A 12-lead ECG showing sinus rhythm with complete right bundle branch block with QRS duration of 160 ms.

BOX 1 Indications for pulmonary valve replacement.

Asymptomatic patients with two or more of the following criteria:

- Right ventricle end-diastolic volume index > 160 mL/m^2
- RV end-systolic volume index > 80 mL/m^2
- RV ejection fraction < 45%
- LV ejection fraction < 55%
- QRS duration > 160 ms
- Right ventricle outflow tract obstruction with right ventricle: Left ventricle systolic pressure ≥ 0.7

Symptomatic patients with one or more of the above criteria

guidelines recommend pulmonary valve replacement in patients with progressive reduction in exercise tolerance and a right ventricle end-diastolic volume index of ≥160 mL/m^2 and/or an end-systolic volume index of ≥80 mL/m^2, or a right ventricle ejection fraction of <45% or a left ventricle ejection fraction of <55% or progressive tricuspid regurgitation **(Box 1)**.[23,24] Replacement can be accomplished either surgically or via transcatheter procedure depending on the anatomic considerations and concomitant lesions requiring surgical correction/revision. Over the last two decades, percutaneous pulmonary valve replacement has emerged as an alternative to surgery with a procedural success reaching 95%. With a diverse range of balloon-expandable and self-expandable percutaneous prosthetic valves, majority of the right ventricle outflow tracts can be addressed via transcatheter intervention barring a few native valve with a diameter > 35 mm and absence of tubular landing zone. Albeit pulmonary valve replacement reverses right ventricle enlargement and improves symptoms, replacing the valve does not abolish anatomic substrate for ventricular tachycardia warranting provocative testing and ablation in high-risk individuals.[20]

Another common lesion is residual or restenosis of right ventricle outflow which can be encountered at multiple levels including valvular, subvalvular, pulmonary artery, individual branches, or in the right ventricle to pulmonary artery conduit. Reintervention for right ventricle outflow tract obstruction is recommended for severe stenosis or symptomatic patients with moderate stenosis. The risk of intervention for right ventricle outflow obstruction correlates well with the residual gradient at the time of surgery. Level of the lesion, severity of obstruction and concomitant abnormalities guides the nature of intervention whether transcatheter or surgical.

MULTIMODALITY IMAGING

Multimodality imaging plays a crucial role in monitoring of repaired tetralogy of Fallot with the aim of identifying anatomic and hemodynamic derangements, assessing their severity, risk stratification, and aiding in timing of intervention. A single imaging modality is not enough to delineate the consequences of repaired tetralogy. The choice of imaging or an amalgamation of them is guided by the clinical examination, patient-related considerations, expertise, strength, and weakness of individual modality.[15,25] An annual assessment is recommended which may be tailored according to the functional status and severity of residual lesions.[25]

Echocardiography

Echocardiography is a reliable noninvasive tool for surveillance of corrected tetralogy of Fallot. Anatomic, functional, and hemodynamic abnormalities of both right- and left-sided heart structures can be assessed which is essential for a complete evaluation. Right ventricle being a retrosternal structure, a focused right ventricle four chamber view is imperative for assessment of right ventricle function, degree, mechanism of tricuspid regurgitation, and chamber size. A gamut of parameters including tricuspid annular plane systolic excursion, right ventricle fraction area change, tissue Doppler velocity, and Tie index are used for evaluation of systolic function, although all these indices are either load or angle dependent **(Figs. 5 and 6)**. Speckle-tracking echocardiography has the advantage of being less angle reliant and is also used to assess electromechanical dyssynchrony which is characterized by early activation of apex and septum and late activation of right ventricle free wall **(Fig. 7)**.[15,25] None of the above indices take into account the aneurysmal and dyskinetic outflow portions of the right ventricle, which is common in patients with repaired tetralogy of Fallot. Three-dimensional (3D) echocardiography holds promise in this regard as it incorporates right ventricle outflow tract while assessing global ventricular function **(Fig. 8)**. 3D derived right ventricle function and volumes correlate well with cardiac magnetic resonance imaging

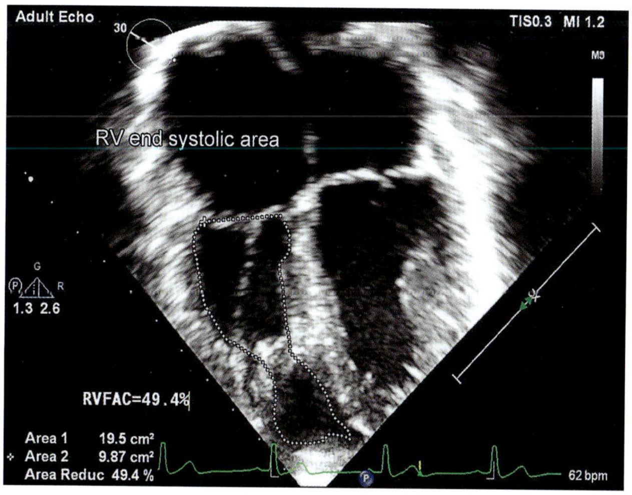

FIG. 5: Echocardiogram demonstrating end systolic area and calculation of right ventricle fractional area change (RVFAC) in four-chamber view.

values.[15,25] Diastolic function should be evaluated using a combination of parameters including antegrade flow during late diastole in main pulmonary artery, right atrial dilatation, flow reversal in hepatic veins, and inferior vena cava variation. A note should be made of the presence and severity of tricuspid regurgitation which can be primary or secondary to annular dilatation. Right ventricle outflow tract analysis warrants a color, continuous, and a pulsed wave Doppler interrogation. Pulmonary regurgitation manifesting as diastolic flow reversal from branch pulmonary arteries, regurgitant jet occupying more than half of the annulus or a pressure half time < 100 ms is termed as severe.[15,25] Left ventricle dysfunction is an independent prognostic factor for sudden cardiac death in corrected tetralogy of Fallot and is vital in surveillance of these patients. Multiple views should be used to assess left ventricular size, regional, and global systolic function. Systolic function estimation should be done both by 2D and 3D echocardiography. Speckle-tracking helps in the early detection of left ventricle systolic dysfunction. Residual shunts estimation should be accomplished via color and continuous Doppler imaging. Transesophageal echocardiography is vital in guiding transcatheter interventions, in cases with limited transthoracic images or in suspected infective endocarditis.

Cardiac Magnetic Resonance Imaging

Cardiac magnetic resonance imaging is considered as the gold standard in estimation of right ventricle size, volume, function, and severity of pulmonary regurgitation.[15,23,25] The phase contrast sequence provides measurement of anterograde and retrograde flow to establish residual shunts and pulmonary regurgitant fraction; with regurgitant fraction > 40% being considered as severe.[15,25] Contrast-enhanced magnetic resonance angiography is essential for assessment of pulmonary artery and venous tree, particularly the

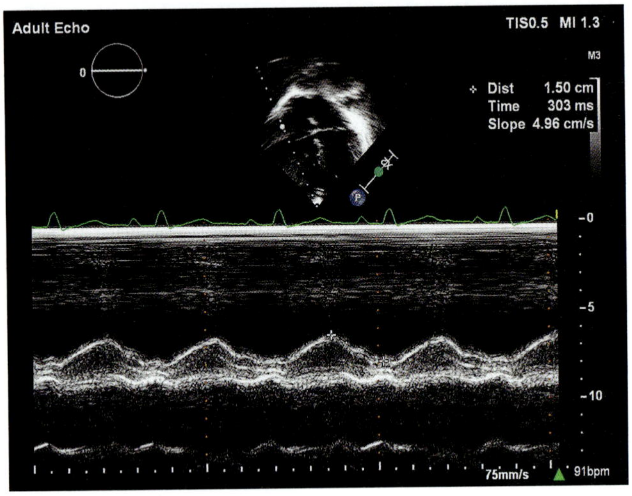

FIG. 6: M-mode echocardiogram demonstrating tricuspid annular plane systolic excursion (TAPSE).

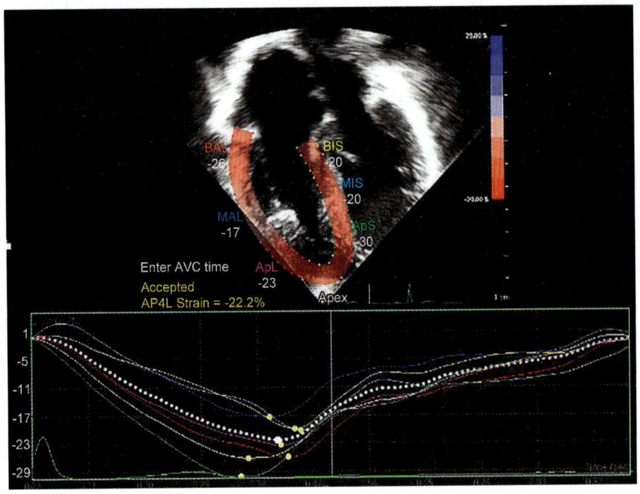

FIG. 7: Echocardiogram demonstrating right ventricle global longitudinal strain using two dimensional speckle tracking.

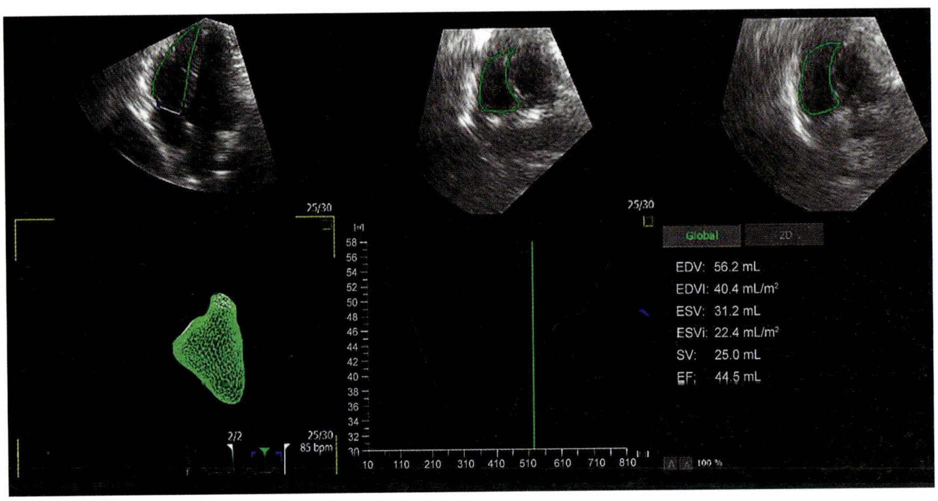

FIG. 8: Echocardiogram demonstrating 3D right ventricle volume and function assessment.

pulmonary arteries for residual stenosis. In these situations, phase contrast sequences aid in estimation of differential pulmonary artery branch flow and planning intervention. Tissue characterization can be established via various cardiac magnetic resonance sequences. Focal myocardial fibrosis which is a substrate for monomorphic ventricular tachycardia can be detected by late gadolinium enhancement. This myocardial fibrosis is found at surgical sites (septal defect patch, resected muscle bundle) and remote regions such as right ventricle free wall or interventricular septum **(Fig. 9)**.[25] Abnormal myocardial loading conditions in repaired tetralogy of Fallot result in expansion of extracellular matrix as a consequence of excessive collagen deposition manifesting as diffuse (interstitial) fibrosis. Increased extracellular matrix can be detected noninvasively by measuring extracellular volume and T1 mapping. This extracellular remodeling correlates with the risk of arrythmia and sudden cardiac death.

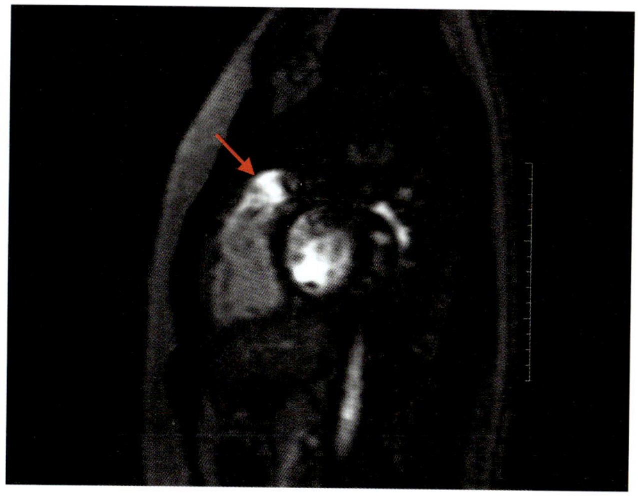

FIG. 9: Postcontrast delayed PSIR short axis view of RVOT showing fibrosis in the form enhancement (red arrow) at the area of transannular patch.

Cardiovascular Computed Tomography

Cardiovascular computed tomography although not frequently used in corrected tetralogy of Fallot, because of high spatial resolution, is vital for detailed assessment of small vessel anatomy, including pulmonary veins, distal pulmonary artery branches, coronary arteries, and aorto-pulmonary collaterals.[15,25] Cardiovascular computed tomography has an indispensable role in preprocedure planning in percutaneous pulmonary valve implantation where accurate assessment of right ventricle outflow tract, landing zone and proximity to the coronary arteries is essential imaging pulmonary artery stenosis after surgical correction for planning stenting of the pulmonary artery is another important indication **(Fig. 10)**. It can be used alternatively in patients where cardiac magnetic resonance imaging is not feasible. The use is, however, limited in view of limited hemodynamic information, use of ionizing radiation, and use of contrast in those with impaired renal function.

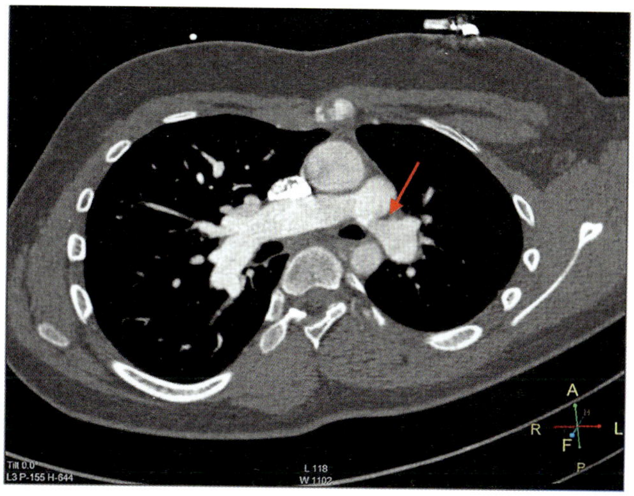

FIG. 10: Axial computed tomography showing left pulmonary artery ostial stenosis (red arrow).

PREGNANCY

Preconception counseling is important in patients with repaired tetralogy of Fallot. The recurrence rate of congenital heart disease of about 3%. The risks during pregnancy depend upon the hemodynamic sequelae with minimal risk in patients with no significant residual. However, patients with significant right ventricle outflow tract obstruction, severe pulmonary regurgitation, severe tricuspid regurgitation, or ventricular dysfunction warrant a multidisciplinary approach during pregnancy.

CONCLUSION

Repaired tetralogy of Fallot has a good long-term survival during the initial decades of follow-up. A lifelong follow-up is necessary as even after complete repair there are a number of complications that can affect these patients later on in life. Reintervention may be required in hemodynamically significant lesions.

ONLINE REFERENCES

Please scan the QR code provided at the end of the table of contents for References of this chapter.

CHAPTER

97

Approach to Adults with Congenital Heart Defects

Ranjit K Nath, Bhushan Tile

ABSTRACT

Adult congenital heart disease (ACHD) represents a complex and evolving field of cardiology, characterized by the management of cardiac abnormalities initially diagnosed in childhood that persist into adulthood.

This chapter outlines a comprehensive approach to ACHD, emphasizing the integration of advanced diagnostic techniques, therapeutic strategies, and holistic ongoing care.

Keywords: ACHD, ASD, VSD, PDA, TOF, TGA, Eisenmenger, Fontan, Ebstein

INTRODUCTION

Adult congenital heart disease (ACHD) presents distinct challenges due to a wide range of cardiac abnormalities and their evolving impacts as individuals move from childhood to adulthood.

Although there is evidence of a rise in the prevalence of CHD at birth—from approximately 1 to 2% of all live births—this rise is likely due to improved detection of milder cases. Nowadays, 97% of children with CHDs survive into adulthood, and 70% of those who reach 18 years of age are expected to live to 70 years of age.[1]

However, an extended life span also brings a greater likelihood of developing acquired cardiovascular diseases, and ACHD patients frequently face complex, multisystemic conditions.

CLINICAL APPROACH

Physical examination in ACHD patients can reveal details about previous procedures, especially when the medical history is incomplete. For instance, the presence of surgical scars can indicate whether a patient has undergone lateral thoracotomy, such as those performed for PDA ligation or aortic coarctation repair. Additionally, if radial pulse is missing in the same arm as thoracotomy scar, it may suggest that the subclavian artery was compromised during surgery (e.g., previous Blalock-Taussig-Thomas shunt or subclavian flap repair for aortic coarctation).

Physical examination can also uncover specific signs in ACHD patients, such as wide fixed split S2 in individuals with unrepaired ASD or reduced pulse in the lower limbs of those with aortic coarctation. In patients with pulmonary stenosis, a notable physical examination finding is a systolic ejection click that diminishes with inspiration.

The electrocardiogram (ECG) provides insights into heart rhythm, rate, and atrioventricular (AV) conduction. Additionally, chest X-rays (CXR) are valuable for evaluating CHD patients.

While echocardiography is fundamental to cardiac imaging, its effectiveness can diminish with age due to suboptimal acoustic windows. In such cases, other imaging methods like CMR or cardiac CT become useful. Cardiopulmonary exercise testing (CPET) and biomarker measurements are important for monitoring, intervention timing, and reintervention.

Cardiac catheterization is advised for ACHD patients showing signs of increased pulmonary artery (PA) pressure to assess pulmonary vascular resistance (PVR).

Ambulatory ECG monitoring is helpful for investigating palpitations and detecting hidden arrhythmias. In individuals with tetralogy of Fallot (TOF), asymptomatic, nonsustained ventricular tachycardia (VT) detected on Holter monitoring may predict clinical VT.

The need for invasive electrophysiology studies should be evaluated on an individual basis. Inducible sustained VT is a known risk factor for clinical VT and sudden death in patients with repaired TOF. The prognostic significance of programmed electrical stimulation is unclear for other types of CHD and may not be relevant in some conditions like transposition of the great arteries (TGA).[2]

SPECIFIC DEFECTS

See **Table 1**.

Ebstein Anomaly

Prevalence

Ebstein anomaly is present in 1/200,000 live births.[3]

Clinical Features and Diagnostic Testing

Clinical manifestations are variable:

- *Adult presentation*: Asymptomatic or severe tricuspid regurgitation with RV dysfunction, exercise intolerance, arrhythmia, fatigue, paradoxical embolism, or cyanosis
- JVP is usually normal even with significant TR because of large and compliant RA
- *ECG*: Tall peaked P waves (>2.5 mm) in leads II and V1/"Himalayan" P waves (>5 mm height), complete/incomplete RBBB, prolonged PR interval or short PR interval and delta wave reflective of pre-excitation, atrial fibrillation/flutter
- *CXR*: "Box-shaped" heart

TABLE 1: Left-to-right shunt lesions.

	ASD	VSD	AVSD	PDA
Prevalence	0.88/1,000 adults (PFO persists in 25% of adults)	2.62/1,000	0.24–0.31/1,000	0.87/1,000[3,4]
Types	OS-ASD, OP-ASD, SV-ASD, CS-ASD	*CHS classification*: Perimembranous, subarterial, inlet, muscular	• Rastelli A, B, C • Balanced/unbalanced • Complete/intermediate/transitional/partial	*Krichenko classification*: A, conical; B, window; C, tubular; D, complex
Clinical features	• Incidentally discovered mostly • *Symptoms*: Exercise intolerance, fatigue, palpitations • Supraventricular arrhythmias by 40 years of age in 10% • *Cyanosis*: ○ Eisenmenger ○ Prominent Eustachian valve directing flow via ASD toward LA • *Examination*: Wide fixed S2, flow murmurs • *ECG*: RBBB, right axis, crochetage sign • *CXR*: Jug-handle appearance	• *Restrictive VSDs*: ○ Asymptomatic mostly ○ Harsh holosystolic murmur, thrill • *Small muscular VSDs*: Early systolic murmur • *Large VSDs*: Mostly repaired in childhood, else present with PH • *Symptoms*: Dyspnea, palpitations, exercise intolerance, chest pain • LA/LV volume overload • RV pressure overload • *ECG*: Katz–Wachtel phenomenon	• Most adult AVSDs are postoperative patients • *Presentation*: Residual AV regurgitation/stenosis, LVOT obstruction, atrial arrhythmias	• LA/LV volume overload • RV pressure overload • Wide pulse pressure, collapsing pulse, hyperdynamic apex, Gibson's continuous murmur, mitral MDM • *Differential cyanosis/clubbing*: PH • *Symptoms*: Dyspnea, palpitations, exercise intolerance, LV dysfunction • *ECG*: LA/LV volume overload • *CXR*: Cardiomegaly, comma-shaped density
Repair	• L > R shunt with: ○ RA/RV enlargement ○ Qp/Qs >1.5 ○ PASP <50% SBP ○ PVR < 1/3 SVR	• *L > R shunt with*: ○ LV volume overload ○ Qp/Qs >1.5 ○ PASP <50% SBP ○ PVR <1/3 SVR	Same as ASD	Same as VSD
	• *OS-ASD*: Device closure (Amplatz/Occlunix/Gore cardioform/Coccon/Helex/Nit-Occlud ASD-R)/surgery • *Other ASDs*: Surgery	• *Gold standard*: Surgery • Device closure in selected muscular/perimembranous VSDs	Surgery may be required for residual AV regurgitation/stenosis, LVOT obstruction	*Transcatheter*: Gianturco/Nit-Occlud coil, ADO I/II device, plugs, or surgery
Long-term outcomes, complications	• *Repair <25 years*: Favorable outcomes • *After 40 years*: 4.5%/year mortality • Annual echo monitoring postrepair	• Annual echo monitoring postrepair • Arrythmias, LV dysfunction, AR, IE, PH	Patch dehiscence, septal defects, CHB	• IE prophylaxis for 6 months post–device closure • Annual echo monitoring for possible recanalization

- *Echocardiography*: To characterize the valve leaflets and subvalvular apparatus, any ASD/PFO, and quantify TR
- CMR to assess the degree of tricuspid valve displacement and quantify TR, RV systolic function, cardiac output, and Qp:Qs for measurement of cardiac shunt[5]

Long-term Outcomes and Complications

Unrepaired Ebstein Anomaly

Factors associated with unfavorable outcomes include younger age at diagnosis, male sex, cardiothoracic ratio ≥0.65, and severity of valve displacement.[6] The most prevalent arrhythmia in these patients is AVRT. For patients experiencing symptomatic arrhythmias/pre-excitation, electrophysiological testing followed by ablation is recommended.[7]

Tricuspid Valve Repair and Replacement Surgery

Surgery is recommended for symptoms of heart failure attributed to tricuspid valve disease. It may also be considered for progressive RV enlargement, desaturation from right-to-left shunt, paroxysmal embolism, or atrial tachyarrhythmia.

Tricuspid valve repair (DaSilva's cone reconstruction) is preferred.

Transcatheter ASD/PFO Closure

It is considered for paradoxical embolism and cyanosis but requires careful evaluation to exclude RA pressure increase or fall in cardiac output.

Cardiac Transplantation

It is considered for patients with severe biventricular dysfunction.

Pulmonary Stenosis

Prevalence

It Pulmonary stenosis is prevalent in 0.50/1,000 live births.[4]

Associated conditions: Noonan syndrome, William's syndrome, Trisomy 13/18.[8]

Clinical Features and Diagnostic Testing

- Often asymptomatic
- Progressive exercise intolerance and signs and symptoms of heart failure due to RV dysfunction
- Associated PFO/ASD may lead to right-to-left shunting and cyanosis, particularly with exercise.
- *Physical findings*: Crescendo-decrescendo systolic ejection murmur, systolic ejection click (becomes softer with inspiration), parasternal heave, prominent jugular a wave, hepatomegaly
- Mixed disease leads to a "to-and-fro" murmur of pulmonary stenosis and regurgitation.
- *Echocardiography*: In patients with moderate/severe stenosis, TTE is appropriate to perform yearly.[9]
- CMR can quantify RV function and size. CPET is recommended every 2 years for moderate valve disease.

Indications for Intervention/Reintervention

For moderate/severe PS in the presence of symptoms including heart failure, exercise intolerance, or cyanosis, the 2018 ACC/AHA guidelines recommend intervention as class I indication.

Primary intervention by balloon valvuloplasty is recommended, with surgical repair recommended for patients having contraindication or failing transcatheter intervention. For asymptomatic severe PS patients, intervention is considered reasonable as class IIa indication.

Pulmonary valve replacement is indicated for patients with symptoms and at least moderate regurgitation and RV dilation.

Long-term Outcomes and Complications

Patients with mild pulmonary stenosis rarely progress or require intervention. More significant valve dysfunction can lead to impairment of RV systolic and diastolic function.

Tetralogy of Fallot

Prevalence

Tetralogy of Fallot is prevalent in 0.34/1,000 live births[4] (most common cyanotic ACHD).

Clinical Features and Diagnostic Testing

- *Symptoms*: Dyspnea, palpitations, or syncope
- *Clinical examination*: Normal oxygen saturations, diastolic to-and-fro murmur in the pulmonary area, RV heave, and single S2 signify pulmonary regurgitation.
- *Signs of RV failure*: Hepatomegaly, raised JVP, and edema are uncommon.
- ECG commonly shows RBBB. BNP is predictive of mortality.[10]
- *Echocardiography*: To assess RVOT obstruction, tricuspid regurgitation, and diastolic dysfunction and residual VSD
- *CMR*: To assess RV volume/function, pulmonary regurgitation, RVOT including branch PAs and the course of the proximal coronaries, aortic root, and ascending aorta, and quantification of tricuspid and aortic regurgitation. RVOT akinetic area length predicts the onset of sustained ventricular arrhythmia.
- *CPET*: For objective measure of exercise capacity which facilitates decision making regarding valve replacement
- Ambulatory ECG monitoring and diagnostic EP study are used in patients with arrhythmia symptoms.
- Cardiac catheterization for diagnostic purposes alone is rarely indicated for asymptomatic patients. Preoperative assessment of TOF with pulmonary atresia with MAPCAs usually includes delineation of the arterial supply to both lungs and angiography to show the course and segmental supply from the collateral arteries and central PAs.

Surgical Repair

Most patients have typically undergone surgical repair with closure of the VSD and relief of pulmonary stenosis with resection of RV muscle bundles in the RVOT with/without RVOT reconstruction. Since surgical repair of TOF was introduced in the 1950s,[11] survival rates of >90% are expected beyond 40 years from repair. The surgical strategy for repair has evolved with time: Previously, many infants received BTT shunt prior to repair but now early primary repair is common **(Box 1)**.

BOX 1 Long-term complications in repaired TOF.

- *RV volume overload*: Tricuspid/pulmonary regurgitation
- *Left-to-right shunt*:
  - ASD/VSD
  - Systemic-to-pulmonary collaterals
- RV/LV systolic or diastolic dysfunction
- Aortic regurgitation
- Ventricular conduction delay and dyssynchrony
- *Arrhythmias*:
  - VT
  - Atrial fibrillation
  - Atrial flutter

Transposition of the Great Arteries

Prevalence

Transposition of the great arteries is prevalent in 0.31/1,000 live births.[4]

Clinical Features

Unrepaired TGA in adults is rare. The physical examination will reveal profound cyanosis and erythrocytosis. The physical findings of the repaired patient depend on the type of repair **(Table 2)**.

Congenitally Corrected Transposition of the Great Arteries

L-TGA/congenitally corrected TGA (ccTGA) is uncommon, accounting for <1% of ACHD.[3]

Clinical Features

Patients with ccTGA and no associated cardiac defects may remain asymptomatic. Those with ventricular dysfunction may have exercise intolerance and signs of heart failure.

- *Physical examination*: May be nearly normal with the exception of a single S2 (as the pulmonic closure sound is obscured by its posterior location)

TABLE 2: Complications following TGA repair.

Surgery	Complication	Clinical features	Evaluation	Treatment
Atrial switch Mustard/ Senning	Baffle leak	Exercise intolerance, cyanosis, erythrocytosis, paradoxical embolism	TTE with agitated saline, TEE, CMR, cardiac CT	*Transcatheter closure*: Covered stent/ASD device
	Pathway obstruction	Asymptomatic, facial swelling, headache	CT/MR angiography	Angioplasty with stenting if symptomatic
	IART	Palpitations, syncope	ECG, Holter, EP study	Ablation, antiarrhythmics
	Sinus node dysfunction	Exercise intolerance, syncope	ECG, Holter	Pacemaker
	Ventricular dysfunction	Exercise intolerance, congestive heart failure	TTE, CMR	GDMT
Arterial switch	Ostial coronary stenosis	Angina, ventricular arrythmias	Stress tests, CT/invasive angiography	PCI/CABG
	Branch pulmonary artery stenosis	Exercise intolerance, systolic murmur	TTE, CT/MR angiography	Balloon angioplasty with stenting/surgery
	Neoaortic root dilation	None	TTE, CMR	Surgery
	Neoaortic regurgitation	Exercise intolerance, diastolic murmur	TTE, CMR	Surgery
Rastelli operation	RV-PA conduit stenosis	Exercise intolerance, systolic murmur, RV dysfunction	TTE	Transcatheter pulmonary valve implantation/surgical conduit replacement
	RV-PA conduit regurgitation	Exercise intolerance, diastolic murmur, RV dysfunction	TTE, CMR	Transcatheter pulmonary valve implantation/surgical conduit revision

- *ECG*: Absent septal Q-waves, AV block
- *Chest radiograph*: Narrow and straight mediastinal silhouette

Surgical Repairs

Patients with no associated cardiac anomalies do not necessarily require surgery, although this would leave them with a systemic RV.

The double-switch operation is a technically complex surgery which results in the LV in the subaortic position. In patients without VSD, this consists of an atrial switch procedure and an arterial switch procedure. In patients with VSD, the double switch can be achieved via an atrial switch and Rastelli operation.

Double-outlet Right Ventricle

Common physiological variations of DORV are:
- *VSD physiology:* DORV with subaortic VSD and no PS
- *TOF physiology:* DORV with subaortic VSD and PS
- *TGA physiology:* DORV with subpulmonary VSD with/without aortic obstruction
- *Single ventricle physiology:* DORV with mitral atresia, severely unbalanced AVSD

Clinical Features

The clinical presentation of DORV patients depends on the lesion with the most similar anatomy and physiology (TOF/TGA physiology).

Repairs

In the most common form (subaortic VSD), the goal includes establishing LV–aortic continuity by patching the VSD to tunnel the LV to the aorta. In case of pulmonary stenosis, relief of obstruction is accomplished by either valvotomy or patch enlargement of the RVOT.

For patients with DORV and a subpulmonary VSD, the surgical repair is similar to that for patients with D-TGA with a baffle from the LV-to-pulmonary valve and arterial switch operation.

For patients with unfavorable anatomy for a biventricular repair, Fontan palliation is performed.

Truncus Arteriosus

Without treatment, the mean age of mortality is 2.5 months, mostly from heart failure. Rarely, isolated cases of survival into adulthood with unrepaired truncus arteriosus have been reported, and these patients usually have Eisenmenger's syndrome.

Repairs

The surgical repair involves removal of PAs from the truncal root, VSD patch closure, and placement of a conduit between RV and PAs. In cases where the truncal valve is dysfunctional, repair/replacement with a homograft is performed.

Long-term Outcomes and Complications

Important risk factors for perioperative mortality are severe truncal valve regurgitation, interrupted aortic arch, coronary artery anomalies, and age at initial surgery > 100 days. Patients with only one PA are especially prone to early development of severe pulmonary vascular disease.

Coarctation of the Aorta

Prevalence

Coarctation of the aorta is prevalent in 0.34/1,000 live births.[4]

Clinical Features and Diagnostic Testing

- Mostly asymptomatic
- Systemic hypertension is common even after repair.[12]
- *Symptoms*: Headache, chest pain, leg claudication
- *Signs*: Brachiofemoral delay, SBP gradient between the right arm and the lower limb ≥20 mm Hg indicating significant coarctation, continuous interscapular murmurs (Suzman's sign)
- *Fundoscopy*: Hypertensive retinopathy
- *ECG*: LVH, ischemia
- *CXR*: Rib notching (2nd to 9th ribs), "figure 3" sign
- *Echocardiography*: To assess aortic valve/root, coarctation site (suprasternal views), LV function
- *CMR*: Evaluating the entire aorta for hypoplasia/Gothic angulation, severity of coarctation, quantification of collaterals, complications post repair (aneurysms/pseudoaneurysms, recoarctation/residual stenosis), and morphology/function of the aortic valve
- *Cardiac CT*: Assessing stent lumen/fracture and coronaries
- *Cardiac catheterization*: Peak-to-peak gradient ≥20 mm Hg in the absence of well-developed collaterals is considered significant.

Repair and Long-term Outcomes

In adults, surgery is rarely needed and stenting is the treatment of choice when technically feasible. Coarctation/recoarctation repair (endovascular/surgical) is indicated in hypertensive patients with an invasive peak-to-peak gradient ≥ 20 mm Hg. Coarctation stenting is also considered when feasible for hypertensive patients with a coarctation diameter ≤ 50% of the aortic diameter at the diaphragm regardless of peak-to-peak gradient and in normotensive coarctation with peak-to-peak gradient ≥ 20 mm Hg.

Balloon dilatation can result in aneurysm formation at the site of coarctation or dissection. These complications are reduced by primary stenting.

Lifelong surveillance is essential with cross-sectional imaging at intervals of at least 3–5 years.[13] Hypertension is a major determinant of late mortality after coarctation repair.[14]

Single Ventricle

Single ventricle heart disease comprises several distinct anatomic lesions, which may represent a true anatomic/functional single ventricle lesion.

- Tricuspid atresia (1.2/10,000 live births)[3]
- HLHS (1.6/10,000 live births)[3]
- Double-inlet LV
- Double-inlet/double-outlet RV
- Unbalanced complete AVSD

Surgical Palliation

Nearly all adults with single ventricle heart disease will have received a Fontan palliation.[15]

The present surgical approach includes neonatal surgery to achieve a stable systemic outflow and balance between systemic and pulmonary circulation to provide adequate oxygenation but protect the pulmonary circulation from pressure/volume overload, followed by superior cavopulmonary anastomosis (bidirectional Glenn) later in the first year of life.

This is finally followed by the Fontan procedure that is usually performed between 18 months and 4 years of age. The three most commonly seen versions of Fontan circuit in adults include the extracardiac Fontan, lateral tunnel Fontan, and direct right atrial to PA anastomosis.

Clinical Features and Diagnostic Testing

Adults with Fontan circulation may present with chronotropic incompetence, dyspnea, palpitations, and symptoms related to end-organ damage from long-term impaired cardiac output.

- *Signs*: Chronic cyanosis, clubbing, single S1 and S2, hepatomegaly, ascites, edema
- *ECG*: Intra-atrial reentrant tachycardia, PVC/PAC

Imaging assessment with either echocardiography or CMR is considered Class I indication annually for these patients, with CMR performed in lieu of echo typically every 2–3 years.[9]

CT scanning overcomes artifacts related to coils and other implants and can also provide excellent visualization of the Fontan pathway and PAs.

Exercise testing is recommended every 1–3 years depending on the severity of the patient's disease state.[9]

Patients undergoing revision Fontan surgery should have a preoperative catheterization. For symptomatic patients, cardiac catheterization is considered as Class IIa indication if imaging does not provide adequate information.[9]

Basic metabolic profile testing, PT/INR, BNP, total cholesterol, and complete blood count are considered class IIa indication for Fontan patients and can be performed every 1–2 years. Liver ultrasound/MRI is indicated to assess the status of Fontan-associated liver disease (FALD) every 1–2 years.[16]

Long-term Outcomes

In two large series, overall 20-year survival following the Fontan surgery was 61% and 74%.[17,18] Over time, survival has improved, and it is estimated that the current 30-year survival for children undergoing a Fontan surgery is approximately 85%.

Complications

- Ventricular dilation, dysfunction, and heart failure
- Arrhythmia:
  - Atrial tachyarrhythmias
  - IART
  - Atrial fibrillation
  - Sinoatrial node dysfunction
- *Cyanosis:* Due to:
  - Patent fenestration/leak in lateral tunnel Fontan baffle
  - Increased PVR
  - Development of systemic vein–pulmonary vein collaterals (if indicated, venovenous collaterals can be closed with embolization coils/devices by catheterization)
- Pulmonary arteriovenous malformations
- Protein-losing enteropathy
- Plastic bronchitis
- Abnormalities of the aorta and pulmonary arteries:
  - Aortic coarctation/aneurysm
  - PA: Discrete narrowing/diffuse hypoplasia
- FALD

Eisenmenger Syndrome

Eisenmenger syndrome is a multiorgan systemic disease.

Exercise capacity is markedly reduced in patients with Eisenmenger syndrome, worse than all other forms of ACHD.

Symptoms are usually nonspecific and include dyspnea, fatigue, arthralgias, chest pain, syncope, hemoptysis, headache, or stroke **(Table 3)**.

The prognosis of patients with Eisenmenger syndrome is variable but better than other forms of severe PAH. Mortality during childhood is rare but becomes more common during the fourth decade of life.[19] The most common causes of mortality include sudden death, congestive heart failure, and pulmonary hemorrhage. Patients are at risk from death during noncardiac surgery or infections (particularly brain abscess). Antibiotic prophylaxis is indicated in all patients with Eisenmenger syndrome.

Management of Eisenmenger Syndrome

The management is mostly supportive. Patients should be seen at least annually with laboratory assessment and imaging.

TABLE 3: Physical and laboratory findings typical for Eisenmenger syndrome.

Vital signs	Hypoxemia
Physical examination	• Central cyanosis • Hypertrophic osteoarthropathy • Prominent jugular venous a wave • Right parasternal heave • Loud P2 • S3/S4 • High-pitched diastolic murmur of pulmonary regurgitation • *Systolic murmurs*: Faint/absent
Laboratory	• Erythrocytosis • Iron deficiency • Thrombocytopenia • Leukopenia • Elevated BNP • Hyperuricemia
Chest radiograph	• Dilation of pulmonary arteries • Peripheral pulmonary artery pruning • RA/RV enlargement
ECG	• RA enlargement • Right-axis deviation • Biventricular hypertrophy • ST-T abnormalities
Transthoracic echocardiography	• RV enlargement/hypertrophy • Pulmonary artery enlargement • Pulmonary hypertension • Large shunt defect with low-velocity flow; PDA may be difficult to visualize

Patients should be particularly counseled against extreme exercise, heat, and volume depletion as these can worsen hyperviscosity.

Pregnancy is absolutely contraindicated in Eisenmenger syndrome as it is associated with very high levels of fetal loss and maternal mortality (>30%).[20]

Most patients with Eisenmenger syndrome develop secondary erythrocytosis as an adaptive response to chronic cyanosis. Routine phlebotomy is contraindicated in asymptomatic patients as it increases the risk of stroke.

For patients experiencing symptoms suggestive of hyperviscosity (visual disturbances, headache, paresthesia, lethargy, myalgia), iron deficiency and volume depletion should first be excluded. In patients who are volume replete and iron replete but still have moderate-to-severe symptoms of hyperviscosity, there is a limited role for therapeutic phlebotomy. Phlebotomy should be accompanied by simultaneous volume expansion with saline and frequent hemodynamic monitoring.

Pulmonary vasodilators should be recommended for Eisenmenger syndrome. The BREATH-5 trial[21] demonstrated that bosentan improved exercise capacity and hemodynamics compared to placebo in Eisenmenger syndrome related to ASD, VSD, or PDA. However, the recent MAESTRO trial[22] did not show similar benefits with macitentan in a more diverse group of patients with Eisenmenger syndrome. Epidemiological data and smaller trials suggest that sildenafil may offer benefits in Eisenmenger syndrome. Calcium channel blockers are contraindicated due to their negative inotropic effects.

For patients with Eisenmenger syndrome who do not respond to medical treatment, combined heart–lung transplantation/lung transplantation combined with cardiac defect repair may be considered.

CONCLUSION

Adult CHD patients need proper clinical evaluation and detailed investigations before taking a decision of operative treatment. All patients, both operated and nonoperated, require close follow-up to look for arrhythmias, ventricular dysfunction, pulmonary hypertension, and other noncardiac long-term sequelae. Periodic echocardiography, Holter evaluation, CXR, CMR, and if required CT angiography are the chief investigation modalities needed time to time. With proper follow-up and treatment, the long-term survival can be improved with good quality of life.

ONLINE REFERENCES

Please scan the QR code provided at the end of the table of contents for References of this chapter.

CHAPTER

98

Coarctation of Aorta in Infants, Children, Adolescents, and Adults

Jayranganath M, Sabyasachi Pandey

ABSTRACT

Coarctation of the aorta (CoA) is a common congenital defect that can present at any age, from neonates to adults. Ever since Dr Clarence Crafoord's pioneering surgical repair in 1944, various surgical techniques have been developed. Today, transcatheter stent placement is the preferred treatment, especially in older children and adults. Despite advancements, recoarctation remains a concern, and patients require lifelong follow-up due to ongoing risks. This chapter discusses the optimal management of CoA across all age groups and offers insights into this straightforward yet challenging condition.

Keywords: Coarctation of the aorta, neonatal coarctation, surgical techniques, transcatheter intervention, balloon angioplasty, coarctation stenting

INTRODUCTION

The term "coarctation" originates from the Latin word "*coarctatus*" which means contracted or tightened. Typical coarctation of the aorta (CoA) is described as congenital narrowing of the upper descending thoracic aorta (DTA) at the isthmus adjacent to ductal insertion site, immediate distal to the origin of the left subclavian artery (LSCA) **(Fig. 1)**. On rare occasions coarctation may be in the arch proximal to LSCA, in DTA below the ductal insertion site and even sometimes may involve abdominal aorta. In most cases, involvement of the aorta is discrete, but occasionally it can be tubular long-segment narrowing. CoA can present in a variety of ways from neonatal age to adulthood. Either in isolation or in association with other cardiac defects, CoA accounts for approximately 4–8% of all congenital heart defects (CHDs) and occurs more commonly in males, with a male-to-female ratio of 2:1.[1] Clinical features and outcomes vary based on age, severity, and associated defects. Approximately 10% of CoA patients present in early infancy with high mortality if left untreated. Three-quarters of adult patients with CoA die by the fifth decade of life without intervention.[2] Despite advances reducing mortality, lifelong follow-up is essential due to risks of hypertension, aortopathy, and reintervention.

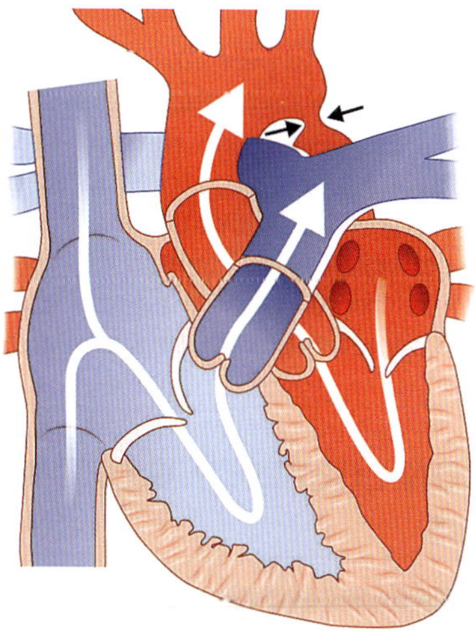

FIG. 1: Coarctation of the aorta.

EMBRYOGENESIS OF COA

The development of CoA during fetal life is disputed among researchers, leading to the coexistence of multiple theories which can be summarized as follows:

- *Edwards hypothetical totipotential double arch hypothesis*: Juxtaductal CoA is due to abnormal development of the embryonic fourth and sixth aortic arches as they connect to the dorsal aorta.[3]
- *The ductus arteriosus theory*: Coarctation is a result of incorporation of ductal tissue into the aortic isthmus

with subsequent constriction leading to narrowing of the aortic lumen.[4]

- *The hemodynamic theory*: In fetal circulation, aortic isthmus is the narrowest part of the DTA, receiving only 8% of the combined cardiac output. When associated with certain intracardiac lesions, such as a restrictive patent foramen ovale (PFO), left superior vena cava (LSVC) draining through the coronary sinus, congenital mitral stenosis, posteriorly malaligned ventricular septal defect (VSD), or left ventricular outflow tract obstruction (LVOTO), reduced flow through the aortic isthmus can lead to the development of coarctation.[5]
- *Neural crest theory*: Abnormal neural crest cell migration leads to an atypical tunica media and changes in the carotid body in the precoarctation aorta.

In Turner syndrome patients, lymphatic obstruction leads to a distended thoracic duct, which hinders aortic flow. This same mechanism causes neck webbing, making CoA more common in Turner syndrome patients with neck webbing.

GENETICS AND SYNDROMIC ASSOCIATION

Multiple single gene mutations have been detected in association with CoA. Nonsyndromic CoA is often linked to genes such as NOTCH1, MCTP2, and MATR-3, with NOTCH1 also being associated with familial bicuspid aortic valve disease.[6,7] Most common syndromic association of CoA is with Turner syndrome. Incidence of Turner syndrome in women with CoA is 12% whereas 10% of Turner syndrome candidates will have associated coarctation.[8] Therefore, it is advisable to screen for Turner syndrome in female babies with CoA and vice versa. CoA is also occasionally seen in other syndromes, such as neurofibromatosis, Kabuki syndrome, Williams syndrome, Noonan syndrome, and PHACES syndrome.

PATHOANATOMY

For localized coarctation, a 50% reduction in the cross-sectional diameter of the aortic isthmus is needed to be considered hemodynamically significant.[9] In tubular coarctation, even a smaller reduction can be significant. Classic coarctation features a ridge on the posterolateral wall of the aorta, made up of hypertrophied aortic media with an abnormal intimal layer. Postintervention, this abnormal tissue can proliferate, potentially leading to recurrent stenosis.[10] Occasionally, the DTA may kink due to the pull of the ligamentum arteriosum, a condition known as "pseudocoarctation", which does not necessarily create a significant pressure gradient.

Recent evidence shows that the prestenotic proximal aorta remains stiffer and has a dysfunctional endothelial layer, regardless of age or intervention type. This persistent stiffness increases the risk of systemic hypertension, left ventricular hypertrophy (LVH), ischemic heart disease, and stroke, even after successful repair.[11]

Collateral circulation between proximal and distal aorta is striking feature of coarctation which gets well developed by 5–6 years **(Fig. 2)**. This is responsible for some well-known clinical and radiological signs of CoA. Inflow to these collaterals predominantly comes from SCA which is responsible for classic rib notching seen in chest X-ray. Unilateral rib notching is seen if the contralateral SCA flow is limited by coarctation.

Aneurysmal dilation commonly occurs distal to the coarctation segment and sometimes at the proximal LSCA due to low pressure and high-velocity blood flow. The prevalence of these aneurysms increases with age, reaching up to 20% by the third decade of life.[12] CoA can also coexist with intracranial aneurysms (IAs), mainly involving the circle of Willis. The overall prevalence of IAs in follow-up patients with repaired CoA is 3.8% in normotensive patients and 10% in those with persistent systemic hypertension.[13] Routine screening for IAs in asymptomatic patients with repaired CoA is generally of low yield, but screening may be more prudent for those with risk factors such as older age or uncontrolled hypertension.

Hemodynamic Consequences of CoA; Illustration from Neonate to Adulthood

In fetal life, only 8% of left ventricular cardiac output passes through the aortic isthmus, with the majority of DTA circulation maintained by RV output via a right-to-left shunt through PDA. Therefore, severe CoA does not significantly disrupt circulation during fetal development. When the baby is born with critical coarctation following hemodynamic sequences take place **(Flowchart 1)**.

The clinical impact of coarctation is exacerbated by presence of a VSD potentially increasing the risk of heart failure during early infancy. As the child grows beyond infancy, the LV develops concentric hypertrophy along with other compensatory circulatory changes. They remain asymptomatic through childhood, adolescence, and young adulthood. However, upper extremity systemic hypertension is a key clinical finding that often reveals the presence of coarctation in them.

The mechanisms of hypertension in coarctation have been debated, leading to various theories on its pathogenesis. Long-term risk of hypertension persists throughout life, even after early neonatal repair. Studies indicate that about one-third of CoA patients develop hypertension during adolescence, despite having undergone early and effective surgical repair. Accepted theories explaining pathogenesis of hypertension can be summarized as follows **(Flowchart 2)**.[14]

COMMON COEXISTING CARDIAC LESIONS

The CoA is usually an isolated anomaly, but in 18–35% of cases, it is associated with other cardiac lesions. The most common coexisting anomaly is a bicuspid aortic valve, found in about

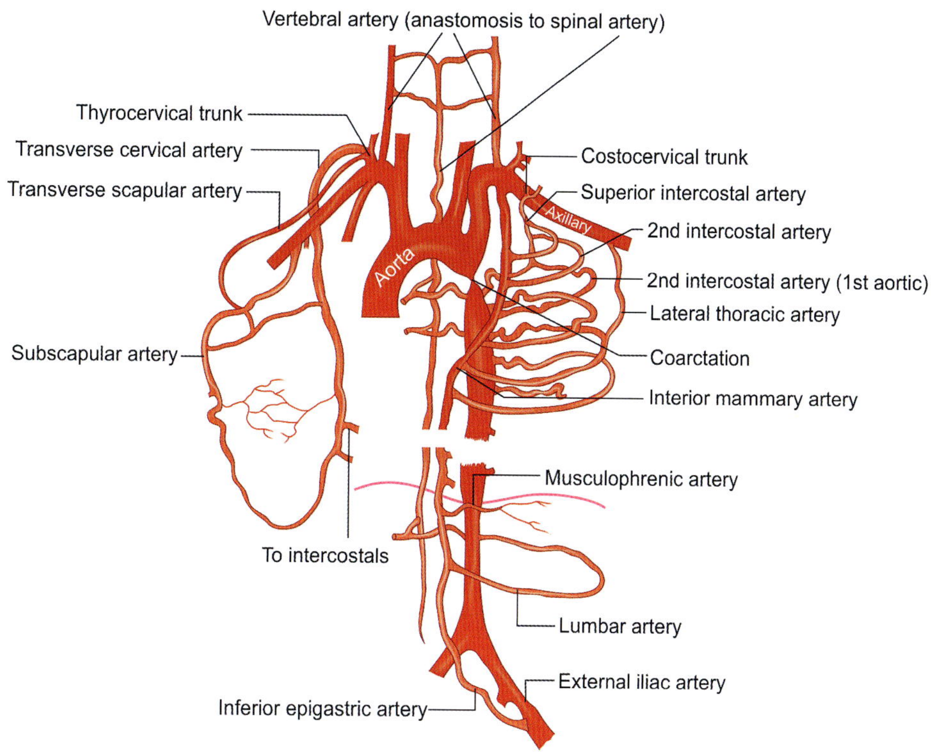

FIG. 2: The intercostal, internal mammary, scapular, and lumbar vessels' collaterals are depicted in the figure.

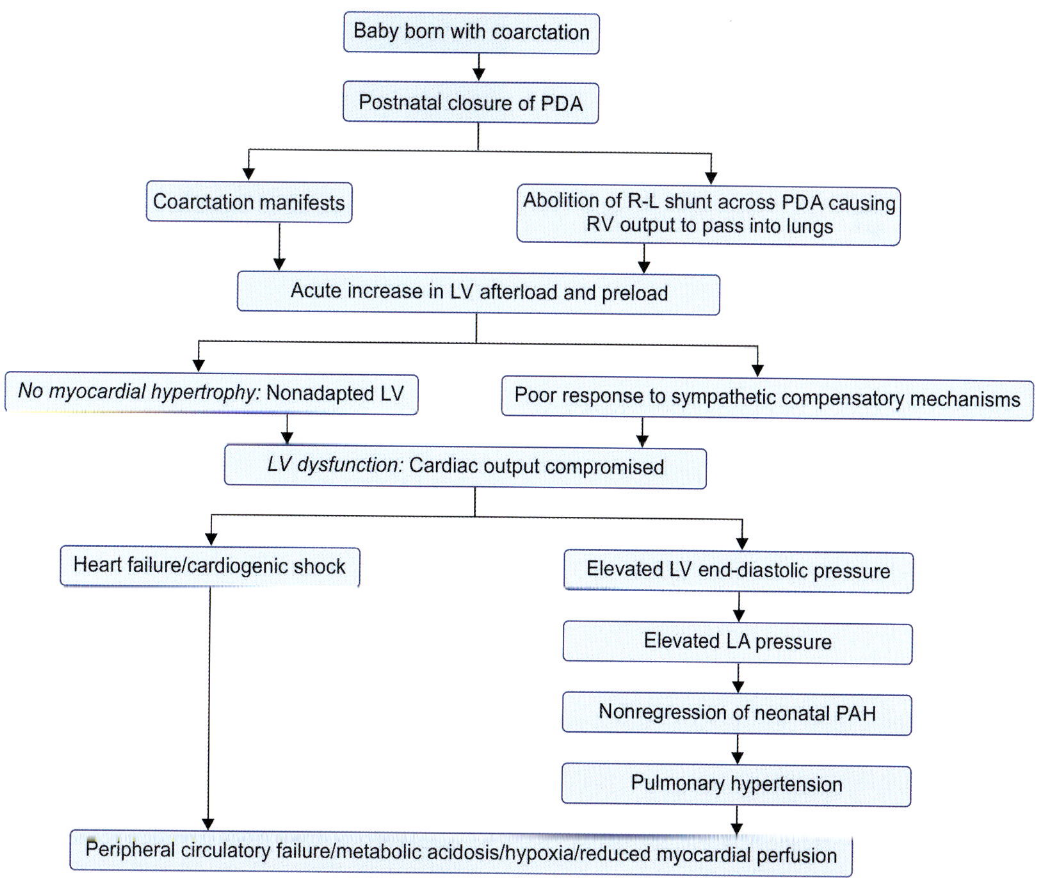

FLOWCHART 1: Sequence of hemodynamic in neonate.

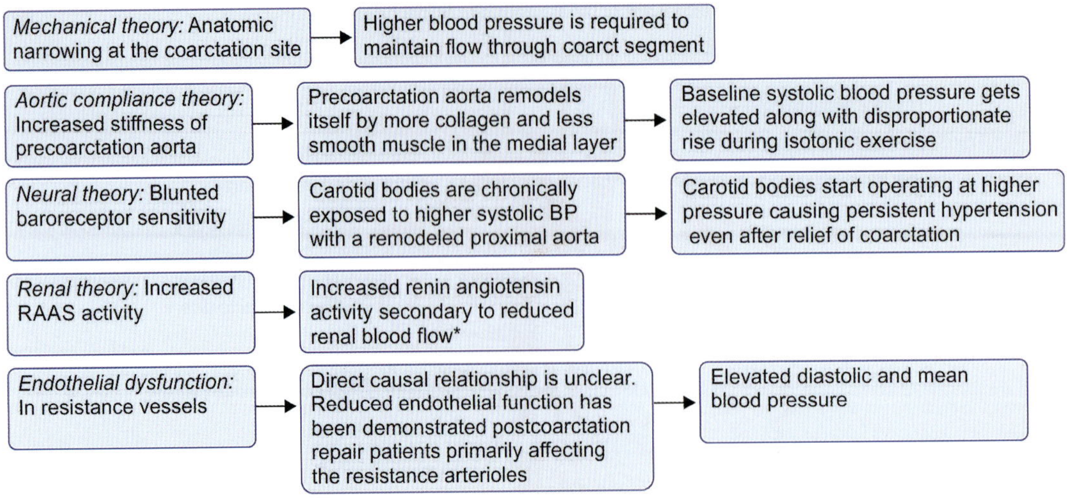

*Measurement of plasma renin activity in human subjects did not show consistently elevated plasma renin level in multiple studies. Recent animal models have shown increased expression of angiotensin II receptors in brain persisting even after successful CoA repair.[15]

FLOWCHART 2: Pathogenesis of hypertension.

50% of cases.[16] A VSD, which may be perimembranous, muscular, or malaligned outlet, is the next most frequent coexisting anomaly.[16]

Left-sided obstructive lesions, such as those seen in classic or partial Shone's complex, are frequently linked with CoA or even a tubular hypoplasia of the aortic arch.[17] Other anomalies that can reduce aortic flow and present with CoA include Taussig-Bing anomaly, tricuspid atresia with d-TGA, and hypoplastic left heart syndrome.

ARSA originating below the site of coarctation is seen in about 5% of cases and is considered a risk factor for early recurrence of CoA after initial repair.[18]

CLINICAL FEATURES

Critical CoA with a right-to-left shunt across the ductus arteriosus can sometimes be detected at birth through pulse oximetry screening. However, most cases of coarctation only become apparent after the ductus arteriosus closes, typically manifesting symptoms within 1–2 weeks after birth. Key clinical signs include cardiogenic shock—characterized by irritability, pallor, tachycardia, tachypnea, and increasing metabolic acidosis—as well as clinically impalpable femoral pulses. Without prompt intervention, these infants face a significant risk of mortality. Similar presentations can occur throughout early infancy.

Beyond infancy, children with isolated coarctation typically remain asymptomatic. During adolescence to young adulthood, symptoms such as headaches, lower limb claudication, or the detection of an incidental murmur can reveal the presence of coarctation. If left untreated, the risk of mortality increases beyond the third decade of life.[2] The primary causes of death are heart failure, aortic dissection or rupture, infective endarteritis, and rupture of an IA.

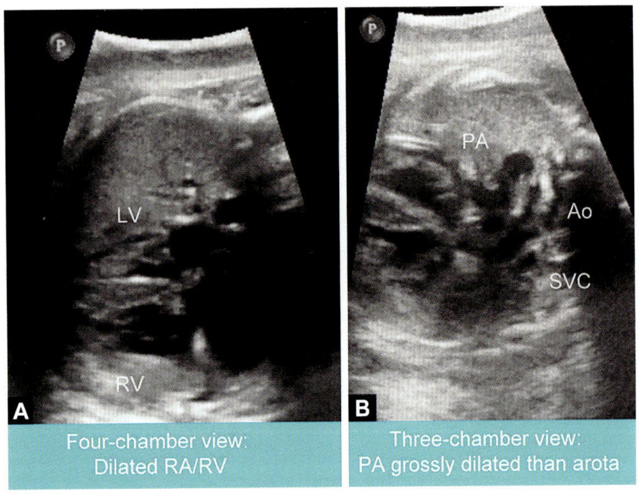

FIGS. 3A AND B: Fetal echo showing features of coarctation.

DIAGNOSTIC EVALUATION

Fetal Diagnosis

CoA often eludes a prenatal echocardiographic screening and manifests in the first few days of life as critical CHD. However, there are certain imaging pearls that should make the physician strongly suspect an evolving coarctation like:

- RV:LV ratio > 1.5 in four chamber view **(Fig. 3A)**.[19]
- In three-vessel view, a marked size difference between the pulmonary artery (PA) and aorta (Ao) with a ratio of ≥1.7 **(Fig. 3B)**.[19]
- *The carotid-subclavian artery index (CSAI)*: A ratio of the aortic arch diameter at the level of LSCA, to distal transverse arch length, smaller value suggests a higher risk of coarctation **(Figs. 4A and B)**.[20]

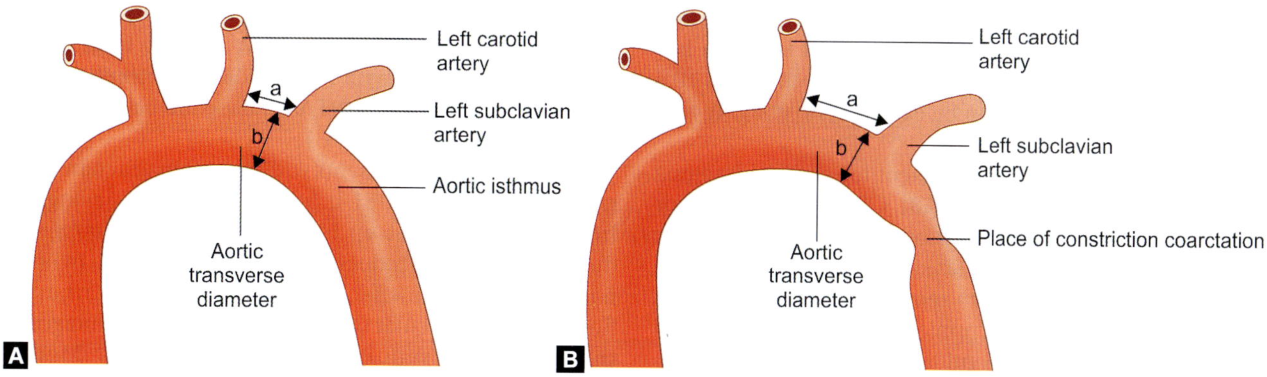

FIGS. 4A AND B: CSAI is a ratio between b/a. A value < 0.78 predicts risk of coarctation.

- Persistent LSVC is seen in association with coarctation in 21% of cases.[21]

Diagnosis in Neonatal and Infantile Presentation

Transthoracic echocardiography (TTE) typically confirms the diagnosis, showing localized stenosis with a fibrous posterior ductal shelf beyond the LSCA origin. Significant obstruction occurs when the artery is narrowed by >50%. Measurements of all arch segments should follow American Society of Echocardiography guidelines **(Fig. 5)**. Right ventricular dominance, LV dysfunction, and pulmonary hypertension are common findings. Continuous-wave Doppler in CoA usually shows peak systolic acceleration and diastolic tailing. An echo gradient of 20 mm Hg with diastolic tailing indicates significant CoA, though the gradient may be underestimated in cases such as LV dysfunction, coexisting aortic stenosis, large ductus, or extensive collaterals.[22] Coarctation may only appear after ductal closure if a large PDA with a narrow isthmus is present **(Fig. 6)**.

Computed tomography (CT) aortogram may be done in selective cases for surgical planning when transthoracic echo images are suboptimal.

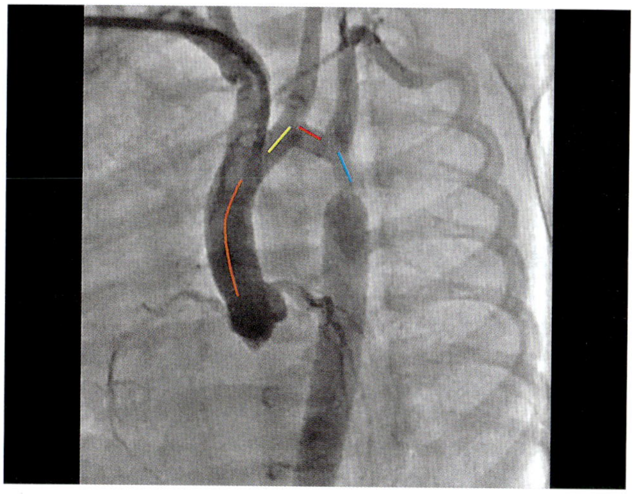

FIG. 5: Aortogram showing parts of aorta: Ascending Aorta (orange line), proximal transverse arch (yellow line), distal transverse arch (red line), and isthmus (blue line). Aortic diameter and z scores should be measured at all these parts.

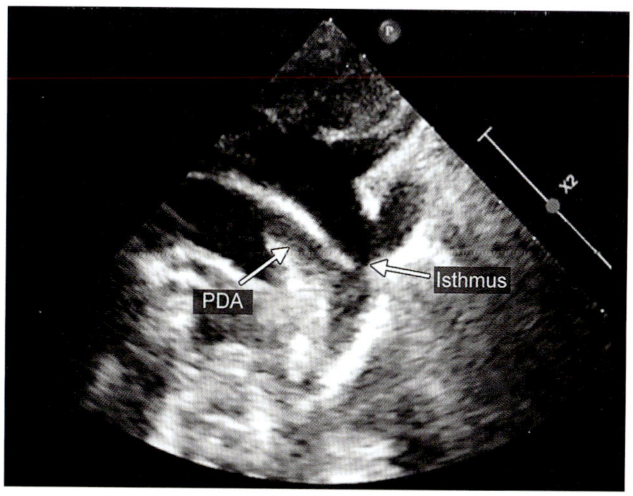

FIG. 6: Coarctation in a neonate with prominent anterior ductal shelf, narrow isthmus, and large PDA.

Diagnosis in Childhood to Adult Age Presentation

Understanding the anatomic extent of coarctation, including details of aneurysms, arch vessel branching pattern, and collateral circulation, is crucial for treatment planning. In isolated coarctation, ECG typically shows left ventricular pressure overload. The classic radiological appearance of bilateral notching from the third to eighth posterior ribs becomes apparent after 5–6 years of age **(Fig. 7)**. These collaterals arise from the ipsilateral subclavian artery (SCA). When the left or right SCA is involved by the coarctation, ipsilateral collaterals fail to develop.

TTE may not provide detailed imaging of the aorta in adults, but it can effectively assess the pressure gradient across the coarctation **(Fig. 8)** and detect associated anomalies like a bicuspid aortic valve. LVH is also a key marker of the disease. Occasionally, complications like endarteritis may be picked up by careful echo imaging also **(Figs. 9A and B)**.

CT aortogram is usually sufficient for optimal imaging and management planning **(Fig. 10)**. CT is also essential for follow-up after repair. Complications such as recoarctation, aortic aneurysm, pseudoaneurysm, and aortic dissection can occur years after primary repair.[23,24] Screening for IA should be considered during primary CT aortogram (class 2B recommendation; 2022 AHA guidelines) **(Box 1)**.[22]

MANAGEMENT

In Neonates with Critical Coarctation

In presence of critical CoA, hemodynamic stability of the baby relies on right to left blood flow through the PDA.

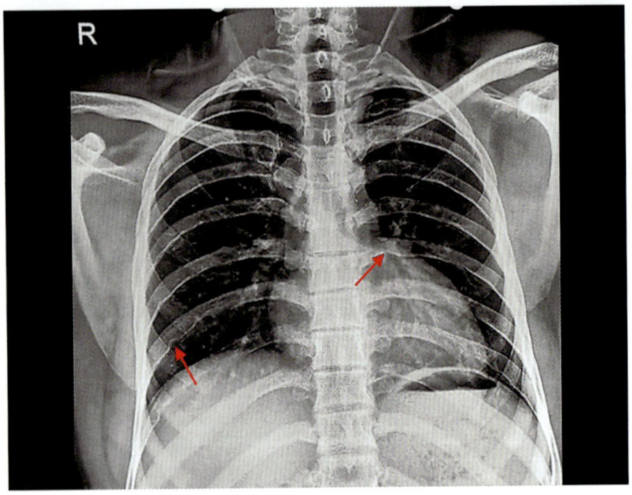

FIG. 7: Chest X-ray showing bilateral rib notching (red arrows).

In presence of narrow isthmus with ductal shelf, there is usually no obstruction in DTA flow as long as PDA remains open. The closure of the ductal ampulla leads to severe obstruction in the DTA, causing the baby to become symptomatic **(Figs. 11A to C)**.

When a neonate presents with symptomatic coarctation, rapid initiation of PGE1 infusion can be life-saving. The infusion can start at up to 50 ng/kg/min to reopen the ductus and then be reduced to 5–10 ng/kg/min to maintain patency.[25] Adverse effects such as apnea, hyperthermia, flushing, and muscular twitching are generally manageable, though apnea requires close monitoring. Medical stabilization may also require inotropic support and diuretics until definitive intervention can be performed.

Surgery is the preferred definitive treatment for infants with coarctation, offering a 98% survival rate and a 90% freedom from reintervention at a median follow-up of 4.8 years.[26] Surgical repair is also feasible in preterm infants weighing < 2.5 kg, though this group faces higher risks of surgical mortality and early reintervention.[27]

Commonly performed surgical techniques are as follows **(Figs. 12A to D)**:

- Resection with end-to-end anastomosis
- Prosthetic patch aortoplasty
- Interposition graft insertion across the area of coarctation
- Subclavian flap aortoplasty

Resection with end-to-end anastomosis initially showed high recurrence rates.[28] To address this, Waldhausen and associates introduced subclavian flap aortoplasty to avoid circumferential suturing.[29] However, later studies did not show a significant advantage in reducing recurrence with this technique. Additionally, risks such as limb length shortening and vertebrobasilar steal were noted.[30] As a result, this technique is no longer commonly practiced.

Prosthetic patch aortoplasty carries a risk of aneurysmal degeneration over time, making it less suitable for infants.[31] Tubular interposition grafts are also not ideal because they

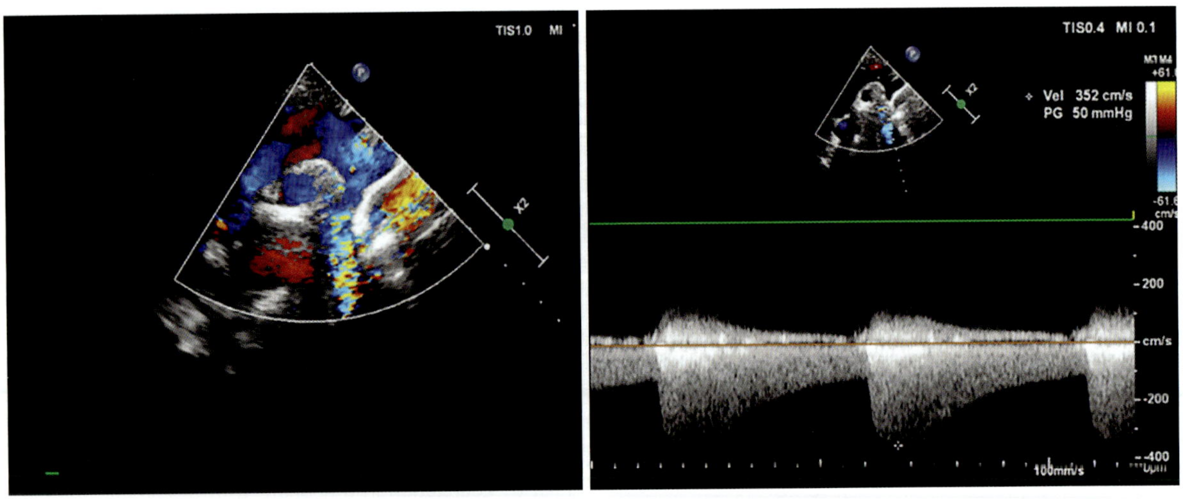

FIG. 8: Color Doppler and continuous wave Doppler images from suprasternal view showing continuous flow with significant pressure gradient and diastolic tailing.

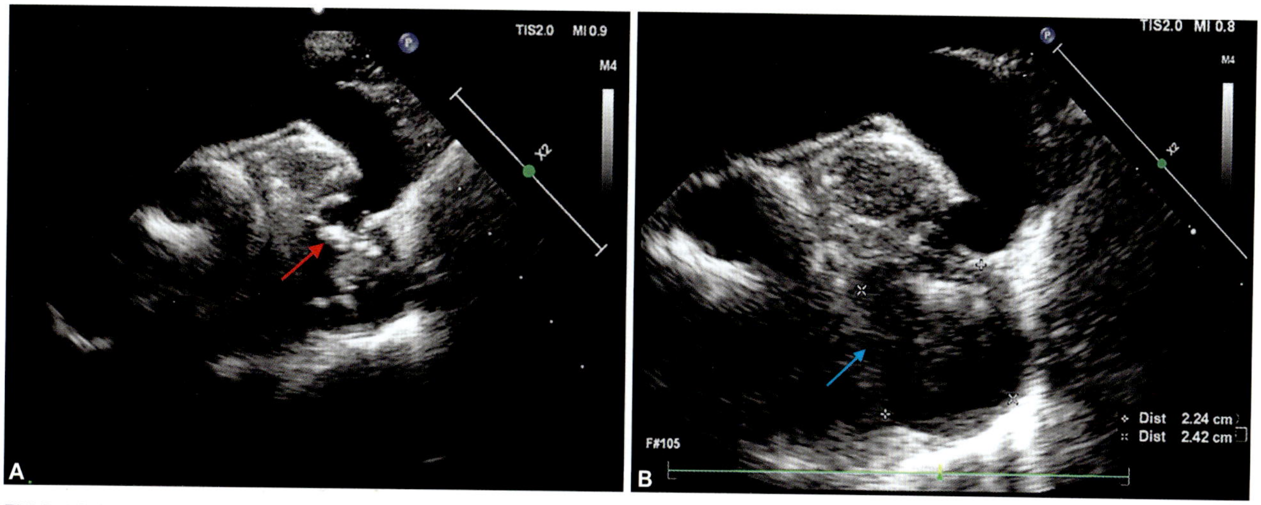

FIGS. 9A AND B: End-arteritis showing a vegetation (red arrow) and a large aneurysm (blue arrow) in an adolescent boy.

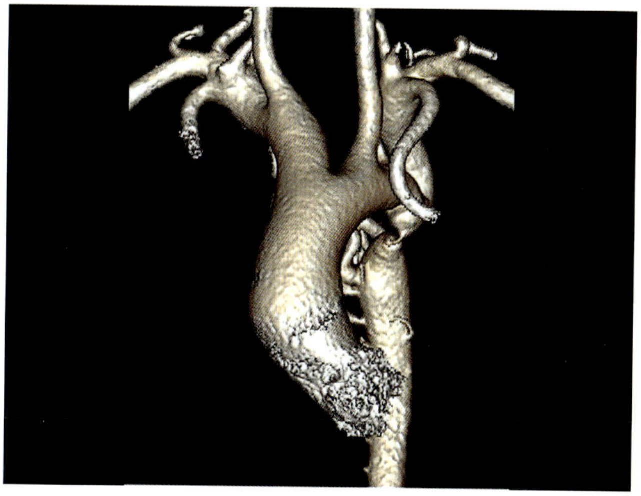

FIG. 10: CT aortogram with 3D reconstruction image showing discrete postsubclavian coarctation.

BOX 1 **Diagnostic criteria for significant coarctation in adult as per AHA 2022 guideline.**

The presence of significant CoA is based on evidence of upper extremity hypertension (at rest, on ambulatory BP monitoring, or with pathologic blood pressure response to exercise) or left ventricular hypertrophy and evidence for one of these gradient measurements.

- A noninvasive blood pressure difference of >20 mm Hg between the upper and lower extremities
- A peak-to-peak gradient of 20 mm Hg across the coarct by catheterization; or a peak-to-peak gradient of 10 mm Hg across the coarctation by catheterization in the setting of decreased left ventricular systolic function or significant collateral flow
- A mean gradient of >20 mm Hg across the coarct by Doppler echocardiography; or a mean gradient of 10 mm Hg across the coarct by Doppler echocardiography in the setting of decreased left ventricular systolic function or significant collateral flow

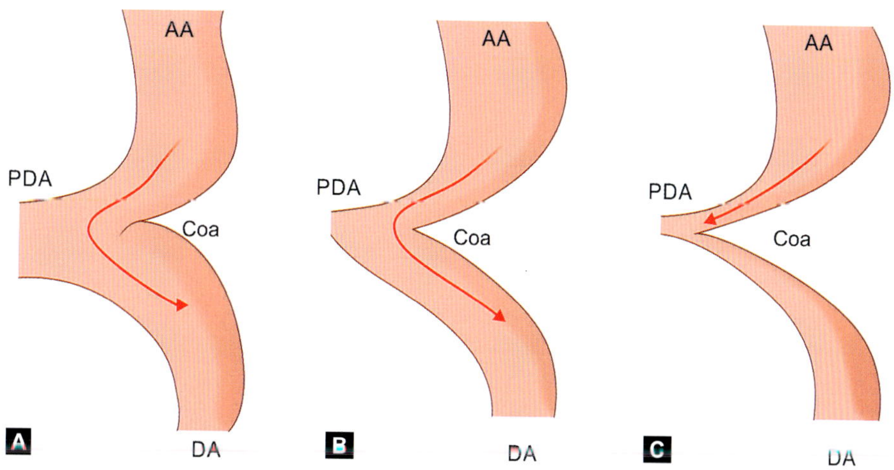

FIGS. 11A TO C: Closure of the ductal ampulla leads to severe obstruction in neonate.

do not grow with the child. In 1977, Dr Amato introduced the extended end-to-end anastomosis technique, which has become the primary surgical method for addressing aortic coarctation.[32] This technique offers a wider suture area compared to the classic Crafoord method, reducing the risk of stricture and restenosis. Studies have shown relatively low recoarctation rates, ranging from 4 to 13%.[33]

A rare but serious complication after surgery in neonates is postcoarctectomy syndrome, which involves gastrointestinal symptoms due to paradoxical hypertension; it typically occurs within the first 3–4 days after surgery and requires close monitoring.

Transcatheter balloon angioplasty (BA) plays a limited but important role in managing neonates and infants with aortic coarctation. Angiographic images often picks up associated arch anomalies very well **(Figs. 13A and B)**. This intervention works by inducing a controlled tear in the intima and media layers of the constricted vessel, allowing for remodeling of the aortic wall and resolution of the coarctation. Measurements of the DTA at the coarctation site, as well as proximal and distal to the lesion, guide the selection of an appropriately sized balloon for dilation. Typically, the balloon diameter should match the DTA diameter at the diaphragm level, with a maximum balloon diameter not exceeding three times the width of the coarctation segment.

Despite its utility, BA is not usually the first choice for primary intervention due to a high recurrence rate (nearly 50%) and potential vascular complications.[34] It is generally reserved for cases with associated ventricular dysfunction to stabilize patients before definitive surgical repair. However, some centers have recently reported success with BA as a primary treatment in late infancy.[35] BA remains a preferred option for infants with postsurgical restenosis.

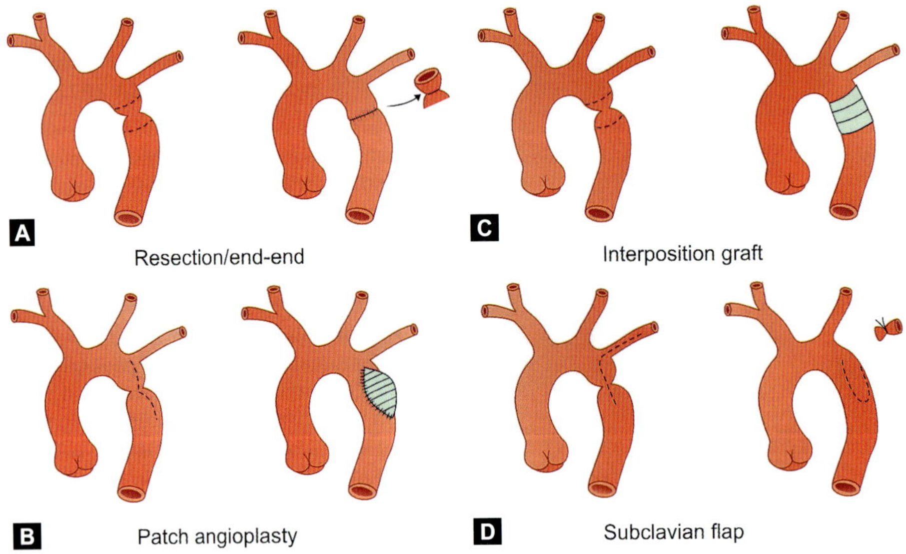

FIGS. 12A TO D: Major surgical techniques for coarctation repair.

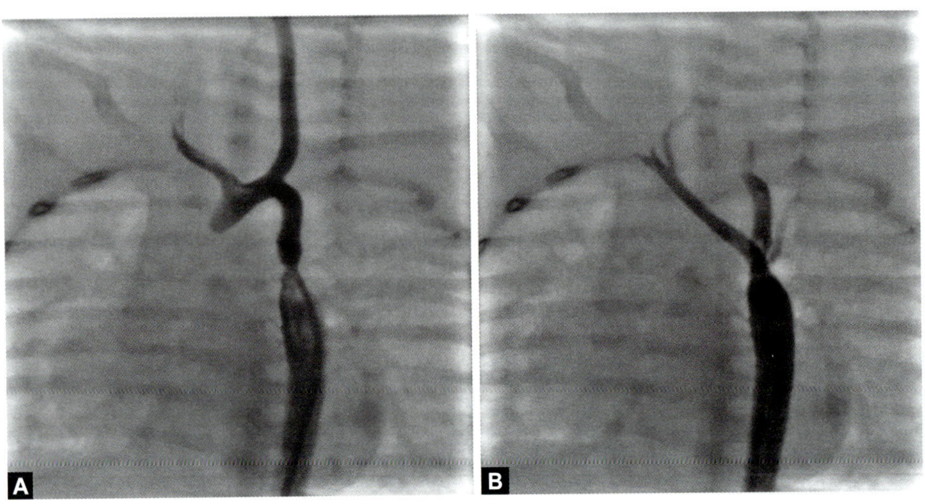

FIGS. 13A AND B: Aortogram of a neonate taken during balloon coarctoplasty showing presence of ARSA.

Endovascular stenting is generally not an option for infants, though some case reports exist in the literature. The novel "Renata Minima" stent, designed for treating coarctation in infants, has shown promising results in early feasibility studies.[36] This stent can be dilated up to 24 mm in diameter and is designed to accommodate the somatic growth of the baby, allowing for multiple dilations without compromising its structural integrity.

Management in Children

Traditionally, surgery is considered the standard treatment for CoA. For children over one year and under 20 kg, balloon angioplasty (BA) is commonly used as the primary procedure in some centers with experience. Endovascular stenting is generally avoided in smaller children due to the technical challenges posed by the large sheath size required to implant adult-sized stents. However, some centers now perform stenting as the primary procedure even in children weighing as little as 10 kg.

A large multicenter retrospective study of transcatheter interventions in 1,187 CoA patients found that 19% of children weighing ≤10 kg and 43% of those weighing between 10 and 20 kg underwent stent implantation as a primary procedure. Percutaneous stenting has a higher reintervention rate compared to surgery with an advantage of significantly low acute procedural complication. With advances in technology, endovascular stenting is increasingly being adopted as a preferred option for smaller children, whether for native CoA or restenosis cases.

Stents, balloon angioplasty, and surgical repair remain viable treatment options for children. Parents and caregivers should be informed of the benefits and risks of each procedure to make an informed decision about the mode of therapy.

Management in Adolescents and Adults

For adolescents and adults, transcatheter stent implantation is the preferred treatment for both native and recurrent CoA. The Congenital Cardiovascular Interventional Study Consortium (CCISC) and the Coarctation of Aorta Stent Trial (COAST) trials reported excellent acute procedural success rates of 96% and 99%, respectively.[38,39] Long-term follow-up data showed a restenosis rate of 4% predominantly in younger patients.

The COAST II trial highlighted the effectiveness of the covered Cheatham-Platinum stent in preventing or treating acute aortic wall injury, leading to its FDA approval in 2016.[40] Multiple other types of open cell and hybrid cell stents have been used in treatment coarctation (Genesis XD, Zephyr, IntraStent LD, Andra stent, etc.) **(Figs. 14A and B)**. The US IMPACT registry indicated that covered stents are increasingly used, with their use rising to 23% overall, particularly in older patients.[41] Aortic pseudoaneurysms associated with CoA are almost exclusively treated with covered stents. Covered stents are also employed to address aortic wall injury from BA or bare-metal stents, as their fabric reduces shear stress and prevents restenosis and long-term stent fracture. BA plays a role in case of restenosis **(Figs. 15A and B)**.

LONG-TERM OUTCOME AND FOLLOW-UP

After surgical or percutaneous repair of CoA, long-term outcomes must be carefully monitored. Key complications to watch for include hypertension, restenosis, and aneurysms at the site of intervention. Lifelong follow-up is crucial, involving regular monitoring and management of hypertension. Periodic echocardiography and CT/MR aortograms are necessary to detect and address any issues that may arise.

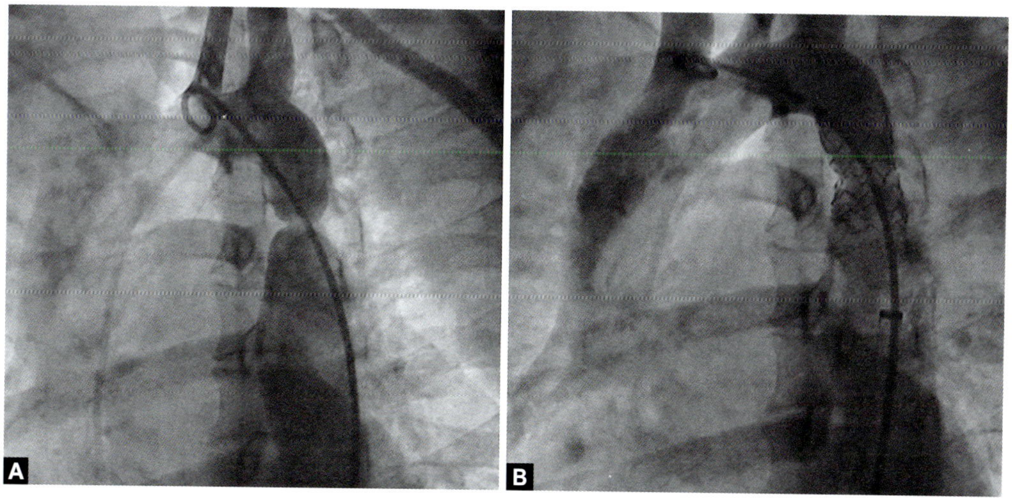

FIGS. 14A AND B: Coarctation stenting in a 35-year-old female using Zephyr XL stent.

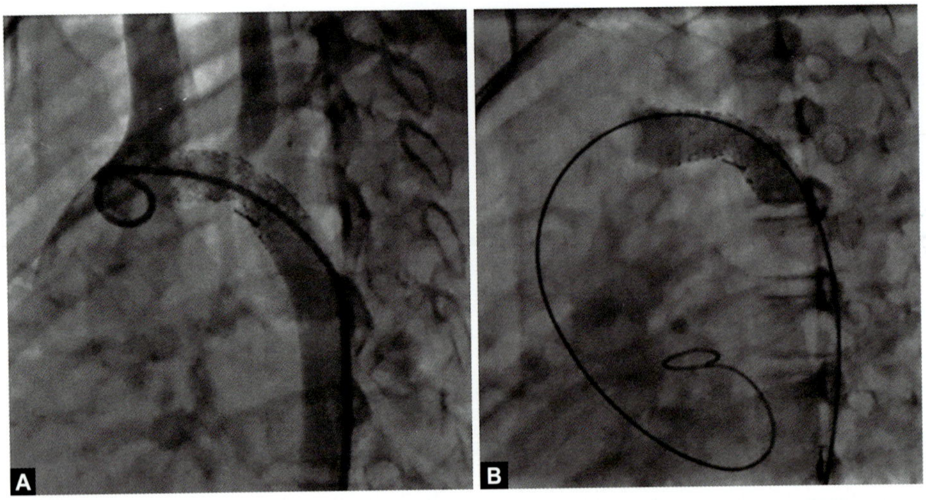

FIGS. 15A AND B: Balloon dilation of DTA stent for restenosis after coarctation stenting at 5 years follow-up.

CONCLUSION

The CoA is a common congenital heart disease that requires lifelong follow-up regardless of the severity of the lesion, age of intervention, or type of intervention. Despite advances in early diagnosis and various treatment options, patients with CoA continue to face cardiovascular risks compared to the general population. Continued improvements in procedural techniques and strategies to minimize long-term complications are essential for better managing this condition and enhancing patient outcomes.

ONLINE REFERENCES

Please scan the QR code provided at the end of the table of contents for References of this chapter.

CHAPTER

99

Diagnosis and Management of Fetal Heart Disease

Chandan Kumar Das

ABSTRACT

Congenital heart disease (CHD) is on the rise due to multifactorial causes. Many of such diseases can be diagnosed prenatally by fetal imaging like fetal echocardiography, magnetic resonance imaging (MRI), magnetocardiography, and fetal electrocardiography. Some of fatal arrhythmias can be addressed with maternal pharmacological interventions or direct fetal pharmacological intervention. Certain congenital cardiac lesions evolve in utero due to faulty circulation, which can be corrected prenatally by fetal percutaneous and pharmacological interventions.

Keywords: Congenital heart disease, echocardiography, magnetocardiography, percutaneous intervention

INTRODUCTION

Amidst the various diversities of culture, education, level of health awareness, and availability of health services, India shares the incidences of congenital heart disease (CHD) almost at par with other parts of the world. Needless to say, when a child is born with CHD, the entire family irrespective of its socioeconomic status gets gripped by a never-ending grim. With the advent of science today, many corners of such underaccessed twig of medical tree have been illuminated. Although the prevalence of CHD does not differ much in developed and developing countries, most children with CHD are diagnosed early and undergo timely intervention in countries like the United States. Hence, there is a long way to go. Earlier, the diagnosis used to be suspected clinically at the postnatal stage and then the plan of evaluation by echocardiography was managed accordingly. By that time, many irreversible changes used to take place in the course of fetal heart disease. Now, with the advent of newer technology in the field of cardiac imaging, CHD can be diagnosed well in advance in the fetal stage as early as 12th week of intrauterine life. In this chapter, we shall be going through the burden of fetal heart diseases, optimal approach to diagnose them with logistics, and, of course, the feasibility of pharmacological, percutaneous, and surgical interventions to treat them in utero.

EPIDEMIOLOGY

Congenital heart disease is the most frequently occurring congenital disorder comprising almost 28% of all congenital birth defects. In India, CHD has a birth prevalence of 8/1,000 resulting in almost 200,000 children born with CHD every year.[1] Out of these, nearly 50,000 children would require intervention during infancy or earlier. Among the fetus detected with CHD, the most severe form is seen in almost 1.5–1.7/1,000 live births.[2] Most of these data are reported from various pediatric centers. As such, there is no strong database system in India to get live birth with CHD reporting. All these data are from full-term babies. It could be 10 times higher in preterm infants (8.3%). In general practice, the referral for fetal echocardiography (FE) is recommended when the probability of fetal CHD is greater than about three times the background population risk, or >1%.

SPECTRUM OF FETAL HEART DISEASES

Many CHD lesions do not need correction or one can wait for natural course without any complication. Lesions like atrial septal defect (ASD) < 5 mm, patent ductus arteriosus < 2 mm with left ventricular volume overload, ventricular septal defect (VSD) with a gradient of >30 mm Hg, aortic stenosis

(AS)/pulmonic stenosis with gradients of <25 mm Hg, and pulmonary artery branch stenosis with gradients of <20 mm Hg are likely to normalize within 6 weeks of postnatal life. Those which may require early intervention are ASD with defect > 5 mm, PDA size > 2 mm with left ventricular volume overload, restrictive VSD, and valvular aortic/pulmonary stenosis with gradients < 25 mm Hg (in addition to major CHD). Some cyanotic lesions like tetralogy of Fallot (TOF) need repairs by 6 months of postnatal life.[3] Apart from the structural cardiac defect in the fetus, there are fetal arrhythmias; some of them may be fatal. If detected prenatally, their correction may prevent secondary cardiac changes. All such anomalies can be studied in the fetus by magnetic resonance imaging (MRI), FE with M-mode, magnetocardiography, and electrocardiography of the fetus.

DIAGNOSIS: ASSESSMENT OF PRETEST PROBABILITY

Maternal Factors

Diabetes Mellitus

Diabetes mellitus (DM) is one of the commonly affecting maternal factors during pregnancy which can complicate the ingrowing fetus. There is almost a fivefold increase of risk for fetal CHD in pregestational diabetic mothers. In such cases, higher incidences of single ventricle, transpositions of great vessels, heterotaxy, and truncus arteriosus have been reported.[4]

Phenylketonuria

It is found that there is a 10- to 15-fold increased risk of CHD in the fetus with maternal serum levels of phenylalanine (>15 mg/dL). CHDs like coarctation of aorta (CoA), VSD, TOF, and hypoplastic left heart syndrome (HLHS) are associated with maternal phenylketonuria.[5]

Positive Autoantibody and Autoimmune Disease

Congenital complete heart block (CHB) in the fetus with maternal lupus and other connective tissue disorders have been reported.[6]

Maternal Medication Effect

Many studies have reported the commonly toxic drugs that are used by the pregnant mother causing various CHDs in the fetus. These are angiotensin-converting enzyme inhibitors (ACEI), retinoic acid, anticonvulsants, lithium, nonsteroidal anti-inflammatory agents (NSAIDs), and selective serotonin reuptake inhibitors (SSRIs). Maternal exposure to ACEI after the first trimester has been reported to cause fetal CHD like ASD and PDA.[7] A vitamin A analog, retinoic acid, is teratogenic. Maternal exposure to this drug has been reported to cause CHDs like conotruncal defects and aortic arch anomalies in the fetus.[8] Vitamin K antagonists like warfarin and other coumadin derivatives are supposed to be teratogenic. A recent multicenter prospective study reported no risk of CHD in the fetus, although other birth defects have been observed.[9] Maternal use of NSAIDs during the first trimester has been reported to cause fetal cardiac malformations like septal defects.[10]

Maternal Infection

Maternal infections with fever (viral like rubella, cytomegalovirus, parvovirus, herpes, varicella, and *Enterovirus*) were associated with cardiac malformations like pulmonary arterial stenosis, PDA, and VSD in the fetus in a population-based study.[11]

Assisted Reproduction Technology

Today, with the advent of modern technology, there is a surge of infertility clinics where artificial inseminations and assisted pregnancy are on the rise. There are few observations with increased incidences of fetal cardiac malformations like ASD and VSD, especially in monozygotic twinning.[12]

Maternal CHD

If the pregnant mother is a known case of a CHD, there is a chance of inheritance by the fetus. CHDs likely to be carried by the ingrowing fetus are heterotaxy, atrioventricular septal defect (AVSD), AS 10–18%, and TOF or dTGA up to 3%.[13]

Paternal CHD

Despite variance, few studies have shown a 2–3% risk of inheritance of CHDs from the father, especially bicuspid aortic valve and other nonsyndromic CHDs.[14]

Siblings with CHD

If more than one sibling in a family carry CHD, there is a fair chance (2–6%) of the fetus to get affected with cardiac malformation.

Fetal Factors

Based on Abnormal Obstetric Ultrasound Study

During the obstetric ultrasound study, the four-chamber view of fetal heart is sometimes reported to be abnormal. About 40% of such cases have been detected to have fetal CHD.[15]

Based on Abnormal Heart Rate or Rhythm

An abnormal fetal heart is suspected when a fetal tachycardia is detected. But to confirm the presence of a fetal bradycardia, one has to rule out congenital CHB or long QT syndrome (LQTS).[16] It is very important to understand the nature of the ectopics in fetal cardiac rhythm. It is difficult to differentiate atrial premature contraction (APC) from ventricular premature contraction (VPC). If it persists for >2 weeks, one should be careful to rule out CHD like cardiomyopathy or stressful situations; fetal anemia, acardiac twins, and other arteriovenous malformations; and twin-to-twin transfusion syndrome (TTTS).

Presence of Noncardiac Anomaly

Obstetric ultrasound-detected fetal anomaly may carry cardiac malformation in some cases. Multiple studies have found 20–45% cardiac malformations with more than one extracardiac anomaly.[17] Apart from these, fetal CHDs have been detected in various fetal anomalies like *known or suspected chromosomal abnormality, increased nuchal translucency on first trimester screening,*[18] *abnormalities of the umbilical cord and venous system, monochorionic twinning, nonimmune hydrops fetalis, and effusions.*

Assessment of Some Extracardiac Factors of the Fetus with CHD

Genetic assessment reveals abnormality in many cases of fetal CHD. Almost 15% of infants born with CHD have chromosomal abnormalities. Most of these are aneuploidies, with trisomies 21, 13, and 18 and monosomy X.

INDICATIONS FOR FETAL HEART IMAGING

Apart from the clinical background, drug history, and family history of the maternal side, some fetal factors should also be considered. Imaging of the fetal heart is done to assess the fetal heart structure as well as its function. The fetal circulation, structure of the fetal heart, its physiology, rhythm, and performances can be assessed by FE **(Fig. 1)** and MRI. The potential indications for FE have been briefed in **Table 1**.

Figures 2 to 8 show some fetal cardiac anomalies that one commonly comes across.

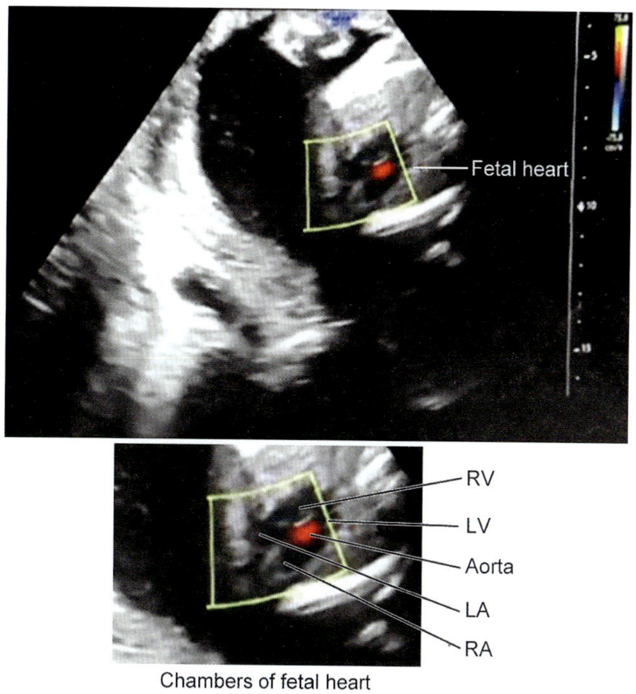

FIG. 1: Normal fetal heart.

TABLE 1: Potential indications for fetal echocardiography.

	ASE (2023) recommendation	AIUM (2020)	AHA (2014)
Maternal factors (absolute risk)			
Pregestational diabetes (3–5%)	Is indicated	Is indicated	I (indicated)
Gestational diabetes diagnosed after second trimester (<1%)	Not indicated	Not indicated	III (no benefit)
Phenylketonuria (12–14%)	Is indicated	Is indicated	I (indicated)
Autoimmune disease: SSA/SSB positive (1–5%)	Is indicated	Is indicated	IIa (probably indicated)
In vitro fertilization (1.1–3.3%)	May be considered	Is indicated	IIa (probably indicated)
Maternal infection: Rubella (3–4%)	Is indicated	Is indicated	I (indicated)
Family history of CHD: First-degree relative (3–20%)	Is indicated	Is indicated	I (Indicated)
Family history of CHD: Second-degree or more distant relative (<2%)	Not indicated	May be indicated	IIb (may be indicated)
Obesity (BMI > 30 kg/m^2) (1–2%)	Not indicated	Not indicated	–
Retinoid (8–20%)	Is indicated	Is indicated	I (indicated)
ACE inhibitors (3%)	May be considered	May be indicated	IIa (probably indicated)
Selective serotonin reuptake inhibitors (1–2%)	Not indicated	Not indicated	III (no benefit)
Anticonvulsants (1–2%)	Not Indicated	May be indicated	IIb (may be indicated)

Continued

Continued

	ASE (2023) recommendation	AIUM (2020)	AHA (2014)
Maternal factors (absolute risk)			
Lithium (1–2%)	Not indicated	May be indicated	IIb (may be indicated)
Warfarin (<1%)	Not indicated	Not indicated	III (no benefit)
Fetal factors identified during screening (absolute risk)			
Fetal hydrops (15–20%)	Is indicated	Is indicated	I (indicated)
Extracardiac anomaly (20–45%)	Is indicated	Is indicated	I (indicated)
Chromosomal abnormalities (10–90%)	Is indicated	Is indicated	I (indicated)
Monochorionic twinning (2–10%)	Is indicated	Is indicated	I (indicated)
Nuchal translucency 3.0–3.4 mm (3%)	May be considered	May be indicated	IIa (probably indicated)
Single umbilical artery in isolation (1.2–1.8%)	Not indicated	Not indicated	IIb (may be indicated)

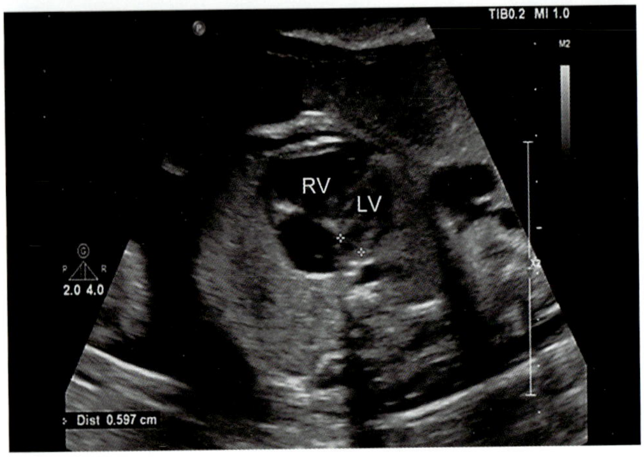

FIG. 2: Hypoplastic left heart.

Courtesy: Dr Bhabani Pegu, Fetal Medicine Faculty, Associate Professor, Department of Obstetrics and Gynecology, JIPMER, Puducherry; Dr Sataroopa Mishra, Assistant Professor, Department of Cardiology, JIPMER, Puducherry.

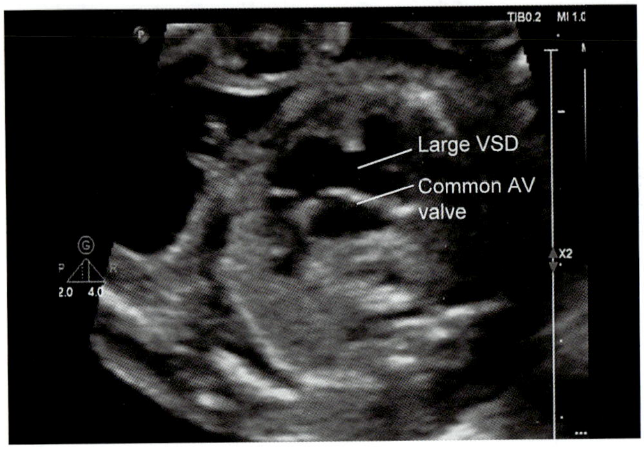

FIG. 4: Common AV valve with large VSD.

Courtesy: Dr Bhabani Pegu, Fetal Medicine Faculty, Associate Professor, Department of Obstetrics and Gynecology, JIPMER, Puducherry; Dr Sataroopa Mishra, Assistant Professor, Department of Cardiology, JIPMER, Puducherry.

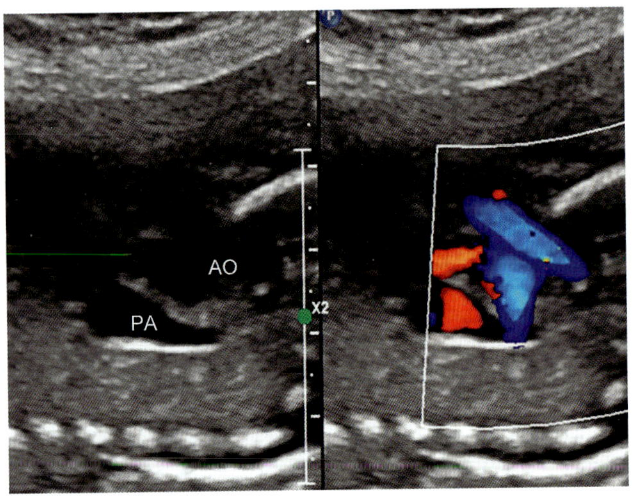

FIG. 3: Transposition of the great arteries (TGA)—parallel running great arteries.

Courtesy: Dr Bhabani Pegu, Fetal Medicine Faculty, Associate Professor, Department of Obstetrics and Gynecology, JIPMER, Puducherry; Dr Sataroopa Mishra, Assistant Professor, Department of Cardiology, JIPMER, Puducherry.

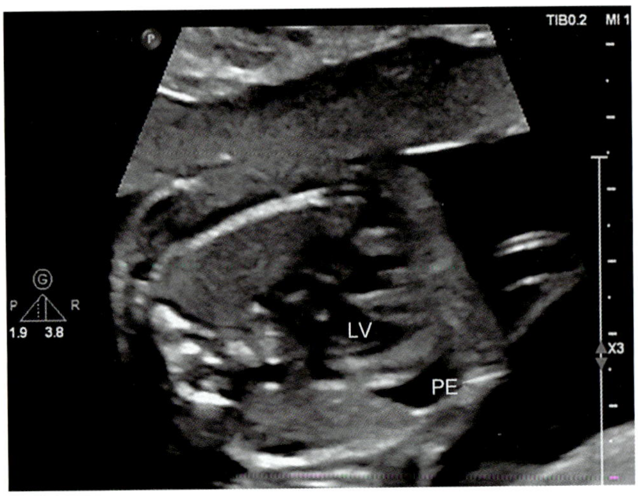

FIG. 5: Fetal HCM with pericardial effusion.

Courtesy: Dr Bhabani Pegu, Fetal Medicine Faculty, Associate Professor, Department of Obstetrics and Gynecology, JIPMER, Puducherry; Dr Sataroopa Mishra, Assistant Professor, Department of Cardiology, JIPMER, Puducherry.

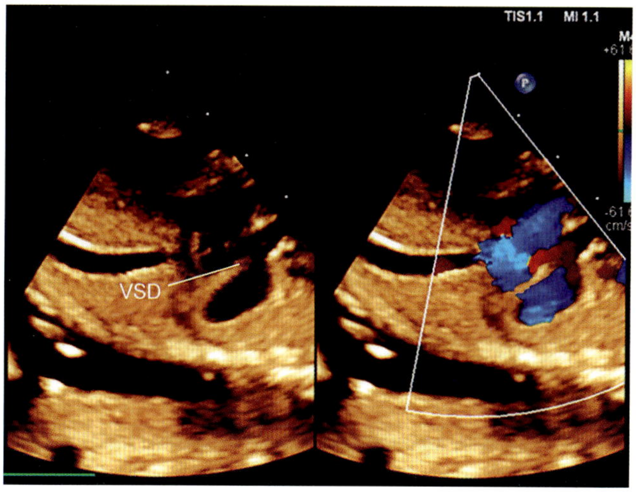

FIG. 6: Tetralogy of Fallot (TOF) with subaortic VSD and aortic override.

Courtesy: Dr Bhabani Pegu, Fetal Medicine Faculty, Associate Professor, Department of Obstetrics and Gynecology, JIPMER, Puducherry; and Dr Sataroopa Mishra, Assistant Professor, Department of Cardiology, JIPMER, Puducherry.

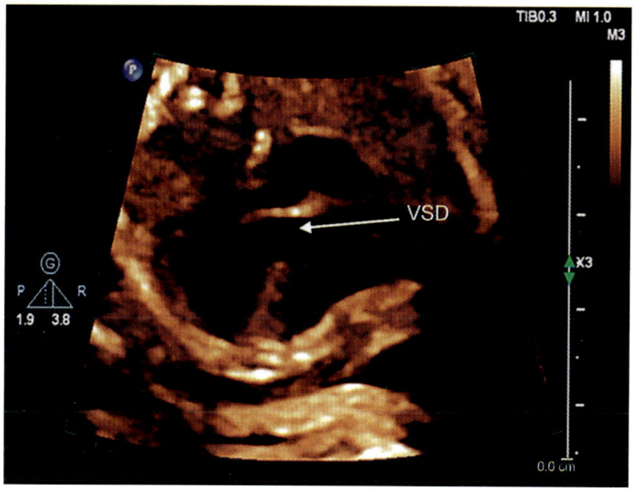

FIG. 7: Large inlet VSD.

Courtesy: Dr Bhabani Pegu, Fetal Medicine Faculty, Associate Professor, Department of Obstetrics and Gynecology, JIPMER, Puducherry; Dr Sataroopa Mishra, Assistant Professor, Department of Cardiology, JIPMER, Puducherry.

INDICATIONS FOR MRI STUDY OF FETAL HEART

- *CHD*: Circulatory patterns, hemodynamic consequences
- *MRI techniques*: Cine phase contrast MRI flow quantification

Congenital Heart Disease

Cine 2D PC MR has been used to assess the redistribution of blood flow in human fetuses with various subtypes of CHD despite obstructions leading to dramatic changes in other

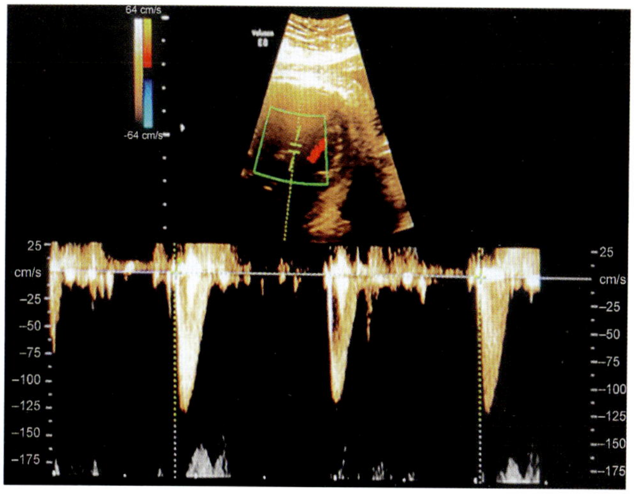

FIG. 8: Fetal complete heart block.

Courtesy: Dr Bhabani Pegu, Fetal Medicine Faculty, Associate Professor, Department of Obstetrics and Gynecology, JIPMER, Puducherry; Dr Sataroopa Mishra, Assistant Professor, Department of Cardiology, JIPMER, Puducherry.

parts of the circulatory system. Superior vena cava (SVC) flow is a surrogate for cerebral blood flow. In fetuses with right heart obstructions, such as TOF and tricuspid atresia, main pulmonary artery and ductus arteriosus flows are reduced. Conversely, in fetuses with hypoplastic left hearts, ascending aorta flow is dramatically reduced and supply to the brain is provided by an increase in ductus arteriosus flow via retrograde flow through the aortic isthmus and arch. Cerebral oxygen consumption is found to be lower in fetuses with CHD and associated with lower brain weight, a predictor of neonatal brain development. In a study of coarctation of the aorta, the combination of reduced flow in the ascending aorta and changes in arch anatomy in 3D MRI in utero was found to be predictive of the need for neonatal surgical repair.

MRI Techniques

Flow quantification with nontriggered 2D PC MR in fetuses with CHD has been employed to reveal direction of blood flow to support diagnosis of left SVC and anomalous pulmonary venous connections. In vitro 4D flow MR in 3D printed phantom models of patient-specific fetal hearts with normal and hypoplastic left ventricle geometries has also been reported.[19]

PHARMACOLOGICAL INTERVENTION IN THE FETUS

Maternal Injections for Fetal Heart Ailments

For treating fetal heart ailments, it is difficult to approach independently. Pregnancy is a unique state, where treating

TABLE 2: Common pharmacological agents.

Drug	Fetal indication	Doses	Maternal effects	Fetal effects
Digoxin	SVT, AF, CHF	• Loading dose: 0.5 mg q12h over 2 days • Maintenance dose: 0.375–0.75 mg/day	Nausea, anorexia, blurred vision, fatigue, sinus bradycardia, first-degree block	No reports available
Flecainide	SVT, AF, VT	200–400 mg/day in 2–3 divided doses	Proarrhythmia, negative inotropy, blurred vision, nausea, paresthesia, headache	Proarrhythmia, negative inotropy
Sotalol	SVT, AF, VT	160–480 mg/day in 2–3 divided doses	Bradycardia, fatigue, hypotension, headache, nausea, dizziness, proarrhythmia	Proarrhythmia, bradycardia
Amiodarone	SVT, VT	• Loading dose: 1.6–2.4 g/day for 2–7 days • Maintenance dose: 0.2–0.4 g/day • Direct: 2.5–5 mg/kg fetal weight IV slowly over 10 minutes	QT prolongation, bradycardia, thrombocytopenia, rash Long term use: Lung fibrosis, thyroid dysfunction, hepatitis; corneal microdeposits, neuropathy, myopathy	Proarrhythmia, bradycardia, transient thyroid dysfunction, growth restriction, bradycardia
Lidocaine	VT	• Loading dose: 1–1.5 mg/kg IV bolus fb • Maintenance dose: 1–4 mg/min	Numbness, drowsiness	CNS depression
Propranolol	Thyrotoxicosis	50–200 mg/day	Bradycardia, fatigue	Bradycardia, growth restriction
Beta-agonist	Fetal CHB, fetal HR <50/min	• Salbutamol: 30–40 mg/day • Terbutaline: 10–20 mg/day	Palpitation, tremor, sweating	Neonatal hypoglycemia

through maternal circulation carries potential risk for both. Pharmacological intervention includes administration of pharmaceutical agents via the maternal circulation or directly into the fetus to treat tachyarrhythmias, cardiac inflammation, and/or congestive heart failure (CHF) and to promote lung maturation.

Antiarrhythmic Fetal Treatment

Fetal arrhythmias of concern are commonly supraventricular tachyarrhythmia. These are atrioventricular reentrant tachycardia (AVRT), permanent junctional reciprocating tachycardia (PJRT), atrial ectopic tachycardia (AET), and atrial flutter (AFl) due to a circular macro-reentrant pathway. Pharmacological agents commonly used are shown in **Table 2**.

Direct Fetal Treatment

If maternal injections fail to tackle fatal arrhythmias, direct fetal injections may be tried. These can be given intramuscularly, intravenously, or intraperitoneally. Drugs like amiodarone, digoxin, and adenosine have been tried.[20]

PERCUTANEOUS INTERVENTION IN THE FETUS

Indications

Basically fetal intervention has been done for the following lesions: pulmonary atresia with intact ventricular septum (PA/IVS), severe AS/HLHS and evolving hypoplastic right heart syndrome (HRHS), and established HLHS with intact or highly restrictive atrial septum (IAS).[21]

Technique

The technique for percutaneous fetal intervention for AS with HLHS is shown in **Figure 9**.

Percutaneous Fetal Intervention for Established Hypoplastic Left Heart Syndrome with Intact or Highly Restrictive Atrial Septum

Under ultrasound guidance, an 18/19-gauge needle is inserted through the right or left atrium with a similar

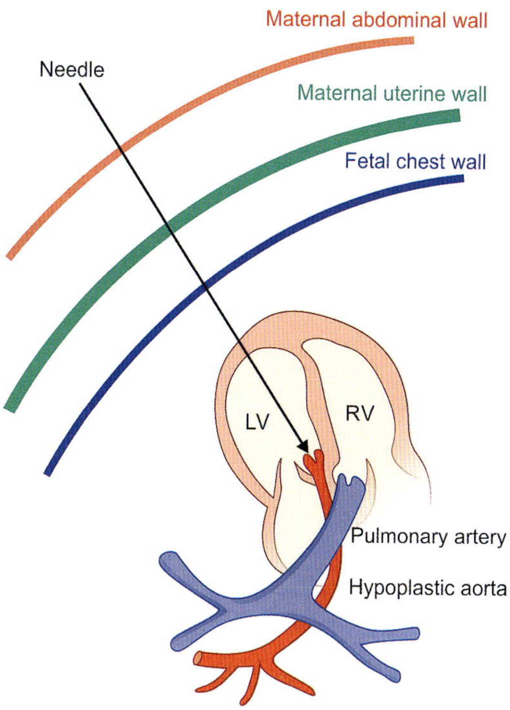

Percutaneous fetal intervention for Severe aortic stenosis with hypoplastic left heart syndrome

Technique: A 19-gauge cannula and a stylet needle are advanced under ultrasound guidance into fetal LV apex. A 0.014 angioplasty wire is manipulated through the LV outlet to cross the Aortic valve into ascending aorta.

Then a coronary angioplasty balloon is used to dilate the Aortic Valve annulus. Demonstration of antegrade broader jet flow indicates successful procedure.

Similar approach is done for *pulmonary atresia with intact ventricular septum and evolving hypoplastic right heart syndrome.*

FIG. 9: Schematic representation of percutaneous fetal intervention for AS with HLHS.

approach. Stylet or Chiba needle is used to puncture the interatrial septum followed by implantation of a balloon-mounted stent of 3 mm to establish a constant communication to save the life.

CONCLUSION

It is not impossible to develop an ideal platform to address the fetal heart diseases in India. The national policy should provide (1) a diagnosing strategy for screening the suspected or high-risk cases; (2) a standard tool, which should be available at the smaller health service provider unit of the government; (3) higher centers at districts and cities that should be equipped with skilled health team and modern machineries to go ahead with requisite intervention for such detected abnormalities; (4) multiple training centers for FE to increase the experts to detect basic defects of fetal heart disease; and (5) incorporation of artificial intelligence in this field that will certainly help in this project. The challenges that prevail include financial constraints, health-seeking behavior of community, and lack of awareness. Hence, a global social awareness drive is highly indispensable today.

ONLINE REFERENCES

Please scan the QR code provided at the end of the table of contents for References of this chapter.

CHAPTER

100

Fontan Circulation: An Overview

Sakshi Sachdeva, Saurabh Kumar Gupta

ABSTRACT

A few congenital heart diseases, often known as functionally univentricular hearts, cannot be corrected but can only be palliated by surgically establishing cavopulmonary or Fontan circulation. While Fontan surgery normalizes oxygen saturation, the lack of a subpulmonary ventricle establishes a passive pulmonary circulation with elevated systemic venous pressure. A sustained elevation of systemic venous pressure, progressive age-related increase in pulmonary vascular resistance, and decline in ventricular function have adverse long-term impacts and necessitate lifelong follow-up and active surveillance for complications.

Keywords: Functionally univentricular heart, total cavopulmonary connection, Fontan circulation

INTRODUCTION

Mammalian circulation consists of pulmonary circulation and systemic circulation, which are in series. Right and left ventricles respectively support the pulmonary and systemic circulation. Nonetheless, morphologic aberrations in certain congenital heart diseases (CHDs) preclude optimal biventricular circulation in series. Besides hearts with only a single ventricle, some morphologic characteristics such as hypoplasia of either of the ventricles or atresia of either of the atrioventricular (AV) valves also preclude biventricular circulation. These "functionally univentricular hearts" are characterized by an admixture of oxygenated and deoxygenated blood causing arterial desaturation. This univentricular arrangement also poses the risk of progressive impairment of ventricular function and reduced life expectancy.[1,2]

First conceived in 1958 by William Glenn and furthered by Francis Fontan in 1968, cavopulmonary circulation has improved the outcome of patients with univentricular hearts.[3-5] This total cavopulmonary connection (TCPC) or Fontan connection separates the pulmonary and systemic circulation to reestablish circulation in series, thus improving oxygen saturation and functional capacity. However, in the absence of a subpulmonary ventricle, systemic venous hypertension poses long-term hemodynamic challenges. This chapter provides an overview of Fontan circulation with emphasis on long-term outcomes.

HEMODYNAMICS OF FONTAN CIRCULATION

Fontan circulation is a surgically created total TCPC that diverts blood from the superior vena cava (SVC) and inferior vena cava (IVC) directly to the pulmonary arteries. In this altered state, the deoxygenated systemic venous blood reaches the lungs for oxygenation directly without passing through the heart. This effectively eliminates the right-to-left shunt, thus nearly normalizing arterial oxygen saturation. Additionally, the functionally single ventricle is saved from volume overload as blood from the systemic veins no longer needs to flow through the heart.

However, in this newly attained Fontan circuit, there is no ventricular pump to propel systemic venous blood to the lungs. Instead, blood in the pulmonary circuit is driven by the pressure in the systemic veins, which must overcome the resistance within the pulmonary circuit. The resistance to flow in Fontan circulation is the cumulative effect of resistances in the overall cavopulmonary circuit, pulmonary arteries, arterioles, pulmonary veins, and the cardiac chamber receiving the pulmonary venous return. Blood flow across the lungs is primarily determined by the pressure difference between the pulmonary artery (PA) and pulmonary vein (transpulmonary gradient). The higher the pressure in the atrium receiving the pulmonary veins, the greater the pressure needed in the systemic veins to drive blood through the Fontan circuit. Consequently, unlike normal circulation, the systemic venous pressure in Fontan circulation is always higher than that of the pulmonary arteries (Fontan paradox). Further, devoid of a subpulmonary ventricle, any change in the characteristics of the pulmonary circuit or the downstream ventricular chamber directly affects the efficiency of Fontan circulation.[6]

INDICATIONS OF FONTAN OPERATION

Fontan surgery can be considered for all hearts with functionally univentricular hearts having single-ventricle physiology. As is now well known, a true single ventricle with a complete absence of one of the ventricles is extremely rare. Instead, most cases with functionally univentricular hearts have either absence or hypoplasia of one of the AV valves (tricuspid or mitral atresia) or one of the ventricles, as seen in hypoplastic left or right ventricle (LV or RV). Further, certain complex CHDs, where the risks of achieving biventricular surgical repair are unacceptably high, are also managed as functional univentricular hearts with Fontan operation providing a much safer palliative option. **Box 1** lists cardiac malformations commonly labeled as functionally univentricular heart.[7]

PATIENT SELECTION FOR FONTAN SURGERY

Since there is no ventricle to pump systemic venous blood through the lungs in Fontan circulation, the blood flow relies on elevated systemic venous pressure. Maintaining a low transpulmonary gradient is crucial for a well-functioning TCPC circuit. Any abnormalities in the lung vasculature, lung tissue, or left-sided heart chambers can hinder pulmonary blood flow, causing systemic venous pressure to rise to nonphysiological levels and eventually leading to Fontan circuit failure. Even in a functioning Fontan circulation, chronic systemic venous hypertension has detrimental long-term effects. Therefore, selecting a suitable patient is important for favorable long-term outcomes.

In 1977, Choussat and colleagues listed 10 morphologic and physiologic characteristics to identify an ideal candidate for a successful Fontan procedure **(Box 2)**.[8] These strict criteria were aimed to select the best candidates. However, over decades, with improving surgical and medical management, these traditional guidelines are no longer followed. Age under four is no longer considered a contraindication, and systemic venous variabilities and AV valvar regurgitation can be managed surgically during the cavopulmonary connection. Surgical advances have also minimized the need for having a normal right atrium (RA) size. In most cases, small or distorted pulmonary arteries can also be addressed surgically or through percutaneous interventions. Similarly, rhythm disturbances such as bradycardia and tachycardia can also be managed with pacemakers or antiarrhythmic medications.

BOX 1 Conditions representing the functionally univentricular heart.

- *Absence of two adequately sized atrioventricular valves*:
  - Tricuspid atresia
  - Mitral atresia
  - Hypoplastic left heart
- *Hypoplasia of one of the ventricles*:
  - Single ventricle
  - Double inlet left ventricle
  - Straddling of one AV valve
  - Unbalanced atrioventricular septal defect
- *Difficult biventricular repair*: CHD with large or multiple or nonroutable VSDs

(AV: atrioventricular; CHD: congenital heart disease; VSD: ventricular septal defect)

BOX 2 Ten commandments for successful Fontan operation.[8]

Original 10 commandments:
1. Age > 4 years
2. Sinus rhythm
3. Normal systemic venous return
4. Normal right atrial volume
5. Mean pulmonary artery pressure <15 mm Hg
6. Pulmonary vascular resistance <4 WU m^2
7. Pulmonary artery-aorta ratio >0.75
8. Left ventricular ejection fraction >0.60
9. Competent mitral valve
10. Absence of pulmonary artery distortion

Hence, in contemporary practice, only two of the original 10 commandments, namely: (1) preoperative ventricular function and (2) preoperative PA pressure below 15 mm Hg, are considered necessary before a patient is considered suitable for Fontan operation. Hoscin and colleagues, in a retrospective analysis of 406 patients, found only these two factors to be the key predictors of both early and late outcomes.[9] In clinical practice, the goal is to identify patients with the most favorable hemodynamics to minimize the risk of Fontan failure. An ideal candidate for Fontan surgery should have good-sized pulmonary arteries (preferably with a McGoon ratio >1.5), low pulmonary vascular resistance index (PVRI <2 WU m^2), unobstructed pulmonary veins, no or mild AV valve regurgitation, and normal or near-normal ventricular function. In other words, the more parameters of the original 10 commandments are met, the higher the likelihood of a successful outcome following Fontan surgery. Additional factors that can reduce ventricular compliance or increase PA pressures such as left ventricular outflow obstruction, coarctation of the aorta, and aortopulmonary collaterals should also be evaluated before making a final decision about managing patients with univentricular hearts.

STEPS TO ACHIEVE UNIVENTRICULAR PALLIATION/FONTAN PATHWAY

The morphological and physiological conditions in a functionally univentricular heart vary significantly. In hearts with unrestricted blood flow to the lungs, the PA pressure is elevated. Conversely, patients with severe pulmonary stenosis (PS) have low PA pressure. As emphasized, the success of Fontan circulation depends heavily on the transpulmonary gradient, with low PA pressure being the most critical factor. Thus, protecting the lungs for future cavopulmonary connections is essential.

Patients with functionally univentricular hearts are carefully assessed, particularly to determine the status of their PA pressure. In cases with no pulmonary blood flow obstruction, a PA banding is initially performed to control pulmonary hypertension. Patients with PS, on the other hand, are initially managed medically. For those with severe PS and significant hypoxemia, an aortopulmonary shunt or stenting of the patent ductus arteriosus may be required. It is also vital to identify and treat any associated lesions that interfere with blood flow to the heart, within the cardiac chambers, or systemic circulation. In cases with a hypoplastic, absent, or obstructed AV valve, surgery should also include creating adequate interatrial communication to allow proper blood mixing. Anomalous obstructed pulmonary venous connections are simultaneously corrected. Lesions that obstruct systemic outflow, such as aortic stenosis or coarctation of the aorta, must also be addressed. The goal of this initial intervention is to protect the pulmonary vasculature and prepare the patient for future TCPC **(Flowchart 1)**.

The second stage of surgery is performed once the child is a few months old and their PVR has decreased. At this point, a partial cavopulmonary connection is established through the bidirectional Glenn (BDG) operation, in which the SVC is anastomosed end-to-side to the right pulmonary artery (RPA). This procedure redirects deoxygenated blood from the upper body directly to the lungs, improving oxygen saturation and allowing time for the child to grow before TCPC is performed later. The increased pulmonary blood flow also promotes PA growth. During surgery, associated lesions that might interfere with future TCPC are also addressed.

In the final stage, blood from the IVC is directed to the pulmonary arteries, achieving TCPC. Considering the need for accurate measurement of PA pressure and PVR, preoperative cardiac catheterization is performed. The decision to perform TCPC is individualized, but a patient is generally considered suitable if the mean PA pressure is <15 mm Hg and the indexed PVR is below 2 WU m^2. In borderline cases, it is advisable to leave a fenestration between the Fontan circuit and the atrium during surgery. Fenestration is also recommended for patients over 10 years old, especially if they have not undergone a prior BDG and are undergoing a primary Fontan procedure.[10]

STAGED VERSUS PRIMARY TOTAL CAVOPULMONARY CONNECTION

The staged approach of performing a BDG first, followed by TCPC later, allows for a gradual reduction in the ventricle's workload. In contrast, direct or primary TCPC results in an abrupt reduction in volume, causing a sudden decrease in preload to a hypertrophied ventricle. This preload–afterload mismatch and resultant altered ventriculoarterial coupling during the early postoperative period may limit the cardiac output adversely. The prior BDG procedure also promotes the growth of pulmonary arteries, especially if the flow across the pulmonary valve is not eliminated. Besides, with less blood going through the lungs, BDG is better tolerated even among those with borderline suitability. This staged approach of BDG followed by TCPC offers significant benefits, including improved cardiac function, fewer arrhythmias, and enhanced long-term survival. Additionally, BDG provides an opportunity for interim interventions, such as correcting AV valve regurgitation, addressing PA distortion, or treating left ventricular outflow tract obstruction, optimizing the patient's condition for future TCPC.[11]

It is currently recommended to perform the BDG procedure at 6–12 months of age, with the TCPC being completed around 4–5 years of age. In select cases, patients older than 6 years can undergo a single-stage TCPC, provided they have good-sized branch pulmonary arteries (preferably McGoon ratio >2.0), normal ventricular function, and low PVR. However, for some patients with borderline hemodynamics or relatively small pulmonary arteries, the BDG is the final palliative procedure.[12] **Flowchart 1** outline a simplified algorithmic approach for decision-making in patients with a functionally univentricular heart.

TYPES OF FONTAN CIRCULATION

In 1949, Rodbard and Wagner successfully performed the first right ventricular bypass by anastomosing the right atrial appendage (RAA) to the PA and ligating the MPA in dogs.[13] Glenn and colleagues followed it in 1958 with the first successful cavopulmonary connection (SVC to right PA) in a child with a functional single ventricle. Then, in 1968, Fontan and Baudet performed the first Fontan procedure on an adult with tricuspid atresia.[5]

The original Fontan procedure involved five key steps: (1) End-to-side anastomosis of the RPA to the SVC, (2) end-to-end anastomosis of the RAA to the LPA using an aortic valve homograft, (3) closure of the atrial septal defect (ASD), (4) placement of a pulmonary valve homograft into the IVC, and (5) ligation of the main MPA. In a similar operation, Kreutzer differed systemic venous blood by anastomosing the RA directly to the MPA without Glenn anastomosis or IVC valve, while keeping the branch pulmonary arteries in continuity **(Fig. 1)**.[14]

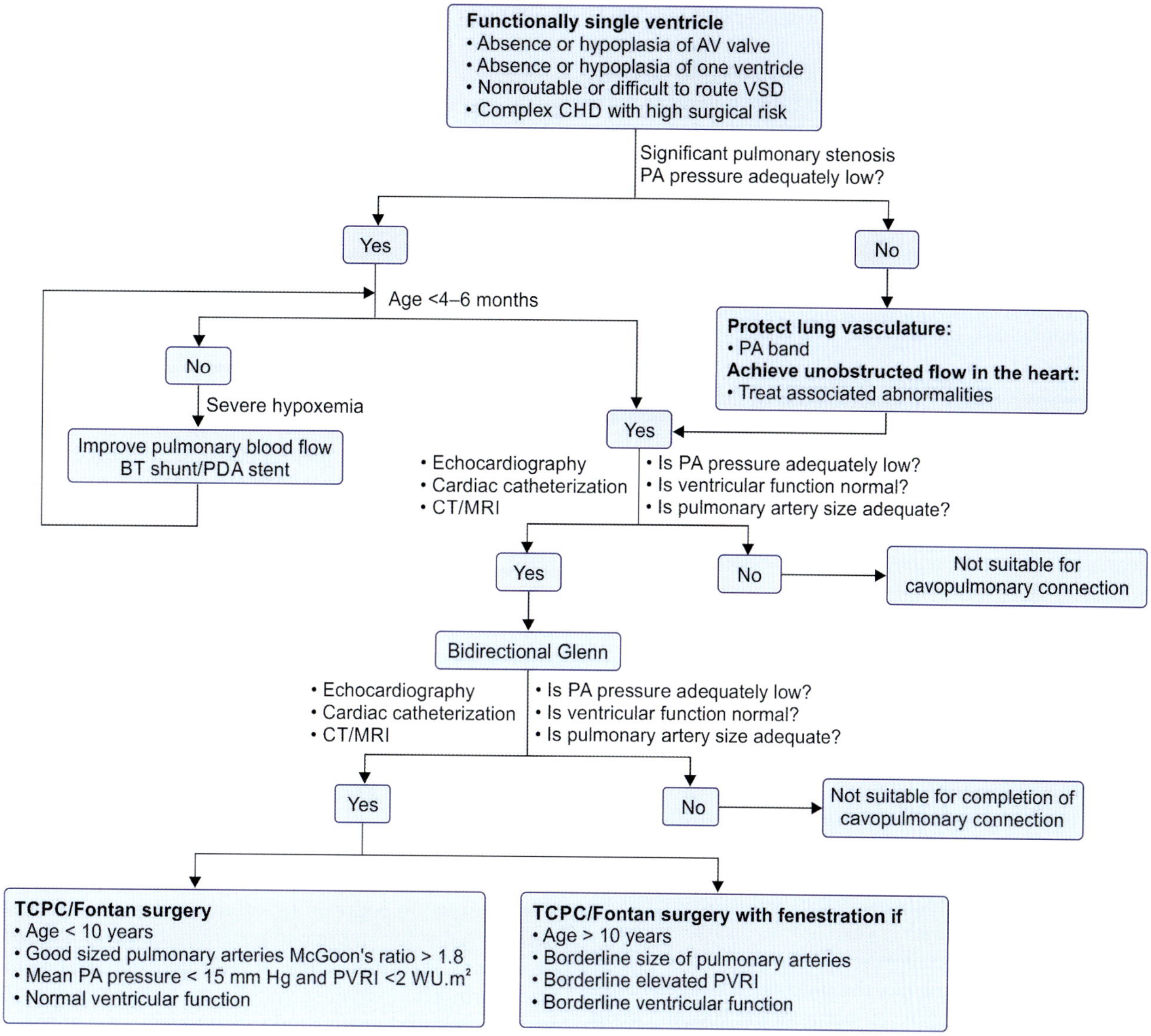

FLOWCHART 1: Flow diagram indicating the decision-making process and timing of surgery and interventions in functionally single ventricle.

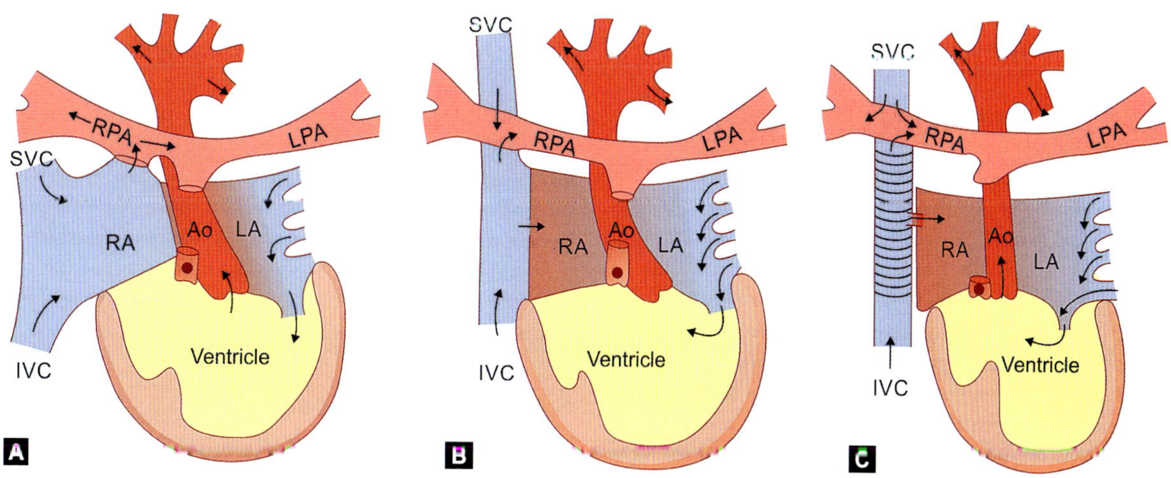

FIGS. 1A TO C: Cartoon showing the various types of Fontan surgery in a univentricular heart (A) atriopulmonary Fontan, (B) bidirectional Glenn and lateral tunnel Fontan, and (C) bidirectional Glenn and extracardiac Fontan.

In the decade following Fontan and Kreutzer's innovations, several modifications emerged. Initially, the RA was thought to boost pulmonary blood flow due to its pulsatile nature, aided by valve homografts. However, it became clear that maintaining PA continuity was essential for better outcomes. Issues with conduit and valve durability also surfaced.

In 1988, de Leval based on flow dynamics studies introduced the lateral tunnel variant of TCPC (LT TCPC) to improve flow efficiency by (1) end-to-side SVC anastomosis to the undivided RPA, (2) constructing an intra-atrial tunnel using the posterior wall of RA, and (3) using a prosthetic patch to channel IVC blood to the SVC orifice anastomosed to the PA **(Fig. 1)**.[15]

The extracardiac TCPC (EC TCPC), introduced by Humes and Marcelletti in 1990, is the latest modification of the Fontan procedure wherein IVC is connected to RA using a conduit.[16,17] This conduit can be made of polytetrafluoroethylene (PTFE) or fashioned from the patient's pericardium. PTFE conduits are preferred for their simplicity, but they lack growth potential, so a conduit larger than the IVC is typically chosen (conduit-to-IVC ratio >1.5). Pericardial conduits, on the other hand, offer some growth potential and carry a lower risk of thrombosis and infection **(Fig. 1)**.

Extracardiac TCPC and LT TCPC both allow for smoother blood flow, reducing energy loss compared to the older atriopulmonary connection. These newer modifications also minimize the risk of interference with pulmonary venous drainage and the AV valve. The LT TCPC approach also has the advantage of accommodating growth and is suitable for patients of all ages, whereas EC TCPC is easier to perform in cases of complex congenital heart defects and minimal handling of atrial tissue, thus reducing the risk of postoperative arrhythmias.

In some cases, especially where there are concerns about the patient's ability to tolerate the procedure, a fenestration (an intentional opening) is left between the Fontan circuit and the atrium.[18] This allows for decompression in case of elevated PA pressures, aiding in postoperative recovery. Fenestrations usually close spontaneously, but if persistent hypoxemia occurs, they may require closure, following a test occlusion to ensure safe closure.

EFFECTS OF FONTAN CIRCULATION

The Fontan circulation results in near-normal oxygen saturation levels at rest, leading to significant improvements in quality of life for most. Nevertheless, the Fontan circuit is limited by its nonpulsatile nature and resultant inability to reduce PVR during exercise. Consequently, an increase in the cardiac output during exercise is significantly impaired, limiting the functional capacity. Nonpulsatile flow also leads to adverse remodeling of the pulmonary vasculature, including increased intimal thickness and reduced medial thickness of the intra-acinar vessels. These structural changes further elevate PVR and contribute to the progressive deterioration of ventricular compliance, compounding the limitations in exercise capacity and overall cardiovascular function as patients age.[19]

EARLY POSTOPERATIVE COMPLICATIONS

In modern Fontan procedures, improved patient selection, a staged surgical approach, and enhanced perioperative care have improved early postoperative mortality to <2%. However, certain high-risk patients—those with elevated PA pressure, a common AV valve, hypoplastic left heart syndrome, more than moderate AV valvar regurgitation, or more than moderate ventricular dysfunction—experience high mortality and morbidity following surgery.

A subset of patients may develop complications such as low cardiac output, pleural effusion, and other signs of Fontan circulation failure and mandate careful management of preload and afterload. Pleural effusions are sometimes persistent in the postoperative period. While many cases can be managed with chest tube drainage and somatostatin analogs, some effusions prove refractory and may require more invasive interventions such as pleurodesis and creation or dilatation of existing fenestration in the Fontan conduit.[20,21]

LATE COMPLICATIONS

Ventricular Dysfunction

Despite advances in surgical techniques, patients who undergo the Fontan procedure are predisposed to progressive ventricular dysfunction due to the underlying CHD. Initially, this dysfunction is driven by volume overload, but later, a chronic reduction in preload becomes the dominant issue. In a cross-sectional study of 546 children post-Fontan operation, 27% exhibited systolic dysfunction, while 72% had diastolic dysfunction, indicating a significant prevalence of ventricular dysfunction after surgery.[22] This ventricular dysfunction tends to worsen with age, especially in patients with a morphological RV functioning as the systemic ventricle and those who have had previous ventriculotomy incisions.

Treatment options for ventricular dysfunction in Fontan patients are largely empirical and are typically guided by general heart failure management protocols. However, conventional heart failure medications, such as inotropes, afterload-reducing agents, vasodilators, and beta-blockers, have shown limited effectiveness in these patients primarily, because these medications do not address the root issue of reduced preload, which is a key factor limiting cardiac function in the Fontan circulation. Consequently, managing ventricular dysfunction in this population remains a challenge.

Systemic Complications

Fontan patients face various long-term complications that can impact their growth, cardiovascular function, and organ systems, making their postoperative care complex.

Growth Restriction

Fontan patients often experience growth restriction, particularly in achieving their full height potential. Difficulty in gaining weight can be an early sign of inadequate cardiac output, necessitating a thorough hemodynamic evaluation to optimize care and growth.[23]

Cyanosis

Even after TCPC, mild resting desaturation can occur, because the coronary sinus continues to drain into the atrium. In some cases, hepatic veins may also directly drain into the atrium. A fenestration in the Fontan circuit can cause persistent right-to-left shunting, resulting in persistent arterial desaturation. The development of systemic vein to left atrium collaterals can also result in desaturation.[22,23]

Arrhythmias

Atrial arrhythmias occur in up to 45% of patients within 10 years of the Fontan procedure, especially those with atrial manipulation or suture lines (as seen in the atriopulmonary connection). The risk of arrhythmias is the lowest in those with EC TCPC. Other arrhythmias, including sinus node dysfunction, AV block, and sudden arrhythmic death, can also exist, with ventricular arrhythmias contributing to about 10% of sudden deaths.[22,23]

Thrombosis and Thromboembolism

Low-velocity blood flow, atrial scarring, arrhythmias, dehydration, and a hypercoagulable state increase the risk of thromboembolism, with an incidence between 6 and 20%. Prophylactic strategies vary, but aspirin has been shown to reduce the risk of thromboembolic events from 18.6% to 8.6%.[24] Oral anticoagulants are typically reserved for those at high risk for thromboembolism.

Protein-losing Enteropathy

Protein-losing enteropathy affects 1–15% of Fontan patients and is characterized by excessive protein loss into the intestines, leading to symptoms of hypoproteinemia such as edema, ascites, malabsorption, and immunodeficiency. Diagnosis can be confirmed through stool tests for alpha-1 antitrypsin, and treatment includes dietary modifications, corticosteroids, unfractionated heparin, and octreotide.[25,26]

Plastic Bronchitis

This rare complication (1–2% of cases) involves the formation of rubbery bronchial casts that obstruct the airways. The exact cause is unclear, but it possibly results from lymphatic leakage due to elevated venous pressures or surgery-related trauma. Plastic bronchitis is often associated with significant hemodynamic derangements and ventricular dysfunction, contributing to poor outcomes.[27]

Hepatic Dysfunction

Chronic congestion from elevated venous pressure and reduced oxygen delivery after the Fontan operation leads to progressive liver fibrosis, which is almost universal. Over time, patients are at risk of complications such as portal hypertension and hepatocellular carcinoma. Monitoring liver function through periodic screening is recommended, though the optimal strategy remains uncertain.[28,29] For severe cases, combined cardiac and liver transplantation has been successfully performed.

These complications highlight the need for continuous monitoring and proactive management in patients who have undergone Fontan procedures, as these issues can significantly affect long-term outcomes.[23]

Chronic Fontan Failure

Fontan circulation is characterized by a gradual decline in cardiac function over time, marked by a progressive reduction in cardiac output and rising central venous pressure. This decline typically becomes noticeable during adolescence when exercise capacity drops to around 66% of predicted levels. Beyond adolescence, exercise tolerance decreases further at a rate of about 2.6% per year. By the third decade of life, exercise capacity falls to around 45% of expected, at which point hospitalization rates and symptoms tend to increase significantly.[30]

MANAGEMENT OF FONTAN FAILURE

Fontan failure can be multifactorial, and the management depends upon the underlying etiology. Hence, it requires a multifaceted approach, with careful consideration of each patient's hemodynamics, anatomic lesions, and overall health status to determine the most appropriate strategy.

- *Medical management*: Select cases with elevated PA pressure patients with Fontan failure may improve with pulmonary vasodilators. Others with arrhythmia benefit from antiarrhythmic medications with some requiring radiofrequency ablation.
- *Correction of obstructive lesions*: Patients with residual obstructive anatomic lesions, such as those in the pulmonary arteries, pulmonary veins, subaortic area, or aortic arch, should be considered for early corrective surgery to alleviate obstructions that exacerbate Fontan failure.
- *Valve surgery*: More than moderate AV valvar regurgitation is an indication of surgical intervention, either through repair or replacement of the valve.
- *Ventricular dysfunction*: Fontan failure due to ventricular dysfunction is particularly challenging to manage. Treatment options are limited, but some reports have indicated a potential benefit from the use of ventricular assist devices (VADs) to support failing ventricular function.

- *Lymphatic interventions*: In recent years, there has been a growing understanding of lymphatic dysfunction in patients with Fontan circulation. In select cases, lymphatic interventions have been proven useful albeit with limited data on long-term success.
- *Conversion to EC TCPC*: For patients with failed atriopulmonary Fontan circulation, conversion to EC TCPC has shown success in improving hemodynamics and reducing symptoms.
- Heart transplantation is the final option for patients with Fontan failure who do not respond to other treatments. However, coexisting multiorgan dysfunction and HLA sensitization from previous surgeries complicate transplantation outcomes. Early posttransplant outcomes in Fontan patients are generally suboptimal, although medium and long-term survival rates are like those seen in patients with other CHD.[30]

OUTCOME OF FONTAN SURGERY

While early mortality rates have significantly decreased, and long-term survival has improved, the life expectancy following Fontan surgery remains below the population average. Estimates from various studies provide a perspective on survival rates across different periods. Mayo Clinic study has estimated survival rates of 74%, 61%, and 43% at 10, 20, and 30 years following TCPC.[31] On the other hand, the Australian-New Zealand registry of 1,006 post-Fontan patients suggests better survival rates with 93%, 90%, and 83% surviving at 10, 20, and 30 years, respectively.[32]

These improved outcomes reflect advancements in surgical techniques, patient selection, and postoperative management. However, despite these gains, Fontan patients continue to face long-term challenges, and survival rates still fall short of the general population. The long-term decline in exercise capacity, increasing risk of complications, and eventual heart failure contribute to these limitations. Lifelong surveillance for early identification and monitoring of complications is a must to ensure optimal outcomes.[33]

CONCLUSION

The circulation of blood following a TCPC or Fontan operation relies heavily on maintaining a low transpulmonary gradient. The key factors determining the success of the Fontan circuit are PA pressure and ventricular function. Elevated PVR or poor ventricular function can significantly compromise hemodynamics in the Fontan circuit.

Although arterial oxygen saturation approaches near-normal levels in these patients, exercise tolerance remains suboptimal and declines progressively with age. Long-term survival for Fontan patients is also improving but is significantly lower than that of the general population. These patients are at risk for various complications, including ventricular dysfunction, arrhythmias, thrombosis, and organ dysfunction, which contribute to their reduced life expectancy thus mandating regular follow-up.

ONLINE REFERENCES

Please scan the QR code provided at the end of the table of contents for References of this chapter.

Interventional Palliation for Cyanotic Congenital Heart Disease in Cath Lab

CHAPTER 101

Deepa S Kumar

ABSTRACT

Cyanotic heart diseases can be classified into biventricular repair and univentricular palliation. Biventricular repair is possible for tetralogy of Fallot (TOF) with pulmonary atresia and other TOF variants, while univentricular palliation is recommended for conditions with AV valve atresia.

Keywords: Heart, repair, biventricular

INTRODUCTION

Cyanotic heart diseases can be broadly classified as those conditions where biventricular repair is possible and those where univentricular palliation is advised. Biventricular repair is possible for tetralogy of Fallot (TOF) with pulmonary atresia and other TOF physiology variants such as DORV, VSD, and PS. It is also possible for admixture lesions with increased pulmonary blood flow such as TAPVC, common atrium, common arterial trunk, DORV with large subaortic, or subpulmonic VSD. Univentricular palliation is recommended in those conditions with AV valve atresia, single ventricle, and DORV with remote VSD.

PALLIATIVE INTERVENTIONS FOR CYANOTIC HEART DISEASE

Balloon Atrial Septostomy

Indications

- To improve intercirculatory mixing in transposition of great arteries with intact ventricular septum
- To maintain unrestrictive systemic and pulmonary venous return respectively in cases with tricuspid atresia or mitral atresia and restrictive ASD
- Pulmonary atresia with intact ventricular septum and restrictive ASD
- As palliation in severely obstructed TAPVC (at the ASD level) in poor surgical candidates

Procedure

The procedure can be done under sedation or general anesthesia; in the bedside with transthoracic echocardiographic imaging or in cardiac catheterization laboratory under fluoroscopic guidance. Balloon atrial septostomy catheters currently available are the dual lumen NuMED Z-5 and the Z-6 BAS catheter (NuMED Inc). A thorough TTE should be done to assess the segmental anatomy and to ensure that there is no juxtaposition of right atrial appendage. Femoral venous or umbilical venous access can be used for septostomy. 6–7 Fr short sheath is used in the femoral access; but catheter can be introduced directly through the umbilical vein. The catheter is advanced over the wire through the foramen ovale into the right atrium, inflated with 1.8 mL diluted contrast and withdrawn sharply into the right atrium and then pushed back into the RA to allow IVC venous return **(Video 1, Figs. 1A and B)**. A successful septostomy results in increase in saturation by at least 10%, with laminar flow through the ASD and no significant gradient between LA and RA. Complications such as cardiac perforation, injury to AV valves, rhythm abnormalities, embolization of balloon fragments or torn atrial septum, injury to systemic, or pulmonary veins are rare. Failure to improve oxygen saturation could be due to inadequate septostomy or due to nonregression of pulmonary vascular resistance. Nonregression of PVR may be managed by pulmonary vasodilators, oxygen, and by continuing low dose PGE1 till surgery.[1,2]

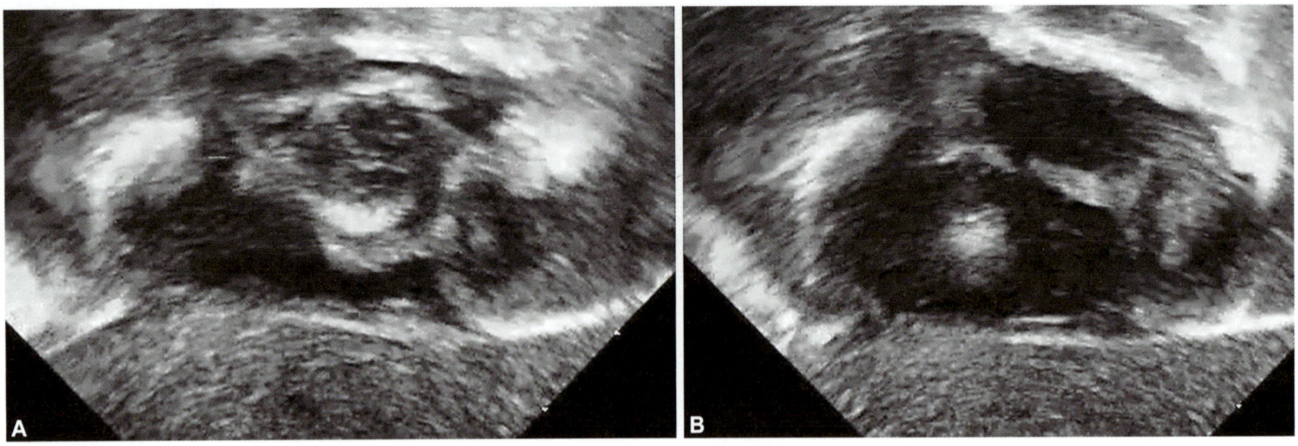

FIGS. 1A AND B: (A) Subcostal four-chamber view showing inflated balloon in left atrium; (B) The balloon has been tugged into the right atrium across the atrial septa defect.

PATENT DUCTUS ARTERIOSUS STENTING

Indications

Duct-dependent Pulmonary Circulation

Assessment and Technique

Patent ductus arteriosus (PDA) is assessed by transthoracic echocardiography for its place of origin [undersurface of arch, descending thoracic aorta (DTA), or base of innominate artery], point of insertion, size of pulmonary end, and tortuosity. Highly tortuous PDA (more than two turns or alpha looping PDA) and presence of confluence stenosis are relative contraindications for PDA stenting.[3,4] Care must be taken to avoid jailing branch pulmonary arteries particularly in cases of univentricular heart as PA distortion and poor branch PA growth is detrimental to future BDG and Fontan. PDA stenting is planned if the newborn needs PGE1 to maintain duct patency. The patient should be assessed for presence of other complications like sepsis or NEC. PGE1 is usually continued till the patient is shifted to cath lab, especially if the duct is very sensitive to PGE1. There is a high risk of PDA stent embolism if PDA size is >2.4 mm. The procedure is usually done under general anesthesia, though it can also be done under sedation, and local anesthesia. Dual antiplatelets are loaded prior to the procedure. Bare metal stents are ideal; however, if they are not available, drug eluting stents may also be used with no significant risk. Size of stent is decided based on the weight of the newborn:

- <2.5 kg—3 mm stent
- 2.5-3.5 kg—3.5 mm stent
- >3.5 kg—4 mm stent

In B/L PDA stent in cases of nonconfluent PDA with bilateral ducts, 3 mm stents are chosen to prevent pulmonary overflow. Access site is chosen based on the aortic origin of the arterial duct:

- *Duct from the undersurface of the arch*:
  - Right or left axillary artery access **(Video 2, Figs. 2A and B)**
  - Transvenous access: This may be difficult if it is a double outlet right ventricle, especially if the VSD is predominantly in the inflow
- *Duct from the DTA*: Femoral arterial approach **(Video 3, Fig. 3)**
- *Duct from the base of the innominate artery*: Femoral artery approach. The duct is cannulated in a similar manner as for BT shunt interventions **(Video 4, Fig. 4)**.
- *Duct at the junction of arch and DTA*: This is the most difficult duct to cannulate. Left axillary approach with right Judkins catheter and femoral arterial approach with cut pigtail are options to cannulate this duct.

We use a 4–5 slender (Glidesheath Slender, Terumo Inc) short sheath at the access site which has an outer diameter of 4 Fr, but permits 5 Fr catheters. After heparinization with 100 IU/kg of UFH, arch angiograms through 5 Jr guide catheter are taken in various views to profile the pulmonary and aortic end of the duct. Care is taken not to engage the duct deeply as it may cause duct spasm or dissection. Then the duct is cannulated with 0.014' wire and approximate length of the duct is measured based on the length of the radio-opaque marker of the wire used. The stent is positioned taking care to cover both pulmonary and aortic ends without too much protrusion at either end. After stent deployment, angiogram is taken to ensure good flow into both branch pulmonary arteries. If a branch PA flow is cut off, the branch has to be recrossed through the stent and the stent struts dilated with small coronary balloons. The wire is usually kept for 10–15 minutes to ensure that there is no early stent thrombosis. After securing access site bleeding, heparin infusion is started at 20–25 IU/kg/h aiming to maintain aPTT of

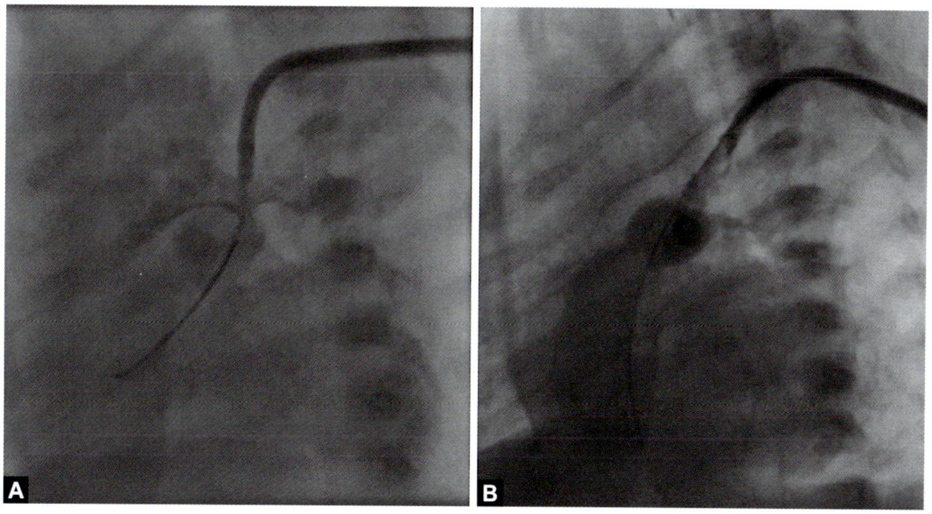

FIGS. 2A AND B: (A) Guide catheter introduced through the left axillary access and the duct is wired. The duct is arising from the undersurface of the arch; (B) A stent has been placed across the duct and dilated. Good flow is seen in branch pulmonary arteries.

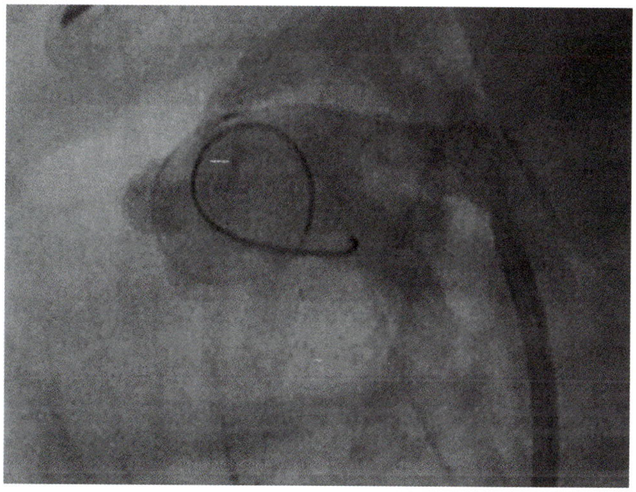

FIG. 3: Guide catheter in descending thoracic aorta (DTA). Duct arising from DTA has been stented through femoral arterial access.

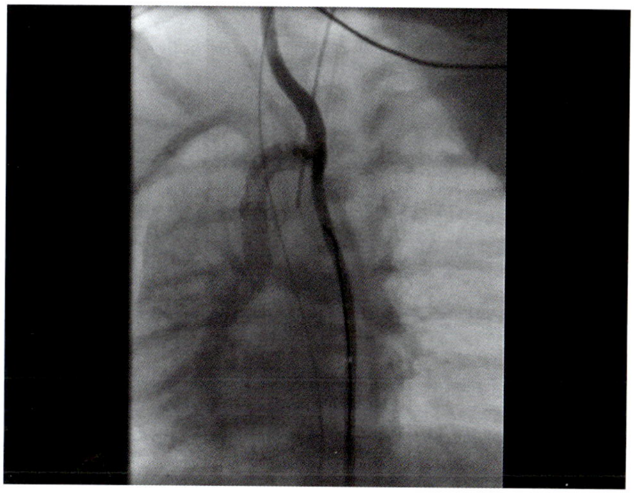

FIG. 4: The arterial duct arising from the base of left innominate artery has been stented using the femoral arterial access.

50–70 seconds and is continued for 12 hours. We continue dual antiplatelets till definitive repair or BDG. Early complications include vascular injury, stent thrombosis, uncovered aortic or pulmonary end, and pulmonary overflow. Close follow-up is mandatory to look for stent flow, growth of branch PA, to monitor overall growth, and to adjust dose of antiplatelets according to weight gain.

Duct-dependent Systemic Circulation

In hypoplastic left heart syndrome, hybrid Norwood procedure consists of bilateral PA banding by the surgeon followed by PDA stenting and balloon atrial septostomy (if ASD is restrictive) by the interventionist. After bilateral PA banding, PDA stenting can be performed in the hybrid theatre by passing a short sheath into the main pulmonary artery by the surgeon and the stent placed under monoplane fluoroscopy. It can also be performed electively under cover of PGE1 through femoral venous access. The duct is cannulated with JR catheter. Angiogram is taken in lateral and RAO views and pulmonary and aortic ends are identified. Stent size between 7 and 10 mm is chosen depending on the weight of the baby and the size of the PDA **(Video 5, Fig. 5)**. Self-expanding and balloon expandable stents have been used with each having advantages and disadvantages. Self-expanding stents have lower radial strength and less capacity for redilatation. Balloon expandable stents are preferred when we want to dilate the duct to a greater size. Sinus-SuperFlex-DS stents (premounted on 4 Fr delivery systems) or renal/biliary bare metal stents (Cook, Formula) can be used through the venous route. Stenting can also be

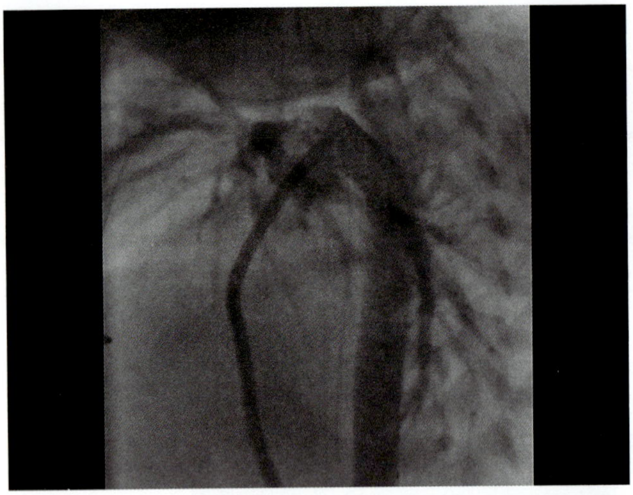

FIG. 5: 7 mm stent placed across the duct through a long sheath passed from the venous access in a duct-dependent systemic circulation as part of hybrid Norwood procedure after bilateral pulmonary artery banding.

performed retrogradely if SS-DS stents are available. The stent is positioned to cover both ends taking care to avoid excess protrusion into the arch. Dual antiplatelets are continued till the second stage of Norwood procedure. Interstage mortality is 5–10%, hence very close monitoring is needed to identify stent overflow, coronary ischemia, development of arch obstruction, and other complications. The second stage is planned by 4th month of life.[5]

RIGHT VENTRICULAR OUTFLOW TRACT STENTING

Indications

- Severe cyanotic spell with hemodynamic decompensation
- TOF with poor PA anatomy
- Syndromic patient, patient with other severe comorbidities

As palliation in cases of TOF with coronary crossing right ventricular outflow tract (RVOT) till the patient attains suitable size for conduit.

Once the decision has been made to stent the RVOT, careful transthoracic echocardiography is done in subcostal and parasternal short axis views. RVOT stenting is contraindicated if the VSD is doubly committed, as there will be lack of infundibular muscle to hold the stent. Femoral or internal jugular venous access can be used. After introducing a long sheath into the RV, angiograms are performed with a Gensini or NIH catheter in lateral and RAO views. The hardware should be prepared before passing wire across RVOT. If the stenosis is very severe, two wires may sometimes be needed, or it may require additional support with microcatheter. If the valve is near atretic, CTO wires of RFA is needed to create an opening. The wire is then parked deep in RPA or LPA through a 4 or 5 Fr JR catheter. The long sheath is advanced over the wire into the RPA/LPA. The wire is then exchanged for one appropriate for the stent planned. Stenting can be done in a valve sparing manner if the pulmonary annulus size is >–2 Z scores. The stent size is decided by multiple factors such as (1) size of pulmonary annulus, particularly if we are planning to stent across the pulmonary valve, (2) duration of palliation needed, (3) age of the patient, (4) presence of MAPCAs, and (5) need for redilatation. For newborns, coronary stents are usually chosen, while in infants and older children, larger balloon expandable bare metal stents are chosen. The size chosen in infants varies between 5 and 8 mm usually **(Videos 6A and B, Figs. 6A to C)**. Covered stents are chosen in older patients. The stent is then deployed in a controlled manner with multiple side arm injections through the long sheath. A push should be maintained on the stent while deploying from the femoral route as there is a tendency for the stent to slip proximally. If valve sparing procedure was done, it is better to dilate the pulmonary valve with the same balloon or with bigger balloon after stent deployment. BPV should never be done before RVOT stent placement as it increases the risk of stent migration. After the balloon is removed, angiograms, and transthoracic echocardiogram is done to ensure that RVOT is fully covered and there are no complications like TR or pericardial effusion. It is better to wait for few minutes to ensure hemodynamic stability before removing the wire. Complications include RVOT perforation, pericardial effusion, TR, conduction defects due to splinting of tricuspid valve, and arrythmias. Cyanotic spells may occur during induction and has to be managed with beta blockers, morphine, IV fluids, and other spell medication. Spells are infrequent once the wire is across the RVOT. Acute reperfusion injury or pulmonary edema can occur due to stent overflow, which should be anticipated if saturation increases by >25% after stenting. Delayed extubation after treatment with diuretics may prevent this complication. Distal stent embolization can be managed by reinflating the balloon and repositioning the stent if the wire is still in place. Proximal embolization into the RV is more difficult to manage and surgeon has to be alerted for possible surgical retrieval. In cases of double outlet right ventricle, stent embolization may happen into the aorta, and it may be best to deploy it in descending aorta if safe retrieval is not possible. Tricuspid valve damage may be related to injury by long sheath entangling in the chordae. If the course of the sheath is in doubt, it is best to withdraw and cross again.[6,7]

PULMONARY VALVE PERFORATION

Indication

This procedure is performed if there are well-formed pulmonary sinuses with discrete membranous valvar atresia with or without ventricular septal defect. Right ventricular infundibulum should be well developed, tricuspid valve

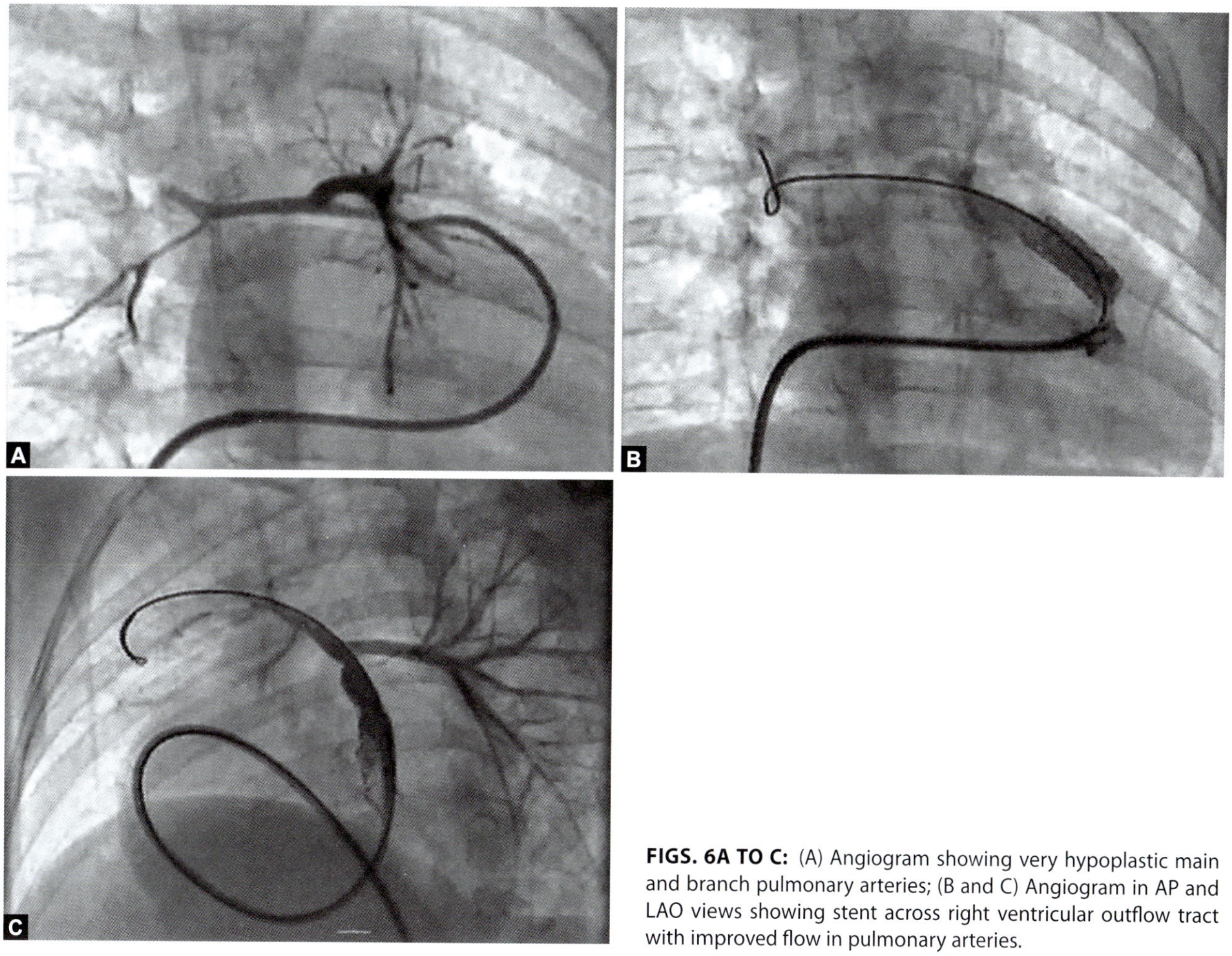

FIGS. 6A TO C: (A) Angiogram showing very hypoplastic main and branch pulmonary arteries; (B and C) Angiogram in AP and LAO views showing stent across right ventricular outflow tract with improved flow in pulmonary arteries.

Z scores should ideally be >–2 and there should be no RV-dependent coronary circulation. Femoral venous and arterial access are secured and RV angiogram done with JR catheter in lateral and AP views. The valve maybe perforated with RFA or the stiff end of the CTO wire. For perforation with wire, the guide catheter is positioned underneath the pulmonary valve taking care to be coaxial to the valve to avoid RV perforation. The position of the wire and catheter maybe confirmed by arterial duct injections through the femoral artery route. Once the wire perforates the valve, the position in the MPA lumen is confirmed by arterial angiograms. The valve is serially dilated with coronary balloons and later by low profile balloons like the Tyshak balloon with the diameter of the balloon not exceeding 1.2–1.4 times the pulmonary valve annulus **(Video 7, Fig. 7)**. In cases of pulmonary atresia with intact ventricular septum and severe TR, care must be taken to avoid causing significant PR as this may cause circular shunt and reduced cardiac output particularly in the presence of large PDA. RVOT perforation and tamponade are the most dreaded complications. Sometimes, PDA stenting or RVOT stenting maybe required if there is inadequate improvement of pulmonary blood flow and saturation.[8,9]

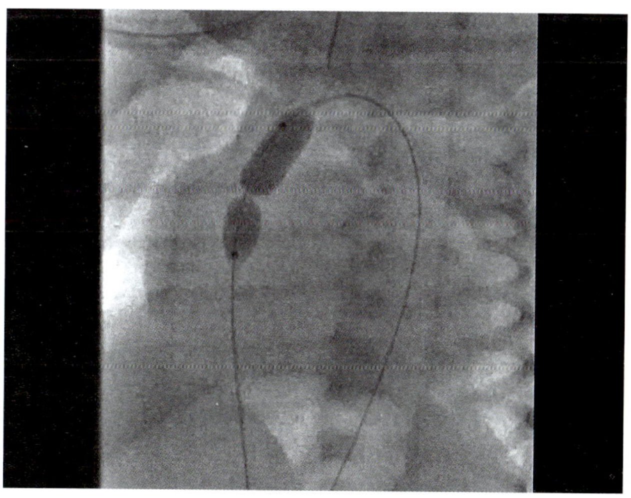

FIG. 7: Fluoroscopic image showing guidewire passed from venous access through the main pulmonary artery and the duct to the descending thoracic aorta. Balloon is inflated across the pulmonary valve.

INTERVENTIONS IN THE UNIVENTRICULAR PATHWAY

Branch PA Stenting

Even the most ideal Fontan pathway functions at a higher systemic venous pressure and will fail if there is any obstruction in the pathway. No gradient is acceptable in the branch pulmonary arteries or BDG or Fontan anastomosis. Branch PA size has to be optimal and any stenosis tackled by stenting. Balloon expandable stents are used and the size is determined by the size of the PA at the hilum **(Video 8, Fig. 8)**. Ideally the size should not exceed three times the narrowest diameter or >1 mm more than the largest diameter at the hilum. There should be a covered stent back-up in case of PA perforation.[10,11]

Aortopulmonary Collaterals

All aortopulmonary collaterals have to be identified prior to univentricular or biventricular repair and have to be tackled prior to definitive surgery in cases of nonessential MAPCAs (communicating MAPCAS or noncommunicating MAPCAs with good native PA arborization). Aortopulmonary collaterals are a cause of prolonged chest drainage in early postoperative period after Fontan completion and ideally they should be tackled prior to Fontan. They are closed with coils or vascular plugs.[12,13]

Systemic Venous Collaterals

Venovenous collaterals have to be looked for in pre-Fontan catheterization. Their presence may indicate raised BDG pressure as they usually develop as a pop-off when the venous pressure is high. The venovenous collaterals need not be tackled if they are draining to IVC or other tributaries of IVC, as ultimately they will be redirected to the Fontan circuit. But they may need to be closed if they are very large, to improve saturation if there is delay in Fontan completion. Balloon occlusion of these collaterals may be needed at times to see if the Glenn pressure increases after occlusion which may indicate underlying high PA pressure. Porto-systemic shunts may develop in patients with left isomerism and if present, it has to be closed with vascular plugs as it may cause hepatopulmonary syndrome resulting in PAVM or PAH. Venoatrial collaterals connect the Glenn circuit to the atrium or pulmonary veins and these may act as natural fenestration for the Fontan circuit. They have to be closed if they cause significant desaturation.[12-14]

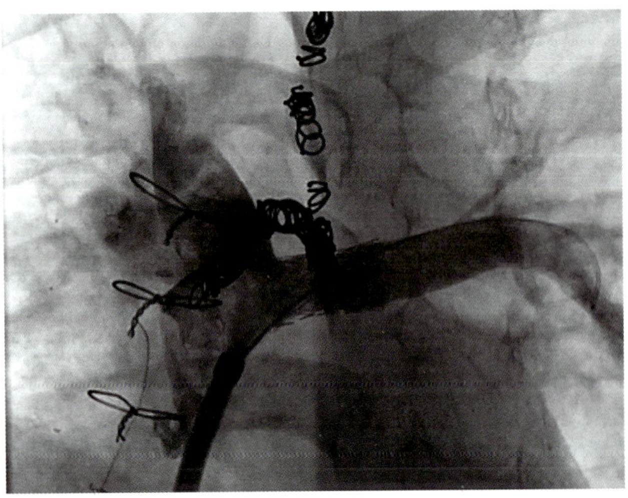

FIG. 8: LPA stenting done in a post Fontan patient.

Fontan Fenestration Stenting

Fenestrating the Fontan circuit is an accepted way of reducing the elevated systemic venous pressure in high-risk cases. Routine fenestration of low-risk Fontan cases is no longer practiced in most centers. Elevation of pulmonary artery pressures can cause elevated Fontan pressures and this may necessitate creating a fenestration in the Fontan circuit. Sometimes surgically created fenestration can close off spontaneously. The procedure can be done under sedation or general anesthesia. Femoral venous access or internal jugular venous access is chosen to create a fenestration with Brockenbrough needle after delineating the conduit with angiograms. Good amount of force is needed to puncture the PTFE conduit into the atrium. Once the entry into the atrium is confirmed with injection of contrast, a coiled tip wire (commonly used for left atrial entry in balloon mitral valvotomy) is passed into the atrium. The fenestration is dilated initially with the dilator the Brockenbrough sheath and then a catheter is passed over the wire into the atrium. The wire is then exchanged for a stiff 0.035 wire over which semi-compliant balloons of size 6 is passed and the fenestration dilated. Then a long sheath with its dilator is introduced into the atrium and an appropriate sized stent (8–10) is placed across the fenestration and dilated slowly. This slow dilatation results in flaring of the two ends of the stent giving it a diabolo shape. The stent is inflated till a small waist of approximately 6 mm is maintained **(Figs. 9A to F)**. Transthoracic echocardiogram is done to rule out pericardial effusion. Creation of fenestration results in clinical improvement at the cost of desaturation.[12,15-17]

Fontan Fenestration Closure

In certain instances, exercise or resting desaturation in a fenestrated Fontan patient maybe disabling enough to warrant closure of the fenestration. Surgically created fenestrations can be closed with septal occluders or ductal occluders. Stented fenestration can be made smaller by crimping the fenestration percutaneously using snares. The snare is introduced through the fenestration to the distal edge of the stent in the atrium and the snare is manipulated over the stent and drawn toward the waist of the stent. The snare is then tightened to crimp the waist of the stent.[18]

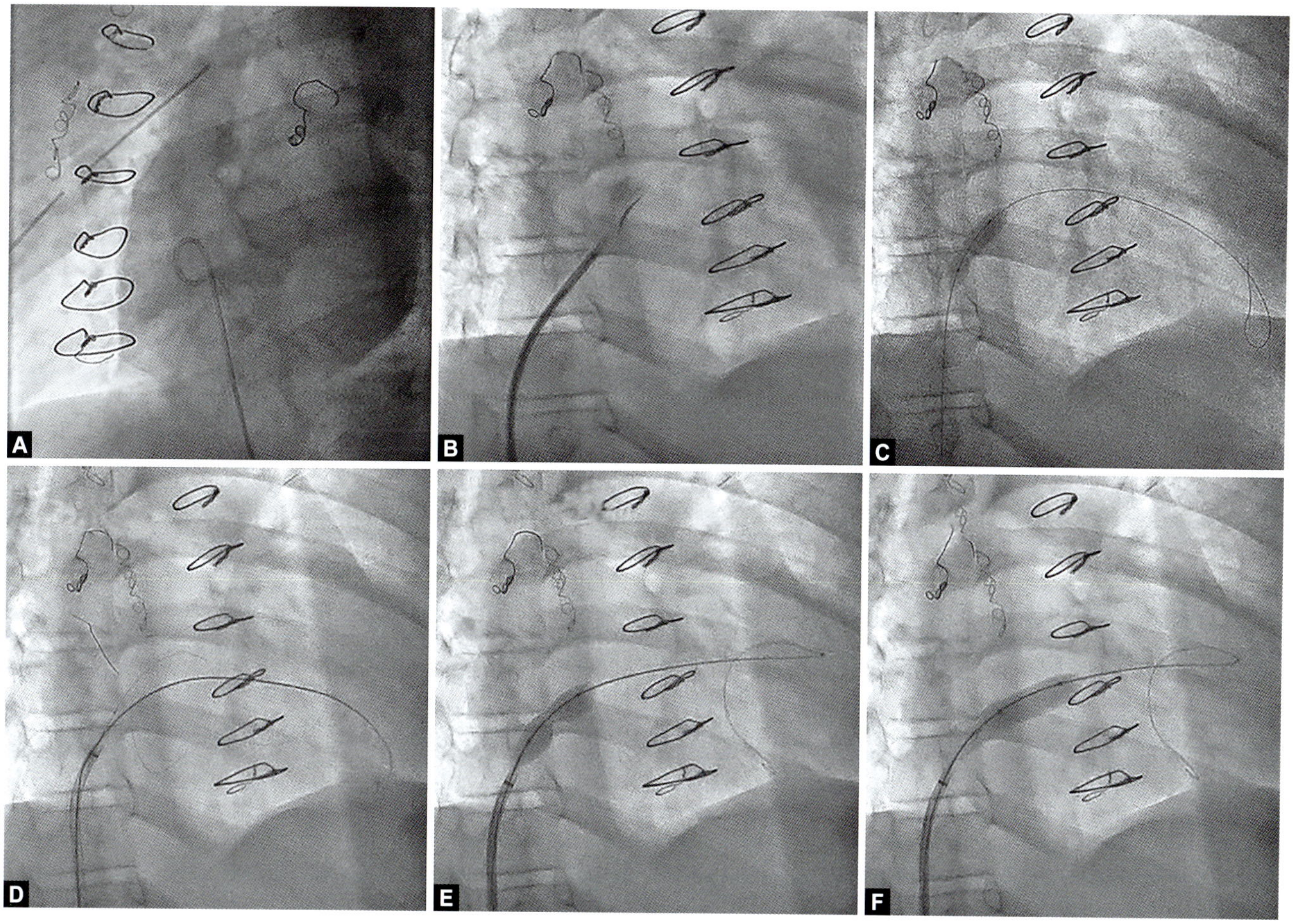

FIGS. 9A TO F: Angiogram done in the Fontan circuit followed by creation of Fontan fenestration by a Brockenbrough needle. The fenestration is then dilated with balloon and then stented.

Fontan Pathway Stenting

Narrowing of SVC/PA anastomosis and IVC-conduit anastomosis are best managed by stenting. Uncovered balloon expandable stents are commonly used.[12]

Fontan Takedown

Percutaneous Fontan takedown can be attempted by putting a covered stent from the IVC into the atrium. The Fontan conduit to PA connection may also be closed using muscular VSD occluders or vascular plugs and the IVC flow connected to the atrium by fenestrating the conduit and stenting from the conduit to the atrium.[19]

Occlusion of Pulmonary Antegrade Flow

Most institutions interrupt antegrade pulmonary blood flow at the time of Fontan completion. If there is persistence of antegrade pulmonary blood flow, it may be advisable to occlude it to reduce PA pressure to optimal levels. Occlusion is done across a pre-existing PA band using ductal occluder with the retention disc on the proximal MPA side or symmetrical devices like muscular VSD occlude **(Videos 9A and B, Fig. 10)** or Konar device if the valve has to be occluded.[20]

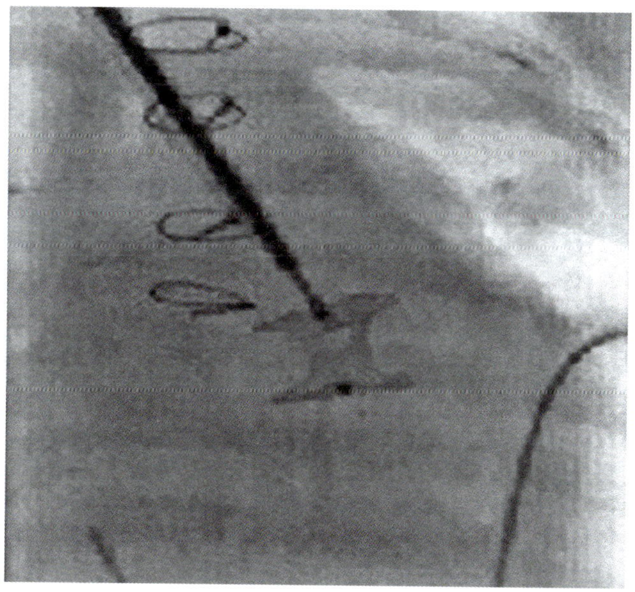

FIG. 10: Interruption of antegrade pulmonary blood flow by a muscular VSD occlude through the internal jugular vein access.

CONCLUSION

Complex congenital heart disease needs the collaborative efforts of the interventional cardiologist and the surgeon for effective management. Newer developments in imaging, newer devices and stents have greatly advanced the role of percutaneous interventions in cyanotic congenital heart disease.

VIDEO LEGENDS

Video 1: Subcostal four-chamber view showing inflated balloon in left atrium and the balloon has been tugged into the right atrium across the atrial septa defect.

Video 2: Guide catheter introduced through the left axillary access and the duct is wired. The duct is arising from the undersurface of the arch. A stent has been placed across the duct and dilated. Good flow is seen in branch pulmonary arteries.

Video 3: Guide catheter in descending thoracic aorta (DTA). Duct arising from DTA has been stented through femoral arterial access.

Video 4: The arterial duct arising from the base of left innominate artery has been stented using the femoral arterial access.

Video 5: 7 mm stent placed across the duct through a long sheath passed from the venous access in a duct dependent systemic circulation as part of hybrid Norwood procedure after bilateral pulmonary artery banding.

Videos 6A and B: (A) Angiogram showing severe right ventricular outflow tract obstruction; (B) Angiogram in AP view showing stent across right ventricular outflow tract with improved flow in pulmonary arteries.

Video 7: Fluoroscopic image showing guidewire passed from venous access through the main pulmonary artery and the duct to the descending thoracic aorta. Balloon is inflated across the pulmonary valve.

Video 8: LPA stenting done in a post Fontan patient.

Videos 9A and B: (A) Creation of Fontan fenestration by a Brockenbrough needle; (B) The fenestration is then dilated with balloon and stented.

Scan the QR CODE to access the above listed videos.

ONLINE REFERENCES

Please scan the QR code provided at the end of the table of contents for References of this chapter.

CHAPTER 102

Congenital Complete Heart Block: Management in Fetus, Childhood, and Beyond

Sanjeev Hanumantacharya Naganur, Abhishek Mallick

ABSTRACT

Congenital atrioventricular heart block is relatively a rare occurrence. The clinical presentation varies with described cases of incidental diagnosis made in adulthood. It is usually consequent to the placental transfer of maternal antibodies and is often associated with high mortality and morbidity. The diagnosis is conclusively made during fetal echocardiography. Maternal therapy with variety of drugs including hydroxychloroquine, steroids, intravenous immunoglobulins alone or in combinations have been tried with varying success rate. Postnatal management includes pacing according to the clinical and hemodynamic needs.

Keywords: Congenital heart block, fetal echocardiography, medications, pacing

INTRODUCTION

The mature adult electrical conduction system of the heart has been well studied and described in humans. Though the origin of the conduction system is subject to discrepancies, Wenink's model of development of the conducting system is the most widely accepted theory regarding its embryogenesis.[1]

The basic layout of the conduction system or the His Tawara system **(Fig. 1)**, as is known after the pathologists who described it, is as follows:

- Sinoatrial (SA) node
- Internodal pathways
- Atrioventricular (AV) node
- His bundle and its branches
- Purkinje fibers

The SA node is a cluster of cells located in the upper part of the right atrium near its connection with the superior vena cava. The SA node serves as the heart's natural pacemaker, controlling the heart rate. It produces electrical signals on its own, which then travel to both the right and the left atria via internodal pathways. These signals prompt the atrial muscle to contract, with the atrial muscle conducting at a relatively rapid speed of 0.5 m/s. The AV node is located in the AV septum in the triangle of Koch and is comprised of specialized cells. It is responsible for receiving electrical impulses from the atria and transmitting them to the ventricles. With a conduction velocity of 0.05 m/s, the AV node temporarily slows the conduction and allows for maximal ventricular filling before ventricular systole. The His bundle consists of specialized heart muscle cells responsible for electrical conduction. These cells receive signals from the AV node.

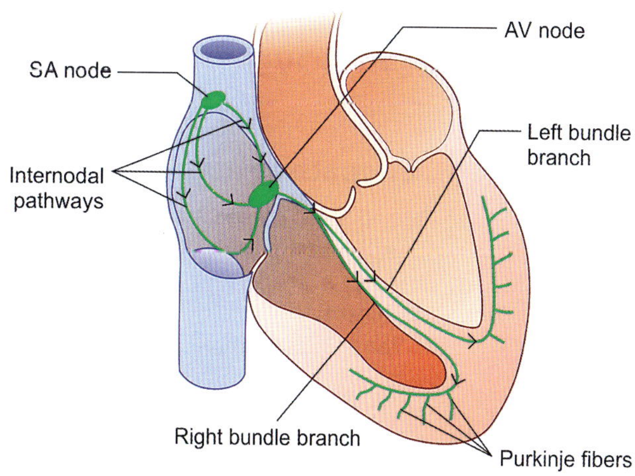

FIG. 1: Basic layout of the conduction system.

From the His bundle, the left and right bundle branches extend down the interventricular septum. The branches of the His bundle transmit electrical impulses to the left and right ventricles at 1 m/s. Each branch ends in multiple Purkinje fibers. Purkinje fibers are located in the subendocardium and are responsible for conducting the electrical impulse to the ventricular myocardium at speeds of 4 m/s, ultimately leading to ventricular contraction.

ATRIOVENTRICULAR BLOCK

Atrioventricular blocks are disturbances in the electrical conduction between the atria and the ventricles of the heart. They are categorized into three main types based on severity and the impact on heart function:

1. *First-degree AV block*: This is the mildest form, where the electrical impulses are delayed but still reach the ventricles.
    - *Electrocardiogram (ECG) characteristics*: Prolonged PR interval (>200 ms) without dropped beats
2. *Second-degree AV block*:
    - *Type I (Mobitz I or Wenckebach)*: The PR interval progressively lengthens until a beat is dropped (a QRS complex is missed).
        - *ECG characteristics*: Progressive PR interval prolongation followed by a nonconducted P wave
    - *Type II (Mobitz II)*: Some impulses are conducted, but others are blocked without a preceding change in PR interval.
        - *ECG characteristics*: Constant PR interval with intermittent nonconducted P waves
3. *Third-degree AV block or complete heart block (CHB)*: No atrial impulses reach the ventricles, resulting in independent atrial and ventricular rhythms.
    - *ECG characteristics*: No correlation between P waves and QRS complexes; the atria and ventricles beat independently.

CONGENITAL ATRIOVENTRICULAR BLOCK

Definition and Etiopathogenesis

Congenital CHB is defined as an AV block occurring prenatally, at birth, or within the first month of life. Congenital CHB affects nearly 1 in every 20,000 live births.[2] It commonly manifests as fetal bradycardia, which is defined as heart rate < 110 beats/min. The causes are broadly classified into two. Nonimmunological causes of CHB include heterotaxy, corrected congenital transposition of great arteries, etc. Immunological processes involve passage of maternal autoantibodies such as anti-Ro/La across the placenta and damage to the cardiac conducting system. Mothers with these antibodies have a 2–5% risk of delivering a baby with CHB. This risk increases to 12–25% in case of a previously affected child.[3] The occurrence of tissue injury in the fetus is believed to be linked to the transplacental passage of maternal IgG autoantibodies. Specifically, anti-SSA/Ro and anti-SSB/La antibodies attach to fetal cardiocytes, impeding the normal elimination of apoptotic cells. This disruption leads to an inflammatory response and fibrosis within the cardiac conduction system. Additional potential mechanisms include the cross-reactivity of SSA/SSB antibodies and the downregulation or inhibition of L-type calcium channels by autoantibodies. Some researchers have delved into the electrophysiological and molecular aspects of congenital heart block, suggesting that anti-SSA/Ro antibodies may directly induce arrhythmias.[4,5] Ultimately, these processes contribute to myocarditis, hemorrhage, fibrosis, calcification, and necrosis in the conduction system, culminating in the manifestation of varying degrees of heart block, myocardial dysfunction, and/or endocardial fibroelastosis (EFE). A recent investigation by Jaeggi et al.[6] revealed that the risk of developing CHB was 85% when a fetus was exposed to anti-Ro antibody titers > 100 U/mL. The study also found that pregnancies with anti-Ro levels < 50 U/mL did not show cardiac involvement. Additionally, fetal and neonatal cardiac manifestations were found to be independent of anti-La antibody titers.[6] In contrast, Gordon et al. discovered that the children of anti-Ro positive mothers had a 2% risk of having AVB, which increased to 3.1% if the mother was anti-La positive as well.[7] However, these antibodies alone do not fully explain the development of cardiac neonatal lupus erythematosus (NLE), as most women with anti-Ro and La (positive and/or high) have normal pregnancy outcomes. Given that cardiac involvement is the most serious complication of NLE, routine screening of anti-SSA/Ro and anti-SSB/La antibodies in mothers with autoimmune disorders such as SLE and Sjögren's syndrome should be conducted during the antenatal period for early detection and successful management. Maternal autoantibodies, as aforementioned, are commonly believed to be the main cause of CHB in NLE; some studies suggest that they are not the sole factor. Research has indicated that cardiac issues may develop in only one of the twins or two of the triplets exposed to maternal SSA/Ro and SSB/La autoantibodies.[8,9] Various environmental, intrauterine, fetal, or maternal factors, along with genetic predisposition, could also influence the development of CHB in neonatal lupus.

INVESTIGATIONS

Fetal Echocardiography

Fetal echocardiography helps in the assessment of heart rate (bradycardia defined as heart rate <110 beats/min) and in the diagnosis of nonimmunological causes of CHB, which include heterotaxy, corrected congenital transposition of great arteries, etc. The American Heart Association (AHA)

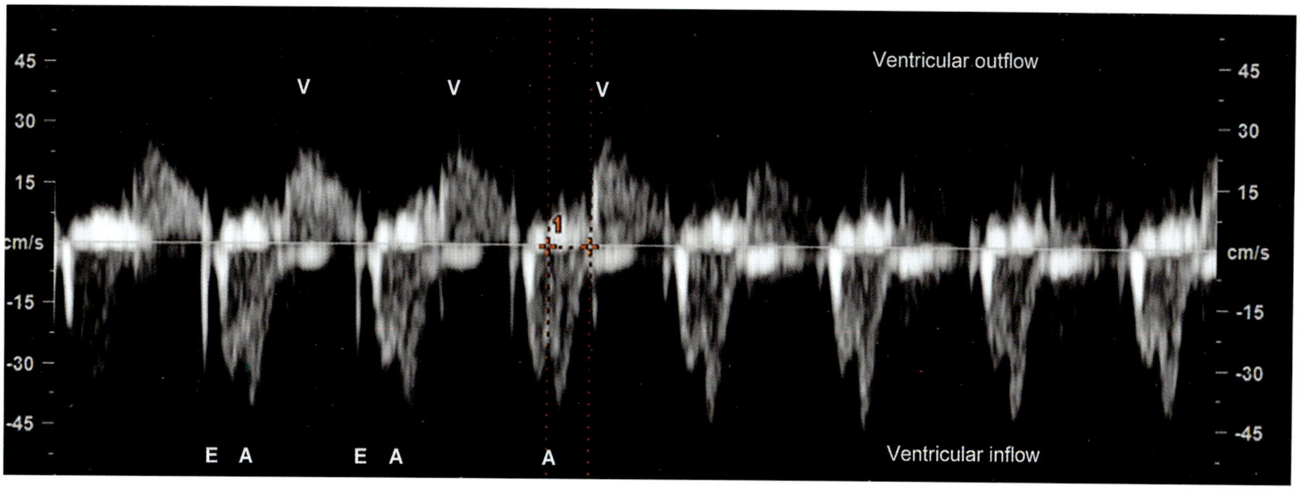

FIG. 2: Fetal echocardiography: Pulse wave doppler interrogation of mitral valve and aortic valve (left ventricular inflow-outflow) measuring the mechanical PR interval.

recommends screening of pregnant women with anti-Ro/anti-La positive status with a fetal echocardiography commencing at 16–18 weeks. Serial evaluation is recommended to be conducted at an interval of 1–2 weeks, till 28 weeks of gestation.[10] In echocardiography, pulsed wave Doppler interrogation with the sample in superior vena cava-aorta (SVC-Ao) view or mitral valve inflow-aortic valve outflow (MV-AoV) view or the pulmonary artery-pulmonary vein (PA-PV) view is taken to calculate the mechanical PR interval, defined as the interval from the beginning of atrial contraction to the onset of ejection across the semilunar valves **(Fig. 2)**. The normal PR interval is 0.12 ± 0.02 second, and a value > 0.15 second is considered abnormal.[11] Other parameters assessed on fetal echocardiography are tricuspid or mitral regurgitation, chamber dimensions, right and left ventricular (LV) systolic function, and fetal hydrops (pericardial effusion, pleural effusion, ascites, skin/scalp edema).

Postnatal evaluation for congenital AV block: Neonates, infants, and toddlers exhibit a varied clinical presentation. Some of them may be totally asymptomatic (incidentally detected bradycardia), whereas others may present with vague symptoms such as unusual fatigue, disturbed sleep, and growth failure. In some cases, the first presentation of congenital AV block may be a seizure/syncope, heart failure, or sudden death. As with fetal evaluation, the scan focuses on structural defects and the consequences of CHB such as systolic dysfunction or associated pulmonary hypertension.

Electrocardiogram

A 12-lead ECG is diagnostic in the evaluation of bradycardia due to congenital AV block in children and adults. The "p" versus "QRS" rate, rhythm, and morphology of escape rhythm are crucial. It is important to differentiate between congenital heart block and prolonged QT interval and those with congenital long QT syndrome who might have a pseudo 2:1 AV block. The latter group has normal AV conduction (differentiating factor), but due to prolonged ventricular repolarization, alternate P wave occurs during the ventricular refractory period and therefore does not lead to ventricular depolarization. The two proposed mechanisms for the development of QT prolongation in patients with congenital AV block are: (1) Conduction disorder, which results in bradycardia, could be the initial event that later causes altered repolarization, and (2) a phenotypic expression of latent congenital long QT syndrome.

Twenty-four Hours Holter

This study helps to assess the mean heart rate and the documentation of episodes of RR prolongation. The risk of sudden cardiac death during sleep is high if one has episodes of long R-R intervals (3,000–6,000 ms).[12]

Echocardiography

Postnatal echocardiography is required to assess the ventricular size and function apart from ruling out structural abnormalities such as heterotaxy and congenitally corrected transposition of the great arteries.

MANAGEMENT

Maternal–Fetal Management

For maternal benefits, the European League Against Rheumatism (EULAR) has suggested hydroxychloroquine (HCQ) for managing disease activity and preventing flare-ups during pregnancy in SLE patients.[13] One of the small observation groups has found HCQ to be potentially beneficial in preventing CHB in fetuses at risk from antibody-positive pregnant women or who have had a previous affected child.[14] However, a large prospective trial is necessary to validate its efficacy. HCQ hinders toll-like receptor signaling, which is crucial in the immune response against the conduction system. The treatment of first-degree and second-degree AV block is still a debatable topic. The effect of fluorinated steroids on the conversion from first-degree block to normal sinus rhythm cannot be definitively determined based on the available information as of today. Though used in some centers, a recent meta-analysis did not show any advantages of antenatal corticosteroids alone or in combination with other medications for second-degree AV block in terms of disease progression, disease stability at birth, postnatal pacing, fetal survival, and neonatal survival.[15] A commonly used fluorinated steroid, dexamethasone is known to reduce maternal autoantibody burden. Dexamethasone can be administered orally or intravenously, with a tapering regimen. The initial dosage is 4–8 mg/day for 2–4 weeks, followed by 2 mg/day until delivery. The side effects in fetuses and pregnant women are of major concern.[16] One of the large randomized studies has found a higher incidence of cerebral palsy after prolonged dexamethasone use. Other side effects include growth restriction and oligohydramnios, whereas maternal side effects include hypertension, diabetes mellitus, mood changes, and an increased susceptibility to infections.[17] In fetuses with CHB, heart rate < 55 beats/min, a combination of β-sympathomimetic agent with dexamethasone has been found to increase fetal heart rate and reduce morbidity and mortality. Commonly used agents are oral salbutamol (10 mg every 8 hours with a maximum daily dose of 30 mg) and terbutaline (2.5–7.5 mg every 4–6 hours with a maximum daily dose of 30 mg), which can increase the fetal ventricular rate by approximately 5–10 beats/min. Some retrospective studies have shown that combination therapy can have a positive effect on the fetal heart, reducing myocardial damage. The efficacy of β-sympathomimetic agents alone in increasing heart rate and preventing heart failure has been documented in several case reports. Additionally, there is a lack of evidence demonstrating that the use of these medications can impact the survival of fetuses. Maternal untoward effects may include tremors, palpitations, and sweating.[18] IVIg and plasmapheresis have been studied with an aim to reduce the levels of circulating maternal autoantibodies to minimize damage to the fetal heart. One small nonrandomized study has found that IVIg (400 mg/kg every 3 weeks from 12 to 24 weeks of gestation) is a potential candidate in preventing the recurrence of CHB among pregnant women who have previously had a child with CHB.[19] Plasmapheresis and IVIg combined with a corticosteroid have been shown to revert second-degree AVB to first-degree AVB and stabilize the progression of complete AV block, especially in fetuses with cardiomyopathy/EFE with or without complete AV block.[20] Novel approaches like percutaneous implantation of a cardiac pacemaker have been successfully placed in utero in experimental studies.[21] However, the procedure poses serious risks.

Postnatal Management of Complete Heart Block

Beta agonists such as IV isoprenaline may be administered in symptomatic neonates with very low heart rates till the pacemaker is deployed. The chronotropic effect of isoprenaline is better than other sympathomimetics making it the agent of choice in this situation.

Complete heart block poses a substantial risk of morbidity and mortality, particularly during the first few months of life. Mortality rates for infants born with CHB exceeded 80% in the presence of hydrops.[22] Factors contributing to a poor prognosis include hydrops fetalis, low heart rate, EFE, dilated cardiomyopathy, valvular dysfunction, low birth weight, male sex, premature delivery, and complications from prematurity or neonatal lupus. The significant echocardiographic predictors of mortality are hydrops and EFE.[23]

Indications for Pacing

There are two guidelines that can be followed for the timing and indication for postnatal pacing, and both are very similar to each other:

1. 1998 ACC/AHA Guidelines for Implantation of Cardiac Pacemakers and Antiarrhythmia Devices: Executive Summary[24]
2. 2021 PACES Expert Consensus Statement on the Indications and Management of Cardiovascular Implantable Electronic Devices in Pediatric Patients.[25] The guidelines are shown in **Table 1**.

Pacing Strategies

Pacing strategy can vary significantly with different centers. Children who present with complete AV block and normal ventricular function may initially be paced in the VVIR mode, with a potential upgrade to the VDD/DDD mode during adolescence, or they may receive a dual-chamber pacemaker as the initial treatment. Epicardial systems are typically chosen for the youngest children, while endocardial pacing is delayed until the child weighs > 10 kg or is at least 2 years old (varies across centers). Some centers postpone endocardial implantation until the child is at least 5–8 years old. Several

TABLE 1: Guidelines for timing and indications for postnatal pacing.

Indications	COR	LOE
Permanent pacemaker implantation is indicated for patients with CHB with symptomatic bradycardia	I	B-NR
Permanent pacemaker implantation is indicated for patients with CHB with a wide QRS escape rhythm, complex ventricular ectopy, or ventricular dysfunction	I	B-NR
Permanent pacemaker implantation is indicated for CHB in asymptomatic neonates or infants when the mean ventricular rate is 50 beats/min. Ventricular rate alone should not be used as implant criteria as symptoms due to low cardiac output may occur at faster heart rates	I	C-LD
Permanent pacemaker implantation is reasonable for asymptomatic CHB beyond the first year of life when the mean ventricular rate is 50 beats/min, or there are prolonged pauses in the ventricular rate	IIa	B-NR
Permanent pacemaker implantation is reasonable for CHB with left ventricular dilation (Z score ≥ 3) associated with significant mitral insufficiency or systolic dysfunction	IIa	C-LD
Permanent pacemaker implantation may be considered for CHB in asymptomatic adolescents with an acceptable ventricular rate, a narrow QRS complex, and normal ventricular function, based on an individualized consideration of the risk/benefit ratio	IIb	C-LD

(COR: class of recommendation; LD: limited data; LOE: level of evidence; NR: nonrandomized)

factors are considered when choosing between an epicardial and an endocardial approach to pacing, including:

- Family's preference and local expertise
- Concerns about high initial and long-term capture thresholds of epicardial leads have been minimized, thanks to the introduction of epicardial leads with steroid-eluting tips, as they appear to perform similar to endocardial leads, prolonging battery life and reducing the need for repeat operations.
- Transvenous pacing in younger kids has a concern about the risk of vascular or valvular injury and the likelihood of a mismatch between leads and recipients due to somatic growth.
- Potentially fatal complications associated with the extraction of transvenous leads, making it a relatively high-risk procedure
- Functional and hemodynamic potential advantages of epicardial LV placement in small children compared to right ventricular (RV) apical pacing are also part of the decision-making process.

Prognosis

Congenital AV block carries a high mortality (20–30%, mostly fetal/neonatal) and morbidity (67% require permanent pacing before reaching adolescence).[2,26] The associated structural abnormalities (ranges from 30 to 53%) significantly increase the risk of mortality.[27,28] The survival of congenital AV block with structural abnormalities is only 14%, compared to 85% of the autoimmune isolated congenital complete AV block beyond the neonatal period.[27] The major risk factors for mortality in isolated CHB are low birth weight, prematurity, hydrops fetalis, EFE, and depressed ventricular function.[29]

Combining several CCHB studies, risk factors for CHF, Stokes–Adams attacks, or sudden death includes:[2,30-32]

- Low newborn ventricular rate (<55 beats/min)
- Low fetal atrial rate (<120 beats/min)
- Wide QRS complex on ECG
- Corrected QT interval prolongation > 460 ms
- Atrial enlargement on ECG or cardiomegaly by chest X-ray (risk factor for CHF)
- Ventricular ectopy in combination with a wide QRS complex or structural heart disease
- Presence of complex structural heart disease

In the Indian context, the existing awareness (2.2%)[33] about the prenatal evaluation of congenital heart diseases in high-risk population, especially rhythm disturbances, is alarmingly low and needs a lot of work. It is noteworthy that the awareness is similar across different demographies and social backgrounds. The combined efforts of obstetrics-gynecology, cardiology, and rheumatology-immunology along with supporting paramedical teams involved in the care are crucial in our setup. The counseling of families for making them aware about the role of fetal echocardiography and maternal workup in the early recognition of AV block, associated structural heart defects helps in the timely management, thereby significantly improving the clinical outcome in the affected fetus.

CONCLUSION

To summarise, complete heart block once diagnosed in intrauterine period is highly unlikely to revert with medication. The outcome of pregnancy depends on the myocardial function of the fetus. If diagnosed antenatally, most of the neonates go on to have a surgically implanted epicardial pacemaker. However, late recognition is common and then the pacemaker insertion is guided by symptomatology and expertise of the treating facility.

ONLINE REFERENCES

Please scan the QR code provided at the end of the table of contents for References of this chapter.

SECTION 10

Valvular Heart Disease/Miscellaneous

Section Outline

CHAPTER 103

Top 10 Papers in Valvular Heart Disease 2023–2024

Rajeev Garg, Vardhini Vijaykumar

ABSTRACT

Recent advancements in valvular heart disease research highlight significant papers on diagnosis, management, and outcomes. This chapter focuses on collating the top 10 research articles between 2023 and 2024 based on the late-breaking sessions of recent conferences and trial design, sourced from high-impact journals, collectively contributing to shaping clinical practice guidelines and improving patient outcomes in valvular heart diseases.

Keywords: Valvular heart disease, aortic stenosis, transcatheter aortic valve replacement, surgical aortic valve replacement, transcatheter aortic valve implantation, transcatheter edge-to-edge repair

INTRODUCTION

Valvular heart disease (VHD) remains a significant contributor to cardiovascular morbidity and mortality worldwide, impacting millions of individuals and posing substantial challenges to healthcare systems. Advances in diagnostic modalities, surgical techniques, and interventional therapies have transformed the management of VHD, necessitating a continuous update of the latest research and clinical practices. This chapter aims to provide a comprehensive summary of the top 10 seminal papers in the field of VHD, highlighting groundbreaking studies that have shaped current understanding, influenced treatment protocols, and paved the way for future innovations. By synthesizing these pivotal findings, this chapter provides clinicians, researchers, and students a valuable resource for staying abreast of the most influential developments in VHD, fostering informed clinical decision-making and inspiring ongoing research endeavors.

TRILUMINATE PIVOTAL

Tricuspid regurgitation (TR) is frequently seen and is linked to a lower quality of life (QOL) and reduced survival rates. The main treatment is diuretics, with surgery reserved for a restricted group of patients who are frequently associated with a significant surgical risk. In right-sided valvular disease, there is a shortage of evidence, and knowledge is commonly extrapolated from left-sided comprehension. Although transcatheter tricuspid therapies are relatively new, a randomized controlled clinical trial has not been conducted to evaluate their benefits. The purpose of the TRILUMINATE Pivotal trial was to compare the safety and efficacy of medical therapy alone (control group) versus transcatheter tricuspid repair with the TriClip™ device in symptomatic patients with severe TR, who are estimated to be at intermediate or higher risk of dying from tricuspid valve surgery (device group).[1] This was a multicenter, prospective, randomized controlled study.

The patient group had severe, symptomatic TR and had been receiving device therapy or stable GDMT for heart failure for >30 days. TriClip™ therapy reduced TR to mild or below in 87% of cases, compared to 4.8% in the control group. This reduction persisted until the 1-year follow-up. The device was shown to be superior, as evidenced by the significant improvement in QOL, which drove the primary endpoint to be reached ($p = 0.02$). The degree of TR reduction was found to be correlated with the degree of QOL improvement. The 30-day MAE rate was only 1.7%, and 0.6% of cases had pacemaker implantation and mortality. At 1 year, both groups had high survival rates (almost 90%), free of both TV surgery and mortality.

Due to the open-label nature of this trial, bias may be a possibility. Nonetheless, to reduce bias, the follow-ups were carried out by staff members who were not aware of the group assignments and used standardized scripts. The groups were known to the staff in the echocardiography core laboratory. The experiment was also carried out during the COVID-19 pandemic, which would have had an impact on clinical outcomes; nonetheless, a COVID-19 sensitivity analysis of the primary endpoint produced findings that were in line with the primary analysis. These outcomes validated the device's approval by the US Food and Drug Administration in April 2024.

The imaging substudy, which comprised 93 patients (mean age 78.6 years; 55.9% women) from 10 US sites, was mandated by the FDA as part of the trial. The researchers used baseline and 30-day CT and MRI scans, followed by a 12-month CT scan. 231 CT scans and 171 MRIs were included in the substudy overall. Based on those scans, patients with higher TR volumes by MRI at baseline had larger tricuspid valve annulus regions, larger right ventricles (RVs), and poorer effective RV ejection percentages ($p < 0.0001$ for all). TR volume on MRI in patients treated with medical therapy alone did not change significantly from baseline to 30 days, but it was dramatically reduced with tricuspid transcatheter edge-to-edge repair (T-TEER), decreasing from a mean of 50 to 18 mL ($p < 0.0001$). Patients with the largest reductions saw the greatest beneficial changes in RV size and function.

SMART TRIAL

In transcatheter aortic valve replacement (TAVR) patients with severe symptomatic aortic stenosis (AS) and a tiny aortic valve annulus, the SMART trial was designed to assess the efficacy and safety of the intra-annular SAPIEN valve [balloon-expanding valve (BEV)] versus the supra-annular Evolut valve [self-expanding valve (SEV)].[2] This postmarket study was a prospective, randomized controlled trial carried out at 83 different foreign locations. All-comer trials include patients with bicuspid valves and all surgical risk categories. The SMART trial is the biggest and most rigorous TAVR trial to date, enrolling primarily women, and randomly assigned patients to the two most popular TAVR devices. At 1 year, the supra-annular SEV showed no worse clinical results than BEV.

Superior valve performance was seen at 1 year with standard hemodynamic measures (EOA, DVI, severe PPM, mean grad > 20 mm Hg) in terms of reduced BVD incidence by 32.2%, 0.5 cm^2 more effective orifice area, 0.19 bigger Doppler velocity index, 6.8% lower incidence of severe PMM, and an 8 mm Hg lower mean gradient. Hemodynamic parameters were comparable at baseline and consistently favored SEV. There were better QOL and less overall aortic regurgitation (AR) according to the KCCQ ordinal outcome. The outcomes held true for women, individuals under and beyond 80 years of age, and the whole spectrum of aortic annuli < 430 mm^2.

The SMART trial shows that differences in clinical parameters, such as stroke volume index, should be taken into account when deciding the optimal treatment for each patient, in addition to selecting the optimum hemodynamic valve for patients with tiny aortic annuli. Additionally, over the whole spectrum of tiny annulus regions, there was a notable reduced bioprosthetic valve dysfunction with the SEV in comparison to the BEV. These results emphasize SEV as the ideal and preferred choice for patients (mostly women) with a small aortic annulus.

TRANSCATHETER OR SURGICAL AORTIC VALVE IMPLANTATION: 10-YEAR OUTCOMES OF THE NOTION TRIAL

In patients with severe isolated aortic valve stenosis who are at a decreased surgical risk, this is the first trial to compare TAVR versus surgical aortic valve replacement (SAVR) with the longest follow-up (at 10 years) data.[3] Following either SAVR or transcatheter aortic valve implantation (TAVI), major clinical outcomes, such as all-cause mortality, stroke, or myocardial infarction, were comparable. While the rates of bioprosthetic valve failure were comparable, SAVR patients exhibited significant structural valve degeneration. After TAVR as opposed to SAVR, there was a decreased chance of severe bioprosthesis structural valve deterioration, but there was no difference in the risk of BVF. Following TAVR, there were increased incidences of pacemaker insertion and prosthetic regurgitation. According to the NOTION trial, individuals with isolated severe aortic valve stenosis who are at lower surgical risk may find TAVR to be a safe therapy option. To prevent paravalvular leakage and conduction anomalies, advancements in TAVR valve prosthesis and implantation methods are necessary. However, since these subgroups were not included in the study, these results do not apply to substantial coronary artery disease, prohibitively high-surgical risk, or technological unsuitability.

TRANSCATHETER AORTIC VALVE IMPLANTATION IN LOW-RISK TRICUSPID OR BICUSPID AORTIC STENOSIS: NOTION-2 TRIAL

Current trials, which compare TAVR with SAVR in low surgical risk individuals, included patients older than 70–75 years and excluded bicuspid aortic valves. This is the first RCT that compared TAVR with SAVR in patients with bicuspid aortic valves (35%), who are truly young AS patients (age ≤ 70 years).[4] In the tricuspid cohort, there was clinical equipoise between TAVR and SAVR for the primary composite objective at 1 year. Nonetheless, the results of TAVR for juvenile bicuspid AS patients were not as favorable. TAVR in bicuspid AS patients had low risk of major bleeding, higher incidence of nondisabling stroke, and paravalvular regurgitation compared to surgery. The findings of the NOTION-2 study should be used cautiously and could influence future randomized controlled trials that compare TAVR with SAVR in bicuspid AS (e.g., bicuspid phenotype selection, cerebral embolic protection).

PARTNER 3 TRIAL

The trial's objective was to assess the effectiveness of TAVR in low-risk patients with symptomatic severe AS in comparison to SAVR.[5] At 1 year, TAVR outperformed SAVR in preventing death, stroke, or rehospitalization in low-risk patients with AS. The duration of this benefit was 5 years. Adverse cardiovascular events at 5 years were comparable across therapy groups. Compared to SAVR, TAVR was linked to a decreased incidence of atrial fibrillation and significant bleeding. SAVR was linked to either milder or more severe paravalvular regurgitation and a decreased incidence of valve thrombosis as compared to TAVR. Nonetheless, there were no differences in bioprosthetic valve failure or valve function (mean gradient) across the therapy groups.

At 30 days, hypoattenuating leaflet thickening (HALT) was higher with TAVR than SAVR, but not at 1 year. In 1 year, HALT resolved on its own in over 50% of patients, with new cases developing in 21% of cases. HALT seems to be a dynamic process. TAVR seemed to be cost-dominant in the majority of cases based on cost-effectiveness analysis (over a 2-year horizon). The long-term cost-effectiveness of TAVR was also predicted, provided that late mortality did not differ between TAVR and SAVR.

This groundbreaking trial significantly increased the number of patients for whom TAVR is a viable therapy option for severe AS. This trial focused on valve durability and longer term clinical results to alleviate some of those limitations. Future studies are scheduled to look at long-term results and valve durability, including the effect of HALT, with a 10-year clinical and electrocardiograph follow-up planned.

LANDMARK TRIAL

The balloon-expandable Myval transcatheter heart valve (THV) series can be precisely sized with the aortic annulus by increasing its diameter in increments of 1.5 mm instead of the customary 3 mm valve size increments. The goal of the LANDMARK trial was to demonstrate that the Myval THV series was not inferior to the more recent Sapien Series THVs.[6] This is a prospective, multinational, randomized, open-label, noninferiority trial across 31 hospitals in 16 countries. The primary endpoint was a composite of all-cause mortality, all stroke, bleeding (types 3 and 4), acute kidney injury (stages 2–4), major vascular complications, moderate or severe prosthetic valve regurgitation, and conduction system disturbances resulting in permanent pacemaker implantation. The principal outcome demonstrated that the Myval (25%) was not inferior to the modern THV (27%), with a risk difference of –2.3% (one-sided upper 95% CI, $p_{\text{noninferiority}} < 0.0001$). The Myval THV achieved its primary goal in 30 days in patients with severe symptomatic native AS.

PROACT XA TRIAL

Vitamin K antagonists are the only oral anticoagulants approved to prevent valve thrombosis and valve-related thromboembolism in patients with mechanical heart valves. Compared to mechanical mitral valves, mechanical aortic valves are less likely to experience thrombotic problems due to their higher flow velocity. The safety of apixaban in patients with an On-X mechanical aortic valve for anticoagulation is unknown. Hence, this trial analyzed the noninferiority of apixaban 5 mg twice daily to warfarin in patients with an On-X mechanical valve in the aortic position.[7] This was a prospective, randomized, open-label study with blinded endpoint adjudication. In patients with an On-X mechanical aortic valve, apixaban was found to be less efficacious than warfarin in preventing valve thrombosis or thromboembolism and also failed to show noninferiority to warfarin. The trial was stopped after 863 participants were enrolled owing to an excess of thromboembolic events in the apixaban group.

TREATMENT OF LATE PARAVALVULAR REGURGITATION AFTER TRANSCATHETER AORTIC VALVE IMPLANTATION: PROGNOSTIC IMPLICATIONS

Paravalvular regurgitation (PVR) post TAVI is linked to higher rates of morbidity and mortality. The effectiveness of transcatheter therapies for PVR following TAVI is discussed in this study.[8] Subsequent treatment with redo-TAVI (n = 87, 43%), plug-closure (n = 79, 39%), or balloon valvuloplasty (n = 35, 18%) following the index TAVI, the PVR ≥ moderate persisted in 17.4% (n – 33) of the patients overall. The rate of persistent AR and mortality was more favorable in patients treated with redo-TAVI as compared to those treated with plug closure or valvuloplasty. It is beyond the scope of this retrospective analysis to recognize whether these variances derive from procedural efficacy differences or bias. Patients with improved prognosis and less AR had lower 1-year mortality. However, since this is an observational study, the patient population had been carefully chosen. The local heart team decided on timing and treatment technique, which likely reflected the patient's features and appropriate anatomy for a particular transcatheter reintervention. Imaging data (i.e., jet measures and number, valve expansion and position, aortic root measures, and root and left ventricular outflow tract calcification) crucial to PVR mechanism recognition and therapy assortment were not available. There was also a lack of an independent adjudication of events or an independent core laboratory imaging analysis. The small number of cases and events (mortality and persistent AR) can lead to erroneous conclusions as well as restrict the capacity to identify modest variations in outcomes that may nevertheless be clinically important. It is not appropriate to interpret results, particularly mortality risk, as solely attributable to the procedural strategy. More research is needed to determine the best PVR treatment technique in this set of population.

OUTCOMES OF TRANSCATHETER AORTIC VALVE REPLACEMENT IN PATIENTS WITH CARDIOGENIC SHOCK

In patients with cardiogenic shock (CS), the safety and effectiveness of TAVR with modern balloon-expandable transcatheter valves are still mostly unclear. This study showed that in 97.9% of patients, the valve was successfully placed.[9] CS was linked to greater 30-day, 1-year, and in-hospital mortality in a propensity-matched analysis as compared to patients receiving TAVR without CS. In the historical analysis conducted 30 days later, the 1-year mortality risk of the two groups was comparable. Even though CS is associated with a high death rate, >90% of patients made it through their initial hospital stay, and most of them were still alive 1 year later, with marked improvements in their QOL and functional status. Similar death rates were observed in patients who survived the first 30 days following TAVR as compared to those who were not in CS. For the majority of CS patients, who are anatomically suitable candidates and do not have debilitating comorbidities that might limit long-term survival, TAVR should be regarded as the ultimate course of treatment. Patients with AS who present with CS can benefit from the safe and efficient TAVR treatment, according to this extensive observational real-world study.

HEART FAILURE MEDICAL THERAPY PRIOR TO MITRAL TRANSCATHETER EDGE-TO-EDGE REPAIR: THE STS/ACC TRANSCATHETER VALVE THERAPY REGISTRY

Mitral transcatheter edge-to-edge repair (MTEER) is recommended in heart failure with severe functional mitral regurgitation; however, if MTEER is done with a background of optimized GDMT is unknown. Out of the 4,199 patients, 19.2% were prescribed triple therapy pre-MTEER with beta blockers predominating the treatment regimen and the proportion of patients ranged from 0 to 61%. Triple and double therapy were associated with lower risks of 1-year heart failure hospitalization or mortality compared to no or single therapy. It was identified that majority of the patients undergoing MTEER were not prescribed comprehensive GDMT with angiotensin receptor neprilysin inhibitors (ARNIs) being underutilized and triple therapy varied widely across sites.[10] Further, this study did not capture the use of sodium-glucose co-transporter 2 inhibitor (SGLT2-i) in patients from the TVT registry and paves way for future exploration of SGLT2-i in HF patients undergoing MTEER. Comprehensive GDMT pre-MTEER was associated with superior outcomes 1 year after intervention. Future quality improvement efforts should target GDMT optimization prior to and after MTEER.

CONCLUSION

These studies encompass a broad spectrum of topics, from novel diagnostic techniques and refined surgical procedures to innovative interventional therapies and comprehensive guidelines for clinical practice. As the field continues to evolve, staying informed of these key developments will be crucial in delivering optimal care and advancing the science of VHD.

ONLINE REFERENCES

Please scan the QR code provided at the end of the table of contents for References of this chapter.

CHAPTER

104

Rheumatic Fever and Rheumatic Heart Disease in India: Current Status

Anita Saxena

ABSTRACT

Rheumatic fever (RF) and rheumatic heart disease (RHD) continue to be major public health problems in India and other developing countries. The exact pathogenesis of RF is not clear; it appears to have an autoimmune basis. Untreated RF can lead to RHD, where progressive damage occurs to cardiac valves, with mitral valve being most commonly affected. Ultimately, it leads to heart failure and other complications, including death. RHD is an important cause of premature mortality and an important contributor to maternal morbidity and mortality in India.

Several epidemiological studies have shown that India has a high burden of RHD. It has indeed declined in some of the states with better economic status such as Kerala. Data from some of the poor states of India are not available, and RHD prevalence may be high since RHD is a disease of poverty. Echocardiographic studies further suggest a much higher prevalence of RHD in India and other developing countries when compared with clinical assessment based on auscultation. RHD is a preventable heart disease, and all efforts must be made for its eradication. Control of RF and RHD is complex and requires a multipronged approach. An early diagnosis and treatment of streptococcal sore throat is a useful strategy for primary prevention. For those diagnosed with RF and/or RHD, an effective secondary prophylaxis is the most cost-effective strategy for arresting the progress of heart valve damage. All efforts must be made to treat the complications of RHD to prolong life in patients with advanced disease.

Keywords: Rheumatic fever, rheumatic heart disease, valve disease, prevention

INTRODUCTION

Rheumatic heart disease (RHD) results from valvular damage caused by acute rheumatic fever (RF). RF is an acute, diffuse, and nonsuppurative autoimmune disease that occurs as a delayed response to untreated or partially treated group A beta-hemolytic *Streptococcus* infection. The infection triggers immune-inflammatory injury to the heart. Injury to pericardium and myocardium is mostly transient and self-limiting, but the cardiac valve injury leads to permanent damage and is the main cause of long-term morbidity and mortality in young patients. The exact pathogenesis of RF is not completely understood. Many patients with RHD do not recall having a history of RF. In regions with a high burden of RHD, most patients are diagnosed in an advanced stage when symptoms develop. A number of patients present for the first time with one of the complications such as heart failure, endocarditis, stroke, and/or cardiac arrhythmias.[1,2] RHD, although considered preventable, continues to be a major public health problem worldwide, with the heaviest burden borne by low and middle-income countries.[3,4] As the disease affects children and young adults, the results are devastating, because these patients are in their most productive years of life.

A spectacular success has been achieved in the control of RHD in high-income countries over the past six decades or so except in some pockets of indigenous population in these regions. This has been possible primarily due to improved living conditions, socioeconomic progress, less overcrowding, better personal sanitation, and better access to healthcare.

Rheumatic heart disease is an important cause of premature mortality, and almost all such deaths are preventable. Global age-standardized death rates have declined from 9.2/100,000 in 1990 to 4.8/100,000 in 2015 (48%), in the last quarter of a century, but the rates of decline vary widely between countries and regions.[4] For example, between 1990 and 2015, age-standardized mortality from RHD in India declined by just 18% (15.5–12.7), whereas China saw a much larger decline (71%).[5] In the same time period, countries in Southeast Asia had RHD mortality rates similar to those in the high-income countries.[5] Most deaths are from low and middle-income countries or in marginalized populations within high-income countries.[4]

BURDEN OF RHEUMATIC FEVER AND RHEUMATIC HEART DISEASE IN INDIA

The last decade has dramatically changed our understanding of the prevailing burden of RHD. It is estimated that 40.5 million people live with RHD and 306,000 die of this disease every year, representing 1.6% of mortality from all cardiovascular deaths. Since most children who are vulnerable to RF live in developing countries, a decline in RF and RHD has occurred for <20% of the world population.[6] A number of reports give the impression that RF and RHD are declining in India.[7,8] However, as per the GBD study, over 13.17 million cases of clinical RHD live in India.[4] There is a decline in DALYs and deaths due to RHD expressed as per 100,000 population. This may point to a reduction in the overall severity of RHD. However, in terms of absolute numbers, disease burden (DALY) as well as mortality is increasing.[9] Furthermore, RF occurs at a relatively younger age in India, affecting children as young as 3 years old. The incidence of carditis in an episode of RF is also higher compared with that in other countries. In addition, the disease progresses very rapidly with almost a malignant course.

Regional Differences

Rheumatic fever/rheumatic heart disease is strongly related to the socioeconomic and cultural factors of the region. It is therefore not surprising that there are large variations in RHD burden within India. Various states of India are at different levels of transition in urbanization and economic growth, and the quality and access to healthcare services vary widely across the states and regions. Unfortunately, very little data on RF RHD burden is available from states with poor health indicators. GBD data shows that the absolute burden is highest in some of the most populous states of India, such as Bihar and Uttar Pradesh, and in some other states such as Assam, Chhattisgarh, Madhya Pradesh, and Odisha.[3] The number of DALYs per 100,000 is over 300 in these states compared to some other regions, such as Goa where it is 100.[9] Physicians practicing in metro cities of India, especially those in private healthcare facilities, may perceive that RF/RHD has greatly declined, but the actual scenario is likely to be very different. There is a dire need for surveys and surveillance in states of India with lower health parameters.

MEASURES OF BURDEN OF RHEUMATIC FEVER/RHEUMATIC HEART DISEASE IN INDIA

A number of reports on the burden of RHD in India have been published over the last six to seven decades. The data is reported as population-based surveys, school-based surveys, and hospital data, the last one being the least reliable. RHD remains largely silent until patients become symptomatic with the advanced form of the disease. Almost all reports on RHD burden published earlier were based on clinical diagnosis. In more recent reports, evaluation has been done by clinical examination followed by echocardiographic confirmation. However, in the past decade or so, the focus has shifted to echocardiographic screening for all.

Subclinical Rheumatic Heart Disease by Echocardiography

Echo screening, which has been one of the most important advancements in our understanding of the global burden of RHD, has resulted from school, community, and clinical echo screening to define the epidemiological burden.[10] Several studies from various parts of the world have shown a very high prevalence of RHD when all children are screened by echocardiography, irrespective of their clinical status. Such screening studies in school children reported from India are shown in **Table 1**. Screening echocardiography has the potential to detect early RHD lesions, perhaps enabling timely commencement of treatment (secondary prophylaxis) to halt disease progression.

Currently, the significance of subclinical RHD as diagnosed by echo-Doppler is not well understood. Whether these cases should be prescribed secondary prophylaxis is also not clear. A recent study concluded that secondary

TABLE 1: Echocardiographic prevalence of rheumatic heart disease amongst school children in India.

Author, year	Site	Sample size	Age group (years)	Prevalence/1,000
Bhaya et al., 2010[12]	Rajasthan	1,059	6–16	51.0
Saxena et al., 2011[13]	Delhi	6,270	5–15	20.4
Rama Kumari et al., 2013[14]	Andhra	4,213	5–16	7.6
Nair et al., 2015[15]	Kerala	2,060	5–15	5.6
Saxena et al., 2017[16]	Multisite	16,294	5–15	7.7

antibiotic prophylaxis for latent RHD is beneficial. This GOAL trial showed that among children and adolescents 5–17 years of age with latent RHD, secondary antibiotic prophylaxis reduced the risk of disease progression at 2 years.[11] 33 out of 400 not given secondary prophylaxis progressed compared to 3 out of 399 who were given secondary prophylaxis. This new evidence may further justify echocardiographic screening of school children so as to prevent the progression of RHD in asymptomatic children and young adults. In an Indian setting, screening in schools may not be a feasible option due to the PCPNDT Act, which restricts the use of portable echocardiography.

Rheumatic Heart Disease Patient Registries

The WHO recommends maintaining RHD registries not only for surveillance, but also as a supplement for prevention and control of RHD. A number of national and regional registries are reported from various parts of the world, a recent one being the REMEDY registry.[17] The REMEDY registry is a multinational prospective follow-up study of patients with RF/RHD; it included a small number of patients from India. The HP-RF/RHD registry is a single-center tertiary care hospital-based prospective registry in the hill state of northern India, Himachal Pradesh, initiated in 2011. Recently, the findings of an 8-year follow-up of this registry were published.[18] About one-fifth of the patients with RF/RHD from this registry had major adverse outcomes; all-cause mortality, hospitalizations for heart failure, and/or stroke/peripheral embolism during the median follow-up of 5.4 years. The adverse outcomes were less in this registry compared to REMEDY. One of the reasons could be that more advanced cases were recruited in the REMEDY registry. A pediatric RHD registry from India included 451 children <18 years of age.[19] Females were reported to have greater severity of lesions.

It must be noted that registries tend to cover a small part of the affected population. Establishing registries helps in optimizing the care of patients with RHD and is known to improve secondary prophylaxis rates. In the Indian Pediatric RHD registry, mean adherence to penicillin prophylaxis among 274 patients with clinic follow-up was 93.6%.[19]

Registry-based care is undoubtedly of great value, but its maintenance is a complex process requiring manpower and financial resources. Since most RHD endemic countries are resource-limited, registry-based care may be more suitable for most endemic regions of India.

RHEUMATIC HEART DISEASE IN PREGNANCY

With declining maternal mortality from infections and other preventable causes, preexisting rheumatic and to some extent congenital heart disease are becoming major contributors to maternal mortality, more so in low and middle-income countries.[20] RHD has a higher prevalence in women and its recognition is important even before pregnancy is planned as it poses a significant risk during pregnancy. In one of the large studies, 0.4% of 14,275 pregnant women in India were diagnosed to have RHD when screened.[21] In the recently published MPAC registry, 433 of 1,029 pregnant women with heart disease had RHD.[22] Mitral valve was most commonly involved. Combined mitral stenosis and mitral regurgitation were present in 30% of cases and isolated mitral stenosis in 17%. Balloon mitral valvotomy has been shown to be safe during pregnancy with good maternal and fetal outcomes. In the MPAC registry, almost 23% of these patients had undergone prior surgical or interventional procedures. A total of 65 women have had prosthetic valve replacement requiring proper anticoagulation.[22] Anticoagulation management during pregnancy is quite complex and challenging. Bioprosthetic valves may be the preferred option for those planning to get pregnant as they circumvent the need for anticoagulation. However, the downside of bioprosthetic valve is the limited durability and need for reoperation.

DIAGNOSIS OF RHEUMATIC FEVER

There is no specific test for diagnosing RF; the diagnosis is clinical. The probability of diagnosing RF should vary according to the location and social factors. A child with fever and joint pains is very likely to have RF in India compared with a similar case in a Western country such as North America. Fortunately, most physicians in India are sensitive to this disease and hence the diagnosis is rarely missed. Dr T Duckett Jones published guidelines in 1944 to help physicians make a diagnosis of the first episode of RF. The criteria divided the clinical features of RF into major and minor manifestations based on their prevalence and specificity. Since then, several modifications of these criteria have been made. These modifications have been primarily made keeping in mind populations where RF and RHD are declining and are at a low risk. The latest modification was published in 2015, where the criteria have been separated for high- and low-risk populations to avoid overdiagnosis and underdiagnosis of RF.[23] These criteria take into account the variability in clinical presentation in these high- and low-risk populations. Echocardiography and Doppler have also been incorporated for the first time in Jones criteria. Echo-Doppler is able to diagnose cardiac involvement in cases with subclinical carditis, which has been included as a major criterion. The authors suggested that echocardiography should be performed in all suspected or confirmed cases of RF to assess whether carditis is present or not, particularly in moderate- and high-risk populations. The group also felt that monoarthritis should be considered as part of the RF spectrum in patients from moderate- and high-risk populations only after careful consideration and exclusion of other causes such as autoimmune, viral, or reactive polyarthritis. Evidence of preceding infection with group A-beta hemolytic *Streptococcus* is required for all cases except for those presenting with chorea.

As per available data, India is likely to fall into the category of moderate/high-risk population (prevalence of RHD >1/1,000 population or incidence of RF >2/100,000 school children). A diagnosis of RF in India by revised Jones criteria is as follows:

- All patients must have evidence of preceding group A beta-hemolytic streptococcal infection: This could be in the form of positive throat culture for the bacteria, high or rising antistreptolysin O (ASO) titer, or other streptococcal antibodies (anti-DNase B).
- For diagnosis of the first episode of RF, the following should be present:
  - Two major criteria
  - One major plus two minor criteria
- For diagnosis of recurrence of RF, the following should be present:
  - Two major criteria
  - One major plus two minor criteria
  - Three minor criteria

Major and minor criteria are given in **Table 2**.

Joint manifestations can be considered only in either the major or the minor categories but not in both categories in the same patient.

Subclinical carditis indicates echocardiographic valvulitis.

C-reactive protein value must be greater than the upper limit of normal for laboratory.

Challenges in Diagnosis of Rheumatic Fever

The established guidelines, although useful, cannot substitute the physician's experience and common sense. Several other conditions can fulfill the Jones criteria. Diagnosis of recurrences can also be challenging. Recurrences may be suspected in those presenting with worsening of previous valvular lesions, pericardial rub, or unexplained recent onset heart failure. In a recently published study from India, recent worsening of NYHA class (dyspnea) was the commonest feature (48%) in children presenting with rheumatic carditis.[24] An evidence-based scoring system has been devised by the same authors where scores have been given to age, NYHA class, severity of mitral regurgitation, presence of nodules, high ESR, and ASO titer. A score of 5 was associated with a sensitivity of 76% and specificity of 79% for diagnosing rheumatic carditis.[25]

TABLE 2: Jones criteria for diagnosis of rheumatic fever.

Major criteria	Minor criteria
Carditis: Clinical and/or subclinical	Monoarthralgia
Arthritis: Monoarthritis or polyarthritis or polyarthralgia	Fever (≥38°C)
Chorea	ESR ≥ 30 mm/h and/or CRP ≥ 3.0 mg/dL
Erythema marginatum	Prolonged PR interval, after accounting for age variability (unless carditis is a major criterion)
Subcutaneous nodules	

(CRP: C-reactive protein; ESR: erythrocyte sedimentation rate)

PREVENTION AND CONTROL OF RHEUMATIC FEVER/RHEUMATIC HEART DISEASE

The prevention of RF/RHD is essential for addressing the significant health, social, and economic burdens of RHD. There are four levels of prevention of RF/RHD: (1) Reducing group A streptococcal (GAS) infections through improvements in housing, living conditions, and sanitation (primordial prevention); (2) treatment of GAS throat infections and possibly GAS skin infections (primary prevention of RF); (3) prevention of recurrence of RF through antibiotic prophylaxis (secondary prevention of RHD onset and progression); and (4) treatment of the complications of RHD via medications including anticoagulants, and cardiac interventions including surgery (tertiary prevention).

Rheumatic fever and rheumatic heart disease are preventable and have been nearly eliminated in high-income countries. In developing parts of the world, RF and RHD continue to be a devastating illness that not only produces considerable morbidity and mortality but also significant social and economic burden. Once valvular damage is severe, heart surgery is often required to replace the damaged valve. Most patients receive prosthetic mechanical valves and require lifelong anticoagulation therapy. Surgery is expensive, and most developing countries where RHD is rampant do not have the resources to provide this facility. Furthermore, patients with prosthetic mechanical valves continue to have adverse events due to valve thrombosis, bleeding, neurological stroke, etc. Their survival is much inferior to that of the healthy population. The best approach to deal with RF and RHD is to prevent it.

All four levels of prevention are important; however, a recent modeling study of scale-up of RHD services in the African Union found that in the short term, the costs of secondary prevention and secondary and tertiary care for RHD would be lower than for primary prevention, with more rapid accrual of benefit.[26]

The incidence of RF and prevalence of RHD are quite variable within a particular country such as India. Keeping in mind the limited resources available in most regions that have high prevalence rates, the preventive programs should cater to high-risk populations as the returns are going to be much higher.

Primary prevention is achieved by treatment of group A streptococcal throat infections in a timely and proper manner. The various antibiotics which should be used for primary prevention are given in **Table 3**.

Secondary prevention is achieved by long-term intramuscular administration of antibiotics, long-acting penicillin (benzathine penicillin G, BPG) in most cases, every 3 weeks to those who have had one or more episodes of RF and to those who have an established RHD. It aims to prevent recurrent episodes of RF in a person who already has the disease. By doing this, the disease progression as well as its complications are prevented. Drugs used for secondary prophylaxis are given in **Table 4**.

Duration of secondary prophylaxis depends on the severity of cardiac involvement and age of onset of RF and is given in **Table 5**.

Tertiary prevention refers to interventions in patients who have RHD to reduce symptoms and disability from associated complications. The aim is to prevent premature death from RHD. Treatment includes medicines to treat heart failure, abnormal heart rhythms, etc. The only definitive treatment is heart surgery, which is to either replace or repair the heart valve. Surgery is expensive and is not curative in nature. Management of patients after surgery is also complicated because patients with a prosthetic valve

TABLE 3: Antibiotics for treatment of streptococcal pharyngitis.

Drug	Dose	Frequency and duration
Benzathine penicillin G (deep IM injection). To be given after the sensitivity test. Contraindicated if penicillin allergy present	• *For those >27 kg (>10 years)*: 1.2 million units • *For those ≤27 kg (≤10 years)*: 0.6 million unit	• Single dose • Single dose
Penicillin V (oral). Contraindicated if penicillin allergy present	• *Children*: 250 mg • *Adults*: 500 mg	• TID for 10 days • TID for 10 days
Amoxicillin (oral). Contraindicated if penicillin allergy present	• *Children*: 10–15 mg/kg/dose • *Adults*: 500 mg	• TID for 10 days • TID for 10 days
Erythromycin ethylsuccinate (oral)	• *Children*: 20 mg/kg/dose (maximum dose: 800 mg) • *Adults*: 800 mg	• BD for 10 days • BD for 10 days
Erythromycin estolate (oral)	• *Children*: 7–13 mg/kg/dose • *Adults*: Not recommended	TID for 10 days
Cefadroxil (oral)	15 mg/kg/dose	BD for 10 days
Azithromycin (oral)	12.5 mg/kg/day	OD for 5 days
Cephalexin (oral)	15–20 mg/kg/dose	BID for 10 days

TABLE 4: Drugs used for secondary prophylaxis.

Drug	Dose	Interval between doses
Benzathine penicillin G (deep IM injection). To be given after the sensitivity test. Contraindicated if penicillin allergy present	• *For those >27 kg (>10 years)*: 1.2 million units • *For those ≤27 kg (≤10 years)*: 0.6 million unit	• 21 days • 21 or 14 days
Penicillin V (oral). Contraindicated if penicillin allergy present	• *Children*: 250 mg • *Adults*: 500 mg	• Daily, twice a day • Daily, twice a day
Erythromycin (oral). Contraindicated in liver disease	20 mg/kg/dose. Maximum of 500 mg	Daily, twice a day

TABLE 5: Recommended duration of secondary prophylaxis.

Group	Duration of secondary prophylaxis
Rheumatic fever with no proven carditis	• Minimum of 5 years after the last RF episode • Until age 18 years (*whichever is longer)* (21 years as per the Australian guidelines)[27]
Mild carditis (or healed carditis)	• Minimum 10 years after last RF • Until age 25 years (*whichever is longer)* (21 years as per the Australian guidelines)[27]
Moderate or severe RHD and following cardiac surgery	Lifelong (or up to 40 years of age) (Australian guidelines: moderate RHD: 10 years or age 35 whichever is longer, severe: 10 years or age 40 years whichever is longer)[27]

need treatment with anticoagulants. Penicillin prophylaxis with BPG should continue after surgery.

The availability of penicillin has been a long pending issue in most states in India. Usage of intramuscular long-acting penicillin has been banned in some states of India. Physicians' fear of anaphylaxis is another major reason for discontinuation of BPG prophylaxis.[28] Healthcare personnel involved in providing injections must be educated about proper technique, and be prepared to deal with allergic reactions, if any. This would result in an improvement in the secondary prophylaxis rates.

Overall, there are several complexities that pose barriers to the elimination of RHD in India. A comprehensive and systematic approach along with concerted efforts by all stakeholders including cardiologists, pediatricians, community physicians, microbiologists, biomedical scientists, and public health advocates are required. All levels of prevention and control should be included in the universal health program of the Indian government. This can be the only way to control the ongoing burden of RHD.

CONCLUSION

Rheumatic heart disease has been forgotten by Western developed countries, and there is a clear-cut decline in new research on RF RHD from the West. The good news is that there is a resurgence of interest in RHD with a number of publications coming from regions of high prevalence, being published by local researchers, indicating that RHD is no more such a neglected reality. These studies should help policymakers implement cost-effective interventions aimed at preventing RHD, especially targeting vulnerable groups of children, adolescents, and women of reproductive age. Whether RHD is here to stay forever or otherwise would only be decided by our future efforts.

ONLINE REFERENCES

Please scan the QR code provided at the end of the table of contents for References of this chapter.

CHAPTER

105

Multivalvular Heart Disease: Clinical Assessment of Severity and Management

T Govindan Unni

ABSTRACT

Multivalvular heart disease is usually due to rheumatic heart disease or degenerative disease. The clinical findings depend on the severity of the valve disease, left ventricular and right ventricular function, and pulmonary artery hypertension. There can be various combinations of valvular diseases and this chapter summarizes the clinical findings of various combinations in detail.

Keywords: Multivalvular disease, valvular disease, rheumatic heart disease, mitral stenosis, mitral regurgitation, aortic stenosis, aortic regurgitation, tricuspid stenosis, tricuspid regurgitation

INTRODUCTION

Multivalvular heart disease was commonly the result of rheumatic heart disease (RHD) until a few decades ago. Now, with socioeconomic development, RHD has become rare even in developing countries. Currently, the most common cause of multivalvular heart disease is degenerative in developed countries, while RHD continues to be an important problem in developing countries. Other common causes include functional valve disease, infiltrative cardiomyopathies, congenital heart diseases (CHD), and infectious endocarditis (IE). Mitral stenosis (MS) is the most common valvular heart disease in RHD. Aortic stenosis (AS) and mitral regurgitation (MR) are the most common degenerative valvular heart diseases, especially in the elderly. With the increasing population of the elderly, we can expect more of these diseases in older and sicker patients. With the fast and impressive progress in imaging modalities and the developments in surgical as well as catheter-based techniques, the scenario is getting interesting. In the presence of combined valvular diseases, it is important to understand their hemodynamic interactions, and here multimodality imaging will be of great help.

AORTIC STENOSIS

Patients with AS can present with angina (35% of patients), syncope (15% of patients), or dyspnea (50% of patients).[1] The reason for angina is multifold. Associated coronary artery disease (CAD) is very common. The left ventricular hypertrophy (LVH) that occurs is initially compensatory to maintain the left ventricular (LV) wall stress in the presence of increased afterload. However, the LVH results in reduced capillary density (fewer capillaries per gram of muscle) resulting in angina in spite of normal coronary arteries. The venturi effect, produced by the jet of blood coming out of the LV through the stenotic aortic valve, can suck blood from coronary arteries causing angina.

Physical findings of AS depend on the severity of AS, LV function, and severity of valve calcification. Pulsus parvus et tardus consists of a pulse which is rising slowly and having a low peak. This is best appreciated in the carotid artery. When the vessels become rigid and lose their elasticity, as in the elderly, this may not be appreciated. A systolic thrill may be palpable in the carotids. Jugular venous pulse (JVP) is usually not elevated. A prominent "a" wave may be seen. This is due to the thick, hypertrophied interventricular septum (IVS) bulging into the right ventricle (RV) and reducing the RV compliance. Apex beat may not be displaced as there is hypertrophy, but no dilatation of LV. However, as LV dysfunction sets in, apex beat can be shifted out and down. Apex beat is sustained, suggesting the pressure overload. The split of second heart sound (S2) gradually reduces as severity of AS increases, finally becoming a single sound. When there is LV dysfunction and left bundle branch block (LBBB), a paradoxical split can occur, which widens on expiration, suggesting that aortic component of S2 (A2) is coming after the pulmonary component of S2 (P2). The hypertrophied LV is dependent on a good preload to maintain stroke volume. Atrial kick is, thus, very important. A fourth heart sound (S4) may be palpable and audible. The systolic murmur of AS is crescendo decrescendo. The intensity of the murmur has no relation to severity of AS, but the length of the murmur is directly related to severity of AS. When there is associated aortic regurgitation (AR), an early diastolic murmur may also be heard along the left sternal border. An ejection systolic click suggests bicuspid aortic valve but disappears as calcification sets in. When LV fails in the course of the disease, cardiomegaly occurs, third heart sound (S3) appears, JVP gets raised, and the murmur may reduce in intensity (but maintains its length), reflecting low stroke volume.[1]

All symptomatic patients require aortic valve replacement (AVR). Asymptomatic patients with LV dysfunction also require AVR. Asymptomatic patients going for other heart surgeries such as coronary artery bypass grafting (CABG) also require AVR. Severe valve calcification and rapid progression are other indications for AVR. The choice between transcatheter aortic valve replacement (TAVR) and surgical AVR is evolving as the procedure of TAVR, and its success rate and durability are improving.

AORTIC REGURGITATION

Rheumatic heart disease continues to be the most common cause of AR in developing countries. In developed countries, disease of aortic root and ascending aorta have become more common. In chronic AR, both preload and afterload on LV increase. The volume overload due to AR increases the preload. The elevated end-diastolic volume increases the LV wall stress and thus the afterload. The systolic BP is high due to the increased stroke volume, which also increases the afterload. Finally, the LV fails due to the increased preload and afterload. The eccentric LVH in early phases of AR is a compensatory phenomenon as the LV wall stress is reduced. LV failure in initial stages is reversible. However, if ignored, the LV dysfunction becomes irreversible.

Physical findings of severe AR reflect the high output state, the aortic runoff, and the volume overload on LV. The increased stroke volume results in a wide pulse pressure. The pulse wave rises rapidly and falls equally rapidly resulting in the collapsing pulse or water hammer pulse. Bisferiens pulse, pistol shot sounds in the femoral arteries, and capillary pulsation in the fingertips, lips, and tongue are other signs of a high output state. Cardiomegaly is evidenced by an apex beat that is shifted down and out. The apex beat will be hyperdynamic and ill sustained, reflecting the volume overload. As LV dysfunction develops, the apex beat may become more sustained. A2 may be loud when there is dilatation of the aortic root. If the AR is due to valve leaflet abnormalities, A2 will be soft. An aortic ejection click may suggest a bicuspid aortic valve. The classic murmur of AR is a blowing, high-frequency, decrescendo early diastolic murmur, best heard at the aortic area or along the left sternal border. The length of the murmur is directly related to the severity of AR. The exception is when the LV fails. The murmur, when LV failure occurs, may get shortened even in severe AR because the diastolic pressure gradient between aorta and LV is reduced due to the increased LV end-diastolic pressure (LVEDP). An acute AR also will have a short murmur in spite of severe AR. A low pitched mid-diastolic murmur may also be heard at the apex beat even without MS (Austin Flint murmur). This may be due to the AR jet preventing full opening of anterior mitral leaflet (AML). Alternatively, the vibrations of the AML may be the cause of the murmur.[2]

Acute AR is usually catastrophic. There is no time for LV to dilate. The LV end-diastolic pressure increases rapidly; hence, the diastolic gradient between aorta and LV diminishes. The murmur may be very soft and short or even absent. Tachycardia, tachypnea, and hypotension will be the cardinal findings.

Chronic AR remains asymptomatic for many years. The rate of progression to asymptomatic LV systolic dysfunction is <3.5% per year; the development of symptoms or LV dysfunction is <6% per year; and the risk of sudden death is <0.2% per year.[3] Close follow-up is required for these patients and AVR is recommended if they become symptomatic or LV dysfunction sets in. On serial follow-up, if there is a progressive increase in LV dimensions or a reduction in LVEF, consideration of AVR is necessary as these are high-risk patients.

MITRAL REGURGITATION

The mitral apparatus consists of the mitral annulus, mitral leaflets, the chordae tendinae, papillary muscles, and the underlying myocardium. Disorders of any of these structures can lead to MR. While RHD is the leading cause of MR in developing countries, degenerative disease is the leading cause in developed countries. Another increasingly important cause of MR is "secondary MR" due to severe LV dysfunction, annular dilatation, and papillary muscle malalignment due to LV remodeling. The compensatory changes in the LV, secondary to severe chronic MR, are LV dilatation, eccentric hypertrophy, and left atrial (LA) dilatation. The changes in LV are similar to chronic AR because of the volume overload. While there is an increase in preload as in AR, the afterload is significantly reduced in chronic MR because the LV is partly ejecting into the low-pressure LA. The LV ejection fraction (EF) will thus be spuriously high, and subtle LV dysfunction is likely to be missed. LA dilatation helps the LA to accommodate the large regurgitant volume without increasing the LA pressure.[4]

Physical findings depend on the LV function. In compensated MR, the pulse may be low to normal volume, but the upstroke will be brisk. As LV fails, the brisk upstroke disappears. The volume overload results in a dilated LV and apex displaced laterally and down. Apex beat will be brisk and hyperdynamic. The first heart sound (S1) is usually soft but may be loud when there is associated MS and when MR is due to mitral valve prolapse (MVP). The LV ejection time is shortened as LV is partly ejecting into low pressure LA. Hence, A2 comes earlier and S2 becomes widely split. S3 indicates rapid LV filling and does not suggest LV dysfunction. A mid-diastolic rumble is due to the large flow across a normal mitral orifice. The murmur is typically confined to mid-diastole. This diastolic rumble disappears as LV dysfunction sets in. The systolic murmur is usually holosystolic, best heard at the apex and the radiation will depend upon the etiology. The murmur may get shortened and become early systolic as LVEDP rises. An early systolic short murmur is also characteristic of acute MR. In MVP and papillary muscle dysfunction, the murmur can be late systolic.

Patients with chronic severe MR can be asymptomatic for a long time. Even LV dysfunction can occur without much symptoms. LV systolic dysfunction in severe MR is defined as an ejection fraction of 60% or less or an end-systolic dimension of 40 mm or greater. Such patients require mitral valve replacement/repair (MVR). Mitral valve repair is always preferred to replacement. If durable repair can be expected, even asymptomatic severe MR can be considered for intervention. Symptoms, atrial fibrillation (AF), pulmonary hypertension, and LV dysfunction are other indications for MVR (replacement or repair).[5,6]

In secondary MR, the time and role of surgery is still evolving. Percutaneous techniques are revolutionizing the field. Which patient and at what time to undergo mitral clip and other procedures is still in a fluid state.

MITRAL STENOSIS

Mitral stenosis is almost always rheumatic in origin. Fibrosis, calcification and fusion of commissures, leaflet thickening, and chordal fusion characterize rheumatic MS. Symptoms depend on mitral valve orifice area and body surface area. Indians with low body surface may tolerate even an orifice <1 cm^2. LA pressure increases first, gets reflected to the pulmonary veins, and patients go into pulmonary edema. Long standing pulmonary venous hypertension leads to pulmonary arterial hypertension (PAH). At this stage, pulmonary edema is replaced with low cardiac output state. Symptoms like dyspnea are replaced by fatigue. Symptoms usually develop when the mitral orifice is below 1 cm^2. But symptoms can develop earlier when the cardiac output is increased as in pregnancy, anemia, thyrotoxicosis, etc. When AF develops, patients go into pulmonary edema. AF can lead to LA thrombus, especially in appendage and lead to systemic embolism. MS with AF is an indication for vitamin K antagonists. Direct oral anticoagulants are contraindicated in this setting.

Physical findings include a normal sized heart, as the LV is not involved. However, as PAH develops, RV hypertrophy can be appreciated as a sustained left parasternal heave. P2 may be palpable in the case of pulmonary artery hypertension. S1 is loud in general, but can be soft if there is extensive calcification. When the valve is pliable an opening snap (OS) may herald the typical mid-diastolic murmur. The time from S1 to OS is an important marker of the severity of MS. The mid-diastolic murmur is low pitched, rough, and rumbling and its length directly correlates with the severity of MS. Presystolic accentuation of the murmur is appreciated in sinus rhythm. In AF, if the murmur extends to presystole in long cycles, it is a reliable sign of the severity of MS.

All symptomatic patients should be considered for percutaneous balloon mitral valvulotomy if the anatomy is suitable for the procedure. Patients with severe MR, severely thickened or highly calcified MV leaflets, and/or subvalvular apparatus are unsuitable for this procedure. In such patients, MVR is the treatment of choice. Rheumatic mitral valves can seldom be repaired.

MULTIVALVULAR HEART DISEASE[4]

In RHD, the most common combination is MS and AR or AS. In a small percentage, MS is associated with tricuspid stenosis (TS). Functional tricuspid regurgitation (TR) occurs in severe MS with PAH and RV dilatation. Simultaneous MR and AR occur in connective tissue disorders. In these cases, there may be TR also. The most common multivalvular disease in developed countries is AS and MR. Functional MR can occur in about 63% of patients with severe AS.[7] Functional TR is seen in around 40% of patients with severe AS.[8] The pressure overload on left ventricle (LV) secondary to severe AS can lead to LV systolic dysfunction, eccentric remodeling, which can result in leaflet tethering and annular dilation with resulting MR. Associated CAD is very common. LV dysfunction can also result from concomitant CAD. Severe AS can also produce LV diastolic dysfunction, increased left atrial (LA) pressure, leading to pulmonary venous and subsequently pulmonary artery hypertension, right ventricular (RV) dysfunction, and functional TR. AF is another complication leading to both functional MR and TR. In RHD, AS is always associated with MS. MR and AR are also usually seen in RHD.

Aortic stenosis is associated with pressure overload; hence, we may not expect cardiomegaly. When AS and MR coexist, because of the volume overload due to MR, cardiac size can increase. In MR, there are two outlets for LV, into the LA and into the aorta. Since LA is a low-pressure chamber compared to aorta, preferential streaming will occur to LA, and due to the low forward flow, AS may be underestimated. Also, presence of MR reduces overall afterload and the LVEF may be overestimated. Subclinical myocardial dysfunction will be missed.[9]

Aortic stenosis with MR is the least common form of RHD. This combination produces very undesirable hemodynamics. While AS murmur may be faint, MR murmur is usually very prominent. S3 is heard if MR is significant but can be heard when there is severe AS with LV dysfunction.

When AS is associated with TR and RV dysfunction, a low output state ensues and AS will be underestimated.

Combination of stenosis of mitral valve and aortic valve is usually of rheumatic origin. This combination is poorly tolerated and patients become symptomatic early in the course of the disease. In AS, LV is hypertrophied and depends on an adequate preload to maintain stroke volume. When MS reduces the preload, they go into a low output stage. Systemic emboli and AF are more common in AS with MS than in isolated AS. Angina and syncope are more common in severe AS. As always, the proximal lesion hides the clinical findings of the distal lesion. Hence, the clinical findings will be of severe MS. The presence of an LV apex and ejection systolic murmur in the base are suggestive of associated AS. In MS, LV is underfilled and an LV apex should make one consider other associated lesions such as AS or AR or MR. Severe LA enlargement and AF are more common when there is associated MS.[5,6] Correction of severe MS without first dealing with the aortic valve can be catastrophic as the hypertrophied LV with a stenosed aortic valve will not be able to accept the sudden increase in filling pressure, resulting in pulmonary edema.

Aortic stenosis and aortic regurgitation are quite commonly associated. Common underlying diseases are RHD and bicuspid aortic valve. The increased stroke volume due to AR results in overestimating AS. The systolic murmur will be harsher and longer. The stenosis prevents augmentation of stroke volume. So, the normal compensation cannot occur as happens in isolated AR. Usually, the clinical findings of AR are modified and severity underestimated. Clinical findings of AS are accentuated. A brisk carotid upstroke and widened pulse pressure are clues for significant AR in patients with severe AS. A displaced apical impulse, in the absence of LV dysfunction, also means significant AR.

Commissural fusion and loss of tissue are hallmarks of RHD. Hence a combination of MS and MR is very common. Both these lesions together or in isolation can produce PAH and AF. The intensity of the systolic murmur will not help in identifying the more dominant lesion. Many of these patients will have associated TR. The pansystolic murmur of TR should not be confused with MR. The MDM heard in MR is usually short and only heard in mid diastole. When the murmur extends to presystole, significant MS should be considered. Loud S1 and OS suggest associated MS but do not give a clue about its severity. The presence of an S3 or S4 rules out significant MS. It must be kept in mind that an RV S3 or S4 may be present in the presence of severe PAH and RV dysfunction. LV enlargement, evidenced by an apex beat shifted down and out, signifies severe MR. Severe AR or LV dysfunction due to other causes, such as hypertension, can also produce a shifted apex beat.

Combination of severe AR and MS is uncommon. The early diastolic murmur heard at left sternal border in severe MS (60–70%) is usually considered due to hypertensive PR (Graham Steell murmur). But most of these murmurs are due to mild AR. Conversely, patients with severe AR can have a mid-diastolic murmur (Austin Flint) at the apex. A wide pulse pressure and a dilated LV suggest associated significant AR. However, these findings may be absent in a significant number of patients with severe AR, because the proximal lesion masks the effect of the distal lesion.

Combined MR and AR can be due to RHD or connective tissue diseases and infective endocarditis. When MR is the dominant lesion, mild AR is well tolerated. But when AR is significant, the resulting LV dilatation distorts the papillary muscles and leads to worsening MR. A competent mitral valve protects LA and pulmonary veins from the effects of severe AR. Severe AR can also lead to end diastolic MR. The characteristic systolic and diastolic murmurs are present. LV will be dilated. Mid-diastolic murmurs are common. S3 is also common. Presence of an S4 suggests either an acute MR or significant AR. Severe AR produces LV dilatation and can produce functional MR without any mitral valvular disease. The MR is usually mild, but pansystolic murmur may be well heard.

Isolated TS is usually not seen. The most common cause of TS is RHD and is associated with significant MS. Carcinoid syndrome and endomyocardial fibrosis are other causes. Relative paucity of pulmonary symptoms in patients with severe MS should make one carefully look for TS. Giant "a" waves are an important finding. In AF, the "a" waves disappear, but the "v" wave will be characterized by a slow "y" descent because of the incomplete opening of tricuspid valve. Inspiratory splitting of S2 will not be heard as the inspiratory increase in RV filling is hampered by TS. The mid-diastolic murmur is best heard at the lower left sternal border and characteristically increases on inspiration.

Tricuspid regurgitation may be due to organic tricuspid valve disease or functional in severe PAH and RV dysfunction. Organic TR is almost always RHD and is associated with mitral and aortic valve disease. Isolated TR can be congenital due to Ebstein's anomaly or carcinoid disease. The classical pansystolic murmur is heard at left sternal border and increases on inspiration. The increase in inspiration may not be appreciated in pulmonary hypertension.

CONCLUSION

Multivalvular heart diseases present interesting clinical scenarios. The findings have to be analyzed carefully to determine the dominant lesion.

ONLINE REFERENCES

Please scan the QR code provided at the end of the table of contents for References of this chapter.

CHAPTER

106

Latest Guidelines for Infective Endocarditis

Joy M Thomas, Arun Arul David

ABSTRACT

Infective endocarditis (IE), a multifaceted disease involving practically every organ in the body, has been the subject of several studies and research. This has led to an ever-changing field with respect to diagnosing, investigating, managing, following up, and preventing the disease. The 2023 ESC guidelines on IE have given the latest leg up in the management of IE, bringing to the fore multi-imaging modality advances, endocarditis team, and finally outpatient antibiotic treatment.

Keywords: Infective endocarditis, endocarditis team, multi-imaging modality, vegetation, antibiotic prophylaxis

INTRODUCTION

Infective endocarditis (IE), "an inflammatory process that affects the inner layer of the heart, by infective or noninfective origin," was first described by Lazare Riviere in 1646, and "vegetation" was first used by Jean-Nicolas Corvisart to describe mitral valve IE. William Osler (Gulstonian Lectures—1885) and Emmanuel Libman brought the disease into focus in patients with fever **(Fig. 1)**.

The regions affected are the heart valves, implanted devices, transcatheter implanted valves, and congenital heart defects and the condition leads to substantial morbidity and mortality. IE caused the death of 66,300 people worldwide in 2019 and the estimated incidence

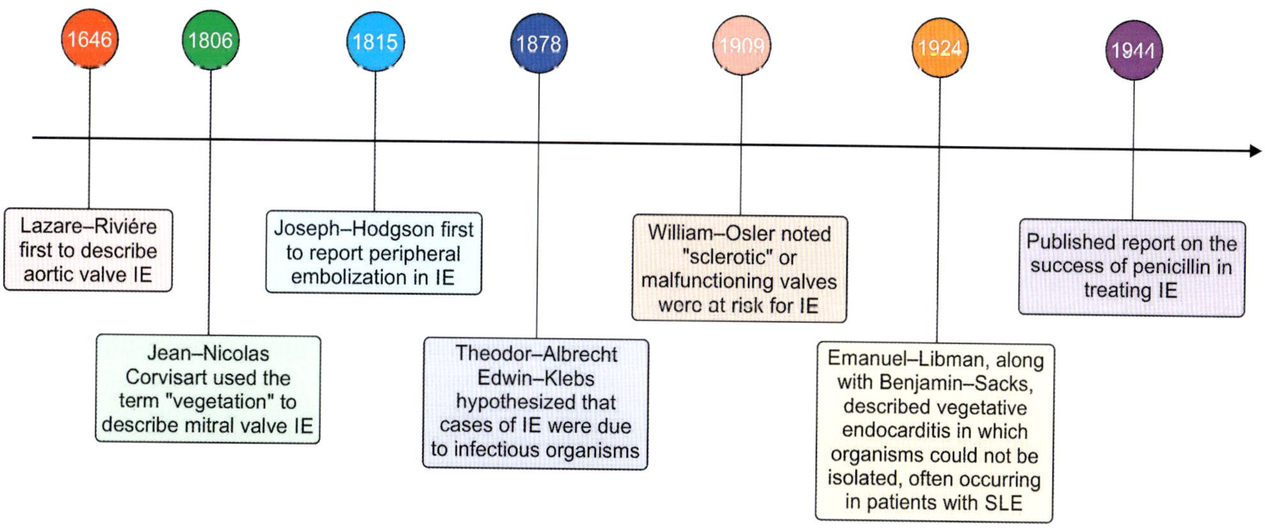

FIG. 1: Timeline of major events in infective endocarditis.[1]

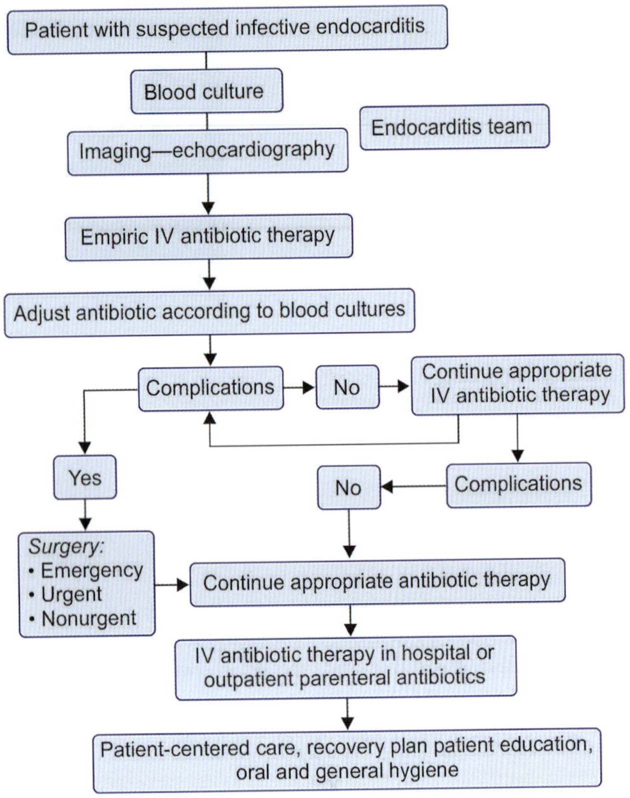

FLOWCHART 1: Management of patients with infective endocarditis.[4]

was 13.8 cases per 100,000 subjects.[2] The European Society of Cardiology (ESC) published guidelines in 2015[3] for the management of patients with IE.[4] This chapter focuses on the latest 2023 ESC guidelines on IE **(Flowchart 1)** and adapted several of its tables and recommendations for the benefit of the readers.

PROPHYLAXIS OF INFECTIVE ENDOCARDITIS

The need for antibiotic prophylaxis (AP) prior to surgical or interventional procedures is questionable because of the poor evidence of the use of bacteremia as surrogate evidence for the presence of IE.[5-7] While the rise of antibiotic resistance has been attributed to the blanket prescription of AP, the emergence of increased incidence and types of IE has been attributed to the inadequate AP prior to high-risk procedures.[8]

The predisposing risk factors that favor the development of IE[9] are:

- The presence of an endothelial surface amenable to colonization when a bacteremia occurs—valve leaflets with turbulent blood flow, as in stenosis or regurgitation, postoperative or percutaneous valve replacements, congenital heart disease (CHD) conditions, medical devices, both occlusion devices or cardiac implantable electronic device (CIED).[9]
- Pathogens entering the blood stream during surgical or interventional procedures
- A compromised host defense system

The usefulness of AP against IE was not statistically significant in low-risk cases.[10]

Patients at high risk of IE and who must receive AP are:

- History of IE or of recurrent IE as in patients with prosthetic heart valves or those who have prosthetic material or people who use injectable drugs (PWID).
- Prosthetic valve endocarditis (PVE) patients are at increased mortality risk, twice as high compared to those with native valve endocarditis (NVE) **(Flowcharts 2 and 3)**. Patients who receive atrial appendage closure, vascular grafts, vena cava filters, and central venous system ventriculoatrial shunts should also be considered for AP.
- Patients with CHD, untreated cyanotic CHD, those with surgically created conduits, patches with prosthetic materials, valved conduits, and transcatheter closure of defects.
- Ventricular assist devices used as destination therapy pose a high risk and needs AP.

In *patients with intermediate risks* such as those with rheumatic heart disease (RHD), nonrheumatic degenerative valvular disorders, congenital valve abnormalities such as bicuspid aortic valve, CIED, and hypertrophic cardiomyopathy AP have to be considered on an individual basis; however, stringent general preventive measures (GPM) are to be employed **(Box 1)**.

Patients undergoing solid organ transplantation (SOT) are at risk of IE from the nosocomial pathogens—*Staphylococcus aureus* (*S. aureus*) followed by *Aspergillus fumigatus*. AP prior to orodental procedure **(Table 1)** is of questionable benefit as the organism isolated has mostly been non-streptococci. However, IE caused by fungi in these patients can be disastrous.

Dental procedures at risk of contracting IE are dental extraction, oral surgical procedures such as periodontal surgery, oral biopsies and implant surgery, and dental procedures involving manipulation of the gingival or periapical region of the tooth (scaling and root canal treatment) and dental implants. Adverse reactions are least with amoxycillin, but due to the risk of *Clostridioides difficile* infections, recent 2023 ESC guidelines **(Table 2)** do not recommend clindamycin.

Nondental medical procedures associated with increased risk of IE are cardiovascular procedures and implants, gynecological examination and procedures, skin procedures and wound management, urological manipulations, bone marrow punctures, and endoscopic procedures. Preoperative screening of nasal carriers of *S. aureus* with nasal swabs or by the rapid gene amplification tests and their treatment with mupirocin or chlorhexidine is recommended prior to surgical or transcatheter valve replacement. Dental hygiene should be assessed by trained dental surgeons and any septic foci in the teeth or gingiva should be treated 2 weeks prior to the procedure **(Tables 3 and 4)**.

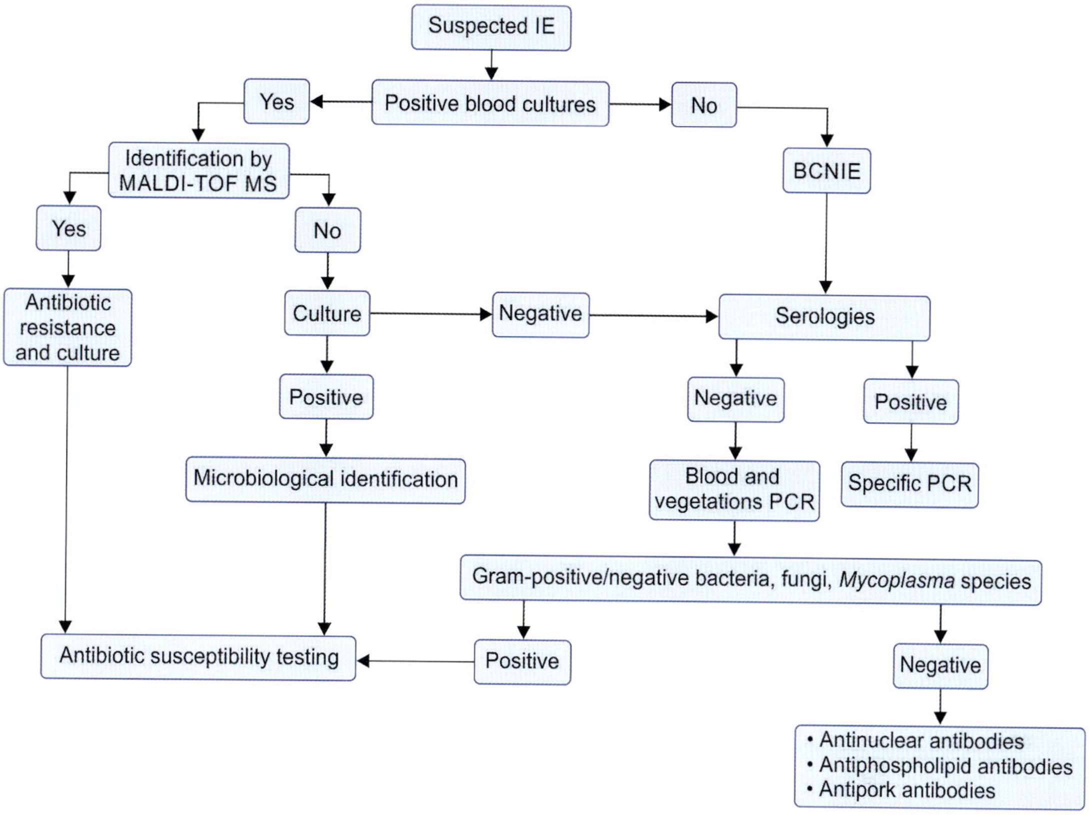

FLOWCHART 2: Microbiological workup schema in a case of suspected IE.[4]

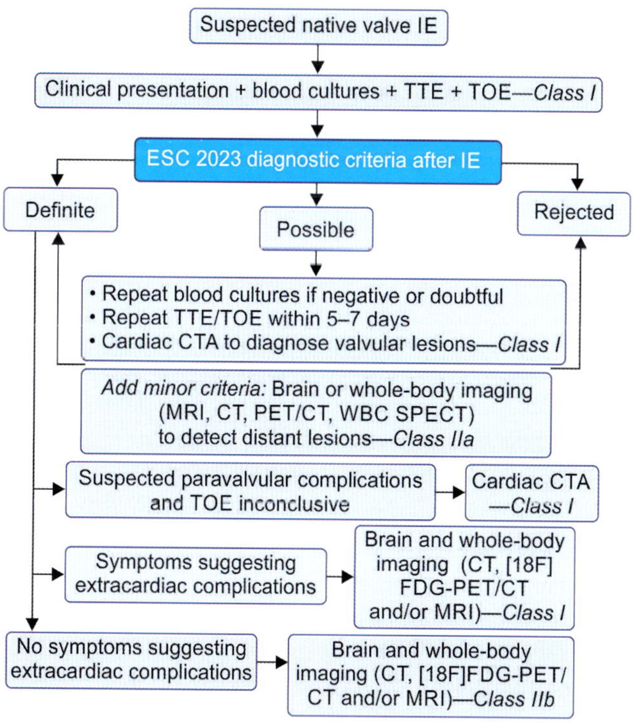

FLOWCHART 3: Workflow in diagnosing native valve endocarditis.[4]

BOX 1 General preventive measures for high- and intermediate-risk patients.

- Twice-daily teeth brushing and yearly dental visit and cleaning; twice yearly for high risk
- Strict cutaneous hygiene and prompt treatment of skin conditions
- Disinfection of wounds
- Curative antibiotics for any focus of bacterial infection
- No self-medication with antibiotics
- Strict infection control measures for any at risk procedures
- Strictly no tattooing
- Limit invasive lines and procedures to an absolute minimum possible
- Strict adherence to care procedures for central and peripheral cannulae

ENDOCARDITIS TEAM

A new concept that has emerged in recent years is that of the endocarditis team (ET) **(Tables 5 and 6)** for the early and accurate diagnosis of the primary disease for the effective management of IE and its complications.[11-15]

TABLE 1: AP in CVD patients undergoing orodental procedures at high risk for IE.

Recommendations	Class	Level
GPM are recommended in patients with high and intermediate risk	I	C
AP is recommended in patients with previous IE	I	B
AP for patients with surgically implanted prosthetic cardiac valves and in surgery where prosthetic material is used	I	C
AP for patients with transcatheter implanted aortic and pulmonary valve prosthesis	I	C
AP in patients with untreated CHD and patients treated with surgery or transcatheter procedures with postoperative palliative shunts, conduits, or other prostheses. AP is recommended for first 6 months only after procedure only for patients after surgical repair in the absence of residual defects or valve prostheses	I	C
AP for patients with ventricular assist devices	I	C
AP for patients with transcatheter mitral or tricuspid valve repair	IIa	C
AP for heart transplant recipients	IIb	C
AP is not recommended for other patients at low risk for IE	III	C

TABLE 2: Recommendations for antibiotic use in high-risk dental procedures.

AP for high-risk dental procedures			
		Single dose 30–60 minutes before procedure	
Situation	Antibiotic	Adults	Children
No allergy to penicillin or ampicillin	Amoxycillin	2 g orally	50 mg/kg orally
	Ampicillin	2 g IM or IV	50 mg/kg IV or IM
	Cefazolin/ceftriaxone	1 g IM or IV	50 mg/kg IV or IM
Allergy to penicillin or ampicillin	Cephalexin	2 g orally	50 mg/kg orally
	Cefazolin/ceftriaxone	1 g IM or IV	50 mg/kg IV or IM
	Azithromycin/clarithromycin	500 mg orally	15 mg/kg orally
	Doxycycline	100 mg orally	<45 kg: 2.2 mg/kg orally; >45 kg: 100 mg orally

TABLE 3: 2023 ESC recommendations for prevention of IE in high-risk patients.

Recommendations	Class	Level
AP for dental extractions, oral surgery procedures, and in procedures requiring manipulation of the gingival and periapical regions of the tooth	I	B
Systemic AP for invasive diagnostic or therapeutic procedure of the gastrointestinal tract, pulmonary, genitourinary tract, skin or musculoskeletal system	IIb	C

TABLE 4: 2023 ESC recommendation for IE prevention in cardiac procedures.

Recommendations	Class	Level
Preoperative screening and treatment of nasal carriers of *Staphylococcus aureus* prior to surgical or transcatheter valve implantation	I	A
Perioperative AP before CIED placement	I	A
Optimal preprocedural aseptic preparation of the implant site to prevent CIED infections	I	B
Periprocedural AP for surgical or transcatheter prosthetic valve implantation, intravascular prosthetic or other foreign material	I	B
Surgical standard aseptic measures during catheterization procedures in the catheterization laboratory	I	C
Elimination of potential sources of sepsis 2 weeks prior to implant of prosthetic valve or intravascular foreign material except in emergencies	IIa	C
AP against common skin pathogens prior to transcatheter valve procedures	IIa	C
Systematic skin or nasal decolonization without screening for *Staphylococcus aureus* is not recommended	III	C

TABLE 5: Constituents of the endocarditis team.

	Heart valve center
Core members	• Cardiologists • Cardiac imaging experts • Cardiovascular surgeons • Infectious disease specialist • Microbiologist • Specialist in outpatient parenteral antibiotic treatment
Adjunct specialists	• Radiologist and nuclear medicine specialist pharmacologist • Nephrologist • Neurologist and neurosurgeon • Anesthesiologist • Critical care • Multidisciplinary addiction medicine teams • Nurses • Social worker • Pathologist

TABLE 6: 2023 ESC recommendation for the endocarditis team.

Recommendations	Class	Level
Diagnosis and management of complicated IE are to be done at an early stage at a heart valve center where surgical expertise and an endocarditis team are available	I	B
Uncomplicated IE can be managed in a referring center with early and regular communication with the endocarditis team of heart valve center to improve the management	I	B

DIAGNOSIS OF INFECTIVE ENDOCARDITIS

Infective endocarditis should be suspected in patients with prolonged fever and positive blood cultures, where no clear focus of infection is identified in patients at risk for contracting IE. Fever is seen in 77.7%, a cardiac murmur in 64.5%, and congestive heart failure (HF) in 27.2% according to the European Infective Endocarditis Registry (EURO-ENDO).[16] Embolic complications are seen in 25.3% and cardiac conduction abnormalities in 11.5%. Vascular and immunological phenomena such as splinter hemorrhages, Roth spots, and glomerulonephritis are common. A low threshold for investigations is needed for atypical presentations as in the elderly, immunocompromised, and in high-risk groups such as those with CHD and prosthetic heart valves.

Laboratory Findings

Biomarkers such as C-reactive protein (CRP) or procalcitonin are not specific enough for diagnosis but are useful for risk stratification in critically ill patients.

Microbiological Diagnosis

The most frequent microorganisms causing IE reported in 2009 in the International Collaboration on Endocarditis Prospective Cohort Study were *S. aureus* (31%), oral *streptococci* (17%), and CoNS (11%).[17]

Infective Endocarditis Culture

Three sets of blood collection with each set targeting different venipuncture sites at least 1 hour apart. When three sets are used, with each set consisting of two 10 mL bottles for aerobic and anaerobic cultures, cultured over 24 hours, the maximum yield is 96–98%. The yield can be increased to 99.8% when four sets are used.[18] Rapid identification of bacterial susceptibility can be provided in a day or two with the matrix-assisted laser desorption ionization time of flight mass spectrometry (MALDI-TOF MS).[19,20] The gold standard still continues to be the determination of minimal inhibitory concentration (MIC).[21]

Blood culture-negative IE (BCNIE) occurs when blood culture is after antibiotic therapy. Repeat blood cultures after withdrawal of antibiotics may be helpful. BCNIE can be caused by fungi or intracellular obligatory bacteria such as *Coxiella burnetii*, *Bartonella* species *Aspergillus* species *Brucella* species *Mycoplasma pneumonia*, and *Legionella pneumophila*. 16S and 18S ribosomal ribonucleic nucleic acid (rRNA) sequencing improves diagnostic yield in prosthetic valve BCNIE by about 30%.[22] Where all cultures are negative, assays for antinuclear antibodies as well as antiphospholipid syndrome (APLS), anticardiolipin antibodies [immunoglobulin G (IgG)], and anti-ß2-glycoprotein 1 antibodies (IgG and IgM) should be done. Pathological and histopathological examination of tissues excised during surgery or biopsy by staining techniques is the gold standard for IE diagnosis and excludes noninfectious causes of IE such as tumors or autoimmune disorders.

IMAGING TECHNIQUES

Echocardiography assesses the structural and functional damage, evaluates the effectiveness of antibiotic treatment, and the result of surgical treatment. Transesophageal echocardiography (TOE), with 3D imaging and intracardiac echocardiography (ICE) are additional tools. TOE is recommended when damage to intracardiac structures is noticed during a clinical examination or a TTE. In right-sided NVE, good quality TTE examination is conclusive. The maximum length of the vegetation is a useful measurement for assessing the effectiveness of treatment and follow-up. Risk scores have been developed recently to assess which patient group (native valve, prosthetic valve, previous IE, or CIED) is at risk of *S. aureus* IE and needs echocardiography.[23,24] The 2023 ESC guidelines recommended multimodality imaging techniques **(Table 7)**.

Computed tomography (CT) is better than TOE in perivalvular and periprosthetic complications of IE to decide about cardiac surgery and presurgery coronary angiography for detecting distant lesions, mycotic aneurysms, and the sources of bacteremia. In emergency situations, CT is preferred to magnetic resonance imaging (MRI) scanning as its sensitivity is 90% and specificity is 96% in neurological situations for detecting ischemic and hemorrhagic lesions. Whole-body CT scan or [18F]FDG PET-CT is useful for detecting extracardiac IE.

Magnetic resonance imaging is useful in the diagnosis of IE and complications. Brain MRI can correctly diagnose 25% of previously undiagnosed IE. Gradient echo T2 images can identify cerebral microbleeds. MRI of the spine is 89–94% accurate in diagnosing spondylodiscitis and vertebral osteomyelitis.

TABLE 7: 2023 ESC guidelines for echocardiography in IE.

Recommendation	Class	Level
Diagnosis		
TTE first-line imaging modality in suspected IE	I	B
TOE in all suspected IE with negative or nondiagnostic TTE	I	B
TOE in all suspected IE with prosthetic heart valve or intracardiac device	I	B
Repeat TTE/TOE in 5–7 days in high-suspicion IE, initial negative scan	I	C
TOE in suspected IE with positive TTE, except in right-sided NVE with good TTE	I	C
Echo in bacteremia of *S. aureus*, *E. faecalis*, and *Streptococcus* species bacteremia	IIa	B
Follow-up under medical treatment		
Repeat TTE/TOE with suspected new IE complications—murmur, abscess, AVB, fever, or bacteremia	I	B
TOE in stable IE patient when switching for IV to oral antibiotic treatment	I	B
In uncomplicated IE, repeat TTE/TOE to detect new silent complications	IIa	B
Intraoperative echocardiography		
Intraoperative echo is required in all cases at surgery	I	C
Following completion of therapy		
TTE/TOE for patients on medical therapy who have completed treatment	I	C

Nuclear imaging positron emission tomography (PET)/CT (angiography) and single-photon emission CT (SPECT) help in the diagnosis of IE and its cardiac complications. [18F] FDG PET-CT and white blood cell (WBC) SPECT yield 84% sensitivity and 86% specificity in diagnosing PVE. In cases of periprosthetic abscesses, the WBC SPECT is useful. ^{99m}Technetium-hexamethoniumpropyleneamine oxime (^{99m}TcHMPAO)-SPECT CT helps to improve diagnosis by 27%. The reduced inflammatory component in NVE reduces sensitivity to 31% in PET-CT and SPECT CT but with a greater specificity at 98%. Detection of distant lesions, source of bacteremia, and location of septic emboli and the monitoring of treatment is possible with whole body [18F]FDG PET-CT; however, its limitation to detect these in the brain where there is a high uptake of [18F]FDG must be borne in mind **(Table 8)**.

Diagnostic Criteria

The modified Duke criteria, adopted since 2000,[25] had some limitations when prosthetic material was present, reducing diagnostic yield by 30%. The 2023 ESC guidelines has incorporated multimodality imaging **(Box 2)**. **Flowchart 3** explains the workflow for diagnosing NVE and this can be modified to include [18F]FDG PET/CT (A) as a Class I recommendation and WBC SPECT as a Class IIa recommendation while defining diagnostic criteria for PVE. Dahl et al.[26] in a prospective study used *E. faecalis* as a typical endocarditis pathogen, and this significantly improved the sensitivity to correctly identify definite IE from 70 to 96%.

TABLE 8: Recommendations for role of CT, nuclear imaging, and magnetic resonance in IE.

Recommendations	Class	Level
Cardiac CTA in possible NVE to detect valvular lesions and confirm IE	I	B
[18F]FDG PET-CT(A) and cardiac CTA in possible PVE to detect valvular lesions and confirm IE	I	B
Cardiac CTA for NVE/PVE for paravalvular and periprosthetic complications	I	B
Brain and whole-body imaging (CT, [18F]FDG PET-CT, MRI for NVE and PVE to detect peripheral lesions and to add minor criteria)	I	B
WBC SPECT/CT in highly suspected PVE, where TTE/TOE is noncontributory and PET/CT is not available	IIa	C
[18F]FDG PET/CT(A) in possible CIED-related IE to confirm IE	IIb	B
Brain and whole-body imaging (CT, [18F] FDG PET-CT, MRI for NVE and PVE to look for peripheral lesions in asymptomatic)	IIb	B

BOX 2 Revised 2023 ESC Modified Diagnostic Criteria for IE.[4]

Major criteria:

(i) Blood cultures positive for IE:

(a) Typical microorganisms consistent with IE from two separate blood cultures: Oral *streptococci*, *Streptococcus gallolyticus* (formerly *S. bovis*), HACEK group, *S. aureus*, *E. faecalis*

(b) Microorganisms consistent with IE from continuously positive blood cultures:

- >2 positive blood cultures of blood samples drawn >12 hours apart
- All of 3 or a majority of ≥4 separate cultures of blood (with first and last samples drawn ≥1 hour apart)

(c) Single positive blood culture for *C. burnetii* or phase I IgG antibody titer > 1:800

(ii) Imaging positive for IE: Valvular, perivalvular/periprosthetic, and foreign material anatomic and metabolic lesions characteristic of IE detected by any of the following imaging techniques:

- Echocardiography (TTE and TOE)
- Cardiac CT
- [18F]FDG-PET/CT(A)
- WBC SPECT/CT

Minor criteria:

(i) Predisposing conditions (i.e., predisposing heart condition at high or intermediate risk of IE or PWIDs)

(ii) Fever defined as temperature > 38°C

(iii) Embolic vascular dissemination (including those asymptomatic detected by imaging only):

- Major systemic and pulmonary emboli/infarcts and abscesses
- Hematogenous osteoarticular septic complications
- Mycotic aneurysms
- Intracranial ischemic/hemorrhagic lesions
- Conjunctival hemorrhages
- Janeway's lesions

(IV) Immunological phenomena:

- Glomerulonephritis
- Osler nodes and Roth spots
- Rheumatoid factor

(V) Microbiological evidence:

- Positive blood culture but does not meet a major criterion as noted earlier
- Serological evidence of active infection with organism consistent with IE

IE classification (at admission and during follow-up)

Definite:

- Two major criteria
- One major criterion and at least three minor criteria
- Five minor criteria

Possible:

- One major criterion and one or two minor criteria
- Three minor criteria

Rejected:

- Does not meet criteria for definite or possible at admission with or without a firm alternative diagnosis

Note: A diagnosis of IE is rejected when there is an alternate diagnosis, when signs and symptoms resolve within 4 days, when there is absence of pathological evidence at the time of surgery (with antibiotic therapy of <4 days), and when criteria for possible IE are not met.

Microbiological Criteria

Molecular biology (16S/18S rRNA PCR sequencing) in cardiac or embolic tissue has improved the sensitivity of diagnosing IE between 41 and 96% and the specificity between 90 and 100%.

ANTIMICROBIAL THERAPY

Bactericidal drugs or combination are preferred to bacteriostatic drugs. Aminoglycosides synergize with cell wall inhibitors (beta-lactams and glycopeptides) **(Table 9)** to make them bactericidal, but the nephrotoxicity of aminoglycosides makes the combinations of ampicillin and ceftriaxone a better alternative as they are effective against *E. faecalis*, despite their high-level aminoglycoside resistance (HLAR).[27]

Biofilms, around PVE and medical devices, are a challenge to microbial eradication of IE bacteria, and bactericidal drug combinations have to be given for 6 or more weeks. Present 2023 ESC guidelines on antibiotic therapy success draw on the 2022 EUCAST MIC breakpoint tables,[28] which define susceptibility as high possibility of success with standard dosing, susceptible with higher dosing, and resistant where there is a high chance of failure of treatment.

Oral antibiotic treatment for IE followed the POET trial[29] which showed that after an initial period of successful IV therapy, further treatment can be completed by oral treatment. In the initial IV antibiotic phase, surgery as well as removal of infected prosthetic material and abscesses should be done. Daptomycin in high doses can be used in Staphylococcal and Enterococcal endocarditis by combining it with a second antibiotic beta-lactam or fosfomycin **(Tables 10 and 11)**.

TABLE 9: Recommendations for oral *Streptococcus* and *Streptococcus gallolyticus* infection.

Recommendations	Level	Class
Penicillin susceptible NVE for 4 weeks and PVE for 6 weeks		
Penicillin, amoxycillin, and ceftriaxone	I	B
Standard 2-week treatment for NVE with normal renal function		
Penicillin G, amoxycillin, ceftriaxone, and gentamycin	I	B
Allergy to beta-lactam treatment for 4 weeks NVE and 6 weeks for PVE		
Vancomycin	I	C
Oral Streptococcus and Streptococcus gallolyticus infection increased exposure, penicillin resistance		
NVE—penicillin, amoxycillin, ceftriaxone × 4 weeks and gentamycin × 2 weeks	I	B
PVE—penicillin, amoxycillin, ceftriaxone × 6 weeks and gentamycin × 2 weeks	I	B
Allergy to beta-lactams		
NVE vancomycin for 4 weeks	I	C
PVE—vancomycin for 6 weeks and gentamycin for 2 weeks	I	C

TABLE 10: Recommendation for *Staphylococcus* species IE treatment.

Recommendation	Class	Level
IE by methicillin-susceptible staphylococci		
NVE (flu) cloxacillin or cefazolin for 4–6 weeks	I	B
PVE (flu) cloxacillin or cefazolin with rifampin for 4–6 weeks and gentamycin for 2 weeks	I	B
Allergy to beta-lactams		
NVE cefazolin for 4–6 weeks	I	B
PVE cefazolin with rifampin for 4–6 weeks and gentamycin for 2 weeks	I	B
NVE *allergic* to penicillin—daptomycin with ceftaroline or fosfomycin for 6 weeks	IIb	C
PVE allergic to penicillin—daptomycin with ceftaroline or fosfomycin or gentamycin with rifampin for 6 weeks and gentamycin for 2 weeks	IIb	C
IE by methicillin-resistant Staphylococci		
NVE—vancomycin for 4–6 weeks	I	B
PVE—vancomycin with rifampin for 4–6 weeks and gentamycin for 2 weeks	I	B
NVE—daptomycin with cloxacillin, ceftaroline, or fosfomycin for 4–6 weeks	IIb	C

TABLE 11: Recommendations for IE due to *Enterococcus* species.

Recommendations	Class	Level
Beta-lactam and gentamycin-susceptible strains		
NVE due to HLAR *Enterococcus* species—ampicillin or amoxycillin with ceftriaxone for 6 weeks or with gentamycin for 2 weeks	I	B
PVE and patients with complicated NVE or >3 months symptoms due to HLAR *Enterococcus* species—ampicillin or amoxycillin with ceftriaxone for 6 weeks or with gentamycin for 2 weeks	I	B
High-level aminoglycoside resistance (HLAR)		
NVE and PVE—ampicillin or amoxycillin with ceftriaxone for 6 weeks	I	B
Beta-lactam-resistant Enterococcus species		
Vancomycin for 6 weeks combined with gentamycin for 2 weeks	I	C
Vancomycin-resistant Enterococcus species		
Daptomycin combined with beta-lactams (ampicillin, ertapenem, and ceftaroline) or fosfomycin	I	C

Recommendations for Gram-negative Bacteria

Gram-negative HACEK microorganisms standard treatment is by ceftriaxone 2 g/day for 4 weeks in NVE and 6 weeks in PVE. If they do not produce beta-lactamase ampicillin for 4–6 weeks plus gentamycin for 2 weeks to be considered. In non-HACEK microorganisms, early surgery followed by 6-week treatment with beta-lactams and aminoglycosides sometimes requiring quinolones or cotrimoxazole.[30]

Fungi such as *Candida* responds to high-dose echinocandin or liposomal amphotericin B with or without flucytosine. *Aspergillus* responds to voriconazole.

Initial empirical treatment while awaiting results of blood culture and sensitivity are given in **Table 12**.

Outpatient parenteral or oral antibiotic therapy (OPAT) using a two-drug combination is an excellent alternative to inpatient IV antibiotic treatment, particularly in the elderly,[31,32] and should be instituted after clinical improvement is seen; complications such as HF, abscesses, septic emboli, and stroke are controlled and the patient stable **(Table 13)**. Careful assessment of home environment to ascertain that adequate self-care facilities exist, educating the patient and the care giver in the meticulous care of IV lines, daily temperature monitoring, assessment of the patient's progress, and identifying complications.

TABLE 12: Recommendations for antibiotic regimens for initial empirical treatment.

Recommendations	Class	Level
Community acquired NVE or late PVE (>12 months postsurgery)—ampicillin with ceftriaxone or flucloxacillin and gentamycin	IIa	C
Early PVE (<12 months postsurgery) or healthcare-associated IE—vancomycin or daptomycin with gentamycin and rifampin	IIb	C
Allergy to beta-lactams		
Community-acquired NVE or late PVE (>12 months postsurgery) who are allergic to penicillin—cefazolin or vancomycin with gentamycin	IIb	C

TABLE 13: Recommendation for outpatient antibiotic treatment for IE.

Recommendation	Class	Level
Clinically stable left-side IE caused by *Streptococcus* species, *E. faecalis*, *S. aureus*, or CoNS treated appropriately by IV antibiotics for at least 10 days (or at least 7 days after cardiac surgery) and who do not have complications that need surgery	II	A
Outpatient parenteral treatment not recommended in difficult-to-treat microorganisms, liver cirrhosis, large abscesses, severe CNS emboli, heart valve complications, or any complication that requires surgical intervention	III	C

INDICATION FOR SURGERY AND MANAGEMENT OF COMPLICATIONS IN INFECTIVE ENDOCARDITIS

The main reasons for surgery in IE are HF, uncontrolled infection, and prevention of septic embolization. Surgery could be *an emergency—where it is done within 24 hours, urgent—within 3–4 days, and nonurgent—beyond 4 days* **(Box 3; Tables 14 and 15)**. Most of the scoring systems used by surgeons are hardly used in clinical practice.[33]

COMPLICATIONS OF INFECTIVE ENDOCARDITIS

Neurological Complications

Up to 35% of IE patients have symptomatic neurological complications, while up to 80% have silent ones, and recommendations for their management are given in **Table 16**.

Heart Rhythm and Conduction Disturbances

Conduction system disturbances were observed at the time of diagnosis in 11.5% of IE patients, including 8.1% with first-degree, 0.6% with second-degree, and 2.8% with third-degree AV block which require pacemakers **(Table 17)**. New-onset AV block demands urgent valve surgery.[16]

BOX 3 Clinical conditions needing surgical valve intervention.

- Anterior mitral vegetation larger than 10 mm
- More than one embolic events during the first fortnight of antimicrobial treatment
- Persistence of vegetation following systemic embolization
- Increase in size of vegetation despite appropriate antimicrobial therapy
- Acute mitral or aortic regurgitation with heart failure
- Heart failure unresponsive to medical therapy
- Valvular dehiscence, rupture, or fistula formation
- Paravalvular leak
- Abscess unresponsive to medical treatment
- New heart block

TABLE 14: Timing and indications for surgery—ESC 2023 IE guidelines.

Type of surgery	Indications		
	Heart failure[34]	**Uncontrolled infections[35]**	**High risk of embolism[36-38]**
Nonurgent	Hemodynamically stable (Class I)	• Resistant bacteria/fungi • PVE not caused by *S. aureus* or non-HACEK gram-negative bacilli (Class I)	
Urgent	Poor hemodynamic tolerance (Class I)	• Local complications—abscess, false aneurysm, enlarging vegetation (Class I) • Persistent positive blood cultures (Class IIa) • Resistant bacteria/fungi (Class I) • PVE caused by *S. aureus* or non-HACEK gram-negative bacilli (Class IIa)	• Vegetation > 10 mm (Class I) • Embolic episodes despite therapy (Class I)
Emergency	Cardiogenic shock or pulmonary edema (Class I)[34]		

TABLE 15: Recommendations for surgery in NVE and PVE—ESC 2023 IE guidelines.

Recommendation	Class	Level
Heart failure		
Emergency surgery for aortic and mitral valve NVE and PVE with severe acute regurgitation, obstruction, fistula-causing pulmonary edema, or cardiogenic shock	I	B
Urgent surgery for aortic and mitral valve NVE and PVE with severe acute regurgitation or obstruction causing HF or echocardiographic signs of poor hemodynamic tolerance	I	B
Uncontrolled infection		
Urgent surgery for local uncontrolled IE—abscesses, false aneurysm, fistula, enlarging vegetation, prosthetic dehiscence, new AVB	I	B
Urgent or nonurgent surgery according to hemodynamics in IE by fungi and multiresistant organisms	I	C
Urgent surgery for persistent blood culture and persistent sepsis	IIa	B
Urgent surgery in PVE by *Staphylococcus aureus* and non-HACEK gram negatives	IIa	C
Urgent surgery for prevention of embolism		
In aortic and mitral NVE or PVE with persistent vegetation > 10 mm after one or more embolic episodes	I	B
In IE with vegetation > 10 mm and other indications for surgery	I	C
In aortic or mitral IE with vegetation > 10 mm and without severe valve dysfunction or without clinical evidence of embolism and low surgical risk	IIb	B

TABLE 16: Recommendation for the treatment of neurological complications.

Recommendation	Class	Level
Brain CT or MRA in IE with suspected infective cerebral aneurysms	I	B
Neurosurgery or endovascular therapy for large aneurysms, ruptured intracranial infective aneurysms, and those with continuous growth despite optimum antibiotics	I	C
Invasive angiography in suspected infective aneurysm where noninvasive tests are negative	IIa	B
Mechanical thrombectomy in a timely manner in embolic stroke	IIb	C
Thrombolytic therapy not recommended in embolic stroke	III	C

TABLE 17: Recommendations for pacemaker implantation in IE patients with complete heart block (CHB).

Recommendations	Class	Level
Immediate epicardial pacemaker implantation for patients undergoing surgery for valvular IE and complete AV block if one of the following predictors of persistent CHB are present:[39] Aortic root abscess, preoperative conduction system disturbance, *Staphylococcus aureus* infection, tricuspid valve involvement, or prior valve surgery	IIa	C

Musculoskeletal Manifestations

Infective endocarditis occurs in 20–30% of spondylodiscitis patients; thus, in patients with pyogenic spondylodiscitis, TEE/TOE must be done to exclude IE[40] and managed as in **Table 18**.

TABLE 18: Recommendations for patients with musculoskeletal manifestations and IE.

Recommendation	Class	Level
MRI or PET/CT for patients with vertebral osteomyelitis and suspected spondylodiscitis complicating IE	I	C
In patients with spondylodiscitis and/or septic arthritis with positive blood culture for typical IE microorganisms and TTE/TOE to be done to rule out IE	I	C
More than 6-weeks of antibiotic treatment is needed for complicated osteoarticular infections and difficult-to-treat microorganisms such as *Staphylococcus aureus*	IIa	C

TABLE 19: Recommendations for preoperative coronary angiography.

Recommendation	Class	Level
For stable high risk for CAD patients who have aortic valve vegetation, multislice CT angiography is preferred to invasive CAG	I	B
For high risk for CAD patients without aortic valve vegetation, needing cardiac surgery invasive CAG is preferred	I	B
In emergencies, valvular surgery should be done without CAG	IIa	C
Invasive CAG despite aortic valve vegetations in select patients with CAD or high risk for significant CAD	IIb	C

SURGICAL THERAPY IN PATIENTS WITH INFECTIVE ENDOCARDITIS

Grafting noncritical lesions during a valve surgery for IE can have a negative impact on perioperative outcomes.[41] Hemoadsorption filters have no beneficial role.[42] The feasibility and long-term success of mitral valve repair procedures is doubtful.[43] The need for preoperative angiography **(Table 19)**, the indications and timing of surgery, and the choice of bioprosthetic valve are given in **Tables 20 and Box 4**.

Ischemic and Hemorrhagic Stroke (Flowchart 4)

Early surgery offers better outcome and survival benefits in patients of IE who had stroke,[44] particularly in patients more than 75 years of age, where in-hospital mortality increases by 10–20% due to comorbidities and complications. Postdischarge follow-up is to be done meticulously to look for recurrence **(Table 21)**.

Specific Situations

Prosthetic valve endocarditis is found in 31% from earlier rates of about 20%. Treatment is replacement with new valve with complete debridement—Class IB recommendation **(Flowchart 3)**.

Infective endocarditis in the elderly is caused frequently by *Enterococci* and *S. aureus* and they have a lower incidence of embolic episodes.[45] In the elderly, surgery is less often considered and less often done, although the 1-year mortality without surgery is higher.[46]

Transcatheter PVE following TAVI ranges from 0.3 to 1.9 per 100 patient-years[47] but lesser than surgical treatment.[48] TOE findings in TAVI: 38–60% have no vegetations, 12–19% have vegetations on stent frame only, and in one third, the vegetations are mural.[49] Nuclear imaging, CT, [18F]FDG PET/CT, CTA, and intracardiac echo have improved diagnostic accuracy by 31%.[50] Surgical treatment is preferable in the presence of large vegetations or large abscesses.

TABLE 20: Indications and timing of cardiac surgery in IE patients.

Recommendations	Class	Level
Post-TIA cardiac surgery is indicated without delay	I	B
Poststroke surgery indicated without delay in HF, uncontrolled infection, abscess or persistent high embolic risk provided there is no coma or cerebral hemorrhage excluded by CT or MRI	I	B
After intracranial hemorrhage delaying cardiac surgery >1 month with frequent reassessment of the clinical condition with imaging if need be	IIa	C
Patients with intracranial hemorrhage and unstable status due to heart failure, uncontrolled infection or persistent high embolic risk, urgent or emergency surgery for a meaningful recovery is recommended	IIa	C

BOX 4 Choice of bioprosthetic valve for IE.

- Early surgery after recent ischemic stroke
- Evidence of intracranial bleeding
- Women of childbearing age
- High likelihood of prolonged mechanical circulatory support
- Advanced age or frailty
- Poor or unknown medical compliance
- Expected complicated and prolonged postoperative course
- Patient preference

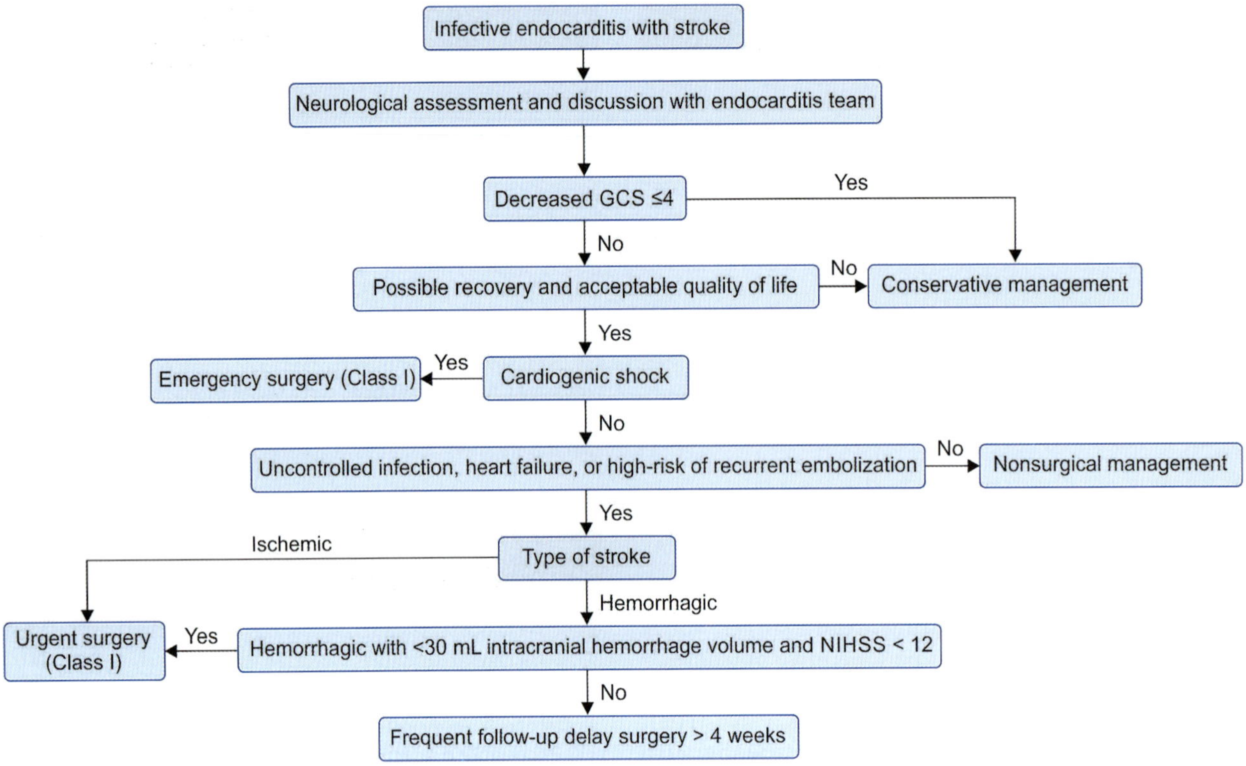

FLOWCHART 4: Workflow for IE with stroke and management based on type of stroke, Glasgow Coma Scale (GCS), and complications of IE, such as shock, heart failure, and embolization.[4]

TABLE 21: Recommendation for postdischarge follow-up.

Recommendation	Class	Level
Patient education on risks of recurrence, and preventive measures with emphasis on dental health and based on individual risk profile	I	C
Addiction treatment for patients with PWID-related IE	I	C
Cardiac rehabilitation including physical exercise based on patient assessment	IIa	C
Psychosocial support, screening for depression and anxiety and psychiatry	IIb	C

Infective Endocarditis Affecting Cardiac Implantable Electronic Devices (Table 22; Flowcharts 5 and 6)

Diagnosis of CIED-related IE by [18F]FDG PET/CT has good sensitivity and specificity. Washing the pocket with antibiotic solution is ineffective.[51] Antibiotic mesh containing minocycline and rifampin is effective in preventing CIED IE in select cases.[52]

Infective Endocarditis in Patients Admitted to ICU

Patients in ICU with IE have a mortality rate[53] of 32%; *S. aureus* is the main causative organism and TOE is essential for diagnosis. Surgery is the treatment of choice, but postoperative recovery can be problematic.

Right-sided Infective Endocarditis (Table 23)

Infective endocarditis in congenital heart diseases (CHD) occurs in multiple defects and more complex CHD. High-risk conditions are prosthetic valves and conduits, transcatheter valves, valve rings, previous IE, unrepaired cyanotic CHD, and any CHD repaired with prosthetic material for up to 6 months after the procedure or lifelong if residual shunt or valvar regurgitation is present.[54] Mortality rates for CHD with IE range from 6 to 15%.[55]

Infective Endocarditis in Rheumatic Heart Disease

In those affected by oral bacteria-related IE linked to RHD, *Streptococcus* species infection was the main organism due to poor oral hygiene. IE causes an enhanced risk of death in patients of RHD undergoing mitral valve replacement.

Infective Endocarditis in Pregnancy

Several recent reports of IE in pregnancy[56,57] have shown an 18% maternal mortality mostly due to HF and embolic events, 55.7% preterm birth, and 29% fetal mortality. Urgent surgery under cardiopulmonary bypass should be done despite the risk to the fetus.

TABLE 22: Recommendation for CIED-related IE.

Recommendation	Class	Level
Antibiotic prophylaxis covering *Staphylococcus aureus* for CIED implantation	I	A
TTE and TOE to identify CIED IE-related vegetations	I	B
Complete system extraction without delay in CIED IE under empirical antibiotic treatment	I	B
Three sets of blood cultures before starting empirical antibiotics	I	C
Reimplant at a distal site after negative cultures for 72 hours in patients without vegetation and for 2 weeks in those with vegetations	I	C
Considering the pathogen and the need for cardiac surgery, complete CIED extraction should be done even though leads are not involved	IIa	C
Where fungemia or gram-positive bacteremia are seen in CIED-related IE, complete system removal is needed if the infection persists	IIa	C
Septic emboli or prosthetic valves antibiotic treatment after device removal for 4–6 weeks	IIa	C
Antibiotic envelope in select patients undergoing CIED reimplantation	IIb	B
Complete system removal in antibiotic unresponsive occult gram-negative bacteremia	IIb	C
In non-*Staphylococcus aureus* CIED IE 2 weeks antibiotics after device extraction if cultures are negative	IIb	C
Removal of CIED after a single positive blood culture and no other evidence of infection is *not* recommended	III	C

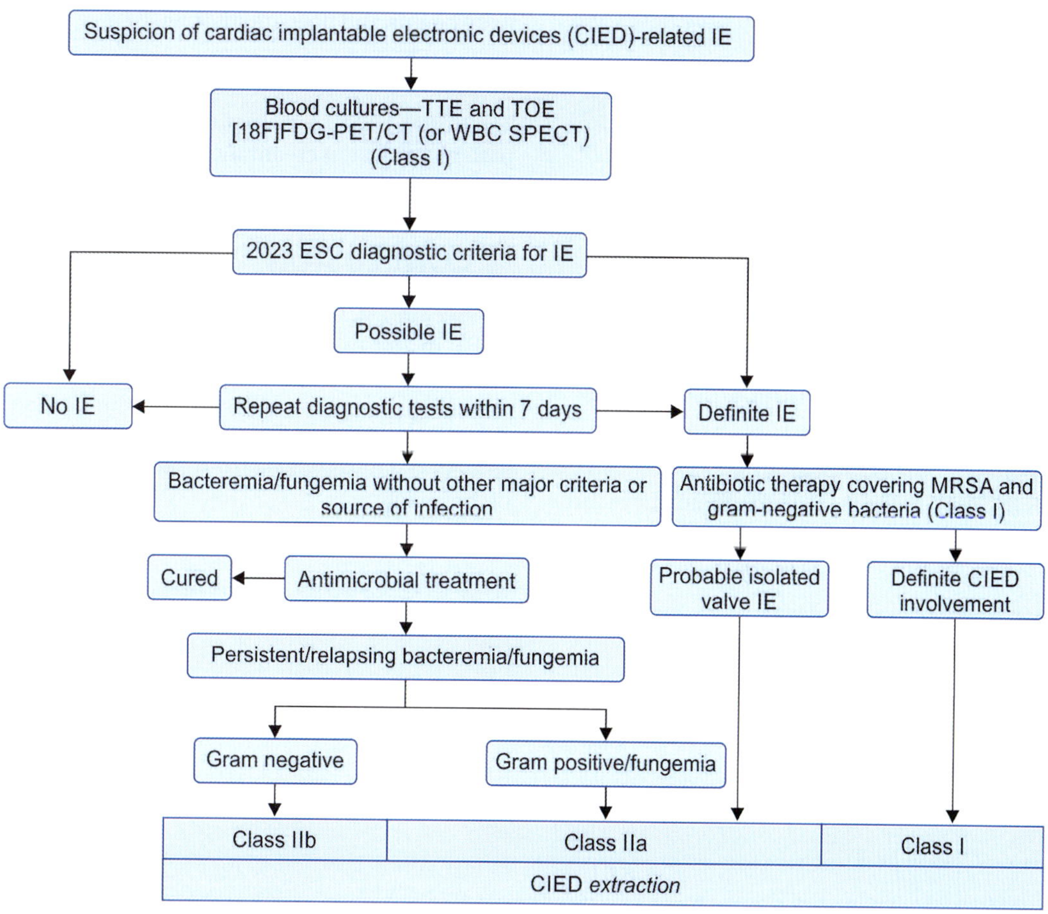

FLOWCHART 5: Workflow for CIED-related IE. Diagnosis of cardiac implantable electronic devices- (CIED)-related IE and line of management-based certainty of the disease.[4]

TABLE 23: Recommendations for surgery for right-sided IE.

Recommendations	Class	Level
Surgery in right-sided IE who are receiving appropriate antibiotic therapy is for		
Right ventricular dysfunction due to severe TR unresponsive to diuretics	I	B
Persistent vegetation with respiratory insufficiency needing ventilation and recurrent pulmonary emboli	I	B
Large residual tricuspid vegetations > 20 mm after recurrent pulmonary emboli	I	C
Simultaneous involvement of left heart structures	I	C
Tricuspid valve repair before replacement whenever feasible	IIa	B
Persistent bacteremia after 1 week of appropriate antibiotic therapy	IIa	C
Prophylactic epicardial pacing lead at the time of tricuspid valve surgery	IIa	C
Debulking of intra-atrial septic masses by aspiration in high-risk cases	IIb	C

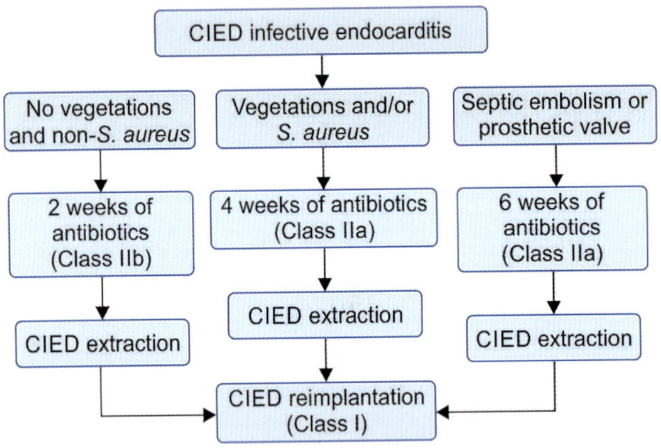

FLOWCHART 6: Workflow for CIED extraction and reimplantation in IE. Reimplantation is planned after 72 hours of negative blood culture reports after appropriate therapy at a different site from the initial site.[4]

Infective Endocarditis in Immunocompromised Patients

The incidence of IE in SOT patients[58] is renal 72%, liver 17%, and pancreas 8%. SOT patients more frequently have atrial and ventricular vegetations without valvar involvement—*mural IE*.[59] The two most frequent organisms are *S. aureus* 34% and *Enterococcus* species 17%. In heart transplant patients with IE, the mitral valve is most frequently affected with mortality figures approaching 45%. HIV patients with IE should be managed as in non-HIV. In neutropenic patients, antibiotics such as cloxacillin and ceftaroline worsen the neutropenia and need monitoring.[60]

Infective Endocarditis and Malignancy

The EURO-ENDO registry found malignancy in 11.6% of IE patients. Elevated creatinine (>2 g/dL), congestive HF, and unperformed cardiac surgery are the predictors of mortality.[61]

CONCLUSION

The recent 2023 ESC guidelines lay stress on involvement of ET in the management of IE patients. Information is shared with all concerned—the patient, their family, and the caregiver—about all aspects of the disease and shared decision-making whether at hospital or home regarding surgery or conservative, irrespective of the gender and age of the patient.

ONLINE REFERENCES

Please scan the QR code provided at the end of the table of contents for References of this chapter.

CHAPTER

107

Venous Thromboembolism: Recent Advancements and Future Perspectives

Vipin Kumar, Arvind Kumar

ABSTRACT

Venous thromboembolism (VTE) includes two entities, deep venous thrombosis (DVT) and pulmonary embolism (PE) with similar pathophysiological mechanisms, but different clinical presentations. DVT formation usually starts in calf vein valve pockets due to sluggish blood flow, local hypoxia, and hypercoagulability in predisposed individuals. Risk factors for developing VTE can be transient, like in surgical patients undergoing knee or hip arthroplasty, or persistent like in patients with cancer, antiphospholipid syndrome (APS), or in hereditary disorders of coagulation. About 20% of calf vein thrombi can propagate to more proximal veins, some of which can lead to PE after dislodgment. Traditional therapy of VTE included unfractionated or low molecular weight heparin (LMWH) or vitamin K antagonists (VKAs). With the advent of direct oral anticoagulants (DOACs), therapy of VTE has become simpler, obviating the need for subcutaneous injections or regular monitoring of INR. The current review aims to overview the recent advances in the understanding of the pathogenesis of VTE, discuss current approaches for the management of VTE, and the future perspectives.

Keywords: Venous thromboembolism, pulmonary embolism, deep venous thrombosis, VTE, PE, DVT, D-dimer

INTRODUCTION

Venous thromboembolism (VTE), encompasses two interrelated conditions, deep venous thrombosis (DVT) and pulmonary embolism (PE) with varying clinical presentation. PE is most commonly caused by embolization of thrombus in lower extremity deep veins into pulmonary arteries, which is treated as VTE. Due to the availability of highly sensitive tests and imaging techniques, the incidence of VTE has been reported to increase over time.[1] The mainstay of treatment and secondary prevention of VTE is anticoagulation therapy. With the advent of direct oral anticoagulants (DOACs), the management of VTE is much simplified. Some of the DOACs have been used as a single drug approach without administering intravenous anticoagulants,[2-4] in low-risk patients which would be more suitable for early hospital discharge or outpatient treatment of VTE. The current review is aimed at an overview of the recent advances in VTE management and discussing the future perspective of VTE.

EPIDEMIOLOGY OF VENOUS THROMBOEMBOLISM

Annual incidence of VTE was 123 per 100,000 persons in the USA and 131 per 100,000 persons in European countries, which increases with older age. Incidence of VTE is 6.1 and 7.3% in Indian patients undergoing major surgery or orthopedic surgery respectively and 20% in Indian cancer patients.[5]

PATHOGENESIS OF VENOUS THROMBOEMBOLISM

Deep venous thrombosis usually starts in the valve pockets of deep veins of the calf, 20% of which propagates into the more proximal veins.[6] These more proximal clots have a risk of breaking off and producing PE. The interplay among hypercoagulability of the blood, sluggish blood flow, and damage of the vessel wall (Virchow triad) causes

VTE.[7] Systemic increase in thrombin generation due to hypercoagulability of the blood and local factors like stasis and damage of the vessel wall leading to the preferential occurrence of DVT in the deep veins of the leg.

Both hereditary and acquired risk factors have been identified, which are associated with systemic activation of coagulation and increased risk of VTE. Among hereditary disorders, antithrombin, protein C, and protein S deficiencies are potent risk factors, whereas other genetic risk factors, such as factor (F) V Leiden and the prothrombin gene mutation moderately increase the risk of VTE. The role of these inherited thrombophilic disorders in recurrent VTE is less clear than in the first episode of VTE. Hence, routine thrombophilia testing does not influence long-term management and is not recommended.[8]

Among acquired risk factors for VTE, major persistent risk factors are cancer and antiphospholipid syndrome (APS), while minor factors include advanced age, obesity, renal impairment, and chronic inflammatory disorders such as inflammatory bowel disease and rheumatoid arthritis. There can be some transient risk factors, which increase the risk of VTE, such as surgery and trauma, immobilization, long-distance travel, pregnancy, and estrogen therapy.

DIAGNOSIS OF VENOUS THROMBOEMBOLISM

Rapid and accurate diagnosis of suspected VTE is essential for initiation of anticoagulant therapy to prevent thrombus extension and fatal PE. Imaging tests are often required to reliably diagnose VTE. Compression ultrasound can diagnose patients with DVT, whereas computed tomography (CT) pulmonary angiography, or ventilation-perfusion (VQ) lung scanning is used for the diagnosis of PE. As positive diagnosis is confirmed in only about 20% and 5%, respectively, of those with suspected DVT and PE, subjecting a large number of suspected VTE patients to imaging is not cost-effective.[9] Hence, clinical prediction rules have been developed to determine the pretest probability of VTE. With the introduction of sensitive and rapid assays for D-dimer,[10] it is possible now to rule out VTE when used in combination with clinical prediction scores. D-dimer is a plasmin-derived breakdown product of cross-linked fibrin, and its levels are elevated in most patients with VTE. Wells and colleagues derived clinical prediction rules that can classify patients with suspected VTE into low, intermediate, and high pretest probability categories on the basis of clinical features.[11] Patients with a high pretest probability of VTE require imaging for confirmation, whereas patients with a low pretest probability require D -dimer levels to be measured in plasma. A negative D-dimer test, defined as a D-dimer level below 500 μg/L, in a patient with a low or intermediate pretest probability of VTE effectively rules out VTE. In contrast, imaging is required to rule out VTE in these patients and a positive D-dimer test.

D-dimer levels increase with age, hence instead of using a fixed cut-off of 500 μg/L, the D-dimer cut-off can be adjusted on the basis of patient age or pretest probability of VTE to increase its specificity.[12,13] For age adjustment, the cut-off is set at 10 times the patient's age for those over 50 years of age.[12] To reduce the need for diagnostic imaging, the D-dimer cutoff can also be adjusted on the basis of pretest probability. For this approach, a cut-off of 500 μg/L is retained for patients with an intermediate pretest probability but increased to 1,000 μg/L for those with a low pretest probability. In patients with suspected DVT or PE, the use of a graduated D-dimer cut-off has been shown to reduce the need for diagnostic imaging.[13,14]

The diagnosis of upper extremity deep vein thrombosis (UEDVT) and recurrent DVT is challenging. UEDVT occurs mainly in patients with central venous catheters or secondary to thoracic outlet syndrome. The use of the clinical prediction rule or D-dimer alone cannot safely rule out UEDVT, which usually requires compression ultrasound imaging.[15]

Recurrent DVT reduces the specificity of D-dimer measurement and increases pretest probability. However, the sensitivity of a low pretest probability and a normal D-dimer level in ruling out recurrent DVT in patients not taking anticoagulants remains high. Because of residual ultrasound abnormality in patients of prior DVT on compression ultrasonography, its diagnostic efficacy is also reduced. Hence, compression ultrasonography is compared to previous examinations and the involvement of new venous segments can be useful. Inflammatory cells, accumulated in fresh thrombus preferentially take up fluorodeoxyglucose which enables differentiation of new thrombus from old thrombus by 18F-fluorodeoxyglucose positron emission tomography/CT (FDG-PET/CT).[16] Magnetic resonance direct thrombus imaging (MRDTI) can also differentiate fresh thrombus from old thrombus, by detecting paramagnetic signal induced by the release of methemoglobin from fresh thrombus.[17]

RISK STRATIFICATION OF PULMONARY EMBOLISM

Clinical presentations of PE vary widely across patients ranging from incidental asymptomatic PE to fatal PE. Risk stratification of patients is recommended at initial diagnosis to identify high-risk patients, who require more aggressive therapy including thrombolysis,[18] and low-risk patients, who might be considered for outpatient treatment.[19] Risk stratification models for PE have been developed, such as the Pulmonary Embolism Severity Index (PESI) and Hestia criteria to select patients with low-risk PE patients. Later, the simplified PESI score **(Table 1)** was developed,[20] which was successfully validated for similar prognostic accuracy and described as a major risk stratification model in the latest 2019, European Society of Cardiology (ESC) guideline.[18] Other predictors of poor outcomes are raised troponin,

TABLE 1: Simplified Pulmonary Embolism Severity Index (sPESI).[20]

Variables	Points
Age > 80 years	1
History of cancer	1
History of chronic lung disease	1
Pulse rate ≥ 110 beats/min	1
Systolic blood pressure < 100 mm Hg	1
Arterial blood saturation < 90%	1

Note: Total points = 0: Low risk; ≥1: High risk

B-type natriuretic peptide (BNP), and N-terminal pro-B-type natriuretic peptide (NT-proBNP) or right ventricular dysfunction by echocardiography and CT examination.

PRIMARY PREVENTION OF VENOUS THROMBOEMBOLISM

Surgical Patients

Patients undergoing elective hip or knee arthroplasty are at the highest risk for the development of VTE. These patients require thromboprophylaxis, for which traditionally low molecular weight heparin (LMWH) was used. DOACs obviated the need for daily subcutaneous injections and provided an attractive alternative. The DOACs were found to be at least as effective as LMWH for the prevention of symptomatic VTE without increased risk of major bleeding[21] in major trials. Based on these results, the DOACs are recommended for initial and extended thromboprophylaxis in patients undergoing elective hip or knee arthroplasty by various guidelines.[22] Recent trials have re-examined the role of extended DOAC thromboprophylaxis after elective major orthopedic surgery.[23] EPCATII trial, compared initial 5-day course of rivaroxaban, followed by extended thromboprophylaxis with low-dose aspirin for up to 30 days with extended prophylaxis with rivaroxaban in patients undergoing major orthopedic surgery. In this trial, a short course of rivaroxaban followed by extended aspirin was non-inferior to extended prophylaxis with rivaroxaban for the prevention of symptomatic VTE. On the basis of this, the most recent guidelines suggest either aspirin or an anticoagulant (DOAC or LMWH) for extended thromboprophylaxis after elective hip or knee arthroplasty.[24] Whether upfront aspirin is non-inferior to anticoagulant prophylaxis is being examined in ongoing trials (PEPPER and EPCAT-3).

Medically Ill Patients

Hospitalized medically ill patients are at risk of VTE, though lower than that in surgical patients undergoing hip or knee arthroplasty. Hence thromboprophylaxis is offered only to high-risk hospitalized medical patients identified by using risk assessment models or by an elevated D-dimer level. Recent American Society of Hematology guidelines recommend LMWH over DOACs for thromboprophylaxis in hospitalized medically ill patients and do not recommend routine extension of thromboprophylaxis after hospital discharge.[25]

High-risk Cancer Patients

Patients undergoing cancer treatment are at high risk of developing VTE. Their risk of thrombosis is predicted by the Khorana score, based on the type of cancer, body mass index, and blood counts. A score over 2 is associated with a VTE risk of at least 6% at 3 months. In the CASSINI trial and AVERT trial, rivaroxaban and apixaban respectively were compared with placebo in cancer patients identified as being at risk of VTE by a Khorana score of 2 or higher.[26,27] Compared with placebo, rivaroxaban or apixaban prophylaxis significantly reduced the risk of VTE by about 60% without a significant increase in major bleeding.[26,27] In high-risk ambulatory patients undergoing cancer therapy with no risk factors for bleeding, primary prophylaxis with rivaroxaban or apixaban for up to 6 months is recommended.[28]

Antiphospholipid Syndrome

Antiphospholipid syndrome is considered to be a potent risk factor for the development of VTE and patients with diagnosed APS should receive indefinite anticoagulation therapy[18] and VKAs are preferred anticoagulation in these patients rather than DOACs. Trials with DOACS in APS showed more thromboembolic events than with VKAs. The TRAPS study compared rivaroxaban with warfarin in 120 triple-positive APS patients[29] and needed to stop early because of more venous and arterial thromboembolic events and major bleeding events with rivaroxaban. Therefore, high risk APS patients require treatment with VKAs and DOACS is contraindicated in these patients.

SYSTEMIC THROMBOLYSIS FOR ACUTE PULMONARY EMBOLISM

Systemic thrombolysis rapidly improves hemodynamic instability and reduces mortality in high-risk PE patients, with insignificant effect in hemodynamically stable patients.[30] At present ESC recommends systemic thrombolysis in Intermediate to high-risk patients of acute PE with hemodynamically decompensation and does not recommend its routine use.[18] Other strategies to reduce the risk of bleeding with thrombolysis are the use of lower-dose thrombolytic drugs or catheter-directed thrombolysis (CDL).[31]

CATHETER-BASED TREATMENT OF PULMONARY EMBOLISM

Pharmacomechanical means can be used to rapidly decrease thrombus burden by using various means namely, by CDL and catheter-based embolectomy. In CDL, a thrombolytic drug is directly infused into the PA circulation via a multiside hole catheter to decrease the required dose and thereby reduce the rate of major and intracranial bleeding. An alternative to these simple infusion catheters is ultrasound-assisted thrombolysis (USAT), which has two lumens, one for drug delivery and the other lumen with an ultrasonic transducer. Low-energy ultrasound is delivered at the thrombus site, which facilitates the dissociation of fibrin strands, thereby allowing more effective thrombolysis at lower doses. Catheter-based embolectomy involves the use of a specialized device to remove a thrombus. Catheter-based thrombus maceration may be performed with a pigtail catheter with a guide wire or, with peripheral smaller size balloons to establish some forward flow in hypotensive patients with totally occluded proximal PA branches and partially decompress the RV. Actual extraction of thrombus from the pulmonary vasculature can be done by means of a large sheath or a straight guide catheter or by way of specialized catheters (FlowTriever or Penumbra device). Percutaneous mechanical thrombectomy with the FlowTriever System and Indigo Penumbra aspiration system led to significant improvement in RV/LV ratio and minimal major bleeding in patients with acute intermediate-risk PE.[31] FDA has approved the EKOSonic endovascular system and the FlowTriever embolectomy device for use in acute PE.[31]

INFERIOR VENA CAVA FILTERS

In patients at high risk with acute proximal DVT, permanent IVC filter placement in addition to standard anticoagulation therapy reduces PE development, but with an increase in recurrent DVT and no difference in overall mortality (PREPIC study).[32] The PREPIC-2 study evaluated the effect of removable IVC filters in patients with high-risk PE and showed no benefit in the use of removable IVC filters with standard anticoagulation therapy compared with anticoagulation therapy alone.[33] Hence 2019 ESC guidelines do not recommend the routine use of IVC filters and recommend only in patients of acute PE with absolute contraindication to anticoagulation therapy or recurrence of PE even after therapeutic anticoagulation.[18]

ANTICOAGULATION THERAPY WITH DIRECT ORAL ANTICOAGULANTS FOR VENOUS THROMBOEMBOLISM

Until recently, patients with acute VTE were treated initially with a rapidly acting parenteral anticoagulant (usually LMWH) overlapped and followed by VKAs. DOACs have streamlined VTE treatment obviating the need for subcutaneous injections with LMWH or regular INR monitoring with VKAs. DOACs for VTE can be given as a sequential approach, i.e., initial treatment with heparin followed by DOACs, or as a single drug approach with DOACs alone. DOACs were found to be non-inferior to conventional treatment (heparin followed by VKA) in large randomized controlled trials.[2,3,34,35] Despite ease of use, DOACs may not be suitable for some subsets of patients with VTE and VKAs remain an important treatment option for patients with severe renal insufficiency, APS.[36]

In the placebo-controlled trials evaluating extended VTE treatment, full-dose treatment with apixaban, dabigatran or rivaroxaban reduced the risk of VTE by at least 80% but increased the risk of clinically relevant bleeding by about twofold.[3,37,38] To reduce of bleeding, low-dose regimens of apixaban or rivaroxaban were studied in two trials. Recurrent VTE risks were similar in low-dose regimens as compared to high-dose regimens, with less clinically relevant bleeding.[39] Hence, lower-dose regimens of rivaroxaban or apixaban can be used in suitable patients.

Aspirin reduced the rate of recurrent VTE by 32% with similar rates of major bleeding; when compared with placebo for secondary VTE prevention with unprovoked VTE after at least 3 months of anticoagulant therapy.[40] However, when compared to rivaroxaban, rivaroxaban reduced the rate of recurrent VTE by 70% without increasing the risk of major bleeding.[41] Therefore, DOACs are more effective than aspirin for extended VTE treatment and are given preference in the guidelines over VKAs for initial, long-term, and extended VTE treatment in patients without active cancer. Lower-dose regimens of apixaban or rivaroxaban can be used for extended VTE treatment, which has a better benefit-risk profile than the usual-dose regimens.

ANTICOAGULATION THERAPY FOR CANCER-ASSOCIATED VENOUS THROMBOEMBOLISM

Cancer is a strong risk factor for VTE, with a higher risk of recurrence, as well as bleeding. Trials comparing LMWH and VKAs for cancer-associated VTE such as the CLOT trial and CATCH trial, showed better reduction of recurrent VTE in patients with LMWH compared with warfarin. Hence LMWH is preferable to anticoagulation therapy than VKAs in cancer-associated VTE.

Patients treated with edoxaban or rivaroxaban had less recurrent VTE with increased major bleeding when compared to dalteparin in the Hokusai VTE Cancer study,[42] and in the SELECT-D study,[43] respectively. Whereas, patients treated with apixaban showed a lower risk of recurrent VTE with a low incidence of major bleeding[44] in the ADM VTE study. These trials proved the efficacy of DOACs for the prevention of recurrence in VTE patients with active cancer with increased bleeding risk, especially in patients with gastrointestinal cancers. Hence both DOACs and LMWH can be used for the treatment of cancer-associated VTE.[45] For patients with a high risk of gastrointestinal or genitourinary bleeding, LMWH is still preferred.

OPTIMAL DURATION OF ANTICOAGULATION THERAPY

The recurrence risk of VTE can be reduced by anticoagulation therapy. Depending on the risk of recurrence, different guidelines recommend the specific durations of anticoagulation therapy.[18,46,47] Various risk scoring algorithms like the Vienna Risk Model, and DASH Prediction Score were developed, to evaluate the risk of recurrence in a particular patient. These scores considered various factors like male sex, elevated D-dimer, presence of post-thrombotic syndrome, obesity, increasing age, location of thrombus, and presence of provoking factors, that may increase the risk of recurrence. The current guidelines suggest anticoagulation therapy for 3 months for low-risk patients and anticoagulation therapy of extended duration (sometimes indefinite) for high-risk patients including patients with active cancer.

HOME TREATMENT OF ACUTE VENOUS THROMBOEMBOLISM

Acute VTE management traditionally required hospitalization and initial parenteral anticoagulation therapy followed by VKAs. DOACs have been used as a single-drug approach without the use of injectable anticoagulants in low-risk patients, which provides the feasibility of home treatment for VTE. No significant difference was observed in terms of mortality, recurrent VTE, or major bleeding in patients of low-risk acute PE, between home treatment or early discharge versus standard hospitalization.[19] Hence home treatment or early discharge with DOACs in appropriately selected low-risk patients seem to be feasible and safe.[18,46]

ISOLATED SUBSEGMENTAL PULMONARY EMBOLISM AND ISOLATED DISTAL DEEP VEIN THROMBOSIS

After the advent of highly sensitive CT scans, subsegmental PE is increasingly diagnosed, the significance of which is uncertain. According to the second update of the CHEST guideline, anticoagulation may not be required in patients with subsegmental PE in the absence of proximal DVT and risk factors of recurrent VTE.[48]

Thrombosis in veins distal to the popliteal vein is referred to as distal DVT, which poses a low risk of extension and development of PE.[49] Low-risk patients with isolated distal DVT (without active cancer or previous VTE) was evaluated in the CACTUS trial, which reported similar incidence of symptomatic VTE with either LMWH or placebo, whereas more bleeding was observed with LMWH.[50] Hence, isolated distal DVT without severe symptoms or risk factors for extension does not require anticoagulation therapy. Serial imaging of the deep veins for 2 weeks is recommended for these patients by the latest updated CHEST guideline.[48]

EMERGING TREATMENTS

Factor XI (FXI) is thought to be less crucial for hemostasis and instead functions to stabilize the thrombus and inhibit its further growth.[51] Hence, inhibiting FXI may prevent thrombus formation with reduced bleeding risk. Monoclonal antibodies (abelacimab and osocimab), which inactivates FXIa by binding to it were found to be effective for the prevention of VTE with less bleeding risk.[52] Antisense oligonucleotide agents block FXI synthesis in the liver and have also been found to be effective in the prevention of VTE in patients undergoing total knee replacement surgery with less risk of bleeding in phase 2 studies when compared to enoxaparin.[53,54]

CONCLUSION

Traditional management of VTE with heparin, either unfractionated or low molecular weight, and oral Vitamin K antagonists have changed dramatically after the advent of DOACs. Despite DOACs use, bleeding remains the major concern of anticoagulant therapy, especially in older patients and in those with chronic kidney disease or cancer. Therefore, there remains a need for safer anticoagulants with less bleeding risk and acceptable efficacy. FXI inhibitors are in development, which have shown to be efficacious with less bleeding risk.

ONLINE REFERENCES

Please scan the QR code provided at the end of the table of contents for References of this chapter.

CHAPTER 108

Constrictive Pericarditis—Diagnosis and Management

Rajesh Thachathodiyil, C Rohit Swaminathan, Meenu Nair

ABSTRACT

Constrictive pericarditis is a common, significant clinical condition characterized by fibrotic and calcified thickening of the pericardium leading to impaired diastolic filling and heart failure. This chapter delves into the contemporary approaches to diagnosing and managing constrictive pericarditis. This remains a potentially curable form of disease, thus providing good quality of life for the patient. Hence, the diagnosis/management is of prime importance. Early and accurate diagnosis is critical and relies on a combination of clinical evaluation, imaging techniques such as echocardiography, cardiac MRI, and CT, as well as invasive hemodynamic assessment. Pericardiectomy remains the definitive treatment for this condition.

Keywords: Constrictive pericarditis, constrictive physiology, constrictive versus restrictive

INTRODUCTION

Constrictive pathophysiology of the pericardium results from an extended insult to the structure over a few months to years with the end result being a fibrotic, calcified pericardium. In the developed world, the main causes are idiopathic, postsurgical, and radiation. But in developing countries, tuberculosis (TB) remains till date to be the predominant cause ranging from 22 to 91% in varied analysis globally (developing countries). Since the clinical characteristics are suggestive of diastolic heart failure, there is a diagnostic dilemma between constrictive pericarditis and restrictive cardiomyopathy. Fibrous casing of the pericardium results in ineffective cardiac filling and a subsequent low output state. The resultant clinical picture/symptomatology is of right heart failure.[1]

NORMAL CARDIAC/PERICARDIAL HEMODYNAMICS

Diastolic filling is dependent on both factors external such as vascular load on the cardia and the nature of pericardium, as well as internal factors such as myocardial properties/stiffness. The ventricular diastole though complicated in actual physiological interplay can be largely simplified into three stages—(1) ventricular relaxation, (2) filling by passive means, and (3) atrial systole contributing to ventricular filling.

Early and passive fillings are contributed mainly by ventricular relaxation, elevated left atrial pressure, interventricular dependance, and myocardial compliance. The atrial contraction distends the ventricle, providing the nidus for further ventricular systole.

Structures within the Pericardium

Left and right ventricles, right atrium, and majority of the left atrium are intrapericardial. The pulmonary venous system, SVC, and IVC are extrapericardial. In addition to this, the SVC and IVC are outside the thoracic cavity, while the pulmonary venous system is largely intrathoracic. The effects of respiration are largely applicable to the pulmonary veins, but not the SVC and IVC.

Hence, during inspiration, there is augmentation of right-sided filling as there is a decrease in thoracic cavitary pressure of approximately 10 mm Hg with the systemic venous pressure being constant. There is a gradual yet not a significant decrease in left-sided heart filling as the pulmonary veins are largely intrathoracic.

HEMODYNAMICS OF CONSTRICTIVE PERICARDITIS: FIXED CARDIAC VOLUME

The hemodynamic hallmark of constrictive pericarditis is equal and raised diastolic pressures in the left and right sides and fixed intracardiac volume during the diastolic phase throughout the respiratory cycle.

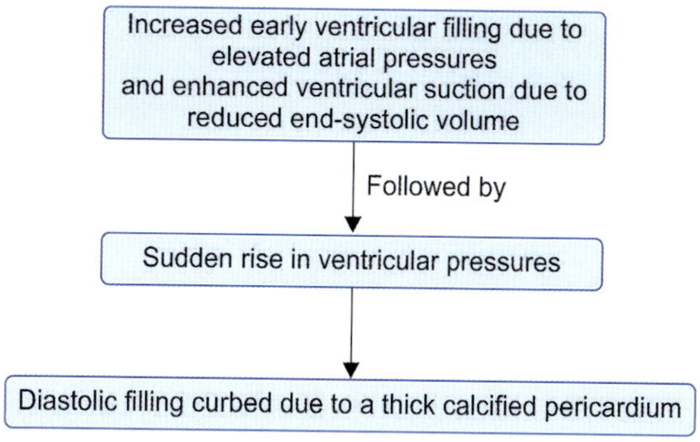

The rapid ventricular filling is accounted by the rapid "Y descent" on JVP and the square root sign during invasive hemodynamic assessment.

The rigid pericardium detaches the cardia from changes in the respiratory variations in intrathoracic pressure. On inspiration, the intrathoracic pressures are transmitted to the pulmonary venous system as they are intrathoracic, but not the left side. As there is a fixed total cardiac volume by the thick pericardium, there is increased right-sided filling with the interventricular septum moving toward the left side.

INSPIRATORY INTERVENTRICULAR SEPTAL MOTION TOWARD LEFT VENTRICLE

Kussmaul's Sign

During inspiration there is an increase in IVC inflow to right side, which is accentuated by enhanced transdiaphragmatic pressures, this competes with SVC inflow into the high pressure RA.

With expiration there is increase in intrathoracic pressures, which are transmitted to the pulmonary venous/capillary system thus increasing the inflow to the left side, pushing the IVS to the right side and thereby reducing RV inflow.

DIAGNOSIS—CLINICAL

The clinical picture depicts predominant presentation with right heart failure symptoms:

- Lower extremity edema
- Ascites

Progressing to:

- Congestive hepatopathy
- Anasarca

Can have features of extreme low cardiac output such as:

- Fatigue
- Cachexia

HALLMARK CLINICAL SIGNS

- Sudden and rapidly collapsing Y descent, with normal X descent resulting in M-shaped venous pressure contour
- Kussmaul's sign—inspiratory increase in JVP
- *Pulsus paradoxus*—in effusive constrictive pericarditis

Classically defined as an exaggerated inspiratory decline in systolic blood pressure > 10 mm Hg. This phenomenon was first explained by Kussmaul in 1873. The paradox being, total obliteration of Korotkoff sounds on inspiration, while there is cardiac activity. Cardiac tamponade is the prototype of this phenomenon, while other conditions such as acute exacerbation of COPD/constrictive pericarditis can exhibit this.

Mechanism of pulsus paradoxus: The exact mechanism of pulsus paradoxus in CCP is not known,[2] but multiple theories have been published.

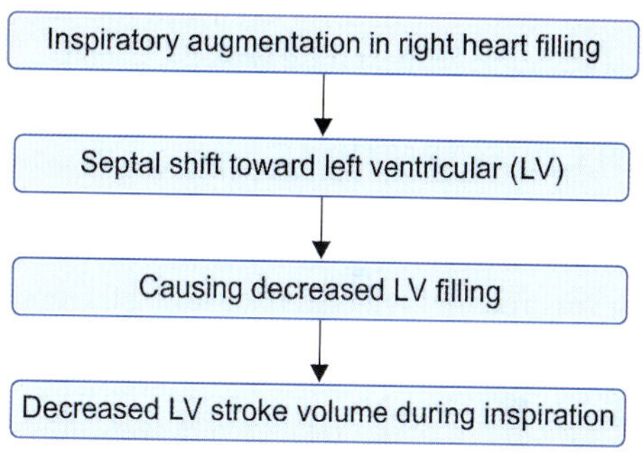

Ling et al. documented this sign in 19% of patients with CCP.[3] It is more common in effusive constrictive pericarditis, as observed by Sagrista et al. in up to 66% of patients.[4]

Pericardial knock on auscultation: Early, high-pitched diastolic sound

CHEST X-RAY IN CONSTRICTIVE PERICARDITIS

X-rays play a limited but useful role in diagnosing CP. It can reveal signs such as pericardial calcification which appears as dense, curvilinear shadows along heart borders. Enlarged cardiac silhouette and the pleural effusions may also be observed. However, X-ray lacks the specificity and detail of advanced imaging modalities like CT. Despite these limitations, chest X-rays are valuable for initial assessment and can prompt further, more detailed investigations if CP

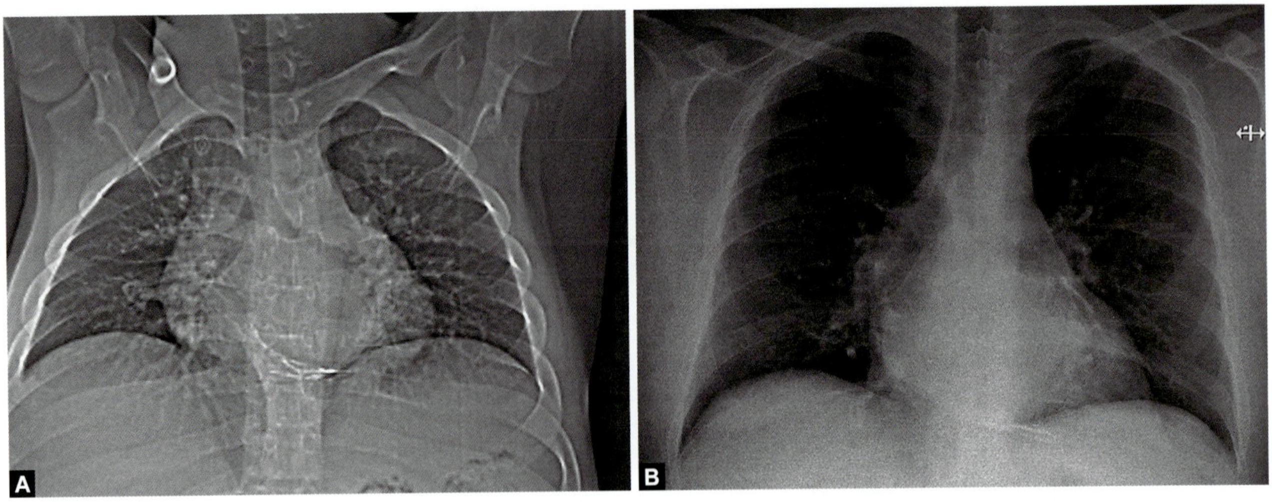

FIGS. 1A AND B: Pericardial calcification seen on chest X-ray.

is suspected based on clinical and radiographic findings **(Figs. 1A and B)**.

TRANSTHORACIC ECHOCARDIOGRAPHY

Noninvasive and extremely accurate for diagnosing pericardial pathology/thickening **(Fig. 2)**.

General Considerations

- Accurate assessment of septal motion with respect to the respiratory cycle (ventricular interdependence), to obtain long record (>12 beats), covering the entire cycle.
- While attempting to demonstrate constrictive physiology on echocardiography, the use of respirometry should be mandatory and a prerequisite while recording Dopplers of mitral/tricuspid inflow, hepatic vein, SVC, and while looking for septal motion.
- Hepatic vein Doppler assessment is important, as it can be dilated in both constrictive and restrictive physiology.[5]

Ventricular Septal Bounce and Interventricular Dependance

Septal bounce and inspiratory leftward septal shift along with expiratory rightward septal shift are typical in CP. The respirophasic septal movement provides the initial differential whether we are dealing with a constrictive physiology.

Septal bounce is simply reflective of the early LV and RV differential diastolic filling and its sudden cessation due to the pericardial nature in CP. IVS bounce is sensitive, it is not specific for CP and it can arise from various conditions such as postsurgery or conduction/pacing-associated septal movements. This is associated with septal notch on M-Mode and diastolic flattening of posterior wall in CP, but are still far less sensitive and specific.

In a series of patients with constrictive pericarditis, the septal shift suggestive of interventricular dependence had 92% PPV and 94% NPV.

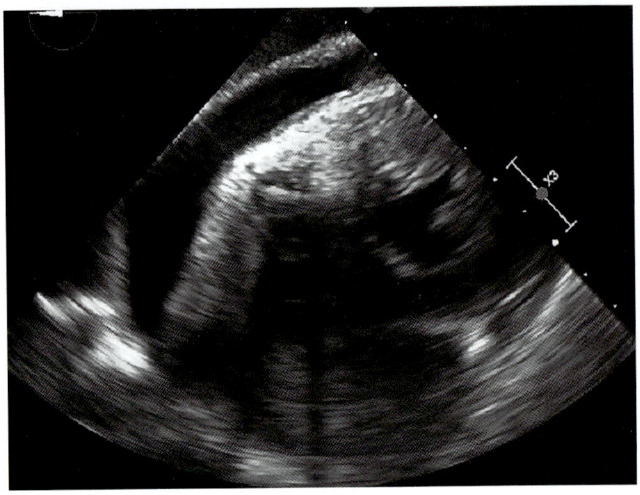

FIG. 2: Echocardiogram showing: Thickened pericardium with localized pericardial effusion alongside right ventricle.

Tissue Doppler Imaging on Echocardiography

The early mitral annulus velocity (E') is a marker of adequate LV relaxation/diastolic function. Normally, the lateral mitral annular velocity is higher than the medial velocity due to unrestricted movement. In constrictive physiology due to lateral pericardial adhesions, there is a restraint on the movement of cardia. Hence the mitral annular E' is more than lateral annular E'—*"annulus reversus"*.

In view of the adhesions and restriction of the lateral LV myocardium, LV filling is more dependent on the septal relaxation.

In a small series by Welch et al., medial $E' > 9$ cm/s and the ratio of medial and lateral E' of >0.91 had a positive predictive value of 90%. Hence in a patient with known myocardial pathology and congestive cardiac failure, a high medial E' should alert the physician whether constrictive physiology is at play.[6]

HEPATIC PULSE VEIN DOPPLER

The most specific sign for constrictive pericarditis on echocardiography is the accentuated expiratory flow reversal in hepatic vein. The specificity and positive predictive value are >90%.

Mechanism for Hepatic Vein Expiratory Flow Reversal

During expiration increase in left-sided filling, curbs the filling of the right side due to interventricular dependence. This reduces the forward hepatic vein outflow and accentuates the normal late diastolic velocity **(Fig. 3)**.

The hepatic vein expiratory diastolic reversal velocity as calculated by:

$$\frac{\text{Late diastolic reversal velocity}}{\text{Systolic forward flow velocity}}$$

If >0.79, positive predictive value is >95%.

Mitral and Tricuspid Inflow Respiratory Variations

More than 25% variation in mitral inflow Doppler with increased velocity during expiration is noted with >40% occurring on the tricuspid inflow Doppler. The tricuspid respiratory variations that so occur, do so while on inspiration **(Figs. 4 and 5)**.

The specificity and positive predictive value are <80%.

Two-dimensional Speckle Tracking

Additional and new tool in differentiation of CP from RCM/myocardial pathologies. Torsional and circumferential strain, both predominantly from subepicardial myocardium are decreased in constrictive pericarditis compared to restrictive cardiomyopathy. On the other hand, longitudinal strain is markedly affected in cardiac amyloidosis.[7]

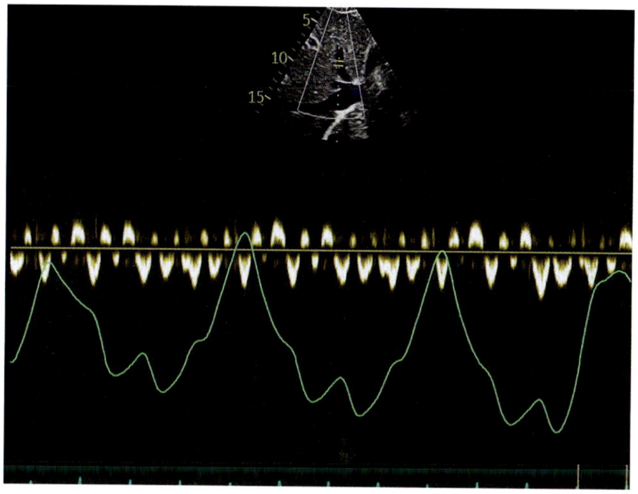

FIG. 3: Echocardiogram—hepatic vein expiratory flow reversal.

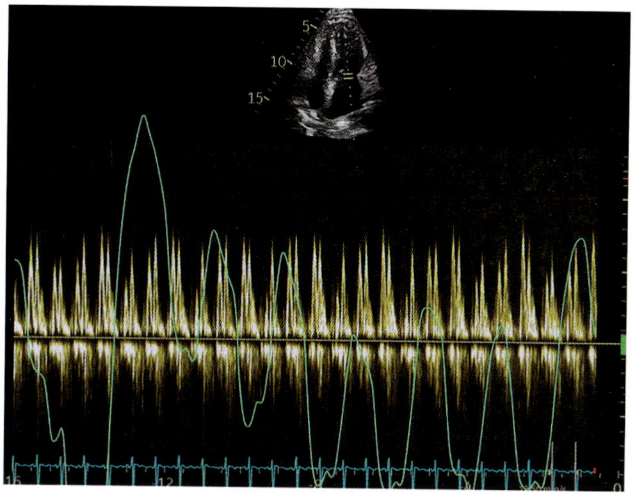

FIG. 4: Echo: Mitral expiratory increase in inflow on PW Doppler.

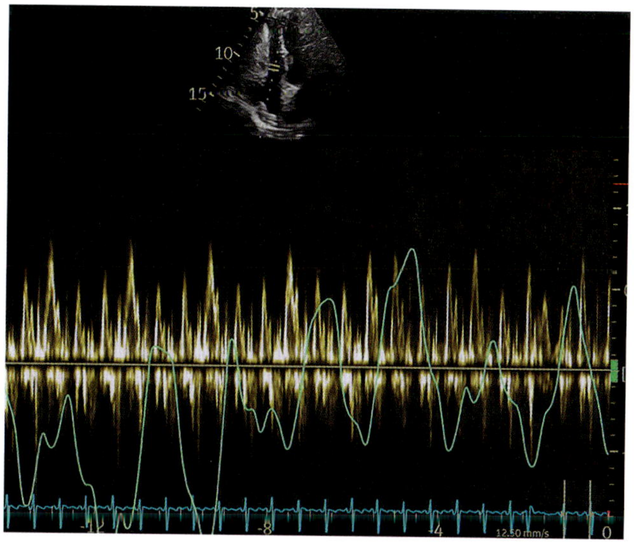

FIG. 5: Echo: Tricuspid inspiratory increase in inflow on PW Doppler.

COMPUTED TOMOGRAPHY

The CT scanning, particularly using MDCT, is highly effective in evaluating the structural aspects of CP. It proven to be highly effective in evaluating the structural aspects of CP. It provides high-resolution images that can detail the extent of pericardial thickening and calcification. The advantages of CT in diagnosing CP include **(Fig. 6)**:

- *Pericardial thickening and calcification*: CT can precisely measure the pericardial thickness, with values > 4 mm typically suggestive of CP. Calcifications, commonly seen in CP, are well visualized on CT often appearing as dense, bright areas within the pericardium.
- *Evaluation of pericardial effusion*: CT can assess presence and size of pericardial effusions, which may coexist with CP. It also aids distinguishing between CP and other causes of effusion.
- *Cardiac chamber morphology*: It can reveal secondary signs of CP, such as abnormal septal motion and changes in the size and shape of the cardiac chambers.
- *Vascular assessment*: Vena caval enlargement or hepatic vein congestion, providing a comprehensive view of the circulatory impact of CP
- *Coronary status*: Coronary atherosclerosis/graft patency can also be checked while doing the CT.[8]

MRI IMAGING IN CONSTRICTIVE PERICARDITIS

An MRI has achieved great strides in diagnosing various cardiac especially myocardial disorders, providing a wealth of information in every dimension possible. The temporal and spatial resolution achieved from CMRI allows us to examine every little detail of cardiac anatomy and physiology. With various sequences that can be used, cardiac structures can be noninvasively characterized to a great extent. In the strata of pericardial disorders too, CMRI has a place in the diagnostic tree.

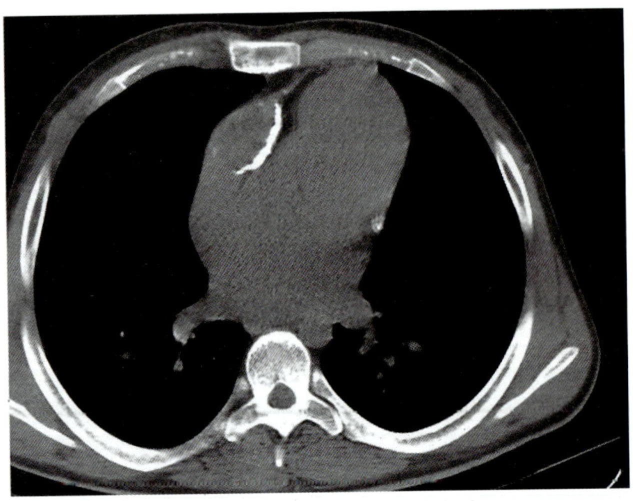

FIG. 6: CT chest showing: Thickened pericardium with interspersed calcium.

Cardiac Anatomy

Interestingly biatrial dilatation can be seen in both RCM and CP, but the relative ratio (left atrial to right atrial volumes) is found to be higher with CP. The ratio of 1.32 is found to have higher specificity and sensitivity. In such cases, a fibrotic pericardium and thickened pericardium (>4 mm) increase the positive predictive value to >90%.

Myocardial Characterization

LGE might not be present in a pure constrictive pericarditis, but pericardial LGE could be a feature of myopericarditis.

Hemodynamic Evaluation

Hemodynamic assessment is possible similar to echocardiography. Mitral/tricuspid inflow phase contrast sequences are possible. 3D/4D imaging has supported study of intracardiac flow patterns and abnormalities associated with it.

Real-time, breathing CMRI allows recording of respirophasic septal shift.

Septal shift on MRI is defined as the maximal difference in expiratory and inspiratory position of IVS. A baseline cut-off of 11.8 % has been published to distinguish CP and RCM **(Figs. 7A and B)**.

HEMODYNAMIC CATHETERIZATION

Constrictive pericarditis or physiology though has an array of echocardiographic signs, it is still to date a hemodynamic diagnosis. Cardiac catheterization is done to differentiate from restrictive cardiomyopathy, which is a close mimicker as there is equalization of diastolic pressures with subtle but important signs **(Fig. 8)**.

Square Root/Dip and Plateau Sign

There is rapid increase in early ventricular filling pressures followed by a plateau due to the pericardial restraint on cardiac filling. This can be noted in both RCM and CP, but a LV filling curve of height > 7 mm Hg points more toward CP **(Fig. 9)**.

Kussmaul's Sign

Observed as <5 mm Hg decrease in inspiratory RA pressures, can be present in both CP and RCM.

Equalization of Diastolic Pressures

A difference in RV and LV end-diastolic pressures of <5 mm Hg results from fixed cardiac volume and from ventricular interdependence **(Fig. 10)**.

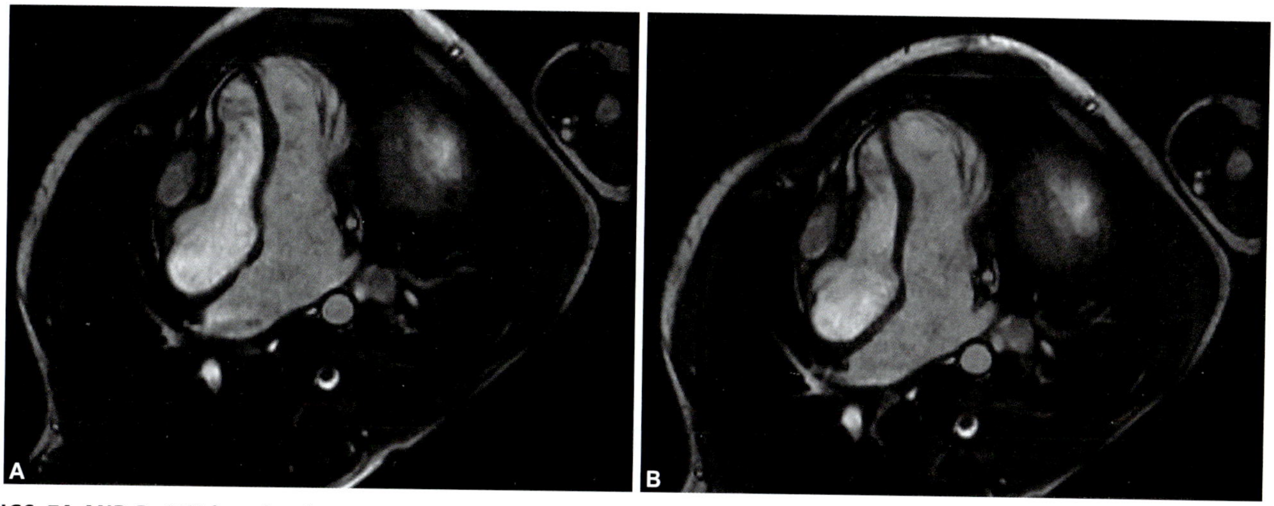

FIGS. 7A AND B: MRI four-chamber cine showing interventricular dependence. (A) The septal shift toward to the LV during inspiration. (B) The septal shift toward the RV during expiration.

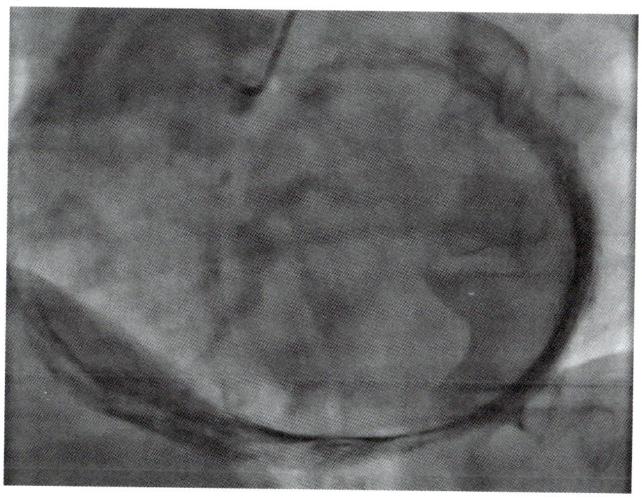

FIG. 8: Cine image of a calcific thickened pericardium while performing cardiac catheterization.

MANAGEMENT

A multidisciplinary heart team approach is always key in managing such patients with complex diagnosis where both hemodynamic physiology and anatomy is at question.

Surgical pericardiectomy remains the treatment of choice.

Pericardiectomy

The first pericardiectomy done by Rehn in 1913 in Germany and by Churchill in 1929 in the United States.

Risk factors for poor post operative outcomes include:
- Radiation associated constrictive pericarditis
- Medical comorbidities
- COPD/renal disease
- LV dysfunction
- Higher NYHA class

Diuretics and salt restriction though help in relieving congestive symptoms are not mainstay. Since sinus tachycardia is a protective mechanism to maintain forward output, it is best not to administer rate control medications.

Pericardiectomy is mostly performed through median sternotomy or bilateral thoracotomy with or without CP bypass. More extensive involvement of the epicardium has been handled with "waffle procedure" by means of longitudinal incisions in the epicardium. Symptomatic and physiological improvement is dramatic after pericardiectomy, which happens in a few patients, can appear after few weeks to months in others. The 5-year survival rates have been satisfactory, >80% and 10 year survival rates 50–80%.

INDIAN CONTEMPORARY DATA

Follow-up outcomes of patients with constrictive pericarditis and who have undergone pericardiectomy were studied by Bashi et al. in CMC Vellore. Though this study was done in 1988 reviewing patients done prior, the outcomes and results still hold valid in today's era. About 118 patients were included, of which males were predominant (86 males). Preoperatively >95% patients fell under NYHA III to IV for breathlessness and 100 patients had anasarca. TB was the proven predominant cause of the pathology with 72 patients affected. However in contrast to modern literature, anterolateral thoracotomy was done in 107 cases. Median sternotomy was done in three patients. Postoperatively a low output state was observed in 34 patients, in which 12 patients expired. At follow-up, there were 72 patients, among whom 63 patients were in Class I/II NYHA.[9]

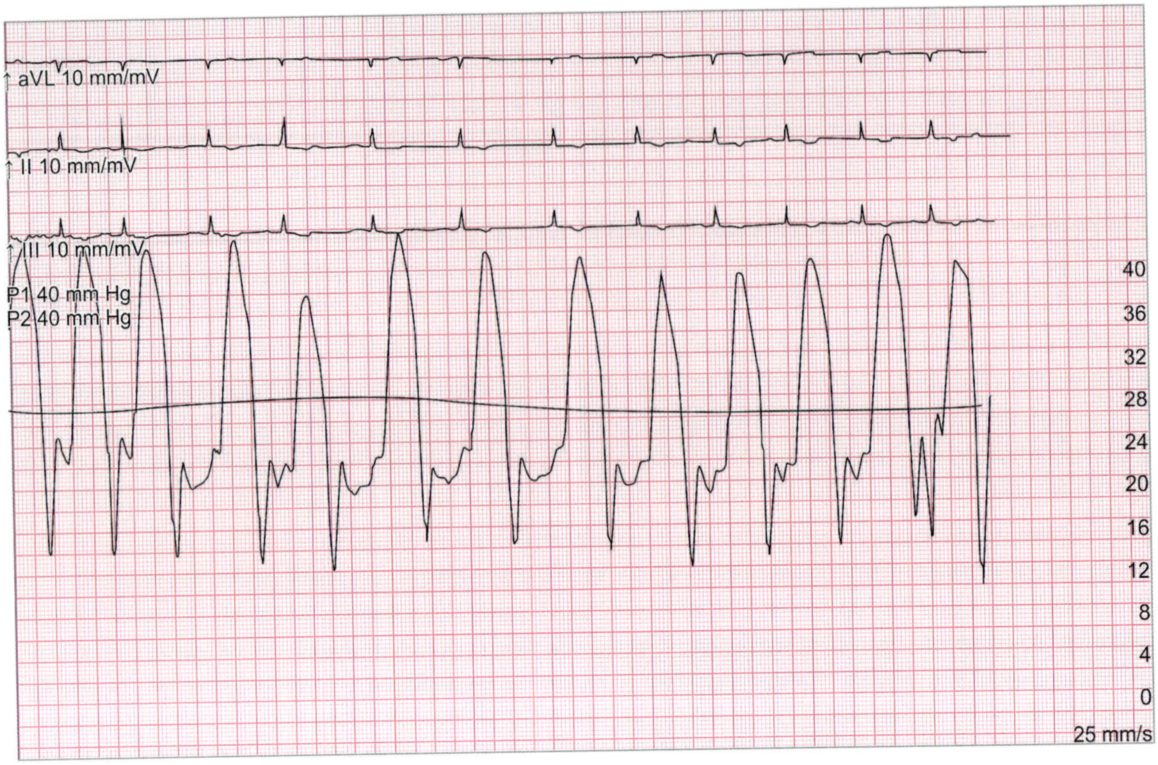

FIG. 9: Square root sign/dip and plateau sign.

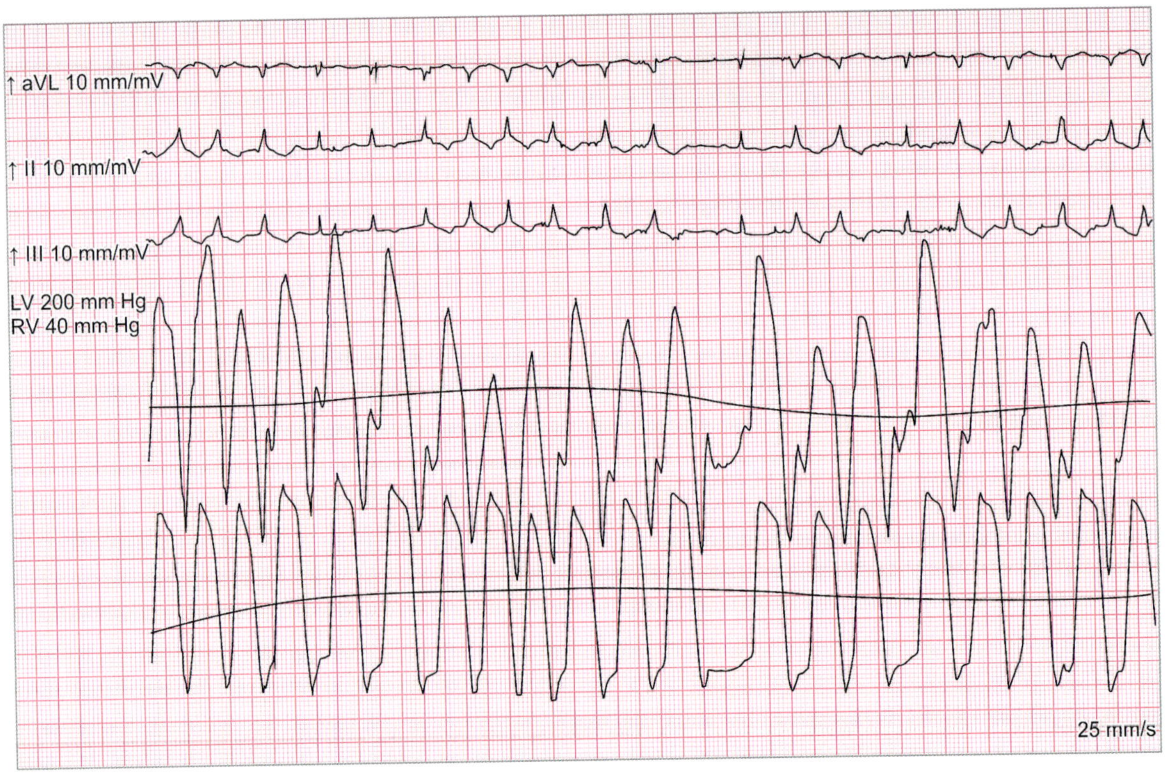

FIG. 10: Respirophasic changes in LV/RV pressures.

COMPREHENSIVE META-ANALYSIS

Tzani et al. conducted a comprehensive meta-analysis search of the MEDLINE, Embase, and Cochrane databases up to April 1, 2020, for studies assessing pericardiectomy outcomes. Studies with patients enrolled before 1985, pediatric patients, or those including >10% of cases with tuberculous pericarditis were excluded. They analyzed 27 eligible studies encompassing 2,114 patients. The most common etiology of constrictive pericarditis was idiopathic (50.2%), followed by postcardiac surgery (26.2%), and radiation (6.9%). The patient population was predominantly male (76%) with a mean age of 58 years and advanced symptoms (NYHA class III/IV in 70.1%). Advanced heart failure (NYHA class III-IV) was present in 70.1% of patients, and 33.1% had ascites. Peripheral edema (64.7%) and hepatomegaly (35.6%) were common, but not consistently reported.[10]

The surgical approach favored total pericardiectomy (85.8%) with midline sternotomy with a significant proportion undergoing concomitant cardiac surgeries (23.8%). The operative mortality was 6.9%, while the 5-year mortality was 32.7%. The 10-year survival rate for patients who underwent pericardiectomy for constrictive pericarditis, according to the meta-analysis, was 55%.

The analysis revealed that pericardiectomy practices have evolved over the years, with an increasing preference for complete pericardiectomy and concomitant cardiac surgeries post-2000. The inpatient and 30-day all-cause mortality rates had not significantly changed over the years, indicating a persistent high-risk profile for these patients. Long-term outcomes, including reoperation and rehospitalization for heart failure, remain concerns, with pooled rates of 8% and 11%, respectively.

PERSONAL EXPERIENCE

In our setting, we have had 20 patients in the past 25 years diagnosed to have constrictive physiology and undergone pericardiectomy, out of which three patients had pericardiectomy done in the pediatric age group (<14 years), etiology in two being TB and one patient idiopathic. All patients were males. About 17 patients had features suggestive of right heart symptoms, ascites along with fever and constitutional symptoms. About 19 patients were in NYHA class III dyspnea on exertion prior to the surgery. On echocardiogram, features suggestive of septal bounce and interventricular dependence could be seen in >90%. Hepatic vein systolic reversal on PW doppler proved to be specific sign which could be noted in all patients. Four patients had dense circumferential calcification while others had thickened pericardium with varying degrees of pericardial effusion with interspersed calcium.

All patients underwent pericardiectomy through midline sternotomy. Three patients had concomitant revascularization done with one graft in each patient. About 12 patients had undergone complete pericardiectomy. Eight patients had proven TB from tissue/MTB PCR. Three patients had expired in immediate postoperative period. Two patients died due to a low cardiac output state, while other cause was sepsis associated multiorgan dysfunction. At follow-up, 15 patients are currently still under follow-up, in functional class I to II.

CONCLUSION

Constrictive pericarditis and its different forms remain a potentially curable form of cardiac disease, with postsurgery patients having good quality of life. The most common cause in developing countries continues to be TB, whereas in the West it is idiopathic pericarditis. Multimodality noninvasive imaging and the latest advancements in the field of imaging do help increase the diagnostic power, and provide an insight toward the diagnosis, and planning an efficient surgical procedure.

ONLINE REFERENCES

Please scan the QR code provided at the end of the table of contents for References of this chapter.

CHAPTER

109

Cardiac Rehabilitation Postcoronary Artery Bypass Graft

Chandra Bhan Meena, Aishwarya Vyas

ABSTRACT

This comprehensive chapter underscores the critical role of structured, phased, and personalized cardiac rehabilitation (CR) programs in enhancing the recovery and long-term health of patients with postcoronary artery bypass graft (CABG). By addressing the barriers to participation and optimizing the protocols, healthcare providers can significantly improve patient outcomes and quality of life.

Keywords: Coronary artery bypass graft, barriers, protocols, patient

INTRODUCTION

Cardiac rehabilitation (CR) is a cornerstone of secondary prevention for patients who have undergone coronary artery bypass graft (CABG) surgery. Think of it as your heart's very own spa retreat, designed to rejuvenate, strengthen, and pamper your cardiovascular system after the heavy lifting of surgery. This chapter provides an in-depth exploration of the evidence supporting CR, the various phases of CR, the specific protocols used, and the multifaceted benefits it offers to post-CABG patients.

EVIDENCE SUPPORTING CARDIAC REHABILITATION

Cardiopulmonary Function Improvements

A comprehensive meta-analysis involving 806 subjects across 13 randomized controlled trials (RCTs) has demonstrated that CR significantly enhances cardiopulmonary function in post-CABG patients.[1] It is like a turbo boost for your heart and lungs. Key improvements include the following:

- *Peak oxygen uptake (peak VO_2)*: Peak VO_2 is a critical measure of cardiovascular health and endurance. The meta analysis showed a significant increase in peak VO_2 among CR participants, reflecting improved oxygen utilization during exercise. Essentially, your heart becomes a high-performance engine, and your lungs become the best air filters money cannot buy.
- *6-minute walk distance (6MWD)*: The distance a patient can walk in 6 minutes significantly increased in the CR group, indicating better functional capacity and endurance. Imagine transforming your daily stroll from a lazy turtle pace to a brisk power walk.
- *Resting heart rate (HR)*: A significant reduction in resting HR was observed, which is associated with improved autonomic function and reduced cardiovascular stress. It is like telling your heart to "chill out" and it actually listens.

These improvements are crucial as they translate to better physical performance, enhanced quality of life, and lower mortality rates.

Timing and Duration of Cardiac Rehabilitation

The timing and duration of CR are pivotal in maximizing its benefits. The meta-analysis highlighted that patients who participated in more than 1,000 minutes of CR or started CR within 1 week after CABG showed the most significant improvements in cardiopulmonary function. Early initiation helps counteract the adverse effects of prolonged inactivity and promotes faster recovery. It is like starting a good habit early; the sooner you begin, the better the results.

Long-term Outcomes and Mortality

Cardiac rehabilitation's impact extends beyond immediate cardiopulmonary benefits. Studies have shown that higher levels of peak VO_2 are strongly linked with improved long-term survival:

- *Carbone et al.*:[2] They identified peak VO_2 as an independent predictor of long-term survival. Higher peak VO_2 levels were associated with a reduced mortality risk [hazard ratio (HR) = 0.84]. It is like finding the secret to a longer, healthier life in a VO_{2max} chart.
- *De Schutter et al.*:[3] Each 1 mL/kg/min increment in peak VO_2 corresponded to a 10% reduction in all-cause mortality. Imagine earning a 10% discount on death—a pretty good deal, right?
- *Vanhees et al.*:[4] A 1% increase in peak VO_2 resulted in a 2% decrease in cardiovascular mortality. So, every little improvement in VO_2 is like getting a BOGO offer on years of life.

Autonomic Function and Cardiovascular Events[5,6]

Cardiac rehabilitation has a beneficial effect on the autonomic nervous system, crucial for patients with cardiovascular diseases (CVDs) who often suffer from autonomic dysfunction characterized by increased sympathetic activity and reduced vagal tone. Improved autonomic function leads to:

- *Reduced resting HR*: Lower resting HR is associated with better cardiovascular outcomes and reduced risk of adverse events. Think of it as your heart mastering the art of Zen.
- *Fewer arrhythmic events*: CR reduces the frequency of arrhythmic events, contributing to better heart rhythm stability. Your heart stops breakdancing and starts waltzing smoothly.

PHASES OF CARDIAC REHABILITATION (FIG. 1)[7,8]

Cardiac rehabilitation programs are structured into pre-CABG and three post-CABG phases, each targeting specific aspects of recovery and health improvement. Consider these phases as levels in a video game, each one bringing you closer to the ultimate goal: A strong, resilient heart.

Precoronary Artery Bypass Graft Procedure

The goal of pre-CABG rehabilitation is to prevent post-CABG complications, particularly pulmonary ones. Benefits include reduced ventilator use, fewer pulmonary complications, and improved lung function. Rehabilitation programs are individualized based on patient needs.

Six-Minute Walk Test

Patients are evaluated using the 6-minute walk test (6MWT) to determine functional ability in METs units. The test measures the distance walked in 6 minutes, converted to VO_{2max} and METs values. This assessment helps prescribe

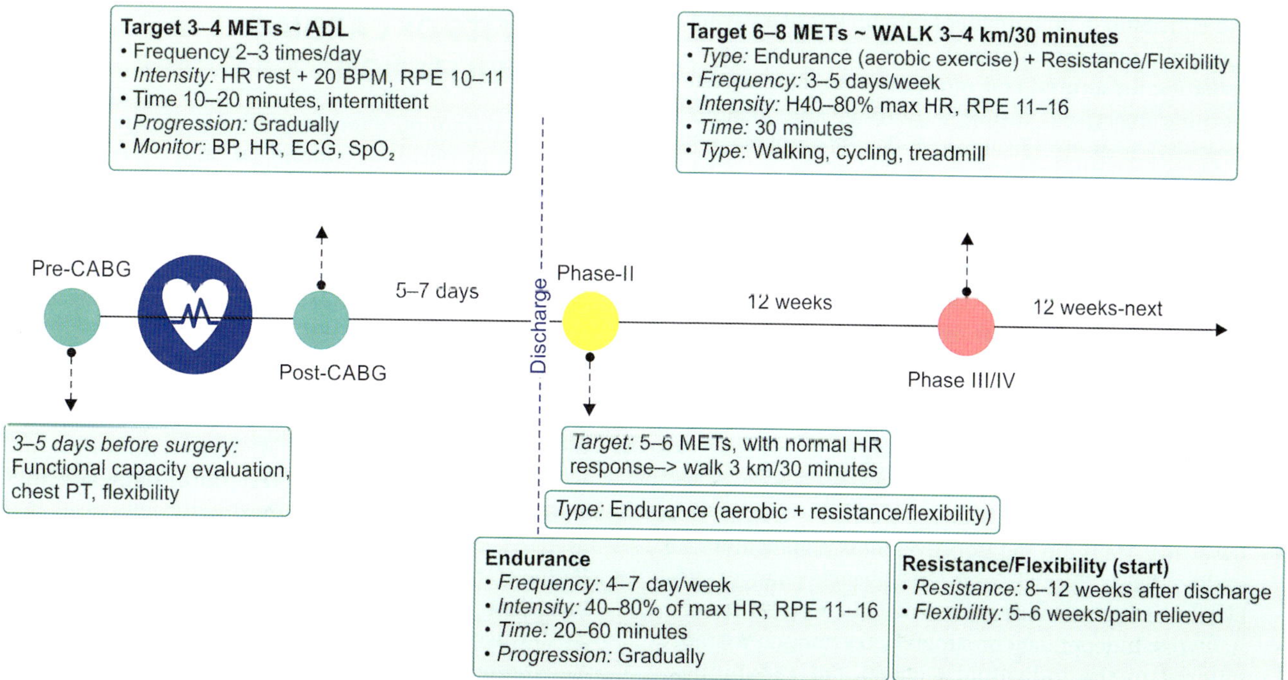

FIG. 1: Phases of cardiac rehabilitation. MET—the oxygen demand in individuals who are awake at rest. MET is equal to 3.5 mL/kg body weight/min, RPE—rating of perceived exertion.

an appropriate exercise program. MET is equal to 3.5 mL/kg body weight/min.

Precoronary Artery Bypass Graft Rehabilitation Activities

- Chest physiotherapy
- *Breathing exercises*: Deep and diaphragmatic breathing exercises
- Incentive spirometry exercises
- Cough exercises
- *Flexibility exercises*: For head, neck, shoulder joints, and extremities

Phase I: Inpatient Cardiac Rehabilitation

- *Objective*: Initiate early mobilization and education during the hospital stay. Think of it as a gentle wake-up call for your heart.
- *Activities*: Light physical activities, such as sitting up, standing, and short walks; education on heart-healthy lifestyle changes, medication adherence, and the importance of CR.
- *Duration*: Typically lasts for the duration of the hospital stay, usually 1–2 weeks postsurgery. Just long enough to get you off the couch but not so long that you start naming the hospital plants.
- *Benefits*: Prevents complications, encourages early recovery, and prepares patients for discharge.

Phase II: Outpatient Cardiac Rehabilitation

- *Objective*: Continue recovery with supervised exercise and education in an outpatient setting. It is like having a personal trainer for your heart.
- *Activities*: Structured and monitored exercise sessions (aerobic exercises, strength training, and flexibility exercises), ongoing education on diet, lifestyle changes, stress management, and smoking cessation; regular monitoring of HR, blood pressure, and ECG.
- *Duration*: Usually lasts 3–6 months, with 2–3 sessions per week. Long enough to develop a routine but short enough to still remember what life was like before.
- *Benefits*: Enhances cardiovascular fitness, reduces risk factors, improves physical and mental well-being, and supports long-term lifestyle changes.

Phase III: Maintenance Cardiac Rehabilitation

- *Objective*: Maintain the improvements achieved in the earlier phases through long-term lifestyle changes. It is like the maintenance phase in a diet but for your heart.
- *Activities*: Independent or supervised exercise programs tailored to the individual's needs and capabilities; ongoing support and education to reinforce healthy habits; periodic health assessments to monitor progress and adjust the program.
- *Duration*: Lifelong commitment to a heart-healthy lifestyle. This is where you make your heart's newfound fitness a permanent fixture, like keeping a New Year's resolution past February.
- *Benefits*: Sustains improvements in cardiovascular health, reduces the risk of future cardiac events, and promotes overall well-being.

EXERCISE RECOMMENDATIONS

International guidelines recommend a combination of moderate-to-vigorous-intensity aerobic exercises and resistance training for major muscle groups. Specific recommendations include the following:

- *Aerobic exercise*:[6] Moderate-intensity cardiopulmonary exercise for at least 150 min/week or vigorous-intensity exercise for at least 75 min/week, achieving a total energy expenditure of 500–1,000 MET-min/week. Think of it as giving your heart a regular workout to keep it in top shape.
- *Resistance training*:[9] Exercise for major muscle groups at least 2–3 days/wk because even your heart likes to show off its muscle gains.
- *Neuromotor exercises*:[10] Activities involving balance, agility, and coordination 2–3 days/week. It is like yoga for your heart and body.

Personalizing CR programs to fit individual capabilities and health status is crucial for maximizing benefits and minimizing risks. After all, one size does not fit all, especially when it comes to heart health.

BENEFITS OF CARDIAC REHABILITATION

Cardiac rehabilitation offers a multitude of benefits, categorized into physical, psychological, and social aspects. Think of it as a triple threat for your heart health, mind, and social life.

Physical Benefits

- *Enhanced cardiovascular health*:[1] Improved heart function, reduced resting HR, lower blood pressure, and increased peak VO_2. It is like turning your heart into a finely tuned machine.
- *Improved functional capacity*:[6] Better endurance and strength, enabling patients to perform daily activities with greater ease. Imagine breezing through tasks that used to leave you winded.
- *Reduced risk of recurrent cardiac events*:[11-13] Lower incidence of myocardial infarction, stroke, and other cardiovascular events by addressing risk factors such as hypertension, hyperlipidemia, and obesity. It is like having a personal bodyguard for your heart.

- *Better weight management*:[14] Structured exercise and dietary counseling help patients achieve and maintain a healthy weight. Think of it as a dual-purpose plan: Getting fit and staying healthy.

Psychological Benefits

- *Reduced anxiety and depression*:[11-13] Regular physical activity and group support within CR programs alleviate symptoms of anxiety and depression. It is like getting a mood booster with every workout.
- *Enhanced quality of life*:[15] Improved physical health and emotional well-being contribute to a better overall quality of life. You will feel like a new person, ready to take on the world.
- *Increased confidence*: Patients gain confidence in their ability to manage their health and engage in physical activities. It is like getting your groove back, one step at a time.

Social Benefits

- *Supportive environment*: CR programs provide a supportive environment where patients can share experiences and encouragement with others facing similar health challenges. It is like joining a heart health club with lifelong membership.
- *Improved social interaction*: Group activities and educational sessions foster social connections and reduce feelings of isolation. Because a healthy heart is even better when shared with friends.

BARRIERS TO CARDIAC REHABILITATION PARTICIPATION[16]

Despite its proven benefits, participation in CR programs remains low, especially in low/middle-income countries (LMICs). Factors contributing to low participation include the following:

- *Patient-related factors*: Older age, low socioeconomic status, lack of awareness. Sometimes, it is hard to get motivated, especially if you are not sure what CR is all about.
- *Physician-related factors*: Inadequate knowledge of CR and failure to recommend CR to patients. Even doctors need a reminder now and then about the importance of CR.
- *System-related factors*: Limited availability of CR facilities, financial difficulty, and lack of medical insurance. Because no one should miss out on heart health due to logistics.

Addressing these barriers requires a multifaceted approach, including patient education, improving physician awareness and training, and enhancing the accessibility and affordability of CR programs.

LIMITATIONS

This chapter acknowledges several limitations, including heterogeneity among the included studies regarding CR protocols, small sample sizes, and reliance on secondary data. Future multicenter, large-scale clinical trials are necessary to validate these findings and refine CR guidelines for post-CABG patients.

CONCLUSION

Cardiac rehabilitation significantly improves cardiopulmonary function, reduces mortality, and enhances the overall quality of life in post-CABG patients. The variability in exercise modalities and program durations highlights the need for personalized and long-term CR strategies. Increasing CR participation through patient education and improving accessibility, particularly in LMICs, is essential for maximizing the benefits of CR.

ONLINE REFERENCES

Please scan the QR code provided at the end of the table of contents for References of this chapter.

SECTION 11

Pulmonary Vascular Disease

Section Outline

CHAPTER

110

Pulmonary Thromboembolism: Recent Advances in Management

A Kader Sahib, AD Arun Mohan, M Shanmathi

ABSTRACT

Pulmonary embolism (PE) is a life-threatening illness that requires immediate diagnosis and treatment. Recent breakthroughs in management have resulted in better patient outcomes. This chapter covers the most recent breakthroughs in PE management, such as thrombolytic therapy and catheter-based therapies. We also look into improvements in imaging and biomarkers, which have improved diagnosis and risk stratification. Catheter-based therapies, including the rotational pigtail catheter, Fogarty balloon embolectomy catheter, cleaner rotational thrombectomy system, rheolytic catheter, and AngioJet, have showed potential in lowering thrombus load and increasing pulmonary perfusion. Furthermore, surgical embolectomy has emerged as a potential treatment option for high-risk individuals. Despite these developments, PE remains a major public health concern, and additional research is required to address outstanding challenges. This chapter focuses on the current condition of PE management.

Keywords: Pulmonary embolism, thrombectomy, catheter-based therapy, thrombolytic therapy, surgical embolectomy

INTRODUCTION

A pulmonary embolism (PE) develops when a blood clot gets into the blood vessels in the lungs, disrupting regular blood flow. Gas exchange is impeded by this blockage. Depending on its size and the number of afflicted vessels, a blood clot may pose a serious threat to life.

EPIDEMIOLOGY

With an incidence rate of 60–70 cases per 100,000 population, more than one-third of patients present with acute PE which could be fatal. With the highest incidence in women more than in men, genetic predisposition also plays a part in tendencies to form thrombus.[1] It is estimated that 10% of patients with acute PE die during the first 1–3 months.[1] 10% of all hospital deaths are due to PE and are often sudden, due to right heart failure and multiorgan involvement causing ventricular tachycardias, pulseless electrical activities, and asystole. There is also a high 30-day hospital readmission rate and a high 6-month mortality rate among elderly PE patients. The incidence is higher in women, especially during pregnancy and postpartum states.[2]

RECENT ADVANCES IN THE MANAGEMENT OF PULMONARY EMBOLISM

Traditional pharmacological management of PE remains the mainstay with parenteral anticoagulants following oral anticoagulants forming the basis in treating PE patients. Recently, various invasive and semi-invasive methods have been developed that can help in reducing the thrombus load, improve pulmonary perfusion, restore right ventricular function, and reduce symptoms and length of hospital stay.

All these recent advances have more role in managing high-risk massive PE patients who are in shock and with multiorgan involvement. The images of catheter-based therapies for acute PE are shown in **Figures 1A to J**.[3]

CATHETER-BASED THERAPIES

The mechanism of catheter-based therapies is shown in **Figures 2A to D**.[3]

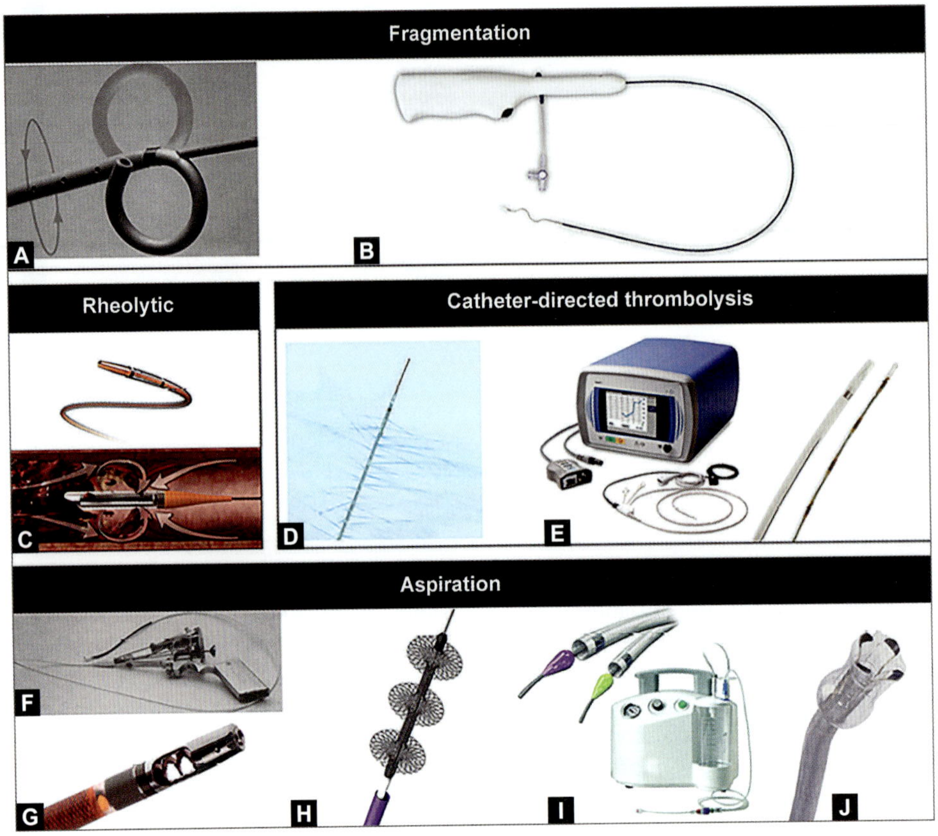

FIGS. 1A TO J: Images of catheter-based therapies for acute PE are shown: (A) Rotational pigtail catheter, (B) Cleaner XT, (C) AngioJet, (D) Unifuse, (E) EkoSonic, (F) Greenfield, (G) Aspirex S, (H) FlowTriever, (I) Indigo, and (J) AngioVac.

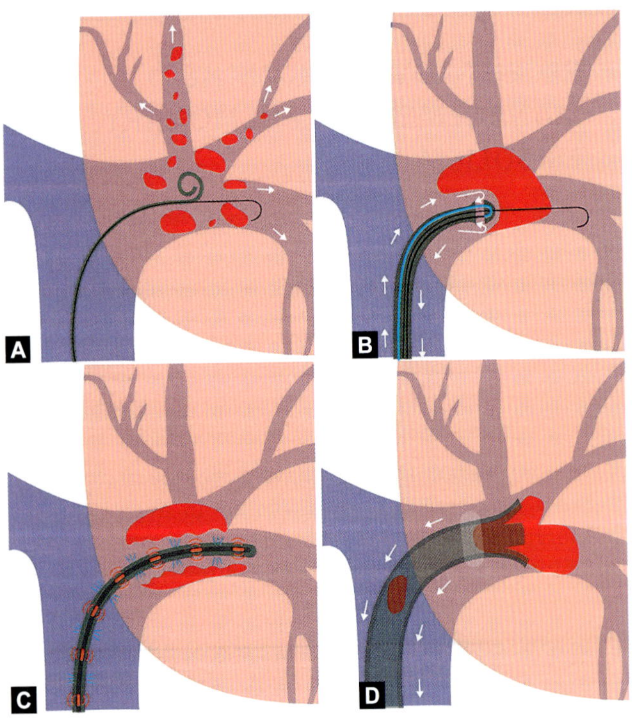

FIGS. 2A TO D: Illustration of the four mechanisms of catheter-based therapy: (A) Fragmentation, (B) Rheolytic therapy, (C) Catheter-directed thrombolysis, and (D) Aspiration.

Rotational Pigtail Catheter

A pigtail catheter has been altered with a side hole that can allow a guidewire to pass through. This guidewire can be used as an axis from which the pigtail catheter can be rotated. As the guidewire crosses the embolus, the pigtail edge of the catheter is rotated leading to mechanical fragmentation of the embolus leading to the breakage of a single bolus into multiple tiny fragments, thus reducing the PA pressure and improving flow. This procedure is quite simple to use and available in most centers. There is an obvious reduction in the amount of mechanical obstruction. The broken-down fragments are more prone to spontaneous thrombolysis. One risk is the fragments may embolize and block distal pulmonary vessels which can increase pulmonary vascular resistance and increase the risk of microinfarction of RV and RV strain. A rotational pigtail catheter is shown in **Figure 3**.[4]

Fogarty Balloon Embolectomy Catheter

In this procedure, the catheter is passed through the embolus in the pulmonary artery and the balloon is inflated. This causes recanalization of the pulmonary artery. The major risk of this procedure is pulmonary artery rupture which can be prevented by using an undersized balloon. There are also chances of residual thrombus being in situ and distant

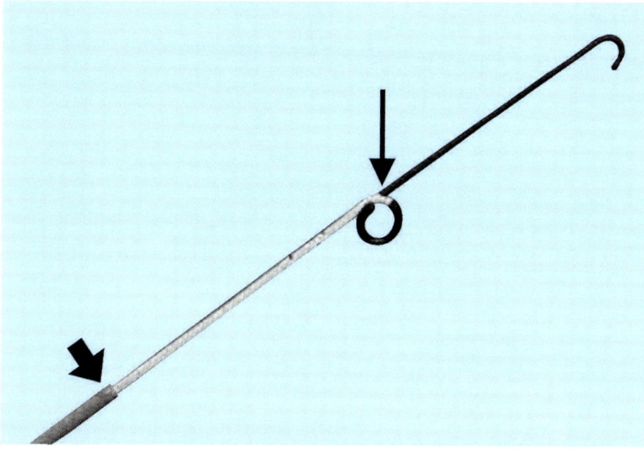

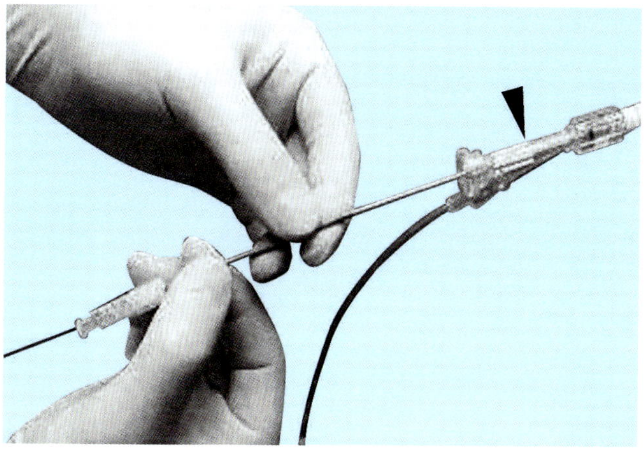

FIG. 3: Rotational pigtail catheter.

embolization into smaller pulmonary arteries. To avoid the risks, balloon angioplasty for PE should be accompanied by catheter-directed thrombolysis or aspiration.[5] Fogarty balloon embolectomy catheter is shown in **Figure 4**.

Cleaner Rotational Thrombectomy System

It is passed into the thrombus and a flexible sinusoidal tip is deployed distal to the embolus. This deployed distal end can be rotated with a battery-driven motor. Then the catheter must be withdrawn slowly and removed via the sheath. The risks involved are fragmentation and distal embolization. Also, the difficulty of aspirating a thrombus via a thin sheath has to be overcome.[6] Cleaner rotational thrombectomy system is shown in **Figure 5**.

Rheolytic Catheter

These catheters have a small lumen with a hairpin loop at the end of the catheter. Under some pressure, some agent such as mostly heparinized saline is injected into the thrombus at a high velocity and flow rate into a larger exhaust, producing a vortex. Using a vacuum created by the Venturi effect, the embolus may get disrupted and aspirated via a catheter.[7] A pulmonary angiogram in a patient with massive bilateral PE and multiple filling defects and repeat angiography after mechanical rheolytic thrombectomy shows improvement in pulmonary perfusion.

A rheolytic catheter is shown in **Figures 6A and B**.

AngioJet

It operates by the rheolytic principle. It was primarily designed to be used for thrombus removal of peripheral vessels. Severe adverse effects have been noted such as bradyarrhythmias, hemoglobinuria, hemorrhagic tendencies, hemoptysis, and renal damage. The FDA has

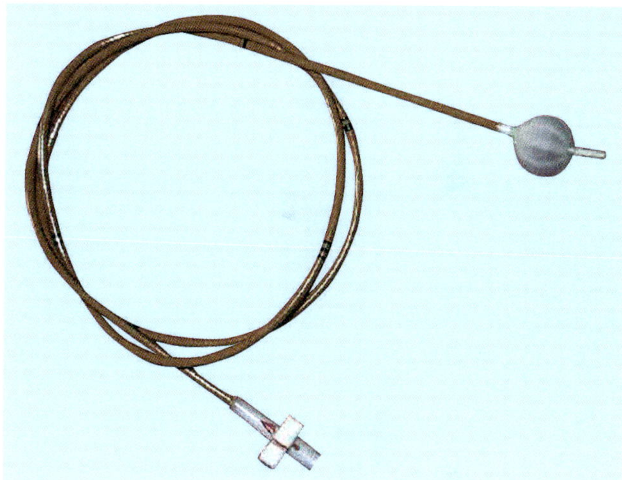

FIG. 4: Fogarty balloon embolectomy catheter.

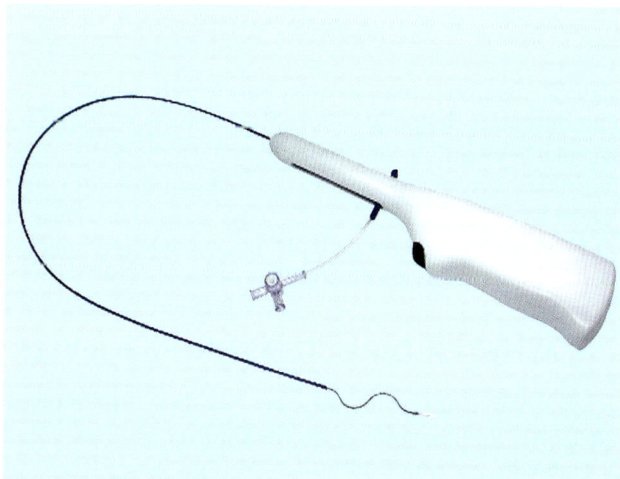

FIG. 5: Cleaner rotational thrombectomy system.

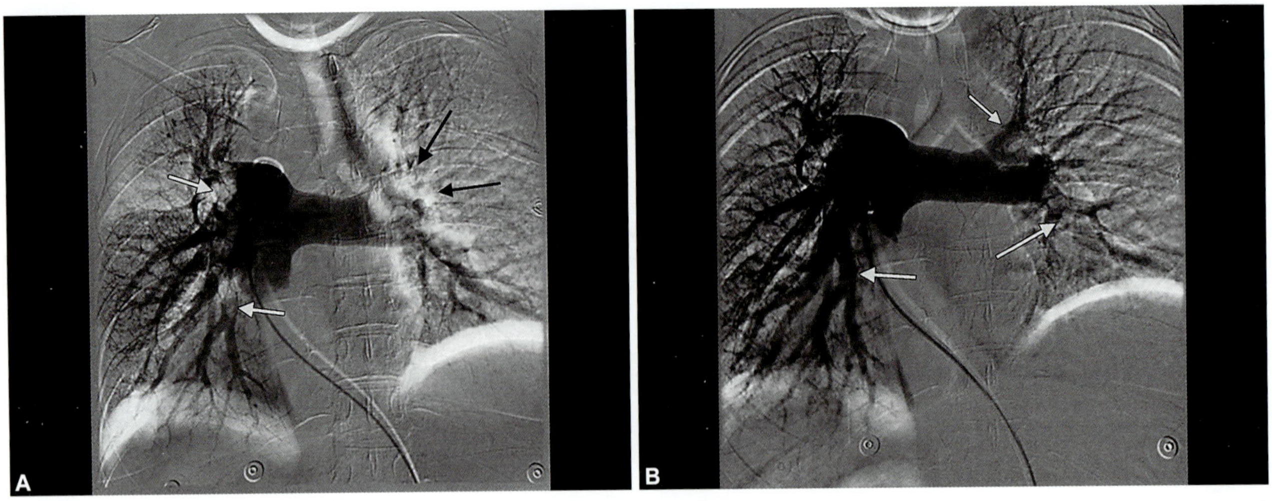

FIGS. 6A AND B: (A) Pulmonary angiogram in patient with massive bilateral PE and multiple filling defects. (B) Repeat angiography after mechanical rheolytic thrombectomy shows improvement in pulmonary perfusion.

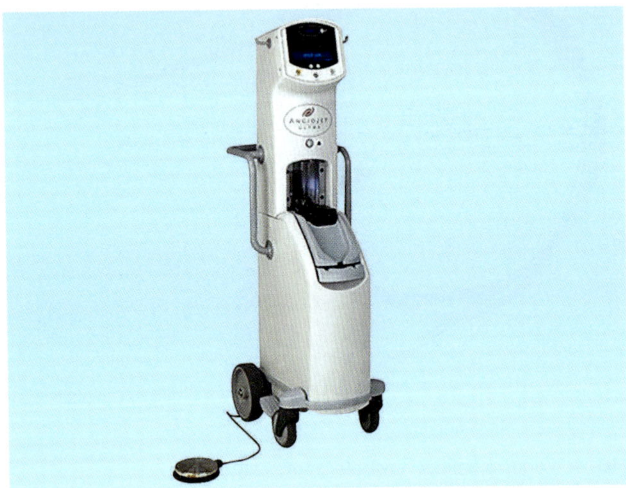

FIG. 7: AngioJet.

labeled AngioJet with a black box warning when used in the pulmonary circulation. Despite adverse effects, a temporary pacemaker insertion with monitoring of vitals, electrolytes, and renal parameters is essential.[8] AngioJet is shown in **Figure 7**.

Figures 8A to D show multiple fragmentation techniques used in catheter-based embolectomy.[9]

CATHETER-DIRECTED THROMBOLYSIS

In this, there is direct delivery of a low-dose thrombolytic drug into the pulmonary artery directly at the site of thrombus. Since there is disturbance of flow during the event of PE, the drug should be delivered into the thrombus, or the thrombus must be fragmented before the drug is delivered. In most cases, catheter-based therapies should be combined with fragmentation techniques (rotational pigtail catheter) for best results. The drug used here is alteplase, with infusion into the main or one of the main branches of the pulmonary artery for 24 hours at a dosage of 0.5–1 mg/hour. Total drug dosage given is 30 mg which is much lesser than the dosage used for systemic thrombolysis (100 mg).

Ultrasound-assisted Catheter-directed Thrombolysis

Here, the ultrasonic waves are purposely used to disturb the integrity of the thrombus to provide more binding sites for thrombolysis to work on. The EkoSonic endovascular system is a FDA-approved device evaluated through randomized control trials. In the ULTIMA trial comparing the effectiveness of USAT with alteplase and heparin alone, the group treated with USAT with alteplase was found to come out with decreased RV dysfunction.[10] There are no added benefits noted in patients with DVT in this study.

ASPIRATION DEVICES

The principle is to aspirate and reduce the mechanical thrombus burden in the pulmonary arteries leading to better flow patterns and RV function, with risk of distal embolization that comes with CDT techniques.

- Greenfield suction catheter
- Aspirex and Rotarex
- FlowTriever
- Indigo
- AngioVac

The Greenfield Suction Catheter

The device was developed in 1969. This device is equipped with a plastic cup in its tip. Through passing the catheter

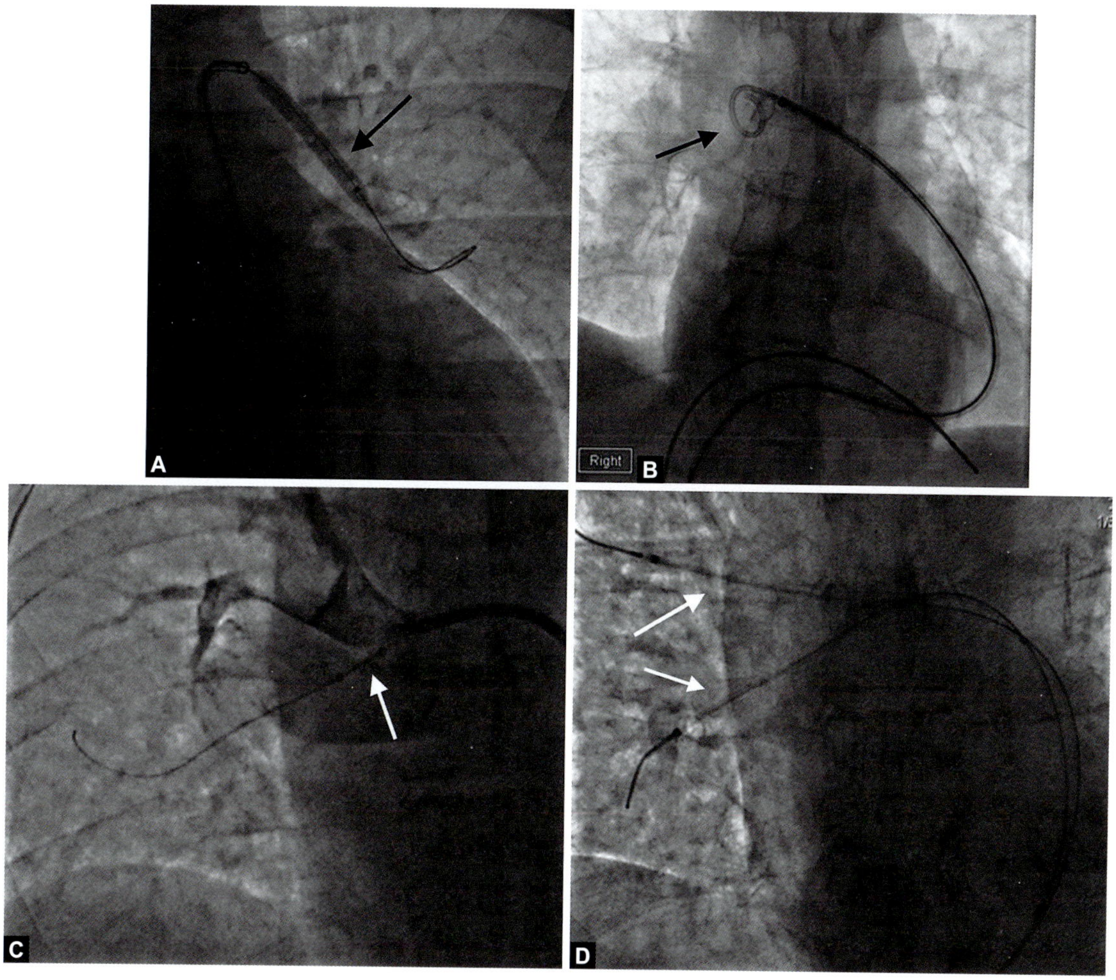

FIGS. 8A TO D: (A) Balloon angioplasty of venous thrombus in the left pulmonary artery; (B) A pigtail catheter; (C) An AngioJet rheolytic catheter performing thrombectomy in the right pulmonary artery; and (D) After mechanical fragmentation, infusion catheters are placed in pulmonary arteries.

into the PA, placing the suction cup at the thrombus, and aspirating it, the thrombus could be taken out in total without distal embolization or with minimal distal embolization. This catheter cannot be passed through conventional sheaths and hence surgical venotomy is needed to pass the catheter. The stiff cup is practically difficult to maneuver into the pulmonary artery along with a guidewire. It has a high success rate of 76%. It has not achieved a broad use in clinical practice.[11]

Aspirex and Rotarex

These are provided with a metal helix that can be rotated inside the catheter to create a vacuum at the tip of the catheter. This is based on Archimedes screw principle. The thrombus material is then pulled toward the catheter, and fragmented and broken pieces are transported back via side holes in the catheter. The tip is blunt to avoid fragmentation leading to distal embolization. This device is suitable for use only in fresh thrombus.

In Rotarex, the tip is faceted and rotates along with the catheter, which is useful in the fragmentation of old thrombus but there is a risk of damaging the pulmonary artery. In both Aspirex and Rotarex, a major setback is there is a large volume of blood loss, up to 130 mL/min, with a large catheter. **Figures 9A and B** show Rotarex and Aspirex.[12]

FlowTriever

The FlowTriever system has an aspiration catheter and a flow restoration catheter. Aspiration catheter is to be passed through thrombus first followed by a flow restoration catheter. Flow restoration catheter has three self-expanding nitinol wire discs that are expanded within the thrombus. Thrombus is trapped between discs and then aspirated by pulling back the catheter. The main challenges here are limited thrombus

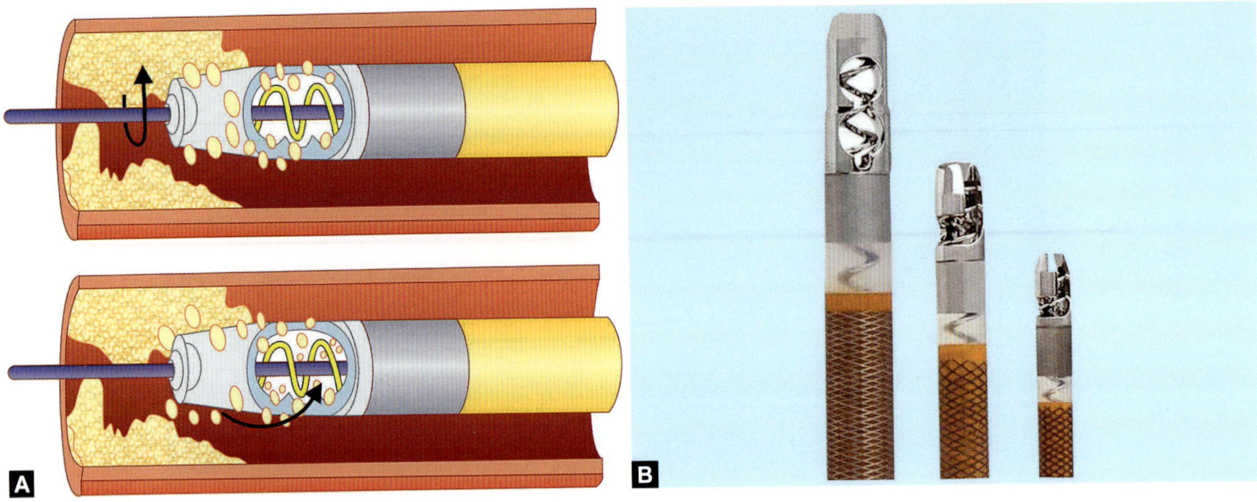

FIGS. 9A AND B: (A) Rotarex and (B) Aspirex.

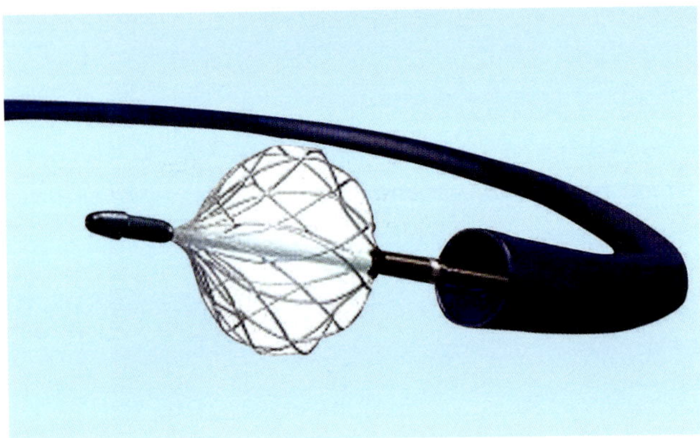

FIG. 10: FlowTriever.

removal and maneuverability of the catheter. The FLARE study (FlowTriever Pulmonary Embolectomy Clinical Study) is going on to evaluate the safety of FlowTriever in 150 patients with acute PE.[13] **Figure 10** shows FlowTriever.

Indigo

The indigo mechanical thrombectomy system includes an aspiration catheter, a pump providing suction, and a separator wire. Aspiration catheter in thrombus and the suction pump create a vacuum for aspiration of thrombus. The catheter could be advanced into a thrombus more distally to engage and remove more thrombus. The separator wire can be passed into the aspiration catheter to clear off the obstructing material. The catheter is provided with three different tips, with varying angles to provide better maneuverability. Catheter diameter is relatively small, which is good for maneuvering through the thrombus;

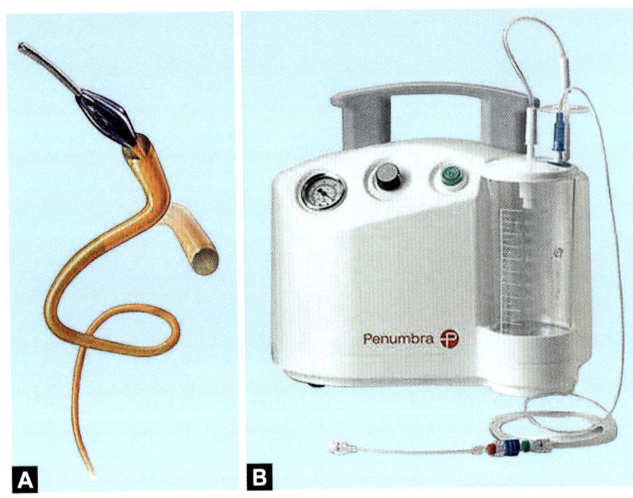

FIGS. 11A AND B: Penumbra.

hence, the amount of thrombus that could be aspirated is limited compared to other devices. The pump must be turned off when the catheter is outside the thrombus to reduce the amount of blood loss.[14] **Figures 11A and B** show Penumbra.

Thrombus removed after the procedure using Penumbra catheter is shown in **Figure 12**.[9]

AngioVac

This is a cannula which is made for the total removal of venous thrombi during extracorporeal venous bypass procedures to aspirate the thrombus before reintroducing the vein into the systemic circulation. The catheter tip is tulip shaped, which can be expanded with a balloon after its placement proximal

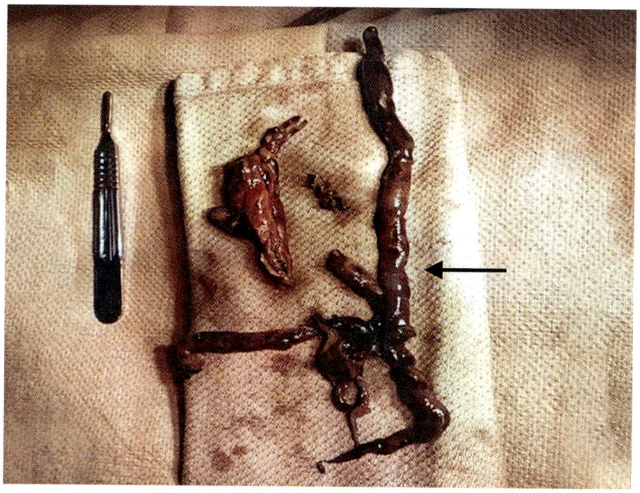

FIG. 12: Thrombus removed after procedure.

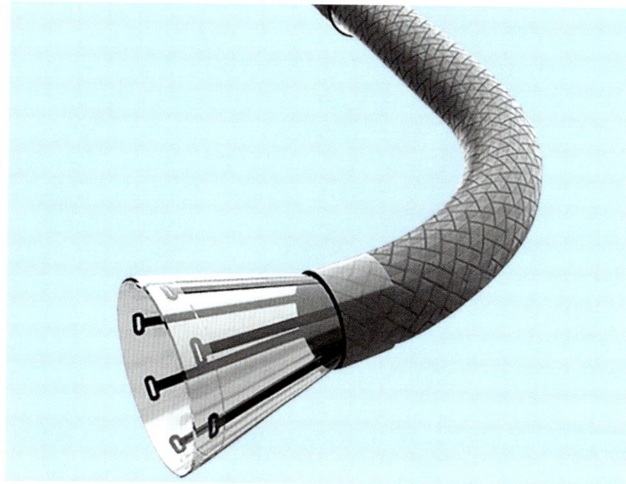

FIG. 13: The AngioVac device.

to the thrombus. Through the design, it allows aspiration of larger thrombi without clotting of the catheter. Due to the size of the catheter, it is difficult to maneuver, and hence there is an increased risk of bleeding.[15] The AngioVac device is shown in **Figure 13**.

LIMITATIONS OF CDT

A major factor is limited availability and expertise. Most hospitals still use systemic thrombolysis and anticoagulation alone in PE management with success rates. Guidelines recommend CDT in patients at high risk for bleeding post-thrombolysis or in patients who have major bleeding risk, post-major surgeries. Besides, CDT therapies are expensive. A vast number of CDT procedures are either ultrasound-assisted or in combination with mechanical fragmentation. More research regarding safety, indications, and efficacy is needed.

SURGICAL EMBOLECTOMY

It is a surgical procedure performed with median sternotomy and then cardiopulmonary bypass being applied. Following this, venae cavae are snared and the pulmonary trunk is opened near the proximity of the pulmonary valve. The type of incision over the pulmonary trunk depends on the location of the thrombus. The left PA thrombus is reached with a hockey stick incision, whereas the right trunk is incised between the aorta and the SVC. The thrombus is visualized and aspirated mostly directly. In some cases, bilateral pleura is opened and the peripheral clot is extruded via manual compression of lung parenchyma. This manual compression carries various risks such as mechanical injury to the arterial wall and lung parenchyma, extrabronchial bleeding, and critical lung bleeding. The opened pulmonary arteriotomy is sutured back directly or a bovine pericardial patch is used in case of a thin or fragile pulmonary artery.

The decision regarding surgical embolectomy is taken by a multidisciplinary team considering the onset, severity, and condition of the patient. Patients who benefit most from surgical embolectomy are the ones with RV dysfunction without shock. The surgical approach is useful in patients who have a high risk of bleeding due to thrombolysis, recent head injury, ischemic/hemorrhagic strokes, and recent surgeries. Surgical embolectomy has been found to have lower mortality rates, lesser recurrence, and less hemorrhagic events than medical therapy. This demonstrates the increased role of surgical management as an evolving option in the management of PE **(Figs. 14A to C)**.[16]

CONCLUSION

To summarize, pulmonary thromboembolism remains a complex and problematic illness, but recent breakthroughs in care have considerably improved patient outcomes. The development of new anticoagulants, the improvement of thrombolytic therapy, and the introduction of catheter-based therapies have all increased our treatment choices. Furthermore, breakthroughs in imaging and biomarkers have improved our capacity to diagnose and risk-group patients. Despite these developments, pulmonary thromboembolism remains a serious public health concern, and more research is needed to address unresolved topics such as the best treatment length, the relevance of aspirin, and the management of particular populations. However, with continuing innovation and collaboration, we can anticipate to lessen the morbidity and death associated with this dreadful disease.

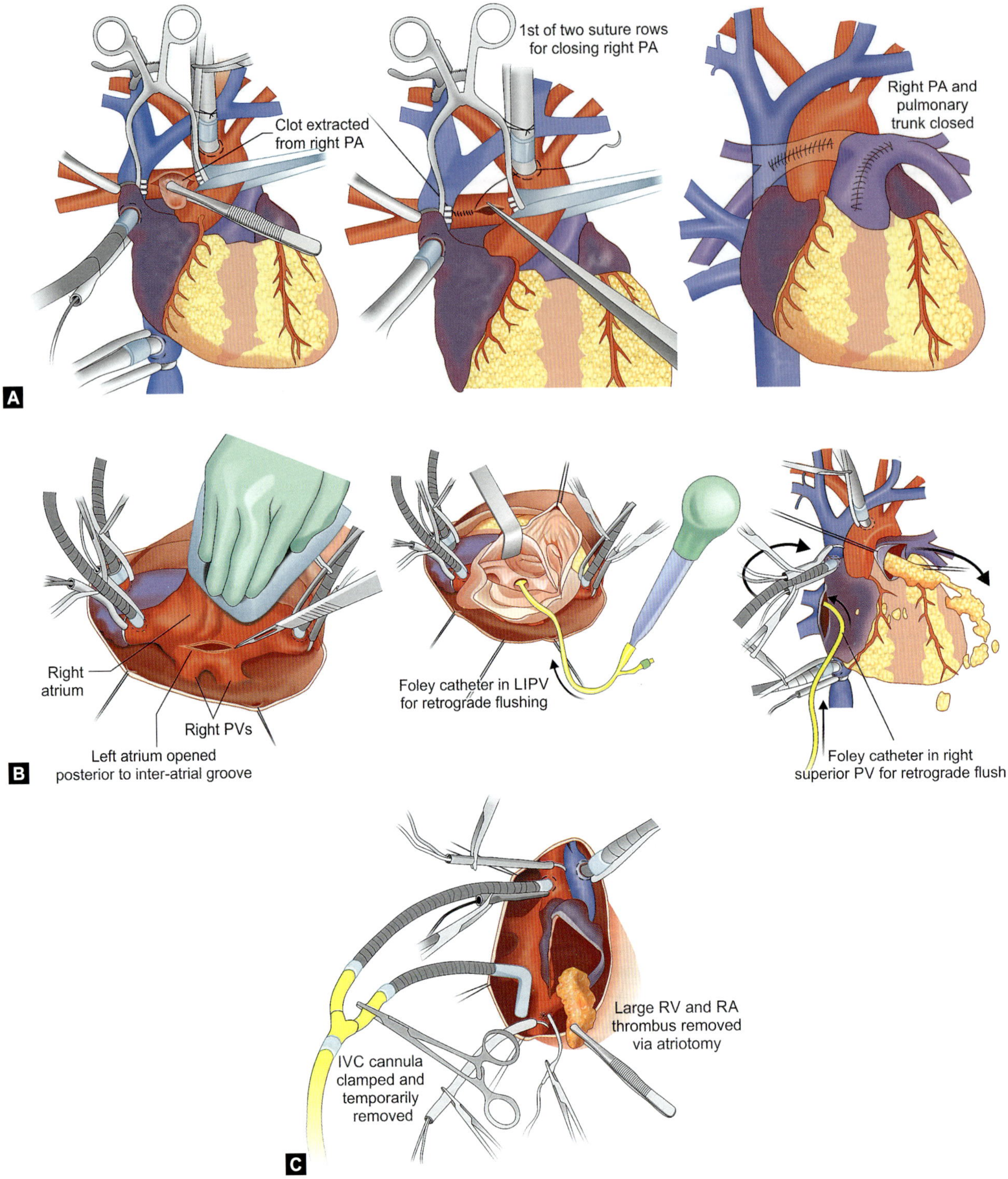

FIGS. 14A TO C: (A) Longitudinal insertion in the main pulmonary artery extending to the left pulmonary artery and thrombus is removed. (B) A retrograde pulmonary vein flush is used in combination with manual compression of pleura in the distant thrombus's removal. (C) Right atrium right ventricular thrombus removed via atriotomy after instituting cardiopulmonary bypass.

ONLINE REFERENCES

Please scan the QR code provided at the end of the table of contents for References of this chapter.

CHAPTER

111

Pediatric Pulmonary Arterial Hypertension: An Overview

Satish Kumar, Prashant Bobhate

ABSTRACT

Pulmonary hypertension (PH) in children is a progressive and debilitating disease that is associated with diverse etiology and with variable onset at any age. The distribution of etiologies in pediatric PH is quite different from that of adults. Pediatric PH management remains difficult because treatments have long relied on evidence-based adult studies and the clinical experience of pediatric experts. This article provides updates on the current definition, epidemiology, classification, diagnostics, risk stratification, and treatment of pediatric PAH.

Keywords: PAH, PPHN, BPD, risk stratification, targeted therapy

INTRODUCTION

Pulmonary hypertension (PH) in children is a rare progressive disease. As compared to the adult population, pediatric PH has diverse etiology and variable onset that can present at any age. Pediatric PH differs from adult patients by etiological, age, and gender distribution. Idiopathic pulmonary arterial hypertension (IPAH), pulmonary arterial hypertension (PAH) associated with congenital heart disease (PAH-CHD), persistent PH of the newborn syndrome (PPHN), and developmental lung disorders have greater predominance in children. These differences in etiological distribution, variable onset, atypical presentation, and variable long-term prognosis warrant the need for a unique approach in pediatric PH management.[1] However, currently used treatment modalities are largely dependent on adult studies and clinical expertise. This chapter mainly focusses on an overview of updated pediatric guidelines, including current definitions, classifications, special pediatric PH groups, and a unique approach in managing pediatric PAH.

DEFINITIONS

Pulmonary hypertension in children is defined as mean pulmonary arterial pressure (mPAP) > 20 mm Hg beyond 3 months of age.[1] In the normal fetal circulation, PA pressure is similar to systemic pressure and rapidly falls after birth. Adult levels usually reach by 2–3 months. Due to variability in pulmonary hemodynamics during postnatal transition, pediatric PH has been defined after 3 months of age. In pediatric PH, especially in association with CHD, it is recommended to use pulmonary vascular resistance indexed to body surface area (PVRI) to differentiate pulmonary vascular disease from hyperkinetic PAH secondary to a post-tricuspid left-to-right shunt, which normalizes after closure of the shunt lesion. PVRI > 3 WU m^2 is considered abnormal.[1] **Table 1** shows definitions of various types of PH.

TABLE 1: Definition of pulmonary hypertension.

Definition	Hemodynamics
Precapillary PH	• mPAP ≥ 20 mm Hg • PAWP ≤ 15 mm Hg • PVRI > 2 WU m^2
Isolated postcapillary PH	• mPAP ≥ 20 mm Hg • PAWP ≥ 15 mm Hg • PVRI < 2 WU m^2
Combined pre- and postcapillary PH	• mPAP ≥ 20 mm Hg • PAWP ≥ 15 mm Hg • PVRI > 2 WU m^2

EPIDEMIOLOGY

Current epidemiological data on pediatric PH are mainly derived from North American or European cohorts. A study done in Europe showed an estimated incidence of 4–10 cases per million children per year with a prevalence of 20–40 cases per million, and a USA study showed an incidence of 5–8 cases per million children per year and 26–33 per million children.[2-4] Although the exact load of pediatric PH in India is unknown, it is estimated that this could be much higher than the western countries due to the higher prevalence of untreated CHD, rheumatic heart disease, and other causes of PH such as HIV and sickle cell disease. The estimated 1, 3, and 5 year survival rates of pediatric PH according to North American and European registries are 96%, 84%, and 74%, respectively.[1,5]

CLASSIFICATION

Box 1 shows updated classification from the 2022 ESC/ERS guidelines.[6] The main changes from previous 2015 guidelines are as follows:

- The subgroups "nonresponders at vasoreactivity testing" and "acute responders at vasoreactivity testing" have been added to IPAH as compared with the 2015 ESC/ERS guidelines for the diagnosis and treatment of PH. In addition to IPAH patients, some patients with heritable PAH (HPAH) or drug- or toxin-associated PAH (DPAH) might be acute responders.
- The groups "PAH with features of venous/capillary [pulmonary veno-occlusive disease/pulmonary capillary hemangiomatosis (PVOD/PCH)] involvement" and "PPHN" have been included in group 1 (PAH) as compared with the 2015 ESC/ERS guidelines.

BOX 1 Classification of pulmonary hypertension.

Group 1—pulmonary arterial hypertension (PAH):
1.1 Idiopathic:
  1.1.1 Nonresponders at vasoreactivity testing
  1.1.2 Acute responders at vasoreactivity testing
1.2 Heritable
1.3 Associated with drugs and toxins
1.4 Associated with:
  1.4.1 Connective tissue disease
  1.4.2 HIV infection
  1.4.3 Portal hypertension
  1.4.4 Congenital heart disease
  1.4.5 Schistosomiasis
1.5 PAH with features of venous/capillary (PVOD/PCH) involvement
1.6 Persistent PH of the newborn
Group 2—PH associated with left heart disease:
2.1 Heart failure:
  2.1.1 With preserved ejection fraction
  2.1.2 With reduced or mildly reduced ejection fraction
2.2 Valvular heart disease
2.3 Congenital/acquired cardiovascular conditions leading to postcapillary PH
Group 3—PH associated with lung diseases and/or hypoxia:
3.1 Obstructive lung disease or emphysema
3.2 Restrictive lung disease
3.3 Lung disease with mixed restrictive/obstructive pattern
3.4 Hypoventilation syndromes
3.5 Hypoxia without lung disease (e.g., high altitude)
3.6 Developmental lung disorders
Group 4—PH associated with pulmonary artery obstructions:
4.1 Chronic thromboembolic PH
4.2 Other pulmonary artery obstructions
Group 5—PH with unclear and/or multifactorial mechanisms:
5.1 Hematological disorders
5.2 Systemic disorders
5.3 Metabolic disorders
5.4 Chronic renal failure with or without hemodialysis
5.5 Pulmonary tumor thrombotic microangiopathy
5.6 Fibrosing mediastinitis

SPECIAL PEDIATRIC PH CATEGORIES

Persistent PH of the Newborn Syndrome

Persistent PH of the newborn syndrome is not very uncommon, with an estimated incidence of 30.1 cases per million children per year.[4] PPHN often goes undiagnosed due to its similar presentation to respiratory distress syndrome (RDS). Its transient course makes it different from other PH subgroups. As compared to preinhaled nitric oxide therapy era, the incidence of PPHN is significantly increased, mainly due to better neonatal survival and improved awareness among neonatologists.[7] The occurrence of PPHN is inversely related to gestational period, with an incidence of 18.5% (range 15.2–22.4%) for neonates born at 22–24 weeks compared with 4.4% (range 3.8–5.2%) for those born at 27 weeks.[8] PPHN origin is multifactorial, lung parenchymal conditions such as meconium aspiration syndrome (MAS), pneumonia, RDS, and sepsis contribute in most cases. Other etiological factors include oligohydramnios, pulmonary hypoplasia, infants born to diabetic mothers, in utero closure of ductus arteriosus, small and large for gestational age, and any event leading to uteroplacental insufficiency increases the risk of PPPN and even higher risk of developing PAH later in life.[9]

PH: DEVELOPMENTAL LUNG DISORDERS

This subgroup accounts for a significant proportion of PH in the long-term preterm survival group, especially with bronchopulmonary dysplasia (BPD), which is a major complication seen in premature neonates. BPD-PH pathogenesis includes alveolar diffusion impairment, abnormal vascular remodeling, and rarefication of pulmonary vessels (vascular growth arrest), which lead to increased pulmonary vascular resistance, high PA pressures, and right heart failure. Netherlands epidemiological data showed that 34% of pediatric patients with sustained PH showed developmental lung disease. The incidence is inversely proportional to gestational age and directly proportional to severity of lung disease and duration of respiratory support.[10,11] BPD-PH can improve over time with optimal respiratory therapy and targeted pulmonary vasodilator therapy; however, the morbidity and mortality of BPD-PH remain high, especially in advanced cases. Recent meta-analyses showed that the BPD-PH in neonates was strongly associated with high mortality (risk ratio 4.7) and with early mortality of 16% and late mortality of 40% on follow-up.[12]

PAH ASSOCIATED WITH CHD (CHD-APAH) AND EISENMENGER PHYSIOLOGY

Untreated CHD often accounts for severe PAH with an estimated incidence of 10%. The onset and severity of CHD-APAH depend on multiple factors such as level of shunt, size of the shunt, and presence of comorbidities.[13] Also apart from shunt lesions, left heart obstructive lesions such as aortic stenosis, mitral stenosis lead to postcapillary PH.[14,15] Overall, pretricuspid shunt lesions (ASD and PAPVC) very rarely lead to severe PH due to low pressure, which usually does not damage the pulmonary vascular bed as long as ventricular compliance is intact. However, associated left heart disease can increase the risk of PH. Unlike pretricuspid lesions, post-tricuspid shunts can cause early damage of pulmonary vascular bed, resulting in vascular remodeling. PH can occur as early as 6 months, especially with shunt at great artery level (aorta pulmonary window and persistent ductus arteriosus). VSD natural history shows that most of the moderate-to-large-sized patients develop PAH (one-fourth) in infancy. Follow-up studies have shown that even after surgical correction, PAH can develop due to persistent ongoing remodeling at the pulmonary vascular bed despite intervention. However, long-term data shows that early intervention is associated with less risk of PAH. Specifically, there has been much interest in PH after the Fontan operation due to its complex pathophysiology, resulting from a complex series of interactions such as poor pulmonary arborization, lack of normal pulsatile flow, and elevated diastolic pressure secondary to ventricular dysfunction. Ultimately, unintervened PAH in this group leads to Eisenmenger complexes due to irreversible vascular remodeling. Histology of such patients showed medial hypertrophy, extensive intimal injury leading to fibrosis and plexiform lesions in advanced cases.[16]

ABERNATHY MALFORMATION AND PAH

Abernathy malformation is a rare developmental congenital extrahepatic portosystemic shunt (CEPS) anomaly of the mesenteric vasculature in which the portal venous system (intestinal and splenic veins) bypass the liver and drain directly into the inferior vena cava (IVC), the left hepatic vein, or the left renal vein.[17-19] PAH is a well-known complication extrahepatic portosystemic shunts. The pathophysiology includes hepatic circulation bypass of vasoactive substances present in the intestinal circulation (e.g., serotonin, histamine, estrogen, and glucagon). These unmetabolized substances induce pulmonary vasoconstriction and pulmonary bed remodeling, resulting in PAH. Closing these malformation can potentially help to normalize the pulmonary artery pressure.[18,19]

DIAGNOSIS OF PEDIATRIC PH

Diagnosis of pediatric PAH is quite challenging due to its atypical presentation and diverse etiology. Moreover, IPAH is a diagnosis of exclusion that can be made only by excluding known causes of PH (refer to **Box 1** classification). Special conditions that predispose to the development of PAH should be considered. **Flowchart 1** shows the algorithm for evaluating pediatric patients with PH.

CLINICAL PRESENTATION

Symptoms of PH are mainly linked to right ventricle (RV) dysfunction. The cardinal symptom is dyspnea on exertion. Other common symptoms are palpitations, syncope, hemoptysis, failure to thrive, and weight gain in the advanced stage due to fluid retention.

Chest Radiography

The characteristic radiological features include altered cardiac silhouette due to the right heart (right atrium), and the prominent MPA segment due to its significant enlargement. In severe cases, pruning of the peripheral vessels is often seen. In addition, signs of the underlying cause of PH, such as left heart disease or lung parenchymal disease, can be made out **(Fig. 1)**.

ELECTROCARDIOGRAM

Electrocardiogram (ECG) changes **(Fig. 2)** such as right axis deviation, tall P waves (P pulmonale), right ventricular hypertrophy with ST changes, and deep q wave in right precordial often help in diagnosing and assessing the severity of disease. Certain features, especially right axis deviation, provide important prognostic information.

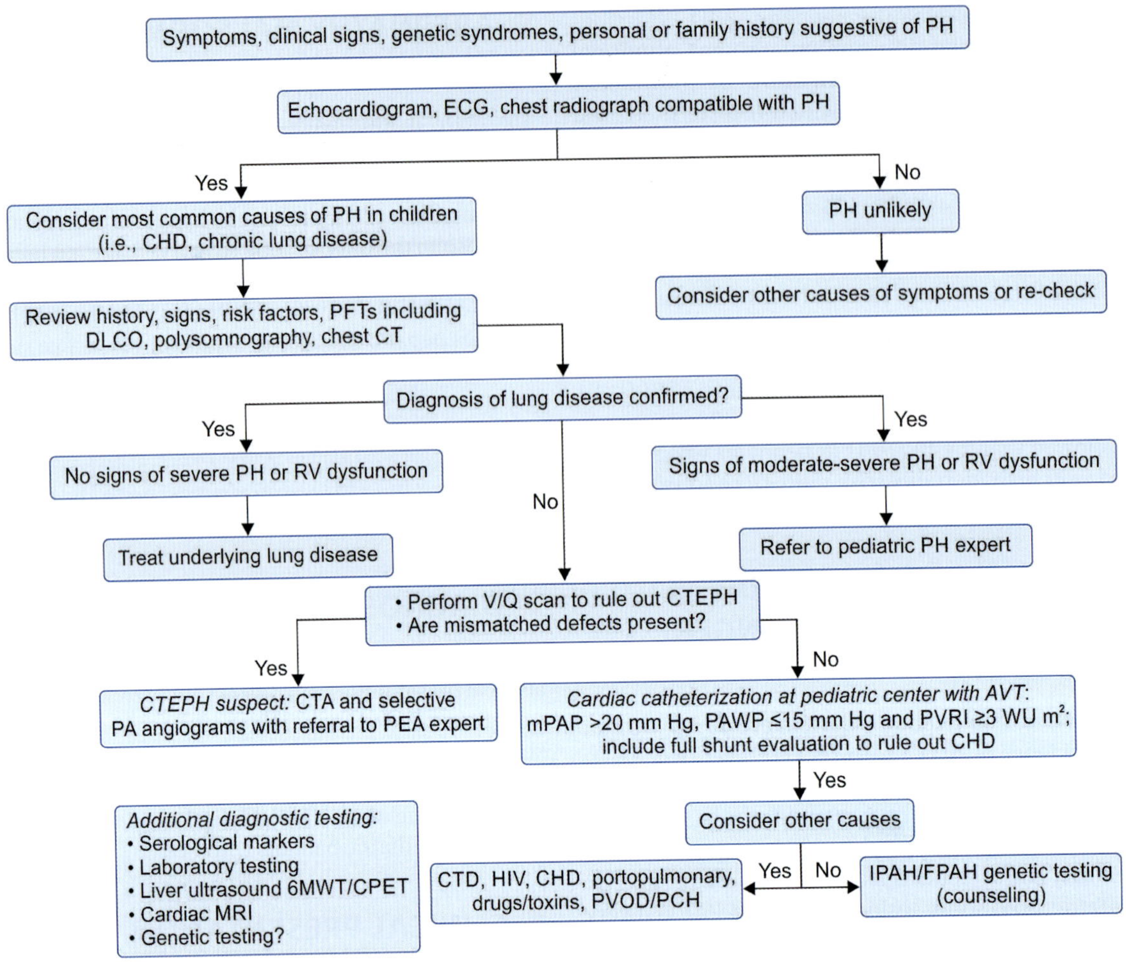

FLOWCHART 1: Diagnostic algorithm for pulmonary hypertension in children.
(AVT: acute vasodilator testing; CHD: congenital heart disease; CTD: connective tissue disease; CPET: cardiopulmonary exercise test; CT: computed tomography; CTA: CT angiography; CTEPH: chronic thromboembolic; mPAP: mean pulmonary arterial pressure; 6MWT: 6-min walk test; MRI: magnetic resonance imaging; DLCO: diffusing capacity of the lung for carbon monoxide; PA: pulmonary artery; PAWP: pulmonary arterial wedge pressure; PEA: pulmonary endarterectomy; PFT: pulmonary function test; PVRI: pulmonary vascular resistance index; WU: Wood Units; PVOD: pulmonary veno-occlusive disease; RV: right ventricular; V/Q: ventilation/perfusion)

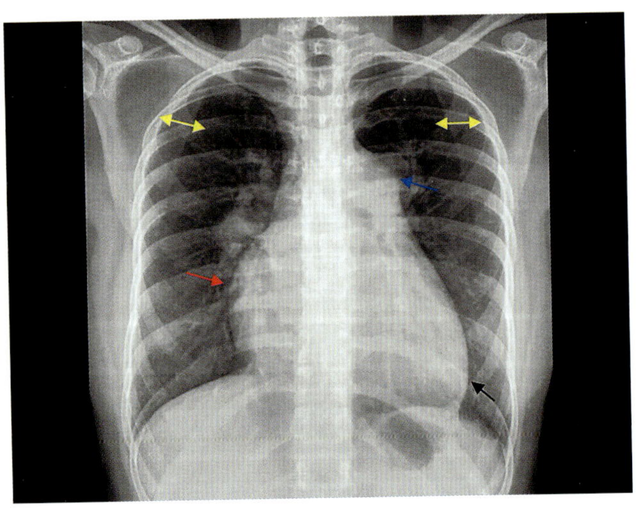

FIG. 1: Radiographic signs of PH include right atrium (red arrow) and PA enlargement (blue arrow), pruning of the peripheral vessels (yellow arrows), and RV apex (black arrow).

ECG may also provide valuable information in diagnosing PAH due to left heart disease. It is important to note that a normal ECG does not exclude the presence of PH, but in the case of a normal ECG in combination with normal PH biomarkers (NT-proBNP), the PAH is unlikely **(Box 2)**.

Right Heart Catheterization

Cardiac catheterization is the gold standard for the definitive diagnosis of PAH. Especially acute vasodilatory testing provides useful information, which plays a vital role in management. However, due to associated risks such as PH crisis it is strongly recommended to be performed in advanced PH centers.[20] Vasoreactivity test should be considered before starting PH therapy, as positive responsive patients would benefit from CCB treatment. Cardiac catheterization also plays an important role in assessing operability in CHD PAH patients with borderline

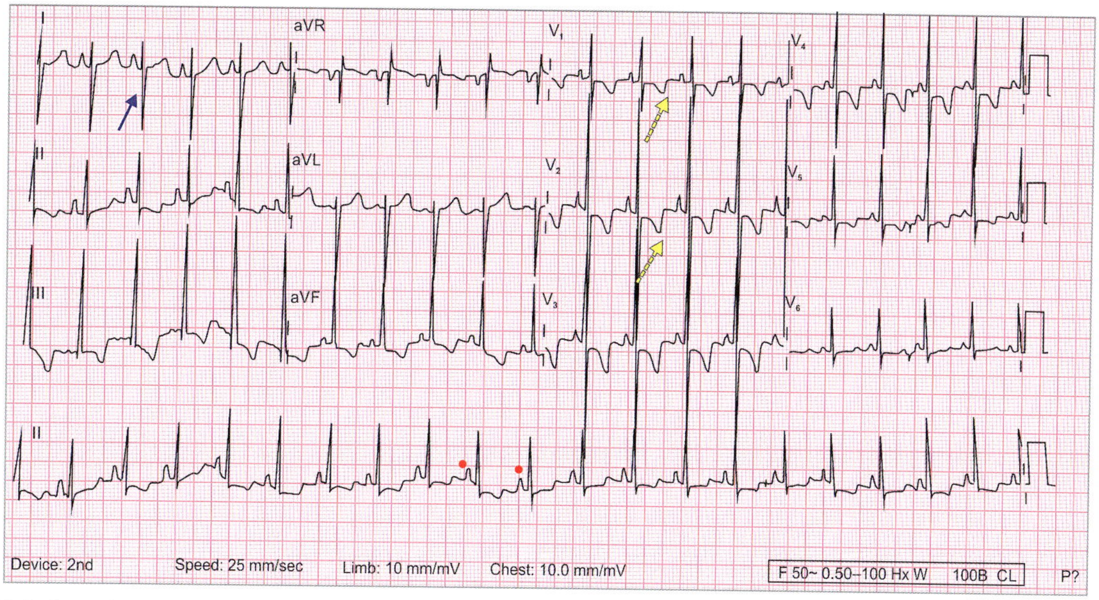

FIG. 2: ECG finding of PH: Right axis deviation (blue arrow), right atrial enlargement (red dots), and right ventricular hypertrophy with RV strain pattern (yellow dotted arrows).

BOX 2 ECG abnormalities.

- P pulmonale (P > 3 mm in V_1)
- Right axis deviation (QRS axis > 90°)
- RV hypertrophy (R/S > 1, with R > 6 mm in V_1); R in V_1 + S in lead V_5 > 10.5 mm
- Right bundle branch block—complete or incomplete (qR or rSR patterns in V_1)
- RV strain pattern (ST depression/T-wave inversion in the right precordial V_1– V_4) and inferior II, III, and aVF leads
- Prolonged QTc interval

operability **(Flowchart 2)**. Vasodilator testing should be done with an agent which has minimal effect on systemic circulation. Ideally, inhaled nitric oxide should be used, however, due to its limited availability sildenafil can also be potentially used for the same. Moreover, it is important to avoid oxygen due to its profound effects on systemic circulation thus leading to a confusing picture.[20,21] Repeat cardiac catheterization guides in assessment of response to treatment, detection of early disease progression, so that early drug escalation and listing for lung transplantation can be considered.

ECHOCARDIOGRAPHY

Echocardiography plays an important role as an initial evaluation tool in diagnosing and assessing PAH. Performing comprehensive echo study in children is quite challenging. When performed accurately, it provides very useful information such as heart morphology, RV and LV function, and valvular abnormalities, also, certain echo hemodynamic parameters (IVCCI, GLS, TAPSE, S/D ratio, septal position, and effusion) can define PAH severity **(Figs. 3 and 4)**. However, echocardiography alone is insufficient to confirm or exclude a diagnosis of PH.

RISK STRATIFICATION AND TREATMENT STRATEGIES

Initial PAH therapy in children should be based on risk stratification. Predictors of worse include clinical evidence of RV failure, progression of symptoms, worsening of functional class, increased NT-Pro BNP level, and decreased 6-minute walk test distance.[22] Further prognosticators identified in pediatric PAH are failure to thrive and hemodynamic variables, such as RAP > 10 mm Hg, the ratio of mean pulmonary-to-systemic blood pressure.0.75, and PVRI > 11 WU m^2 **(Table 2)**. Currently, goal-orientated drug therapy is recommended for the treatment of pediatric PAH. General measures such as diuretics, oxygen, anticoagulation, and digoxin should be considered on a case-by-case basis. If possible, cardiac catheterization should be considered in all patients before initiation of therapy. In cases of a positive AVT response, oral CCBs should be considered. If there is a sustained and improved response, CCBs should be continued along with other general measures, in case of inadequate response or clinical deterioration, repeat detailed evaluation and additional therapy are required **(Flowchart 3)**. Risk stratification should determine the further therapy in children with a negative AVT test or in the children who are nonresponsive to CCBs **Table 2**.

Determinants of higher risk in children include clinical evidence of right ventricular failure (TAPSE < 12 mm, RVFAC: < 25%, and RVGLS: < –14%), failure to thrive, WHO FC III or IV, significantly elevated or rising NT-proBNP level (>1,200 ng/L), severe right atrial enlargement or dysfunction, and pericardial effusion. Additional hemodynamic parameters that predict higher risk include mPAP/mSAP ratio > 0.75, mRAP > 10 mm Hg, and PVRI > 11 WU m^2. In cases of negative acute vasoreactivity and lower risk, oral monotherapy should be considered. Commonly recommended drugs include endothelin receptor antagonists (bosentan and ambrisentan) or phosphodiesterase type 5 (PDE5) inhibitors

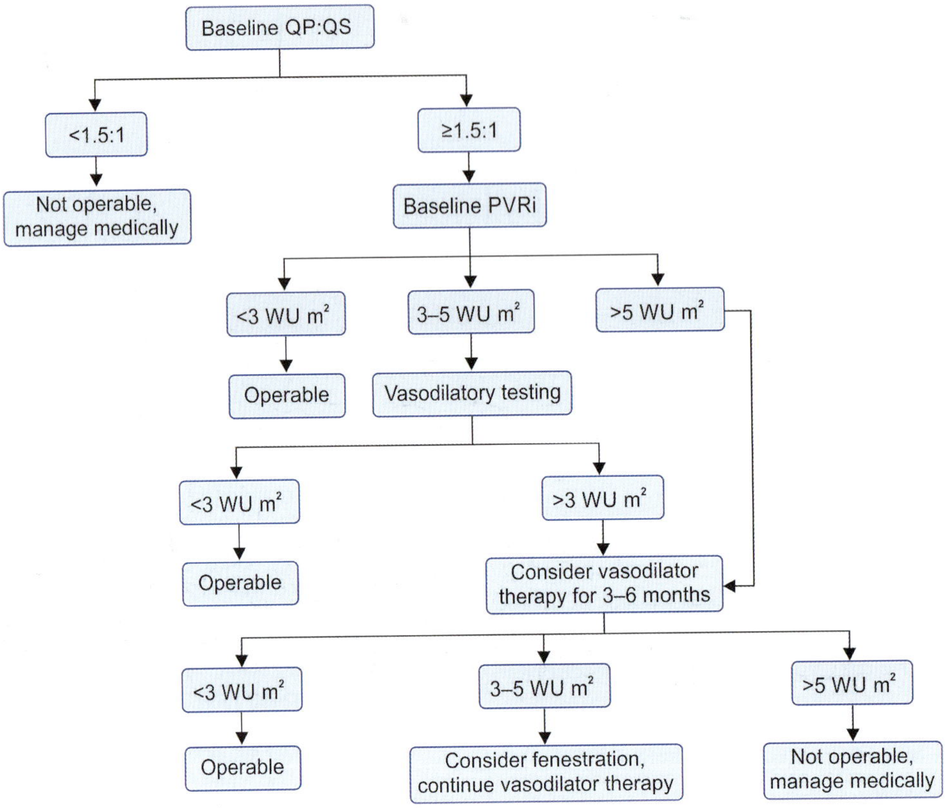

FLOWCHART 2: Approach to operability in pulmonary arterial hypertension associated with congenital heart disease.
(PVRi: pulmonary vascular resistance index; QP:QS: pulmonary and systemic blood flow ratio; WU: Wood Units)

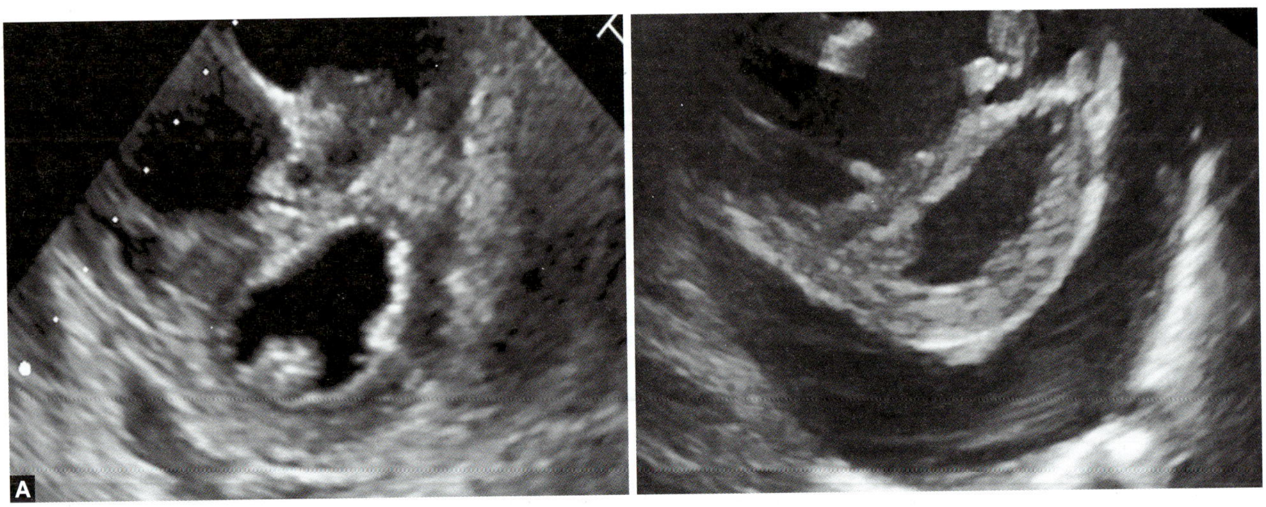

FIGS. 3A TO C: *Continued*

Continued

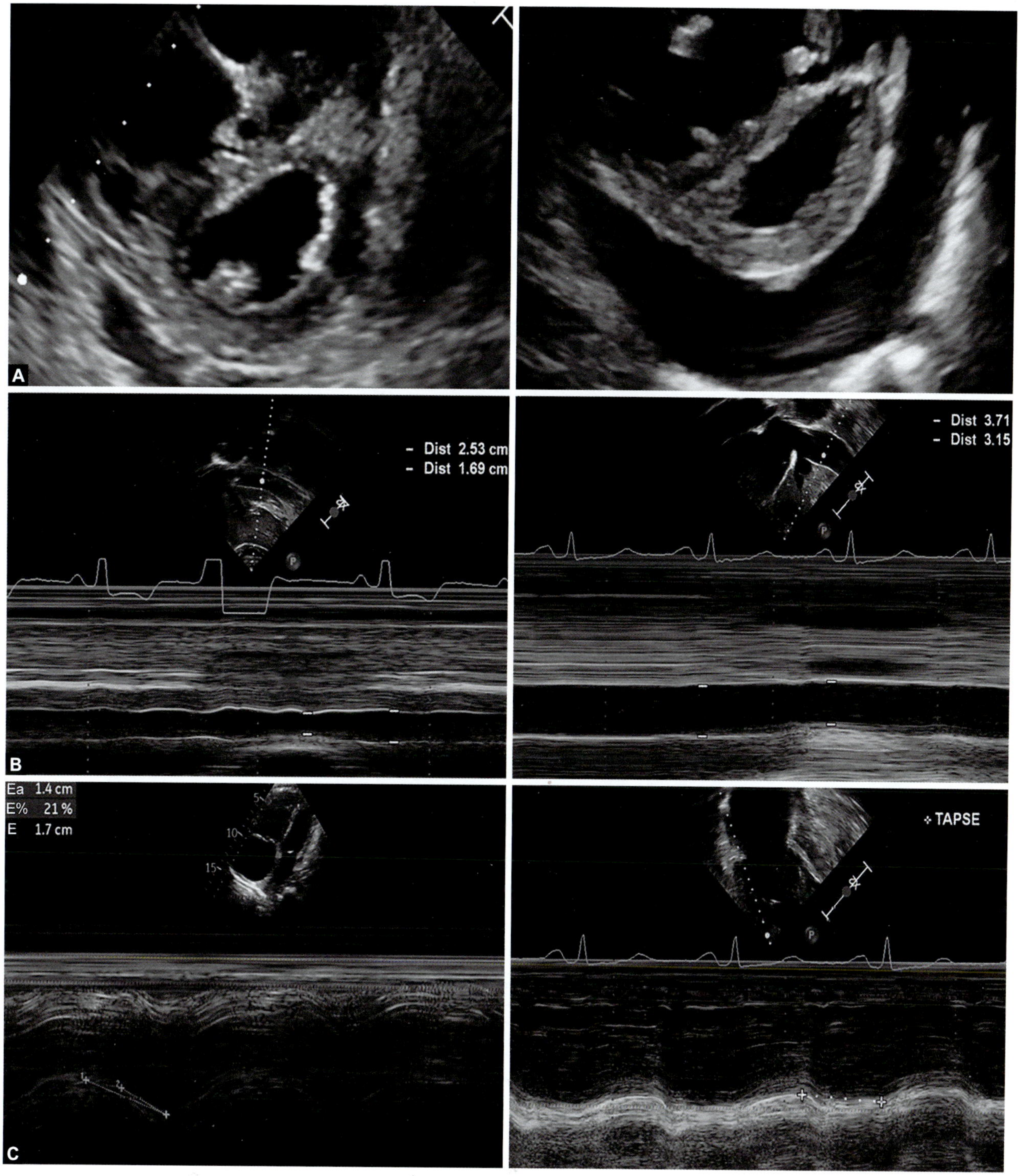

FIGS. 3A TO C: Echo assessment of severity: Left figure shows mild disease and right figure shows severe disease.
From top to bottom: (A) Pericardial effusion, (B) IVC collapsibility, and (C) TAPSE.
Top left: No effusion; *Top right*: Severe effusion.
Middle left: IVC mildly dilated and collapsing; *Middle right*: IVC severely dilated and not collapsing.
Lower left: TAPSE 1.7 cm with good right ventricular function; *Lower right*: TAPSE 0.3 cm with poor function.

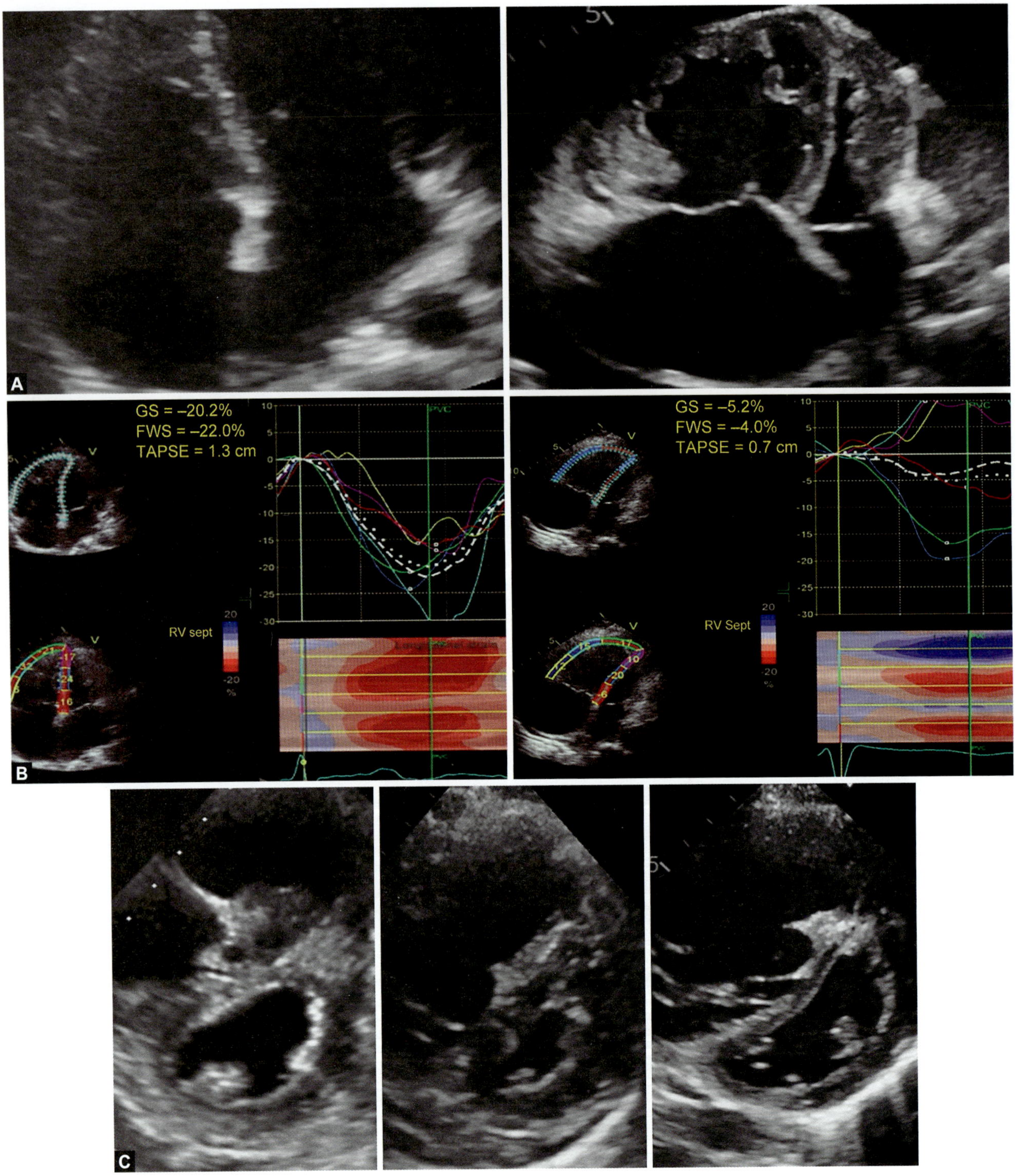

FIGS. 4A TO C: Echo assessment of severity: Left figure shows mild disease and right figure shows severe disease.

From top to bottom: (A) RA RV size, (B) Ventricular strain pattern, and (C) Septal position.

Top left: Mild RA RV dilatation.

Top right: Hugely dilated RA RV.

Middle left: Good strain pattern of –20.2%; *Middle right*: Poor strain pattern of –5.2%.

Lower left: Ventricular septum bowing towards RV suggesting subsytemic RV pressures.

Lower middle: Septum at midline suggesting systemic RV pressures.

Lower right: Ventricular septum bowing toward LV suggesting suprasytemic RV pressures.

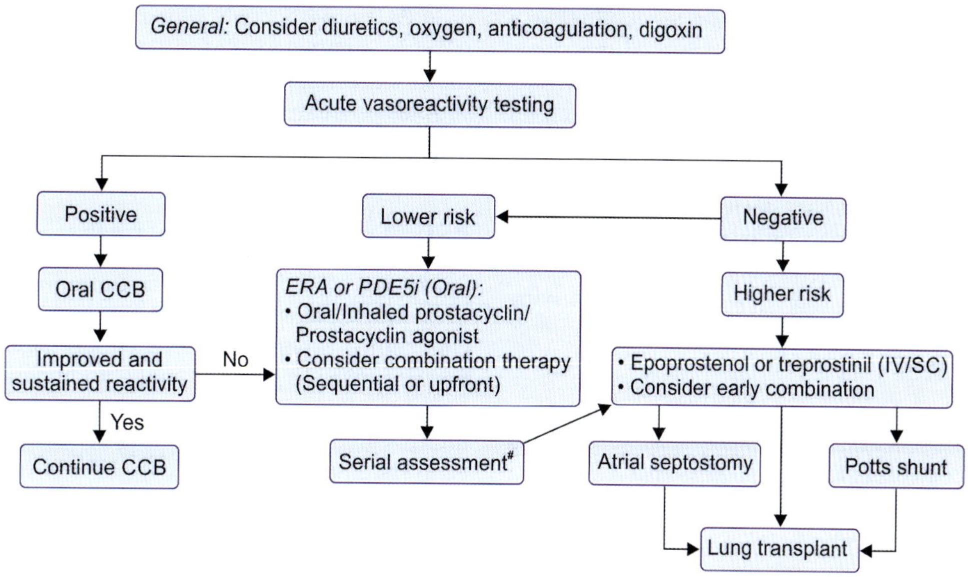

Deterioration or not meeting treatment goals.

FLOWCHART 3: Pediatric pulmonary arterial hypertension treatment algorithm.

(CCB: calcium channel blocker; ERA: endothelin receptor agonist; PDE5i: phosphodiesterase type 5 inhibitor)

TABLE 2: 2024 Updated pediatric risk stratification tool by task force 15.

Lower risk	Determinant	High risk
• Older • No • No	• Age • Clinical evidence of RV failure • Progression of symptoms	• Younger • Yes • Yes
• Height z-score ≥ −2 • Weight z-score ≥ −2 • I, II • >350 m	• Growth, failure to thrive • WHO functional class • 6MWT (>6 years)	• Height z-score < −2 • Weight z-score < −2 • III, IV • < 350 m
<300 ng/L	NT-ProBNP	>1,200 ng/L
• TAPSE ≥ 12 mm • RVFAC > 25% • RVLS free wall ≥ −17% • Global ≥ 14% • RVd/LVd ≤ 1 • RA area ≤ 18 cm^2 • Pericardial effusion: No	Echocardiography	• TAPSE <12 mm • RVFAC < 25% • RVLS free wall < −17% • Global < −14% • RVd/LVd > 1 • RA area > 18 cm^2 • Pericardial effusion: Yes
• PVRI ≤ 11 WU m^2 • mRAP < 10 mm Hg • Systemic CI ≥ 2.5 L/min/m^2 • PACi ≥ 0.9 mL/mm Hg/m^2 • SVO_2 ≥ 65% • Acute response Sitbon criteria: Yes	Hemodynamics	• PVRI > 11 WU m^2 • mRAP > 10 mm Hg • Systemic CI < 2.5 L/min/m^2 • PACi < 0.9 mL/mm Hg/m^2 • SVO_2 < 65% • Acute response Sitbon criteria: No
• RVEF ≥ 44% • RVMi ≤ 80 g/m^2	Cardiac MRI	• RVEF < 44% • RVMi > 80 g/m^2

(sildenafil and tadalafil) (**Table 3** details the medications in pediatric PAH). Children who deteriorate on the above therapy should be considered for early combination therapy (add-on or up-front). The addition of inhaled prostacyclin (iloprost) to background therapy may be helpful.[23] In the high-risk category, children IV epoprostenol or IV/SC treprostinil should be considered. In refractory high-risk children, early consideration of lung transplantation and interventions such as atrial septostomy and revered Pott shunt is recommended. In case BPD-PH, the underlying lung disease should primarily be addressed. The commonly used PAH drugs include sildenafil and bosentan; however, there is insufficient data in the infant population, and these are not approved by the EMA. This subgroup of PH should be treated by multidisciplinary teams including pediatric cardiologists, neonatologists, pulmonologists, and nutritionists.[24]

TABLE 3: PAH drug therapy.

Drug	European Medicines Agency approval for use in children with PAH
Phosphodiesterase 5 inhibitors (oral)	
Sildenafil	Yes, for ≥1 year of age recommended dosing: • <20 kg: 30 mg/day in three doses; ≥20 kg: 60 mg/day in three doses • Avoid higher dosing in children (3 mg/kg/day)
Tadalafil	No Suggested dosing: • 0.5–1 mg/kg/day in one dose max.: 40 mg/day • Evaluated only in children aged > 3 years
Endothelin receptor antagonists (oral)	
Bosentan	• Yes, for ≥1 year of age pediatric formulation • Recommended dosing: 4 mg/kg/day in two doses • Max: 250 mg/day
Ambrisentan	• Yes, for children aged > 8 years • Recommended dosing: 2.5–10 mg/day in one dose
Macitentan	No
Prostacyclin analogues (IV/SC)	
Epoprostenol IV	No Suggested dosing: • Starting dose: 1–2 ng/kg/min without a known maximum • In children, a stable dose is usually 40–80 ng/kg/min • Dose increases may be required
Treprostinil IV/SC	No Suggested dosing: • Starting dose: 2 ng/kg/min without a known maximum • In children, a stable dose is usually 50–100 ng/kg/min • Dose increases may be required

Selexipag in Pediatric PAH

Safety and efficacy of selexipag have not been established in pediatric patients, nor FDA-approved for pediatric use. Our center experience in 12 children [median age was 8.5 years (3.2–18 years), 7 male, 8 idiopathic PAH, 4 PAH out of proportion to CHD] 9 out of 12 patients (75%) showed improvement in functional class, NT-Pro BNP level and in echo parameters, three (25%) patients were deteriorated (one patient died, one patient underwent transcatheter Pott's Shunt, and one patient required drug escalation). None of the patients had any significant side effects except mild epistaxis in one patient. Selexipag initiation dose was of 50 µg, 100 µg and 200 µg every 12 hourly in children weighing < 15 kg, 16–30 kg and >30 kg respectively and rapidly titrated up in 50–100 µg per dose per day increments until the target dose was achieved.[25,26]

INTERVENTIONAL PALLIATIVE BRIDGE THERAPIES IN ADVANCED PAH

Atrial Septostomy

It should be considered in children with worsening of disease despite of triple combination therapy. Atrial septostomy improves cardiac output and systemic oxygen carrying capacity. It acts as a bridge to transplant, increasing the chance for survival while waiting for a donor organ. It is relatively safe procedure with survival rates being 87%, 61%, and 32%, respectively at 30 days, 1 year, and 5 years.[27]

Reversed Potts Shunt

It involves creation of a palliative shunt between left pulmonary artery and descending aorta. It has been considered as a new option for severely ill children with suprasystemic IPAH.[28] It helps in decompressing failing RV through right-to-left shunting, similar to a patient with patent ductus arteriosus-related Eisenmenger syndrome. As compared to atrial septostomy, reversed Potts shunt provides high oxygen saturated blood to the coronary arteries and the central nervous system, and only causes desaturation of the lower body. It also improves left ventricular function as a result of reduction in shifting of the interventricular septum toward the left ventricle.[29,30] Recently several centers have demonstrated successful catheter-based creation of reversed Potts shunt[31] (in our center we have performed 8, including one pediatric). In adult patients, Salna et al.[32] demonstrated a novel, successful approach to the Potts shunt using a unidirectional valved shunt from the main pulmonary artery to the descending aorta, which has the advantage of unidirectional flow and prevents back flow from the descending aorta to PA when the PA pressures are subsystemic and during diastole.

LUNG TRANSPLANT

Bilateral lung transplant or heart and lung transplant may be an option for some children with PH. However, despite improvement in immunosuppression medications, the overall survival after lung transplant remains limited. Besides, it is limited by its availability and financial constraints in a medium- and low-income country like India. Among all causes for a lung transplant, the patients with PAH as an indication for transplant have the worst survival. Median survival after lung transplantation has been reported to be 4.9 years.[33]

CONCLUSION

In spite of many unique characteristics, pediatric PH patients are often assessed and managed based on adult PH management guidelines. Currently, the WSPH Pediatric Task Force recommends pediatric-specific risk stratification and drug therapy. Still, there is a strong need for pediatric-specific clinical trials in order to develop pediatric management guidelines.

ONLINE REFERENCES

Please scan the QR code provided at the end of the table of contents for References of this chapter.

CHAPTER

112

Pulmonary Embolism: Current Status and Update

Gaurav Singhal, Aishwarya Gaur

ABSTRACT

Pulmonary embolism (PE) is a common and fatal disease in the community. It is the result of complications of venous thrombosis and is one of the leading causes of death worldwide. There are no guidelines that clearly tell which patients should be evaluated for PE. Few probability scores are available which can only predict eligible patients for further workup. Physician's familiarity with these "rule out scores" is important to diagnose PE at an early stage. D-dimer may be used for screening purposes but cannot be solely relied upon, as elevated levels may be seen in other conditions such as sepsis, postsurgery, and pregnancy. Ultrasound of bilateral lower limbs should be considered in suspects. Early diagnosis is key to management to prevent morbidity and mortality. A multidisciplinary team should be available for the best treatment to prevent mortality. Treatment includes novel oral anticoagulant therapy, intravenous systemic thrombolysis, catheter-directed low-dose thrombolysis, and surgical embolectomy.

Keywords: Pulmonary embolism, venous thromboembolism (VTE), low-molecular-weight heparin (LMWH), unfractionated heparin (UFH), right ventricle (RV), left ventricle (LV), ventilation–perfusion (V/Q) scan, computed tomography pulmonary angiography (CTPA), pulmonary arterial hypertension (PAH), chronic thromboembolic pulmonary hypertension (CTPEH), catheter-directed thrombolysis (CDT)

INTRODUCTION

A thrombus is formed when there is endothelial injury, hypercoagulability, and stasis or turbulence of blood flow. All these factors are well known as the "Virchow triad." This thrombus may progress and dislocate, leading to embolism in distant circulation. Pulmonary embolism (PE) is one of the most common cardiovascular emergencies all over the world.[1] It is a leading cause of death in the United States. The incidence of PE ranges from 39 to 115 per 100,000 general population.[2] The incidence increases with age and is equal in men and women. Pregnancy increases the risk of venous thromboembolism (VTE) fivefold, and this risk persists in the postpartum period at least for 12 weeks.

When thrombosis of any deep vein occurs, most commonly lower limb veins, part of the thrombus may detach and reach the right side of the heart and then to main pulmonary artery. When thrombi are small, they occlude distal pulmonary circulation leading to pleuritic chest pain and pulmonary infarction. Pleuritic chest pain may be present due to an inflammatory response of the parietal pleura; hence, clinical presentation of PE is nonspecific, and the diagnosis may be delayed or missed. If the thrombi burden is large, it lodges in the main pulmonary artery or its major branches, causing hemodynamic instability. Its diagnosis and urgent management (medical or intervention) are crucial at this time to prevent mortality. Sudden death may occur after massive PE.

Obstruction to major pulmonary vessels leads to a sudden rise in pulmonary pressure resulting in stretching of the thin-walled right atrium and right ventricle (RV afterload)—IVS is shifted toward left ventricle (LV), leading to underfilling of LV, which in turn causes systolic and diastolic dysfunction.[3] Hypotension results in reduced coronary perfusion and myocardial ischemia. Simultaneously, there are abnormal respiratory functions in the form of hyperventilation, hypoxemia and V/Q mismatch, regional loss of surfactant, and lung infarction. The cross-sectional area of the pulmonary vascular bed is reduced, resulting in an increment in pulmonary vascular resistance and the RV afterload. All these humoral and reflex mechanisms lead to the sudden development of cardiovascular collapse, hypotension, and shock. If this stage is not identified early, then mortality may occur within 1–2 hours of disease onset. Early administration of anticoagulants prevents hemodynamic compromise. If there is massive PE with hypotension, then thrombolysis should be considered. This therapy is most successful in the first 2 weeks. When the initial thrombus fails to undergo lysis or recurrent thrombosis occurs, chronic thromboembolic syndrome may be established.

In this chapter, we shall discuss recent updates in the management of PE.

ETIOLOGY AND PREDISPOSING FACTORS

The causes of PE are multifactorial and may not be readily apparent. The risk factors which are described in the literature include the following **(Box 1)**.[4] These factors interact with patients' comorbidities and increase the risk of development of PE. Prolonged immobilization leads to local venous stasis by accumulation of clotting factors and fibrin, resulting in blood clot formation. In various predicted risk scores, immobilization is one of the major risk factors. Trauma, surgical conditions,[5] and severe burns are major factors that are independent of immobilization. The incidence of thromboembolic disease in pregnancy has been reported to range from 1 case in 200 deliveries.[6] Fatal events are rare, with 1–2 cases occurring per 100,000 pregnancies. There is a strong association between pregnancy duration and high level of activated platelets with decreased fibrinolytic activity. Moreover, there is venous stasis due to the gravid uterus, leading to an increased risk of left lower limb deep vein thrombosis (DVT). Estrogen-containing oral contraceptive pills (OCPs) are associated with increased occurrence of VTE in healthy women. The risk is proportional to the estrogen content and is increased in postmenopausal women on hormonal replacement therapy.[7] Third-generation OCPs are more prone to PE than second-generation OCPs. Pulmonary emboli have been reported to occur in association with solid tumors, leukemias, and lymphomas.[8] Hereditary factors associated with the development of PE include, most commonly, factor V Leiden and prothrombin gene mutation. Acquired thrombophilia includes antiphospholipid syndrome, which is also responsible for arterial and venous thrombosis.

BOX 1 Risk factors of PE.

Strong risk factors (OR >10):
- Fracture of lower limb
- Hospitalization for heart failure or atrial fibrillation/flutter (within the previous 3 months)
- Hip or knee replacement
- Major trauma
- Myocardial infarction (within the previous 3 months)
- Previous VTE
- Spinal cord injury

Moderate risk factors (OR 2–9):
- Arthroscopic knee surgery
- Autoimmune diseases
- Blood transfusion
- Central venous lines
- Intravenous catheters and leads
- Chemotherapy
- Congestive heart failure or respiratory failure
- Erythropoiesis-stimulating agents
- Hormone replacement therapy (depends on formulation)
- In-vitro fertilization
- Oral contraceptive therapy
- Postpartum period
- Infection (specifically pneumonia, urinary tract infection, and HIV)
- Inflammatory bowel disease
- Cancer (highest risk in metastatic disease)
- Paralytic stroke
- Superficial vein thrombosis
- Thrombophilia

Weak risk factors (OR <2):
- Bedrest >3 days
- Diabetes mellitus
- Arterial hypertension
- Immobility due to sitting (e.g., prolonged car or air travel)
- Increasing age
- Laparoscopic surgery (e.g., cholecystectomy)
- Obesity
- Pregnancy
- Varicose veins

DIAGNOSIS

Diagnosis of PE is difficult because of nonspecific clinical features. Many other diseases may present similarly in the emergency department such as accelerated hypertension, cardiomyopathy, acute coronary syndrome, pneumonia, bronchitis, pericarditis, and aortic dissection; however, such diseases can be ruled out eventually by investigations.

It is critical to start early treatment to prevent mortality. History is very important for risk factors assessment. History of recent travel, limb swelling, prolonged immobilization, and malignancy can point toward PE.

In the emergency room, one should look for proximal limb swelling, tachycardia, tachypnea, chest pain, etc. Dyspnea is the most common symptom of PE. It may be acute and severe or mild and transient, depending upon the location of the emboli. In patients with preexisting heart failure or lung disease, worsening dyspnea may be the presentation of PE. Chest pain and tachypnea are other common symptoms of

BOX 2 Clinical features—signs and symptoms.

The common symptoms are:
- Dyspnea—82%
- Abrupt onset of chest pain—49–66%
- Cough—20–37%
- Hemoptysis—13%

The most common presenting signs of PE are as follows:
- Tachypnea
- Crackles
- Tachycardia
- Low-grade fever, diaphoresis
- Neck veins distension
- RV heave and loud P2 and right side S3, etc.

Patients with massive PE may present with the following:
- Severe dyspnea and cyanosis
- Syncope
- Hypotension
- Pulseless cardiac electrical activity
- Death

PE, and it is usually secondary to pulmonary infarction. Main clinical features are given in **Box 2**.

In addition to these signs and symptoms, physicians should have knowledge of predisposing risk factors for PE, but up to 40% of PE patients may not have any symptoms.[9]

Pulmonary embolism is classified mainly into three categories: Massive, submassive, and small to moderate PE.

Massive Pulmonary Embolism

Massive pulmonary embolism is mainly characterized by the presence of acute-onset breathing difficulty with pallor, poor perfusion of the extremities, diaphoresis, oliguria, tachycardia with tachypnea with impaired mentation, hypotension, and shock. Hemodynamic parameters along with the anatomic extent of thrombus can define massive PE. Delay in treatment results in cardiogenic shock with multisystem organ dysfunction.

Submassive Pulmonary Embolism

Such patients are usually hemodynamically stable (SBP > 90 mm Hg) with tachypnea and tachycardia. This category is further divided into high risk and low risk. High-risk patients present with typical signs and symptoms plus RV hypokinesia with RV enlargement and increased cardiac markers such as troponin, brain natriuretic peptide (BNP), and NT-proBNP, while the low-risk category will have either elevated cardiac markers or RV dysfunction but not both.

Small to Moderate Pulmonary Embolism

Such patients are hemodynamically stable, and cardiac markers are normal with normal biventricular functions. The main symptoms are acute onset of chest pain and breathlessness, without or with hemoptysis. If a patient presents only with pleuritic chest pain, it indicates that the thrombus is smaller and the obstruction is at the peripheral site. Fever and leukocytosis are common associated findings. ECG findings are normal. Pleural friction rub may be audible or palpable.

MAIN DIAGNOSTIC TESTS

Nonimaging Methods

Electrocardiogram

Electrocardiogram is helpful to exclude acute myocardial infarction and acute pericarditis. The most common ECG finding in PE is sinus tachycardia. Few patients show a classical S1Q3T3 pattern. Other findings include new-onset right bundle branch block and T-wave inversion in inferior/anterior leads due to RV strain (V1–V4).[10] Some changes are not classical; hence, they are labeled as nonspecific ST-T changes.

D-dimer Level

Plasma D-dimer assay should be considered for screening purposes, if suspicion of PE or DVT is present.[11] Negative results exclude VTE because of its high sensitivity. D-dimer is elevated in myocardial infarction, sepsis, malignancy, almost every systemic illness, and pregnancy; hence, positive predictive value and specificity are low.

Arterial Blood Gas

Arterial blood gas shows hypoxemia (low pO_2), hypocapnia, and respiratory alkalosis. It only provides supportive evidence.

Serum Troponin Levels

More than 50% of patients with moderate PE may demonstrate elevated troponin levels due to acute RV myocardial stretch. Increased mortality in PE is correlated with elevated troponin levels.[12]

Brain Natriuretic Peptide

High levels of BNP or NT-proBNP in PE are correlated with an increased risk of subsequent complications and mortality. A meta-analysis showed that more than 50% patients with PE on admission have elevated BNP and NT-proBNP.[13] Elevated markers do not predict early mortality in normotensive PE patients, but normal levels may correlate with good clinical outcomes. Hence, BNP testing can be used as a prognostic marker.[14]

Imaging Studies

Chest Radiography

Initially, the chest radiographic findings were normal in most cases. However, in later stages, radiographic signs may include Westermark sign (dilatation of pulmonary vessels and a sharp cutoff), atelectasis, small pleural effusion, an elevated hemidiaphragm, and Hampton hump (wedge-shaped, pleura-based triangular opacity with an apex pointing toward the hilum).

Venous Ultrasonography

Compression venous ultrasonography of lower limb veins has a sensitivity of >90% and specificity of >95% for establishing diagnosis of DVT.[15,16] However, in many studies, it has been found that in confirmed cases, around 50% of cases do not have imaging evidence of DVT, probably due to complete dislodgement of thrombus in the pulmonary artery.

Ventilation/Perfusion Scanning

In massive PE, a common finding in V/Q scanning (pulmonary radionuclide scintigraphy) is multiple perfusion defects. Most of the time, the findings are nonconfirmatory in preexisting lung diseases. Also, there may be observer bias. Hence, there are limited indications for this test. This imaging modality is used in cases where radiation and contrast are contraindicated, such as pregnancy, renal dysfunction, and contrast allergy. A normal V/Q scan may rule out PE in the absence of pulmonary disease.[17]

Computed Tomography Pulmonary Angiography

If the patient has a high probability of PE and no signs of DVT, then one should go directly for computed tomography pulmonary angiography (CTPA) without any further delay. In the current health care system, CTPA has replaced V/Q scan due the better sensitivity, high specificity, and validity.[18] CTPA also has replaced pulmonary angiography, which was previously the gold standard as it is comparatively less invasive with better diagnostic yield. It measures RV size and volume along with a diagnosis of other lung diseases. Hence, this test can also be used for prognosis.

2D Echocardiography

2D echocardiography is a rapid bedside test to find out the RV's size and function. However, almost 50% of PE cases have normal echo findings. RV dilation is present in almost 25% of cases of patients with PE on 2D echo.[19] RV dilation is associated with a worse prognosis. There are other parameters that also help in risk stratification in PE like TAPSE (tricuspid annular plane systolic excursion), pulmonary ejection acceleration time, and tricuspid valve velocity.

Magnetic Resonance Angiography

Magnetic resonance angiography is less sensitive than a CT scan to detect distal segmental PE. It can also assess RV function, size, and pulmonary artery branches. It is safe in pregnancy, so it can be considered in case of the absence of a CT scan facility.

DIFFERENTIAL DIAGNOSIS

Diagnosis of PE is challenging because of a wide spectrum of diseases presenting similarly. It can range from benign (anxiety neurosis) to fatal diseases such as acute myocardial infarction. Differential diagnoses are given in **Box 3**.

MEDICAL MANAGEMENT OF PULMONARY EMBOLISM

Early evaluation and management of PE are very important because the majority of deaths occur in the first 1–2 hours of massive and high-risk submassive PE. Rapid risk stratification **(Table 1)**[4] should be done based on history, clinical features and physical examination, and analysis of cardiac markers and cardiopulmonary imaging. Management depends upon clinical features and risk stratification.

In hemodynamically stable patients, if the diagnosis of PE is established, therapeutic anticoagulation must be started. In massive PE, hemodynamic and respiratory stabilization is paramount. This includes fluid administration, inotropic support, oxygen therapy, mechanical ventilation, and other measures. A rapid fluid challenge test may be given in hypotension while monitoring central venous pressure (CVP). If CVP cannot be measured, then echo-guided inferior vena cava (IVC) size may be checked for indirect measurement. If there are signs of raised CVP, fluid should be stopped. In such cases, definitive therapy, i.e., anticoagulation with systemic thrombolysis or catheter-directed thrombolysis (CDT) (if no contraindication), should be initiated along with inotropic support. Hemodynamic collapse and cardiac arrest leave clinicians with limited alternative options **(Table 2)**.[20,21] In refractory cases, patients may be advised for mechanical circulatory support (VA-ECMO) along with surgical embolectomy.

BOX 3 Differential diagnosis.

- Acute coronary syndrome
- Acute valvular dysfunction
- Aortic dissection
- Cardiac tamponade
- Pneumonia, pneumothorax, pleurisy
- Hypovolemia
- Acute respiratory distress syndrome
- Cardiomyopathy
- Congestive heart failure
- Idiopathic pulmonary hypertension
- Anxiety neurosis

TABLE 1: PESI score and risk stratification.

Parameter	Original	Modified/Simplified
Age	Age in years	1 point (if age >80 years)
Male sex	+10 points	–
Cancer	+30 points	1 point
Chronic heart failure	+10 points	
Chronic pulmonary disease	+10 points	1 point
PR > 110 bpm	+20 points	1 point
Systolic BP < 100 mm Hg	+30 points	1 point
Respiratory rate > 30 breaths per minute	+20 points	–
Temperature < 36°C	+20 points	–
Altered mental status	+60 points	–
Arterial oxyhemoglobin saturation < 90%	+20 points	1 point
Risk strata (based on the sum of points)		
	Class I: <65 points Very low 30-day mortality risk (0–1.6%)	*0 point:* 30-day mortality risk 1.0% (95% CI 0.0–2.1%)
	Class II: 66–85 points Low mortality risk (1.7–3.5%)	
	Class III: 86–105 points Moderate mortality risk (3.2–7.1%)	*>1 point(s)* = 30-day mortality risk 10.95 (95% CI 8.5–13.2%)
	Class IV: 106–125 points High mortality risk (4.0–11.4%)	
	Class V: >125 points Very high mortality risk (10.0–24.5%)	

TABLE 2: Society guidelines and statements for management of high-risk PE.

Society	Recommendations for high-risk PE management	Grade, level of evidence
ESC (2019)	Systemic thrombolysis	I, B
	Surgical embolectomy (when systemic thrombolysis fails or contraindicated)	I, C
	Catheter-based therapy (when systemic thrombolysis fails or contraindicated)	IIa, C
	ECMO	IIb, C
AHA	Systemic thrombolysis	IIa, B
Scientific Statement (2011)	Surgical embolectomy (when systemic thrombolysis fails or contraindicated)	IIb, C
Consensus Statement (2019)	Catheter-based therapy (when systemic thrombolysis fails or contraindicated)	IIb, C
CHEST 2021 Update	Systemic thrombolysis	Weak, low certainty
	Catheter-based therapy (when systemic thrombolysis fails or contraindicated)	Weak, low certainty
PERT Consortium Consensus Practice (2019)	• Systemic thrombolysis • Catheter-based therapy (when systemic thrombolysis fails or contraindicated) • Surgical embolectomy (when systemic thrombolysis failed or contraindicated) • MSC (with refractory shock or cardiac arrest)	N/A
Society of Interventional Radiology Position Statement (2018)	Catheter-based therapy in highly selected patients	N/A

SYSTEMIC THROMBOLYTIC THERAPY FOR THE MANAGEMENT OF PULMONARY EMBOLISM

- *Alteplase*: 100 mg IV over 2 hours infusion
- *Streptokinase*: 250,000 IU as a loading dose over 30 minutes followed by 100,000 IU/h over 12–24 hours
- *Urokinase*: 4,400 IU/kg as a loading dose over 10 minutes followed by 4,400 IU/kg/h over 12–24 hours
- *Tenecteplase*: IV bolus 30–50 mg depending on weight

The most preferred thrombolytic agent is alteplase. Other agents such as tenecteplase, streptokinase, and urokinase can be used depending on availability and cost factors. Intracranial bleeding is the most feared complication. Hence, it should be avoided in hemodynamic stable patients despite RV dysfunction. One study compared thrombolysis with anticoagulant therapy in submassive PE patients. In case of absolute contraindication of systemic thrombolysis, alternative treatment strategies such as percutaneous low-dose CDT or aspiration or surgical embolectomy/thrombectomy should be considered. In certain situations where anticoagulation is contraindicated and the patient has a history of recurrent PE, an IVC filter may be implanted.

ANTICOAGULATION FOR PULMONARY EMBOLISM

- Unfractionated heparin (UFH) is the preferred anticoagulation of choice if there is high suspicion of PE or confirmed PE where any intervention is required. The short half-life of IV UFH allows for temporary cessation of anticoagulation with reduced bleeding risk. The use of UFH is now restricted in patients with renal dysfunction and hemodynamic instability. Low-molecular-weight heparin (LMWH) and fondaparinux have many advantages over UFH. These have greater bioavailability, lesser incidence of bleeding and heparin-induced thrombocytopenia, ease of administration, and a longer duration of action. The fixed dose can be used, without the need of monitoring.[22] The CHEST guidelines suggest that patients with low-risk PE and who have acceptable home circumstances be discharged early from the hospital (i.e., before the first 5 days of treatment). Direct oral anticoagulants (DOACs) are now considered the first-line treatment for PE and are preferred over vitamin K antagonists (VKAs) (e.g., warfarin) for nearly all patients. Apixaban, edoxaban, and rivaroxaban inhibit factor Xa, whereas dabigatran is a direct thrombin inhibitor. DOACs have now been proven to be noninferior to VKAs in efficacy and are superior in safety without the requirement of regular laboratory monitoring.[23-27] On the other hand, for VKAs, the peak effect does not occur until 36–72 hours after drug administration, and dosage is difficult to titrate, and frequent monitoring of prothrombin time and ratio is required.
- *Duration of anticoagulation therapy*: All patients with a first thromboembolic event should receive oral anticoagulant therapy for at least 3 months. Studies compared the recurrence of embolic events in patients who received 3 versus 6 months of anticoagulant therapy; no difference in the rate of recurrence was observed.[28] The current recommendation is anticoagulation for at least 3 months in all patients. The need for extending the duration of anticoagulation should be evaluated. The current CHEST and ASH guidelines recommend that all patients with unprovoked PE should receive 3 months of treatment with anticoagulation with an assessment of the risk–benefit ratio of extended therapy at the end of 3 months. Indefinite antithrombotic therapy should also be given to patients with recurrent unprovoked PE. Patients who have PE and preexisting irreversible risk factors, such as deficiency of antithrombin III, proteins S and C, factor V Leiden mutation, or the presence of antiphospholipid antibodies, should be kept on long-term anticoagulation. In patients who will receive long-term anticoagulants, their hepatic, renal function, bleeding risk, drug adherence, and tolerance should be assessed at regular intervals.

CATHETER-DIRECTED INTERVENTIONS

Catheter-directed interventions are evaluated in high-risk and intermediate-risk PE cases. The main goal is to achieve better results in terms of mortality, clinical symptoms, and hemodynamics. Studies suggest that CDT was associated with a lower incidence of major bleeding and intracranial hemorrhage (ICH) as compared to systemic thrombolysis.[20] In general, one-fourth dose of a thrombolytic agent is required for CDT as in few cases of massive PE where high bleeding risk is present, CDT may be considered via femoral vein access directly into main pulmonary or branch pulmonary arteries. Many types of catheters are available which are used for thrombolysis, thrombus suction and aspiration,[29] clot fragmentation, mechanical disruption of thrombus, etc. In some recent studies, ultrasound-directed thrombus fragmentation followed by low-dose CDT was better than low-dose thrombolysis alone. All studies done with catheter interventions were either single-center studies or nonrandomized.[29,30] All these studies showed that CDT in high-risk PE was better than anticoagulant alone.[31] There is no data showing better outcomes with CDT than systemic thrombolysis except for lower bleeding risk with catheter interventions. CDT may give more rapid correction of RV afterload and RV/LV ratio. The most common and early method is to use a pigtail catheter in the pulmonary circulation and with rotatory movement to disrupt the clot which leads to restoring the circulation to some extent to stabilize the hemodynamics. Other dedicated systems are large French sizes which are very expensive and require skill. Smaller-size aspiration catheters are available and used in high-volume centers but data to support of their routine use is lacking. Hence, no cardiac society gave CDT or mechanical aspiration or thrombectomy as class I recommendations.[20] Few trials are going on to see the long-term safety and effectiveness of mechanical aspiration catheters (STRIKE-PE).[32] PEERLESS trial is studying the outcome of CDT and mechanical thrombectomy in intermediate- and high-risk stable PE patients. Still, there is a need for more studies and research to find the efficacy of interventions in PE.

Surgical Embolectomy[33]

Surgical embolectomy consists of a cardiopulmonary bypass followed by an incision of both pulmonary arteries and removal or aspiration of clots from the pulmonary circulation. There are favorable results observed in high-risk PE with or without cardiac arrest. Studies say that if the patient requires ECMO in PE cases, then surgical embolectomy should be combined for positive ECMO results.[34]

Current Status of Inferior Vena Cava Filter in Pulmonary Embolism[35]

Inferior vena cava filters are not recommended in all cases. Many studies have been done which do not advocate IVC filter implantation routinely. There is a 50% decrease in recurrent PE but around 60–70% increased chances of recurrent DVT by putting an IVC filter.[36] Also, there was no mortality difference between patients who received IVC filters and those who did not. At present, there are only a few indications—intolerance for anticoagulation, recurrent PE despite therapeutic anticoagulation, high bleeding risk patients, presence of free-floating thrombi, etc.

Management during Pregnancy

At present, parenteral anticoagulation is the preferred modality in pregnant patients with hemodynamic stability. There is a lack of data regarding the safety of DOACs, and warfarin is well documented for its teratogenicity. In hemodynamically unstable patients, systemic thrombolysis should be considered after the assessment of the risk–benefit ratio.[37] Supportive measures such as compression stockings are recommended for varicose veins in pregnancy.

CONCLUSION

Pulmonary embolism is a fatal disease and one of the major causes of cardiovascular death worldwide. Its symptoms and signs are not specific; hence, a delay in diagnosis is common. In the emergency room, patients with acute-onset dyspnea with or without chest pain with normal ECG and chest X-ray, and workup for PE should be considered which includes evaluation of risk factors of PE and application of probability risk score and bleeding risk calculation followed by other investigations. D-dimer is a screening test, but it does not rule out PE. 2D echo is a good screening test to find out massive or submassive PE and rule out other acute conditions like LV dysfunction, valvular heart diseases, pericardial effusion, and tamponade. Immediate anticoagulant should be administered if no contraindication is seen. CTPA is the investigation of choice in high-probability cases. Systemic thrombolysis should be started in massive PE as early as possible. In certain high bleeding risk cases, catheter-directed interventions are the only choice to save the patients. Surgical pulmonary embolectomy should be considered if failure of alternative therapy or thrombolysis is contraindicated. However, its results are not validated in all high-risk or massive PE patients. Further research is required to see the long-term efficacy in high-risk patients. A fully equipped multidisciplinary team is required for the management of high-risk cases. Nonvitamin K antagonists are the main drugs for long-term treatment and for prophylaxis. Follow-up should be done at regular intervals to assess drug compliance, adherence, and side effects. If persistent and new-onset dyspnea develops, a workup for chronic thromboembolic pulmonary hypertension (CTEPH) should be done. Recurrence is common in the absence of long-term anticoagulant therapy. The duration of oral anticoagulant therapy should be evaluated against the bleeding risk. At the time of discharge, the risk of recurrent PE should be assessed. CTEPH syndrome is a major sequela of PE with unsatisfactory outcomes.

ONLINE REFERENCES

Please scan the QR code provided at the end of the table of contents for References of this chapter.

Index

Page numbers followed by *b* refer to box, *f* refer to figure, *fc* refer to flowchart, and *t* refer to table.

A

D

E

I

J

K

L

M

N

O

P

Q

R

S

T

S

T

U

V